Stedman's

MEDICAL
SPELLER

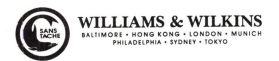

WILLIAMS & WILKINS
BALTIMORE · HONG KONG · LONDON · MUNICH
PHILADELPHIA · SYDNEY · TOKYO

Editor: Harriet Felscher
Staff: Jane Sellman
　　　Christopher Muldor
　　　Julie Rodowski
Production Coordinator: Cordelia Slaughter
Cover Design: Carla Frank

Copyright © 1992
Williams & Wilkins
428 East Preston Street
Baltimore, Maryland 21202, USA

Printed in the United States of America

Library of Congress Cataloging-in-Publication Data

Stedman's medical speller.
　　p.　　cm.
　ISBN 0-683-07938-7
　1. Medicine—Terminology.　I. Title: Medical speller.
　[DNLM: 1. Nomenclature.　W 15 S812]
R123.S7　　1992
610'.14—dc20
DNLM/DLC
for Library of Congress　　　　　　　　　　　　　　　91-40215
　　　　　　　　　　　　　　　　　　　　　　　　　　　　CIP

　　　　　　　　　　　　　　　　　92　93　94　95　96
　　　　　　　　　　　　1　2　3　4　5　6　7　8　9　10

Acknowledgments

This speller is the result of the efforts of a number of people working on the Williams & Wilkins Reference Division staff, to all of whom thanks are due. In particular, I would like to thank Jane Sellman who not only contributed enormously to the final stage of research and work but also to an exchange of ideas, shared aggravation, and hilarity about the arcane subject of hyphenation. We are all "hyphenators" now.

Harriet Felscher

•*Among the publications consulted in determining hyphenation are the following:*
Webster's Third New International Dictionary of the English Language: Unabridged. Gove PB, ed. 3rd ed. Springfield, Massachusetts: Merriam-Webster; 1986.
Webster's New International Dictionary of the English Language: Unabridged. Nielson WA, Knott TA, Carhart PW, eds. 2nd ed. Springfield, Massachusetts: G&C Merriam Company; 1934.
Webster's Ninth New Collegiate Dictionary. Springfield, Massachusetts: Merriam-Webster; 1990.
Webster's Medical Speller. Springfield, Massachusetts: Merriam-Webster; 1975.
Webster's New Biographical Dictionary. Springfield, Massachusetts: Merriam-Webster; 1988.
Webster's New Geographical Dictionary. Springfield, Massachusetts: Merriam-Webster; 1988.

•*Another group was consulted for comparison and verification of pronunciation as a basis for hyphenation:*
Churchill's Illustrated Medical Dictionary. New York: Churchill Livingstone; 1989.
Dorland's Medical Dictionary. 27th ed. Philadelphia: WB Saunders; 1988.
Stedman's Medical Dictionary. 25th ed. Baltimore: Williams & Wilkins; 1990.
USAN and the USP Dictionary of Drug Names. Rockville Maryland: United States Pharmacopeial Convention; 1989.

•*The GPO was consulted for help with foreign language pronunciation:*
United States Government Printing Office Style Manual. Washington, DC: US Government Printing Office; 1984.

•These technical manuals were also consulted for background:

Dodd JS, ed. *The ACS Style Guide.* Washington, DC: American Chemical Society; *1986*
ASM Style Manual. Washington, DC: American Society for Microbiology; 1985.
CBE Style Manual Committee. *CBE Style Manual. 5th ed.* Bethesda, Maryland: Council of Biology Editors; 1983.
Huth EJ. *Medical Style and Format.* Philadelphia: ISI Press; 1987.
Iverson C, et al. *American Medical Association Manual of Style. 8th ed.* Baltimore: Williams & Wilkins, 1989;120-126.
Publication Manual of the American Psychological Association. Washington, DC: American Psychological Association; 1983 rev. 1984.

•Finally, one other group was consulted for background—historical and current, British and American—on styles of hyphenation and on problems and solutions:

Divisions in Boldface Words. In: *Webster's New International Dictionary. 3rd ed.* Springfield, Massachusetts: Merriam-Webster; 1986:19a,20a
Fawthrop D. *Hyphenation by Algorithm.* London: *Computer Hyphenation*; 1990.
Follett W. *The Hyphen: Splitting Words.* In: Follett W. *Modern American Usage: A Guide.*
Barzun J, et al. New York: Hill & Wang; 1966:455-459.
Fowler HW. *A Dictionary of Modern English Usage. 2nd ed.* Gowers E, ed. Oxford: Oxford University Press; 1965.
Irmscher WF. *The Holt Guide to English.* New York: Holt, Rinehart and Winston; 1972.
Walsh JM, Walsh AK. *Plain English Handbook: A Complete Guide to Good English. 6th ed.* Cincinnatti, Ohio; 1972.
Warriner JE. *English Grammar and Composition: Complete Course.* Franklin ed. New York: Harcourt Brace Jovanovich; 1982.
McIntosh R. *Hyphenation.* London: Computer Hyphenation; 1990.

Preface

Stedman's Medical Speller was developed from the *Stedman's-25* database as a means of offering all the wordsmiths of the health care professions—medical transcriptionists, medical editors and copy editors, medical coders, and medical records managers as well as the many other users and producers of medical writing—their most authoritative assurance of quality and exactness in the records, reports, and articles for which they have responsibility.

Comprehensiveness in a compact book was the first goal. More than 127,000 words and phrases have been built from a base of nearly 76,000 terms. This is nearly double the base vocabulary of any currently available speller. About 50,000 cross-references of adjectival and noun phrases complete the list.

To avoid overloading the list unnecessarily with esoteric biochemical terminology and *Nomina Anatomica* Latin entries, both of these groups of terms were taken out of the database for this speller. (Complete Latin entries including the *Nomina Anatomica* are available in our *Stedman's Anatomy & Physiology Words*.) Abbreviations, which only represented a small portion of those used in medicine, were also removed from this database. (A complete listing of such abbreviations is available in our *Stedman 's Abbreviations, Acronyms & Symbols Words*.)

The second goal was to provide a user-friendly format. Our thanks go to transcriptionists at The Johns Hopkins Hospital, Baltimore, Maryland and Baltimore County General Hospital, Randallstown, Maryland who reviewed page format designs and helped us determine the final design. Taking a cue from their suggestions, we tried to keep space on the page for notations without dictating where the notations should be placed. We also followed their preference for a combination **boldface**/lightface type that breaks up the density of the page and allows easier tracking of a desired term.

Finally, with this speller we offer the largest hyphenated medical vocabulary available in print—or electronically. When hyphenation is needed or required for a finished presentation, this speller gives the basis for the best decision on end-of-line breaks.

Speller Organization

Three simple organizational features are used to order the information contained in this speller:

1. The words in the list are alphabetized letter by letter.

   NOTE: Articles, prepositions, chemical prefixes, and the letters used to abbreviate nours in subentries are disregarded in alphabetization.

2. The list itself is set up like an index, with main entries followed by a listing of their related subentries.

3. Main entries appear in **boldface** and may be nouns (or any word used as a noun) or adjectives (or any word used as an adjective). Subentries relating to the main entry are shown in lightface type.

   A noun main entry-subentry is set up as follows:

   foramen
       alveolar foramina
       foramina alveolaria
       aortic f.
       apical dental f.
       f. apices dentis
       f. of Arnold

   NOTE: The abbreviations in the example above show the location of the noun before or after its adjectives or adjectival phrases:

   The noun may occur first in Latin grammatical order: f. apices dentis
   An English noun may be followed by an adjectival phrase: f. of Arnold.
   The normal position of a noun in English is after its adjective: aortic f.

   An adjectival main entry-subentry is set up as follows:

   abdominal
       brain
       canal
       cavity
       fissure
       part

NOTE: The noun subentries listed in lightface do not repeat the main entry adjective in an abbreviation, because the normal position of English adjectives is before the noun.

The proper names in eponymic entries (eponyms are terms named after one or more persons) should not be broken at the ends of lines except at the hyphen in hyphenated names.

	ACCEPTABLE
McCune-Albright syndrome	McCune- Albright syndrome

This speller also includes information about correct use of the possessive for eponymic entries:

Down's syndrome	Downs' analysis
(John L. H. Down)	(William B. Downs)

The information given for correct possessives may be useful in cases in which a specific preference for their use is expressed or requested.

NOTE: The official style of the American Association of Medical Transcriptionists (AAMT) recommends avoidance of the possessive in order to maintain consistency of presentation. To follow this recommendation while using this speller, simply exclude any apostrophe "s" (Down's / Down) or apostrophe following an "s" (Downs' / Downs) used to show possession with an eponym. The AAMT recommendation prefers Down (not Down's) and Downs (not Downs').

Hyphenation: The Mark of Quality

Today, work printed from computer-generated files is often unhyphenated—especially if lines can be automatically justified. Nevertheless, hyphenation is necessary and useful in many cases.

End-of-line hyphenation tends to serve as a measurement of the care with which a given document—page, letter, book, journal, or other written record—has been produced. It also serves as a measure of overall quality.

Some medical words are so long that they must occasionally be broken to avoid a very obvious space at the right of the page. Sometimes, setting up narrow columns, tables, or graphs necessitates breaking words. Finally, formal publication in a journal or book always requires decisions about end-of-line breaks.

DETERMINING END-OF-LINE BREAKS

When guidance on hyphenation is available, choices still need to be made among the possible end-of-line breaks available for a particular word. Determining which to choose is usually a simple process that involves accepted pronunciation and readability.

How Pronunciation Affects Hyphenation

Pronunciation is generally, but not always, the most widely accepted factor used in setting end-of-line hyphenation in the United States. However, pronunciations vary, so even when dictionaries show more than one pronunciation for a word, they will still show a single version of the end-of-line break for the word.

Hyphenate for Readability

Think from the reader's point of view. Keep the broken word as intelligible as possible. Be sure that the chosen break will not mislead the reader by suggesting another word.

FIVE MAJOR RULES OF HYPHENATION

Rule 1:   *A word pronounced as a single sound may not be broken.*

NOT PERMITTED

cast   ca-
                                           st
cause   cau-
                                           se

Rule 2:   *Do not leave a single letter at the end of a line or at the beginning of a line.*

NOT PERMITTED

a#car*di*ac   a-
                                           cardiac
car*di*o*pho*bi#a   cardiophobi-
                                           a

Rule 3:   *Use at least two letters for an end-of-line break.*

NOTE: Three or four letters increase readability and are strongly recommended.

	MINIMUM	BETTER
car*bol*ic	carbol-	car-
	ic	bolic

Rule 4:   *When a spelling hyphen is part of the word being broken, use the spelling hyphen as the end-of line break if at all possible.*

NOTE: Very long compound medical words may force a break at a place other than at the spelling hyphen. When this is necessary, be sure to consider readability first.

	BEST	OR (see Rule 5)
car*bo*hy*drate-in*duced	carbohydrate-	carbo-
	induced	hydrate-induced
cli*ent-cen*tered	client-	
	centered	
McCune-Albright	McCune-	
	Albright	

Rule 5:   *For words without composed of one or more combining forms, but which do not include spelling hyphens, hyphenate at the end of a combining form.*

NOTE: Very long medical words may occasionally force a break at a place other than between combining forms. When this is necessary, be sure to consider readability first.

	BEST	OR
car*di*o*ky*mo*gram	cardio-	cardiokymo-
	kymogram	gram

NOTE: Some societies have developed hyphenation patterns peculiar to their subject area. The American Chemical Society's **ACS Style Guide** lists hyphenated chemical prefixes which can be used as building blocks to find acceptable breaks for otherwise unlisted chemical terms.

A

A
- bands
- bile
- cells
- chain
- disks
- fi·bers
- wave

A-
- es·o·tro·pia
- ex·o·tro·pia
- stra·bis·mus

Aaron's
- sign

Aarskog-Scott
- syn·drome

abac·te·ri·al throm·bot·ic
- en·do·car·di·tis

Abadie's
- sign of ex·oph·thal·mic goi·ter
- sign of ta·bes dor·sa·lis

ab·am·pere

abap·i·cal
- pole

abar·og·no·sis

ab·ar·tic·u·lar
- gout

aba·si·a
- atac·tic a.
- atax·ic a.
- cho·re·ic a.
- spas·tic a.
- a. tre·pi·dans

aba·si·a-asta·si·a

aba·sic

abat·ic

ab·ax·i·al

ab·ax·ile

ab·bau

Abbe
- flap
- op·er·a·tion

Abbé's
- con·dens·er

Abbé-Zeiss
- ap·pa·ra·tus

Abbé-Zeiss count·ing
- cham·ber

Abbott's
- meth·od
- stain for spores
- tube

ABC
- leads

A.B.C.
- pro·cess

ab·do·men
- acute a.
- boat-shaped a.
- car·i·nate a.
- na·vic·u·lar a.
- a. ob·sti·pum
- pen·du·lous a.
- pro·tu·ber·ant a.
- scaph·oid a.
- sur·gi·cal a.

ab·dom·i·nal
- an·gi·na
- ap·o·plexy
- brain
- ca·nal
- cav·i·ty
- drop·sy
- fi·bro·ma·to·sis
- fis·sure
- fis·tu·la
- guard·ing
- her·nia
- hys·ter·ec·to·my
- hys·ter·o·pex·y
- hys·ter·ot·o·my
- mi·graine
- my·o·mec·to·my
- ne·phrec·to·my
- pad
- part
- pool
- preg·nan·cy
- pres·sure
- pulse
- re·flex·es
- re·gions
- res·pi·ra·tion
- ring
- sac
- sal·pin·gec·to·my
- sal·pin·go-o·o·pho·rec·to·my

ab·dom·i·nal *(continued)*
  sal·pin·got·o·my
  sec·tion
  ty·phoid
  zones
ab·dom·i·nal aor·tic
  plex·us
ab·dom·i·nal ex·ter·nal ob·lique
  mus·cle
ab·dom·i·nal in·ter·nal ob·lique
  mus·cle
ab·dom·i·nal mus·cle de·fi·cien·cy
  syn·drome
ab·dom·i·no·car·di·ac
  re·flex
ab·dom·i·no·cen·te·sis
ab·dom·i·no·cy·e·sis
ab·dom·i·no·cys·tic
ab·dom·i·no·gen·i·tal
ab·dom·i·no·hys·ter·ec·to·my
ab·dom·i·no·hys·ter·ot·o·my
ab·dom·i·no·jug·u·lar
  re·flux
ab·dom·i·no·per·i·ne·al
ab·dom·i·no·plas·ty
ab·dom·i·nos·co·py
ab·dom·i·no·scro·tal
ab·dom·i·no·tho·rac·ic
  arch
ab·dom·i·no·vag·i·nal
  hys·ter·ec·to·my
ab·dom·i·no·ves·i·cal
ab·duce
ab·du·cens
  a. oc·u·li
ab·du·cens
  nu·cle·us
ab·du·cent
  nerve
ab·duct
ab·duc·tion
ab·duc·tor
  mus·cle of great toe
  mus·cle of lit·tle fin·ger
  mus·cle of lit·tle toe
Abegg's
  rule
Abell-Kendall
  meth·od
Abel's
  ba·cil·lus
Abelson mu·rine leu·ke·mia
  vi·rus
ab·em·bry·on·ic
ab·en·ter·ic

Abernethy's
  fas·cia
ab·er·rant
  ar·tery
  bun·dles
  com·plex
  duct
  duc·tule
  gan·gli·on
  goi·ter
  he·mo·glo·bin
  re·gen·er·a·tion
ab·er·rant bile
  ducts
ab·er·rant ven·tric·u·lar
  con·duc·tion
ab·er·ra·tion
  chro·mat·ic a.
  chro·mo·some a.
  col·or a.
  co·ma a.
  cur·va·ture a.
  di·op·tric a.
  dis·tor·tion a.
  lat·er·al a.
  lon·gi·tu·di·nal a.
  men·tal a.
  me·rid·i·o·nal a.
  mon·o·chro·mat·ic a.
  new·to·ni·an a.
  op·ti·cal a.
  spher·i·cal a.
  ven·tric·u·lar a.
ab·er·rom·e·ter
abe·ta·lip·o·pro·tein·e·mia
abey·ance
ab·far·ad
ab·hen·ry
ab·i·ent
abil·i·ty
abi·o·gen·e·sis
abi·o·ge·net·ic
ab·i·o·sis
ab·i·ot·ic
ab·i·ot·ro·phy
ab·ir·ri·tant
ab·ir·ri·ta·tion
ab·ir·ri·ta·tive
ab·lac·ta·tion
ablas·te·mic
ablas·tin
ab·late
ab·la·tion
ab·la·tio pla·cen·tae
ab·la·tio ret·i·nae
ABLB
  test
ableph·a·ria

ablep·si·a
ablep·sy
ab·lu·ent
ab·lu·tion
ab·lu·to·ma·nia
ab·ner·val
ab·neu·ral
ab·nor·mal
  cleav·age of car·di·ac valve
  cor·re·spon·dence
  oc·clu·sion
ab·nor·mal·i·ty
  fig·ure-of-eight a.
ABO
  an·ti·gens.
  fac·tors
ABO blood group
ABO he·mo·lyt·ic
  dis·ease of the new·born
ab·ohm
aboi·e·ment
ab·o·ma·si·tis
ab·o·ma·sum
ab·o·rad
ab·o·ral
abort
abort·ed
  sys·to·le
abort·ed ec·top·ic
  preg·nan·cy
abor·tient
abor·ti·fa·cient
abor·ti·gen·ic
abor·tion
  ac·ci·den·tal a.
  am·pul·lar a.
  bo·vine in·fec·tious a.
  com·plete a.
  con·ta·gious a.
  crim·i·nal a.
  en·zo·ot·ic a. of ewes
  equine vi·rus a.
  ha·bit·u·al a.
  im·mi·nent a.
  in·cip·i·ent a.
  in·com·plete a.
  in·duced a.
  in·ev·i·ta·ble a.
  in·fect·ed a.
  jus·ti·fi·a·ble a.
  men·stru·al ex·trac·tion a.
  missed a.
  sep·tic a.
  spon·ta·ne·ous a.
  ther·a·peu·tic a.
  threat·en·ed a.
  tub·al a.
  vib·ri·on·ic a.

abor·tion
  rate
abor·tion·ist
abor·tive
  neu·ro·fi·bro·ma·to·sis
  trans·duc·tion
abor·tus
  ba·cil·lus
abor·tus-Bang-ring
  test
abouche·ment
abou·lia
ABR
  au·di·om·e·try
abra·chia
abra·chi·o·ce·pha·lia
abra·chi·o·ceph·a·ly
abrade
abrad·ed
  wound
Abrahams'
  sign
Abrams' heart
  re·flex
abra·sion
  brush burn a.
  gin·gi·val a.
  me·chan·i·cal a.
  tooth a.
abra·sive
  strip
abra·sive·ness
ab·re·act
ab·re·ac·tion
  mo·tor a.
abrup·tion
ab·rup·tio pla·cen·tae
Ab·rus
ab·scess
  acute a.
  al·ve·o·lar a.
  ame·bic a.
  ap·i·cal a.
  ap·i·cal per·i·o·don·tal a.
  ap·pen·dic·e·al a.
  Bartholin's a.
  Bezold's a.
  bi·cam·er·al a.
  bone a.
  Brodie's a.
  bur·sal a.
  ca·se·ous a.
  chron·ic a.
  cold a.
  col·lar-but·ton a.
  crypt a.'s
  den·tal a.
  den·to·al·ve·o·lar a.

ab·scess *(continued)*
  dif·fuse a.
  Douglas a.
  dry a.
  Dubois' a.'s
  em·bol·ic a.
  fe·cal a.
  fol·lic·u·lar a.
  gas a.
  gin·gi·val a.
  grav·i·ta·tion a.
  gum·ma·tous a.
  he·ma·tog·e·nous a.
  hot a.
  hy·po·stat·ic a.
  is·chi·o·rec·tal a.
  la·cu·nar a.
  lat·er·al al·ve·o·lar a.
  lat·er·al per·i·o·don·tal a.
  mas·toid a.
  met·a·stat·ic a.
  mi·grat·ing a.
  mil·i·a·ry a.
  Munro's a.
  my·cot·ic a.
  or·bi·tal a.
  otic a.
  pal·a·tal a.
  par·a·fre·nal a.
  par·a·met·ric a.
  par·a·me·trit·ic a.
  par·a·neph·ric a.
  pa·rot·id a.
  Pautrier's a.
  pel·vic a.
  per·fo·rat·ing a.
  per·i·ap·i·cal a.
  per·i·ap·pen·di·ce·al a.
  per·i·ar·tic·u·lar a.
  per·i·ce·men·tal a.
  per·i·cor·o·nal a.
  per·i·neph·ric a.
  per·i·o·don·tal a.
  per·i·rec·tal a.
  per·i·ton·sil·lar a.
  per·i·u·re·ter·al a.
  per·i·u·re·thral a.
  phleg·mon·ous a.
  Pott's a.
  pre·mam·ma·ry a.
  pso·as a.
  pulp a.
  py·e·mic a.
  ra·dic·u·lar a.
  re·sid·u·al a.
  ret·ro·bul·bar a.
  ret·ro·ce·cal a.
  ret·ro·pha·ryn·ge·al a.

  ring a.
  root a.
  sat·el·lite a.
  sep·ti·ce·mic a.
  shirt-stud a.
  stel·late a.
  ster·co·ral a.
  ster·ile a.
  stitch a.
  sub·a·cute a.
  sub·di·a·phrag·mat·ic a.
  sub·ep·i·der·mal a.
  sub·per·i·os·te·al a.
  sub·phren·ic a.
  sub·un·gual a.
  su·do·rip·a·rous a.
  syph·i·lit·ic a.
  the·cal a.
  thy·mic a.'s
  Tornwaldt's a.
  trop·i·cal a.
  tu·ber·cu·lous a.
  tu·bo-o·var·i·an a.
  ver·min·ous a.
  wan·der·ing a.
  worm a.
ab·scis·sa
ab·scis·sion
ab·scon·sio
ab·sco·pal
  ef·fect
ab·sence
  sei·zure
ab·sence
  aton·ic a.
  atyp·i·cal a.
  au·to·mat·ic a.
  com·plex a.
  en·u·ret·ic a.
  ep·i·lep·tic a.
  hy·per·ton·ic a.
  my·o·clon·ic a.
  pure a.
  ret·ro·cur·sive a.
  sim·ple a.
  ster·nu·ta·to·ry a.
  sub·clin·i·cal a.
  tus·sive a.
  typ·i·cal a.
  va·so·mo·tor a.
ab·sent
  state
ab·sen·tia ep·i·lep·ti·ca
Ab·sid·ia
ab·sinthe
ab·sin·thin
ab·sin·thi·um
ab·sin·thol

4

ab·so·lute
    agraph·ia
    al·co·hol
    de·hy·dra·tion
    glau·co·ma
    hem·i·a·nop·sia
    hu·mid·i·ty
    hy·dra·tion
    hy·per·o·pia
    leu·ko·cy·to·sis
    scale
    sco·to·ma
    ste·ril·i·ty
    sys·tem of units
    tem·per·a·ture
    thresh·old
    unit
    vis·cos·i·ty
    ze·ro
ab·so·lute cell
    in·crease
ab·so·lute in·ten·si·ty thresh·old
    acu·i·ty
ab·so·lute re·frac·to·ry
    pe·ri·od
ab·so·lute ter·mi·nal in·ner·va·tion
    ra·tio
ab·sorb
ab·sorb·a·ble gel·a·tin
    film
    sponge
ab·sorb·a·ble sur·gi·cal
    su·ture
ab·sor·bance
    spe·cif·ic a.
ab·sorb·an·cy
    in·dex
ab·sorbed
    dose
ab·sor·be·fa·cient
ab·sorb·en·cy
ab·sor·bent
    cot·ton
    points
    sys·tem
    ves·sels
ab·sorb·er head
ab·sorp·tion
    cu·ta·ne·ous a.
    dis·junc·tive a.
    elec·tron res·o·nance a.
    ex·ter·nal a.
    in·ter·sti·tial a.
    par·en·ter·al a.
    path·o·log·ic a.

ab·sorp·tion
    band
    cell
    chro·ma·tog·ra·phy
    co·ef·fi·cient
    col·lapse
    fe·ver
    lines
    spec·trum
ab·sorp·tive
    cells of in·tes·tine
ab·sorp·tiv·i·ty
    mo·lar a.
ab·sti·nence
    symp·toms
ab·stract
    in·tel·li·gence
    think·ing
ab·strac·tion
ab·stric·tion
ab·ter·mi·nal
ab·trop·fung
abu·lia
abu·lic
abuse
    drug a.
    sub·stance a.
abut·ment
    aux·il·ia·ry a.
    in·ter·me·di·ate a.
    iso·lat·ed a.
    splint·ed a.
ab·volt
a-c
    in·ter·val
aca·cia
acal·cu·lia
acamp·sia
acam·y·lo·phe·nine
acan·tha
acan·tha·me·bi·a·sis
Acan·tha·moe·ba
ac·an·thel·la
acan·thes·the·sia
Acan·thia lec·tu·lar·ia
acan·thi·on
Acan·tho·ceph·a·la
acan·tho·ceph·a·li·a·sis
Acan·tho·chei·lo·ne·ma
acan·tho·cyte
acan·tho·cy·to·sis
acan·thoid
ac·an·thol·y·sis
ac·an·tho·ma
    a. ad·e·noi·des cys·ti·cum
    clear cell a.
    Degos' a.

ac·an·tho·ma *(continued)*
  a. fis·su·ra·tum
  in·tra·ep·i·the·li·al a.
acan·tho·po·dia
acan·thor
acan·thor·rhex·is
ac·an·tho·sis
  gly·co·gen a.
  a. ni·gri·cans
ac·an·thot·ic
acan·thro·cyte
acan·thro·cy·to·sis
acap·nia
acap·ni·al
  al·ka·lo·sis
acar·bia
acar·dia
acar·di·ac
acar·di·o·tro·phia
acar·di·us
  a. aceph·a·lus
  a. amor·phus
  a. an·ceps
ac·a·ri·a·sis
  dem·o·dec·tic a.
  pso·rop·tic a.
  pul·mo·nary a.
  sar·cop·tic a.
acar·i·cide
ac·a·rid
Acar·i·dae
acar·i·dan
ac·ar·i·di·a·sis
Ac·a·ri·na
ac·a·rine
  der·ma·to·sis
ac·ar·i·no·sis
ac·a·ro·der·ma·ti·tis
  a. ur·ti·ca·ri·oi·des
ac·a·roid
ac·a·rol·o·gy
ac·a·ro·pho·bia
Ac·a·rus
  A. bal·a·tus
  A. fol·lic·u·lo·rum
  A. gal·li·nae
  A. hor·dei
  A. rhi·zog·lyp·ti·cus hy·a·
    cin·thi
  A. sca·biei
ac·a·rus
acar·y·ote
acat·a·la·se·mia
acat·a·la·sia
acat·a·ma·the·sia
acat·a·pha·si·a
ac·a·thec·tic
ac·a·thex·ia

ac·a·thex·is
aca·thi·sia
acau·dal
acau·date
ac·cel·er·ans
ac·cel·er·ant
ac·cel·er·at·ed
  con·duc·tion
  erup·tion
  re·ac·tion
  re·jec·tion
ac·cel·er·a·tion
  an·gu·lar a.
  lin·e·ar a.
  ra·di·al a.
ac·cel·er·a·tor
  lin·e·ar a.
  pro·se·rum pro·throm·bin
    con·ver·sion a.
  pro·throm·bin a.
  se·rum a.
  se·rum pro·throm·bin con·
    ver·sion a.
ac·cel·er·a·tor
  fac·tor
  fi·bers
  glob·u·lin
  nerves
ac·cel·er·in
ac·cel·er·om·e·ter
ac·cen·tu·a·tor
ac·cep·tor
  hy·dro·gen a.
ac·cés per·ni·ci·eux
ac·cess
  open·ing
ac·ces·so·ri·us
  a. wil·li·sii
ac·ces·so·ry
  ad·re·nal
  atri·um
  au·ri·cles
  breast
  ca·nal
  car·ti·lage
  chro·mo·some
  cramp
  floc·cu·lus
  gland
  lig·a·ments
  nerve
  or·gans
  or·gans of eye
  pla·cen·ta
  pro·cess
  sign
  spleen
  symp·tom

thy·roid
tu·ber·cle
ac·ces·so·ry ce·phal·ic
vein
ac·ces·so·ry cu·ne·ate
nu·cle·us
ac·ces·so·ry hem·i·az·y·gos
vein
ac·ces·so·ry lac·ri·mal
glands
ac·ces·so·ry na·sal
car·ti·lag·es
ac·ces·so·ry nerve lymph
nodes
ac·ces·so·ry ob·tu·ra·tor
ar·tery
ac·ces·so·ry ol·i·vary
nu·clei
ac·ces·so·ry pan·cre·at·ic
duct
ac·ces·so·ry pa·rot·id
gland
ac·ces·so·ry phren·ic
nerves
ac·ces·so·ry plan·tar
lig·a·ments
ac·ces·so·ry quad·rate
car·ti·lage
ac·ces·so·ry sa·phe·nous
vein
ac·ces·so·ry su·pra·re·nal
glands
ac·ces·so·ry thy·roid
gland
ac·ces·so·ry ver·te·bral
vein
ac·ces·so·ry vo·lar
lig·a·ments
ac·ci·dent
neu·ro·sis
ac·ci·dent
car·di·ac a.
cer·e·bro·vas·cu·lar a.
se·rum a.
ac·ci·den·tal
abor·tion
hy·po·ther·mia
im·age
mur·mur
symp·tom
ac·ci·dent-prone
ac·cli·mat·ing
fe·ver
ac·cli·ma·tion
ac·cli·ma·ti·za·tion
ac·co·lé
forms

ac·com·mo·da·tion
phos·phene
re·flex
ac·com·mo·da·tion
am·pli·tude of a.
a. of eye
his·to·log·ic a.
neg·a·tive a.
a. of nerve
pos·i·tive a.
range of a.
rel·a·tive a.
ac·com·mo·da·tive
as·the·no·pia
con·ver·gence
stra·bis·mus
ac·com·mo·da·tive con·ver·
gence-ac·com·mo·da·tion
ra·tio
ac·com·pa·ny·ing
vein
ac·com·plice
ac·cor·di·on
graft
ac·couche·ment
a. forcé
ac·cou·cheur
ac·cou·cheur's
hand
ac·cre·men·ti·tion
ac·cre·tio cor·dis
ac·cre·tion
lines
ac·cre·tion·ary
growth
ac·cro·chage
ac·e·bu·to·lol
ac·e·car·bro·mal
acec·li·dine
ac·e·dap·sone
acef·yl·line pi·per·a·zine
acel·lu·lar
ace·lom
ace·lo·mate
ace·lo·ma·tous
ace·nes·the·sia
acen·o·cou·ma·rin
acen·o·cou·ma·rol
acen·tric
chro·mo·some
ace·pha·lia
aceph·a·line
aceph·a·lism
aceph·a·lo·bra·chia
aceph·a·lo·car·dia
aceph·a·lo·chei·ria
aceph·a·lo·chi·ria
aceph·a·lo·cyst

aceph·a·lo·gas·ter
aceph·a·lo·gas·ter·ia
aceph·a·lo·po·dia
aceph·a·lor·rha·chia
aceph·a·lo·sto·mia
aceph·a·lo·tho·ra·cia
aceph·a·lous
aceph·a·lus
   a. di·bra·chi·us
   a. di·pus
   a. mon·o·bra·chi·us
   a. mon·o·pus
   a. par·a·ceph·a·lus
   a. sym·pus
aceph·a·ly
acer·vu·line
acer·vu·lus
aces·to·ma
ace·ta
ac·e·tab·u·la
ac·e·tab·u·lar
   ar·tery
   fos·sa
   lip
   notch
ac·e·tab·u·lec·to·my
ac·e·tab·u·lo·plas·ty
ac·e·tab·u·lum
ac·e·tal
   a. phos·pha·ti·date
   a. phos·pha·tide
ac·et·al·de·hyde
acet·a·mide
ac·et·am·i·dine
ac·et·a·min·o·phen
ac·e·tam·in·o·sal·ol
ac·et·an·i·lid
ac·et·ar·sol
ac·et·ar·sone
ac·e·tate
   ac·tive a.
   a. ki·nase
   a. thi·o·ki·nase
ac·e·tate-CoA li·gase
ac·e·tate re·place·ment
   fac·tor
acet·a·zol·a·mide
acet·e·nyl
ace·tic
   fer·men·ta·tion
   so·lu·tion
ace·tic ac·id
   di·lut·ed a. a.
   gla·cial a. a.
ace·tic ac·id am·ide
ace·tic al·de·hyde
ace·tic am·ide
ace·ti·co·cep·tor

ace·tic phos·phor·ic an·hy·dride
ace·ti·fy
ac·e·tim·e·ter
ac·e·to·ac·e·tate
   a. de·car·box·yl·ase
ac·e·to·a·ce·tic ac·id
ac·e·to·a·ce·tyl-CoA
ac·e·to·a·ce·tyl-CoA re·duc·tase
ac·e·to·a·ce·tyl-CoA thi·o·lase
ac·e·to·a·ce·tyl·co·en·zyme A
ac·e·to·a·ce·tyl-suc·cin·ic thi·o·
   phor·ase
ac·e·to·hex·am·ide
ac·e·to·hy·drox·a·mic ac·id
acet·o·in
ac·e·to·ki·nase
ac·e·tol
ac·e·tol·y·sis
ac·e·to·me·naph·thone
ac·e·tom·e·ter
ac·e·tone
   body
   chlo·ro·form
   com·pound
   fix·a·tive
   test
ac·e·tone-in·sol·u·ble
   an·ti·gen
ac·e·ton·e·mia
   bo·vine a.
   ovine a.
ac·e·to·ne·mic
ac·e·to·ni·trile
ac·e·to·nu·ria
ac·e·to-or·ce·in
   stain
ac·e·to·phen·a·zine ma·le·ate
ac·e·to·phe·net·i·din
ac·e·to·sol·u·ble
   al·bu·min
ac·e·to·sul·fone so·di·um
ace·tous
   fer·men·ta·tion
ac·et·phe·no·li·sa·tin
ac·e·tri·zo·ate so·di·um
ace·tum
acet·u·rate
ace·tyl
   a. chlo·ride
   a. phos·phate
   a. trans·ac·yl·ase
ace·tyl
   val·ue
ace·tyl-ac·ti·vat·ing
   en·zyme
ace·tyl·ad·e·nyl·ate
acet·y·lase
acet·y·la·tion

ace·tyl·car·bro·mal
ace·tyl·cho·line
   a. chlo·ride
ace·tyl·cho·lin·es·ter·ase
ace·tyl-CoA
ace·tyl-CoA   ace·tyl·trans·fer·ase
ace·tyl-CoA   ac·yl·ase
ace·tyl-CoA   ac·yl·trans·fer·ase
ace·tyl-CoA   car·box·yl·ase
ace·tyl-CoA   de·ac·yl·ase
ace·tyl-CoA   hy·dro·lase
ace·tyl-CoA   syn·the·tase
ace·tyl-CoA   thi·o·lase
ace·tyl·co·en·zyme A
ace·tyl·cys·te·ine
ace·tyl·dig·i·tox·in
ace·tyl·di·gox·in
acet·y·lene
N-ace·tyl·glu·ta·mate
ace·tyl·or·ni·thin·ase
ace·tyl·or·ni·thine de·a·cet·yl·
   ase
ace·tyl·sal·i·cyl·ic ac·id
ace·tyl·sul·fi·sox·a·zole
ace·tyl·tan·nic ac·id
ace·tyl·trans·fer·ase
acha·la·sia
   esoph·a·ge·al a.
Achard
   syn·drome
Achard-Thiers
   syn·drome
ache
   bone a.
   stom·ach a.
achei·lia
achei·lous
achei·ria
achei·rop·o·dy
achei·rous
Achenbach
   syn·drome
achieve·ment
   age
   mo·tive
   quo·tient
   test
achi·lia
Achilles
   bur·sa
   re·flex
   ten·don
Achilles ten·don
   re·flex
achil·lo·bur·si·tis
achil·lo·dyn·ia
ach·il·lor·rha·phy
achil·lo·ten·ot·o·my

ach·il·lot·o·my
achi·lous
achi·ral
achi·ria
achi·rop·o·dy
achi·rous
achlor·hy·dria
achlor·hy·dric
   ane·mia
achlor·o·phyl·lous
Acho·le·plas·ma
   A. ax·an·thum
   A. gran·u·la·rum
   A. laid·la·wii
Acho·le·plas·ma·ta
acho·lia
achol·ic
achol·u·ria
achol·u·ric
   jaun·dice
achon·dro·gen·e·sis
achon·dro·pla·sia
   avi·an a.
   bo·vine a.
   ho·mo·zy·gous a.
achon·dro·plas·tic
   dwarf·ism
achon·dro·plas·ty
achor·dal
achor·date
acho·re·sis
Acho·ri·on
achres·tic
   ane·mia
achro·a·cyte
achro·a·cy·to·sis
ach·ro·dex·trin
ach·ro·glo·bin
achro·ma·cyte
ach·ro·ma·sia
achro·mate
ach·ro·mat·ic
   ap·pa·ra·tus
   lens
   ob·jec·tive
   thresh·old
   vi·sion
achro·ma·tin
achro·ma·tin·ic
achro·ma·tism
achro·mat·o·cyte
achro·ma·tol·y·sis
achro·mat·o·phil
achro·mat·o·phil·ia
achro·ma·top·sia
   atyp·i·cal a.
   com·plete a.
   cone a.

achro·ma·top·sia *(continued)*
    in·com·plete a.
    rod a.
    typ·i·cal a.
    X-linked a.
achro·ma·top·sy
achro·ma·to·sis
achro·ma·tous
achro·ma·tu·ria
achro·mia
    a. pa·ra·sit·i·ca
    a. un·gui·um
achro·mic
achro·mo·cyte
achro·mo·der·ma
achro·mo·phil
achro·mo·phil·ic
achro·moph·i·lous
achro·mo·trich·ia
ach·ro·o·dex·trin
achy·lia
    a. gas·tri·ca
    a. pan·cre·a·ti·ca
achy·lous
acic·u·lar
ac·id
    bile a.'s
    di·ba·sic a.
    fat·ty a.
    in·or·gan·ic a.
    mon·o·ba·sic a.
    or·gan·ic a.
    pol·y·ba·sic a.
ac·id
    ag·glu·ti·na·tion
    al·co·hol
    car·box·y·pep·ti·dase
    cell
    de·ox·y·ri·bo·nu·cle·ase
    dys·pep·sia
    fuch·sin
    gland
    in·di·ges·tion
    in·tox·i·ca·tion
    malt·ase
    ox·ide
    phos·pha·tase
    rad·i·cal
    re·ac·tion
    rig·or
    salt
    se·ro·mu·coid
    stain
    sul·fate
    tar·trate
    tide
    wave
ac·id·am·i·nu·ria

ac·id-ash
    di·et
ac·id-base
    bal·ance
    equi·lib·ri·um
ac·i·de·mia
ac·id etch ce·ment·ed
    splint
ac·id-etched
    res·to·ra·tion
ac·id-fast
aci·dic
    dyes
acid·i·fied se·rum
    test
acid·i·fy
acid·i·ty
    to·tal a.
ac·i·do·cyte
ac·i·do·phil
    ad·e·no·ma
    cell
    gran·ule
ac·i·do·phile
ac·i·do·phil·ic
    leu·ko·cyte
ac·i·doph·i·lus
    milk
ac·i·do·sis
    car·bon di·ox·ide a.
    com·pen·sat·ed a.
    di·a·bet·ic a.
    lac·tic a.
    met·a·bol·ic a.
    pri·mary re·nal tu·bu·lar a.
    re·nal tu·bu·lar a.
    res·pi·ra·to·ry a.
    sec·on·dary re·nal tu·bu·lar
      a.
    un·com·pen·sat·ed a.
ac·i·dot·ic
ac·id per·fu·sion
    test
ac·id phos·pha·tase
    test for se·men
ac·id re·flux
    test
acid·u·late
acid·u·lous
ac·i·du·ria
ac·i·du·ric
ac·id·yl
ac·i·nar
    car·ci·no·ma
    cell
ac·i·nar cell
    tu·mor

Ac·i·ne·to·bac·ter
   A. cal·co·a·ce·ti·cus
ac·i·ni
acin·ic
acin·ic cell
   ad·e·no·car·ci·no·ma
   car·ci·no·ma
acin·i·form
ac·i·ni·tis
ac·i·nose
   car·ci·no·ma
ac·i·no·tu·bu·lar
   gland
ac·i·nous
   car·ci·no·ma
   cell
   gland
ac·i·nus
   liv·er a.
   pul·mo·nary a.
ack·ee
   poi·son·ing
ac·la·sis
   di·a·phys·i·al a.
aclas·tic
acleis·to·car·dia
ac·me
ac·mes·the·sia
ac·ne
   a. ag·mi·na·ta
   a. al·bi·da
   a. ar·ti·fi·ci·a·lis
   as·bes·tos a.
   bro·mide a.
   a. ca·chec·ti·co·rum
   chlo·rine a.
   a. cil·i·ar·is
   col·loid a.
   a. con·glo·ba·ta
   a. cos·me·ti·ca
   cys·tic a.
   a. de·cal·vans
   a. er·y·the·ma·to·sa
   a. fron·ta·lis
   a. ge·ne·ra·lis
   hal·o·gen a.
   a. hy·per·tro·phi·ca
   a. in·du·ra·ta
   io·dide a.
   a. ke·ra·to·sa
   a. lu·poi·des
   a. me·di·ca·men·to·sa
   a. ne·cro·ti·ca
   a. ne·o·na·to·rum
   a. pa·pu·lo·sa
   po·made a.
   a. punc·ta·ta
   a. pus·tu·lo·sa

   a. ro·dens
   a. ro·sa·cea
   a. scrof·u·lo·so·rum
   a. se·ba·cea
   sim·ple a.
   a. sim·plex
   ste·roid a.
   a. syph·i·li·ti·ca
   tar a.
   a. tar·si
   a. tel·an·gi·ec·to·des
   trop·i·cal a.
   a. ur·ti·ca·ta
   a. va·ri·o·li·for·mis
   a. ve·ne·na·ta
   a. vul·ga·ris
ac·ne
   ba·cil·lus
   ke·loid
ac·ne·form
   syph·i·lid
ac·ne·gen·ic
ac·ne·i·form
ac·ne·mia
ac·ni·tis
ac·o·kan·thera
ac·o·la·sia
aco·lous
aco·mia
acon·a·tive
acon·i·tase
acon·i·tate hy·dra·tase
ac·o·nite
cis-**ac·o·nit·ic ac·id**
acon·i·tine
aco·rea
acor·mus
acorn-tipped
   cath·e·ter
Acosta's
   dis·ease
acou·asm
acous·ma
acous·ma·tam·ne·sia
acous·tic
   agraph·ia
   apha·sia
   ar·ea
   cell
   crest
   lem·nis·cus
   nerve
   neu·ri·le·mo·ma
   neu·ri·no·ma
   neu·ro·ma
   pa·pil·la
   ra·di·a·tion
   schwan·no·ma

acous·tic *(continued)*
  spots
  stri·ae
  tet·a·nus
  tol·er·ance
  tu·ber·cle
  ves·i·cle
acous·ti·co·fa·cial
  crest
  gan·gli·on
acous·ti·co·pal·pe·bral
  re·flex
acous·ti·co·pho·bia
acous·tic ref·er·ence
  lev·el
acous·tics
acous·tic trau·ma
  deaf·ness
ACP-ace·tyl·trans·fer·ase
ACP-mal·o·nyl·trans·fer·ase
ac·quired
  agam·ma·glob·u·lin·e·mia
  char·ac·ter
  cu·ti·cle
  dis·tich·ia
  drives
  hy·per·lip·o·pro·tein·e·mia
  hy·po·gam·ma·glob·u·lin·e·
   mia
  ich·thy·o·sis
  im·mu·ni·ty
  leu·ko·der·ma
  leu·ko·path·ia
  met·he·mo·glo·bi·ne·mia
  ne·vus
  pel·li·cle
  re·flex
  sen·si·tiv·i·ty
  tox·o·plas·mo·sis in adults
  trich·o·ep·i·the·li·o·ma
ac·quired cen·tric
  re·la·tion
ac·quired ec·cen·tric
  re·la·tion
ac·quired enam·el
  cu·ti·cle
ac·quired ep·i·lep·tic
  apha·sia
ac·quired he·mo·lyt·ic
  ane·mia
  ic·ter·us
ac·quired im·mu·no·de·fi·cien·
 cy
  syn·drome
ac·qui·si·tion
ac·quis·i·tus
ac·ral

ac·ral len·tig·i·nous
  mel·a·no·ma
Acra·nia
acra·nia
acra·ni·al
Acrel's
  gan·gli·on
Ac·re·mo·ni·um
ac·ri·bom·e·ter
ac·rid
  poi·son
ac·ri·dine
  dyes
ac·ri·dine
  tet·ra·meth·yl a.
ac·ri·dine or·ange
ac·ri·dine yel·low
ac·ri·fla·vine
ac·ri·mo·ny
ac·ri·nol
ac·ri·sor·cin
acrit·i·cal
ac·ro·ag·no·sis
ac·ro·an·es·the·sia
ac·ro·ar·thri·tis
ac·ro·as·phyx·ia
ac·ro·a·tax·ia
ac·ro·blast
ac·ro·brach·y·ceph·a·ly
ac·ro·bys·ti·tis
ac·ro·cen·tric
  chro·mo·some
ac·ro·ce·pha·lia
ac·ro·ce·phal·ic
ac·ro·ceph·a·lo·pol·y·syn·dac·
 ty·ly
ac·ro·ceph·a·lo·syn·dac·tyl·ia
ac·ro·ceph·a·lo·syn·dac·tyl·ism
ac·ro·ceph·a·lo·syn·dac·ty·ly
  atyp·i·cal a.
  type I a.
  type II a.
  type III a.
  type V a.
  typ·i·cal a.
ac·ro·ceph·a·lous
ac·ro·ceph·a·ly
ac·ro·chor·don
ac·ro·ci·ne·sia
ac·ro·ci·ne·sis
ac·ro·con·trac·ture
ac·ro·cy·a·no·sis
ac·ro·cy·a·not·ic
ac·ro·der·ma·ti·tis
  a. chron·i·ca atroph·i·cans
  a. con·tin·ua
  a. en·ter·o·path·i·ca
  a. hi·e·ma·lis

pap·u·lar a. of child·hood
a. per·stans
a. ve·si·cu·lo·sa tro·pi·ca
ac·ro·der·ma·to·sis
ac·ro·dol·i·cho·me·lia
ac·ro·dont
ac·ro·dyn·ia
ac·ro·dyn·ic
er·y·the·ma
ac·ro·dys·es·the·sia
ac·ro·dys·os·to·sis
ac·ro·dys·pla·sia
ac·ro·e·de·ma
ac·ro·es·the·sia
ac·ro·fa·cial
dys·os·to·sis
syn·drome
acrog·e·nous
ac·ro·ger·ia
ac·rog·no·sis
ac·ro·hy·per·hi·dro·sis
ac·ro·ker·a·to·e·las·toi·do·sis
ac·ro·ker·a·to·sis
par·a·ne·o·plas·tic a.
ac·ro·ker·a·to·sis ver·ru·ci·for·mis
ac·ro·ki·ne·sia
ac·ro·le·ic ac·ids
ac·ro·leu·kop·a·thy
ac·ro·me·ga·lia
ac·ro·me·gal·ic
gi·gan·tism
ac·ro·meg·a·lo·gi·gan·tism
ac·ro·meg·a·loid·ism
ac·ro·meg·a·ly
ac·ro·mel·al·gia
ac·ro·me·lia
ac·ro·mel·ic
dwarf·ism
ac·ro·met·a·gen·e·sis
acro·mi·al
an·gle
ar·tery
ex·trem·i·ty of clav·i·cle
net·work
pro·cess
re·flex
acro·mi·al ar·tic·u·lar
fa·ci·es of clav·i·cle
sur·face of clav·i·cle
ac·ro·mic·ria
acro·mi·o·cla·vic·u·lar
disk
joint
lig·a·ment
acro·mi·o·cor·a·coid
acro·mi·o·hu·mer·al

acro·mi·on
pre·sen·ta·tion
acro·mi·o·scap·u·lar
acro·mi·o·tho·rac·ic
ar·tery
a·crom·pha·lus
ac·ro·my·o·to·nia
ac·ro·my·ot·o·nus
ac·ro·neu·ro·sis
ac·ro·nine
ac·ro·nyx
ac·ro-os·te·ol·y·sis
ac·ro·pachy
ac·ro·pach·y·der·ma
ac·ro·par·es·the·sia
syn·drome
acrop·a·thy
acrop·e·tal
ac·ro·pho·bia
ac·ro·pig·men·ta·tion
ac·ro·pleu·rog·e·nous
ac·ro·pos·thi·tis
ac·ro·pus·tu·lo·sis
in·fan·tile a.
ac·ro·scle·ro·der·ma
ac·ro·scle·ro·sis
ac·ro·sin
ac·ro·so·mal
cap
gran·ule
ves·i·cle
ac·ro·some
ac·ro·so·min
ac·ro·sphe·no·syn·dac·ty·ly
ac·ro·spi·ro·ma
ec·crine a.
ac·ros·te·al·gia
ac·ro·ter·ic
Ac·ro·the·ca
ac·ro·the·ca
acrot·ic
ac·ro·tism
ac·ro·troph·o·dyn·ia
ac·ro·troph·o·neu·ro·sis
ac·ryl·ate
acryl·ic
res·in
acryl·ic ac·ids
acryl·ic res·in
base
tooth
tray
ac·ry·lo·ni·trile
ac·thi·a·zi·dum
ACTH-pro·duc·ing
ad·e·no·ma
ACTH stim·u·la·tion
test

ac·tin
  fil·a·ment
ac·tin
  F-a.
  G-a.
act·ing out
ac·tin·ic
  chei·li·tis
  con·junc·ti·vi·tis
  der·ma·ti·tis
  gran·u·lo·ma
  ker·a·ti·tis
  ker·a·to·sis
  po·ro·ker·a·to·sis
  ray
  re·tic·u·loid
ac·tin·i·de
  el·e·ments
ac·tin·i·des
ac·ti·nism
ac·tin·i·um
  em·a·na·tion
ac·ti·no·bac·il·lo·sis
Ac·ti·no·ba·cil·lus
  A. ac·ti·noi·des
  A. ac·ti·no·my·ce·tem co·
   mi·tans
  A. equ·u·li
  A. lig·ni·er·e·sii
  A. mal·lei
ac·ti·no·der·ma·ti·tis
ac·tin·o·gen
ac·ti·no·gen·e·sis
ac·ti·no·gen·ic
ac·ti·no·gen·ics
ac·tin·o·gram
ac·tin·o·graph
ac·ti·nog·ra·phy
ac·ti·no·he·ma·tin
ac·tin·o·lite
ac·tin·o·lyte
Ac·ti·no·mad·u·ra
ac·ti·nom·e·try
ac·ti·no·my·ce·li·al
Ac·ti·no·my·ces
  A. bo·vis
  A. is·rae·lii
  A. naes·lun·dii
  A. odon·to·ly·ti·cus
  A. vis·co·sus
Ac·ti·no·my·ce·ta·ce·ae
Ac·ti·no·my·ce·ta·les
ac·ti·no·my·cetes
ac·ti·no·my·cin
  a. A
  a. C
  a. D
ac·ti·no·my·co·ma

ac·ti·no·my·co·sis
ac·ti·no·my·cot·ic
  ap·pen·di·ci·tis
Ac·ti·no·myx·id·ia
ac·ti·no·neu·ri·tis
ac·tin·o·phage
ac·ti·no·phy·to·sis
Ac·ti·no·po·da
ac·tin·o·sin
ac·ti·no·ther·a·peu·tics
ac·ti·no·ther·a·py
ac·ti·no·tox·e·mia
ac·tion
  ball valve a.
  ca·lor·i·gen·ic a.
  cu·mu·la·tive a.
  salt a.
  spar·ing a.
  spe·cif·ic a.
  spe·cif·ic dy·nam·ic a.
  ther·mo·gen·ic a.
ac·tion
  cur·rent
  po·ten·tial
  trem·or
ac·ti·vate
ac·ti·vat·ed
  at·om
  char·coal
  ep·i·lep·sy
  hy·dro·gen
  res·in
  sludge
  state
ac·ti·vat·ed par·tial throm·bo·
  plas·tin
  time
ac·ti·vat·ed sludge
  meth·od
ac·ti·va·tion
  anal·y·sis
ac·ti·va·tion
  EEG a.
ac·ti·va·tor
  ca·tab·o·lite gene a.
  plas·min·o·gen a.
  tis·sue plas·min·o·gen a.
ac·tive
  ac·e·tate
  an·a·phy·lax·is
  car·bon di·ox·ide
  car·ies
  con·ges·tion
  elec·trode
  for·myl
  hy·per·e·mia
  im·mu·ni·ty
  im·mu·ni·za·tion

me·thi·o·nine
meth·yl
move·ment
mu·tant
prin·ci·ple
pro·phy·lax·is
psy·cho·a·nal·y·sis
re·pres·sor
site
splint
sul·fate
trans·port
va·so·con·stric·tion
va·so·di·la·tion
ac·tive chron·ic
hep·a·ti·tis
ac·tive ro·sette
test
ac·tiv·i·ty
co·ef·fi·cient
ac·tiv·i·ty
block·ing a.
in·su·lin-like a.
op·ti·cal a.
plas·ma re·nin a.
spe·cif·ic a.
trig·gered a.
ac·to·my·o·sin
plate·let a.
ac·tu·al
cau·tery
Ac·u·a·ria spi·ra·lis
acu·i·ty
ab·so·lute in·ten·si·ty
thresh·old a.
res·o·lu·tion a.
spa·tial a.
ster·e·o·scop·ic a.
Vernier a.
vis·i·bil·i·ty a.
vi·su·al a.
acu·le·ate
acu·mi·nate
acu·mi·nate pap·u·lar
syph·i·lid
ac·u·ol·o·gy
ac·u·punc·ture
an·es·the·sia
acus
ac·u·sec·tion
ac·u·sec·tor
acu·sis
acute
ab·do·men
ab·scess
al·co·hol·ism
an·gle

ap·pen·di·ci·tis
atax·ia
cha·la·zi·on
cho·le·cys·ti·tis
de·lir·i·um
glau·co·ma
glo·mer·u·lo·ne·phri·tis
goi·ter
in·flam·ma·tion
ma·lar·ia
ne·phri·tis
ne·phro·sis
por·phyr·ia
py·e·lo·ne·phri·tis
rhi·ni·tis
rick·ets
try·pan·o·so·mi·a·sis
tu·ber·cu·lo·sis
ur·ti·car·ia
acute adre·no·cor·ti·cal
in·suf·fi·cien·cy
acute Af·ri·can sleep·ing
sick·ness
acute an·te·ri·or
po·li·o·my·e·li·tis
acute as·cend·ing
pa·ral·y·sis
acute atroph·ic
pa·ral·y·sis
acute bac·te·ri·al
en·do·car·di·tis
acute brach·i·al
ra·dic·u·li·tis
acute bul·bar
po·li·o·my·e·li·tis
acute ca·tarrh·al
con·junc·ti·vi·tis
acute cel·lu·lar
re·jec·tion
acute com·pres·sion
tri·ad
acute con·ta·gious
con·junc·ti·vi·tis
acute cres·cen·tic
glo·mer·u·lo·ne·phri·tis
acute cu·ta·ne·ous
leish·man·i·a·sis
acute de·cu·bi·tus
ul·cer
acute dis·sem·i·nat·ed
en·ceph·a·lo·my·e·li·tis
my·o·si·tis
acute ep·i·dem·ic
con·junc·ti·vi·tis
leu·ko·en·ceph·a·li·tis
acute fol·lic·u·lar
con·junc·ti·vi·tis

acute ful·mi·nat·ing me·nin·go·coc·cal
  sep·ti·ce·mia
acute hal·lu·ci·na·to·ry
  par·a·noia
acute hem·or·rhag·ic
  con·junc·ti·vi·tis
  en·ceph·a·li·tis
  glo·mer·u·lo·ne·phri·tis
  pan·cre·a·ti·tis
acute id·i·o·path·ic
  pol·y·neu·ri·tis
acute in·fec·tious non·bac·te·ri·al
  gas·tro·en·ter·i·tis
acute in·ter·mit·tent
  por·phyr·ia
acute in·ter·sti·tial
  ne·phri·tis
  pneu·mo·nia
acute iso·lat·ed
  my·o·car·di·tis
acute lead
  poi·son·ing
acute lym·pho·nod·u·lar
  phar·yn·gi·tis
acute mer·cu·ry
  poi·son·ing
acute mil·i·a·ry
  tu·ber·cu·lo·sis
acute nec·ro·tiz·ing
  en·ceph·a·li·tis
  gin·gi·vi·tis
acute neu·tro·phil·ic
  der·ma·to·sis
acute par·en·chym·a·tous
  hep·a·ti·tis
acute phase
  re·ac·tants
acute post-strep·to·coc·cal
  glo·mer·u·lo·ne·phri·tis
acute pri·mary hem·or·rhag·ic
  me·nin·go·en·ceph·a·li·tis
acute pro·my·e·lo·cyt·ic
  leu·ke·mia
acute pul·mo·nary
  al·ve·o·li·tis
acute ra·di·a·tion
  syn·drome
acute re·cur·rent
  rhab·do·my·ol·y·sis
acute re·flex bone
  at·ro·phy
acute rheu·mat·ic
  ar·thri·tis
acute scalp
  cel·lu·li·tis

acute sit·u·a·tion·al
  re·ac·tion
acute splen·ic
  tu·mor
acute trans·verse
  my·e·li·tis
acute vas·cu·lar
  pur·pu·ra
acute yel·low
  at·ro·phy of the liv·er
acy·a·not·ic
acy·clic
  com·pound
acy·clo·guan·o·sine
acy·clo·vir
ac·yl
ac·yl-ACP de·hy·dro·gen·ase
ac·yl-ACP re·duc·tase
ac·yl-ac·ti·vat·ing
  en·zyme
ac·yl·ad·e·nyl·ate
ac·yl·am·i·dase
n-ac·yl·a·mi·no ac·id
ac·yl·ase
ac·yl·a·tion
ac·yl car·ri·er
  pro·tein
ac·yl-CoA
ac·yl-CoA de·hy·dro·gen·ase (NADPH$^+$)
ac·yl-CoA syn·the·tase
ac·yl·co·en·zyme A
ac·yl-mal·o·nyl-ACP syn·thase
ac·yl·mer·cap·tan
  bond
N-ac·yl·sphin·gol
N-ac·yl·sphin·go·sine
ac·yl·trans·fer·as·es
acys·tia
adac·tyl·ia
adac·tyl·ism
adac·ty·lous
adac·ty·ly
ad·a·man·tine
  mem·brane
ad·a·man·ti·no·ma
  a. of long bones
  pi·tu·i·tary a.
Adams'
  op·er·a·tion for ec·tro·pi·on
Adam's ap·ple
Adams-Stokes
  dis·ease
  syn·drome
ad·an·so·ni·an
  clas·si·fi·ca·tion

ad·ap·ta·tion
  dis·eas·es
  syn·drome of Selye
ad·ap·ta·tion
  dark a.
  light a.
  pho·top·ic a.
  re·al·i·ty a.
  ret·i·nal a.
  sco·top·ic a.
  so·cial a.
adapt·er
adap·tive
  be·hav·ior
  en·zyme
  hy·per·tro·phy
adap·tive be·hav·ior
  scales
ad·ap·tom·e·ter
adap·tor
ad·ax·i·al
ad·der
ad·dict
ad·dic·tion
Addis
  count
Addison-Biermer
  dis·ease
ad·di·so·ni·an
  ane·mia
  cri·sis
Addison's
  ane·mia
  dis·ease
Addison's clin·i·cal
  planes
ad·di·tion
  com·pound
ad·di·tion-de·le·tion
  mu·ta·tion
ad·di·tive
  ef·fect
ad·di·tiv·i·ty
  al·le·lic a.
  caus·al a.
  in·ter·lo·cal a.
ad·du·cent
ad·duct
ad·duc·tion
ad·duc·tor
  ca·nal
  mus·cle of great toe
  mus·cle of thumb
  re·flex
  tu·ber·cle
ade·lo·mor·phous

Aden
  fe·ver
  ul·cer
ad·e·nal·gia
aden·dric
aden·drit·ic
ad·e·nec·to·my
ad·e·nec·to·pia
ad·e·nem·phrax·is
aden·i·form
ad·e·nine
  a. ar·a·bi·no·side
  a. de·ox·y·ri·bo·nu·cle·o·tide
  a. nu·cle·o·tide
  a. sul·fate
ad·e·ni·tis
ad·e·ni·za·tion
ad·e·no·ac·an·tho·ma
ad·e·no·am·e·lo·blas·to·ma
ad·e·no-as·so·ci·at·ed
  vi·rus
ad·e·no·blast
ad·e·no·car·ci·no·ma
  acin·ic cell a.
  bron·chi·o·lar a.
  clear cell a.
  Lucké's a.
  mes·o·neph·ric a.
  a. of Moll
  mu·coid a.
  pap·il·lary a.
  re·nal a.
  a. in si·tu
ad·e·no·cel·lu·li·tis
ad·e·no·chon·dro·ma
ad·e·no·cys·to·ma
ad·e·no·cyte
ad·e·no·di·as·ta·sis
ad·e·no·dyn·ia
ad·e·no·ep·i·the·li·o·ma
ad·e·no·fi·bro·ma
ad·e·no·fi·bro·my·o·ma
ad·e·no·fi·bro·sis
ad·e·no·gen·e·sis
ad·e·nog·en·ous
ad·e·no·hy·po·phy·si·al
ad·e·no·hy·poph·y·sis
ad·e·no·hy·poph·y·si·tis
  lym·pho·cyt·ic a.
ad·e·noid
  dis·ease
  fa·ci·es
  tis·sue
  tu·mor
ad·e·noi·dal-pha·ryn·ge·al-con·junc·ti·val
  vi·rus

ad·e·noid cys·tic
  car·ci·no·ma
ad·e·noid·ec·to·my
ad·e·noi·dism
ad·e·noid·i·tis
ad·e·noids
ad·e·noid squa·mous cell
  car·ci·no·ma
ad·e·no·lei·o·my·o·fi·bro·ma
ad·e·no·li·po·ma
ad·e·no·lip·o·ma·to·sis
  sym·met·ric a.
ad·e·no·lym·pho·cele
ad·e·no·lym·pho·ma
ad·e·nol·y·sis
ad·e·no·ma
  ac·i·do·phil a.
  ACTH-pro·duc·ing a.
  ad·nex·al a.
  adre·no·cor·ti·cal a.
  ap·o·crine a.
  ba·sal cell a.
  ba·so·phil a.
  bron·chi·al a.
  chro·mo·phil a.
  chro·mo·phobe a.
  col·loid a.
  em·bry·o·nal a.
  eo·sin·o·phil a.
  fe·tal a.
  fi·broid a.
  a. fi·bro·sum
  fol·lic·u·lar a.
  Fuchs' a.
  go·nad·o·tro·pin-pro·duc·ing
    a.
  growth hor·mone-pro·duc·ing
    a.
  Hürthle cell a.
  is·let cell a.
  lac·tat·ing a.
  Leydig cell a.
  mac·ro·fol·lic·u·lar a.
  mi·cro·fol·lic·u·lar a.
  mon·o·mor·phic a.
  neph·ro·gen·ic a.
  a. of nip·ple
  null-cell a.
  ovar·i·an tu·bu·lar a.
  ox·y·phil a.
  pap·il·lary cys·tic a.
  pap·il·lary a. of large in·
    tes·tine
  Pick's tu·bu·lar a.
  pi·tu·i·tary a.
  ple·o·mor·phic a.
  pol·yp·oid a.
  pro·lac·tin-pro·duc·ing a.

pros·tat·ic a.
re·nal cor·ti·cal a.
se·ba·ceous a.
a. se·ba·ce·um
sweat duct a.
tes·tic·u·lar tu·bu·lar a.
thy·rot·ro·pin-pro·duc·ing a.
tu·bu·lar a.
un·dif·fer·en·ti·at·ed cell a.
vil·lous a.
ad·e·no·ma·toid
  tu·mor
ad·e·no·ma·toid odon·to·gen·ic
  tu·mor
ad·e·no·ma·to·sis
  ero·sive a. of nip·ple
  fi·bros·ing a.
  plu·ri·glan·du·lar a.
  pul·mo·nary a.
  pul·mo·nary a. of sheep
ad·e·nom·a·tous
  goi·ter
  pol·yp
ad·e·no·mere
ad·e·no·my·o·ma
ad·e·no·my·o·sar·co·ma
ad·e·no·my·o·sis
  a. uteri
ad·e·no·neu·ral
ad·e·nop·a·thy
ad·e·no·phar·yn·gi·tis
ad·e·no·phleg·mon
Ad·e·no·pho·ra·si·da
Ad·e·no·pho·rea
ad·e·no·phy·ma
ad·e·no·sal·pin·gi·tis
ad·e·no·sar·co·ma
  mül·le·ri·an a.
ad·e·no·sat·el·lite
  vi·rus
ad·e·nose
ad·e·no·sin·ase
aden·o·sine
  a. cy·clic phos·phate
  a. de·am·i·nase
  a. di·phos·phate
  a. ki·nase
  a. mon·o·phos·phate
  a. nu·cle·o·si·dase
  a. phos·phate
  a. tet·ra·phos·phate
  a. tri·phos·phate
ad·e·no·sine·tri·phos·pha·tase
ad·e·no·sis
  blunt duct a.
  fi·bros·ing a.
  mi·cro·glan·du·lar a.
  scle·ros·ing a.

aden·o·syl
S-aden·o·syl·ho·mo·cys·te·ine
S-aden·o·syl·me·thi·o·nine
ad·e·not·o·my
ad·e·no·ton·sil·lec·to·my
ad·e·nous
Ad·e·no·vi·ri·dae
ad·e·no·vi·rus
   bo·vine a.'s
   por·cine a.'s
ad·e·nyl
   a. cy·clase
aden·y·late
   a. cy·clase
   a. ki·nase
ad·e·nyl·ic ac·id
   cy·clic a. a.
   a. a. de·am·i·nase
   a. a. ki·nase
ad·e·nyl·o·suc·ci·nase
ad·e·nyl·o·suc·ci·nate ly·ase
ad·e·nyl·o·suc·ci·nate syn·thase
ad·e·nyl·o·suc·cin·ic ac·id
ad·en·yl·py·ro·phos·pha·tase
aden·y·lyl
   a. cy·clase
   a. py·ro·phos·phate
aden·y·lyl·o·suc·ci·nate ly·ase
aden·y·lyl·o·suc·ci·nate syn·thase
aden·y·lyl·o·suc·cin·ic ac·id
a·deps
   a. re·nis
ad·e·qual
   cleav·age
ad·e·quate
   stim·u·lus
ader·mia
ader·mine
ader·mo·gen·e·sis
ad·her·ence
   syn·drome
ad·her·ent
   leu·ko·ma
   per·i·car·di·um
   pla·cen·ta
ad·he·sins
ad·he·sio
ad·he·sion
   am·ni·ot·ic a.'s
   fi·brin·ous a.
   fi·brous a.
   in·ter·tha·lam·ic a.
   pri·mary a.
   sec·on·dary a.
ad·he·sion
   dys·pep·sia

phe·nom·e·non
   test
ad·he·si·o·nes
ad·he·si·ot·o·my
ad·he·sive
   arach·noid·i·tis
   ban·dage
   cap·su·li·tis
   in·flam·ma·tion
   per·i·car·di·tis
   per·i·to·ni·tis
   phle·bi·tis
   pleu·ri·sy
   tape
   vag·i·ni·tis
ad·he·sive ab·sor·bent
   dress·ing
adi·ac·tin·ic
ad·i·ad·o·cho·ci·ne·sia
ad·i·ad·o·cho·ci·ne·sis
ad·i·ad·o·cho·ki·ne·sis
adi·a·pho·re·sis
adi·a·pho·ret·ic
adi·a·pho·ria
adi·ap·neu·stia
adi·a·spi·ro·my·co·sis
adi·a·spore
adi·as·to·le
adi·a·ther·man·cy
Adie
   syn·drome
ad·i·em·or·rhy·sis
ad·i·ent
   be·hav·ior
Adie's
   pu·pil
Adin·i·da
ad·i·pec·to·my
adi·pes
adiph·e·nine hy·dro·chlo·ride
adip·ic ac·id
adi·pis
ad·i·po·cele
ad·i·po·cel·lu·lar
ad·i·po·cer·a·tous
ad·i·po·cere
ad·i·po·cyte
ad·i·po·der·mal
   graft
ad·i·po·gen·e·sis
ad·i·po·gen·ic
ad·i·pog·e·nous
ad·i·poid
ad·i·po·ki·net·ic
   hor·mone
ad·i·po·ki·nin
ad·i·pom·e·ter
ad·i·po·ne·cro·sis

ad·i·po·sal·gia
ad·i·pose
cap·sule
cell
de·gen·er·a·tion
folds of the pleu·ra
fos·sae
in·fil·tra·tion
tis·sue
tu·mor
ad·i·po·sis
a. car·di·a·ca
a. ce·re·bra·lis
a. do·lo·ro·sa
a. or·chi·ca
a. tu·be·ro·sa sim·plex
a. uni·ver·sa·lis
ad·i·pos·i·ty
ad·i·po·so·gen·i·tal
de·gen·er·a·tion
dys·tro·phy
syn·drome
ad·i·po·su·ria
adip·sia
adip·sy
ad·i·tus
a. ad aq·ue·duc·tum ce·re·
bri
a. ad in·fun·dib·u·lum
a. ad sac·cum pe·ri·to·na·ei
mi·no·rum
a. glot·ti·dis in·fe·ri·or
a. glot·ti·dis su·pe·ri·or
a. pel·vis
ad·i·tus
ad·ja·cent
an·gle
ad·just·a·ble
ar·tic·u·la·tor
ad·just·a·ble ax·is
face-bow
ad·just·a·ble oc·clu·sal
piv·ot
ad·just·ment
dis·or·ders
ad·just·ment
oc·clu·sal a.
ad·ju·vant
Freund's com·plete a.
Freund's in·com·plete a.
ad·ju·vant
vac·cine
ad·le·ri·an
psy·cho·a·nal·y·sis
psy·chol·o·gy
Adler's
test

ad·max·il·lary
gland
ad·me·di·al
ad·me·di·an
ad·mi·nic·u·la
ad·mi·nic·u·lum
ad·ner·val
ad·neu·ral
ad·nexa
a. oc·u·li
a. uter·i
ad·nex·al
ad·e·no·ma
car·ci·no·ma
ad·nex·ec·to·my
ad·nex·i·tis
ad·nex·o·pexy
ad·nex·um
ad·o·les·cence
ad·o·les·cent
al·bu·min·ur·ia
cri·sis
med·i·cine
ste·ril·i·ty
ad·o·les·cent round
back
adon·i·tol
adop·tive
im·mu·ni·ty
im·mu·no·ther·a·py
ad·o·ral
ADPase
ad·re·nal
ac·ces·so·ry a.
but·ter·fly a.
Marchand's a.'s
ad·re·nal
an·dro·gen
ap·o·plexy
body
cap·sule
cor·tex
cri·sis
gland
her·maph·ro·dit·ism
hy·per·ten·sion
rest
vir·i·lism
ad·re·nal ascor·bic ac·id de·
ple·tion
test
ad·re·nal cor·ti·cal
car·ci·no·mas
syn·drome
ad·re·nal·ec·to·my
adren·a·line
a. ox·i·dase

adren·a·line
   re·ver·sal
adre·nal·i·tis
adren·a·lone
adre·na·lop·a·thy
ad·re·nal vir·i·liz·ing
   syn·drome
ad·re·nal weight
   fac·tor
ad·ren·ar·che
ad·re·ner·gic
   amine
   block·ade
   fi·bers
   re·cep·tors
ad·re·ner·gic block·ing
   agent
ad·re·ner·gic neu·ro·nal block·
  ing
   agent
adren·ic
adre·no·cep·tive
adre·no·cor·ti·cal
   ad·e·no·ma
   hor·mones
   in·suf·fi·cien·cy
adre·no·cor·ti·co·mi·met·ic
adre·no·cor·ti·co·tro·phic
adre·no·cor·ti·co·tro·pic
   hor·mone
   pep·tide
adre·no·cor·ti·co·tro·pin
adre·no·gen·ic
adre·no·gen·i·tal
   syn·drome
adre·nog·e·nous
adre·no·leu·ko·dys·tro·phy
adre·no·lyt·ic
adre·no·meg·a·ly
adre·no·mi·met·ic
   amine
adre·no·my·e·lo·neu·rop·a·thy
adre·nop·a·thy
adre·no·pri·val
adre·no·re·ac·tive
adre·no·re·cep·tors
adre·nos·ter·one
adre·no·tox·in
adre·no·tro·phic
adre·no·tro·pic
   hor·mone
adre·no·tro·pin
adri·a·my·cin
adro·mia
Adson
   for·ceps
   ma·neu·ver

Adson's
   pro·ce·dure
   test
ad·sorb
ad·sorb·ate
ad·sorb·ent
ad·sorp·tion
   im·mune a.
ad·sorp·tion
   the·o·ry of nar·co·sis
ad·ster·nal
ad·ter·mi·nal
adult
   me·dul·lo·ep·i·the·li·o·ma
   rick·ets
   tu·ber·cu·lo·sis
adul·ter·ant
adul·ter·a·tion
adul·to·mor·phism
adult-on·set
   di·a·be·tes
adult pseu·do·hy·per·tro·phic
  mus·cu·lar
   dys·tro·phy
adult res·pi·ra·to·ry dis·tress
   syn·drome
adult T-cell
   leu·ke·mia
   lym·pho·ma
ad·vanced life sup·port
ad·vance·ment
   cap·su·lar a.
   ten·don a.
ad·vance·ment
   flap
ad·ven·ti·tia
ad·ven·ti·tial
   cell
   neu·ri·tis
ad·ven·ti·tious
   al·bu·min·ur·ia
   bur·sa
   cyst
ad·verse
   re·ac·tion
ad·ver·sive
   move·ment
ady·nam·ia
   a. ep·i·so·di·ca he·re·di·ta·
   ria
ady·nam·ic
   il·e·us
Aeby's
   mus·cle
   plane
Aedes
   A. ae·gyp·ti
   A. al·bo·pic·tus

Aedes *(continued)*
  A. ca·bal·lus
  A. leu·co·ce·lae·nus
  A. pol·y·ne·si·en·sis
  A. sca·pu·la·ris
  A. sol·li·ci·tans
  A. va·ri·e·ga·tus
ae·lu·ro·pho·bia
Aelu·ro·stron·gy·lus
ae·quo·rin
aer·as·the·nia
aer·a·ted
aer·a·tion
aer·e·mia
aer·en·do·car·dia
aer·i·al
  my·ce·li·um
aer·o·as·the·nia
aer·o·at·el·ec·ta·sis
Aer·o·bac·ter
aer·obe
  ob·li·gate a.
aer·o·bic
  de·hy·dro·gen·ase
  res·pi·ra·tion
aer·o·bi·ol·o·gy
aer·o·bi·o·scope
aer·o·bi·o·sis
aer·o·bi·ot·ic
aer·o·cele
Aer·o·coc·cus
aer·o·col·pos
aer·o·cys·tog·ra·phy
aer·o·cys·to·scope
aer·o·cys·tos·co·py
aer·o·der·mec·ta·sia
aer·o·don·tal·gia
  pri·mary a.
  sec·on·dary a.
aer·o·don·tia
aer·o·dy·nam·ics
aer·o·dy·nam·ic size
aer·o·em·phy·se·ma
aer·o·gas·tria
  blocked a.
aer·o·gen
aer·o·gen·e·sis
aer·o·gen·ic
aer·og·e·nous
aer·o·hy·dro·ther·a·py
aer·o·med·i·cine
aer·o·mo·nad
Aer·o·mo·nas
  A. hy·dro·phi·la
aer·o·neu·ro·sis
aer·o-o·don·tal·gia
aer·o-o·don·to·dyn·ia
aer·op·a·thy

aer·o·pause
aer·o·pha·gia
aer·oph·a·gy
aer·o·phil
aer·o·phile
aer·o·phil·ic
aer·oph·i·lous
aer·o·pho·bia
aer·o·pi·e·so·ther·a·py
aer·o·plank·ton
aer·o·ple·thys·mo·graph
aer·o·si·al·oph·a·gy
aer·o·si·nus·i·tis
aer·o·sis
aer·o·sol
  res·pi·ra·ble a.'s
aer·o·sol
  gen·er·a·tor
aer·o·sol·i·za·tion
aer·o·space
  med·i·cine
aer·o·ther·a·peu·tics
aer·o·ther·a·py
aer·o·ti·tis me·dia
aer·o·ton·om·e·ter
aes·cu·lin
aes·ti·val
aes·ti·vo·au·tum·nal
  fe·ver
afe·brile
afe·tal
af·fect
  flat a.
  in·ap·pro·pri·ate a.
  la·bile a.
af·fect
  dis·place·ment
  hun·ger
  mem·o·ry
  spasms
af·fect dis·play
af·fec·tion
af·fec·tive
  dis·or·ders
  psy·cho·sis
  tone
af·fec·tiv·i·ty
af·fec·to·mo·tor
af·fer·ent
  fi·bers
  lym·phat·ic
  nerve
  ves·sel
af·fer·ent glo·mer·u·lar
  ar·te·ri·ole
af·fer·ent loop
  syn·drome

af·fin·i·ty
  chro·ma·tog·ra·phy
  col·umn
af·fin·i·ty
  re·sid·u·al a.
af·fi·nous
af·fir·ma·tion
af·flux
af·flux·ion
af·fu·sion
afi·bril·lar
  ce·men·tum
afi·brin·o·gen·e·mia
  con·gen·i·tal a.
af·la·tox·in
AFORMED
  phe·nom·e·non
Af·ri·can
  his·to·plas·mo·sis
  try·pan·o·so·mi·a·sis
Af·ri·can fu·run·cu·lar
  my·i·a·sis
Af·ri·can hem·or·rhag·ic
  fe·ver
Af·ri·can horse
  sick·ness
Af·ri·can horse sick·ness
  vi·rus
Af·ri·can sleep·ing
  sick·ness
Af·ri·can swine
  fe·ver
Af·ri·can swine fe·ver
  vi·rus
af·ter-
  con·trac·tion
  cur·rent
  dis·charge
  ef·fect
  move·ment
  nys·tag·mus
  pains
  po·ten·tial
  sound
  taste
af·ter·birth
af·ter·care
af·ter·cat·a·ract
af·ter·chrom·ing
af·ter·con·trac·tion
af·ter·cur·rent
af·ter·dis·charge
af·ter·ef·fect
af·ter·gild·ing
af·ter·hear·ing
af·ter·im·age
  neg·a·tive a.
  pos·i·tive a.

af·ter·im·pres·sion
af·ter·load
  ven·tric·u·lar a.
af·ter·load·ing
  screw
af·ter·move·ment
af·ter·pains
af·ter·per·cep·tion
af·ter·po·ten·tial
  di·a·stol·ic a.
af·ter·sen·sa·tion
af·ter·sound
af·ter·taste
af·ter·touch
af·to·sa
afunc·tion·al
  oc·clu·sion
ag·a·lac·tia
  con·ta·gious a.
aga·lac·tor·rhea
ag·a·lac·to·sis
ag·a·lac·tous
ag·a·mete
agam·ic
agam·ma·glob·u·lin·e·mia
  ac·quired a.
  Bruton type a.
  con·gen·i·tal a.
  pri·mary a.
  sec·on·dary a.
  Swiss type a.
  tran·sient a.
  X-linked a.
agam·o·cy·tog·e·ny
Aga·mo·fi·lar·ia
ag·a·mo·gen·e·sis
ag·a·mo·ge·net·ic
ag·a·mog·o·ny
Ag·a·mo·mer·mis cu·li·cis
ag·a·mont
ag·a·mous
agan·gli·on·ic
agan·gli·o·no·sis
agap·ism
agar
  ascit·ic a.
  bile salt a.
  blood a.
  Bordet-Gengou po·ta·to
   blood a.
  brain-heart in·fu·sion a.
  bril·liant green bile salt a.
  choc·o·late a.
  chol·era a.
  Conradi-Drigalski a.
  corn·meal a.
  Czapek's so·lu·tion a.
  Drigalski-Conradi a.

agar *(continued)*
 EMB a.
 Endo a.
 Endo's fuch·sin a.
 eo·sin-meth·yl·ene blue a.
 French proof a.
 fuch·sin a.
 Guarnieri's gel·a·tin a.
 lac·tose-lit·mus a.
 MacConkey a.
 Novy and MacNeal's blood
  a.
 nu·tri·ent a.
 oat·meal-to·ma·to paste a.
 Pfeiffer's blood a.
 po·ta·to dex·trose a.
 rice-Tween a.
 Sabouraud's a.
 se·rum a.
 yeast ex·tract a.
ag·a·ric
 dead·ly a.
 fly a.
agar·ic·ic
agar·i·cin·ic ac·id
Agar·i·cus
ag·a·rose
Ag-AS
 stain
agas·tric
agas·tro·neu·ria
age
 achieve·ment a.
 an·a·tom·i·cal a.
 ba·sal a.
 Binet a.
 bone a.
 child·bear·ing a.
 chro·no·log·ic a.
 de·vel·op·men·tal a.
 emo·tion·al a.
 fe·tal a.
 ges·ta·tion·al a.
 men·tal a.
 phys·i·cal a.
 phys·i·o·log·ic a.
agene
 pro·cess
agen·e·sis
 go·nad·al a.
 re·nal a.
 thy·mic a.
agen·i·tal·ism
agen·o·so·mia
agent
 ad·re·ner·gic block·ing a.
 ad·re·ner·gic neu·ro·nal
  block·ing a.

al·kyl·at·ing a.'s
an·ti·anx·i·e·ty a.
an·ti·foam·ing a.'s
an·ti·psy·chot·ic a.
Bittner a.
block·ing a.
cal·ci·um chan·nel-block·ing
 a.
chim·pan·zee co·ry·za a.
cho·lin·er·gic a.
del·ta a.
Eaton a.
em·bed·ding a.'s
en·ter·o·ki·net·ic a.
F a.
F a.
fer·til·i·ty a.
foamy a.'s
gan·gli·on·ic block·ing a.
in·i·ti·a·ting a.
LDH a.
lut·ing a.
neu·ro·lep·tic a.
neu·ro·mus·cu·lar block·ing
 a.
non·de·po·lar·iz·ing neu·ro·
 mus·cu·lar block·ing a.
Nor·walk a.
Pitts·burgh pneu·mo·nia a.
pro·mot·ing a.
re·o·vi·rus-like a.
scle·ros·ing a.
slow chan·nel-block·ing a.
sym·pa·thet·ic a.
trans·form·ing a.
TRIC a.'s
Agent Or·ange
age·ra·sia
ageu·sia
ageus·tia
ag·ger
 a. per·pen·di·cu·la·ris
 a. val·vae ve·nae
ag·ger·es
ag·glom·er·ate
ag·glom·er·at·ed
ag·glom·er·a·tion
ag·glu·ti·nant
ag·glu·ti·nate
ag·glu·ti·nat·ing
 an·ti·body
ag·glu·ti·na·tion
 ac·id a.
 bac·te·ri·o·gen·ic a.
 cold a.
 cross a.
 false a.
 group a.

im·mune a.
in·di·rect a.
mixed a.
non·im·mune a.
pas·sive a.
spon·ta·ne·ous a.
ag·glu·ti·na·tive
throm·bus
ag·glu·ti·nin
blood group a.'s
chief a.
cold a.
cross-re·act·ing a.
fla·gel·lar a.
group a.
H a.
im·mune a.
ma·jor a.
mi·nor a.
O a.
par·tial a.
plant a.
sa·line a.
se·rum a.
so·mat·ic a.
warm a.'s
ag·glu·tin·o·gen
blood group a.'s
T a.
ag·glu·tin·o·gen·ic
ag·glu·tin·o·phil·ic
ag·glu·tin·o·phore
ag·glu·tin·o·scope
ag·glu·to·gen
ag·glu·to·gen·ic
ag·gre·gate
an·a·phy·lax·is
glands
ag·gre·gat·ed
ag·gre·gat·ed lym·phat·ic
fol·li·cles
nod·ules
ag·gre·ga·tion
fa·mil·i·al a.
ag·gre·gom·e·ter
ag·gres·sin
ag·gres·sion
ag·gres·sive
in·stinct
ag·gres·sive in·fan·tile
fi·bro·ma·to·sis
ag·ing
clo·nal a.
ag·i·tat·ed
de·pres·sion
ag·i·to·graph·ia
ag·i·to·la·lia

ag·i·to·pha·sia
ag·lo·bu·lia
ag·lo·bu·li·o·sis
aglob·u·lism
aglo·mer·u·lar
aglos·sia
aglos·sia-adac·tyl·ia
syn·drome
aglos·so·sto·mia
aglu·con
ag·lu·ti·tion
agly·con
agly·cos·u·ria
agly·cos·u·ric
ag·men
a. pey·er·i·a·num
ag·mina
ag·mi·nate
glands
ag·mi·nat·ed
glands
ag·nail
ag·na·thia
ag·na·thous
ag·nea
Agnew-Verhoeff
in·ci·sion
ag·no·gen·ic
ag·no·gen·ic my·e·loid
met·a·pla·sia
ag·no·sia
au·di·to·ry a.
fin·ger a.
ide·a·tion·al a.
lo·cal·i·za·tion a.
op·tic a.
po·si·tion a.
tac·tile a.
vi·su·al-spa·tial a.
agom·phi·a·sis
agom·pho·sis
ago·nad·al
ag·o·nal
in·fec·tion
leu·ko·cy·to·sis
rhythm
throm·bus
ag·o·nist
ag·o·ny
clot
ag·o·ra·pho·bia
agor·a·pho·bic
agou·ti
agraffe
ag·ram·mat·i·ca
agram·ma·tism
agram·ma·to·lo·gia

agran·u·lar
  cor·tex
  leu·ko·cyte
agran·u·lar en·do·plas·mic
  re·tic·u·lum
agran·u·lo·cyte
agran·u·lo·cyt·ic
  an·gi·na
agran·u·lo·cy·to·sis
  fe·line a.
agran·u·lo·plas·tic
agraph·ia
  ab·so·lute a.
  acous·tic a.
  am·ne·mon·ic a.
  atac·tic a.
  ce·re·bral a.
  lit·er·al a.
  men·tal a.
  mo·tor a.
  mu·si·cal a.
  ver·bal a.
agraph·ic
ag·ri·o·thy·mia
ag·ro·ma·nia
agryp·nia
agryp·no·co·ma
ague
ag·yi·o·pho·bia
agy·ria
A-H
  in·ter·val
A-H con·duc·tion
  time
Ahumada-Del Castillo
  syn·drome
ahy·log·no·sia
Aicardi's
  syn·drome
aich·mo·pho·bia
AIDS
AIDS-re·lat·ed
  com·plex
  vi·rus
ai·le·ron
ai·lu·ro·pho·bia
ai·nhum
air
  al·ve·o·lar a.
  com·ple·men·tal a.
  com·ple·men·ta·ry a.
  func·tion·al re·sid·u·al a.
  liq·uid a.
  min·i·mal a.
  re·serve a.
  re·sid·u·al a.
  sup·ple·men·tal a.

  tid·al a.
  vi·ti·at·ed a.
air
  blad·der
  cells
  con·duc·tion
  dose
  em·bo·lism
  pol·lu·tion
  sac
  sick·ness
  splint
  sy·ringe
  ther·mom·e·ter
  tube
  ves·i·cles
air-bone
  gap
air·bra·sive
  tech·nique
air-con·di·tion·er
  lung
air·plane
  splint
air·sac·cu·li·tis
air·sick·ness
air-slaked
  lime
air·way
  re·sis·tance
air·way
  con·duct·ing a.
  low·er a.
  res·pi·ra·to·ry a.
  up·per a.
Ajel·lo·my·ces cap·su·la·tum
Ajel·lo·my·ces der·ma·tit·i·dis
aj·ma·line
aj·o·wan oil
Ak·a·bane
  vi·rus
ak·a·mu·shi
  dis·ease
akan·thi·on
akar·y·o·cyte
akar·y·ote
aka·ta·ma
akat·a·ma·the·sia
a·ka·thi·sia
akem·be
aker·a·to·sis
Åkerlund
  de·for·mi·ty
aki·ne·sia
  a. al·ge·ra
  a. am·nes·ti·ca
aki·ne·sic
aki·ne·sis

akin·es·the·sia
aki·net·ic
  ep·i·lep·sy
  mut·ism
aki·ya·mi
ak·lo·mide
Aku·rey·ri
  dis·ease
ala
  a. au·ris
  a. ce·re·bel·li
  a. ci·ne·rea
  alae lin·gu·lae ce·re·bel·li
  a. or·bi·ta·lis
  a. tem·po·ra·lis
  a. ves·per·ti·li·o·nis
alac·ri·ma
alac·tic ox·y·gen
  debt
alae
ala·lia
alal·ic
al·a·nine
al·a·nine ami·no·trans·fer·ase
al·a·nine-ox·o·mal·o·nate ami·no·trans·fer·ase
al·a·nine rac·e·mase
al·a·nine trans·am·i·nase
alan·o·sine
Al·an·son's
  am·pu·ta·tion
alan·tin
al·an·tol
al·ant starch
al·a·nyl
alar
  ar·tery of nose
  chest
  folds
  lam·i·na of neu·ral tube
  lig·a·ments
  part
  plate of neu·ral tube
  pro·cess
  spine
alarm
  re·ac·tion
alas·trim
al·ba
Al·bar·ran's
  glands
  test
Al·bar·ran y Dominguez'
  tu·bules
al·be·do
Albers-Schönberg
  dis·ease

Albert's
  dis·ease
  stain
  su·ture
al·bi·cans
al·bi·can·tia
al·bi·du·ria
al·bi·dus
Al·bi·ni's
  nod·ules
al·bi·nism
  cu·ta·ne·ous a.
  oc·u·lar a.
  oc·u·lo·cu·ta·ne·ous a.
  ru·fous a.
  ty·ro·sin·ase neg·a·tive type
  ty·ro·sin·ase pos·i·tive type
al·bi·no
  rats
al·bi·not·ic
al·bi·nu·ria
Al·bi·nus'
  mus·cle
al·bo·ci·ne·re·ous
Albrecht's
  bone
Albright's
  dis·ease
  syn·drome
Albright's he·red·i·tary
  os·te·o·dys·tro·phy
al·bu·gin·ea
al·bu·gin·e·ot·o·my
al·bu·gin·e·ous
al·bu·go
al·bu·men
al·bu·min
  a. A
  ac·e·to·sol·u·ble a.
  a. B
  Bence Jones a.
  blood a.
  bo·vine se·rum a.
  dried hu·man a.
  egg a.
  a. Ghent
  mac·ro·ag·gre·ga·ted a.
  a. Mex·i·co
  a. Nas·ka·pi
  na·tive a.
  nor·mal hu·man se·rum a.
  Patein's a.
  ra·di·o·io·din·at·ed se·rum a.
  a. Read·ing
  se·rum a.
  a. tan·nate
  a. X

al·bu·mi·nate
al·bu·mi·na·tu·ria
al·bu·min-glob·u·lin
  ra·ti·o
al·bu·min·if·er·ous
al·bu·min·ip·ar·ous
al·bu·mi·nized
  iron
al·bu·mi·no·cho·lia
al·bu·mi·no·cy·to·log·ic
  dis·so·ci·a·tion
al·bu·min·og·e·nous
al·bu·mi·noid
  de·gen·er·a·tion
al·bu·mi·nol·y·sis
al·bu·mi·nop·ty·sis
al·bu·mi·nor·rhea
al·bu·min·ous
  cell
  de·gen·er·a·tion
  gland
  swell·ing
al·bu·min·ur·ia
  ad·o·les·cent a.
  ad·ven·ti·tious a.
  a. of ath·letes
  Bamberger's a.
  be·nign a.
  car·di·ac a.
  col·liq·ua·tive a.
  cy·clic a.
  di·e·tet·ic a.
  di·ges·tive a.
  es·sen·tial a.
  false a.
  feb·rile a.
  func·tion·al a.
  in·ter·mit·tent a.
  lor·dot·ic a.
  neu·ro·path·ic a.
  or·tho·stat·ic a.
  phys·i·o·log·ic a.
  post·re·nal a.
  pos·tur·al a.
  pre·re·nal a.
  re·cur·rent a.
  reg·u·la·to·ry a.
  tran·sient a.
al·bu·min·ur·ic
  ret·i·ni·tis
al·bu·moid
al·bu·ter·ol
Al·ca·lig·e·nes
al·cap·ton
al·cap·ton·u·ria
Al·ci·an blue
al·clo·fe·nac
al·clo·met·a·sone

Alcock's
  ca·nal
al·co·gel
al·co·hol
  ab·so·lute a.
  ac·id a.
  an·hy·drous a.
  de·hy·drat·ed a.
  de·na·tured a.
  di·hy·dric a.
  di·lute a.
  fat·ty a.
  grain a.
  mon·o·hy·dric a.
  pri·mary a.
  py·ro·lig·ne·ous a.
  rub·bing a.
  sec·on·dary a.
  sug·ar a.
  ter·ti·ary a.
  tri·hy·dric a.
  un·sat·u·rat·ed a.'s
al·co·hol
  di·u·re·sis
al·co·hol ac·ids
al·co·hol am·nes·tic
  syn·drome
al·co·hol·ate
al·co·hol de·hy·dro·gen·ase
al·co·hol de·hy·dro·gen·ase
  (ac·cep·tor)
al·co·hol de·hy·dro·gen·ase
  (NADP⁺)
al·co·hol de·hy·dro·gen·ase
  (NAD(P)⁺)
al·co·hol·ic
  car·di·o·my·op·a·thy
  cir·rho·sis
  de·te·ri·o·ra·tion
  ex·tract
  hy·a·lin
  psy·cho·ses
  tinc·ture
al·co·hol·ic hy·a·line
  bod·ies
al·co·hol·ism
  acute a.
  al·pha a.
  be·ta a.
  chron·ic a.
  del·ta a.
  ep·si·lon a.
  gam·ma a.
al·co·hol·i·za·tion
al·co·hol·o·pho·bia
al·co·hol-sol·u·ble
  eo·sin
al·co·hol·y·sis

al·cur·o·ni·um chlo·ride
al·da·di·ene
al·dar·ic ac·id
al·de·hol
al·de·hyde
  an·gu·lar a.
  a. re·duc·tase
al·de·hyde
  base
  fuch·sin
  re·ac·tion
al·de·hyde de·hy·dro·gen·ase
al·de·hyde de·hy·dro·gen·
  ase(ac·yl·at·ing)
al·de·hyde → DPN trans·hy·
  dro·gen·ase
al·de·hyde-ly·as·es
al·de·hyde → TPN trans·hy·
  dro·gen·ase
Alder
  bod·ies
Alder's
  anom·a·ly
al·di·tol
al·do·bi·u·ron·ic ac·id
al·do·cor·tin
al·do·hex·ose
al·do·ke·to·mu·tase
al·dol·ase
al·don·ic ac·ids
al·do·pen·tose
al·dose
  a. mu·ta·ro·tase
  a. re·duc·tase
al·do·side
al·dos·ter·one
al·do·ste·ron·ism
  id·i·o·path·ic a.
  pri·mary a.
  sec·on·dary a.
al·do·tet·rose
al·dox·ime
Aldrich
  syn·drome
al·drin
alec·i·thal
  ovum
Alec·to·ro·bi·us ta·la·je
alem·mal
Alep·po
  boil
ale·thia
ale·to·cyte
aleu·ke·mia
aleu·ke·mic
  leu·ke·mia
  my·e·lo·sis
aleu·ke·moid

aleu·kia
aleu·ko·cyt·ic
aleu·ko·cy·to·sis
aleu·ri·o·co·nid·i·um
aleu·ri·o·spore
al·eu·ron
aleu·ro·nate
aleu·ro·noid
Aleu·tian
  dis·ease of mink
Aleu·tian dis·ease of mink
  vi·rus
Alexander's
  deaf·ness
  dis·ease
alex·ia
  in·com·plete a.
  mu·si·cal a.
alex·ic
alex·in
  unit
alex·i·phar·mac
alex·i·thy·mia
aley·dig·ism
Alezzandrini's
  syn·drome
al·fa·cal·ci·dol
al·fad·o·lone ac·e·tate
al·fax·a·lone
al·fen·ta·nil hy·dro·chlo·ride
al·gae
  blue-green a.
al·gal
al·ga·ro·ba
al·ge·do·nic
al·ge·fa·cient
al·ge·sia
al·ge·sic
al·ge·si·chro·nom·e·ter
al·ge·si·dys·tro·phy
al·ge·sim·e·ter
al·ge·si·o·gen·ic
al·ge·si·om·e·ter
al·ges·the·sia
al·ges·the·sis
al·ges·tone ac·e·to·phe·nide
al·get·ic
al·gi·cide
al·gid
  ma·lar·ia
  stage
al·gid per·ni·cious
  fe·ver
al·gin
al·gi·nate
al·gi·o·mo·tor
al·gi·o·mus·cu·lar
al·gi·o·vas·cu·lar

al·go·dys·tro·phy
al·go·ge·ne·sia
al·go·gen·e·sis
al·go·gen·ic
al·goid
  cell
al·go·lag·nia
al·gom·e·ter
al·gom·e·try
al·go·phil·ia
al·go·pho·bia
al·go·psy·cha·lia
al·go·rithm
al·gos·co·py
al·go·spasm
al·go·vas·cu·lar
al·i·ble
Alice in Won·der·land
  syn·drome
al·i·cy·clic
  com·pounds
alien·a·tion
ali·e·nia
alien·ist
al·i·flu·rane
al·i·form
align·ment
  curve
  mark
al·i·ment
al·i·men·ta·ry
  ap·pa·ra·tus
  ca·nal
  di·a·be·tes
  gly·cos·ur·ia
  hy·per·in·su·lin·ism
  li·pe·mia
  os·te·op·a·thy
  pen·to·su·ria
  sys·tem
  tract
al·i·men·ta·ry tract
  smear
al·i·men·ta·tion
  forced a.
  par·en·ter·al a.
  rec·tal a.
al·i·na·sal
aline·ment
al·in·jec·tion
al·i·phat·ic
  com·pound
al·i·phat·ic ac·ids
ali·poid
alip·o·tro·pic
al·i·quant
al·i·quot

al·i·sphe·noid
  car·ti·lage
aliz·a·rin
  in·di·ca·tor
aliz·a·rin
  a. cy·a·nin
  a. pur·pu·rin
  a. red S
al·ka·di·ene
al·ka·le·mia
al·ka·les·cence
al·ka·les·cent
al·ka·li
  caus·tic a.
  fixed a.
  veg·e·ta·ble a.
al·ka·li
  dis·ease
  met·al
  re·serve
  ther·a·py
al·ka·li de·na·tur·a·tion
  test
al·ka·li earth
  met·al
al·ka·lies
al·ka·line
  earths
  phos·pha·tase
  re·ac·tion
  RNase
  tide
  to·lu·i·dine blue O
  wa·ter
  wave
al·ka·line-ash
  di·et
al·ka·line earth
  el·e·ments
al·ka·line milk
  drip
al·ka·lin·i·ty
al·ka·lin·i·za·tion
al·ka·li·nu·ria
al·ka·lis
al·ka·li·ther·a·py
al·ka·li·za·tion
al·ka·liz·er
al·ka·loid
  fixed a.
al·ka·lo·sis
  acap·ni·al a.
  com·pen·sat·ed a.
  met·a·bol·ic a.
  res·pi·ra·to·ry a.
  un·com·pen·sat·ed a.
al·ka·lot·ic
al·ka·lu·ria

al·kane
al·ka·net
al·kan·nan
al·kan·nin
al·kap·ton
al·kap·ton·u·ria
al·ka·tri·ene
al·ka·ver·vir
al·kene
al·ke·nyl
al·kide
al·kyl
  ar·yl·at·ed a.
al·kyl·a·mine
al·kyl·at·ing
  agents
al·kyl·a·tion
al·la·ches·the·sia
  op·ti·cal a.
al·lan·ti·a·sis
al·lan·to·cho·ri·on
al·lan·to·en·ter·ic
  di·ver·tic·u·lum
al·lan·to·gen·e·sis
al·lan·to·ic
  blad·der
  cav·i·ty
  cyst
  di·ver·tic·u·lum
  flu·id
  sac
  stalk
  ves·i·cle
al·lan·toid
  mem·brane
al·lan·toid·o·an·gi·op·a·gous
  twins
al·lan·toid·o·an·gi·op·a·gus
al·lan·to·in
al·lan·to·in·ase
al·lan·to·in·u·ria
al·lan·to·is
al·lax·is
al·lele
  co·dom·i·nant a.
  si·lent a.
al·le·lic
  ad·di·tiv·i·ty
  ex·clu·sion
  gene
al·lel·ism
al·le·lo·ca·tal·y·sis
al·le·lo·cat·a·lyt·ic
al·le·lo·morph
al·le·lo·mor·phic
al·le·lo·mor·phism
al·le·lo·tax·is
al·le·lo·taxy

Allen
  test
Allen-Doisy
  test
  unit
Allen-Masters
  syn·drome
Allen's
  test
al·ler·gen
al·ler·gen·ic
  ex·tract
al·ler·gic
  an·gi·i·tis
  con·junc·ti·vi·tis
  co·ry·za
  ec·ze·ma
  ex·tract
  gran·u·lo·ma·to·sis
  in·flam·ma·tion
  pur·pu·ra
  re·ac·tion
  rhi·ni·tis
al·ler·gic gran·u·lom·a·tous
  an·gi·i·tis
al·ler·gic sa·lute
al·ler·gin
al·ler·gist
al·ler·gi·za·tion
al·ler·gized
al·ler·go·der·mia
al·ler·go·sis
al·ler·gy
  atop·ic a.
  bac·te·ri·al a.
  cold a.
  con·tact a.
  de·layed a.
  drug a.
  im·me·di·ate a.
  la·tent a.
  phys·i·cal a.
  pol·y·va·lent a.
Al·les·che·ria boy·dii
al·les·the·sia
  vi·su·al a.
al·le·thrins
al·leth·ro·lone
al·lied
  re·flex·es
al·li·ga·tion
al·li·ga·tor
  for·ceps
  skin
Allis
  for·ceps
Allis'
  sign

al·lit·er·a·tion
al·li·um
all or none
 law
al·lo·al·bu·mi·ne·mia
al·lo·an·ti·body
al·lo·an·ti·gen
al·lo·arth·ro·plas·ty
al·lo·bar·bi·tal
al·lo·cen·tric
al·lo·chei·ria
al·lo·che·tia
al·lo·che·zia
al·lo·chi·ria
al·lo·cho·lane
al·lo·cho·les·ter·ol
al·lo·chro·ic
al·lo·chro·ism
al·lo·chro·ma·sia
al·lo·cor·tex
al·lo·dip·loid
al·lo·dyn·ia
al·lo·e·rot·ic
al·lo·e·rot·i·cism
al·lo·er·o·tism
al·lo·es·the·sia
al·log·a·my
al·lo·ge·ne·ic
 graft
 in·hi·bi·tion
al·lo·gen·ic
al·lo·go·tro·phia
al·lo·graft
al·lo·group
al·lo·hex·a·ploid
al·lo·i·so·mer
al·lo·ker·a·to·plas·ty
al·lo·ki·ne·sis
al·lo·la·lia
al·lo·ma·le·ic ac·id
al·lom·er·ic
 func·tion
al·lom·er·ism
al·lom·e·tron
al·lo·mor·phism
al·longe·ment
al·lon·o·mous
al·lo·path
al·lo·path·ic
 ker·a·to·plas·ty
al·lop·a·thist
al·lop·a·thy
al·lo·pen·ta·ploid
al·lo·phan·a·mide
al·lo·phan·ic ac·id
al·loph·a·sis
al·lo·phe·nic
al·lo·phore

al·loph·thal·mia
al·lo·pla·sia
al·lo·plast
al·lo·plas·ty
al·lo·ploid
al·lo·ploi·dy
al·lo·pol·y·ploid
al·lo·pol·y·ploi·dy
al·lo·preg·nane
al·lo·psy·chic
al·lo·pu·ri·nol
al·lo·rhyth·mia
al·lo·rhyth·mic
al·lose
al·lo·some
 paired a.
 un·paired a.
al·lo·ste·ric
 site
al·lo·ster·ism
al·lo·ste·ry
al·lo·tet·ra·ploid
al·lo·therm
al·lo·thre·o·nines
al·lo·to·pia
al·lo·trans·plan·ta·tion
al·lo·trich·ia cir·cum·scrip·ta
al·lot·ri·o·don·tia
al·lot·ri·o·geu·stia
al·lot·ri·oph·a·gy
al·lot·ri·os·mia
al·lo·trip·loid
al·lo·trope
al·lo·tro·phic
al·lo·tro·pic
 per·son·al·i·ty
al·lot·ro·pism
al·lot·ro·py
al·lo·type
al·lo·typ·ic
 de·ter·mi·nants
 mark·er
al·lox·an
 di·a·be·tes
al·lox·an·tin
al·lox·a·zine
al·lox·u·re·mia
al·lox·u·ria
al·loy
 chrome-co·balt a.'s
 eu·tec·tic a.
 gold a.
 Raney a.
 sil·ver-tin a.
all-*trans*-ret·i·nal
all·spice oil
ᴅ-al·lu·lose

al·lyl
  a. al·co·hol
  a. cy·a·nide
  a. iso·thi·o·cy·a·nate
  a. sul·fide
al·lyl·a·mine
al·lyl·bar·bi·tal
al·lyl·es·tre·nol
al·lyl·mer·cap·to·meth·yl·pen·i·cil·lin
N-al·lyl·nor·mor·phine
al·ly·sines
Almeida's
  dis·ease
Almén's
  test for blood
al·mond
  nu·cle·us
al·mond oil
  bit·ter a. o.
al·oe
al·oe-em·o·din
al·o·e·tin
alo·gia
al·o·in
al·o·pe·cia
  a. ad·na·ta
  an·dro·gen·ic a.
  a. ar·e·a·ta
  a. ca·pi·tis to·ta·lis
  a. cel·si
  Celsus' a.
  cic·a·tri·cial a.
  a. ci·ca·tri·sa·ta
  a. cir·cum·scrip·ta
  con·gen·i·tal a.
  a. con·ge·ni·ta·lis
  con·gen·i·tal su·tur·al a.
  a. dis·sem·i·na·ta
  a. dy·na·mi·ca
  a. fol·lic·u·la·ris
  a. he·re·di·ta·ria
  Jonston's a.
  a. lep·ro·ti·ca
  a. li·mi·na·ris fron·ta·lis
  li·pe·de·ma·tous a.
  male pat·tern a.
  a. mar·gi·na·lis
  a. me·di·ca·men·to·sa
  moth-eat·en a.
  a. mu·ci·no·sa
  a. neu·ro·ti·ca
  a. par·vi·cu·la·ta
  pat·terned a.
  a. pit·y·ro·des
  post·op·er·a·tive pres·sure a.
  post·par·tum a.

  a. pre·ma·tu·ra
  pre·ma·ture a.
  a. pre·se·ni·lis
  a. se·ni·lis
  a. symp·to·ma·ti·ca
  a. syph·i·li·ti·ca
  a. to·ta·lis
  a. tox·i·ca
  trac·tion a.
  trau·mat·ic a.
  a. tri·an·gu·la·ris con·ge·ni·ta·lis
  a. uni·ver·sa·lis
al·o·pe·cic
alox·i·prin
Alpers
  dis·ease
al·pha
  al·co·hol·ism
  an·gle
  block·ing
  cells of an·te·ri·or lobe of hy·poph·y·sis
  cells of pan·cre·as
  fi·bers
  gran·ule
  par·ti·cle
  ray
  rhythm
  sub·stance
  units
  wave
al·pha am·y·lase
al·pha·bet·i·cal
  ker·a·ti·tis
al·pha-block·er
al·pha·di·one
al·phad·o·lone ac·e·tate
al·pha·pro·dine
al·pha·sone ac·e·to·phe·nide
Al·pha·vi·rus
al·phax·a·lone
al·pho·der·mia
al·phos
Al·pine
  scur·vy
Alport's
  syn·drome
al·praz·o·lam
al·pren·o·lol hy·dro·chlo·ride
al·pros·ta·dil
al·ser·ox·y·lon
Alström's
  syn·drome
ALT:AST
  ra·tio
al·ter

al·ter·a·tion
  mo·dal a.
  qual·i·ta·tive a.
  quan·ti·ta·tive a.
al·ter·a·tive
  in·flam·ma·tion
al·ter·cur·sive
  in·tu·ba·tion
al·ter·e·go·ism
al·ter·nans
  au·di·to·ry a.
  aus·cul·ta·to·ry a.
  con·cor·dant a.
  dis·cor·dant a.
  elec·tri·cal a.
  pul·sus a.
Al·ter·nar·ia
al·ter·nate
  hem·i·an·es·the·sia
al·ter·nate bin·au·ral loud·ness
  bal·ance
  test
al·ter·nate cov·er
  test
al·ter·nate day
  stra·bis·mus
al·ter·nat·ing
  cur·rent
  hem·i·ple·gia
  my·dri·a·sis
  pulse
  stra·bis·mus
  trem·or
al·ter·na·tion
  con·cor·dant a.
  dis·cor·dant a.
  elec·tri·cal a. of heart
  a. of gen·er·a·tions
  a. of the heart
  me·chan·i·cal a.
al·ter·na·tive
  in·her·i·tance
al·ter·noc·u·lar
al·thea
al·ti·tude
  cham·ber
  er·y·thre·mia
  sick·ness
al·ti·tu·di·nal
  hem·i·a·nop·sia
Altmann-Gersh
  meth·od
Altmann's
  fix·a·tive
  gran·ule
  the·o·ry

Altmann's an·i·lin-ac·id fuch·sin
  stain
al·tri·gen·drism
al·trose
al·um
  burnt a.
  cake a.
  chrome a.
  dried a.
  ex·sic·cat·ed a.
  fer·ric a.
  iron a.
  whey a.
al·um
  whey
al·um-he·ma·tox·y·lin
alu·mi·na
  hy·drat·ed a.
alu·mi·nat·ed
alu·mi·non
alu·mi·no·sis
alu·mi·num
  a. ac·e·tate
  a. ac·e·to·tar·trate
  a. ace·tyl·sa·lic·y·late
  a. am·mo·ni·um sul·fate
  a. as·pi·rin
  a. bis·muth ox·ide
  a. car·bon·ate, ba·sic
  a. chlo·rate non·a·hy·drate
  a. chlo·ride hex·a·hy·drate
  a. di·ac·e·tate
  a. hy·drate
  a. hy·drox·ide
  a. hy·drox·ide gel
  a. hy·drox·y·chlo·ride
  a. mag·ne·si·um sil·i·cate
  a. mon·o·ste·a·rate
  a. nic·o·tin·ate
  a. ole·ate
  a. ox·ide
  a. pen·i·cil·lin
  a. phe·nol·sul·fo·nate
  a. phos·phate
  a. phos·phate gel
  a. po·tas·si·um sul·fate
  a. sa·lic·y·late, ba·sic
  a. sa·lic·y·late, ba·sic, sol·u·ble
  a. sil·i·cate
  a. sub·ac·e·tate
  a. sul·fate oc·ta·dec·a·hy·drate
alu·mi·num
  pen·i·cil·lin
alu·mi·num group
al·vei

al·ve·o·al·gia
al·ve·o·lal·gia
al·ve·o·lar
  ab·scess
  air
  an·gle
  arch of man·di·ble
  arch of max·il·la
  at·ro·phy
  body
  bone
  bor·der
  ca·nals
  cell
  crest
  duct
  fo·ram·i·na
  gas
  gin·gi·va
  gland
  in·dex
  mac·ro·phage
  mu·co·sa
  os·te·i·tis
  part of man·di·ble
  per·i·os·te·um
  point
  pro·cess
  ridge
  sac
  sep·tum
  ven·ti·la·tion
  yoke
al·ve·o·lar-ar·te·ri·al ox·y·gen
  dif·fer·ence
al·ve·o·lar cell
  car·ci·no·ma
al·ve·o·lar dead
  space
al·ve·o·lar gas
  equa·tion
al·ve·o·lar hy·da·tid
  cyst
al·ve·o·lar soft part
  sar·co·ma
al·ve·o·lar sup·port·ing
  bone
al·ve·o·late
al·ve·o·lec·to·my
al·ve·o·li
al·ve·o·lin·gual
al·ve·o·li·tis
  acute pul·mo·nary a.
  ex·trin·sic al·ler·gic a.
al·ve·o·lo·buc·cal
  groove
  sul·cus
al·ve·o·lo·cla·sia

al·ve·o·lo·den·tal
  ca·nals
  lig·a·ment
  mem·brane
al·ve·o·lo·la·bi·al
  groove
  sul·cus
al·ve·o·lo·la·bi·a·lis
al·ve·o·lo·lin·gual
  groove
  sul·cus
al·ve·o·lo·na·sal
  line
al·ve·o·lo·pal·a·tal
al·ve·o·lo·plas·ty
  in·ter·ra·dic·u·lar a.
  in·tra·sep·tal a.
al·ve·o·los·chi·sis
al·ve·o·lot·o·my
al·ve·o·lus
al·ve·o·plas·ty
al·ve·us
  a. uro·ge·ni·ta·lis
al·vin·o·lith
alym·phia
alym·pho·cy·to·sis
alym·pho·pla·sia
  Nezelof type of thy·mic a.
  thy·mic a.
Alzheimer's
  de·men·tia
  dis·ease
  scle·ro·sis
am·a·crine
  cell
am·a·dou
amal·gam
  pin a.
  spher·i·cal a.
amal·gam
  car·ri·er
  ma·trix
  strip
  tat·too
amal·ga·mate
amal·ga·ma·tion
amal·ga·ma·tor
Am·a·ni·ta
  A. mus·ca·ria
  A. phal·loi·des
aman·ta·dine hy·dro·chlo·ride
am·a·ra
am·a·ranth
am·a·ran·thum
am·a·rine
am·a·roid
am·a·roi·dal
ama·rum

amas·tia
amas·ti·gote
am·a·tho·pho·bia
am·a·tive·ness
am·au·ro·sis
   a. cen·tra·lis
   a. con·gen·i·ta of Leber
   a. fu·gax
   pres·sure a.
   sa·bur·ral a.
   tox·ic a.
am·au·rot·ic
   my·dri·a·sis
   nys·tag·mus
   pu·pil
am·au·rot·ic cat's
   eye
am·au·rot·ic fa·mil·i·al
   id·i·o·cy
amax·o·pho·bia
ama·zia
am·ba·geu·sia
Ambard's
   con·stant
   laws
am·be·no·ni·um chlo·ride
am·ber
   mu·ta·tion
am·ber·gris
Amberg's lat·er·al si·nus
   line
am·bi·dex·ter·i·ty
am·bi·dex·trism
am·bi·dex·trous
am·bi·ent
   be·hav·ior
   cis·ter·na
am·big·u·ous
   nu·cle·us
am·big·u·ous ex·ter·nal
   gen·i·ta·lia
am·bi·lat·er·al
am·bi·le·vous
am·bi·sex·u·al
am·bi·sin·is·ter
am·bi·si·nis·trous
am·biv·a·lence
am·biv·a·lent
am·bi·vert
am·bly·a·phia
am·bly·geus·tia
Am·bly·om·ma
   A. ame·ri·ca·num
   A. ca·jen·nense
   A. he·bra·e·um
   A. ma·cu·la·tum
   A. va·ri·e·ga·tum

am·bly·o·pia
   an·i·so·me·tro·pic a.
   ax·i·al a.
   dep·ri·va·tion a.
   eclipse a.
   a. ex anop·sia
   func·tion·al a.
   hys·ter·i·cal a.
   in·dex a.
   noc·tur·nal a.
   nu·trit·ion·al a.
   re·frac·tive a.
   rel·a·tive a.
   re·vers·i·ble a.
   sen·so·ry a.
   stra·bis·mic a.
   tox·ic a.
am·bly·o·pic
am·bly·o·scope
   ma·jor a.
   Worth's a.
am·bo·cep·tor
   unit
am·bo·mal·le·al
am·bos
Am·boy·na
   but·ton
am·bro·sin
Am·bu
   bag
am·bu·cet·a·mide
am·bu·lant
   er·y·sip·e·las
   plague
am·bu·la·to·ry
   au·tom·a·tism
   plague
   schiz·o·phre·nia
   sur·gery
   ty·phoid
am·bu·phyl·line
am·bus·tion
am·cin·o·nide
am·di·no·cil·lin
ame·ba
ame·ba·cide
ame·bae
ame·ba·ism
ame·bas
am·e·bi·a·sis
   ca·nine a.
   a. cu·tis
   he·pa·tic a.
ame·bic
   ab·scess
   co·li·tis
   dys·en·tery

gran·u·lo·ma
vag·i·ni·tis
ame·bi·ci·dal
ame·bi·cide
ame·bi·form
am·e·bi·o·sis
ame·bism
ame·bo·cyte
ame·boid
as·tro·cyte
cell
move·ment
ame·boi·did·i·ty
ame·boid·ism
am·e·bo·ma
ame·bu·la
ame·bu·lae
ame·bule
am·e·bu·ria
amel·a·not·ic
mel·a·no·ma
ame·lia
por·cine a.
ame·lio·ra·tion
am·e·lo·blast
am·e·lo·blas·tic
fi·bro·ma
fi·bro·sar·co·ma
lay·er
odon·to·ma
sar·co·ma
am·e·lo·blas·tic ad·e·no·ma·
toid
tu·mor
am·e·lo·blas·to·ma
pig·ment·ed a.
am·e·lo·den·tal
junc·tion
am·e·lo·den·tin·al
junc·tion
am·e·lo·gen·e·sis
a. im·per·fec·ta
ame·nia
amen·or·rhea
di·e·tary a.
emo·tion·al a.
hy·per·pro·lac·ti·ne·mic a.
hy·po·phy·si·al a.
hy·po·tha·lam·ic a.
jog·ger's a.
lac·ta·tion a.
ovar·i·an a.
path·o·log·ic a.
phys·i·o·log·ic a.
post·par·tum a.
pri·mary a.
sec·on·dary a.
trau·mat·ic a.

amen·or·rhea-ga·lac·tor·rhea
syn·drome
amen·or·rhe·al
amen·or·rhe·ic
amen·tia
ne·void a.
phe·nyl·py·ru·vic a.
Stearns al·co·hol·ic a.
amen·ti·al
Amer·i·can
leish·man·i·a·sis
ta·ran·tu·la
am·er·i·ci·um
am·er·ism
am·er·is·tic
Ames
as·say
test
am·e·thop·ter·in
ame·tria
ame·tri·o·din·ic ac·id
am·e·trom·e·ter
am·e·tro·pia
ax·i·al a.
in·dex a.
am·e·tro·pic
am·i·an·ta·ceous
am·i·an·thoid
ami·cro·bic
ami·cro·scop·ic
am·i·dase
am·i·das·es
am·ide
ox·imes
am·i·dine
am·i·di·no·hy·dro·las·es
am·i·din·o·trans·fer·as·es
ami·do·gen
ami·do·hy·dro·las·es
ami·do·naph·thol red
ami·do·py·rine
Am·i·dos·to·mum an·ser·is
am·i·dox·imes
am·i·dox·yl
am·i·ka·cin sul·fate
amil·o·ride hy·dro·chlo·ride
amim·ia
am·i·nac·rine hy·dro·chlo·ride
am·i·nate
amine
ad·re·ner·gic a.
adre·no·mi·met·ic a.
a. ox·i·dase (cop·per-con·
tain·ing)
a. ox·i·dase (fla·vin-con·
tain·ing)
a. ox·i·dase (pyr·i·dox·al-
con·tain·ing)

amine *(continued)*
   pres·sor a.
   sym·pa·thet·ic a.
   sym·pa·tho·mi·met·ic a.
   va·so·ac·tive a.
ami·no
   sug·ars
ami·no ac·id
   a. a. de·hy·dro·gen·as·es
   es·sen·tial a. a.'s
   non·es·sen·tial a. a.'s
   a. a. ox·i·das·es
ami·no·ac·i·de·mia
ami·no·ac·id-tRNA li·gas·es
ami·no·ac·i·du·ria
ami·no·ac·yl
ami·no·ac·yl·a·den·y·late
ami·no·ac·yl·ase
ami·no·ac·yl-tRNA
ami·no·ben·zene
o-ami·no·ben·zo·ic ac·id
p-ami·no·ben·zo·ic ac·id
ami·no·ca·pro·ic ac·id
am·i·no·car·bon·yl
ami·no·glu·teth·i·mide
am·i·no·gly·co·side
p-ami·no·hip·pu·rate
   clear·ance
p-ami·no·hip·pu·ric ac·id
p-ami·no·hip·pu·ric ac·id syn·thase
ami·no·i·so·met·ra·dine
am·i·nol·y·sis
ami·no·met·ra·dine
ami·no·met·ra·mide
ami·no·pep·ti·dase(cy·to·sol)
ami·no·pep·ti·dase(mi·cro·som·al)
ami·no·pep·ti·das·es
ami·no·phen·a·zone
am·i·noph·er·as·es
ami·no·phyl·line
ami·no·pro·ma·zine
p-ami·no·pro·pi·o·phe·none
am·i·nop·ter·in
ami·no·py·rine
amin·o·rex
p-ami·no·sal·i·cyl·ic ac·id
ami·no-ter·mi·nal
ami·no·trans·fer·as·es
ami·no·tri·a·zole
am·i·nu·ria
ami·o·da·rone hy·dro·chlo·ride
am·i·so·met·ra·dine
am·i·thi·o·zone
ami·to·sis
ami·tot·ic

am·i·trip·ty·line hy·dro·chlo·ride
am·i·trole
am·me·ter
am·mo·ne·mia
am·mo·nia
   rash
am·mo·ni·ac
am·mo·ni·a·cal
   urine
am·mo·nia-ly·as·es
am·mo·ni·at·ed
   mer·cu·ric chlo·ride
   mer·cu·ry
   tinc·ture
am·mo·ni·e·mia
am·mo·ni·um
   a. ben·zo·ate
   a. bro·mide
   a. car·bon·ate
   a. chlo·ride
   di·ba·sic a. phos·phate
   a. fer·ric sul·fate
   a. ich·tho·sul·fo·nate
   a. io·dide
   a. man·del·ate
   a. mo·lyb·date
   mon·o·ba·sic a. phos·phate
   a. ni·trate
am·mo·ni·u·ria
am·mo·nol·y·sis
Ammon's
   fis·sure
   horn
   op·er·a·tion
   prom·i·nence
am·ne·mon·ic
   agraph·ia
am·ne·sia
   an·ter·o·grade a.
   la·cu·nar a.
   lo·cal·ized a.
   post·hyp·not·ic a.
   ret·ro·grade a.
am·ne·si·ac
am·ne·sic
   apha·sia
am·nes·tic
   apha·sia
   psy·cho·sis
   syn·drome
am·ni·o·car·di·ac
   ves·i·cle
am·ni·o·cen·te·sis
am·ni·o·cho·ri·al
am·ni·o·cho·ri·on·ic
am·ni·o·em·bry·on·ic
   junc·tion

am·ni·o·gen·e·sis
am·ni·o·gen·ic
  cells
am·ni·og·ra·phy
am·ni·o·ma
am·ni·on
  a. no·do·sum
am·ni·on
  ring
am·ni·on·ic
am·ni·o·ni·tis
am·ni·or·rhea
am·ni·or·rhex·is
am·ni·o·scope
am·ni·os·co·py
Am·ni·o·ta
am·ni·ot·ic
  ad·he·sions
  bands
  cav·i·ty
  cor·pus·cle
  duct
  flu·id
  fold
  ra·phe
  sac
am·ni·ot·ic flu·id
  em·bo·lism
  syn·drome
am·ni·o·tome
am·ni·ot·o·my
am·o·bar·bi·tal
A-mode
am·o·di·a·quine hy·dro·chlo·ride
Amoe·ba
  A. buc·ca·lis
  A. co·li
  A. den·ta·lis
  A. dys·en·te·ri·ae
  A. his·to·lyt·i·ca
  A. me·le·ag·ri·dis
  A. pro·te·us
Amoe·bo·tae·nia
amok
amorph
amor·phag·no·sia
amor·phia
amor·phism
amor·pho·syn·the·sis
amor·phous
  frac·tion of ad·re·nal cor·tex
  phos·pho·rus
amor·phous in·su·lin zinc
  sus·pen·sion
amor·phus

Amoss'
  sign
amo·tio pla·cen·tae
amo·tio ret·i·nae
amox·a·pine
amox·i·cil·lin
AMP de·am·i·nase
am·per·age
am·pere
Ampère's
  pos·tu·late
am·per·om·e·try
am·phe·clex·is
am·phet·a·mine
  a. phos·phate
  a. sul·fate
d-am·phet·a·mine phos·phate
d-am·phet·a·mine sul·fate
am·phi·ar·thro·di·al
am·phi·ar·thro·sis
am·phi·as·ter
am·phi·bar·ic
am·phi·bles·tro·des
am·phi·bol·ic
  fis·tu·la
am·phib·o·lous
  fis·tu·la
am·phi·ce·lous
am·phi·cen·tric
am·phi·chro·ic
am·phi·chro·mat·ic
am·phi·cra·nia
am·phi·cyte
am·phi·ge·net·ic
am·phi·kar·y·on
am·phi·leu·ke·mic
Am·phim·er·us
am·phi·mi·crobe
am·phi·mix·is
am·phi·nu·cle·o·lus
Am·phi·ox·us
am·phi·path·ic
am·phi·phil·ic
am·phi·pho·bic
am·phi·pro·tic
  sol·vent
am·phis·tome
am·phi·thy·mia
am·phit·ri·chate
am·phit·ri·chous
am·phit·y·py
am·phix·en·o·sis
am·pho·chro·mat·o·phil
am·pho·chro·mat·o·phile
am·pho·chro·mo·phil
am·pho·chro·mo·phile
am·pho·cyte
am·pho·dip·lo·pia

am·pho·ge·net·ic
am·pho·lyte
am·pho·my·cin
am·pho·phil
  gran·ule
am·pho·phile
am·pho·phil·ic
am·phoph·i·lous
am·phor·ic
  rale
  res·o·nance
  res·pi·ra·tion
  voice
am·phor·ic voice
  sound
am·pho·ril·o·quy
am·phor·oph·o·ny
am·pho·ter·ic
  elec·tro·lyte
  el·e·ment
  re·ac·tion
am·pho·ter·i·cin
am·pho·ter·i·cin B
am·pho·to·nia
am·phot·o·ny
am·pho·tro·pic
  vi·rus
am·pi·cil·lin
am·plex·us
am·pli·fi·ca·tion
  ge·net·ic a.
am·pli·fi·er
  host
am·pli·tude of
  ac·com·mo·da·tion
  con·ver·gence
am·pli·tude
  a. of ac·com·mo·da·tion
  a. of con·ver·gence
  a. of pulse
am·poule
am·pro·tro·pine phos·phate
am·pul
am·pule
am·pul·la
  Bryant's a.
  a. chy·li
  a. duc·tus la·cri·ma·lis
  du·o·de·nal a.
  Henle's a.
  a. lac·tif·era
  mem·bra·nous a.
  a. of milk duct
  os·se·ous a.
  a. of rec·tum
  Thoma's a.
  a. of uter·ine tube

  a. of vas def·er·ens
  Vater's a.
am·pul·lae
am·pul·lar
  abor·tion
  preg·nan·cy
am·pul·la·ry
  an·eu·rysm
  crest
  limbs of sem·i·cir·cu·lar
    ducts
  sul·cus
am·pul·li·tis
am·pul·lu·la
am·pu·tat·ing
  ul·cer
am·pu·ta·tion
  neu·ro·ma
am·pu·ta·tion
  Alanson's a.
  aper·i·os·te·al a.
  Bier's a.
  birth a.
  blood·less a.
  Callander's a.
  Carden's a.
  cen·tral a.
  cer·vi·cal a.
  Chopart's a.
  cin·e·mat·ic a.
  cin·e·plas·tic a.
  cir·cu·lar a.
  con·gen·i·tal a.
  con·sec·u·tive a.
  a. in con·ti·nu·i·ty
  dou·ble flap a.
  dry a.
  Dupuytren's a.
  ec·cen·tric a.
  el·lip·ti·cal a.
  ex·cen·tric a.
  Farabeuf's a.
  flap a.
  flap·less a.
  fore·quar·ter a.
  Gritti-Stokes a.
  guil·lo·tine a.
  Guyon's a.
  Hancock's a.
  Hey's a.
  hind·quar·ter a.
  im·me·di·ate a.
  in·ter·il·i·o·ab·dom·i·nal a.
  in·ter·me·di·ate a.
  in·ter·pel·vi·ab·dom·i·nal a.
  in·ter·scap·u·lo·tho·rac·ic a.
  in·tra·py·ret·ic a.
  in·tra·u·ter·ine a.

Jaboulay's a.
kin·e·plas·tic a.
Kirk's a.
Krukenberg's a.
Larrey's a.
Le Fort's a.
lin·e·ar a.
Lisfranc's a.
Mackenzie's a.
ma·jor a.
Malgaigne's a.
me·di·o·tar·sal a.
Mikulicz-Vladimiroff a.
mi·nor a.
mul·ti·ple a.
mus·cu·lo·cu·ta·ne·ous a.
ob·lique a.
os·te·o·plas·tic a.
oval a.
path·o·log·ic a.
per·i·os·te·o·plas·tic a.
Pirogoff's a.
pri·mary a.
pulp a.
quad·ru·ple a.
rack·et a.
rect·an·gu·lar a.
root a.
sec·on·dary a.
spon·ta·ne·ous a.
Stokes a.
sub·as·trag·a·lar a.
sub·per·i·os·te·al a.
Syme's a.
tar·so·tib·i·al a.
Teale's a.
ter·ti·ary a.
a. by trans·fix·ion
trans·verse a.
trau·mat·ic a.
Tripier's a.
Vladimiroff-Mikulicz a.
am·pu·tee
am·ri·none lac·tate
Amsler
test
Amsler's
chart
mark·er
Am·ster·dam
syn·drome
amuck
amu·sia
sen·so·ry a.
vo·cal a.
Amussat's
valve
val·vu·la

am·y·cho·pho·bia
amyc·tic
amy·el·en·ce·pha·lia
amy·el·en·ce·phal·ic
amy·el·en·ceph·a·lous
amy·e·lia
amy·el·ic
amy·e·li·nat·ed
amy·e·li·na·tion
amy·e·lin·ic
amy·e·lo·ic
amy·e·lon·ic
amy·e·lous
amyg·da·la
a. ce·re·bel·li
amyg·da·lae
amyg·da·lase
amyg·da·lin
amyg·da·line
amyg·da·loid
com·plex
fos·sa
nu·cle·us
tu·ber·cle
amyg·da·lo·side
am·yl
a. al·co·hol
a. hy·drate
a. ni·trite
ter·ti·ary a. al·co·hol
a. val·er·ate
am·y·la·ceous
cor·pus·cle
am·y·lase
am·y·lase-cre·at·i·nine clear·ance
ra·tio
am·y·la·su·ria
am·y·le·mia
am·yl·ene
a. chlo·ral
a. hy·drate
am·yl·ic
fer·men·ta·tion
am·y·lin
am·y·lo·caine hy·dro·chlo·ride
am·y·lo·clast
am·y·lo·dex·trin
am·y·lo·gen·e·sis
am·y·lo·gen·ic
body
am·y·lo··glu·co·si·dase
am·y·loid
bod·ies of the pros·tate
cor·pus·cle
de·gen·er·a·tion
kid·ney

am·y·loid *(continued)*
  ne·phro·sis
  tu·mor
am·y·loi·do·sis
  a. cu·tis
  fa·mil·i·al a.
  fo·cal a.
  li·chen a.
  mac·u·lar a.
  a. of mul·ti·ple my·e·lo·ma
  nod·u·lar a.
  pri·mary a.
  re·nal a.
  sec·on·dary a.
  se·nile a.
am·y·lol·y·sis
am·y·lo·lyt·ic
am·y·lo·malt·ase
am·y·lo·pec·tin
am·y·lo·pec·tin·o·sis
  branch·ing de·fi·cien·cy a.
am·y·lo·pha·gia
am·y·lo·phos·phor·y·lase
am·y·lo·plast
am·y·lor·rhea
am·y·lose
am·y·lo·su·ria
am·y·lum
am·y·lu·ria
amy·o·car·dia
amy·o·es·the·sia
amy·o·es·the·sis
amy·o·pla·sia
  a. con·gen·i·ta
amy·o·sta·sia
amy·o·stat·ic
amy·os·the·nia
amy·os·then·ic
amy·o·tax·ia
amy·o·taxy
amy·o·to·nia
  a. con·gen·i·ta
amy·o·tro·phia
amy·o·tro·phic
amy·o·tro·phic lat·er·al
  scle·ro·sis
amy·ot·ro·phy
  hem·i·ple·gic a.
  neu·ral·gic a.
  pro·gress·ive spi·nal a.
am·y·ous
amyx·ia
amyx·or·rhea
A-N
  in·ter·val
An·a·bae·na
an·a·bi·o·sis

an·a·bi·ot·ic
  cells
an·a·bol·ic
anab·o·lism
anab·o·lite
an·a·bro·sis
an·a·brot·ic
an·a·camp·tom·e·ter
an·a·car·di·ol
an·a·cat·a·did·y·mus
an·a·cat·es·the·sia
an·a·cid·i·ty
anac·la·sis
an·a·clit·ic
  de·pres·sion
  psy·cho·ther·a·py
an·ac·me·sis
an·a·crot·ic
  limb
  pulse
anac·ro·tism
an·a·cu·sis
an·a·de·nia
  a. ven·tric·u·li
an·a·di·crot·ic
  pulse
an·a·di·cro·tism
an·a·did·y·mus
an·a·dip·sia
an·ad·re·nal·ism
an·aer·obe
  fac·ul·ta·tive a.
  ob·li·gate a.
an·aer·o·bic
  de·hy·dro·gen·ase
  res·pi·ra·tion
an·aer·o·bi·o·sis
an·aer·o·gen·ic
an·aer·o·phyte
an·aer·o·plas·ty
an·a·gen
an·a·gen·e·sis
an·a·ge·net·ic
an·a·ges·tone ac·e·tate
Anagnostakis'
  op·er·a·tion
an·a·go·gy
an·á·khré
an·ak·me·sis
an·a·ku·sis
anal
  atre·sia
  ca·nal
  cleft
  col·umns
  ducts
  er·o·tism
  fas·cia

fis·sure
fis·tu·la
gland
mem·brane
or·i·fice
pec·ten
phase
pit
plate
re·flex
re·gion
sac
si·nus·es
sphinc·ter
tri·an·gle
valves
verge
an·al·bu·mi·ne·mia
an·a·lep·tic
en·e·ma
an·al·ge·sia
a. al·ge·ra
con·duc·tion a.
a. do·lo·ro·sa
in·ha·la·tion a.
spi·nal a.
sur·face a.
an·al·ge·sic
cui·rass
ne·phri·tis
ne·phrop·a·thy
an·al·ge·sim·e·ter
an·al·get·ic
anal·i·ty
an·al·ler·gic
an·a·log
anal·o·gous
an·a·logue
an·al·pha·lip·o·pro·tein·e·mia
anal skin
tag
anal·y·sand
anal·y·ses
anal·y·sis
ac·ti·va·tion a.
bite a.
blood gas a.
bra·dy·ki·net·ic a.
ceph·a·lo·met·ric a.
char·ac·ter a.
clus·ter a.
con·tent a.
di·dac·tic a.
dis·place·ment a.
dis·trib·u·tive a.
Downs' a.
ego a.
gas·tric a.

in·ter·ac·tion pro·cess a.
link·age a.
North·ern blot a.
oc·clu·sal a.
ped·i·gree a.
per·cept a.
qual·i·ta·tive a.
quan·ti·ta·tive a.
sat·u·ra·tion a.
seg·re·ga·tion a.
South·ern blot a.
stra·to·graph·ic a.
train·ing a.
trans·ac·tion·al a.
vol·u·met·ric a.
West·ern blot a.
an·a·lyst
an·a·lyte
an·a·lyt·ic
chem·is·try
psy·chi·a·try
ther·a·py
an·a·lyt·i·cal
psy·chol·o·gy
an·a·lyz·er
cen·trif·u·gal fast a.
ki·net·ic a.
wave a.
an·a·lyz·ing
rod
an·a·lyz·or
an·am·ne·sis
an·am·nes·tic
re·ac·tion
an·am·ni·on·ic
An·am·ni·o·ta
an·am·ni·ot·ic
an·a·mor·pho·sis
an·an·a·phy·lax·is
an·an·a·sta·sia
an·an·casm
an·an·cas·tia
an·an·cas·tic
an·an·dria
an·an·gi·o·pla·sia
an·an·gi·o·plas·tic
an·a·pei·rat·ic
an·a·phase
lag
an·a·phia
an·a·pho·re·sis
an·aph·o·ret·ic
an·a·pho·ria
an·aph·ro·di·sia
an·aph·ro·di·si·ac
an·a·phy·lac·tic
an·ti·body

an·a·phy·lac·tic *(continued)*
  in·tox·i·ca·tion
  shock
an·a·phy·lac·to·gen
an·a·phy·lac·to·gen·e·sis
an·a·phy·lac·to·gen·ic
an·a·phy·lac·toid
  cri·sis
  pur·pu·ra
  shock
an·a·phyl·a·tox·in
an·a·phyl·a·tox·in in·ac·ti·va·
  tor
an·a·phy·lax·is
  ac·tive a.
  ag·gre·gate a.
  an·ti·se·rum a.
  chron·ic a.
  gen·er·al·ized a.
  in·verse a.
  lo·cal a.
  pas·sive a.
  pas·sive cu·ta·ne·ous a.
  re·versed a.
  re·versed pas·sive a.
  sys·tem·ic a.
an·a·phyl·o·tox·in
an·a·pla·sia
An·a·plas·ma
  A. cen·tra·le
  A. mar·gi·na·le
  A. ovis
an·a·plas·mo·sis
an·a·plas·tic
  car·ci·no·ma
  cell
an·a·plas·ty
an·a·poph·y·sis
anap·tic
an·a·rith·mia
an·ar·thria
an·ar·thrit·ic rheu·ma·toid
  dis·ease
an·a·sar·ca
  fe·to·pla·cen·tal a.
an·a·sar·cous
an·a·stig·mat·ic
an·as·to·le
anas·to·mose
anas·to·mosed
  graft
anas·to·mo·ses
anas·to·mos·ing
  fi·bers
anas·to·mo·sis
  an·ti·per·i·stal·tic a.
  ar·te·ri·o·lo·ven·u·lar a.
  ar·te·ri·o·ve·nous a.

Béclard's a.
bev·elled a.
Billroth I a.
Billroth II a.
Braun's a.
cir·cu·lar a.
Clado's a.
con·joined a.
cru·cial a.
cru·ci·ate a.
el·lip·ti·cal a.
Galen's a.
het·er·o·clad·ic a.
Hofmeister-Pólya a.
ho·mo·clad·ic anas·to·mo·
  ses
Hoyer's anas·to·mo·ses
Hyrtl's a.
in·tes·ti·nal a.
iso·per·i·stal·tic a.
Jacobson's a.
mi·cro·neu·ro·vas·cu·lar a.
mi·cro·vas·cu·lar a.
post·cos·tal a.
Potts' a.
pre·cap·il·lary a.
pre·cos·tal a.
Riolan's a.
Roux-en-Y a.
Schmidel's anas·to·mo·ses
Sucquet-Hoyer anas·to·mo·
  ses
Sucquet's anas·to·mo·ses
ter·mi·no-ter·mi·nal a.
trans·u·re·ter·o·u·re·ter·al
  a.
ure·ter·o-il·e·al a.
ure·ter·o·sig·moid a.
ure·ter·o·tub·al a.
ure·ter·o·u·re·ter·al a.
anas·to·mot·ic
  fi·bers
  stric·ture
  ul·cer
  veins
anas·to·mot·i·ca mag·na
an·as·tral
an·a·tom·ic
  ri·gid·i·ty
  teeth
an·a·tom·i·cal
  age
  crown
  el·e·ment
  neck of hu·mer·us
  pa·thol·o·gy
  po·si·tion
  root

sphinc·ter
tu·ber·cle
wart
an·a·tom·i·cal dead
space
an·a·tom·i·cal snuff·box
an·a·tom·i·co·med·i·cal
an·a·tom·i·co·path·o·log·i·cal
an·a·tom·i·co·sur·gi·cal
anat·o·mist
anat·o·my
ap·plied a.
ar·ti·fi·cial a.
ar·tis·tic a.
clas·tic a.
com·par·a·tive a.
den·tal a.
de·scrip·tive a.
de·vel·op·men·tal a.
func·tion·al a.
gen·er·al a.
gross a.
liv·ing a.
mac·ro·scop·ic a.
med·i·cal a.
mi·cro·scop·ic a.
path·o·log·i·cal a.
phys·i·o·log·i·cal a.
plas·tic a.
prac·ti·cal a.
ra·di·o·log·i·cal a.
re·gion·al a.
spe·cial a.
sur·face a.
sur·gi·cal a.
sys·tem·at·ic a.
sys·tem·ic a.
top·o·graph·ic a.
tran·scen·den·tal a.
ul·tra·struc·tur·al a.
anat·o·pism
an·a·tox·ic
an·a·tox·in
an·a·tri·crot·ic
an·a·tric·ro·tism
an·a·trip·sis
an·a·trip·tic
an·a·tro·phic
ne·phrot·o·my
an·a·tro·pia
an·au·dia
an·ax·on
an·ax·one
an·a·zo·tu·ria
an·cho·ne
an·chor
splint

an·chor·age
cer·vi·cal a.
ex·tra·o·ral a.
in·ter·max·il·lary a.
in·tra·max·il·lary a.
in·tra·o·ral a.
mul·ti·ple a.
oc·cip·i·tal a.
re·cip·ro·cal a.
re·in·forced a.
sim·ple a.
sta·tion·ary a.
an·chor·ing
vil·lus
an·chu·sin
an·cil·lary
an·cip·i·tal
an·cip·i·tate
an·cip·i·tous
an·con
an·co·nad
an·co·nal
fos·sa
an·co·ne·al
an·co·ne·us
mus·cle
an·co·ni·tis
an·co·noid
an·crod
An·cy·los·to·ma
A. bra·zi·li·ense
A. ca·ni·num
A. cey·la·ni·cum
A. du·o·de·na·le
an·cy·lo·sto·mat·ic
an·cy·lo·sto·mi·a·sis
cu·ta·ne·ous a.
a. cu·tis
an·cy·lo·sto·mi·a·sis
der·ma·ti·tis
an·cy·roid
Andernach's
os·si·cles
Anders'
dis·ease
Andersch's
gan·gli·on
nerve
Andersen's
dis·ease
Anderson
splint
Anderson-Collip
test
Anderson-Hynes
py·e·lo·plas·ty
an·di·ra
an·di·rine

Andral's
de·cu·bi·tus
an·dre·nos·ter·one
an·dri·at·rics
an·dri·a·try
an·dro·blas·to·ma
an·dro·gen
ad·re·nal a.
an·dro·gen
unit
an·dro·gen·e·sis
an·dro·gen·ic
al·o·pe·cia
hor·mone
zone
an·drog·e·nous
an·drog·y·nism
an·drog·y·noid
an·drog·y·nous
an·drog·y·ny
an·droid
pel·vis
an·drol·o·gy
an·dro·ma·nia
an·drom·e·do·tox·in
an·dro·mor·phous
an·drop·a·thy
an·dro·pho·bia
an·dro·stane
an·dro·stane·di·ol
an·dro·stane·di·one
an·dro·stene
an·dro·stene·di·ol
an·dro·stene·di·one
an·dro·sten·o·lone
an·dros·ter·one
an·e·cho·ic
cham·ber
an·ec·ta·sis
an·e·lec·trode
an·e·lec·tro·ton·ic
an·e·lec·trot·o·nus
Anel's
meth·od
probe
ane·mia
achlor·hy·dric a.
achres·tic a.
ac·quired he·mo·lyt·ic a.
ad·di·so·ni·an a.
Addison's a.
an·gi·o·path·ic he·mo·lyt·ic a.
aplas·tic a.
asid·er·ot·ic a.
au·to·al·ler·gic he·mo·lyt·ic a.

au·to·im·mune he·mo·lyt·ic a.
Bel·gian Con·go a.
Biermer's a.
brick·mak·er's a.
cam·el·oid a.
chlo·rot·ic a.
con·gen·i·tal a.
con·gen·i·tal aplas·tic a.
con·gen·i·tal are·gen·er·a·tive a.
con·gen·i·tal dys·e·ryth·ro·poi·et·ic a.
con·gen·i·tal he·mo·lyt·ic a.
con·gen·i·tal hy·po·plas·tic a.
Cooley's a.
cres·cent cell a.
de·fi·cien·cy a.
Diamond-Blackfan a.
di·lu·tion a.
di·mor·phic a.
di·phyl·lo·both·ri·um a.
dys·he·mo·poi·et·ic a.
Ehrlich's a.
el·lip·to·cyt·ic a.
equine in·fec·tious a.
eryth·ro·blas·tic a.
Faber's a.
false a.
fa·mil·i·al eryth·ro·blas·tic a.
fa·mil·i·al hy·po·plas·tic a.
fa·mil·i·al mi·cro·cyt·ic a.
fa·mil·i·al pyr·i·dox·ine-re·spon·sive a.
fa·mil·i·al splen·ic a.
Fanconi's a.
fish tape·worm a.
ge·net·ic a.
globe cell a.
goat's milk a.
a. gra·vis
ground itch a.
Hayem-Widal a.
he·mo·lyt·ic a.
he·mo·lyt·ic a. of new·born
hem·or·rhag·ic a.
he·mo·tox·ic a.
hook·worm a.
hy·per·chro·mat·ic a.
hy·per·chro·mic a.
hy·po·chro·mic a.
hy·po·chro·mic mi·cro·cyt·ic a.
hy·po·fer·ric a.
hy·po·plas·tic a.
ic·ter·o·he·mo·lyt·ic a.

a. in·fan·tum pseu·do·leu·ke·mi·ca
in·fec·tious a.
in·ter·trop·i·cal a.
iron de·fi·cien·cy a.
iso·chro·mic a.
lead a.
Lederer's a.
leu·ko·e·ryth·ro·blas·tic a.
lo·cal a.
a. lym·pha·ti·ca
mac·ro·cyt·ic a.
mac·ro·cyt·ic achy·lic a.
mac·ro·cyt·ic a. of preg·nan·cy
ma·lig·nant a.
Marchiafava-Micheli a.
Med·i·ter·ra·ne·an a.
meg·a·lo·blas·tic a.
meg·a·lo·cyt·ic a.
met·a·plas·tic a.
mi·cro·an·gi·o·path·ic he·mo·lyt·ic a.
mi·cro·cyt·ic a.
mi·cro·drep·a·no·cyt·ic a.
milk a.
mo·lec·u·lar a.
my·e·lo·path·ic a.
my·e·lo·phthis·ic a.
ne·o·na·tal a.
a. ne·o·na·to·rum
nor·mo·chro·mic a.
nor·mo·cyt·ic a.
nu·trit·ion·al a.
os·te·o·scle·rot·ic a.
oval·o·cyt·ic a.
per·ni·cious a.
phys·i·o·log·ic a.
po·lar a.
post·hem·or·rha·gic a.
pri·mary eryth·ro·blas·tic a.
pri·mary re·frac·to·ry a.
pure red cell a.
ra·di·a·tion a.
re·frac·to·ry a.
sec·on·dary re·frac·to·ry a.
sick·le cell a.
sid·er·o·a·chres·tic a.
sid·er·o·blas·tic a.
slaty a.
spas·tic a.
sphe·ro·cyt·ic a.
splen·ic a.
tar·get cell a.
tox·ic a.
trau·mat·ic a.
trop·i·cal a.
type I

type II
type III
ane·mic
an·ox·ia
ha·lo
hy·pox·ia
in·farct
mur·mur
an·e·mom·e·ter
a·nem·o·nol
an·e·mo·pho·bia
an·e·mot·ro·phy
an·en·ce·pha·lia
an·en·ce·phal·ic
an·en·ceph·a·lous
an·en·ceph·a·ly
par·tial a.
an·en·ter·ous
an·en·zy·mia
a. cat·a·la·sia
aneph·ric
anep·ia
an·ep·i·plo·ic
an·er·ga·sia
an·er·gas·tic
an·er·gia
an·er·gic
leish·man·i·a·sis
an·er·gy
neg·a·tive a.
non·spe·cif·ic a.
pos·i·tive a.
spe·cif·ic a.
an·er·oid
ma·nom·e·ter
an·e·ryth·ro·pla·sia
an·e·ryth·ro·plas·tic
an·e·ryth·ro·re·gen·er·a·tive
an·es·the·ci·ne·sia
an·es·the·ki·ne·sia
an·es·the·sia
ac·u·punc·ture a.
ax·il·lary a.
bal·anced a.
ba·sal a.
block a.
brach·i·al a.
cau·dal a.
cer·vi·cal a.
cir·cle ab·sorp·tion a.
closed a.
com·pres·sion a.
con·duc·tion a.
con·tin·u·ous ep·i·du·ral a.
con·tin·u·ous spi·nal a.
crossed a.
den·tal a.
di·ag·nos·tic a.

an·es·the·sia *(continued)*
dif·fer·en·tial spi·nal a.
dis·so·ci·at·ed a.
dis·so·ci·a·tive a.
a. do·lo·ro·sa
elec·tric a.
en·do·tra·che·al a.
ep·i·du·ral a.
ex·tra·du·ral a.
field block a.
frac·tion·al ep·i·du·ral a.
frac·tion·al spi·nal a.
gen·er·al a.
gir·dle a.
glove a.
gus·ta·to·ry a.
high spi·nal a.
hy·per·bar·ic a.
hy·per·bar·ic spi·nal a.
hy·po·bar·ic spi·nal a.
hy·po·ten·sive a.
hy·po·ther·mic a.
hys·ter·i·cal a.
in·fil·tra·tion a.
in·ha·la·tion a.
in·suf·fla·tion a.
in·ter·cos·tal a.
in·tra·med·ul·lary a.
in·tra·na·sal a.
in·tra·o·ral a.
in·tra·os·se·ous a.
in·tra·spi·nal a.
in·tra·tra·che·al a.
in·tra·ve·nous a.
in·tra·ve·nous re·gion·al a.
iso·bar·ic spi·nal a.
lo·cal a.
low spi·nal a.
mus·cu·lar a.
nerve block a.
non·re·breath·ing a.
ol·fac·to·ry a.
open drop a.
pain·ful a.
par·a·cer·vi·cal block a.
par·a·ver·te·bral a.
per·i·du·ral a.
per·i·neu·ral a.
per·i·o·don·tal a.
pha·ryn·ge·al a.
pre·sa·cral a.
pres·sure a.
pu·den·dal a.
re·breath·ing a.
rec·tal a.
re·frig·er·a·tion a.
re·gion·al a.
ret·ro·bul·bar a.

sa·cral a.
sad·dle block a.
seg·men·tal a.
sem·i-closed a.
sem·i-o·pen a.
spi·nal a.
splanch·nic a.
stock·ing a.
sub·a·rach·noid a.
sur·gi·cal a.
tac·tile a.
ther·a·peu·tic a.
ther·mal a.
ther·mic a.
to-and-fro a.
top·i·cal a.
to·tal spi·nal a.
trau·mat·ic a.
uni·lat·e·ral a.
vis·cer·al a.

an·es·the·sia
ma·chine
rec·ord

an·es·the·si·ol·o·gist
an·es·the·si·ol·o·gy
an·es·the·si·o·phore
an·es·thet·ic
flam·ma·ble a.
gen·er·al a.
in·ha·la·tion a.
in·tra·ve·nous a.
lo·cal a.
pri·mary a.
sec·on·dary a.
spi·nal a.
vol·a·tile a.

an·es·thet·ic
cir·cuit
depth
ether
gas
in·dex
lep·ro·sy
shock
va·por

anes·the·tist
anes·the·ti·za·tion
anes·the·tize
an·es·trous
o·vu·la·tion
an·es·trus
ane·tho·path
an·e·to·der·ma
Jadassohn-Pellizzari a.
Schweninger-Buzzi a.
an·eu·ploid
an·eu·ploi·dy
par·tial a.

an·eu·rine
a. hy·dro·chlo·ride
aneu·ro·lem·mic
an·eu·rysm
am·pul·la·ry a.
a. by anas·to·mo·sis
ar·te·ri·o·scle·rot·ic a.
ar·te·ri·o·ve·nous a.
ath·er·o·scle·rot·ic a.
ax·i·al a.
bac·te·ri·al a.
be·nign bone a.
Bérard's a.
ber·ry a.
car·di·ac a.
cav·ern·ous-ca·rot·id a.
cir·soid a.
com·pound a.
con·gen·i·tal ce·re·bral a.
con·sec·u·tive a.
cyl·in·droid a.
dif·fuse a.
dis·sect·ing a.
ec·tat·ic a.
em·bol·ic a.
em·bo·lo·my·cot·ic a.
false a.
fu·si·form a.
her·nial a.
in·fra·cli·noid a.
in·tra·cra·ni·al a.
mil·i·a·ry a.
mu·ral a.
my·cot·ic a.
Park's a.
pe·riph·e·ral a.
phan·tom a.
Pott's a.
rac·e·mose a.
Rasmussen's a.
sac·cu·lar a.
sac·cu·lat·ed a.
ser·pen·tine a.
su·pra·cli·noid a.
syph·i·lit·ic a.
trac·tion a.
trau·mat·ic a.
true a.
tu·bu·lar a.
var·i·cose a.
ven·tric·u·lar a.
ver·min·ous a.
worm a.
an·eu·rysm
nee·dle
an·eu·rys·mal
bru·it
phthi·sis

sac
var·ix
an·eu·rys·mal bone
cyst
an·eu·rys·mat·ic
an·eu·rys·mec·to·my
an·eu·rys·mo·gram
an·eu·rys·mo·plas·ty
an·eu·rys·mor·rha·phy
an·eu·rys·mot·o·my
an·gel·i·ca root
an·gel's
wing
Angelucci's
syn·drome
Anger
cam·era
Anghelescu's
sign
an·gi·al·gia
an·gi·as·the·nia
an·gi·ec·ta·sia
con·gen·i·tal dys·plas·tic a.
an·gi·ec·ta·sis
an·gi·ec·tat·ic
an·gi·ec·to·my
an·gi·ec·to·pia
an·gi·i·tis
al·ler·gic a.
al·ler·gic gran·u·lom·a·tous a.
con·sec·u·tive a.
cu·ta·ne·ous sys·tem·ic a.
hy·per·sen·si·tiv·i·ty a.
leu·ko·cy·to·clas·tic a.
a. li·ve·do re·tic·u·la·ris
nec·ro·tiz·ing a.
an·gi·leu·ci·tis
an·gi·na
ab·dom·i·nal a.
a. ab·do·mi·nis
agran·u·lo·cyt·ic a.
cre·scen·do a.
a. cru·ris
a. de·cu·bi·tus
a. diph·the·ri·ti·ca
a. ep·i·glot·ti·dea
false a.
Heberden's a.
hy·per·cy·a·not·ic a.
in·tes·ti·nal a.
a. in·ver·sa
Ludwig's a.
lym·phat·ic a.
a. lym·pho·ma·to·sa
mon·o·cyt·ic a.
ne·crot·ic a.

an·gi·na *(continued)*
 neu·tro·pe·nic a.
 a. no·tha
 a. pec·to·ris
 a. pec·to·ris de·cu·bi·tus
 a. pec·to·ris sine do·lore
 a. pec·to·ris va·so·mo·to·ria
 Prinzmetal's a.
 re·flex a.
 a. scar·la·ti·no·sa
 a. sine do·lore
 a. spu·ria
 un·sta·ble a.
 var·i·ant a. pec·to·ris
 va·so·mo·tor a.
 a. va·so·mo·to·ria
 Vincent's a.
 walk-through a.
an·gi·nal
an·gi·ni·form
an·gi·noid
an·gin·o·pho·bia
an·gi·nose
 scar·la·ti·na
an·gi·nous
an·gi·o·ar·chi·tec·ture
an·gi·o·blast
an·gi·o·blas·tic
 cells
an·gi·o·blas·to·ma
an·gi·o·car·di·o·ci·net·ic
an·gi·o·car·di·og·ra·phy
 rap·id bi·plane a.
an·gi·o·car·di·o·ki·net·ic
an·gi·o·car·di·op·a·thy
an·gi·o·car·di·tis
an·gi·o·cho·le·cys·ti·tis
an·gi·o·cho·li·tis
an·gi·o·cyst
an·gi·o·der·ma·ti·tis
an·gi·o·di·as·co·py
an·gi·o·dyn·ia
an·gi·o·dys·ge·net·ic
 my·e·lo·ma·la·cia
an·gi·o·dys·pla·sia
an·gi·o·dys·tro·phia
an·gi·o·dys·tro·phy
an·gi·o·e·de·ma
an·gi·o·el·e·phan·ti·a·sis
an·gi·o·en·do·the·li·o·ma·to·sis
 pro·lif·er·at·ing sys·tem·a·
 tized a.
an·gi·o·fi·bro·li·po·ma
an·gi·o·fi·bro·ma
 ju·ve·nile a.
an·gi·o·fi·bro·sis

an·gi·o·fol·lic·u·lar me·di·as·
 ti·nal lymph node
 hy·per·pla·sia
an·gi·o·gen·e·sis
 fac·tor
an·gi·o·gen·ic
an·gi·o·gli·o·ma
an·gi·o·gli·o·ma·to·sis
an·gi·o·gli·o·sis
an·gi·o·gram
an·gi·o·graph·ic
an·gi·og·ra·phy
 ce·re·bral a.
 closed a.
 dig·i·tal sub·trac·tion a.
 flu·o·res·ce·in a.
 open a.
 ra·di·o·nu·clide a.
 se·lec·tive a.
 spi·nal a.
 ther·a·peu·tic a.
an·gi·o·he·mo·phil·ia
an·gi·o·hy·a·li·no·sis
an·gi·o·hy·per·to·nia
an·gi·o·hy·po·to·nia
an·gi·oid
 streaks
an·gi·o·im·mu·no·blas·tic
 lym·phad·e·nop·a·thy
an·gi·o·in·va·sive
an·gi·o·ker·a·to·ma
 a. cor·po·ris dif·fu·sum
 Fordyce's a.
 Mibelli's a.'s
an·gi·o·ker·a·to·sis
an·gi·o·ki·ne·sis
an·gi·o·ki·net·ic
an·gi·o·lei·o·my·o·ma
an·gi·o·lip·o·fi·bro·ma
an·gi·o·li·po·ma
an·gi·o·lith
an·gi·o·lith·ic
 de·gen·er·a·tion
 sar·co·ma
an·gi·o·lo·gia
an·gi·ol·o·gy
an·gi·o·lu·poid
an·gi·o·lym·phoid
 hy·per·pla·sia with eo·sin·
 o·phil·ia
an·gi·ol·y·sis
an·gi·o·ma
 cap·il·lary a.
 cav·ern·ous a.
 cher·ry a.
 en·ce·phal·ic a.
 a. lym·pha·ti·cum
 pe·te·chi·al a.'s

a. ser·pi·gi·no·sum
spi·der a.
su·per·fi·cial a.
tel·an·gi·ec·tat·ic a.
a. ve·no·sum ra·ce·mo·sum
an·gi·o·ma·toid
tu·mor
an·gi·o·ma·to·sis
ceph·a·lo·tri·gem·i·nal a.
con·gen·i·tal dys·plas·tic a.
cu·ta·ne·o·me·nin·go·spi·nal
a.
en·ceph·a·lo·tri·gem·i·nal a.
oc·u·lo·en·ce·phal·ic a.
ret·i·no·cer·e·bral a.
tel·an·gi·ec·tat·ic a.
an·gi·o·ma·tous
an·gi·o·meg·a·ly
an·gi·om·e·ter
an·gi·o·my·o·car·di·ac
an·gi·o·my·o·fi·bro·ma
an·gi·o·my·o·li·po·ma
an·gi·o·my·o·ma
an·gi·o·my·o·neu·ro·ma
an·gi·o·my·op·a·thy
an·gi·o·my·o·sar·co·ma
an·gi·o·myx·o·ma
an·gi·o·neu·ral·gia
an·gi·o·neu·rec·to·my
an·gi·o·neur·e·de·ma
an·gi·o·neu·ro·my·o·ma
an·gi·o·neu·ro·sis
an·gi·o·neu·rot·ic
ede·ma
he·ma·tu·ria
an·gi·o·neu·rot·o·my
an·gi·o-os·te·o·hy·per·tro·phy
syn·drome
an·gi·o·pa·ral·y·sis
an·gi·o·par·a·lyt·ic
neur·as·the·nia
an·gi·o·pa·re·sis
an·gi·o·path·ic
neur·as·the·nia
ret·i·nop·a·thy
an·gi·o·path·ic he·mo·lyt·ic
ane·mia
an·gi·op·a·thy
ce·re·bral am·y·loid a.
con·gen·i·tal dys·plas·tic a.
con·go·phil·ic a.
an·gi·o·phac·o·ma·to·sis
an·gi·o·phak·o·ma·to·sis
an·gi·o·pla·ny
an·gi·o·plas·ty
per·cu·ta·ne·ous trans·lu·
mi·nal a.
an·gi·o·poi·e·sis

an·gi·o·poi·et·ic
an·gi·o·pres·sure
an·gi·or·rha·phy
an·gi·or·rhex·is
an·gi·o·sar·co·ma
an·gi·o·scope
an·gi·os·co·py
an·gi·o·sco·to·ma
an·gi·o·sco·tom·e·try
an·gi·o·sis
an·gi·o·spasm
lab·y·rin·thine a.
an·gi·o·spas·tic
an·gi·o·stax·is
an·gi·o·ste·no·sis
an·gi·os·to·my
an·gi·o·stron·gy·lo·sis
An·gi·o·stron·gy·lus
A. can·ton·en·sis
A. cos·tar·i·cen·sis
A. ma·lay·si·en·sis
A. va·so·rum
an·gi·os·tro·phy
an·gi·o·tel·ec·ta·sia
an·gi·o·te·lec·ta·sis
an·gi·o·ten·sin
an·gi·o·ten·sin am·ide
an·gi·o·ten·sin·ase
an·gi·o·ten·sin-con·vert·ing
en·zyme
an·gi·o·ten·sin con·vert·ing en·
zyme
in·hib·i·tor
an·gi·o·ten·sin I
an·gi·o·ten·sin II
an·gi·o·ten·sin III
an·gi·o·ten·sin·o·gen
an·gi·o·ten·sin·o·gen·ase
an·gi·o·ten·sin pre·cur·sor
an·gi·ot·o·my
an·gi·o·to·nia
an·gi·o·ton·ic
an·gi·o·tribe
an·gi·o·trip·sy
an·gi·o·tro·phic
an·gi·tis
an·gle
a. of ab·nor·mal·i·ty
acro·mi·al a.
acute a.
ad·ja·cent a.
al·pha a.
al·ve·o·lar a.
a. of anom·a·ly
a. of an·te·ver·sion
a. of ap·er·ture
ap·i·cal a.
ax·i·al a.

an·gle *(continued)*
  bas·i·lar a.
  Bennett a.
  be·ta a.
  bi·or·bit·al a.
  Broca's a.'s
  Broca's bas·i·lar a.
  Broca's fa·cial a.
  buc·cal a.'s
  buc·co-oc·clu·sal a.
  car·di·o·he·pat·ic a.
  car·ry·ing a.
  cav·i·ty line a.
  ca·vo·sur·face a.
  ce·phal·ic a.
  ceph·a·lo·med·ul·lary a.
  cer·e·bel·lo·pon·tile a.
  cer·e·bel·lo·pon·tine a.
  a. of con·ver·gence
  cos·tal a.
  cra·ni·o·fa·cial a.
  crit·i·cal a.
  cusp a.
  Daubenton's a.
  a. of dec·li·na·tion
  a. of de·pres·sion
  a. of de·vi·a·tion
  dis·par·i·ty a.
  du·o·de·no·je·ju·nal a.
  a. of ec·cen·tric·i·ty
  a. of emer·gence
  ep·i·gas·tric a.
  eth·moid a.
  fa·cial a.
  fil·tra·tion a.
  Frankfort-man·dib·u·lar in·ci·sor a.
  fron·tal a. of pa·ri·e·tal
  a. of Fuchs
  gam·ma a.
  hyp·si·loid a.
  im·ped·ance a.
  a. of in·ci·dence
  in·ci·dent a.
  in·ci·sal guide a.
  a. of in·cli·na·tion
  in·fe·ri·or a. of scap·u·la
  in·fra·ster·nal a.
  ir·i·do·cor·ne·al a.
  a. of iris
  Jacquart's fa·cial a.
  a. of jaw
  kap·pa a.
  lat·er·al a. of eye
  lat·er·al a. of scap·u·la
  lat·er·al a. of uter·us
  lim·it·ing a.
  line a.

  Louis' a.
  Lovibond's a.
  Ludwig's a.
  lum·bo·sa·cral a.
  a. of man·di·ble
  mas·toid a. of pa·ri·e·tal
  max·il·lary a.
  me·di·al a. of eye
  me·si·al a.
  met·a·fa·cial a.
  me·ter a.
  a. of mouth
  oc·cip·i·tal a. of pa·ri·e·tal
  ol·fac·to·ry a.
  oph·ry·o·spi·nal a.
  pa·ri·e·tal a.
  pel·vi·ver·te·bral a.
  phre·no·per·i·car·di·al a.
  Pirogoff's a.
  point a.
  a. of po·lar·i·za·tion
  pon·tine a.
  pu·bic a.
  Q a.
  Quatrefages' a.
  Ranke's a.
  a. of re·flec·tion
  re·fract·ing a. of a prism
  a. of re·frac·tion
  Rolando's a.
  Serres' a.
  S-N-A a.
  S-N-B a.
  sphe·noid a.
  sphe·noi·dal a.
  a. of squint
  ster·nal a.
  ster·no·cla·vic·u·lar a.
  sub·pu·bic a.
  sub·ster·nal a.
  su·pe·ri·or a. of scap·u·la
  syl·vi·an a.
  ten·to·ri·al a.
  Topinard's fa·cial a.
  a. of tor·sion
  ve·nous a.
  Virchow-Holder a.
  Virchow's a.
  vi·su·al a.
  Vogt's a.
  Weisbach's a.
  Welcker's a.
  y-a.
an·gle of
  con·ver·gence
an·gle-clo·sure
  glau·co·ma

Angle's
 clas·si·fi·ca·tion of mal·oc·
  clu·sion
an·gor
 a. ani·mi
 a. pec·to·ris
an·gos·tu·ra bark
Ångström
 scale
 unit
ang·strom
Ångström's
 law
An·guil·lu·la
an·gu·lar
 ac·cel·er·a·tion
 al·de·hyde
 ap·er·ture
 ar·tery
 chei·li·tis
 con·junc·ti·vi·tis
 con·vo·lu·tion
 cur·va·ture
 gy·rus
 meth·yl
 notch
 sphinc·ter
 spine
 sto·ma·ti·tis
 vein
an·gu·la·tion
an·gu·li
an·gu·lus
 a. in·fec·ti·o·sus
 a. ir·i·dis
 a. oc·u·li na·sa·lis
 a. oc·u·li tem·po·ra·lis
an·ha·lon·i·dine
an·hal·o·nine
An·ha·lo·ni·um le·win·ii
an·haph·ia
an·he·do·nia
an·hi·dro·sis
an·hi·drot·ic
an·hi·drot·ic ec·to·der·mal
 dys·pla·sia
an·his·tic
an·his·tous
an·hy·drase
 car·bon·ic a.
an·hy·dra·tion
an·hy·dride
an·hy·dro·gi·tal·in
an·hy·dro·leu·cov·o·rin
an·hy·dro·sug·ars
an·hy·drous
 al·co·hol

chlo·ral
lan·o·lin
ani
a·ni·a·cin·am·i·do·sis
a·ni·a·cin·o·sis
an·ic·ter·ic
an·ic·ter·ic vi·rus
 hep·a·ti·tis
an·id·e·an
an·id·e·us
 em·bry·on·ic a.
an·i·dous
an·i·dro·sis
an·i·drot·ic
an·ile
an·i·ler·i·dine
an·i·lide
ani·linc·tion
ani·linc·tus
an·i·line
 fuch·sin
an·i·line blue
ani·lin·gus
an·i·lin·ism
an·i·li·no·phil
an·i·li·no·phile
an·i·li·noph·i·lous
an·il·ism
anil·i·ty
an·i·ma
an·i·mal
 cold-blood·ed a.
 con·trol a.
 con·ven·tion·al a.
 Houssay a.
 nor·mal a.
 sen·ti·nel a.
 warm-blood·ed a.
an·i·mal
 char·coal
 dex·tran
 force
 graft
 mod·el
 pole
 soap
 starch
 tox·in
 vi·rus·es
 wax
an·i·mal black
an·i·mal·cule
an·i·mal pro·tein
 fac·tor
an·i·ma·tion
 sus·pend·ed a.
an·i·mat·ism
an·i·mism

an·i·mus
an·i·on
  gap
an·i·on-ex·change
  res·in
an·i·on ex·change
an·i·on ex·chang·er
an·i·on·ic
  de·ter·gents
an·i·on·ot·ro·py
an·i·rid·ia
an·i·sa·ki·a·sis
an·i·sa·kid
An·i·sa·ki·dae
An·i·sa·kis
an·is·ate
an·ise
an·is·ei·ko·nia
anis·ic
anis·ic ac·id
an·i·sin·di·one
an·i·so·ac·com·mo·da·tion
an·i·so·chro·ma·sia
an·i·so·chro·mat·ic
an·i·so·co·ria
an·i·so·cy·to·sis
an·i·so·dac·ty·lous
an·i·so·dac·ty·ly
an·i·sog·a·my
an·i·sog·na·thous
an·i·so·kar·y·o·sis
an·is·ole
an·i·so·mas·tia
an·i·so·me·lia
an·i·so·me·tro·pia
an·i·so·me·tro·pic
  am·bly·o·pia
an·i·so·pho·ria
an·i·so·pi·e·sis
an·i·sor·rhyth·mia
an·i·so·sphyg·mia
an·i·so·spore
an·i·sos·then·ic
an·i·so·ton·ic
an·i·so·tro·pic
  disks
  lip·id
an·i·so·tro·pine meth·yl·bro·
mide
Anitschkow
  cell
  my·o·cyte
an·kle
  bone
  clo·nus
  jerk
  joint

re·flex
re·gion
an·ky·lo·bleph·a·ron
an·ky·lo·col·pos
an·ky·lo·dac·tyl·ia
an·ky·lo·dac·ty·ly
an·ky·lo·glos·sia
an·ky·lo·glos·sia su·pe·ri·or
  syn·drome
an·ky·lo·me·le
an·ky·lo·poi·et·ic
an·ky·lo·proc·tia
an·ky·losed
  tooth
an·ky·los·ing
  hy·per·os·to·sis
  spon·dy·li·tis
an·ky·lo·sis
  ar·ti·fi·cial a.
  bony a.
  den·tal a.
  ex·tra·cap·su·lar a.
  false a.
  fi·brous a.
  in·tra·cap·su·lar a.
  spu·ri·ous a.
  true a.
An·ky·los·to·ma
an·ky·los·to·ma
an·ky·lo·sto·mi·a·sis
an·ky·lot·ic
an·kyl·u·re·thria
an·ky·roid
an·la·ge
an·la·gen
an·neal
an·neal·ing
  lamp
  tray
an·nec·tent
  gy·rus
An·nel·i·da
an·ne·lids
an·nel·lide
an·nel·lo·co·nid·i·um
an·nexa
an·nex·al
an·nex·ec·to·my
an·nex·i·tis
an·nex·o·pexy
an·ni·hi·la·tion
  ra·di·a·tion
an·not·to
an·nu·lar
  band
  car·ti·lage
  cat·a·ract
  lig·a·ment

lig·a·ment of the ra·di·us
lig·a·ment of the sta·pes
lig·a·ments of the tra·chea
pan·cre·as
pla·cen·ta
plex·us
scle·ri·tis
sco·to·ma
sphinc·ter
staph·y·lo·ma
stric·ture
syn·ech·ia
syph·i·lid
an·nu·late
  la·mel·lae
an·nu·lo·plasty
an·nu·lor·rha·phy
an·nu·lo·spi·ral
  end·ing
  or·gan
an·nu·lus
  a. ab·do·mi·na·lis
  a. cil·i·ar·is
  a. of fi·brous sheath
  Haller's a.
  a. hem·or·rhoi·dal·is
  a. ir·i·dis
  a. ir·i·dis ma·jor
  a. ir·i·dis mi·nor
  a. ova·lis
  a. pre·pu·ti·a·lis
  a. ure·thra·lis
  Vieussens' a.
an·o·chle·sia
an·o·chro·ma·sia
ano·ci·as·so·ci·a·tion
ano·coc·cyg·e·al
  body
  lig·a·ment
  nerves
ano·cu·ta·ne·ous
  line
anod·al
  cur·rent
anod·al clo·sure
  con·trac·tion
  tet·a·nus
anod·al du·ra·tion
  tet·a·nus
anod·al open·ing
  con·trac·tion
  tet·a·nus
an·ode
  rays
an·od·ic
an·o·don·tia
  par·tial a.
an·o·dont·ism

an·o·dyne
an·o·et·ic
ano·gen·i·tal
  band
  ra·phe
anom·a·lad
anom·a·lo·scope
anom·a·lous
  com·plex
  cor·re·spon·dence
  tri·chro·ma·tism
  uter·us
  vis·cos·i·ty
anom·a·lous mi·tral
  ar·cade
anom·a·ly
  Alder's a.
  Aristotle's a.
  Chédiak-Steinbrinck-Higashi
    a.
  de·vel·op·men·tal a.
  Ebstein's a.
  eu·gnath·ic a.
  Freund's a.
  Hegglin's a.
  May-Hegglin a.
  morn·ing glo·ry a.
  Pelger-Huët nu·cle·ar a.
  Peters' a.
  Rieger's a.
  Shone's a.
  Uhl a.
an·o·mer
an·o·mer·ic
  car·bon
ano·mia
anom·ic
  apha·sia
an·o·mie
an·o·nych·ia
an·o·ny·cho·sis
anon·y·ma
anon·y·mous
  ar·tery
  veins
Anoph·e·les
  A. al·bim·a·nus
  A. al·bi·tar·sus
  A. bal·a·ba·cen·sis
  A. cu·li·ci·fa·cies
  A. dar·lingi
  A. flu·vi·a·ti·lis
  A. free·borni
  A. fu·nes·tus
  A. gam·bi·ae
  A. la·bran·chi·ae
  A. ma·cu·la·tus
  A. mac·u·li·pen·nis

Anoph·e·les *(continued)*
A. mi·ni·mus
A. pseu·do·punc·ti·pen·nis
A. quad·ri·ma·cu·la·tus
A. ste·phensi
A. sun·dai·cus
A. su·per·pic·tus
anoph·e·li·cide
anoph·e·li·fuge
Anoph·e·li·nae
anoph·e·line
Anophe·li·ni
anoph·e·lism
an·oph·thal·mia
con·sec·u·tive a.
pri·mary a.
sec·on·dary a.
ano·plas·ty
An·op·lo·ceph·a·la
A. per·fo·li·a·ta
An·o·plu·ra
an·or·chia
an·or·chism
ano·rec·tal
junc·tion
spasm
syn·drome
ano·rec·tal lymph
nodes
an·o·rec·tic
an·o·ret·ic
an·o·rex·ia
a. ner·vo·sa
an·o·rex·i·ant
an·o·rex·ic
an·o·rex·i·gen·ic
an·or·gas·mia
an·or·gas·my
an·or·thog·ra·phy
ano·scope
Bacon's a.
ano·sig·moid·os·co·py
an·os·mia
an·os·mic
ano·so·di·a·pho·ria
ano·sog·no·sia
ano·sog·no·sic
ep·i·lep·sy
sei·zure
ano·spi·nal
cen·ter
an·os·te·o·pla·sia
an·os·to·sis
an·o·tia
ano·ves·i·cal
an·ov·u·lar
men·stru·a·tion

an·ov·u·lar ovar·i·an
fol·li·cle
an·ov·u·la·tion
an·ov·u·la·tion·al
men·stru·a·tion
an·ov·u·la·to·ry
cy·cle
an·ox·e·mia
test
an·ox·ia
ane·mic a.
an·ox·ic a.
dif·fu·sion a.
his·to·tox·ic a.
a. ne·o·na·to·rum
ox·y·gen af·fin·i·ty a.
stag·nant a.
an·ox·ic
an·ox·ia
Anrep
phe·nom·e·non
an·sa
Haller's a.
Henle's a.
a. hy·po·glos·si
len·tic·u·lar a.
an·sae ner·vo·rum spi·na·li·um
pe·dun·cu·lar a.
Reil's a.
a. sa·cra·lis
Vieussens' a.
an·sae
an·sate
an·ser·ine
bur·sa
bur·si·tis
an·si·form
lob·ule
an·sot·o·my
ant
har·vest·er a.
vel·vet a.
ant·ac·id
an·tag·o·nism
bac·te·ri·al a.
an·tag·o·nist
as·so·ci·at·ed a.
cal·ci·um a.
com·pet·i·tive a.
en·zyme a.
fo·lic ac·id a.'s
in·su·lin a.
an·tag·o·nis·tic
mus·cles
re·flex·es
ant·al·ge·sia

ant·al·gic
  gait
ant·al·ka·line
ant·aph·ro·di·si·ac
ant·aph·ro·dit·ic
ant·ar·thrit·ic
ant·as·then·ic
ant·asth·mat·ic
ant·a·tro·phic
an·taz·o·line hy·dro·chlo·ride
an·te·brach·i·al
  fas·cia
an·te·bra·chi·um
an·te·car·di·um
an·te·ced·ent
  plas·ma throm·bo·plas·tin a.
an·te·ced·ent
  sign
an·te ci·bum
an·te·cu·bi·tal
  space
an·te·fe·brile
an·te·flex
an·te·flex·ion
  a. of iris
antegonial
  notch
an·te·grade
  cys·tog·ra·phy
  py·e·log·ra·phy
  urog·ra·phy
an·te·mor·tem
  clot
  throm·bus
an·te·na·tal
  di·ag·no·sis
an·te·par·tum
ant·eph·i·al·tic
an·te·po·si·tion
an·te·pros·tate
an·te·py·ret·ic
an·te·ri·or
  arch of at·las
  asyn·cli·tism
  bor·der
  cells
  cham·ber of eye
  cho·roid·i·tis
  col·umn of me·dul·la ob·
    lon·ga·ta
  col·umn of spi·nal cord
  com·mis·sure
  com·po·nent of force
  cur·va·ture
  cusp
  em·bry·o·tox·on
  ep·i·the·li·um of cor·nea
  ex·trem·i·ty

  ex·trem·i·ty of cau·date
    nu·cle·us
  fon·ta·nel
  fu·nic·u·lus
  guide
  horn
  lay·er of rec·tus ab·do·mi·
    nis sheath
  lig·a·ment of head of fib·u·
    la
  lig·a·ment of mal·le·us
  limb of in·ter·nal cap·sule
  limb of sta·pes
  lip
  lobe of hy·poph·y·sis
  mar·gin
  meg·a·loph·thal·mus
  na·ris
  ne·phrec·to·my
  notch of cer·e·bel·lum
  notch of ear
  nu·clei of thal·a·mus
  oc·clu·sion
  part
  part of pons
  pil·lar of fau·ces
  pil·lar of for·nix
  pi·tu·i·tary
  pole of eye·ball
  pole of lens
  pro·cess of mal·le·us
  pyr·a·mid
  re·cess of tym·pan·ic mem·
    brane
  re·gion of fore·arm
  re·gion of neck
  rhi·nos·co·py
  rhi·zot·o·my
  root
  scle·ri·tis
  scle·rot·o·my
  seg·ment
  si·nus·es
  staph·y·lo·ma
  sur·face
  sur·face of eye·lids
  sur·face of leg
  sur·face of max·il·la
  sur·face of pet·rous part
  sym·bleph·a·ron
  syn·ech·ia
  teeth
  tri·an·gle
  tu·ber·cle of at·las
  tu·ber·cle of cer·vi·cal ver·
    te·brae
  tu·ber·cle of thal·a·mus
  ure·thri·tis

an·te·ri·or *(continued)*
  uve·i·tis
  vein of sep·tum pel·lu·ci·dum
  vit·rec·to·my
  wall of mid·dle ear
  wall of stom·ach
  wall of va·gi·na
an·te·ri·or am·pul·lar
  nerve
an·te·ri·or an·te·brach·i·al
  nerve
an·te·ri·or ar·tic·u·lar
  sur·face of dens
an·te·ri·or at·lan·to-oc·cip·i·tal
  mem·brane
an·te·ri·or au·ric·u·lar
  groove
  mus·cle
  nerves
  vein
an·te·ri·or ax·il·lary
  line
an·te·ri·or ba·sal
  seg·ment
an·te·ri·or cal·ca·ne·al ar·tic·u·lar
  sur·face
an·te·ri·or car·di·ac
  veins
an·te·ri·or car·di·nal
  veins
an·te·ri·or car·pal
  re·gion
an·te·ri·or ce·cal
  ar·tery
an·te·ri·or cen·tral
  con·vo·lu·tion
  gy·rus
an·te·ri·or ce·re·bral
  ar·tery
  vein
an·te·ri·or cer·vi·cal in·ter·trans·verse
  mus·cles
an·te·ri·or cer·vi·cal lymph
  nodes
an·te·ri·or cham·ber
  tra·bec·u·la
an·te·ri·or cham·ber cleav·age
  syn·drome
an·te·ri·or cho·roi·dal
  ar·tery
an·te·ri·or cil·i·ary
  ar·tery
an·te·ri·or cir·cum·flex hu·mer·al
  ar·tery

an·te·ri·or com·mu·ni·cat·ing
  ar·tery
an·te·ri·or con·dy·loid
  ca·nal of oc·cip·i·tal bone
  fo·ra·men
an·te·ri·or con·junc·ti·val
  ar·tery
an·te·ri·or cor·o·nary
  plex·us
an·te·ri·or cor·ti·co·spi·nal
  tract
an·te·ri·or cos·to·trans·verse
  lig·a·ment
an·te·ri·or cra·ni·al
  base
  fos·sa
an·te·ri·or cru·ci·ate
  lig·a·ment
an·te·ri·or cru·ral
  nerve
an·te·ri·or cu·bi·tal
  re·gion
an·te·ri·or de·scend·ing
  ar·tery
an·te·ri·or elas·tic
  lay·er
an·te·ri·or eth·moi·dal
  ar·tery
  nerve
an·te·ri·or fa·cial
  height
  vein
an·te·ri·or fo·cal
  point
an·te·ri·or ground
  bun·dle
an·te·ri·or in·fe·ri·or
  seg·ment
an·te·ri·or in·fe·ri·or cer·e·bel·lar
  ar·tery
an·te·ri·or in·fe·ri·or il·i·ac
  spine
an·te·ri·or in·ter·con·dy·lar
  ar·ea
an·te·ri·or in·ter·cos·tal
  ar·tery
  veins
an·te·ri·or in·ter·me·di·ate
  groove
an·te·ri·or in·ter·os·se·ous
  ar·tery
  nerve
an·te·ri·or in·ter·ven·tric·u·lar
  ar·tery
  groove
an·te·ri·or in·tes·ti·nal
  por·tal

an·te·ri·or in·tra·oc·cip·i·tal
  joint
an·te·ri·or jug·u·lar
  vein
an·te·ri·or jug·u·lar lymph
  nodes
an·te·ri·or la·bi·al
  ar·ter·ies
  com·mis·sure
  nerves
  veins
an·te·ri·or lac·ri·mal
  crest
an·te·ri·or lat·er·al mal·le·o·
  lar
  ar·tery
an·te·ri·or lim·it·ing
  lay·er of cor·nea
  ring
an·te·ri·or lin·gual
  gland
an·te·ri·or lon·gi·tu·di·nal
  lig·a·ment
an·te·ri·or lu·nate
  lob·ule
an·te·ri·or me·di·al mal·le·o·
  lar
  ar·tery
an·te·ri·or me·di·an
  fis·sure of me·dul·la ob·
    lon·ga·ta
  fis·sure of spi·nal cord
  line
an·te·ri·or me·di·as·ti·nal
  lymph
  nodes
an·te·ri·or med·ul·lary
  ve·lum
an·te·ri·or me·nin·ge·al
  ar·tery
an·te·ri·or me·nis·co·fem·o·ral
  lig·a·ment
an·te·ri·or my·o·car·di·al
  in·farc·tion
an·te·ri·or na·sal
  spine
an·te·ri·or oc·u·lar
  seg·ment
an·te·ri·or pal·a·tine
  arch
  fo·ram·i·na
an·te·ri·or pa·ri·e·tal
  ar·tery
an·te·ri·or par·ol·fac·to·ry
  sul·cus
an·te·ri·or pel·vic
  ex·en·ter·a·tion

an·te·ri·or per·fo·rat·ed
  sub·stance
an·te·ri·or per·o·ne·al
  ar·tery
an·te·ri·or pir·i·form
  gy·rus
an·te·ri·or pi·tu·i·tary
  go·nad·o·tro·pin
an·te·ri·or pi·tu·i·tary-like
  hor·mone
an·te·ri·or pon·to·mes·en·ce·
  phal·ic
  vein
an·te·ri·or pri·mary
  di·vi·sion
an·te·ri·or py·ram·i·dal
  tract
an·te·ri·or rec·tus
  mus·cle of head
an·te·ri·or sa·cro·coc·cyg·e·al
  lig·a·ment
an·te·ri·or sa·cro·il·i·ac
  lig·a·ments
an·te·ri·or sa·cro·sci·at·ic
  lig·a·ment
an·te·ri·or sca·lene
  mus·cle
an·te·ri·or scro·tal
  nerves
  veins
an·te·ri·or sem·i·cir·cu·lar
  ca·nals
an·te·ri·or ser·ra·tus
  mus·cle
an·te·ri·or spi·nal
  ar·tery
an·te·ri·or spi·no·cer·e·bel·lar
  tract
an·te·ri·or spi·no·tha·lam·ic
  tract
an·te·ri·or ster·no·cla·vic·u·lar
  lig·a·ment
an·te·ri·or su·pe·ri·or
  seg·ment
an·te·ri·or su·pe·ri·or al·ve·o·
  lar
  ar·tery
an·te·ri·or su·pe·ri·or den·tal
  ar·tery
an·te·ri·or su·pe·ri·or il·i·ac
  spine
an·te·ri·or su·pra·cla·vic·u·lar
  nerve
an·te·ri·or ta·lo·fib·u·lar
  lig·a·ment
an·te·ri·or ta·lo·tib·i·al
  lig·a·ment

an·te·ri·or tem·po·ral
ar·tery
an·te·ri·or tib·i·al
ar·tery
bur·sa
mus·cle
nerve
node
veins
an·te·ri·or tib·i·al com·part·
ment
syn·drome
an·te·ri·or tib·i·al re·cur·rent
ar·tery
an·te·ri·or tib·i·o·fib·u·lar
lig·a·ment
an·te·ri·or tib·i·o·ta·lar
part
an·te·ri·or tym·pan·ic
ar·tery
an·te·ri·or ure·thral
valve
an·te·ri·or ver·te·bral
vein
an·te·ri·or white
com·mis·sure
an·ter·o·ex·ter·nal
an·ter·o·fa·cial
dys·pla·sia
an·ter·o·grade
am·ne·sia
block
con·duc·tion
mem·o·ry
an·ter·o·in·fe·ri·or
an·ter·o·in·fe·ri·or my·o·car·
di·al
in·farc·tion
an·ter·o·in·ter·nal
an·ter·o·lat·er·al
col·umn of spi·nal cord
cor·dot·o·my
fon·ta·nel
groove
sul·cus
sur·face of hu·mer·us
trac·tot·o·my
an·ter·o·lat·er·al cen·tral
ar·ter·ies
an·ter·o·lat·er·al my·o·car·di·
al
in·farc·tion
an·ter·o·lat·er·al stri·ate
ar·ter·ies
an·ter·o·lat·er·al thal·a·mo·
stri·ate
ar·ter·ies

an·ter·o·me·di·al
sur·face of hu·mer·us
an·ter·o·me·di·al cen·tral
ar·ter·ies
an·ter·o·me·di·al thal·a·mo·
stri·ate
ar·ter·ies
an·ter·o·me·di·an
groove
an·ter·o·pos·te·ri·or
di·am·e·ter of the pel·vic
in·let
dys·pla·sia
an·ter·o·pos·te·ri·or fa·cial
dys·pla·sia
an·ter·o·sep·tal my·o·car·di·al
in·farc·tion
an·ter·o·su·pe·ri·or
ant·e·rot·ic
an·te·sys·to·le
an·te·ver·sion
an·te·vert·ed
an·te·ves·i·cal
her·nia
ant·he·lix
an·thel·min·thic
an·thel·min·tic
an·the·lone
a. E
a. U
ant·he·lot·ic
an·the·ma
an·thi·o·li·mine
an·tho·cy·a·nins
An·tho·my·ia
A. ca·ni·cu·la·ris
an·tho·xan·thins
an·thra·ce·mia
an·thra·cene
an·thra·cia
an·thrac·ic
an·thra·cin
an·thra·coid
an·thra·co·sil·i·co·sis
an·thra·co·sis
an·thra·cot·ic
tu·ber·cu·lo·sis
an·thra·lin
an·thra·mu·cin
an·thra·nil·ic ac·id
an·thra·nil·o·yl
an·thra·pur·pu·rin
an·thrax
ce·re·bral a.
cu·ta·ne·ous a.
in·tes·ti·nal a.
pul·mo·nary a.

an·thrax
   pneu·mo·nia
   sep·ti·ce·mia
   tox·in
an·throne
an·thro·po·bi·ol·o·gy
an·thro·po·cen·tric
an·thro·po·gen·e·sis
an·thro·po·ge·net·ic
an·thro·po·gen·ic
an·thro·pog·e·ny
an·thro·pog·o·ny
an·thro·pog·ra·phy
an·thro·poid
   pel·vis
An·thro·poi·dea
an·thro·pol·o·gy
   ap·plied a.
   crim·i·nal a.
   cul·tur·al a.
   phys·i·cal a.
an·thro·pom·e·ter
an·thro·po·met·ric
an·thro·pom·e·try
an·thro·po·mor·phism
an·thro·pon·o·my
an·thro·po·not·ic cu·ta·ne·ous
   leish·man·i·a·sis
an·thro·pop·a·thy
an·thro·po·phil·ic
an·thro·po·pho·bia
an·thro·pos·co·py
an·thro·po·so·ma·tol·o·gy
an·thro·po·zo·o·no·sis
an·ti·ac·id
an·ti·ad·ren·er·gic
an·ti·ag·glu·ti·nin
an·ti·a·lex·in
an·ti·al·ler·gic
an·ti·al·o·pe·cia
   fac·tor
an·ti·an·a·phy·lax·is
an·ti·an·dro·gen
an·ti·a·ne·mic
   prin·ci·ple
an·ti·an·ti·body
an·ti·an·ti·tox·in
an·ti·anx·i·e·ty
   agent
an·ti·a·rach·nol·y·sin
an·ti·ar·rhyth·mic
an·ti·ar·thrit·ic
an·ti·asth·mat·ic
an·ti·au·tol·y·sin
an·ti·bac·te·ri·al
an·ti·base·ment mem·brane
   an·ti·body

glo·mer·u·lo·ne·phri·tis
ne·phri·tis
an·ti·bech·ic
an·ti·ber·i·beri
   fac·tor
   vi·ta·min
an·ti·bi·o·gram
an·ti·bi·ont
an·ti·bi·o·sis
an·ti·bi·ot·ic
   broad spec·trum a.
an·ti·bi·ot·ic
   en·ter·o·co·li·tis
   sen·si·tiv·i·ty
an·ti·bi·ot·ic-re·sis·tant
an·ti·bi·ot·ic sen·si·tiv·i·ty
   test
an·ti·bi·o·tin
an·ti·black-tongue
   fac·tor
an·ti·blen·nor·rhag·ic
an·ti·body
   ag·glu·ti·nat·ing a.
   an·a·phy·lac·tic a.
   an·ti-base·ment mem·brane
     a.
   an·ti-id·i·o·type a.
   an·ti·nu·cle·ar a.
   bi·va·lent a.
   block·ing a.
   blood group a.'s
   cell-bound a.
   CF a.
   com·ple·ment-fix·ing a.
   com·plete a.
   cross-re·act·ing a.
   cy·to·phil·ic a.
   cy·to·tro·pic a.
   flu·o·res·cent a.
   Forssman a.
   het·er·o·cy·to·tro·pic a.
   het·er·o·ge·net·ic a.
   het·er·o·phil a.
   het·er·o·phile a.
   ho·mo·cy·to·tro·pic a.
   id·i·o·type a.
   im·mo·bi·liz·ing a.
   in·com·plete a.
   in·hib·it·ing a.
   lym·pho·cy·to·tox·ic a.'s
   mon·o·clo·nal a.
   nat·u·ral a.
   neu·tra·liz·ing a.
   non·pre·cip·i·ta·ble a.
   non·pre·cip·i·tat·ing a.
   nor·mal a.
   Prausnitz-Küstner a.
   pre·cip·i·tat·ing a.

an·ti·body *(continued)*
  re·a·gin·ic a.
  trep·o·ne·ma-im·mo·bi·liz·
   ing a.
  trep·o·ne·mal a.
  uni·va·lent a.
  Vi a.
  Wassermann a.
an·ti·body
  ex·cess
an·ti·body de·fi·cien·cy
  dis·ease
  syn·drome
an·ti·bra·chi·al
an·ti·bra·chi·um
an·ti·bro·mic
an·ti·cal·cu·lous
an·ti·car·i·ous
an·ti·ca·thex·is
an·ti·ceph·a·lal·gic
an·ti·chol·a·gogue
an·ti·cho·lin·er·gic
an·ti·cho·lin·es·ter·ase
an·tic·i·pate
an·tic·i·pa·tion
an·ti·cli·nal
an·tic·ne·mi·on
an·ti·co·ag·u·lant
  ther·a·py
an·ti·co·don
an·ti·com·ple·ment
an·ti·com·ple·men·ta·ry
  fac·tor
  se·rum
an·ti·con·ta·gious
an·ti·con·vul·sant
an·ti·con·vul·sive
an·ti·cus
an·ti·cy·to·tox·in
an·ti-D
  im·mu·no·glob·u·lin
an·ti·de·pres·sant
  tet·ra·cy·clic a.
  tri·a·zol·o·pyr·i·dine a.
  tri·cyc·lic a.
an·ti·di·a·bet·ic
an·ti·di·ar·rhe·al
an·ti·di·ar·rhet·ic
an·ti·di·u·re·sis
an·ti·di·u·ret·ic
  hor·mone
an·ti·dot·al
an·ti·dote
  chem·i·cal a.
  me·chan·i·cal a.
  phys·i·o·log·ic a.
an·ti·drom·ic
an·ti·dys·en·ter·ic

an·ti·dys·rhyth·mic
an·ti·dys·u·ric
an·ti·e·met·ic
an·ti·e·ner·gic
an·ti·en·zyme
an·ti·ep·i·lep·tic
an·ti·ep·i·the·li·al
  se·rum
an·ti·es·tro·gen
an·ti·fe·brile
an·ti·fi·bri·nol·y·sin
an·ti·fi·bri·no·lyt·ic
an·ti·foam·ing
  agents
an·ti·fo·lic
an·ti·fun·gal
an·ti·ga·lac·ta·gogue
an·ti·ga·lac·tic
an·ti·gen
  ABO a.'s
  ac·e·tone-in·sol·u·ble a.
  Au a.
  Aus a.
  Aus·tra·lia a.
  Be[a] a.'s
  Becker a.
  Bi a.
  Bile's a.
  blood group a.
  By a.
  cap·su·lar a.
  car·ci·no·em·bry·on·ic a.
  C car·bo·hy·drate a.
  CDE a.'s
  cho·les·ter·in·ized a.
  Chr[a] a.'s
  com·mon a.
  com·plete a.
  con·ju·gat·ed a.
  del·ta a.
  Dharmendra a.
  Di a.
  Duffy a.'s
  fla·gel·lar a.
  Forssman a.
  Fy a.'s.
  G a.
  Ge a.
  Good a.
  Gr a.
  group a.'s
  H a.
  He a.'s
  heart a.
  hep·a·ti·tis-as·so·ci·at·ed a.
  hep·a·ti·tis B core a.
  hep·a·ti·tis B e a.
  hep·a·ti·tis B sur·face a.

het·er·o·ge·net·ic a.
het·er·o·gen·ic en·ter·o·bac·
    te·ri·al a.
het·er·o·phil a.
hex·on a.
HL-A a.'s
Ho a.
Hu a.'s
hu·man leu·ke·mia-as·so·ci·
    at·ed a.'s
hu·man lym·pho·cyte a.'s
H-Y a.
I a.'s
i a.'s
in·com·plete a.
in·ter·nal a.
Jk a.'s
Jobbins a.
Js a.
K a.'s
k a.'s
Kveim a.
Kveim-Stilz·bach a.
Lan a.
Le a.'s
Levay a.
Lu a.'s
lym·pho·gran·u·lo·ma ve·
    ne·re·um a.
M a.
Mitsuda a.
MNSs a.'s
Mu a.
mumps skin test a.
O a.
on·co·fe·tal a.'s
or·gan-spe·cif·ic a.
Ot a.
P a.'s
par·tial a.
pen·ton a.
pol·len a.
pri·vate a.'s
pub·lic a.'s
R a.
Rh a.'s
Rhus tox·i·co·den·dron a.
Rhus ve·ne·na·ta a.
S a.
sen·si·tized a.
shock a.
Sm a.
sol·u·ble a.
so·mat·ic a.
spe·cies-spe·cif·ic a.
spe·cif·ic a.'s
Sto·bo a.
Strep·to·coc·cus M a.

Sw^a a.
Swann a.'s
T a.'s
tis·sue-spe·cif·ic a.
Tj a.
Tr^a a.
tu·mor a.'s
tu·mor-spe·cif·ic trans·plan·
    ta·tion a.'s
V a.
Vel a.
Ven a.
Vi a.
Vw a.
Webb a.
Wr^a a.
Wright a.'s
Xg a.
Yt^a a.
an·ti·gen
    ex·cess
    in·ter·fer·on
    unit
an·ti·gen-an·ti·body
    re·ac·tion
an·ti·ge·ne·mia
an·ti·gen·ic
    com·pe·ti·tion
    com·plex
    de·ter·mi·nant
    drift
    shift
an·ti·ge·nic·i·ty
an·ti·gen-pre·sent·ing
    cell
an·ti·gen-re·spon·sive
    cell
an·ti·gen-sen·si·tive
    cell
an·ti·glob·u·lin
    test
an·ti·gon·or·rhe·ic
an·ti·grav·i·ty
    mus·cles
an·ti-HB$_s$
an·ti-HB$_c$
an·ti-HB e
an·ti·he·lix
an·ti·hem·ag·glu·ti·nin
an·ti·he·mo·ly·sin
an·ti·he·mo·lyt·ic
an·ti·he·mo·phil·ic
    fac·tor A
    fac·tor B
    glob·u·lin
    glob·u·lin A
    glob·u·lin B

an·ti·he·mo·phil·ic *(continued)*
 plas·ma
 plas·ma hu·man
an·ti·hem·or·rhag·ic
 fac·tor
 vi·ta·min
an·ti·hi·drot·ic
an·ti·his·ta·mines
an·ti·his·ta·min·ic
an·ti·hor·mones
an·ti·hu·man
 glob·u·lin
an·ti·hu·man glob·u·lin
 test
an·ti·hy·dri·ot·ic
an·ti·hy·drop·ic
an·ti·hy·per·ten·sive
an·ti·hyp·not·ic
an·ti-ic·ter·ic
an·ti-id·i·o·type
 an·ti·body
 au·to·an·ti·body
an·ti-in·flam·ma·to·ry
an·ti·ke·to·gen·e·sis
an·ti·ke·to·gen·ic
an·ti-kid·ney se·rum
 ne·phri·tis
an·ti·leu·koc·i·din
an·ti·leu·ko·tox·in
an·ti·lew·is·ite
an·ti·lip·o·tro·pic
an·ti·lith·ic
an·ti·lo·bi·um
an·ti·lu·te·o·gen·ic
an·ti·lym·pho·cyte
 se·rum
an·ti·ly·sin
an·ti·ma·lar·i·al
an·ti·mer
an·ti·mere
an·ti·mes·en·ter·ic
an·ti·me·tab·o·lite
an·ti·me·tro·pia
an·ti·mi·cro·bi·al
 spec·trum
an·ti·mi·tot·ic
an·ti·mon·gol·oid
an·ti·mo·nid
an·ti·mo·ni·um
an·ti·mo·nous ox·ide
an·ti-Mon·son
 curve
an·ti·mo·ny
 a. chlo·ride
 a. di·mer·cap·to·suc·ci·nate
 a. ox·ide
 a. po·tas·si·um tar·trate
 a. so·di·um glu·co·nate

 a. so·di·um tar·trate
 a. so·di·um thi·o·gly·col·
 late
 tar·trat·ed a.
 a. thi·o·gly·col·lam·ide
 a. tri·chlo·ride
 a. tri·ox·ide
an·ti·mo·nyl
an·ti·mus·ca·rin·ic
an·ti·mu·ta·gen
an·ti·mu·ta·gen·ic
an·ti·my·as·then·ic
an·ti·my·cot·ic
an·ti·na·trif·er·ic
an·ti·nau·se·ant
an·ti·ne·o·plas·tic
an·ti·ne·phrit·ic
an·ti·neu·ral·gic
an·ti·neu·rit·ic
 fac·tor
 vi·ta·min
an·ti·neu·ro·tox·in
an·tin·i·ad
an·tin·i·al
an·tin·i·on
an·tin·o·my
an·ti·nu·cle·ar
 an·ti·body
 fac·tor
an·ti·o·don·tal·gic
an·ti·on·co·gene
an·ti·ox·i·dant
an·ti·par·al·lel
an·ti·par·a·sit·ic
an·ti·pa·ras·ta·ta
an·ti·pe·dic·u·lar
an·ti·pe·dic·u·lot·ic
an·ti·pel·la·gra
 fac·tor
an·ti·pe·ri·od·ic
an·ti·per·i·stal·sis
an·ti·per·i·stal·tic
 anas·to·mo·sis
an·ti·per·ni·cious ane·mia
 fac·tor
an·ti·per·spi·rant
an·ti·phag·o·cyt·ic
an·ti·phlo·gis·tic
an·ti·pho·bic
an·ti·plas·min
an·ti·plate·let
an·ti·pneu·mo·coc·cic
an·tip·o·dal
 cone
an·ti·pode
 op·ti·cal a.
an·ti·port
an·ti·por·ter

an·ti·po·sic
an·ti-Pr cold
   au·to·ag·glu·ti·nin
an·ti·pre·cip·i·tin
an·ti·pro·ges·tin
an·ti·pros·tate
an·ti·pro·throm·bin
an·ti·pru·rit·ic
an·ti·pso·ric
an·ti·psy·chot·ic
   agent
an·ti·py·o·gen·ic
an·ti·py·re·sis
an·ti·py·ret·ic
an·ti·py·rine
   a. ace·tyl·sa·lic·y·late
   a. sal·i·cyl·ac·e·tate
   a. sa·lic·y·late
an·ti·py·rot·ic
an·ti·ra·bies
   se·rum
an·ti·ra·chit·ic
   vi·ta·mins
an·ti·re·flec·tion
   coat·ing
an·ti·re·tic·u·lar cy·to·tox·ic
   se·rum
an·ti·rheu·mat·ic
an·ti·ri·cin
an·ti·ru·mi·nant
an·ti-S
an·ti·scor·bu·tic
   vi·ta·min
an·ti·seb·or·rhe·ic
an·ti·se·cre·to·ry
an·ti·sense
   DNA
an·ti·sep·sis
an·ti·sep·tic
   dress·ing
an·ti·se·rum
   an·a·phy·lax·is
an·ti·se·rum
   blood group a.s
   het·er·ol·o·gous a.
   ho·mol·o·gous a.
   mon·o·va·lent a.
   nerve growth fac·tor a.
   NGF a.
   pol·y·va·lent a.
   spe·cif·ic a.
an·ti·si·al·a·gogue
an·ti·si·al·ic
an·ti·si·der·ic
an·ti·so·cial
   per·son·al·i·ty
an·ti·so·cial per·son·al·i·ty
   dis·or·der

an·ti·spas·mod·ic
an·ti·staph·y·lo·coc·cic
an·ti·staph·y·lol·y·sin
an·ti·ste·ap·sin
an·ti·ste·ril·i·ty
   fac·tor
   vi·ta·min
an·ti·strep·to·coc·cic
an·ti·strep·to·ki·nase
an·ti·strep·tol·y·sin
an·ti·sub·stance
an·ti·su·do·rif·ic
an·ti·te·tan·ic
an·ti·the·nar
an·ti·ther·mic
an·ti·throm·bin
   nor·mal a.
an·ti·thy·roid
an·ti·ton·ic
an·ti·tox·ic
   se·rum
an·ti·tox·i·gen
an·ti·tox·in
   bi·va·lent gas gan·grene a.
   bo·throp·ic a.
   Bo·throps a.
   bot·u·li·num a.
   bot·u·lism a.
   bo·vine a.
   Cro·ta·lus a.
   de·spe·ci·at·ed a.
   diph·the·ria a.
   dys·en·tery a.
   gas gan·grene a.
   nor·mal a.
   pen·ta·va·lent gas gan·grene
     a.
   plant a.
   scar·let fe·ver a.
   staph·y·lo·coc·cus a.
   tet·a·nus a.
   tet·a·nus and gas gan·grene
     a.'s
   tet·a·nus-per·frin·gens a.
an·ti·tox·in
   rash
   unit
an·ti·tox·in·o·gen
an·ti·trag·i·cus
an·ti·tra·go·hel·i·cine
   fis·sure
an·ti·tra·gus
an·ti·trep·o·ne·mal
an·ti·tris·mus
an·ti·trope
an·ti·tro·pic
an·ti·tryp·sic

an·ti·tryp·sin
  de·fi·cien·cy
an·ti·tryp·tic
  in·dex
an·ti·tu·mor·i·gen·e·sis
an·ti·tus·sive
an·ti·ty·phoid
an·ti·ve·nene
  unit
an·ti·ve·ne·re·al
an·ti·ven·in
an·ti·vi·ral
  im·mu·ni·ty
  pro·tein
an·ti·vi·ta·min
an·ti·viv·i·sec·tion
an·ti·xe·roph·thal·mic
an·ti·xe·rot·ic
Antoni type A
  neu·ri·le·mo·ma
Antoni type B
  neu·ri·le·mo·ma
Anton's
  syn·drome
an·tra
an·tral
  pouch
  sphinc·ter
an·trec·to·my
an·tri
an·tro·du·o·de·nec·to·my
an·tro·na·sal
an·tro·phose
an·tro·py·lo·ric
an·tro·scope
an·tros·co·py
an·tros·to·my
  in·tra·o·ral a.
an·trot·o·my
an·tro·to·nia
an·tro·tym·pan·ic
an·trum
  a. au·ris
  a. car·di·a·cum
  an·tra eth·moi·da·le
  fol·lic·u·lar a.
  a. of Highmore
  mas·toid a.
  max·il·lary a.
  py·lor·ic a.
  tym·pan·ic a.
  Valsalva's a.
Antyllus'
  meth·od
an·u·li
an·u·lus
an·u·re·sis
an·u·ret·ic

an·u·ria
an·u·ric
anus
  ar·ti·fi·cial a.
  Bartholin's a.
  a. ce·re·bri
  im·per·fo·rate a.
  a. ve·si·ca·lis
  ves·tib·u·lar a.
  vul·vo·vag·i·nal a.
an·vil
  sound
an·vil
anx·i·e·ty
  cas·tra·tion a.
  free-float·ing a.
  no·et·ic a.
  sep·a·ra·tion a.
  sit·u·a·tion a.
anx·i·e·ty
  dream
  hys·te·ria
  neu·ro·sis
  re·ac·tion
  state
  syn·drome
anx·i·o·lyt·ic
anx·ious
  de·lir·i·um
aor·ta
  a. ab·do·mi·na·lis
  a. an·gus·ta
  a. as·cen·dens
  buck·led a.
  a. de·scen·dens
  dy·nam·ic a.
  kinked a.
  over·rid·ing a.
  prim·i·tive a.
  a. tho·ra·ci·ca
  ven·tral aor·tas
aor·tae
aor·tal
aor·tal·gia
aor·tarc·tia
aor·tar·tia
aor·tec·ta·sia
aor·tec·ta·sis
aor·tec·to·my
aor·tic
  arch
  arch·es
  ar·ea
  atre·sia
  body
  bulb
  dwarf·ism
  fa·ci·es

fo·ra·men
in·com·pe·tence
in·suf·fi·cien·cy
mur·mur
nerve
notch
open·ing
os·ti·um
plex·us
re·flex
re·gur·gi·ta·tion
sac
si·nus
spin·dle
ste·no·sis
sul·cus
valve
ves·ti·bule
win·dow
aor·tic arch
   syn·drome
aor·tic body
   tu·mor
aor·ti·co·pul·mo·nary sep·tal
   de·fect
aor·ti·co·re·nal
   gan·glia
aor·tic sep·tal
   de·fect
aor·tis·mus ab·do·mi·na·lis
aor·ti·tis
   gi·ant cell a.
   syph·i·lit·ic a.
aor·to·cor·o·nary
   by·pass
aor·to·gram
aor·tog·ra·phy
   ret·ro·grade a.
   trans·lum·bar a.
aor·to·il·i·ac
   by·pass
aor·to·il·i·ac oc·clu·sive
   dis·ease
aor·top·a·thy
aor·to·plas·ty
aor·top·to·sia
aor·top·to·sis
aor·to·pul·mo·nary
   sep·tum
aor·to·re·nal
   by·pass
aor·tor·rha·phy
aor·to·scle·ro·sis
aor·to·ste·no·sis
aor·tot·o·my
apall·es·the·sia

apal·lic
   state
   syn·drome
apan·cre·at·ic
apar·a·lyt·ic
apar·a·thy·roid·ism
apa·reu·nia
ap·a·thet·ic
   thy·ro·tox·i·co·sis
ap·a·thism
ap·a·thy
ap·a·tite
   cal·cu·lus
ap·a·zone
A-P-C
   vi·rus
ape
   fis·sure
   hand
ap·ei·do·sis
apel·lous
ap·en·ter·ic
apep·sin·ia
ape·ri·od·ic
aper·i·os·te·al
   am·pu·ta·tion
aper·i·stal·sis
aper·i·tive
Apert-Crouzon
   syn·drome
aper·to·gnath·ia
ap·er·tom·e·ter
Apert's
   hir·sut·ism
   syn·drome
ap·er·tu·ra
   a. pel·vis mi·no·ris
ap·er·tu·rae
ap·er·ture
   an·gu·lar a.
   fron·tal si·nus a.
   in·fe·ri·or tho·rac·ic a.
   lat·er·al a. of the fourth
     ven·tri·cle
   me·di·an a. of the fourth
     ven·tri·cle
   nu·mer·i·cal a.
   sphe·noi·dal si·nus a.
   su·pe·ri·or tho·rac·ic a.
apex
   a. of ar·y·te·noid car·ti·lage
   a. of dens
   a. of head of fib·u·la
   a. of heart
   a. of lung
   or·bi·tal a.
   a. of pa·tel·la

apex *(continued)*
  a. of pet·rous part of tem·po·ral bone
  a. of pros·tate
  root a.
  a. of sa·crum
  a. sat·y·ri
  a. of uri·nary blad·der
apex
  beat
  pneu·mo·nia
apex·car·di·o·gram
apex·i·fi·ca·tion
apex·i·graph
Apgar
  score
apha·gia
  a. al·ge·ra
apha·kia
apha·ki·al
apha·kic
  eye
  glau·co·ma
apha·lan·gia
aphan·i·sis
apha·sia
  acous·tic a.
  ac·quired ep·i·lep·tic a.
  am·ne·sic a.
  am·nes·tic a.
  anom·ic a.
  as·so·ci·a·tive a.
  atax·ic a.
  au·di·to·ry a.
  Broca's a.
  con·duc·tion a.
  ex·pres·sive a.
  func·tion·al a.
  glob·al a.
  graph·ic a.
  graph·o·mo·tor a.
  im·pres·sive a.
  jar·gon a.
  Kussmaul's a.
  mixed a.
  mo·tor a.
  nom·i·nal a.
  pa·the·mat·ic a.
  psy·cho·sen·so·ry a.
  pure a.'s
  re·cep·tive a.
  se·man·tic a.
  sen·so·ry a.
  syn·tac·ti·cal a.
  to·tal a.
  trans·cor·ti·cal a.
  vi·su·al a.
  Wernicke's a.

apha·si·ac
apha·sic
apha·si·ol·o·gist
apha·si·ol·o·gy
aphas·mid
Aphas·mid·ia
aph·e·li·ot·ro·pism
aphe·mes·the·sia
aphe·mia
aphe·mic
aphe·pho·bia
apher·e·sis
aphil·op·o·ny
apho·nia
  hys·ter·i·cal a.
  a. pa·ra·ly·ti·ca
  spas·tic a.
aphon·ic
  pec·to·ril·o·quy
apho·no·ge·lia
aph·o·nous
apho·tes·the·sia
aphra·sia
aph·ro·di·sia
aph·ro·di·si·ac
aph·ro·di·si·o·ma·nia
aph·tha
  Bednar's aph·thae
  con·ta·gious aph·thae
  her·pet·i·form aph·thae
  aph·thae ma·jor
  Mikulicz' aph·thae
  aph·thae mi·nor
  re·cur·rent scar·ring aph·thae
aph·thae
aph·tho·bul·lous
  sto·ma·ti·tis
aph·thoid
aph·thon·gia
aph·tho·sis
aph·thous
  fe·ver
  sto·ma·ti·tis
aphy·lac·tic
aphy·lax·is
ap·i·cal
  ab·scess
  an·gle
  ar·ea
  com·plex
  den·drite
  gland
  gran·u·lo·ma
  in·fec·tion
  lig·a·ment of dens
  per·i·o·don·ti·tis
  pneu·mo·nia

pro·cess
seg·ment
space
ap·i·cal den·tal
fo·ra·men
ap·i·cal ec·to·der·mal
ridge
ap·i·ca·lis
ap·i·cal lymph
nodes
ap·i·cal per·i·o·don·tal
ab·scess
cyst
ap·i·cec·to·my
apic·e·ot·o·my
ap·i·ces
ap·i·cis
ap·i·ci·tis
ap·i·co·ec·to·my
ap·i·co·lo·ca·tor
ap·i·col·y·sis
Api·com·plexa
ap·i·co·pos·te·ri·or
seg·ment
ap·i·co·stome
ap·i·cos·to·my
ap·i·cot·o·my
apic·u·late
apic·u·lus
ap·i·cu·ret·tage
apin·e·al·ism
api·pho·bia
api·tu·i·tar·ism
apla·cen·tal
ap·la·nat·ic
lens
aplan·a·tism
apla·sia
con·gen·i·tal a. of thy·mus
a. cu·tis con·gen·i·ta
ger·mi·nal a.
go·nad·al a.
a. pi·lo·rum pro·pia
pure red cell a.
aplas·tic
ane·mia
lymph
apleu·ria
ap·nea
cen·tral a.
de·glu·ti·tion a.
in·duced a.
ob·struc·tive a.
pe·riph·e·ral a.
sleep a.
sleep-in·duced a.
true a.

va·gal a.
a. ve·ra
ap·ne·ic
ox·y·gen·a·tion
pause
apneu·ma·to·sis
ap·neu·mia
ap·neu·sis
ap·neus·tic
breath·ing
ap·o·bi·o·sis
ap·o·car·ter·e·sis
ap·o·chro·mat·ic
lens
ob·jec·tive
ap·o·clei·sis
ap·o·crine
ad·e·no·ma
car·ci·no·ma
chrom·hi·dro·sis
gland
met·a·pla·sia
mil·i·a·ria
ap·o·crus·tic
ap·o·dal
ap·o·de·mi·al·gia
apo·dia
ap·o·dous
ap·o·dy
ap·o·en·zyme
ap·o·fer·ri·tin
ap·o·gam·ia
apog·a·my
apo·lar
cell
ap·o·lip·o·pro·tein
ap·o·mix·ia
ap·o·mor·phine hy·dro·chlo·ride
ap·o·neu·rec·to·my
ap·o·neu·rol·o·gy
ap·o·neu·ror·rha·phy
ap·o·neu·ro·ses
ap·o·neu·ro·sis
bi·cip·i·tal a.
a. bi·ci·pi·ta·lis
Denonvilliers' a.
ep·i·cra·ni·al a.
ex·ten·sor a.
a. of in·ser·tion
a. of in·vest·ment
lin·gual a.
a. of or·i·gin
pal·a·tine a.
pal·mar a.
Petit's a.
a. pha·ryn·gea
plan·tar a.
Sibson's a.

ap·o·neu·ro·sis *(continued)*
  tem·po·ral a.
  tho·ra·co·lum·bar a.
ap·o·neu·ro·si·tis
ap·o·neu·rot·ic
  fi·bro·ma
  re·flex
ap·o·neu·ro·tome
ap·o·neu·rot·o·my
ap·o·pa·thet·ic
ap·o·phy·lax·is
apoph·y·sary
  point
apoph·y·se·al
apoph·y·ses
ap·o·phys·i·al
  frac·ture
  point
apoph·y·sis
  bas·i·lar a.
  a. con·chae
  a. he·li·cis
  Ingrassia's a.
  len·tic·u·lar a.
  tem·po·ral a.
apoph·y·si·tis
  a. tib·i·a·lis ado·les·cen·ti·
  um
ap·o·plas·mia
ap·o·plec·tic
  cyst
  ret·i·ni·tis
ap·o·plec·ti·form
ap·o·plec·toid
ap·o·plexy
  ab·dom·i·nal a.
  ad·re·nal a.
  bul·bar a.
  cu·ta·ne·ous a.
  em·bol·ic a.
  func·tion·al a.
  heat a.
  in·gra·ves·cent a.
  ne·o·na·tal a.
  pi·tu·i·tary a.
  pon·tile a.
  Raymond type of a.
  se·rous a.
  spas·mod·ic a.
  spi·nal a.
  splen·ic a.
  throm·bot·ic a.
  uter·o·pla·cen·tal a.
ap·o·pro·tein
ap·o·pto·sis
ap·o·re·pres·sor
apo·ria
apo·ri·o·neu·ro·sis

ap·o·some
ap·o·stax·is
apos·thia
ap·o·stilb
ap·o·tha·na·sia
apoth·e·cary
ap·o·them
ap·o·theme
ap·ox·e·sis
ap·o·zem
apoz·e·ma
ap·pa·ra·tus
  Abbé-Zeiss a.
  ach·ro·mat·ic a.
  al·i·men·ta·ry a.
  at·tach·ment a.
  Barcroft-Warburg a.
  Beckmann's a.
  Benedict-Roth a.
  bran·chi·al a.
  cen·tral a.
  chro·mat·ic a.
  chro·mid·i·al a.
  den·tal a.
  di·ges·tive a.
  gen·i·to·u·ri·nary a.
  Golgi a.
  Haldane's a.
  Heyns' ab·dom·i·nal de·
  com·pres·sion a.
  hy·oid a.
  a. hy·oi·de·us
  jux·ta·glo·mer·u·lar a.
  Kirschner's a.
  Kjeldahl a.
  lac·ri·mal a.
  a. lig·a·men·to·sus col·li
  a. lig·a·men·to·sus weit·
  brechti
  mas·ti·ca·to·ry a.
  men·tal a.
  pyr·i·form a.
  res·pi·ra·to·ry a.
  Roughton-Scholander a.
  Sayre's sus·pen·sion a.
  Scholander a.
  sub·neu·ral a.
  a. sus·pen·so·ri·us len·tis
  Taylor's a.
  Tiselius a.
  uri·nary a.
  uro·gen·i·tal a.
  Van Slyke a.
  Warburg's a.
ap·par·ent
  vis·cos·i·ty
ap·par·ent or·i·gin

ap·pend·age
au·ric·u·lar a.
drum·stick a.
ep·i·plo·ic a.
a.'s of eye
a.'s of the fe·tus
left au·ric·u·lar a.
right au·ric·u·lar a.
a.'s of skin
uter·ine a.'s
ver·mi·form a.
ve·sic·u·lar a.
ap·pen·dal·gia
ap·pen·dec·to·my
au·ric·u·lar a.
ap·pen·di·cal
ap·pen·dic·e·al
ab·scess
ap·pen·di·cec·ta·sis
ap·pen·di·cec·to·my
ap·pen·di·ces
ap·pen·di·cis
ap·pen·di·cism
ap·pen·di·ci·tis
ac·ti·no·my·cot·ic a.
acute a.
bil·har·zi·al a.
chron·ic a.
fo·cal a.
gan·gre·nous a.
lum·bar a.
ob·struc·tive a.
ster·co·ral a.
sub·per·i·to·ne·al a.
sup·pu·ra·tive a.
ver·min·ous a.
ap·pen·di·clau·sis
ap·pen·di·co·cele
ap·pen·di·co·en·ter·os·to·my
ap·pen·di·co·li·thi·a·sis
ap·pen·di·col·y·sis
ap·pen·di·cos·to·my
ap·pen·dic·u·lar
ar·tery
col·ic
mus·cle
skel·e·ton
vein
ap·pen·dic·u·lar lymph
nodes
ap·pen·dix
au·ric·u·lar a.
a. ce·ci
a. of ep·i·did·y·mi·dis
fi·brous a. of liv·er
Morgagni's a.
a. ven·tric·u·li la·ryn·gis
ver·mi·form a.

ap·per·cep·tion
ap·per·cep·tive
mass
ap·per·son·a·tion
ap·per·son·i·fi·ca·tion
ap·pe·stat
ap·pe·tite
juice
ap·pe·ti·tion
ap·pet·i·tive
be·hav·ior
ap·pla·na·tion
to·nom·e·ter
ap·pla·nom·e·try
ap·ple jel·ly
nod·ules
ap·ple oil
ap·pli·ance
cra·ni·o·fa·cial a.
edge·wise a.
ex·tra·o·ral frac·ture a.
Hawley a.
in·tra·o·ral frac·ture a.
la·bi·o·lin·gual a.
light wire a.
ob·tu·ra·tor a.
or·tho·don·tic a.
rib·bon arch a.
Roger-Anderson pin fix·a·
tion a.
sur·gi·cal a.
uni·ver·sal a.
ap·pli·ca·tor
ap·plied
anat·o·my
an·thro·pol·o·gy
chem·is·try
ap·pli·qué
forms
ap·po·si·tion
su·ture
ap·po·si·tion·al
growth
ap·proach
id·i·o·graph·ic a.
nom·o·thet·ic a.
re·gres·sive-re·con·struc·tive
a.
ap·proach-ap·proach
con·flict
ap·proach-avoid·ance
con·flict
ap·prox·i·mate
ap·prox·i·ma·tion
su·ture
aprac·tag·no·sia
aprac·tic
aprag·ma·tism

aprax·ia
a. al·ge·ra
cor·ti·cal a.
ide·a·tion·al a.
ide·a·tory a.
ide·o·ki·net·ic a.
ide·o·mo·tor a.
in·ner·va·tion a.
limb-ki·net·ic a.
mo·tor a.
oc·u·lar mo·tor a.
trans·cor·ti·cal a.
aprax·ic
ap·ri·cot ker·nel oil
ap·ro·bar·bi·tal
aproc·tia
ap·ro·fen
ap·ro·fene
ap·ro·phen
ap·ro·pho·ria
apros·ex·ia
apros·o·dy
ap·ro·so·pia
apro·ti·nin
ap·si·thy·ria
ap·ti·tude
test
apty·a·lia
apty·a·lism
APUD
cells
apu·rin·ic ac·id
apyk·no·mor·phous
ap·y·rase
apy·ret·ic
tet·a·nus
ty·phoid
apy·rex·ia
apy·rex·i·al
apy·rim·i·din·ic ac·id
aq·ua
a. re·ga·lis
a. re·gia
aq·ua·co·bal·a·min
aq·uae
aq·ua·gen·ic
pru·ri·tus
aq·ua·pho·bia
aq·ua·punc·ture
Aq·ua·spi·ril·lum
aquat·ic
aq·ue·duct
a. of cer·e·brum
co·chle·ar a.
Cotunnius' a.
fal·lo·pi·an a.
syl·vi·an a.
a. of ves·ti·bule

aq·ue·duct
veil
aq·ue·duct·al
in·tu·ba·tion
aq·ue·duc·tus
a. co·chle·ae
a. co·tun·nii
a. fal·lo·pii
a. syl·vii
aque·ous
cham·bers
flare
hu·mor
phase
vac·cine
vein
aque·ous in·flux
phe·nom·e·non
aquip·ar·ous
aq·uo-ion
aq·uo·co·bal·a·min
aquos·i·ty
ar·a·ban
ar·a·bic
ar·a·bic ac·id
ar·a·bin
ar·a·bi·no·a·den·o·sine
ar·a·bi·no·cy·ti·dine
ar·a·bi·no·fu·ra·no·syl·cy·to·
sine
arab·i·nose
arab·i·no·sis
ar·a·bi·no·su·ria
ar·a·bi·no·syl·ad·e·nine
ar·a·bi·no·syl·cy·to·sine
arab·i·tol
arach·ic ac·id
ar·a·chid·ic ac·id
ar·a·chi·don·ic ac·id
ar·a·chi·don·ic ac·id cas·cade
ar·a·chis oil
arach·ne·pho·bia
Arach·nia
A. pro·pi·o·ni·ca
Arach·ni·da
arach·nid·ism
arach·no·dac·ty·ly
arach·noid
cyst
fo·ra·men
mem·brane
vil·li
ar·ach·noi·dal
gran·u·la·tions
ar·ach·noi·dea
ar·ach·noi·dea en·ceph·a·li
ar·ach·noi·dea spi·na·lis
ar·ach·noi·des

arach·noid·i·tis
  ad·he·sive a.
  ne·o·plas·tic a.
  oblit·er·a·tive a.
arach·no·ly·sin
arach·no·pho·bia
ar·al·kyl
Aran-Duchenne
  dis·ease
ara·ne·ism
Arantius'
  lig·a·ment
  nod·ule
  ven·tri·cle
ara·phia
ar·bor
  a. vi·tae uteri
ar·bo·res
ar·bo·res·cent
  cat·a·ract
ar·bo·ri·za·tion
  block
ar·bo·rize
ar·bo·roid
ar·bor·vi·rus
ar·bo·vi·rus
arc
  au·ric·u·lar a.
  bin·au·ric·u·lar a.
  breg·ma·to·lamb·doid a.
  cra·ter a.
  flame a.
  lon·gi·tu·di·nal a. of skull
  mer·cu·ry a.
  na·so·breg·mat·ic a.
  na·so-oc·cip·i·tal a.
  pul·mo·nary a.
  re·flex a.
arc
  pe·rim·e·ter
ar·cade
  anom·a·lous mi·tral a.
  Flint's a.
  Riolan's a.
ar·cate
arc-flash
  con·junc·ti·vi·tis
arch
  bar
  form
  length
arch
  ab·dom·i·no·tho·rac·ic a.
  al·ve·o·lar a. of man·di·ble
  al·ve·o·lar a. of max·il·la
  an·te·ri·or a. of at·las
  an·te·ri·or pal·a·tine a.
  a. of the aor·ta

aor·tic a.
ar·te·ri·al a.'s of co·lon
ar·te·ri·al a.'s of il·e·um
ar·te·ri·al a.'s of je·ju·num
ar·te·ri·al a. of low·er eye·lid
ar·te·ri·al a. of up·per eye·lid
ax·il·lary a.
bran·chi·al a.'s
car·pal a.'s
cor·ti·cal a.'s of kid·ney
Corti's a.
cos·tal a.
a. of cri·coid car·ti·lage
cru·ral a.
deep pal·mar a.
deep pal·mar ve·nous a.
den·tal a.
dor·sal ve·nous a. of foot
ex·pan·sion a.
fall·en a.'s
fal·lo·pi·an a.
fem·o·ral a.
a.'s of the foot
glos·so·pal·a·tine a.
Goth·ic a.
Haller's a.'s
he·mal a.'s
hy·oid a.
il·i·o·pec·tin·e·al a.
in·fe·ri·or den·tal a.
jug·u·lar ve·nous a.
la·bi·al a.
Langer's a.
lat·er·al lon·gi·tu·di·nal a.
lat·er·al lum·bo·cos·tal a.
lin·gual a.
lon·gi·tu·di·nal a. of foot
ma·lar a.
man·dib·u·lar a.
me·di·al lon·gi·tu·di·nal a.
me·di·al lum·bo·cos·tal a.
na·sal ve·nous a.
neu·ral a.
a. of the pal·ate
pal·a·to·glos·sal a.
pal·a·to·pha·ryn·ge·al a.
pha·ryn·ge·al a.'s
pha·ryn·go·pal·a·tine a.
plan·tar a.
plan·tar ve·nous a.
pos·te·ri·or a. of at·las
pos·te·ri·or pal·a·tine a.
post·o·ral a.'s
prim·i·tive cos·tal a.'s
pu·bic a.
rib·bon a.

arch *(continued)*
su·per·cil·i·ary a.
su·per·fi·cial pal·mar a.
su·per·fi·cial pal·mar ve·
nous a.
su·pe·ri·or den·tal a.
su·pra·or·bit·al a.
tar·sal a.
ten·di·nous a.
ten·di·nous a. of le·va·tor
ani mus·cle
ten·di·nous a. of pel·vic
fas·cia
ten·di·nous a. of so·le·us
mus·cle
a. of tho·rac·ic duct
trans·verse a. of foot
Treitz' a.
ver·te·bral a.
vis·cer·al a.'s
W-a.
wire a.
zy·go·mat·ic a.
ar·cha·ic
ar·cha·ic-par·a·log·i·cal
think·ing
arched
crest
arch·en·ter·ic
ca·nal
arch·en·ter·on
ar·che·o·cyte
ar·che·o·ki·net·ic
ar·che·type
ar·chi·cer·e·bel·lum
ar·chi·cor·tex
ar·chil
ar·chin
ar·chi·pal·li·um
ar·chi·tec·ton·ics
arch length
de·fi·cien·cy
arch-loop-whorl
sys·tem
arch·wire
ar·ci·form
ar·ter·ies.
veins of kid·ney
ar·con
ar·tic·u·la·tor
arc·ta·tion
ar·cu·al
ar·cu·ate
ar·ter·ies of kid·ney
ar·tery
crest
em·i·nence
fas·cic·u·lus

fi·bers
line
nu·clei
nu·cle·us
sco·to·ma
uter·us
veins of kid·ney
zone
ar·cu·ate pop·lit·e·al
lig·a·ment
ar·cu·ate pu·bic
lig·a·ment
ar·cu·a·tion
ar·cus
a. adi·po·sus
a. cor·ne·a·lis
a. cos·ta·rum
a. glos·so·pal·a·ti·nus
a. ju·ve·ni·lis
a. li·poi·des
a. lum·bo·cos·ta·lis la·te·
ra·lis
a. lum·bo·cos·ta·lis me·di·
a·lis
a. pa·la·ti·ni
a. ra·ni·nus
a. se·ni·lis
a. tar·se·us
a. un·gui·um
a. vo·la·ris pro·fun·dus
a. vo·la·ris su·per·fi·ci·a·lis
ard·an·es·the·sia
ar·dent
fe·ver
spir·its
ar·dor
ar·ea
acous·tic a.
a. acus·ti·ca
an·te·ri·or in·ter·con·dy·lar
a.
aor·tic a.
ap·i·cal a.
as·so·ci·a·tion ar·e·as
au·di·to·ry a.
bare a. of liv·er
bare a. of stom·ach
ba·sal seat a.
Broca's a.
Broca's par·ol·fac·to·ry a.
Brodmann's ar·e·as
a. of car·di·ac dull·ness
Celsus' a.
a. cen·tra·lis
co·chle·ar a.
Cohnheim's a.
con·tact a.
crib·ri·form a.

den·ture-bear·ing a.
den·ture foun·da·tion a.
den·ture-sup·port·ing a.
der·ma·tom·ic a.
em·bry·o·nal a.
em·bry·on·ic a.
en·to·rhi·nal a.
ex·cit·a·ble a.
a. of fa·cial nerve
Flechsig's ar·e·as
fron·tal a.
fron·to-or·bit·al a.
fu·sion a.
ger·mi·nal a.
a. ger·mi·na·ti·va
Head's ar·e·as
im·pres·sion a.
in·fe·ri·or ves·tib·u·lar a.
in·su·lar a.
Jonston's a.
Kiesselbach's a.
Little's a.
mac·u·lar a.
Martegiani's a.
mi·tral a.
mo·tor a.
obe·li·ar a.
ol·fac·to·ry a.
a. opa·ca
oval a. of Flechsig
Panum's a.
par·a·stri·ate a.
par·ol·fac·to·ry a.
pear-shaped a.
a. pel·lu·ci·da
per·i·stri·ate a.
pir·i·form a.
Pitres' a.
post·cen·tral a.
post dam a.
pos·te·ri·or in·ter·con·dy·lar
    a.
pos·te·ri·or pal·a·tal seal a.
post·pal·a·tal seal a.
a. po·stre·ma
pre·cen·tral a.
pre·com·mis·sur·al sep·tal
    a.
pre·fron·tal a.
pre·mo·tor a.
pre·op·tic a.
pre·stri·ate a.
pre·tec·tal a.
pri·mary vi·su·al a.
pul·mo·nary a.
re·lief a.
rest a.
re·ten·tion a.

Rolando's a.
sec·on·dary vi·su·al a.
sen·so·ri·al ar·e·as
sen·so·ri·mo·tor a.
sen·so·ry ar·e·as
sep·tal a.
si·lent a.
skip ar·e·as
som·es·thet·ic a.
stress-bear·ing a.
stri·ate a.
Stroud's pec·ti·nat·ed a.
sub·cal·lo·sal a.
su·pe·ri·or ves·tib·u·lar a.
sup·port·ing a.
tis·sue-bear·ing a.
tri·cus·pid a.
trig·ger a.
va·gus a.
a. vas·cu·lo·sa
ves·tib·u·lar a.
vi·su·al a.
Wernicke's a.
ar·e·ae
ar·e·a·ta
ar·e·a·tus
Are·ca
arec·ai·dine
are·caine
arec·o·line
are·flex·ia
ar·e·na·ceous
Are·na·vi·ri·dae
Are·na·vi·rus
are·o·la
    Chaussier's a.
    a. pa·pil·la·ris
    a. um·bil·i·cus
are·o·lae
are·o·lar
    cho·roid·i·tis
    cho·roi·dop·a·thy
    glands
    tis·sue
ar·e·om·e·ter
Argas
    A. per·si·cus
    A. re·flex·us
ar·ga·sid
Argas·i·dae
ar·gen·taf·fin
    cells
    gran·ules
ar·gen·taf·fine
ar·gen·taf·fi·no·ma
ar·gen·ta·tion
ar·gen·ti
ar·gen·tic

ar·gen·tine
Ar·gen·tin·i·an hem·or·rhag·ic
 fe·ver
ar·gen·to·phil
ar·gen·to·phile
ar·gen·tous
ar·gen·tum
ar·gi·nase
ar·gi·nine
 a. am·i·dase
 a. de·im·i·nase
 a. di·hy·dro·lase
 a. glu·ta·mate
 a. hy·dro·chlo·ride
 a. im·i·no·hy·dro·lase
 a. phos·phate
ar·gi·nine
 ox·y·to·cin
 va·so·pres·sin
 va·so·to·cin
ar·gi·ni·no·suc·ci·nase
ar·gi·ni·no·suc·ci·nate ly·ase
ar·gi·ni·no·suc·cin·ic ac·id
ar·gi·ni·no·suc·cin·ic·ac·i·du·
 ria
ar·gin·yl
ar·gi·pres·sin
ar·gon
Argonz-Del Castillo
 syn·drome
Argyll Robertson
 pu·pil
ar·gyr·ia
ar·gy·ri·a·sis
ar·gyr·ic
ar·gy·rism
ar·gyr·o·phil
ar·gyr·o·phile
ar·gyr·o·phil·ic
 cells
 fi·bers
ar·gy·ro·sis
arhin·ia
Arias-Stella
 ef·fect
 phe·nom·e·non
 re·ac·tion
ari·bo·fla·vin·o·sis
aris·to·gen·ics
aris·to·loch·ic ac·id
ar·is·to·te·lian
 meth·od
Aristotle's
 anom·a·ly
arith·me·tic
 mean
arith·mo·ma·nia
A·ri·zo·na

Arlt's
 op·er·a·tion
 si·nus
arm
 bar clasp a.
 brawny a.
 cir·cum·fer·en·tial clasp a.
 clasp a.
 dyn·ein a.
 re·cip·ro·cal a.
 re·ten·tion a.
 re·ten·tive a.
 re·ten·tive cir·cum·fer·en·
 tial clasp a.
 sta·bi·liz·ing cir·cum·fer·en·
 tial clasp a.
arm
 phe·nom·e·non
ar·ma·men·tar·i·um
Armanni-Ebstein
 change
 kid·ney
ar·mar·i·um
armed
 ros·tel·lum
Ar·mil·li·fer
 A. ar·mil·la·tus
ar·mored
 heart
arm·pit
Arndt-Gottron
 syn·drome
Arndt's
 law
Arneth
 clas·si·fi·ca·tion
 count
 for·mu·la
 in·dex
 stag·es
ar·ni·ca
Arnold-Chiari
 de·for·mi·ty
 mal·for·ma·tion
 syn·drome
Arnold's
 bod·ies
 bun·dle
 ca·nal
 gan·gli·on
 nerve
 tract
ar·o·mat·ic
 bit·ters
 cas·tor oil
 com·pound
 se·ries
 wa·ter

ar·o·mat·ic D-amino-ac·id de·
car·box·yl·ase
arous·al
func·tion
re·ac·tion
ar·o·yl
ar·rack
ar·rec·tor
ar·rec·to·res pi·lo·rum
ar·rec·to·res
ar·rest
car·di·ac a.
cir·cu·la·to·ry a.
ep·i·phys·i·al a.
mat·u·ra·tion a.
si·nus a.
ar·rest·ed
tu·ber·cu·lo·sis
ar·rest·ed den·tal
car·ies
ar·rhen·ic
med·i·ca·tion
Arrhenius
doc·trine
equa·tion
law
Arrhenius-Madsen
the·o·ry
ar·rhe·no·blas·to·ma
ar·rhe·no·gen·ic
ar·rhe·no·to·cia
ar·rhi·go·sis
ar·rhin·en·ce·pha·lia
ar·rhin·en·ceph·a·ly
ar·rhin·ia
ar·rhyth·mia
car·di·ac a.
ju·ve·nile a.
non·pha·sic si·nus a.
pha·sic si·nus a.
res·pi·ra·to·ry a.
si·nus a.
ar·rhyth·mic
ar·rhyth·mo·gen·ic
ar·rhyth·mo·ki·ne·sis
ar·row
poi·son
ar·row point
trac·ing
ar·row·root
Arroyo's
sign
Arruga's
for·ceps
ar·sa·ce·tin
ar·sen·a·mide
ar·se·nate
ar·sen·i·a·sis

ar·se·nic
a. tri·hy·dride
a. tri·ox·ide
white a.
ar·se·nic
pig·men·ta·tion
ar·se·nic ac·id
ar·sen·i·cal
ker·a·to·sis
trem·or
ar·sen·i·cal·ism
ar·se·nic-fast
ar·se·nide
ar·se·ni·ous
ar·se·ni·um
ar·sen·iu·ret
ar·sen·iu·ret·ed
hy·dro·gen
ar·se·no·ther·a·py
ar·se·nous
ar·se·nous ac·id
ar·se·nous hy·dride
ar·se·nous ox·ide
ar·se·nox·i·des
ar·sine
ar·son·ic ac·id
ar·so·ni·um
ars·phen·a·mine
ars·thi·nol
ar·te·fact
ar·te·ria
a. ac·e·tab·u·li
a. anas·to·mot·i·ca au·ric·
u·la·ris mag·na
a. anas·to·mot·i·ca mag·na
a. anon·y·ma
ar·te·ri·ae ar·cu·a·tae re·nis
a. ar·ti·cu·la·ris az·y·gos
a. au·di·ti·va in·ter·na
a. bul·bi ure·thrae
a. cal·ca·ri·na
a. ce·li·a·ca
a. cer·vi·co·va·gi·na·lis
a. cho·roi·dea pos·te·ri·or
a. co·mes ner·vi me·di·a·ni
a. co·mes ner·vi phreni·ci
a. de·fe·ren·tia·lis
a. fron·ta·lis
a. gas·tro·ep·i·plo·i·ca dex·
tra
a. gas·tro·ep·i·plo·i·ca si·
nis·tra
a. hy·po·gas·tri·ca
a. in·ter·cos·ta·lis an·ter·o·
su·pe·ri·or
a. in·ter·cos·ta·lis su·pre·
ma
a. in·ter·os·sea vo·la·ris

ar·te·ria *(continued)*
  ar·te·ri·ae in·tes·ti·na·les
  a. is·chi·a·di·ca
  a. is·chi·a·ti·ca
  ar·te·ri·ae la·bi·a·les an·te·
    ri·o·res
  a. lu·so·ria
  ar·te·ri·ae mal·le·o·la·res
    pos·te·ri·o·res la·te·ra·les
  ar·te·ri·ae mal·le·o·la·res
    pos·te·ri·o·res me·di·a·les
  a. mam·ma·ria in·ter·na
  a. max·il·la·ris ex·ter·na
  ar·te·ri·ae me·di·a·sti·na·les
    an·te·ri·o·res
  a. me·ta·tar·sa·lis
  a. pul·mo·na·lis
  a. ra·ni·na
  a. ret·i·nae cen·tra·lis
  a. sca·pu·la·ris de·scen·dens
  a. sper·ma·ti·ca in·ter·na
  ar·te·ri·ae thy·mi·cae
  a. vit·el·li·na
  a. vo·la·ris in·di·cis ra·di·
    a·lis
ar·te·ri·ae
ar·te·ri·al
  arch·es of co·lon
  arch·es of il·e·um
  arch·es of je·ju·num
  arch of low·er eye·lid
  arch of up·per eye·lid
  blood
  bulb
  ca·nal
  cap·il·lary
  cir·cle of cer·e·brum
  cone
  duct
  flap
  for·ceps
  grooves
  he·man·gi·o·ma
  hy·per·e·mia
  hy·po·ten·sion
  lig·a·ment
  line
  mur·mur
  neph·ro·scle·ro·sis
  net·work
  scle·ro·sis
  seg·ments of kid·ney
  spi·der
  ten·sion
  trans·fu·sion
  vein
  wave
ar·te·ri·al·i·za·tion

ar·te·ri·arc·tia
ar·te·ri·ec·ta·sia
ar·te·ri·ec·ta·sis
ar·te·ri·ec·to·my
ar·te·ri·o·at·o·ny
ar·te·ri·o·cap·il·lary
  scle·ro·sis
ar·te·ri·o·coc·cyg·e·al
  gland
ar·te·ri·o·gram
ar·te·ri·o·graph·ic
ar·te·ri·og·ra·phy
  ce·re·bral a.
  spi·nal a.
ar·te·ri·o·la
ar·te·ri·o·lae
ar·te·ri·o·lar
  neph·ro·scle·ro·sis
  scle·ro·sis
ar·te·ri·ole
  af·fer·ent glo·mer·u·lar a.
  cap·il·lary a.
  ef·fer·ent glo·mer·u·lar a.
  in·fe·ri·or mac·u·lar a.
  in·fe·ri·or na·sal a. of ret·
    i·na
  in·fe·ri·or tem·po·ral a. of
    ret·i·na
  me·di·al a. of ret·i·na
  su·pe·ri·or mac·u·lar a.
  su·pe·ri·or na·sal a. of ret·
    i·na
  su·pe·ri·or tem·po·ral a. of
    ret·i·na
ar·te·ri·o·lith
ar·ter·i·o·li·tis
  nec·ro·tiz·ing a.
ar·te·ri·ol·o·gy
ar·te·ri·o·lo·ne·cro·sis
ar·te·ri·o·lo·neph·ro·scle·ro·sis
ar·te·ri·o·lo·scle·ro·sis
ar·te·ri·o·lo·scle·rot·ic
  kid·ney
ar·te·ri·o·lo·ve·nous
ar·te·ri·o·lo·ven·u·lar
  anas·to·mo·sis
  bridge
ar·te·ri·o·ma·la·cia
ar·te·ri·om·e·ter
ar·te·ri·o·mo·tor
ar·te·ri·o·my·o·ma·to·sis
ar·te·ri·o·neph·ro·scle·ro·sis
ar·te·ri·o·pal·mus
ar·te·ri·op·a·thy
  hy·per·ten·sive a.
  plex·o·gen·ic pul·mo·nary a.
ar·te·ri·o·pla·nia
ar·te·ri·o·plas·ty

ar·te·ri·o·pres·sor
ar·te·ri·or·rha·phy
ar·te·ri·or·rhex·is
ar·te·ri·o·scle·ro·sis
  hy·per·plas·tic a.
  hy·per·ten·sive a.
  me·di·al a.
  Mönckeberg's a.
  nod·u·lar a.
  a. ob·li·te·rans
  se·nile a.
ar·te·ri·o·scle·rot·ic
  an·eu·rysm
  gan·grene
  kid·ney
  psy·cho·sis
  ret·i·nop·a·thy
ar·te·ri·o·spasm
ar·te·ri·o·ste·no·sis
ar·te·ri·o·strep·sis
ar·te·ri·o·tome
ar·te·ri·ot·o·my
ar·te·ri·ot·o·ny
ar·te·ri·o·ve·nous
  anas·to·mo·sis
  an·eu·rysm
  fis·tu·la
  nick·ing
  shunt
ar·te·ri·o·ve·nous car·bon di·ox·ide
  dif·fer·ence
ar·te·ri·o·ve·nous ox·y·gen
  dif·fer·ence
ar·te·ri·tis
  cra·ni·al a.
  equine vi·ral a.
  gi·ant cell a.
  gran·u·lom·a·tous a.
  Horton's a.
  a. no·do·sa
  a. ob·li·te·rans
  ob·lit·er·at·ing a.
  rheu·mat·ic a.
  rheu·ma·toid a.
  tem·po·ral a.
ar·tery
  ab·er·rant a.
  ac·ces·so·ry ob·tu·ra·tor a.
  ac·e·tab·u·lar a.
  acro·mi·al a.
  acro·mi·o·tho·rac·ic a.
  a.'s of Adam·kie·wicz
  alar a. of nose
  an·gu·lar a.
  a. of an·gu·lar gy·rus
  anon·y·mous a.
  an·te·ri·or ce·cal a.

an·te·ri·or ce·re·bral a.
an·te·ri·or cho·roi·dal a.
an·te·ri·or cil·i·ary a.
an·te·ri·or cir·cum·flex hu·mer·al a.
an·te·ri·or com·mu·ni·cat·ing a.
an·te·ri·or con·junc·ti·val a.
an·te·ri·or de·scend·ing a.
an·te·ri·or eth·moi·dal a.
an·te·ri·or in·fe·ri·or cer·e·bel·lar a.
a. to an·te·ri·or in·fe·ri·or seg·ment of kid·ney
an·te·ri·or in·ter·cos·tal a.
an·te·ri·or in·ter·os·se·ous a.
an·te·ri·or in·ter·ven·tric·u·lar a.
an·te·ri·or la·bi·al a.'s
an·te·ri·or lat·er·al mal·le·o·lar a.
an·te·ri·or me·di·al mal·le·o·lar a.
an·te·ri·or me·nin·ge·al a.
an·te·ri·or pa·ri·e·tal a.
an·te·ri·or per·o·ne·al a.
an·te·ri·or spi·nal a.
an·te·ri·or su·pe·ri·or al·ve·o·lar a.
an·te·ri·or su·pe·ri·or den·tal a.
a. to an·te·ri·or su·pe·ri·or seg·ment of kid·ney
an·te·ri·or tem·po·ral a.
an·te·ri·or tib·i·al a.
an·te·ri·or tib·i·al re·cur·rent a.
an·te·ri·or tym·pan·ic a.
an·ter·o·lat·er·al cen·tral a.'s
an·ter·o·lat·er·al stri·ate a.'s
an·ter·o·lat·er·al thal·a·mo·stri·ate a.'s
an·ter·o·me·di·al cen·tral a.'s
an·ter·o·me·di·al thal·a·mo·stri·ate a.'s
ap·pen·dic·u·lar a.
ar·ci·form a.'s.
ar·cu·ate a.
ar·cu·ate a.'s of kid·ney
as·cend·ing a.
as·cend·ing cer·vi·cal a.
as·cend·ing pal·a·tine a.
as·cend·ing pha·ryn·ge·al a.
atri·al a.'s
ax·il·lary a.

ar·tery *(continued)*

az·y·gos a. of va·gi·na
bas·i·lar a.
brach·i·al a.
bron·chi·al a.'s
buc·cal a.
buc·ci·na·tor a.
a. of bulb of pe·nis
a. of bulb of ves·ti·bule
cal·ca·ne·al a.'s
cal·ca·rine a.
a. of calf
cal·lo·so·mar·gin·al a.
ca·rot·i·co·tym·pan·ic a.'s
ca·rot·id a.'s
car·pal a.
cau·dal pan·cre·at·ic a.
a. of cau·date lobe
cav·ern·ous a.'s
ce·cal a.'s
ce·li·ac a.
cen·tral a.
cen·tral a. of ret·i·na
a. of cen·tral sul·cus
cer·e·bel·lar a.'s
ce·re·bral a.'s
a. of ce·re·bral hem·or·rhage
cer·vi·co·vag·i·nal a.
Charcot's a.
chief a. of thumb
cir·cum·flex fib·u·lar a.
cir·cum·flex scap·u·lar a.
coiled a. of the uter·us
col·lat·er·al a.
col·lat·er·al dig·i·tal a.
com·mon ca·rot·id a.
com·mon he·pa·tic a.
com·mon il·i·ac a.
com·mon in·ter·os·se·ous a.
com·mon pal·mar dig·i·tal a.
com·mon plan·tar dig·i·tal a.
com·mu·ni·cat·ing a.
com·pan·ion a. to sci·at·ic nerve
con·junc·ti·val a.'s
cor·o·nary a.
cor·ti·cal a.'s
cos·to·cer·vi·cal a.
crem·as·ter·ic a.
cri·co·thy·roid a.
cru·ral a.
cys·tic a.
deep au·ric·u·lar a.
deep brach·i·al a.
deep cer·vi·cal a.

deep cir·cum·flex il·i·ac a.
deep a. of clit·o·ris
deep ep·i·gas·tric a.
deep a. of pe·nis
deep tem·po·ral a.
deep a. of thigh
deep a. of tongue
de·scend·ing a. of knee
de·scend·ing pal·a·tine a.
de·scend·ing scap·u·lar a.
dig·i·tal col·lat·er·al a.
dis·trib·ut·ing a.
dol·i·cho·ec·tat·ic a.
dor·sal a. of clit·o·ris
dor·sal dig·i·tal a.
dor·sal a. of foot
dor·sal in·ter·os·se·ous a.
dor·sal met·a·car·pal a.
dor·sal met·a·tar·sal a.
dor·sal a. of nose
dor·sal pan·cre·at·ic a.
dor·sal a. of pe·nis
dor·sal scap·u·lar a.
dor·sal tho·rac·ic a.
a. of duc·tus def·er·ens
elas·tic a.
end a.
ep·i·scle·ral a.
esoph·a·ge·al a.'s
ex·ter·nal ca·rot·id a.
ex·ter·nal il·i·ac a.
ex·ter·nal mam·ma·ry a.
ex·ter·nal max·il·lary a.
ex·ter·nal a. of nose
ex·ter·nal pu·den·dal a.'s
ex·ter·nal sper·mat·ic a.
fa·cial a.
fem·o·ral a.
fib·u·lar a.
fron·tal a.
gas·tro·du·o·de·nal a.
gla·se·ri·an a.
great anas·to·mot·ic a.
great·er pal·a·tine a.
great pan·cre·at·ic a.
great su·pe·ri·or pan·cre·at·ic a.
hel·i·cine a.
a. of Heubner
high·est in·ter·cos·tal a.
high·est tho·rac·ic a.
hu·mer·al a.
hy·a·loid a.
hy·po·gas·tric a.
il·e·al a.'s
il·e·o·co·lic a.
il·i·o·lum·bar a.
in·fe·ri·or al·ve·o·lar a.

in·fe·ri·or den·tal a.
in·fe·ri·or ep·i·gas·tric a.
in·fe·ri·or glu·te·al a.
in·fe·ri·or hem·or·rhoi·dal a.
in·fe·ri·or hy·po·phy·si·al a.
in·fe·ri·or in·ter·nal pa·ri·e·tal a.
in·fe·ri·or la·bi·al a.
in·fe·ri·or la·ryn·ge·al a.
in·fe·ri·or mes·en·ter·ic a.
in·fe·ri·or pan·cre·at·ic a.
in·fe·ri·or pan·cre·at·i·co·du·o·de·nal a.
in·fe·ri·or phren·ic a.
in·fe·ri·or rec·tal a.
a. of in·fe·ri·or seg·ment of kid·ney
in·fe·ri·or su·pra·re·nal a.
in·fe·ri·or thy·roid a.
in·fe·ri·or tym·pan·ic a.
in·fe·ri·or ul·nar col·lat·er·al a.
in·fe·ri·or ves·i·cal a.
in·fra·or·bit·al a.
in·fra·scap·u·lar a.
in·nom·i·nate a.
in·su·lar a.'s
in·ter·lo·bar a.'s
in·ter·lob·u·lar a.'s
in·ter·me·di·ate tem·po·ral a.
in·ter·nal au·di·to·ry a.
in·ter·nal ca·rot·id a.
in·ter·nal il·i·ac a.
in·ter·nal mam·ma·ry a.
in·ter·nal max·il·lary a.
in·ter·nal pu·den·dal a.
in·ter·nal sper·mat·ic a.
in·ter·nal tho·rac·ic a.
in·tes·ti·nal a.'s
je·ju·nal a.'s
a.'s of kid·ney
Kugel's a.
a. of lab·y·rinth
lac·ri·mal a.
lat·er·al cir·cum·flex a. of thigh
lat·er·al fron·to·ba·sal a.
lat·er·al in·fe·ri·or ge·nic·u·lar a.
lat·er·al na·sal a.
lat·er·al oc·cip·i·tal a.
lat·er·al plan·tar a.
lat·er·al sa·cral a.
lat·er·al splanch·nic a.'s
lat·er·al stri·ate a.'s

lat·er·al su·pe·ri·or ge·nic·u·lar a.
lat·er·al tar·sal a.
lat·er·al tho·rac·ic a.
left col·ic a.
left cor·o·nary a.
left gas·tric a.
left gas·tro·ep·i·plo·ic a.
left gas·tro-o·men·tal a.
left pul·mo·nary a.
len·tic·u·lo·stri·ate a.'s
less·er pal·a·tine a.
li·e·nal a.
lin·gual a.
long cen·tral a.
long pos·te·ri·or cil·i·ary a.
long tho·rac·ic a.
low·est lum·bar a.
low·est thy·roid a.
lum·bar a.
mac·u·lar a.'s
mar·gi·nal a. of co·lon
mas·se·ter·ic a.
mas·toid a.
max·il·lary a.
me·di·al cir·cum·flex a. of thigh
me·di·al fron·to·ba·sal a.
me·di·al in·fe·ri·or ge·nic·u·lar a.
me·di·al oc·cip·i·tal a.
me·di·al plan·tar a.
me·di·al stri·ate a.'s
me·di·al su·pe·ri·or ge·nic·u·lar a.
me·di·al tar·sal a.
me·di·an a.
me·di·an sa·cral a.
me·di·um a.
med·ul·lary a.'s of brain
men·tal a.
met·a·tar·sal a.
mid·dle ce·re·bral a.
mid·dle col·ic a.
mid·dle col·lat·er·al a.
mid·dle ge·nic·u·lar a.
mid·dle hem·or·rhoi·dal a.
mid·dle me·nin·ge·al a.
mid·dle rec·tal a.
mid·dle sa·cral a.
mid·dle su·pra·re·nal a.
mid·dle tem·po·ral a.
mus·cu·lar a.
mus·cu·lo·phren·ic a.
my·o·me·tri·al ar·cu·ate a.'s
my·o·me·tri·al ra·di·al a.'s
Neubauer's a.
nu·tri·ent a.

ar·tery *(continued)*

nu·tri·ent a. of fe·mur
nu·tri·ent a. of fib·u·la
nu·tri·ent a.'s of hu·mer·us
nu·tri·ent a. of the tib·ia
ob·tu·ra·tor a.
oc·cip·i·tal a.
om·pha·lo·mes·en·ter·ic a.
oph·thal·mic a.
or·bi·tal a.
or·bi·to·fron·tal a.
ovar·i·an a.
pal·mar in·ter·os·se·ous a.
pal·mar met·a·car·pal a.
pal·pe·bral a.'s
par·a·cen·tral a.
pa·ri·e·tal a.'s
pa·ri·e·to-oc·cip·i·tal a.
a.'s of pe·nis
per·fo·rat·ing a.'s
per·fo·rat·ing a.'s of foot
per·fo·rat·ing a.'s of hand
per·fo·rat·ing a.'s of in·ter·nal mam·ma·ry
per·fo·rat·ing a. of per·o·ne·al
per·i·cal·lo·sal a.
per·i·car·di·a·co·phren·ic a.
per·i·ne·al a.
per·o·ne·al a.
pipe·stem a.'s
plan·tar met·a·tar·sal a.
a.'s of pons
pon·tine a.'s
pop·lit·e·al a.
post·cen·tral a.
a. of post·cen·tral sul·cus
pos·te·ri·or al·ve·o·lar a.
pos·te·ri·or au·ric·u·lar a.
pos·te·ri·or ce·cal a.
pos·te·ri·or ce·re·bral a.
pos·te·ri·or cho·roi·dal a.
pos·te·ri·or cir·cum·flex hu·mer·al a.
pos·te·ri·or com·mu·ni·cat·ing a.
pos·te·ri·or con·junc·ti·val a.
pos·te·ri·or den·tal a.
pos·te·ri·or de·scend·ing a.
pos·te·ri·or eth·moi·dal a.
pos·te·ri·or in·fe·ri·or cer·e·bel·lar a.
pos·te·ri·or in·ter·cos·tal a.
pos·te·ri·or in·ter·os·se·ous a.
pos·te·ri·or in·ter·ven·tric·u·lar a.

pos·te·ri·or la·bi·al a.'s
pos·te·ri·or lat·er·al na·sal a.'s
pos·te·ri·or me·nin·ge·al a.
pos·te·ri·or pan·cre·at·i·co·du·o·de·nal a.
pos·te·ri·or pa·ri·e·tal a.
pos·te·ri·or per·o·ne·al a.'s
a. to pos·te·ri·or seg·ment of kid·ney
pos·te·ri·or sep·tal a. of nose
pos·te·ri·or spi·nal a.
pos·te·ri·or su·pe·ri·or al·ve·o·lar a.
pos·te·ri·or tem·po·ral a.
pos·te·ri·or tib·i·al a.
pos·te·ri·or tib·i·al re·cur·rent a.
pos·te·ri·or tym·pan·ic a.
pos·ter·o·lat·er·al cen·tral a.'s
pos·ter·o·me·di·al cen·tral a.'s
pre·cen·tral a.
a. of pre·cen·tral sul·cus
pre·cu·ne·al a.
prin·ceps cer·vi·cis a.
prin·ci·pal a. of thumb
prop·er he·pa·tic a.
prop·er pal·mar dig·i·tal a.
prop·er plan·tar dig·i·tal a.
a. of pter·y·goid ca·nal
pu·bic a.'s
pul·mo·nary a.
a. of pulp
py·lor·ic a.
quad·ri·ceps a. of fe·mur
ra·di·al a.
ra·di·al col·lat·er·al a.
ra·di·al in·dex a.
ra·di·al re·cur·rent a.
ra·dic·u·lar a.'s
ra·nine a.
re·cur·rent a.
re·cur·rent in·ter·os·se·ous a.
re·cur·rent ul·nar a.
re·nal a.
ret·ro·du·o·de·nal a.
right col·ic a.
right cor·o·nary a.
right gas·tric a.
right gas·tro·ep·i·plo·ic a.
right gas·tro·o·men·tal a.
right pul·mo·nary a.
a. of round lig·a·ment of uter·us

a. to sci·at·ic nerve
screw a.'s
scro·tal a.'s
seg·men·tal a.
sep·tal a.
sheathed a.
short cen·tral a.
short gas·tric a.'s
short pos·te·ri·or cil·i·ary
  a.
sig·moid a.'s
small a.'s
so·mat·ic a.'s
sphe·no·pal·a·tine a.
spi·ral a.
splen·ic a.
sta·pe·di·al a.
ster·nal a.'s
ster·no·mas·toid a.
sty·lo·mas·toid a.
sub·cla·vi·an a.
sub·cos·tal a.
sub·lin·gual a.
sub·men·tal a.
sub·scap·u·lar a.
sul·cal a.
su·per·fi·cial brach·i·al a.
su·per·fi·cial cer·vi·cal a.
su·per·fi·cial cir·cum·flex
  il·i·ac a.
su·per·fi·cial ep·i·gas·tric a.
su·per·fi·cial pal·mar a.
su·per·fi·cial tem·po·ral a.
su·per·fi·cial vo·lar a.
su·pe·ri·or cer·e·bel·lar a.
su·pe·ri·or cor·o·nary a.
su·pe·ri·or ep·i·gas·tric a.
su·pe·ri·or glu·te·al a.
su·pe·ri·or hem·or·rhoi·dal
  a.
su·pe·ri·or hy·po·phy·si·al
  a.
su·pe·ri·or in·ter·nal pa·ri·
  e·tal a.
su·pe·ri·or la·bi·al a.
su·pe·ri·or la·ryn·ge·al a.
su·pe·ri·or mes·en·ter·ic a.
su·pe·ri·or pan·cre·at·i·co·
  du·o·de·nal a.
su·pe·ri·or phren·ic a.
su·pe·ri·or rec·tal a.
a. to su·pe·ri·or seg·ment
  of kid·ney
su·pe·ri·or su·pra·re·nal a.
su·pe·ri·or tho·rac·ic a.
su·pe·ri·or thy·roid a.
su·pe·ri·or tym·pan·ic a.

su·pe·ri·or ul·nar col·lat·er·
  al a.
su·pe·ri·or ves·i·cal a.
su·pra·du·o·de·nal a.
su·pra·or·bit·al a.
su·pra·scap·u·lar a.
su·pra·troch·le·ar a.
su·preme in·ter·cos·tal a.'s
su·ral a.
ter·mi·nal a.
tes·tic·u·lar a.
tho·ra·co·a·cro·mi·al a.
tho·ra·co·dor·sal a.
trans·verse cer·vi·cal a.
trans·verse fa·cial a.
trans·verse a. of neck
trans·verse pan·cre·at·ic a.
trans·verse scap·u·lar a.
ul·nar a.
um·bil·i·cal a.
ure·thral a.
uter·ine a.
vag·i·nal a.
ve·nous a.
ven·tral splanch·nic a.'s
ven·tric·u·lar a.'s
ver·te·bral a.
vid·i·an a.
vi·tel·line a.
vo·lar in·ter·os·se·ous a.
Wilkie's a.
Zinn's a.
zy·go·mat·i·co-or·bi·tal a.
ar·tery
  nee·dle
arth·rag·ra
ar·thral
ar·thral·gia
  in·ter·mit·tent a.
  pe·ri·od·ic a.
  a. sa·tur·ni·na
ar·thral·gic
ar·threc·to·my
ar·thres·the·sia
ar·thri·fuge
ar·thrit·ic
  at·ro·phy
  cal·cu·lus
ar·thrit·ic gen·er·al
  pseu·do·pa·ral·y·sis
ar·thri·tide
ar·thrit·i·des
ar·thri·tis
  acute rheu·mat·ic a.
  atroph·ic a.
  chla·myd·i·al a.
  chron·ic ab·sorp·tive a.
  chy·lous a.

ar·thri·tis *(continued)*
    a. de·for·mans
    de·gen·er·a·tive a.
    en·ter·o·path·ic a.
    fi·lar·i·al a.
    gouty a.
    he·mo·phil·ic a.
    hy·per·tro·phic a.
    Jaccoud's a.
    ju·ve·nile a.
    ju·ve·nile rheu·ma·toid a.
    Lyme a.
    a. mu·ti·lans
    ne·o·na·tal a. of foals
    neu·ro·path·ic a.
    a. no·do·sa
    ochro·not·ic a.
    pro·lif·er·a·tive a.
    pso·ri·at·ic a.
    rheu·ma·toid a.
    sup·pu·ra·tive a.
    a. ura·ti·ca
Arth·ro·bac·ter
ar·thro·cele
ar·thro·cen·te·sis
ar·thro·chon·dri·tis
ar·thro·cla·sia
ar·thro·co·nid·i·um
ar·throd·e·sis
    tri·ple a.
ar·thro·dia
ar·thro·di·al
    car·ti·lage
    joint
ar·thro·dyn·ia
ar·thro·dyn·ic
ar·thro·dys·pla·sia
ar·thro·en·dos·co·py
ar·thro·e·rei·sis
ar·throg·e·nous
ar·thro·gram
ar·throg·ra·phy
ar·thro·gry·po·sis
    a. mul·ti·plex con·gen·i·ta
ar·thro·ka·tad·y·sis
ar·thro·lith
ar·thro·li·thi·a·sis
ar·thro·lo·gia
ar·throl·o·gy
ar·throl·y·sis
ar·throm·e·ter
ar·throm·e·try
ar·thro·no·sos
ar·thro-on·y·cho·dys·pla·sia
ar·thro-oph·thal·mop·a·thy
    he·red·i·tary pro·gress·ive a.
ar·thro·path·ia
    a. pso·ri·a·ti·ca

ar·thro·pa·thol·o·gy
ar·throp·a·thy
    di·a·bet·ic a.
    Jaccoud's a.
    long-leg a.
    neu·ro·path·ic a.
    stat·ic a.
    ta·bet·ic a.
ar·throph·ly·sis
ar·thro·phy·ma
ar·thro·plas·ty
    Charnley hip a.
    gap a.
    in·ter·po·si·tion a.
    in·tra·cap·su·lar tem·po·ro·
      man·dib·u·lar joint a.
    to·tal joint a.
ar·thro·pneu·mo·roent·gen·og·
  ra·phy
ar·thro·pod
Ar·throp·o·da
ar·thro·po·di·a·sis
ar·thro·po·dic
ar·throp·o·dous
ar·thro·py·o·sis
ar·thro·ri·sis
ar·thro·scle·ro·sis
ar·thro·scope
ar·thros·co·py
ar·thro·sis
    tem·po·ro·man·dib·u·lar a.
ar·thro·spore
ar·thros·te·i·tis
ar·thros·to·my
ar·thro·sy·no·vi·tis
ar·thro·tome
ar·throt·o·my
ar·thro·tro·pic
ar·thro·ty·phoid
ar·throx·e·sis
Arthus
    phe·nom·e·non
    re·ac·tion
ar·ti·ad
ar·tic·u·lar
    cap·sule
    car·ti·lage
    chon·dro·cal·ci·no·sis
    cir·cum·fer·ence of ra·di·us
    cir·cum·fer·ence of ul·na
    cor·pus·cles
    crep·i·tus
    cres·cent
    crests
    disk
    em·i·nence
    fos·sa of tem·po·ral bone
    frac·ture

gout
la·mel·la
lep·ro·sy
lip
mar·gin
me·nis·cus
mus·cle
mus·cle of el·bow
mus·cle of knee
nerve
net·work of el·bow
net·work of knee
pit of head of ra·di·us
pro·cess
rheu·ma·tism
sen·si·bil·i·ty
sur·face of acro·mi·on
sur·face of ar·y·te·noid car·
   ti·lage
sur·face of head of fib·u·la
sur·face of head of rib
sur·face of pa·tel·la
sur·face of tem·po·ral bone
sur·face of tu·ber·cle of rib
tu·ber·cle
ar·tic·u·la·re
ar·tic·u·lar vas·cu·lar
cir·cle
net·work
ar·tic·u·late
ar·tic·u·lat·ed
skel·e·ton
ar·tic·u·lat·ing
pa·per
ar·tic·u·la·tio
a. man·di·bu·la·ris
ar·tic·u·la·tion
at·lan·to-oc·cip·i·tal a.
bal·anced a.
bi·con·dy·lar a.
car·pal a.
con·dy·lar a.
con·flu·ent a.
cri·co·ar·y·te·noid a.
cri·co·thy·roid a.
cu·ne·o·na·vic·u·lar a.
den·tal a.
dis·tal ra·di·o·ul·nar a.
a.'s of foot
a.'s of hand
hu·mer·al a.
hu·mer·o·ra·di·al a.
in·cu·do·sta·pe·di·al a.
in·ter·chon·dral a.'s
in·ter·met·a·tar·sal a.'s
in·ter·pha·lan·ge·al a.'s
in·ter·tar·sal a.'s

met·a·car·po·pha·lan·ge·al
   a.'s
met·a·tar·so·pha·lan·ge·al
   a.'s
peg-and-sock·et a.
a. of pis·i·form bone
prox·i·mal ra·di·o·ul·nar a.
ra·di·o·car·pal a.
sa·cro·il·i·ac a.
sphe·roid a.
ster·no·cos·tal a.'s
su·pe·ri·or tib·i·al a.
ta·lo·cru·ral a.
tem·po·ro·man·dib·u·lar a.
tib·i·o·fib·u·lar a.
trans·verse tar·sal a.
tro·choid a.
ar·tic·u·la·ti·o·nes
ar·tic·u·la·tor
ad·just·a·ble a.
ar·con a.
non-ar·con a.
ar·tic·u·la·to·ry
ar·tic·u·lo·stat
ar·tic·u·lus
ar·ti·fact
ar·ti·fac·ti·tious
ar·ti·fac·tu·al
ar·ti·fi·cial
anat·o·my
an·ky·lo·sis
anus
crown
den·ti·tion
eye
heart
hi·ber·na·tion
in·sem·i·na·tion
kid·ney
mel·a·nin
pace·mak·er
pneu·mo·thor·ax
pu·pil
ra·di·o·ac·tiv·i·ty
res·pi·ra·tion
se·lec·tion
sphinc·ter
stone
tears
ven·ti·la·tion
ar·ti·fi·cial ac·tive
im·mu·ni·ty
ar·ti·fi·cial Carlsbad
salt
ar·ti·fi·cial Kis·sin·gen
salt
ar·ti·fi·cial pas·sive
im·mu·ni·ty

ar·ti·fi·cial Vichy
 salt
Ar·ti·o·dac·ty·la
ar·tis·tic
 anat·o·my
ar·y·ep·i·glot·tic
 fold
 mus·cle
ar·yl
 a. ac·yl·am·i·dase
ar·yl·am·i·dase
ar·yl·ar·son·ic ac·id
ar·yl·at·ed
 al·kyl
ar·yl·sul·fa·tase
ar·y·te·no·ep·i·glot·tid·e·an
 fold
ar·y·te·noid
 car·ti·lage
 glands
 swell·ing
ar·y·te·noi·dal ar·tic·u·lar
 sur·face of cri·coid
ar·y·te·noi·dec·to·my
ar·y·te·noi·de·us
ar·yt·e·noi·di·tis
ar·y·te·noi·do·pexy
as·a·fet·i·da
asaph·ia
Asa·rum
 A. can·a·dense
 A. eu·ro·pae·um
as·bes·toid
as·bes·tos
 ac·ne
 bod·ies
 corn
 li·ner
 wart
as·bes·to·sis
as·ca·ri·a·sis
as·car·i·cide
as·ca·rid
As·car·i·dae
As·car·i·da·ta
As·ca·rid·ia
 A. co·lum·bae
 A. gal·li
as·car·i·di·a·sis
As·ca·rid·i·da
As·ca·rid·i·dae
As·car·i·did·ea
As·car·i·doi·dea
as·car·i·dole
As·car·i·dor·i·da
As·ca·ris
 A. equo·rum
 A. lum·bri·coi·des

As·ca·roi·dea
as·ca·ron
As·ca·rops stron·gy·li·na
as·cen·dens
as·cend·ing
 ar·tery
 co·lon
 cur·rent
 de·gen·er·a·tion
 my·e·li·tis
 neu·ri·tis
 pa·ral·y·sis
 part
 part of aor·ta
 pro·cess
 py·e·lo·ne·phri·tis
as·cend·ing cer·vi·cal
 ar·tery
as·cend·ing fron·tal
 con·vo·lu·tion
 gy·rus
as·cend·ing lum·bar
 vein
as·cend·ing pal·a·tine
 ar·tery
as·cend·ing pa·ri·e·tal
 con·vo·lu·tion
 gy·rus
as·cend·ing pha·ryn·ge·al
 ar·tery
 plex·us
ascen·sus
as·cer·tain·ment
 com·plete a.
 in·com·plete a.
 sin·gle a.
 trun·cate a.
Asc·hel·min·thes
Ascher's
 syn·drome
Ascher's aque·ous in·flux
 phe·nom·e·non
Aschheim-Zondek
 test
Aschner-Dagnini
 re·flex
Aschner's
 phe·nom·e·non
 re·flex
Aschoff
 bod·ies
 nod·ules
as·ci
as·ci·tes
 a. adi·po·sus
 chy·li·form a.
 a. chy·lo·sus
 chy·lous a.

fat·ty a.
ge·lat·i·nous a.
hem·or·rhag·ic a.
milky a.
a. pre·cox
pseu·do·chy·lous a.
ascit·ic
agar
as·ci·tog·e·nous
Asclepias
as·co·carp
as·cog·e·nous
as·co·go·ni·um
Ascoli
re·ac·tion
As·co·my·ce·tes
as·cor·base
ascor·bate
a. ox·i·dase
ascor·bate-cy·a·nide
test
ascor·bic ac·id
ascor·byl pal·mi·tate
as·co·spore
as·cus
ase·cre·to·ry
Aselli's
gland
pan·cre·as
as·e·ma·sia
ase·mia
asep·sis
asep·tate
asep·tic
fe·ver
ne·cro·sis
sur·gery
asep·ti·cism
ase·quence
asex·u·al
dwarf·ism
gen·er·a·tion
re·pro·duc·tion
Ashby
meth·od
ash·en
tu·ber
tu·ber·cle
wing
Asherman's
syn·drome
Ashley's
phe·nom·e·non
Ashman's
phe·nom·e·non
asi·a·lia
asi·a·lism

Asian
in·flu·en·za
Asi·at·ic
chol·era
schis·to·so·mi·a·sis
asid·er·ot·ic
ane·mia
asit·ia
Askanazy
cell
Ask-Upmark
kid·ney
aso·cial
aso·ma
aso·ma·ta
as·pal·a·so·ma
as·par·a·gi·nase
as·par·a·gine
a. li·gase
a. syn·the·tase
as·par·a·gin·ic ac·id
as·pa·rag·i·nyl
As·par·a·gus
as·par·mide
as·par·tame
as·par·tase
as·par·tate
a. ami·no·trans·fer·ase
a. am·mo·nia-ly·ase
a. car·bam·o·yl·trans·fer·ase
a. ki·nase
a. trans·am·i·nase
as·par·tic ac·id
as·par·tyl
as·par·tyl·gly·co·sa·mine
as·par·tyl·gly·cos·a·mi·nu·ria
as·pect
as·per·gil·lic ac·id
as·per·gil·lin
as·per·gil·lo·ma
as·per·gil·lo·sis
bron·cho·pul·mo·nary a.
dis·sem·i·nat·ed a.
in·va·sive a.
pul·mo·nary a.
As·per·gil·lus
A. cla·va·tus
A. fla·vus
A. fu·mi·ga·tus
A. ni·du·lans
A. ni·ger
A. ter·re·us
asper·ma·tism
asper·mat·o·gen·ic
ste·ril·i·ty
asper·mia
as·per·sion

aspher·ic
  lens
as·phyg·mia
as·phyx·ia
  blue a.
  cy·a·not·ic a.
  a. li·vi·da
  lo·cal a.
  a. ne·o·na·to·rum
  a. pal·li·da
  sym·met·ric a.
  trau·mat·ic a.
as·phyx·i·al
as·phyx·i·ant
as·phyx·i·ate
as·phyx·i·at·ing
as·phyx·i·at·ing tho·rac·ic
  chon·dro·dys·tro·phy
  dys·pla·sia
as·phyx·i·a·tion
As·pic·u·lu·ris tet·rap·tera
as·pid·in
as·pid·i·nol
as·pid·i·um
as·pi·do·sam·ine
as·pi·do·sper·mine
as·pi·rate
as·pi·rat·ing
  nee·dle
as·pi·ra·tion
  bi·op·sy
  pneu·mo·nia
as·pi·ra·tion
  me·co·ni·um a.
as·pi·ra·tor
  vac·u·um a.
  wa·ter a.
as·pi·rin
asple·nia
asplen·ic
aspo·rog·e·nous
aspo·rous
aspor·u·late
As·sam
  fe·ver
as·sas·sin bug
as·say
  Ames a.
  clo·no·gen·ic a.
  com·pet·i·tive bind·ing a.
  com·ple·ment bind·ing a.
  dou·ble an·ti·body sand·
    wich a.
  en·zyme-linked im·mu·no·
    sor·bent a.
  Grunstein-Hogness a.
  im·mu·no·chem·i·cal a.
  im·mu·no·ra·di·o·met·ric a.

  in·di·rect a.
  ra·di·o·re·cep·tor a.
  Raji cell ra·di·o·im·mune a.
as·ser·tive
  con·di·tion·ing
  train·ing
Assézat's
  tri·an·gle
as·si·dent
  sign
  symp·tom
as·sim·i·la·ble
as·sim·i·la·tion
  re·pro·duc·tive a.
as·sim·i·la·tion
  pel·vis
  sa·crum
as·sist-con·trol
  ven·ti·la·tion
as·sist·ed
  res·pi·ra·tion
  ven·ti·la·tion
as·sist·ed ce·phal·ic
  de·liv·ery
as·sist·ive
  move·ment
Assmann's tu·ber·cu·lous
  in·fil·trate
as·so·ci·ate
  paired a.'s
as·so·ci·at·ed
  an·tag·o·nist
  move·ment
as·so·ci·a·tion
  ar·e·as
  con·stant
  cor·tex
  fi·bers
  mech·a·nism
  neu·ro·sis
  sys·tem
  test
  time
  tract
as·so·ci·a·tion
  clang a.
  dream a.'s
  free a.
  ge·net·ic a.
as·so·ci·a·tion·ism
as·so·ci·a·tive
  apha·sia
  re·ac·tion
  strength
as·sort·a·tive
  mat·ing
as·sort·ment
  in·de·pen·dent a.

as·ta·coid
　rash
asta·sia
asta·sia-aba·sia
astat·ic
as·ta·tine
aste·a·to·des
aste·a·to·sis
　a. cu·tis
as·ter
　sperm a.
aster·e·og·no·sis
as·te·ri·on
aster·ix·is
aster·nal
aster·nia
As·ter·o·coc·cus
as·ter·oid
　body
　hy·a·lo·sis
as·the·nia
　neu·ro·cir·cu·la·to·ry a.
as·then·ic
as·the·no·pia
　ac·com·mo·da·tive a.
　mus·cu·lar a.
　ner·vous a.
　neur·as·then·ic a.
　ret·i·nal a.
as·the·nop·ic
as·the·no·sper·mia
asth·ma
　atop·ic a.
　bron·chi·al a.
　bron·chit·ic a.
　car·di·ac a.
　ca·tarrh·al a.
　ex·trin·sic a.
　hay a.
　in·trin·sic a.
　mill·er's a.
　min·er's a.
　ner·vous a.
　re·flex a.
　spas·mod·ic a.
　steam-fit·ter's a.
　strip·per's a.
　sum·mer a.
asth·ma
　crys·tals
asth·mat·ic
　bron·chi·tis
asth·ma·toid
　wheeze
asth·ma-weed
asth·mo·gen·ic

as·tig·mat·ic
　di·al
　lens
astig·ma·tism
　a. against the rule
　com·pound hy·per·o·pic a.
　com·pound my·o·pic a.
　cor·ne·al a.
　di·rect a.
　hy·per·o·pic a.
　ir·reg·u·lar a.
　len·tic·u·lar a.
　mixed a.
　my·o·pic a.
　a. of ob·lique pen·cils
　reg·u·lar a.
　re·versed a.
　sim·ple hy·per·o·pic a.
　sim·ple my·o·pic a.
　a. with the rule
as·tig·ma·tom·e·ter
astig·ma·tom·e·try
as·tig·mat·o·scope
as·tig·ma·tos·co·py
astig·mia
as·tig·mom·e·ter
as·tig·mom·e·try
astig·mo·scope
as·tig·mos·co·py
asto·ma·tous
asto·mia
asto·mous
as·trag·a·lar
as·trag·a·lec·to·my
as·trag·a·lo·cal·ca·ne·an
as·trag·a·lo·fib·u·lar
as·trag·a·lo·scaph·oid
as·trag·a·lo·tib·i·al
As·trag·a·lus
as·trag·a·lus
as·tral
　fi·bers
as·tra·po·pho·bia
as·tric·tion
as·trin·gent
as·tro·blast
as·tro·blas·to·ma
as·tro·cele
as·tro·cyte
　ame·boid a.
　fi·bril·lary a.
　fi·brous a.
　ge·mis·to·cyt·ic a.
　pro·to·plas·mic a.
　re·ac·tive a.
as·tro·cy·to·ma
　ge·mis·to·cyt·ic a.
　grade I a.

as·tro·cy·to·ma *(continued)*
  grade II a.
  grade III a.
  grade IV a.
  pi·loid a.
  pro·to·plas·mic a.
as·tro·cy·to·sis
  a. ce·re·bri
as·tro·ep·en·dy·mo·ma
as·trog·lia
  cell
as·troid
as·tro·ki·net·ic
as·tro·sphere
Astwood's
  test
as·ver·in
asyl·la·bia
asy·lum
asym·bo·lia
asym·met·ric
asym·met·ri·cal
  chon·dro·dys·tro·phy
asym·met·ric mo·tor
  neu·rop·a·thy
asym·me·try
asymp·tom·at·ic
  coc·cid·i·oi·do·my·co·sis
asyn·chro·nous pulse
  gen·er·a·tor
asyn·cli·tism
  an·te·ri·or a.
  pos·te·ri·or a.
asyn·de·sis
asyn·ech·ia
asy·ner·gia
asyn·er·gic
asyn·er·gy
asy·ne·sia
asyn·e·sis
asys·tem·at·ic
asys·to·le
asys·to·lia
asys·tol·ic
atac·tic
  aba·si·a
  agraph·ia
atac·til·ia
at·a·rac·tic
at·a·rax·ia
at·a·rax·ic
at·a·vic
at·a·vism
at·a·vis·tic
  epiph·y·sis
at·a·vus
atax·ia
  acute a.

  bo·vine con·gen·i·tal a.
  Briquet's a.
  Bruns a.
  a. of calves
  cer·e·bel·lar a.
  a. cor·dis
  en·zo·ot·ic a.
  equine spi·nal a.
  Friedreich's a.
  he·red·i·tary cer·e·bel·lar a.
  he·red·i·tary spi·nal a.
  ki·net·ic a.
  a. of lambs
  Leyden's a.
  lo·co·mo·tor a.
  Marie's a.
  mor·al a.
  mo·tor a.
  oc·u·lar a.
  spi·nal a.
  stat·ic a.
  a. tel·an·gi·ec·ta·sia
  va·so·mo·tor a.
  ves·tib·u·lo·cer·e·bel·lar a.
atax·i·a·dy·nam·ia
atax·i·a·gram
atax·i·a·graph
atax·i·a·me·ter
atax·i·a·pha·sia
atax·ic
  aba·si·a
  apha·sia
  gait
  nys·tag·mus
  par·a·my·o·to·nia
  par·a·ple·gia
atax·i·o·phe·mia
atax·i·o·pho·bia
ataxy
at·el·ec·ta·sis
  pri·mary a.
  round a.
  sec·on·dary a.
at·e·lec·tat·ic
  rale
ate·lia
atel·i·o·sis
atel·i·ot·ic
  dwarf·ism
atel·op·id·tox·in
aten·o·lol
athe·lia
ather·man·cy
ather·ma·nous
ather·mo·sys·tal·tic
ath·er·o·em·bo·lism
ath·er·o·gen·e·sis
ath·er·o·gen·ic

ath·er·o·ma
  em·bo·lism
ath·er·om·a·tous
  de·gen·er·a·tion
  plaque
ath·er·o·scle·ro·sis
ath·er·o·scle·rot·ic
  an·eu·rysm
ath·er·o·sis
ath·er·o·throm·bo·sis
ath·er·o·throm·bot·ic
ath·e·toid
ath·e·to·sic
ath·e·to·sis
  dou·ble a.
  dou·ble con·gen·i·tal a.
  post·hem·i·ple·gic a.
  pu·pil·lary a.
ath·e·tot·ic
ath·lete's
  foot
ath·let·ic
  heart
athrep·sia
ath·rep·sy
ath·ro·cy·to·sis
athrom·bia
athy·mia
athy·mism
athy·rea
athy·roid·ism
athy·ro·sis
athy·rot·ic
at·lan·tad
at·lan·tal
at·lan·to·ax·i·al
at·lan·to·did·y·mus
at·lan·to·ep·i·stroph·ic
at·lan·to-oc·cip·i·tal
  ar·tic·u·la·tion
  joint
  mem·brane
at·lan·to-odon·toid
at·las
at·lo·ax·oid
at·lo·did·y·mus
at·loid
at·lo-oc·cip·i·tal
at·mol·y·sis
at·mom·e·ter
at·mo·sphere
  a. ab·so·lute
  ICAO stan·dard a.
  stan·dard a.
at·mo·spher·ic
  pres·sure
at·mo·spher·i·za·tion
At·mungs·fer·ment

at·om
  ac·ti·vat·ed a.
  Bohr's a.
  ex·cit·ed a.
  ion·ized a.
  la·beled a.
  nu·cle·ar a.
  qua·ter·na·ry car·bon a.
  ra·di·o·ac·tive a.
  re·coil a.
  stripped a.
  tagged a.
at·om
  me·ter
atom·ic
  core
  heat
  num·ber
  the·o·ry
  vol·ume
  weight
atom·ic ab·sorp·tion
  spec·tro·pho·tom·e·try
atom·ic mass
  unit
at·om·ism
at·om·is·tic
  psy·chol·o·gy
at·om·i·za·tion
at·om·iz·er
ato·nia
aton·ic
  ab·sence
  blad·der
  dys·pep·sia
  ec·tro·pi·on
  en·tro·pi·on
  ep·i·lep·sy
  epiph·o·ra
  im·po·tence
  ul·cer
at·o·nic·i·ty
at·o·ny
at·o·pen
atop·ic
  al·ler·gy
  asth·ma
  cat·a·ract
  con·junc·ti·vi·tis
  der·ma·ti·tis
  ec·ze·ma
  ker·a·to·con·junc·ti·vi·tis
  re·a·gin
atop·og·no·sia
atop·og·no·sis
at·o·py
atox·ic
ATP-di·phos·pha·tase

ATP-mon·o·phos·pha·tase
at·ra·bil·i·ary
   cap·sule
atrac·to·syl·id·ic ac·id
atrac·tyl·ic ac·id
atrac·tyl·i·gen·in
atrac·tyl·in
atra·cu·ri·um be·syl·ate
atrau·mat·ic
   nee·dle
   su·ture
atrep·sy
atre·sia
   anal a.
   a. ani
   aor·tic a.
   bil·i·ary a.
   cho·a·nal a.
   esoph·a·ge·al a.
   a. fol·lic·u·li
   in·tes·ti·nal a.
   a. ir·i·dis
   la·ryn·ge·al a.
   pul·mo·nary a.
   tri·cus·pid a.
   vag·i·nal a.
atre·sic
   ter·a·to·sis
atret·ic
   cor·pus lu·te·um
atret·ic ovar·i·an
   fol·li·cle
atre·to·ble·pha·ria
atre·to·cys·tia
atre·to·gas·tria
atre·top·sia
atria
atri·al
   ar·ter·ies
   au·ri·cle
   au·ric·u·la
   bi·gem·i·ny
   cap·ture
   com·plex
   dis·so·ci·a·tion
   echo
   ex·tra·sys·to·le
   fi·bril·la·tion
   flut·ter
   gal·lop
   kick
   myx·o·ma
   sound
   stand·still
   sys·to·le
   tach·y·car·dia
atri·al cha·ot·ic
   tach·y·car·dia

atri·al fu·sion
   beat
atri·al na·tri·u·ret·ic
   fac·tor
atri·al sep·tal
   de·fect
atri·al syn·chro·nous pulse
   gen·er·a·tor
atri·al trans·port
   func·tion
atri·al trig·gered pulse
   gen·er·a·tor
atri·al-well
   tech·nique
atrich·ia
atri·cho·sis
at·ri·chous
atri·o·ca·rot·id
   in·ter·val
atri·o·dig·i·tal
   dys·pla·sia
atri·o·meg·a·ly
atri·o·nec·tor
atri·o·pep·tin
atri·o·sep·to·pexy
atri·o·sep·to·plas·ty
atri·o·sep·tos·to·my
   bal·loon a.
atri·o·sys·tol·ic
   mur·mur
atri·o·tome
atri·ot·o·my
atri·o·ven·tric·u·lar
   band
   block
   bun·dle
   ca·nal
   con·duc·tion
   dis·so·ci·a·tion
   ex·tra·sys·to·le
   gra·di·ent
   groove
   node
   sep·tum
   sul·cus
   trunk
   valves
atri·o·ven·tric·u·lar ca·nal
   cush·ions
atri·o·ven·tric·u·lar no·dal
   bi·gem·i·ny
   ex·tra·sys·to·le
   rhythm
   tach·y·car·dia
atrip·li·cism
atri·um
   ac·ces·so·ry a.
   a. glot·ti·dis

a. of heart
left a.
a. pul·mo·na·le
right a.
At·ro·pa
atroph·e·de·ma
atro·phia
a. bul·bo·rum he·re·di·tar·
ria
a. cu·tis
a. ma·cu·lo·sa va·ri·o·li·
for·mis cu·tis
a. pi·lo·rum pro·pria
atroph·ic
ar·thri·tis
ex·ca·va·tion
gas·tri·tis
glos·si·tis
het·er·o·chro·mia
in·flam·ma·tion
kid·ney
phar·yn·gi·tis
rhi·ni·tis
rhi·ni·tis of swine
throm·bo·sis
vag·i·ni·tis
atro·phie blanche
at·ro·phied
at·ro·pho·der·ma
a. al·bi·dum
a. bi·o·trip·ti·cum
a. dif·fu·sum
a. ma·cu·la·tum
a. neu·ri·ti·cum
a. of Pasini and Pierini
a. pig·men·to·sum
a. re·ti·cu·la·tum sym·met·
ri·cum fa·ci·ei
se·nile a.
a. se·ni·lis
a. stri·a·tum
a. ver·mi·cu·la·tum
at·ro·pho·der·ma·to·sis
at·ro·phy
acute re·flex bone a.
acute yel·low a. of the liv·
er
al·ve·o·lar a.
ar·thrit·ic a.
blue a.
brown a.
Buchwald's a.
cen·tral are·o·lar cho·roi·dal
a.
cer·e·bel·lar a.
cho·roi·dal vas·cu·lar a.
com·pen·sa·to·ry a.
cy·a·not·ic a.

cy·a·not·ic a. of the liv·er
Erb's a.
es·sen·tial pro·gress·ive a.
of iris
ex·haus·tion a.
fa·ci·o·scap·u·lo·hu·mer·al
a.
fa·mil·i·al spi·nal mus·cu·
lar a.
fat·ty a.
gin·gi·val a.
gray a.
gy·rate a. of cho·roid and
ret·i·na
Hoffmann's mus·cu·lar a.
hor·i·zon·tal a.
Hunt's a.
id·i·o·path·ic mus·cu·lar a.
in·fan·tile mus·cu·lar a.
in·fan·tile pro·gress·ive spi·
nal mus·cu·lar a.
is·che·mic mus·cu·lar a.
ju·ve·nile mus·cu·lar a.
Kienböck's a.
Leber's he·red·i·tary op·tic
a.
lin·e·ar a.
mac·u·lar a.
ma·ran·tic a.
mus·cu·lar a.
my·o·path·ic a.
neu·rit·ic a.
neu·ro·gen·ic a.
neu·ro·tro·phic a.
nu·trit·ion·al type cer·e·bel·
lar a.
ol·i·vo·pon·to·cer·e·bel·lar
a.
per·i·o·don·tal a.
per·o·ne·al mus·cu·lar a.
Pick's a.
post·men·o·pau·sal a.
pres·sure a.
pri·mary id·i·o·path·ic
mac·u·lar a.
pri·mary mac·u·lar a. of
skin
pro·gress·ive cho·roi·dal a.
pro·gress·ive mus·cu·lar a.
pseu·do·hy·per·tro·phic
mus·cu·lar a.
pulp a.
red a.
scap·u·lo·hu·mer·al a.
se·nile a.
se·rous a.
spi·nal a.
stri·ate a. of skin

at·ro·phy *(continued)*
  Sudeck's a.
  trac·tion a.
  trans·neu·ro·nal a.
  troph·o·neu·rot·ic a.
  Vulpian's a.
  yel·low a. of the liv·er
  Zimmerlin's a.
at·ro·pine
  a. meth·o·ni·trate
  a. meth·yl·bro·mide
  a. sul·fate
at·ro·pine
  test
at·ro·pin·ism
at·ro·pin·i·za·tion
at·ro·tox·in
at·tached
  cra·ni·ot·o·my
  gin·gi·va
at·tached cra·ni·al
  sec·tion
at·tach·ment
  ap·pa·ra·tus
at·tach·ment
  bar clip a.
  bar-sleeve a.'s
  ep·i·the·li·al a.
  fric·tion·al a.
  in·ter·nal a.
  key a.
  key·way a.
  mus·cle-ten·don a.
  par·al·lel a.
  per·i·ce·men·tal a.
  pre·ci·sion a.
  slot·ted a.
at·tack
  drop a.
  pan·ic a.
  sa·laam a.
  tran·sient is·che·mic a.
  un·ci·nate a.
  va·gal a.
  va·so·va·gal a.
at·tack
  rate
at·tar of rose
at·tend·ing
at·ten·tion def·i·cit
  dis·or·der
at·ten·u·ant
at·ten·u·ate
at·ten·u·at·ed
  tu·ber·cu·lo·sis
  vi·rus
at·ten·u·a·tion
at·ten·u·a·tor

at·tic
  tym·pan·ic a.
at·ti·co·mas·toid
at·ti·cot·o·my
at·ti·tude
  emo·tion·al a.'s
  fe·tal a.
  pas·sion·al a.'s
at·ti·tu·di·nal
  re·flex·es
at·tol·lens
  a. au·rem
  a. au·ric·u·lam
  a. oc·u·li
at·trac·tion
  cap·il·lary a.
  chem·i·cal a.
  mag·net·ic a.
  neu·ro·tro·pic a.
at·trac·tion
  sphere
at·tra·hens
at·tri·tion
atyp·ia
atyp·i·cal
  ab·sence
  achro·ma·top·sia
  ac·ro·ceph·a·lo·syn·dac·ty·ly
  fi·bro·xan·tho·ma
  in·su·lin
  li·po·ma
  mea·sles
  pneu·mo·nia
  pseu·do·cho·lin·es·ter·ase
atyp·i·cal fa·cial
  neu·ral·gia
atyp·i·cal me·la·no·cyt·ic
  hy·per·pla·sia
atyp·i·cal tri·gem·i·nal
  neu·ral·gia
atyp·i·cal ver·ru·cous
  en·do·car·di·tis
atyp·ism
Au
  an·ti·gen
Aub-DuBois
  ta·ble
Auberger blood group
Aubert's
  phe·nom·e·non
Au blood group
Auch·mer·o·my·ia
  A. lu·te·o·la
au·cu·bin
au·dile
au·di·o·an·al·ge·sia
au·di·o·gen·ic
  ep·i·lep·sy

au·di·o·gram
 pure tone a.
 speech a.
au·di·ol·o·gist
au·di·ol·o·gy
au·di·om·e·ter
 au·to·mat·ic a.
 Békésy a.
 group a.
 lim·it·ed range a.
 pure-tone a.
 speech a.
 wide range a.
au·di·o·met·ric
au·di·o·me·tri·cian
au·di·om·e·trist
au·di·om·e·try
 ABR a.
 au·di·to·ry brain·stem re·sponse a.
 au·to·mat·ic a.
 Békésy a.
 brain·stem evoked re·sponse a.
 BSER a.
 cor·ti·cal a.
 di·ag·nos·tic a.
 elec·tro·der·mal a.
 elec·tro·phys·i·o·log·ic a.
 evoked re·sponse a.
 group a.
 pure-tone a.
 screen·ing a.
 speech a.
au·di·o·vi·su·al
au·di·tion
 chro·mat·ic a.
 gus·ta·to·ry a.
au·di·tive
au·di·to·ry
 ag·no·sia
 al·ter·nans
 apha·sia
 ar·ea
 ca·nal
 cap·sule
 car·ti·lage
 cor·tex
 fa·tigue
 field
 gan·gli·on
 hairs
 hy·per·al·ge·sia
 hy·per·es·the·sia
 lem·nis·cus
 lo·cal·i·za·tion
 nerve
 nu·cle·us

 os·si·cles
 path·way
 pits
 plac·odes
 pore
 pro·cess
 re·flex
 stri·ae
 strings
 syn·es·the·sia
 teeth
 thresh·old
 tract
 tube
 ver·ti·go
 ves·i·cle
au·di·to·ry brain·stem re·sponse
 au·di·om·e·try
au·di·to·ry oc·u·lo·gy·ric
 re·flex
au·di·to·ry re·cep·tor
 cells
Auenbrugger's
 sign
Auer
 bod·ies
 rods
Auerbach's
 gan·glia
 plex·us
Aufrecht's
 sign
Auger
 elec·tron
aug·men·ta·tion
 graft
 mam·ma·plas·ty
aug·ment·ed his·ta·mine
 test
aug·men·tor
 fi·bers
 nerves
aug·na·thus
Aujeszky's
 dis·ease
Aujeszky's dis·ease
 vi·rus
au·ra
 in·tel·lec·tu·al a.
 kin·es·thet·ic a.
 rem·i·nis·cent a.
au·rae
au·ral
 my·i·a·sis
 ver·ti·go
au·ra·mine O

au·ra·mine O flu·o·res·cent
  stain
au·ran·o·fin
au·ran·ti·a·sis cu·tis
au·re·o·lic ac·id
au·res
au·ri·a·sis
au·ric
au·ri·cle
  ac·ces·so·ry a.'s
  atri·al a.
  cer·vi·cal a.
  left a.
  right a.
au·ric·u·la
  atri·al a.
au·ric·u·lae
au·ric·u·lar
  ap·pend·age
  ap·pen·dec·to·my
  ap·pen·dix
  arc
  can·a·lic·u·lus
  car·ti·lage
  com·plex
  ex·tra·sys·to·le
  fi·bril·la·tion
  fis·sure
  flut·ter
  gan·gli·on
  in·dex
  lig·a·ments
  notch
  point
  re·flex
  stand·still
  sur·face of il·i·um
  sur·face of sa·crum
  sys·to·le
  tach·y·car·dia
  tri·an·gle
  tu·ber·cle
  veins
au·ric·u·la·re
au·ric·u·lar·ia
au·ric·u·lo·cra·ni·al
au·ric·u·lo-in·fra·or·bit·al
  plane
au·ric·u·lo·pal·pe·bral
  re·flex
au·ric·u·lo·pres·sor
  re·flex
au·ric·u·lo·tem·po·ral
  nerve
au·ric·u·lo·tem·po·ral nerve
  syn·drome
au·ric·u·lo·ven·tric·u·lar
  groove

au·rid
au·ri·des
au·ri·form
au·rin
au·rin·tri·car·box·yl·ic ac·id
au·ris
au·ri·scope
au·ro·chro·mo·der·ma
au·ro·mer·cap·to·ac·et·an·i·lid
au·rone
au·ro·pal·pe·bral
  re·flex
au·ro·ther·a·py
au·ro·thi·o·glu·cose
au·ro·thi·o·gly·ca·nide
au·rum
Aus
  an·ti·gen
aus·cult
aus·cul·tate
aus·cul·ta·tion
  di·rect a.
  im·me·di·ate a.
  me·di·ate a.
aus·cul·ta·to·ry
  al·ter·nans
  gap
  per·cus·sion
  sound
aus·sa·ge
  test
Austin Flint
  mur·mur
Aus·tra·lia
  an·ti·gen
Aus·tra·li·an X
  dis·ease
  en·ceph·a·li·tis
Aus·tra·li·an X dis·ease
  vi·rus
au·te·cic
au·te·cious
au·te·me·sia
au·then·tic·i·ty
au·thor·i·tar·i·an
  per·son·al·i·ty
au·thor·i·ty
  fig·ure
au·tism
  in·fan·tile a.
au·tis·tic
  par·a·site
au·to·ac·ti·va·tion
au·to·ag·glu·ti·na·tion
au·to·ag·glu·ti·nin
  an·ti-Pr cold a.
  cold a.
au·to·al·ler·gic

au·to·al·ler·gic he·mo·lyt·ic
  ane·mia
au·to·al·ler·gi·za·tion
au·to·al·ler·gy
au·to·a·nal·y·sis
au·to·an·a·lyz·er
  se·quen·tial mul·ti·chan·nel
    a.
au·to·an·a·phy·lax·is
au·to·an·ti·body
  an·ti-id·i·o·type a.
  cold a.
  Donath-Landsteiner cold a.
  he·mag·glu·ti·nat·ing cold a.
  id·i·o·type a.
  warm a.
au·to·an·ti·com·ple·ment
au·to·an·ti·gen
au·to·as·say
au·to·blast
au·to·ca·tal·y·sis
au·to·cat·a·lyt·ic
au·to·cath·e·ter·ism
au·to·cath·e·ter·i·za·tion
au·toch·thon·ous
  ide·as
  ma·lar·ia
  par·a·site
au·to·cla·sia
au·toc·la·sis
au·to·clave
au·to·coid
au·to·crine
  hy·poth·e·sis
au·to·cys·to·plas·ty
au·to·cy·to·ly·sin
au·to·cy·tol·y·sis
au·to·cy·to·tox·in
au·to·der·mic
  graft
au·to·di·ges·tion
au·to·dip·loid
au·to·drain·age
au·to·ech·o·la·lia
au·to·e·rot·ic
au·to·e·rot·i·cism
au·to·er·o·tism
au·to·e·ryth·ro·cyte
  sen·si·ti·za·tion
au·to·e·ryth·ro·cyte sen·si·ti·
  za·tion
  syn·drome
au·to·flu·o·ro·scope
au·tog·a·mous
au·tog·a·my
au·to·ge·ne·ic
  graft
au·to·gen·e·sis

au·to·ge·net·ic
au·to·gen·ic
au·tog·e·nous
  ker·a·to·plas·ty
  un·ion
  vac·cine
au·tog·no·sis
au·to·graft
au·to·graft·ing
au·to·gram
au·tog·ra·phism
au·to·hem·ag·glu·ti·na·tion
au·to·he·mo·ly·sin
au·to·he·mol·y·sis
  test
au·to·he·mo·ther·a·py
au·to·he·mo·trans·fu·sion
au·to·hex·a·ploid
au·to·hyp·no·sis
au·to·hyp·not·ic
au·to·hyp·no·tism
au·to·im·mune
  dis·ease
  throm·bo·cy·to·pe·nia
  thy·roid·i·tis
au·to·im·mune he·mo·lyt·ic
  ane·mia
au·to·im·mu·ni·ty
au·to·im·mu·ni·za·tion
au·to·im·mu·no·cy·to·pe·nia
au·to·in·fec·tion
au·to·in·fu·sion
au·to·in·oc·u·la·ble
au·to·in·oc·u·la·tion
au·to·in·tox·i·cant
au·to·in·tox·i·ca·tion
au·to·i·sol·y·sin
au·to·ker·a·to·plas·ty
au·to·ki·ne·sia
au·to·ki·ne·sis
au·to·ki·net·ic
  ef·fect
au·to·le·sion
au·tol·o·gous
  graft
  pro·tein
au·tol·y·sate
au·to·lyse
au·tol·y·sin
au·tol·y·sis
au·to·lyt·ic
  en·zyme
au·to·lyze
au·to·mal·let
au·to·mat·ed dif·fer·en·tial leu·
  ko·cyte
  count·er

au·to·mat·ic
  ab·sence
  au·di·om·e·ter
  au·di·om·e·try
  beat
  cho·rea
  con·dens·er
  con·trac·tion
  ep·i·lep·sy
  plug·ger
au·tom·a·tism
  am·bu·la·to·ry a.
  im·me·di·ate post·trau·mat·
   ic a.
au·to·mat·o·graph
au·to·mix·is
au·tom·ne·sia
au·to·my·so·pho·bia
au·to·nom·ic
  dis·or·der
  ep·i·lep·sy
  gan·glia
  im·bal·ance
  nerve
  part
  plex·us·es
au·to·nom·ic mo·tor
  neu·ron
  neu·rons
au·to·nom·ic ner·vous
  sys·tem
au·to·nom·ic neu·ro·gen·ic
  blad·der
au·to·nom·o·tro·pic
au·ton·o·mous
  psy·cho·ther·a·py
au·ton·o·my
  func·tion·al a.
au·to-ox·i·da·tion
au·to-ox·i·diz·a·ble
au·to·par·en·chym·a·tous
  met·a·pla·sia
au·to·path·ic
au·to·pen·ta·ploid
au·to·pep·sia
au·to·pha·gia
au·to·pha·gic
  vac·u·ole
au·to·pha·go·ly·so·some
au·toph·a·gy
au·to·phil·ia
au·to·pho·bia
au·toph·o·ny
au·to·plast
au·to·plas·tic
  graft
au·to·plas·ty
au·to·ploid

au·to·ploi·dy
au·to·plug·ger
au·to·pod
au·to·po·dia
au·to·po·di·um
au·to·poi·son·ous
au·to·pol·y·mer
  res·in
au·to·po·lym·er·i·za·tion
au·to·po·ly·mer·iz·ing
  res·in
au·to·pol·y·ploid
au·to·pol·y·ploi·dy
au·top·sy
au·to·ra·di·o·gram
au·to·ra·di·o·graph
au·to·ra·di·og·ra·phy
au·to·reg·u·la·tion
  het·er·o·met·ric a.
  ho·me·o·met·ric a.
au·to·re·in·fec·tion
au·to·re·pro·duc·tion
au·tor·rha·phy
au·to·scop·ic
  phe·nom·e·non
au·to·sen·si·tize
au·to·sep·ti·ce·mia
au·to·se·ro·ther·a·py
au·to·se·rum
  ther·a·py
au·to·sex·u·al·ism
au·to·site
au·tos·mia
au·to·so·mal
  gene
au·to·so·ma·tog·no·sis
au·to·so·ma·tog·nos·tic
au·to·some
au·to·sug·gest·i·bil·i·ty
au·to·sug·ges·tion
au·to·syn·noia
au·to·syn·the·sis
au·to·te·lic
au·to·tem·nous
au·to·tet·ra·ploid
au·to·ther·a·py
au·tot·o·my
au·to·top·ag·no·sia
au·to·tox·e·mia
au·to·tox·ic
au·to·tox·i·co·sis
au·to·tox·in
au·to·trans·fu·sion
au·to·trans·plant
au·to·trans·plan·ta·tion
au·to·trip·loid
au·to·troph
au·to·tro·phic

au·to·vac·ci·na·tion
au·tox·i·da·tion
au·to·zy·gous
au·tumn
  fe·ver
au·tum·nal
  ca·tarrh
aux·an·o·gram
aux·an·o·graph·ic
  meth·od
aux·a·nog·ra·phy
aux·an·ol·o·gy
aux·e·sis
aux·et·ic
  growth
aux·il·ia·ry
  abut·ment
aux·il·i·o·mo·tor
aux·i·lyt·ic
aux·o·car·dia
aux·o·chrome
aux·o·drome
aux·o·flore
aux·o·gluc
aux·om·e·ter
aux·o·ton·ic
aux·o·tox
aux·o·troph
aux·o·tro·phic
  strains
A-V
  block
  con·duc·tion
  dis·so·ci·a·tion
  ex·tra·sys·to·le
  in·ter·val
avail·a·ble arch
  length
av·a·lanche
  con·duc·tion
aval·vu·lar
avas·cu·lar
  ne·cro·sis
avas·cu·lar·i·za·tion
Avellis'
  syn·drome
ave·nin
av·er·age pulse
  mag·ni·tude
aver·sion
  ther·a·py
aver·sive
  be·hav·ior
  con·di·tion·ing
  train·ing
Avi·ad·e·no·vi·rus
avi·an
  achon·dro·pla·sia

diph·the·ria
eryth·ro·blas·to·sis
in·flu·en·za
leu·ko·sis
lym·pho·ma·to·sis
ma·lar·ia
mon·o·cy·to·sis
my·e·lo·blas·to·sis
re·tic·u·lo·en·do·the·li·o·sis
sar·co·ma
spi·ro·che·to·sis
trich·o·mo·ni·a·sis
avi·an en·ceph·a·lo·my·e·li·tis
  vi·rus
avi·an eryth·ro·blas·to·sis
  vi·rus
avi·an in·fec·tious
  en·ceph·a·lo·my·e·li·tis
  la·ryn·go·tra·che·i·tis
avi·an in·fec·tious la·ryn·go·
  tra·che·i·tis
  vi·rus
avi·an in·flu·en·za
  vi·rus
avi·an leu·ke·mia-sar·co·ma
  com·plex
avi·an leu·ko·sis-sar·co·ma
  com·plex
  vi·rus
avi·an lym·pho·ma·to·sis
  vi·rus
avi·an my·e·lo·blas·to·sis
  vi·rus
avi·an neu·ro·lym·pho·ma·to·sis
  vi·rus
avi·an pneu·mo·en·ceph·a·li·tis
  vi·rus
avi·an sar·co·ma
  vi·rus
avi·an vi·ral ar·thri·tis
  vi·rus
avi·a·tion
  med·i·cine
  oti·tis
avi·a·tor's
  dis·ease
  ear
av·i·din
A·vi·pox·vi·rus
avir·u·lent
avi·ta·min·o·sis
  con·di·tioned a.
avive·ment
A-V no·dal
  bi·gem·i·ny
  ex·tra·sys·to·le
  rhythm
  tach·y·car·dia

Avogadro's
  con·stant
  hy·poth·e·sis
  law
  num·ber
  pos·tu·late
avoid·ance
  con·di·tion·ing
avoid·ance-avoid·ance
  con·flict
avoid·ant
  per·son·al·i·ty
av·oir·du·pois
A-V stra·bis·mus
  syn·drome
avulsed
  wound
avul·sion
  frac·ture
avul·sion
  a. of ca·run·cu·la la·cri·
   ma·lis
  nerve a.
  tooth a.
Axenfeld's
  syn·drome
axen·ic
ax·es
ax·i·al
  am·bly·o·pia
  am·e·tro·pia
  an·eu·rysm
  an·gle
  cat·a·ract
  cur·rent
  fil·a·ment
  hy·per·o·pia
  il·lu·mi·na·tion
  mus·cle
  my·o·pia
  neu·ri·tis
  plate
  point
  pro·jec·tion
  skel·e·ton
  sur·face
  view
  walls of the pulp cham·bers
ax·i·al pat·tern
  flap
ax·if·u·gal
ax·il
ax·ile
  cor·pus·cle
ax·il·la
ax·il·lae
ax·il·lary
  an·es·the·sia

  arch
  ar·tery
  cat·a·ract
  cav·i·ty
  fas·cia
  fold
  fos·sa
  glands
  line
  nerve
  plex·us
  re·gion
  space
  tri·an·gle
  vein
ax·il·lary lymph
  nodes
ax·il·lary sweat
  glands
ax·i·o·buc·cal
ax·i·o·buc·co·gin·gi·val
ax·i·o·in·ci·sal
ax·i·o·la·bi·al
ax·i·o·la·bi·o·lin·gual
  plane
ax·i·o·lin·gual
ax·i·o·lin·guo·cer·vi·cal
ax·i·o·lin·guo·clu·sal
ax·i·o·lin·guo·gin·gi·val
ax·i·o·me·si·al
ax·i·o·me·si·o·cer·vi·cal
ax·i·o·me·si·o·dis·tal
  plane
ax·i·o·me·si·o·gin·gi·val
ax·i·o·me·si·o·in·ci·sal
ax·i·on
ax·io-oc·clu·sal
ax·i·o·plasm
ax·i·o·po·dia
ax·i·o·po·di·um
ax·i·o·pul·pal
ax·i·o·ver·sion
ax·ip·e·tal
ax·i·ram·if·i·cate
ax·is
  ba·si·breg·mat·ic a.
  ba·si·cra·ni·al a.
  ba·si·fa·cial a.
  bi·au·ric·u·lar a.
  ce·li·ac a.
  ceph·a·lo·cau·dal a.
  cer·e·bro·spi·nal a.
  con·dy·lar a.
  con·ju·gate a.
  cra·ni·o·fa·cial a.
  elec·tri·cal a.
  em·bry·on·ic a.
  en·ceph·a·lo·my·e·lon·ic a.

ex·ter·nal a. of eye
fa·cial a.
fron·tal a.
hinge a.
in·stan·ta·ne·ous elec·tri·cal
   a.
in·ter·nal a. of eye
a. of lens
long a.
long a. of body
man·dib·u·lar a.
mean elec·tri·cal a.
neu·ral a.
neu·tral a. of straight beam
nor·mal a.
open·ing a.
op·tic a.
or·bi·tal a.
pel·vic a.
prin·ci·pal op·tic a.
pu·pil·lary a.
ro·ta·tion·al a.
sag·it·tal a.
sec·on·dary a.
a. of sym·me·try
tho·rac·ic a.
thy·roid a.
trans·po·ri·on·ic a.
trans·verse hor·i·zon·tal a.
ver·ti·cal a.
vi·su·al a.
Y-a.
ax·is
cor·pus·cle
cyl·in·der
de·vi·a·tion
lig·a·ment of mal·le·us
shift
trac·tion
ax·is-trac·tion
for·ceps
ax·o·ax·on·ic
syn·apse
ax·o·den·drit·ic
syn·apse
ax·of·u·gal
ax·o·graph
ax·o·lem·ma
ax·ol·y·sis
ax·om·e·ter
ax·on
hil·lock
re·flex
ter·mi·nals
ax·o·nal
pro·cess
ax·o·nal ter·mi·nal
bou·tons

ax·o·neme
ax·on·og·ra·phy
ax·o·nom·e·ter
ax·o·nop·a·thy
ax·on·ot·me·sis
ax·op·e·tal
ax·o·plasm
ax·o·plas·mic
trans·port
ax·o·po·dia
ax·o·po·di·um
ax·o·so·mat·ic
syn·apse
ax·o·style
ax·ot·o·my
Ayala's
in·dex
quo·tient
Ayerza's
dis·ease
syn·drome
Ayre
brush
A.-Z.
test
aza·crine
aza·cy·clo·nol hy·dro·chlo·ride
aza·me·tho·ni·um bro·mide
aza·per·one
azap·e·tine phos·phate
aza·pro·pa·zone
azar·i·bine
aza·ser·ine
aza·spi·ro·dec·ane·di·one
azat·a·dine ma·le·ate
az·a·thi·o·prine
aze·o·trope
hal·o·thane-e·ther a.
aze·o·tro·pic
az·ide
az·i·do·thy·mi·dine
azin
dyes
az·lo·cil·lin so·di·um
azo
dyes
itch
az·o·bil·i·ru·bin
az·o·car·mine
dyes
az·o·car·mine B
az·o·car·mine G
azo·ic
az·ole
az·o·lit·min
a·zo·o·sper·mia
az·o·phlox·in
az·o·pro·tein

Azor·e·an
dis·ease
az·o·sul·fa·mide
az·o·te·mia
non·re·nal a.
pre·re·nal a.
az·o·tem·ic
ret·i·ni·tis
az·o·ther·mia
Azo·to·bac·ter
nu·cle·ase
azo·tu·ria
a. of hors·es
az·o·van blue
Az·tec
ear
az·tre·o·nam
az·ul
az·ure
a. A
a. B
a. C
a. I
a. II
az·ure
lu·nu·la of nails
az·u·res·in
az·u·ro·phil
gran·ule
az·u·ro·phile
azy·go·gram
azy·gog·ra·phy
az·y·gos
ar·tery of va·gi·na
vein
az·y·gos vein
prin·ci·ple
az·y·gos ve·nous
line
az·y·gous

B
  bile
  cell
  chain
  fi·bers
  lym·pho·cyte
  vi·rus
  wave
B$_T$
  fac·tor
Babbitt
  met·al
Babcock
  tube
Babès'
  nodes
Babès-Ernst
  bod·ies
Ba·be·sia
  B. ar·gen·ti·na
  B. ber·bera
  B. bi·gem·i·na
  B. bo·vis
  B. ca·balli
  B. ca·nis
  B. di·ver·gens
  B. equi
  B. fe·lis
  B. gib·soni
  B. mi·cro·ti
  B. mo·ta·si
  B. ovis
  B. traut·manni
Ba·be·si·el·la
Ba·be·si·i·dae
ba·be·si·o·sis
  bo·vine b.
  ca·nine b.
  equine b.
  hu·man b.
Babinski
  re·flex
Babinski's
  phe·nom·e·non
  sign
ba·by
  tooth
ba·by
  blue b.

  blue·ber·ry muf·fin b.
  col·lo·di·on b.
  gi·ant b.
  test-tube b.
bac·am·pi·cil·lin hy·dro·chlo·ride
bac·cate
Baccelli's
  sign
bac·ci·form
Bachmann's
  bun·dle
Bachman-Pettit
  test
Ba·cil·la·ce·ae
ba·cil·lar
bac·il·la·ry
  dys·en·tery
  lay·er
Ba·cil·le bi·lié de Calmette-Guérin
bac·il·le·mia
ba·cil·li
ba·cil·li·form
ba·cil·lin
ba·cil·lo·myx·in
bac·il·lo·sis
bac·il·lu·ria
Ba·cil·lus
  B. am·y·lo·li·que·fa·ci·ens
  B. an·thra·cis
  B. bre·vis
  B. ce·re·us
  B. he·mo·lyt·i·cus
  B. his·to·lyt·i·cus
  B. me·ga·te·ri·um
  B. pol·y·myxa
  B. pseu·do·diph·the·ri·ae
  B. sphae·ri·cus
  B. sub·ti·lis
  B. thu·rin·gi·en·sis
ba·cil·lus
  Abel's b.
  abor·tus b.
  ac·ne b.
  Bang's b.
  Battey b.
  blue pus b.
  Bordet-Gengou b.

ba·cil·lus *(continued)*
Calmette-Guérin b.
chol·era b.
co·lon b.
com·ma b.
Döderlein's b.
Ducrey's b.
dys·en·tery b.
Eberth's b.
Flexner's b.
Friedländer's b.
Gärtner's b.
gas b.
Ghon-Sachs b.
glan·ders b.
grass b.
Hansen's b.
hay b.
Hofmann's b.
in·flu·en·za b.
Johne's b.
Kitasato's b.
Klebs-Loeffler b.
Koch's b.
Koch-Weeks b.
lac·tic ac·id b.
lep·ro·sy b.
Loeffler's b.
mist b.
Moeller's grass b.
Morgan's b.
Much's b.
ne·cro·sis b.
par·a·co·lon b.
par·a·dys·en·tery b.
par·a·ty·phoid b.
Park-Williams b.
Pfeiffer's b.
plague b.
Plaut's b.
Plotz b.
Preisz-Nocard b.
Sachs' b.
Schmorl's b.
Schottmüller's b.
Shiga b.
Shiga-Kruse b.
Sonne b.
tim·o·thy hay b.
tu·ber·cle b.
ty·phoid b.
Vincent's b.
vole b.
Weeks' b.
Welch's b.
Whitmore's b.
Ba·cil·lus an·thra·cis
tox·in

ba·cil·lus Calmette-Guérin
vac·cine
bac·i·tra·cin
back
ad·o·les·cent round b.
hol·low b.
pok·er b.
sad·dle b.
back
cross
mu·ta·tion
pres·sure
teeth
back·ache
back-ac·tion
plug·ger
back·board
splint
back·bone
back·cross
back of foot
re·flex
back·ground
ra·di·a·tion
back·ing
back-knee
back·scat·ter
back ver·tex
pow·er
back·ward
cur·va·ture
back·ward heart
fail·ure
back·wash
il·e·i·tis
bac·lo·fen
Bacon's
ano·scope
bac·te·re·mia
bac·te·ria
bac·te·ria-free stage of bac·te·ri·al
en·do·car·di·tis
bac·te·ri·al
al·ler·gy
an·eu·rysm
an·tag·o·nism
cap·sule
end·ar·te·ri·tis
en·do·car·di·tis
he·mo·ly·sin
in·ter·fer·ence
plaque
tox·in
vi·rus
bac·te·ri·al food
poi·son·ing
bac·te·ri·cho·lia

bac·te·ri·cid·al
bac·te·ri·cide
  spe·cif·ic b.
bac·ter·id
bac·te·ri·e·mia
bac·te·ri·o·ag·glu·ti·nin
bac·te·ri·o·chlo·rin
bac·te·ri·o·chlo·ro·phyll
bac·te·ri·o·cid·al
bac·ter·i·o·cide
bac·te·ri·o·cid·in
bac·te·ri·o·cin
  fac·tors
bac·te·ri·o·cin·o·gen·ic
  plas·mids
bac·te·ri·o·cin·o·gens
bac·te·ri·o·cins
bac·te·ri·oc·la·sis
bac·te·ri·o·flu·o·res·cin
bac·te·ri·o·gen·ic
  ag·glu·ti·na·tion
bac·te·ri·og·e·nous
bac·te·ri·oid
bac·te·ri·o·log·ic
bac·te·ri·o·log·i·cal
bac·te·ri·ol·o·gist
bac·te·ri·ol·o·gy
  sys·tem·at·ic b.
bac·te·ri·o·ly·sin
bac·te·ri·ol·y·sis
bac·te·ri·o·lyt·ic
  se·rum
bac·te·ri·o·lyze
bac·te·ri·o·pexy
bac·te·ri·o·phage
  de·fec·tive b.
  fil·a·men·tous b.
  ma·ture b.
  tem·per·ate b.
  ty·phoid b.
  veg·e·ta·tive b.
  vir·u·lent b.
bac·te·ri·o·phage
  im·mu·ni·ty
  re·sis·tance
  typ·ing
bac·te·ri·o·pha·gia
bac·te·ri·o·pha·gol·o·gy
bac·te·ri·o·phe·o·phor·bide
bac·te·ri·o·phe·o·phor·bin
bac·te·ri·o·phe·o·phy·tin
bac·te·ri·o·phor·bin
bac·te·ri·o·phy·to·ma
bac·te·ri·o·pro·tein
bac·te·ri·op·so·nin
bac·te·ri·o·sis
bac·te·ri·o·sta·sis
bac·te·ri·o·stat

bac·te·ri·o·stat·ic
bac·te·ri·o·tox·ic
bac·te·ri·o·tro·pic
  sub·stance
bac·te·ri·ot·ro·pin
bac·te·ri·o·tryp·sin
Bac·te·ri·um
bac·te·ri·um
  Binn's b.
  blue-green b.
  Chauveau's b.
  en·do·ter·ic b.
  ex·o·ter·ic b.
  ly·so·gen·ic b.
  py·o·gen·ic b.
bac·te·ri·u·ria
bac·te·roid
Bac·te·roi·da·ce·ae
Bac·te·roi·des
  B. bi·vi·vus
  B. ca·pil·lo·sus
  B. cor·ro·dens
  B. disiens
  B. frag·i·lis
  B. fur·co·sus
  B. mel·a·nin·o·ge·ni·cus
  B. no·do·sus
  B. ora·lis
  B. oris
  B. pneu·mo·sin·tes
  B. prae·a·cu·tus
  B. pu·tre·di·nis
  B. ur·o·lyt·i·cus
bac·te·roi·do·sis
bac·u·li·form
Bac·u·lo·vi·ri·dae
bac·u·lum
Baehr-Lohlein
  le·sion
Baelz'
  dis·ease
Baer's
  law
  ves·i·cle
Baeyer's
  the·o·ry
bag of
  wa·ters
bag
  Am·bu b.
  breath·ing b.
  co·los·to·my b.
  Douglas b.
  nu·cle·ar b.
  Petersen's b.
  Plummer's b.
  Politzer b.

bag *(continued)*
  res·er·voir b.
  b. of wa·ters
bag·as·so·sis
Bag·dad
  boil
bag-gel
  im·plant
Baggenstoss
  change
Bagolini
  test
bah·nung
Baillarger's
  bands
  lines
Bailliart's
  oph·thal·mo·dy·na·mom·e·ter
Bainbridge
  re·flex
baked
  tongue
Baker's
  cyst
bak·er's
  ec·ze·ma
  itch
Baker's ac·id
  he·ma·te·in
Baker's pyr·i·dine
  ex·trac·tion
bak·ing
  so·da
bal·ance
  the·o·ry
  the·o·ry of sex
bal·ance
  ac·id-base b.
  gen·ic b.
  oc·clu·sal b.
  Wilhelmy b.
bal·anced
  an·es·the·sia
  ar·tic·u·la·tion
  bite
  oc·clu·sion
  pol·y·mor·phism
  trans·lo·ca·tion
bal·anc·ing
  con·tact
  side
bal·anc·ing oc·clu·sal
  sur·face
ba·lan·ic
  hy·po·spa·di·as
Ba·la·ni·tes ae·gyp·ti·a·ca

bal·a·ni·tis
  b. cir·ci·na·ta
  b. cir·cum·scrip·ta plas·ma·cel·lu·la·ris
  b. di·a·be·ti·ca
  plas·ma cell b.
  b. xe·ro·ti·ca ob·li·te·rans
  b. of Zoon
bal·a·no·blen·nor·rhea
bal·a·no·cele
bal·a·no·plas·ty
bal·a·no·pos·thi·tis
bal·a·no·pre·pu·tial
bal·a·nor·rha·gia
bal·a·nor·rhea
bal·an·tid·i·al
  dys·en·tery
bal·an·ti·di·a·sis
Ba·lan·ti·di·um
  B. co·li
  B. su·is
bal·an·ti·do·sis
bal·a·nus
BALB
  test
bald
  tongue
bald·ness
  con·gen·i·tal b.
  male pat·tern b.
  pu·bic b.
Baldy's
  op·er·a·tion
Balint's
  syn·drome
Bal·kan
  beam
  frame
  ne·phrop·a·thy
  splints
ball
  throm·bus
  valve
  var·i·ance
ball
  chon·drin b.
  dust b.
  food b.
  b. of the foot
  fun·gus b.
  hair b.
  wool b.
Ballance's
  sign
ball-and-sock·et
  joint
bal·le·ri·na-foot
  pat·tern

Ballet's
  dis·ease
  sign
bal·ling gun
bal·ling iron
bal·lism
bal·lis·mus
bal·lis·to·car·di·o·gram
bal·lis·to·car·di·o·graph
bal·lis·to·car·di·og·ra·phy
bal·lis·to·pho·bia
bal·loon
  atri·o·sep·tos·to·my
  cell
bal·loon cell
  ne·vus
bal·loon·ing
  col·li·qua·tion
  de·gen·er·a·tion
bal·loon·sep·tos·to·my
bal·loon-tip
  cath·e·ter
bal·lot·ta·ble
bal·lotte·ment
  re·nal b.
Ball's
  op·er·a·tion
ball valve
  ac·tion
ball-valve
  throm·bus
balm
  b. of Gil·e·ad
  moun·tain b.
  sweet b.
bal·ne·o·ther·a·peu·tics
bal·ne·o·ther·a·py
Baló's
  dis·ease
bal·sam
  Can·a·da b.
  b. of co·pai·ba
  Mec·ca b.
  b. of Pe·ru
  To·lu b.
bal·sam·ic
Bamberger-Marie
  dis·ease
  syn·drome
Bamberger's
  al·bu·min·ur·ia
  dis·ease
  sign
bam·boo
  hair
ba·meth·an sul·fate
ba·mif·yl·line hy·dro·chlo·ride
bam·i·pine

ban·croft·i·an
  fil·a·ri·a·sis
ban·crof·ti·a·sis
ban·crof·to·sis
band
  A b.'s
  ab·sorp·tion b.
  am·ni·ot·ic b.'s
  an·nu·lar b.
  ano·gen·i·tal b.
  atri·o·ven·tric·u·lar b.
  Baillarger's b.'s
  Bechterew's b.
  Broca's di·ag·o·nal b.
  chro·mo·some b.
  Clado's b.
  b.'s of co·lon
  con·trac·tion b.
  cor·o·nary b.
  Essick's cell b.'s
  Gennari's b.
  b. of Giacomini
  H b.
  His' b.
  Hunter-Schreger b.'s
  I b.
  il·i·o·tib·i·al b.
  b. of Kaes-Bechterew
  Ladd's b.
  Lane's b.
  M b.
  Mach's b.
  Maissiat's b.
  ma·trix b.
  Meckel's b.
  mod·er·a·tor b.
  or·tho·don·tic b.
  pec·ten b.
  per·i·op·lic b.
  Q b.'s
  Reil's b.
  Simonart's b.'s
  Soret b.
  Streeter's b.'s
  un·cus b. of Giacomini
  ven·tric·u·lar b. of lar·ynx
  Z b.
  zo·nu·lar b.
band
  cell
  neu·tro·phil
ban·dage
  sign
ban·dage
  ad·he·sive b.
  Barton's b.
  cap·e·line b.
  cir·cu·lar b.

ban·dage *(continued)*
  cra·vat b.
  cru·cial b.
  dem·i·gaunt·let b.
  Desault's b.
  elas·tic b.
  four-tailed b.
  gaunt·let b.
  gauze b.
  Gibney's fix·a·tion b.
  Gibson's b.
  ham·mock b.
  im·mov·a·ble b.
  many-tailed b.
  Martin's b.
  ob·lique b.
  plas·ter b.
  roll·er b.
  scarf b.
  Scultetus' b.
  spi·ca b.
  spi·ral b.
  sus·pen·so·ry b.
  T-b.
  tri·an·gu·lar b.
  Velpeau's b.
band·box
  res·o·nance
band·ing
  BrDu-b.
  C-b.
  G-b.
  high-res·o·lu·tion b.
  NOR-b.
  pro·met·a·phase b.
  Q-b.
  R-b.
  re·verse b.
Bandl's
  ring
band-shaped
  ker·a·top·a·thy
ban·dy-leg
bane
Bang's
  ba·cil·lus
  dis·ease
ba·nis·te·rine
Bannister's
  dis·ease
Banti's
  dis·ease
  syn·drome
bar
  clasp
bar
  arch b.
  b. of blad·der

  clasp b.
  con·nec·tor b.
  la·bi·al b.
  lin·gual b.
  me·di·an b. of Mercier
  Mercier's b.
  oc·clu·sal rest b.
  pal·a·tal b.
  Passavant's b.
  ster·nal b.
  ter·mi·nal b.
bar·ag·no·sis
Bárány's
  sign
Bárány's ca·lor·ic
  test
bar·ba
Bar·ba·dos
  leg
barb·al·o·in
barbed
  broach
bar·ber's
  itch
bar·ber's pi·lo·ni·dal
  si·nus
bar·bi·e·ro
bar·bi·tal
bar·bi·tu·rate
bar·bi·tu·ric ac·id
bar·bi·tu·rism
bar·bo·tage
bar·bu·la hir·ci
bar clasp
  arm
Barclay-Baron
  dis·ease
bar clip
  at·tach·ments
Bar·coo
  rot
  vom·it
Barcroft-Warburg
  ap·pa·ra·tus
  tech·nique
Bardet-Biedl
  syn·drome
Bardinet's
  lig·a·ment
Bard's
  sign
bare
  ar·ea of liv·er
  ar·ea of stom·ach
bare lym·pho·cyte
  syn·drome
bar·es·the·sia
bar·es·the·si·om·e·ter

bar·i·at·ric
bar·i·at·rics
ba·ric
ba·ric·i·ty
ba·ri·lla
bar·i·to·sis
bar·i·um
  b. chlo·ride
  b. hy·drox·ide
  b. mon·ox·ide
  b. ox·ide
  b. sul·fate
  b. sul·fide
bar·i·um
  en·e·ma
bar joint
  den·ture
bark
  cin·cho·na b.
  Jes·u·its' b.
  Pe·ru·vi·an b.
Barkan's
  op·er·a·tion
Barkman's
  re·flex
Barkow's
  lig·a·ment
Barlow
  syn·drome
Barlow's
  dis·ease
barn
Barnes'
  curve
  dys·tro·phy
  zone
bar·o·cep·tor
bar·o·graph
bar·o·met·ric
  pres·sure
bar·o·met·ro·graph
bar·o·phil·ic
bar·o·re·cep·tor
  nerve
bar·o·re·flex
bar·o·scope
bar·o·si·nus·i·tis
bar·o·stat
bar·o·tax·is
bar·o·ti·tis me·dia
bar·o·trau·ma
  otic b.
  si·nus b.
bar·ot·ro·pism
Barraquer's
  dis·ease
  meth·od

Barr chro·ma·tin
  body
bar·rel
  chest
bar·ren
Barré's
  sign
Barrett
  esoph·a·gus
  syn·drome
Barrett's
  ep·i·the·li·um
bar·ri·er
  blood-air b.
  blood-aque·ous b.
  blood-brain b.
  blood-ce·re·bro·spi·nal flu·id b.
  blood-CSF b.
  in·cest b.
  pla·cen·tal b.
bar-sleeve
  at·tach·ments
Bartels'
  spec·ta·cles
bar·tho·lin·i·tis
Bartholin's
  ab·scess
  anus
  cyst
  cys·tec·to·my
  duct
  gland
Barth's
  her·nia
Bar·ton·el·la
  B. ba·cil·li·for·mis
bar·ton·el·lo·sis
Barton's
  ban·dage
  for·ceps
  frac·ture
Bart's
  syn·drome
Bartter's
  syn·drome
Baruch's
  law
bar·u·ria
bar·ye
bar·y·glos·sia
bar·y·la·lia
bar·y·ma·zia
bar·y·pho·nia
ba·ry·ta
  wa·ter
ba·sad

ba·sal
  age
  an·es·the·sia
  body
  bone
  cell
  cor·pus·cle
  di·et
  gan·glia
  gran·ule
  lam·i·na
  lam·i·na of cho·roid
  lam·i·na of neu·ral tube
  lay·er
  lay·er of cho·roid
  lay·er of cil·i·ary body
  me·tab·o·lism
  part of oc·cip·i·tal bone
  part of pul·mo·nary ar·tery
  plate of neu·ral tube
  ridge
  rod
  seat
  sphinc·ter
  stri·a·tions
  sur·face
  tu·ber·cu·lo·sis
  vein of Rosenthal
  veins
ba·sal cell
  ad·e·no·ma
  car·ci·no·ma
  ep·i·the·li·o·ma
  hy·per·pla·sia
  lay·er
  ne·vus
  pap·il·lo·ma
ba·sal cell ne·vus
  syn·drome
ba·sal·i·o·ma
ba·sa·lis
ba·sal joint
  re·flex
ba·sal met·a·bol·ic
  rate
ba·sa·loid
  car·ci·no·ma
  cell
ba·sa·lo·ma
ba·sal seat
  ar·ea
ba·sal skull
  frac·ture
ba·sal squa·mous cell
  car·ci·no·ma
Basan's
  syn·drome

base
  com·po·si·tion
  def·i·cit
  ex·cess
  line
  ma·te·ri·al
  met·al
  pair
  plate
  pro·jec·tion
  units
  view
base
  acryl·ic res·in b.
  al·de·hyde b.
  an·te·ri·or cra·ni·al b.
  b. of ar·y·te·noid car·ti·lage
  b. of blad·der
  b. of brain
  Brønsted b.
  cav·i·ty prep·a·ra·tion b.
  ce·ment b.
  b. of co·chlea
  cra·ni·al b.
  den·ture b.
  b. of heart
  hex·one b.'s
  his·tone b.'s
  in·ter·nal b. of skull
  b. of lung
  b. of man·di·ble
  b. of met·a·car·pal bone
  met·al b.
  b. of met·a·tar·sal bone
  b. of mo·di·o·lus
  nu·cle·ic ac·id b.
  nu·cle·in·ic b.
  b. of pa·tel·la
  b. of pha·lanx
  pres·sor b.
  b. of pros·tate
  rec·ord b.
  b. of re·nal pyr·a·mid
  b. of sa·crum
  Schiff b.
  shel·lac b.
  b. of skull
  b. of sta·pes
  tem·po·rary b.
  tint·ed den·ture b.
  b. of tongue
  tooth-borne b.
  tri·al b.
  veg·e·ta·ble b.
base·ball
  fin·ger
bas·e·doid

ba·se·dow·i·an
in·san·i·ty
Basedow's
dis·ease
pseu·do·par·a·ple·gia
base·line
to·nus
var·i·a·bil·i·ty of fe·tal
heart rate
base·line fe·tal heart
rate
base·ment
lam·i·na
mem·brane
base·plate
wax
base·plate
sta·bi·lized b.
Basex's
syn·drome
bas-fond
ba·si·a·lis
ba·si·al·ve·o·lar
ba·si·breg·mat·ic
ax·is
ba·sic
di·et
dyes
es·o·tro·pia
ex·o·tro·pia
fuch·sin
met·al
ox·ide
per·son·al·i·ty
salt
stain
ba·sic fuch·sin-meth·yl·ene blue
stain
ba·sic·i·ty
ba·sic life sup·port
ba·sic per·son·al·i·ty
type
ba·si·cra·ni·al
ax·is
flex·ure
ba·sid·ia
Ba·sid·i·ob·o·lus
Ba·sid·i·o·my·ce·tes
ba·sid·i·o·spore
ba·sid·i·um
ba·si·fa·cial
ax·is
ba·si·hy·al
ba·si·hy·oid
bas·i·lar
an·gle
apoph·y·sis
ar·tery

bone
car·ti·lage
cell
crest of co·chle·ar duct
im·pres·sion
in·dex
in·vag·i·na·tion
lam·i·na
lep·to·men·in·gi·tis
mem·brane
men·in·gi·tis
part of pons
plex·us
pro·cess
prog·na·thism
si·nus
sul·cus
ver·te·bra
bas·i·la·ris
ba·si·lat·er·al
ba·si·lem·ma
ba·sil·ic
vein
ba·sil·i·cus
ba·sin
em·e·sis b.
kid·ney b.
pus b.
ba·si·na·sal
line
ba·si·oc·cip·i·tal
bone
ba·si·o·glos·sus
ba·si·on
ba·sip·e·tal
ba·si·pha·ryn·ge·al
ca·nal
bas·i·pho·bia
ba·sis
b. ce·re·bri
b. pe·dun·cu·li
ba·si·sphe·noid
bone
ba·si·squa·mous
car·ci·no·ma
ba·si·tem·po·ral
ba·si·ver·te·bral
vein
bas·ket
cell
bas·ket
fi·bril·lar b.'s
stone b.
ba·so·cyte
ba·so·cy·to·pe·nia
ba·so·cy·to·sis
ba·so·e·ryth·ro·cyte
ba·so·e·ryth·ro·cy·to·sis

ba·so·graph
ba·so·lat·er·al
ba·so·met·a·chro·mo·phil
ba·so·met·a·chro·mo·phile
ba·so·pe·nia
ba·so·phil
  tis·sue b.
ba·so·phil
  ad·e·no·ma
  cell of an·te·ri·or lobe of
    hy·poph·y·sis
  gran·ule
  sub·stance
ba·so·phile
ba·so·phil·ia
  Grawitz' b.
  pi·tu·i·tary b.
  punc·tate b.
ba·so·phil·ic
  de·gen·er·a·tion
  leu·ke·mia
  leu·ko·cyte
  leu·ko·cy·to·sis
  leu·ko·pe·nia
ba·soph·i·lism
  Cushing's b.
  pi·tu·i·tary b.
ba·so·phil·o·cyte
ba·so·phil·o·cyt·ic
  leu·ke·mia
ba·so·plasm
ba·so·squa·mous
  car·ci·no·ma
Bassen-Kornzweig
  syn·drome
Bassini's
  op·er·a·tion
Bassler's
  sign
Bas·so·ra
  gum
bas·sor·in
Bastedo's
  sign
bat
  vam·pire b.
bath
  col·loid b.
  con·trast b.
  douche b.
  dous·ing b.
  elec·tric b.
  elec·tro·ther·a·peu·tic b.
  Greville b.
  ha·fussi b.
  hy·dro·e·lec·tric b.
  light b.
  Nau·heim b.

  nee·dle b.
  oil b.
  sand b.
  sitz b.
  wa·ter b.
bath
  itch
  pru·ri·tus
bath·ing trunk
  ne·vus
bath·mic
  ev·o·lu·tion
bath·mo·tro·pic
  neg·a·tive·ly b.
  pos·i·tive·ly b.
bath·o·chro·mic
bath·o·flore
bath·o·pho·bia
bath·y·an·es·the·sia
bath·y·car·dia
bath·y·es·the·sia
bath·y·gas·try
bath·y·hy·per·es·the·sia
bath·y·hyp·es·the·sia
Batson's
  plex·us
Batten-Mayou
  dis·ease
bat·tered child
  syn·drome
bat·tery
  Halstead-Reitan b.
Battey
  ba·cil·lus
bat·tle
  fa·tigue
  neu·ro·sis
bat·tle·dore
  pla·cen·ta
Battle's
  sign
Baudelocque's
  di·am·e·ter
  op·er·a·tion
Baudelocque's uter·ine
  cir·cle
Bauer's
  syn·drome
Bauer's chro·mic ac·id leu·co·
  fuch·sin
  stain
Bauhin's
  gland
  valve
Baumé
  scale
Baumès
  symp·tom

Baumgarten's
  glands
  veins
baux·ite
  pneu·mo·co·ni·o·sis
bay
  sore
bay
  ce·lom·ic b.'s
  lac·ri·mal b.
bay·ber·ry bark
Bayes
  the·o·rem
Bayle's
  dis·ease
Bayley
  Scales of In·fant De·vel·op·
  ment
bay·o·net
  hair
Bazett's
  for·mu·la
Bazin's
  dis·ease
BCG
  vac·cine
Be^a
  an·ti·gens
bead·ed
  hair
bead·ing
  b. of the ribs
beak
beaked
  pel·vis
beak·er
  cell
Beale's
  cell
Béal's
  con·junc·ti·vi·tis
beam
  Bal·kan b.
  can·ti·le·ver b.
  con·tin·u·ous b.
  re·strained b.
  sim·ple b.
bean
bear·ing
  cen·tral b.
bear·ing-down
  pain
beat
  apex b.
  atri·al fu·sion b.
  au·to·mat·ic b.
  cap·ture b.
  com·bi·na·tion b.

  cou·pled b.'s
  de·pen·dent b.
  Dressler b.
  dropped b.
  echo b.
  ec·top·ic b.
  es·cape b.
  es·caped b.
  forced b.
  fu·sion b.
  heart b.
  in·ter·fer·ence b.
  mixed b.
  paired b.'s
  par·a·sys·tol·ic b.
  pre·ma·ture b.
  pseu·do·fu·sion b.
  re·cip·ro·cal b.
  ret·ro·grade b.
  sum·ma·tion b.
  ven·tric·u·lar fu·sion b.
beat-to-beat
  var·i·a·tion of fe·tal heart
  rate
Beau's
  lines
Beau·var·ia
be·can·thone hy·dro·chlo·ride
Bechterew-Mendel
  re·flex
Bechterew's
  band
  dis·ease
  nu·cle·us
  sign
Becker
  an·ti·gen
Becker's
  dis·ease
  ne·vus
  stain for spi·ro·chetes
Becker type tar·dive mus·cu·lar
  dys·tro·phy
Beckmann's
  ap·pa·ra·tus
Beck's
  meth·od
  tri·ad
Beckwith-Wiedemann
  syn·drome
Béclard's
  anas·to·mo·sis
  her·nia
  tri·an·gle
be·clo·meth·a·sone di·pro·pi·o·
nate
Becquerel
  rays

bec·que·rel
bed
  cap·il·lary b.
  frac·ture b.
  Gatch b.
  mud b.
  nail b.
  wa·ter b.
bed
  sore
bed·bug
bed·lam
Bednar
  tu·mor
Bednar's
  aph·thae
Bed·so·nia
bed·sore
bed-wet·ting
beech oil
beech·wood
  sug·ar
beech·wood tar
beer
  heart
beer-drink·er's
  car·di·o·my·op·a·thy
Beer's
  knife
  law
  op·er·a·tion
bees·wax
  white b.
beet
  sug·ar
beet-tongue
bee·tu·ria
Beevor's
  sign
Begbie's
  dis·ease
Begg light wire dif·fer·en·tial force
  tech·nique
Béguez César
  dis·ease
be·hav·ior
  chain
  dis·or·der
  ge·net·ics
  mod·i·fi·ca·tion
  re·flex
  ther·a·py
be·hav·ior
  adap·tive b.
  ad·i·ent b.
  am·bi·ent b.
  ap·pet·i·tive b.

aver·sive b.
hook·e·an b.
mo·lar b.
mo·lec·u·lar b.
ob·ses·sive b.
op·er·ant b.
pas·sive-ag·gres·sive b.
re·spon·dent b.
rit·u·al·is·tic b.
tar·get b.
type A b.
type B b.
be·hav·ior·al
  im·mu·no·gen
  man·i·fes·ta·tion
  med·i·cine
  path·o·gen
  psy·chol·o·gy
be·hav·ior·ism
be·hav·ior·ist
Behçet's
  dis·ease
  syn·drome
be·hen·ic ac·id
Behring's
  law
Behr's
  dis·ease
  syn·drome
BEI
  test
bej·el
Békésy
  au·di·om·e·ter
  au·di·om·e·try
belch·ing
bel·em·noid
Bel·gian Con·go
  ane·mia
bell
  sound
bel·la·don·na
bel·la·don·nine
bell-crowned
belle in·dif·fer·ence
Bellini's
  ducts
  lig·a·ment
Bell-Magendie
  law
bell·met·al
  res·o·nance
bel·lows
  mur·mur
Bell's
  law
  mus·cle
  pal·sy

phe·nom·e·non
spasm
bell-shaped
crown
Bell's res·pi·ra·to·ry
nerve
bel·ly
b.'s of di·gas·tric mus·cle
fron·tal b.
oc·cip·i·tal b.
b.'s of omo·hy·oid mus·cle
prune b.
bel·ly·ache
bel·ly but·ton
bel·o·ne·pho·bia
Belsey
op·er·a·tion
belt
test
bem·e·gride
ben·ac·ty·zine hy·dro·chlo·ride
Bence Jones
al·bu·min
cyl·in·ders
my·e·lo·ma
pro·tein
pro·tein·u·ria
re·ac·tion
ben·da·zac
Bender ge·stalt
test
bend·ing
frac·ture
ben·dro·flu·a·zide
ben·dro·flu·me·thi·a·zide
bends
ben·e·cep·tor
Benedek's
re·flex
Benedict-Hopkins-Cole
re·a·gent
Benedict-Roth
ap·pa·ra·tus
cal·o·rim·e·ter
Benedict's
so·lu·tion
test for glu·cose
Benedikt's
syn·drome
be·nign
al·bu·min·ur·ia
ce·ment·o·blas·to·ma
dys·ker·a·to·sis
gly·cos·ur·ia
hy·per·ten·sion
lym·phad·e·no·sis
lym·pho·cy·to·ma cu·tis
lym·pho·ma of the rec·tum

mes·o·the·li·o·ma of gen·i·tal tract
neph·ro·scle·ro·sis
stu·por
tet·a·nus
tu·mor
be·nign bone
an·eu·rysm
be·nign bo·vine
thei·le·ri·o·sis
be·nign chron·ic bul·lous
der·ma·to·sis of child·hood
be·nign dry
pleu·ri·sy
be·nign es·sen·tial
trem·or
be·nign fa·mil·i·al
ic·ter·us
be·nign in·oc·u·la·tion
lym·pho·re·tic·u·lo·sis
re·tic·u·lo·sis
be·nign ju·ve·nile
mel·a·no·ma
be·nign lym·pho·ep·i·the·li·al
le·sion
be·nign me·di·as·ti·nal lymph node
hy·per·pla·sia
be·nign mes·en·chy·mo·ma
be·nign mi·gra·to·ry
glos·si·tis
be·nign mu·co·sal
pem·phi·goid
be·nign my·al·gic
en·ceph·a·lo·my·e·li·tis
be·nign par·ox·ys·mal
per·i·to·ni·tis
be·nign pros·tat·ic
hy·per·tro·phy
be·nign ter·tian
ma·lar·ia
Béniqué's
sound
ben·ne oil
Bennett
an·gle
move·ment
Bennett's
frac·ture
Bennhold's Con·go red
stain
Benois
scale
ben·ox·a·pro·fen
ben·ox·in·ate hy·dro·chlo·ride
ben·per·i·dol
Bensley's spe·cif·ic
gran·ules

Benson's
dis·ease
ben·tir·o·mide
test
ben·ton·ite
ben·ton·ite floc·cu·la·tion
test
ben·zal·ac·e·to·phe·none
benz·al·de·hyde
ben·zal·ko·ni·um chlo·ride
benz·am·ide
ben·zan·threne
ben·zene
b. bro·mide
ben·zene
nu·cle·us
ring
ben·zene·a·mine
ben·zes·trol
benz·e·tho·ni·um chlo·ride
ben·zi·dine
test
benz·im·id·az·ole
ben·zin
ben·zin·da·mine hy·dro·chlo·ride
ben·zine
ben·zi·o·da·rone
ben·zo·ate
ben·zo·at·ed
ben·zo·caine
ben·zoc·ta·mine hy·dro·chlo·ride
ben·zo·di·az·e·pine
ben·zo·ic
ben·zo·ic ac·id
ben·zo·ic al·de·hyde
ben·zo·in
ben·zol
ben·zo·mor·phan
ben·zo·na·tate
ben·zo·qui·no·ni·um chlo·ride
ben·zo·res·in·ol
ben·zo·sul·fi·mide
ben·zo·thi·a·di·a·zides
ben·zox·i·quine
ben·zox·y·line
ben·zo·yl
b. chlo·ride
b. hy·drate
b. per·ox·ide
ben·zo·yl·cho·lin·es·ter·ase
ben·zo·yl·pas cal·ci·um
benz·per·i·dol
benz·phet·a·mine hy·dro·chlo·ride
benz·pyr·in·i·um bro·mide
benz·quin·a·mide

benz·stig·mi·num bro·mi·dum
benz·thi·a·zide
benz·tro·pine mes·y·late
ben·zyd·a·mine hy·dro·chlo·ride
ben·zyl
b. al·co·hol
b. ben·zo·ate
b. ben·zo·ate-chlo·ro·phe·no·thane-eth·yl ami·no·ben·zo·ate
b. car·bi·nol
b. cin·na·mate
b. fu·ma·rate
b. man·del·ate
b. suc·ci·nate
ben·zyl·ic
ben·zyl·i·dene
ben·zyl·ox·y·car·bon·yl
ben·zyl·pen·i·cil·lin
be·phen·i·um hy·drox·y·naph·tho·ate
Beradinelli's
syn·drome
Bérard's
an·eu·rysm
Béraud's
valve
ber·ber·ine
Berger
cells
rhythm
Berger's
par·es·the·sia
space
Berger's fo·cal
glo·mer·u·lo·ne·phri·tis
Bergmann's
cords
fi·bers
Bergmeister's
pa·pil·la
Berg's
stain
ber·i·beri
dry b.
wet b.
berke·li·um
Ber·lin blue
Ber·lin's
ede·ma
ber·lock
der·ma·ti·tis
ber·loque
der·ma·ti·tis
Bernard-Cannon
ho·me·o·sta·sis
Bernard-Horner
syn·drome

Bernard's
ca·nal
duct
punc·ture
Bernard-Sergent
syn·drome
Bernard-Soulier
syn·drome
Bernays'
sponge
Bernhardt-Roth
syn·drome
Bernhardt's
dis·ease
for·mu·la
Bernheim's
syn·drome
Bernoulli
ef·fect
Bernoulli's
law
prin·ci·ple
the·o·rem
Bernstein
test
ber·ry
an·eu·rysm
cell
Berry's
lig·a·ment
Berson
test
Berthelot
re·ac·tion
Berthollet's
law
ber·ti·el·lo·sis
Bertin's
bones
col·umns
lig·a·ment
os·si·cles
be·ryl·li·o·sis
be·ryl·li·um
gran·u·lo·ma
Besnier-Boeck-Schaumann
dis·ease
syn·drome
Besnier's
pru·ri·go
Bes·noi·tia
B. ben·netti
B. bes·noiti
B. ta·ran·di
bes·noi·ti·a·sis
Bes·noi·ti·i·dae
bes·noi·ti·o·sis

bes·ti·al·i·ty
Best's
dis·ease
Best's car·mine
stain
be·ta
al·co·hol·ism
an·gle
cell of an·te·ri·or lobe of
hy·poph·y·sis
cell of pan·cre·as
fi·bers
gran·ule
par·ti·cle
ra·di·a·tion
ray
rhythm
sub·stance
wave
beta-
ox·i·da·tion
be·ta-block·er
be·ta·cism
be·ta·cy·a·ni·nu·ria
be·ta·his·tine hy·dro·chlo·ride
be·ta·ine
b. al·de·hyde
b. hy·dro·chlo·ride
**be·ta·ine-al·de·hyde de·hy·dro·
gen·ase**
be·ta·meth·a·sone
be·tan·i·dine sul·fate
**be·ta-ox·i·da·tion-con·den·sa·
tion**
the·o·ry
be·ta·tron
be·tax·o·lol hy·dro·chlo·ride
be·ta·zole hy·dro·chlo·ride
be·tel
can·cer
be·tel nut
be·tha·ne·chol chlo·ride
be·than·i·dine sul·fate
Be·thes·da
unit
Bethesda-Ballerup Group
Betke-Kleihauer
test
Bettendorff's
test
bet·u·la oil
Betz
cells
Beuren
syn·drome
Bevan-Lewis
cells

bev·el
    ca·vo·sur·face b.
    re·verse b.
bev·elled
    anas·to·mo·sis
be·vo·ni·um meth·yl sul·fate
be·zoar
Bezold-Jarisch
    re·flex
Bezold's
    ab·scess
    gan·gli·on
    mas·toid·i·tis
    per·fo·ra·tion
    sign
    symp·tom
    tri·ad
BH
    in·ter·val
bhang
Bi
    an·ti·gen
bi·a·lam·i·col hy·dro·chlo·ride
Bial's
    test
Bianchi's
    nod·ule
    valve
bi·ar·tic·u·lar
bi·as·te·ri·on·ic
bi·au·ric·u·lar
    ax·is
bi·ax·i·al
    joint
bi·ba·sic
bi·ben·zo·ni·um bro·mide
bi-bi
    re·ac·tion
bib·li·o·ma·nia
bib·u·lous
bi·cam·er·al
    ab·scess
bi·can·a·lic·u·lar
    sphinc·ter
bi·cap·su·lar
bi·car·bon·ate
    stan·dard b.
bi·car·di·o·gram
bi·cel·lu·lar
bi·ceph·a·lus
bi·ceps
    mus·cle of arm
    mus·cle of thigh
    re·flex
bi·ceps fe·mo·ris
    re·flex
Bichat's
    ca·nal

    fat-pad
    fis·sure
    fo·ra·men
    fos·sa
    lig·a·ment
    mem·brane
    pro·tu·ber·ance
    tu·nic
bi·chlo·ride
bi·cho
bi·chro·mate
bi·cil·i·ate
bi·cip·i·tal
    ap·o·neu·ro·sis
    bur·si·tis
    fas·cia
    groove
    rib
    ridg·es
    tu·ber·os·i·ty
bi·cip·i·to·ra·di·al
    bur·sa
Bickel's
    ring
bi·clo·nal
    gam·mop·a·thy
bi·clon·al·i·ty
bi·clo·nal peak
bi·con·cave
    lens
bi·con·dy·lar
    ar·tic·u·la·tion
    joint
bi·con·vex
    lens
bi·cor·nate
    uter·us
bi·cor·nous
bi·cor·nu·ate
bi·cou·date
    cath·e·ter
bi·cron
bi·cus·pid
    tooth
    valve
bi·cus·pi·di·za·tion
bi·dac·ty·ly
bi·det
bi·di·rec·tion·al ven·tric·u·lar
    tach·y·car·dia
bi·dis·coi·dal
    pla·cen·ta
bid·u·ous
Biebl
    loop
Biebrich scar·let red
Biederman's
    sign

Bielschowsky's
dis·ease
sign
stain
Biemond
syn·drome
Biermer's
ane·mia
dis·ease
sign
Biernacki's
sign
Bier's
am·pu·ta·tion
hy·per·e·mia
meth·od
Biesiadecki's
fos·sa
bi·fas·cic·u·lar
bi·fid
cra·ni·um
pe·nis
rib
tongue
uter·us
uvu·la
Bi·fi·do·bac·te·ri·um
B. bi·fi·dum
bif·i·dus
fac·tor
bi·fo·cal
lens
spec·ta·cles
bi·fo·rate
uter·us
bi·fo·ve·al
fix·a·tion
bi·fur·cate
bi·fur·cat·ed
lig·a·ment
bi·fur·ca·tio
bi·fur·ca·tion
b. of aor·ta
b. of pul·mo·nary trunk
b. of tra·chea
bi·fur·ca·tion lymph
nodes
Bigelow's
lig·a·ment
sep·tum
bi·gem·i·na
bi·gem·i·nal
bod·ies
preg·nan·cy
pulse
rhythm
bi·gem·i·ni
bi·gem·i·num

bi·gem·i·ny
atri·al b.
atri·o·ven·tric·u·lar no·dal b.
A-V no·dal b.
es·cape-cap·ture b.
no·dal b.
re·cip·ro·cal b.
ven·tric·u·lar b.
bi·ger·min·al
big-head
bi·git·a·lin
big liv·er
dis·ease
bi·labe
bi·lam·i·nar
blas·to·derm
bi·lat·er·al
hem·i·a·nop·sia
her·maph·ro·dit·ism
left-sid·ed·ness
li·thot·o·my
syn·chro·ny
bi·lat·er·al·ism
bile
A b.
B b.
C b.
white b.
bile
ac·ids
cap·il·lary
cyst
duct
pa·pil·la
per·i·to·ni·tis
pig·ments
salts
throm·bus
bile ac·id tol·er·ance
test
bile pig·ment
he·mo·glo·bin
Bile's
an·ti·gen
bile salt
agar
Bil·har·zia
bil·har·zi·al
ap·pen·di·ci·tis
dys·en·tery
gran·u·lo·ma
bil·har·zi·a·sis
bil·har·zi·o·ma
bil·har·zi·o·sis
bil·i·ary
atre·sia
cal·cu·lus

bil·i·ary *(continued)*
  can·a·lic·u·lus
  cir·rho·sis
  col·ic
  duct
  duc·tules
  dys·ki·ne·sia
  fe·ver of dogs
  fe·ver of hors·es
  fis·tu·la
  ste·a·tor·rhea
  xan·tho·ma·to·sis
bil·i·fac·tion
bil·if·er·ous
bil·i·fi·ca·tion
bil·i·gen·e·sis
bil·i·gen·ic
bi·lin
bi·line
bil·ious
  head·ache
  ty·phoid of Griesinger
bil·ious·ness
bil·ious re·mit·tent
  fe·ver
  ma·lar·ia
bil·ip·ty·sis
bil·i·ra·chia
bil·i·ru·bin
  con·ju·gat·ed b.
  di·rect re·act·ing b.
  in·di·rect re·act·ing b.
  un·con·ju·gat·ed b.
bil·i·ru·bin
  en·ceph·a·lop·a·thy
bil·i·ru·bi·ne·mia
bil·i·ru·bin·glob·u·lin
bil·i·ru·bin-glu·cu·ron·o·side
  glu·cu·ron·o·syl·trans·fer·ase
bil·i·ru·bin·oids
bil·i·ru·bi·nu·ria
bil·i·ther·a·py
bil·i·u·ria
bil·i·ver·din
bil·i·ver·dine
bil·i·ver·din·glo·bin
Billroth I
  anas·to·mo·sis
Billroth II
  anas·to·mo·sis
Billroth's
  cords
  op·er·a·tion I
  op·er·a·tion II
  ve·nae ca·ver·no·sae
Bill's
  ma·neu·ver
bi·lo·bate

bi·lobed
  flap
bi·lob·u·lar
bi·loc·u·lar
  joint
  stom·ach
bi·loc·u·lar fem·o·ral
  her·nia
bi·loc·u·late
bi·loph·o·dont
bi·man·u·al
  per·cus·sion
  ver·sion
bi·mas·toid
bi·max·il·lary
  pro·tru·sion
bi·max·il·lary den·to·al·ve·o·lar
  pro·tru·sion
bi·max·il·lary pro·tru·sive
  oc·clu·sion
bi·mod·al
bi·mo·lec·u·lar
bin·an·gle
  chis·el
bi·na·ry
  com·bi·na·tion
  fis·sion
  no·men·cla·ture
bi·na·sal
  hem·i·a·nop·sia
bin·au·ral
  steth·o·scope
bin·au·ral al·ter·nate loud·ness
  bal·ance
  test
bin·au·ric·u·lar
  arc
bind
  dou·ble b.
bind·er
  ob·stet·ri·cal b.
  T-b.
bind·ing
  en·er·gy
Binet
  age
  scale
  test
Binet-Simon
  scale
Bingham
  mod·el
  plas·tic
Bing's
  re·flex
Binn's
  bac·te·ri·um

bin·oc·u·lar
 fix·a·tion
 hem·i·a·nop·sia
 het·er·o·chro·mia
 loupe
 mi·cro·scope
 oph·thal·mo·scope
 par·al·lax
 ri·val·ry
 vi·sion
bi·no·mi·al
 dis·tri·bu·tion
 no·men·cla·ture
bin·ot·ic
bin·ov·u·lar
Binswanger's
 dis·ease
 en·ceph·a·lop·a·thy
bi·nu·cle·ar
bi·nu·cle·ate
bi·nu·cle·o·late
Binz'
 test
bi·o·a·cous·tics
bi·o·as·say
bi·o·as·tro·nau·tics
bi·o·a·vail·a·bil·i·ty
bi·o·ce·no·sis
bi·o·chem·i·cal
 ge·net·ics
 me·tas·ta·sis
 phar·ma·col·o·gy
 pro·file
bi·o·chem·i·cal path·way
bi·o·chem·is·try
bi·o·che·mor·phic
bi·o·che·mor·phol·o·gy
bi·o·cid·al
bi·o·cli·ma·tol·o·gy
bi·o·cy·tin
bi·o·cy·tin·ase
bi·o·de·grad·a·ble
bi·o·deg·ra·da·tion
bi·o·dy·nam·ic
bi·o·dy·nam·ics
bi·o·e·col·o·gy
bi·o·e·lec·tric
 po·ten·tial
bi·o·en·er·get·ics
bi·o·en·gi·neer·ing
bi·o·feed·back
bi·o·fla·vo·noids
bi·o·gen·e·sis
bi·o·ge·net·ic
 law
bi·o·ge·o·chem·is·try
bi·o·grav·ics
bi·o·in·stru·ment

bi·o·ki·net·ics
bi·o·log·ic
 ev·o·lu·tion
 he·mol·y·sis
 time
bi·o·log·i·cal
 chem·is·try
 co·ef·fi·cient
 con·trol
 half-life
 vec·tor
bi·o·log·i·cal stan·dard
 unit
bi·ol·o·gist
bi·ol·o·gy
 cel·lu·lar b.
 mo·lec·u·lar b.
 oral b.
 ra·di·a·tion b.
bi·o·lu·mi·nes·cence
bi·ol·y·sis
bi·o·lyt·ic
bi·o·mass
bi·ome
bi·o·me·chan·ics
 den·tal b.
bi·o·med·i·cal
 en·gi·neer·ing
bi·om·e·ter
bi·o·me·tri·cian
bi·om·e·try
bi·o·mi·cro·scope
bi·o·mi·cros·co·py
Bi·om·pha·la·ria
bi·on
Biondi-Heidenhain
 stain
bi·o·ne·cro·sis
bi·on·ic
bi·on·ics
bi·o·nom·ics
bi·on·o·my
bi·o·phage
bi·oph·a·gism
bi·oph·a·gous
bi·oph·a·gy
bi·o·phar·ma·ceu·tics
bi·o·phil·ia
bi·o·pho·tom·e·ter
bi·o·phy·lac·tic
bi·o·phy·lax·is
bi·o·phys·ics
 den·tal b.
bi·o·plasm
bi·o·plas·mic
bi·op·sy
 as·pi·ra·tion b.
 brush b.

bi·op·sy *(continued)*
  en·do·scop·ic b.
  ex·ci·sion b.
  in·ci·sion b.
  nee·dle b.
  open b.
  punch b.
  shave b.
  sponge b.
  tre·phine b.
  wedge b.
bi·op·sy
  nee·dle
bi·o·psy·chol·o·gy
bi·op·ter·in
bi·o·py·o·cul·ture
bi·or·bit·al
  an·gle
bi·o·rhe·ol·o·gy
bi·o·rhythm
bi·o·roent·gen·og·ra·phy
bi·ose
bi·o·side
bi·o·sis
bi·o·so·cial
bi·o·spec·trom·e·try
bi·o·spec·tros·co·py
bi·o·spe·le·ol·o·gy
bi·o·sphere
bi·o·stat·ics
bi·o·sta·tis·tics
bi·o·syn·the·sis
bi·o·syn·thet·ic
bi·o·sys·tem
bi·o·ta
bi·o·tax·is
bi·o·te·lem·e·try
bi·ot·ic
  com·mu·ni·ty
  fac·tors
  po·ten·tial
bi·ot·ics
bi·o·tin
  b. ox·i·dase
bi·o·tin·i·dase
bi·ot·i·nides
bi·o·tin·yl·ly·sine
bi·o·tope
bi·o·tox·i·col·o·gy
bi·o·tox·in
bi·o·trans·for·ma·tion
bi·o·tro·pism
Biot's
  breath·ing
  res·pi·ra·tion
bi·o·type
bi·o·var

bi·o·vu·lar
bi·pal·a·ti·noid
bi·par·a·sit·ism
bi·pa·ren·tal
bi·pa·ri·e·tal
  di·am·e·ter
bip·a·rous
bi·par·tite
  uter·us
bi·ped
bi·ped·al
bi·ped·i·cle
  flap
bi·pen·nate
  mus·cle
bi·pen·ni·form
bi·per·fo·rate
bi·per·i·den
bi·pha·sic
  in·su·lin
  re·sponse
bi·phen·a·mine hy·dro·chlo·ride
bi·phe·no·ty·pic
bi·phe·no·ty·py
bi·phen·yl
  pol·y·chlo·rin·at·ed b.
bi·po·lar
  cau·tery
  cell
  dis·or·der
  lead
  neu·ron
  tax·is
  ver·sion
bi·po·ten·ti·al·i·ty
bi·ra·mous
Birbeck's
  gran·ule
Birch-Hirschfeld
  stain
birch tar
birch tar oil
bird
  face
  unit
bird-breed·er's
  dis·ease
  lung
bird-fan·ci·er's
  lung
Bird's
  sign
bird shot
  ret·i·no·cho·roid·i·tis
bi·re·frin·gence
bi·re·frin·gent
bi·ro·ta·tion

birth
  cross b.
  pre·ma·ture b.
birth
  am·pu·ta·tion
  ca·nal
  con·trol
  frac·ture
  pal·sy
  rate
  trau·ma
  weight
birth·mark
  straw·ber·ry b.
bis·ac·o·dyl
bis·a·cro·mi·al
bis·al·bu·mi·ne·mia
bi·salt
bis·ax·il·lary
Bischof's
  my·e·lot·o·my
bis·cuit
  bite
bis·cuit-bake
bis·cuit-fir·ing
bis·de·qua·lin·i·um chlo·ride
bis in die
bi·sex·u·al
bis·fer·i·ous
  pulse
Bishop's
  sphyg·mo·scope
bis·hy·drox·y·cou·ma·rin
bis·il·i·ac
Bis·kra
  but·ton
Bismarck brown R
Bismarck brown Y
bis·muth
  b. alu·mi·nate
  b. am·mo·ni·um cit·rate
  b. car·bon·ate
  b. chlo·ride ox·ide
  b. cit·rate
  b. io·dide
  b. ox·ide
  b. ox·y·car·bon·ate
  b. ox·y·chlo·ride
  b. ox·y·ni·trate
  b. sa·lic·y·late
  b. so·di·um tar·trate
  b. so·di·um tri·gly·col·la·
  mate
  b. sub·car·bon·ate
  b. sub·gal·late
  b. sub·ni·trate
  b. sub·sa·lic·y·late
  b. tri·bro·mo·phe·nate

  b. tri·bro·mo·phe·nol
  b. tri·chlo·ride
  b. tri·i·o·dide
bis·muth
  line
bis·mu·tho·sis
bis·muth·yl
  b. car·bon·ate
  b. chlo·ride
bis·ox·a·tin ac·e·tate
bi·ste·phan·ic
bi·ste·roid
bis·tou·ry
bi·stra·tal
bi·sul·fate
bi·sul·fide
bi·sul·fite
bi·tar·trate
bitch
bite
  bal·anced b.
  bis·cuit b.
  close b.
  closed b.
  deep b.
  edge-to-edge b.
  end-to-end b.
  jump·ing the b.
  locked b.
  nor·mal b.
  open b.
  rest b.
  work·ing b.
bite
  anal·y·sis
  fork
  gauge
  plane
  rim
bi·tem·po·ral
  hem·i·a·nop·sia
bite·plane
bite·plate
bites
bite·wing
  film
  ra·di·o·graph
bi·thi·o·nol
bit·ing
  louse
  pres·sure
  strength
bi·tol·ter·ol mes·y·late
Bitot's
  spots
bi·tro·chan·ter·ic
bi·tro·pic

bit·ter
  al·mond oil
  or·ange peel
  or·ange peel, dried
  or·ange peel, fresh
  or·ange peel oil
  ton·ic
  wa·ter
bit·ter ap·ple
bit·ters
  ar·o·mat·ic b.
Bittner
  agent
Bittner's milk
  fac·tor
Bittorf's
  re·ac·tion
bi·un·du·lant
  me·nin·go·en·ceph·a·li·tis
bi·u·ret
  re·ac·tion
  re·a·gent
  test
bi·va·lence
bi·va·len·cy
bi·va·lent
  an·ti·body
  chro·mo·some
bi·va·lent gas gan·grene
  an·ti·tox·in
bi·valve
  spec·u·lum
bi·ven·ter
  b. cer·vi·cis
  b. man·dib·u·lae
bi·ven·tral
  lob·ule
bix·in
bi·zy·go·mat·ic
Bizzozero's
  cor·pus·cle
Bizzozero's red
  cells
Bjerrum
  screen
Bjerrum's
  sco·to·ma
  sign
Bjornstad's
  syn·drome
BK
  vi·rus
B-K mole
  syn·drome
black
  cat·a·ract
  death
  dis·ease

  eye
  fe·ver
  jaun·dice
  lead
  line
  lung
  mea·sles
  mus·tard
  pie·dra
  plague
  sick·ness
  spore
  ta·ran·tu·la
  tongue
  urine
  vom·it
  wa·ter
black cur·rant
  rash
black-dot
  ring·worm
black·head
black·leg
black·out
  vi·su·al b.
Black's
  clas·si·fi·ca·tion
  for·mu·la
black-tongue
  dis·ease
black·wa·ter
  fe·ver
blad·der
  re·flex
  schis·to·so·mi·a·sis
blad·der
  air b.
  al·lan·to·ic b.
  aton·ic b.
  au·to·nom·ic neu·ro·gen·ic
    b.
  cord b.
  fas·cic·u·late b.
  gall b.
  il·e·al b.
  low-com·pli·ance b.
  ner·vous b.
  neu·ro·gen·ic b.
  pseu·do·neu·ro·gen·ic b.
  re·flex neu·ro·gen·ic b.
  swim b.
  un·in·hib·i·ted neu·ro·gen·
    ic b.
  uri·nary b.
blad·der·worm
blade
  bone
blade·vent

Blagden's
law
blain
Blainville
ears
Blair-Brown
graft
Blalock-Hanlon
op·er·a·tion
Blalock-Taussig
op·er·a·tion
bland
di·et
em·bo·lism
in·farct
Blandin's
gland
blan·ket
su·ture
Blasius'
duct
Blaskovics'
op·er·a·tion
blast
cell
chest
cri·sis
in·ju·ry
blas·te·ma
neph·ric b.
blas·tem·ic
blas·to·cele
blas·to·cel·ic
blas·to·coele
blas·to·coel·ic
Blas·to·co·nid·i·um
blas·to·cyst
blas·to·cyte
blas·to·cy·to·ma
blas·to·derm
bi·lam·i·nar b.
em·bry·on·ic b.
ex·tra·em·bry·on·ic b.
tri·lam·i·nar b.
blas·to·der·ma
blas·to·der·mal
blas·to·der·mic
disk
lay·ers
ves·i·cle
blas·to·disk
blas·to·gen·e·sis
blas·to·ge·net·ic
blas·to·gen·ic
blas·tol·y·sis
blas·to·lyt·ic
blas·to·ma
blas·to·mere

blas·to·mer·ot·o·my
blas·to·mo·gen·ic
Blas·to·my·ces der·ma·tit·i·dis
blas·to·my·ce·tic
der·ma·ti·tis
blas·to·my·cin
blas·to·my·co·sis
North Amer·i·can b.
South Amer·i·can b.
blas·to·neu·ro·pore
blas·to·phore
blas·to·pore
blas·to·por·ic
ca·nal
blas·to·spore
blas·tot·o·my
blas·tu·la
blas·tu·lar
blas·tu·la·tion
Blatin's
syn·drome
Blat·ta
Blat·tel·la
Blat·ti·dae
bleached
wax
bleach·ing
pow·der
blear
eye
bleb
bleed
bleed·er
bleed·ing
dys·func·tion·al uter·ine b.
oc·cult b.
bleed·ing
pol·yp
time
blem·ish
blend·ing
in·her·i·tance
blen·nad·e·ni·tis
blen·ne·me·sis
blen·no·gen·ic
blen·nog·e·nous
blen·noid
blen·noph·thal·mia
blen·nor·rha·gia
blen·nor·rhag·ic
blen·nor·rhea
b. con·junc·ti·va·lis
in·clu·sion b.
b. ne·o·na·to·rum
Stoerk's b.
blen·nor·rhe·al
con·junc·ti·vi·tis
blen·nos·ta·sis

blen·no·stat·ic
blen·nu·ria
ble·o·my·cin sul·fate
bleph·ar·ad·e·ni·tis
bleph·a·ral
bleph·a·rec·to·my
bleph·ar·e·de·ma
bleph·a·ri·tis
    b. acar·i·ca
    b. an·gu·la·ris
    cil·i·ary b.
    dem·o·dec·tic b.
    b. fol·lic·u·la·ris
    mar·gi·nal b.
    b. mar·gi·na·lis
    mei·bo·mi·an b.
    b. ole·o·sa
    b. pa·ra·sit·i·ca
    pe·dic·u·lous b.
    b. phthi·ri·a·ti·ca
    pus·tu·lar b.
    b. ro·sa·cea
    seb·or·rhe·ic b.
    b. sic·ca
    b. squa·mo·sa
    b. ul·ce·ro·sa
bleph·a·ro·ad·e·ni·tis
bleph·a·ro·ad·e·no·ma
bleph·a·ro·chal·a·sis
bleph·a·ro·chro·mi·dro·sis
bleph·a·roc·lo·nus
bleph·a·ro·col·o·bo·ma
bleph·a·ro·con·junc·ti·vi·tis
bleph·a·ro·di·as·ta·sis
bleph·a·ro·ker·a·to·con·junc·ti·
    vi·tis
bleph·a·ro·me·las·ma
bleph·a·ron
bleph·a·ro·pach·yn·sis
bleph·a·ro·phi·mo·sis
bleph·a·ro·phy·ma
bleph·a·ro·plast
bleph·a·ro·plas·tic
bleph·a·ro·plas·ty
bleph·a·ro·ple·gia
bleph·ar·op·to·sia
bleph·a·rop·to·sis
    b. adi·po·sa
    false b.
bleph·a·ror·rha·phy
bleph·a·ro·spasm
bleph·a·ro·spas·mus
bleph·a·ro·stat
bleph·a·ro·ste·no·sis
bleph·a·ro·syn·ech·ia
bleph·a·rot·o·my
Blessig's
    cysts

blight·ed
    ovum
blind
    boil
    en·e·ma
    fis·tu·la
    fo·ra·men of fron·tal bone
    fo·ra·men of the tongue
    gut
    head·ache
    spot
    stag·gers
    study
    test
blind·ing
    dis·ease
    glare
blind loop
    syn·drome
blind na·so·tra·che·al
    in·tu·ba·tion
blind·ness
    ca·nine he·red·i·tary b.
    col·or b.
    cor·ti·cal b.
    day b.
    eclipse b.
    flash b.
    flight b.
    func·tion·al b.
    le·gal b.
    let·ter b.
    mind b.
    moon b.
    mu·sic b.
    night b.
    note b.
    ob·ject b.
    riv·er b.
    sign b.
    smell b.
    snow b.
    so·lar b.
    taste b.
    text b.
    word b.
blis·ter
    blood b.
    fe·ver b.
    fly b.
    fly·ing b.
blis·ter·ing
    col·lo·di·on
blis·ter·ing
bloat
bloat·ing
Bloch's
    re·ac·tion

Bloch-Sulzberger
dis·ease
syn·drome
block
an·es·the·sia
ver·te·brae
block
an·ter·o·grade b.
ar·bo·ri·za·tion b.
atri·o·ven·tric·u·lar b.
A-V b.
bone b.
bun·dle-branch b.
com·plete A-V b.
de·po·lar·iz·ing b.
en·trance b.
ep·i·du·ral b.
ex·it b.
fas·cic·u·lar b.
field b.
first de·gree A-V b.
heart b.
in·tra-a·tri·al b.
in·tra·ven·tric·u·lar b.
I-V b.
Mobitz types of atri·o·ven·
tric·u·lar b.
nerve b.
non·de·po·lar·iz·ing b.
peri-in·farc·tion b.
phase I b.
phase II b.
pro·tec·tive b.
ret·ro·grade b.
sec·ond de·gree A-V b.
si·no·a·tri·al b.
si·no·au·ric·u·lar b.
si·nus b.
spi·nal b.
stel·late b.
su·pra·his·i·an b.
uni·di·rec·tion·al b.
Wilson b.
Wolff-Chaikoff b.
block·ade
ad·re·ner·gic b.
cho·lin·er·gic b.
gan·gli·on·ic b.
my·o·neu·ral b.
nar·cot·ic b.
sym·pa·thet·ic b.
vi·rus b.
block de·sign
test
blocked
aer·o·gas·tria
block·er
Macintosh b.'s

block·ing
al·pha b.
block·ing
ac·tiv·i·ty
agent
an·ti·body
block-out
Blocq's
dis·ease
blood
agar
al·bu·min
blis·ter
cal·cu·lus
cap·il·lary
cast
cell
cir·cu·la·tion
clot
cor·pus·cle
count
cri·sis
crys·tals
cyst
disk
dys·cra·sia
fac·tor
gas·es
group
is·land
is·let
lymph
mole
motes
plas·ma
plas·tid
plate
poi·son·ing
pres·sure
quo·tient
re·la·tion·ship
se·rum
spav·in
spots
sub·sti·tute
sug·ar
tu·mor
type
typ·ing
ves·sel
blood
ar·te·ri·al b.
cord b.
laky b.
oc·cult b.
sludged b.
straw·ber·ry-cream b.

blood *(continued)*
  ve·nous b.
  whole b.
blood-air
  bar·ri·er
blood-aque·ous
  bar·ri·er
blood bank
blood-brain
  bar·ri·er
blood-ce·re·bro·spi·nal flu·id
  bar·ri·er
blood count
  com·plete b. c.
  dif·fer·en·tial white b. c.
  Schilling's b. c.
blood-CSF
  bar·ri·er
blood dust
blood gas
  anal·y·sis
blood group
  ag·glu·ti·nins
  ag·glu·tin·o·gens
  an·ti·bod·ies
  an·ti·gen
  an·ti·se·rums
  sub·stance
  sys·tems
blood group·ing
blood group-spe·cif·ic
  sub·stanc·es A and B
blood·less
  am·pu·ta·tion
  de·cer·e·bra·tion
  op·er·a·tion
  phle·bot·o·my
blood·let·ting
  gen·er·al b.
  lo·cal b.
blood plas·ma
  frac·tions
blood puz·zles
blood·shot
blood·stream
blood urea
  ni·tro·gen
blood-vas·cu·lar
  sys·tem
blood vol·ume
  nom·o·gram
blood·worm
Bloom's
  syn·drome
blot
blotch
Blount-Barber
  dis·ease

Blount's
  dis·ease
blow·fly
blow·ing
  wound
blow-out
  frac·ture
blue
  as·phyx·ia
  at·ro·phy
  ba·by
  cat·a·ract
  dis·ease
  ede·ma
  fe·ver
  line
  ne·vus
  pus
  scle·ra
  spot
  vi·sion
blue·bag
blue·ber·ry muf·fin
  ba·by
blue·comb
  dis·ease of chick·ens
  dis·ease of tur·keys
  vi·rus
blue cone
  mon·o·chro·ma·sy
blue dome
  cyst
blue-green
  al·gae
  bac·te·ri·um
blue pus
  ba·cil·lus
blue rub·ber-bleb
  nevi
blue·tongue
  vi·rus
Blumberg's
  sign
Blumenau's
  nu·cle·us
Blumenbach's
  cli·vus
Blumer's
  shelf
blunt duct
  ad·e·no·sis
blush
B-mode
boat
  con·for·ma·tion
  form
boat-shaped
  ab·do·men

bob·bing
in·verse oc·u·lar b.
oc·u·lar b.

Bochdalek's
fo·ra·men
gan·gli·on
gap
her·nia
mus·cle
valve

Bockhart's
im·pe·ti·go

Bock's
gan·gli·on
nerve

Bodansky
unit

Bödecker
in·dex

Bodian's cop·per-PRO·TAR·GOL
stain

Bo·do
B. cau·da·tus
B. sal·tans
B. uri·na·ri·us

body
ac·e·tone b.
ad·re·nal b.
al·co·hol·ic hy·a·line b.'s
Alder b.'s
al·ve·o·lar b.
am·y·lo·gen·ic b.
am·y·loid b.'s of the pros·tate
ano·coc·cyg·e·al b.
aor·tic b.
Arnold's b.'s
as·bes·tos b.'s
Aschoff b.'s
as·ter·oid b.
Auer b.'s
Babès-Ernst b.'s
Barr chro·ma·tin b.
ba·sal b.
bi·gem·i·nal b.'s
Bollinger b.'s
Borrel b.'s
brassy b.
Cabot's ring b.'s
Call-Exner b.'s
can·cer b.'s
ca·rot·id b.
cav·ern·ous b. of clit·o·ris
cav·ern·ous b. of pe·nis
cell b.
cen·tral b.
chro·maf·fin b.
chro·ma·tin b.

cil·i·ary b.
Civatte b.'s
b. of clav·i·cle
b. of clit·o·ris
coc·cyg·eal b.
col·loid b.'s
com·press·i·ble cav·ern·ous b.'s
con·choi·dal b.'s
Councilman b.
Councilman hy·a·line b.
Cowdry's type A in·clu·sion b.'s
Cowdry's type B in·clu·sion b.'s
cre·o·la b.'s
cy·toid b.'s
Cy·to·plas·mic in·clu·sion b.'s
cy·to·plas·mic in·clu·sion b.'s
Deetjen's b.'s
dem·i·lune b.
Döhle b.'s
Donovan b.
Ehrlich's in·ner b.
el·e·men·ta·ry b.'s
b. of ep·i·did·y·mis
ep·i·the·li·al b.
fat b. of cheek
fat b. of is·chi·o·rec·tal fos·sa
fat b. of or·bit
fer·ru·gi·nous b.'s
for·eign b.
b. of for·nix
fuch·sin b.'s
b. of gall·blad·der
Gamna-Favre b.'s
Gamna-Gandy b.'s
Gandy-Gamna b.'s
ge·nic·u·late b.
glass b.
glo·mus b.
Guarnieri b.'s
Halberstaedter-Prowazek b.'s
Hassall-Henle b.'s
Hassall's b.'s
Heinz b.'s
Heinz-Ehrlich b.
he·ma·tox·y·lin b.'s
he·ma·tox·y·phil b.'s
Herring b.'s
Highmore's b.
Howell-Jolly b.'s
hy·a·line b.'s
hy·a·line b.'s of pi·tu·i·tary
hy·a·loid b.

body *(continued)*

b. of hy·oid bone
b. of il·i·um
im·mune b.
in·clu·sion b.'s
b. of in·cus
in·fra·pa·tel·lar fat b.
in·ter·ca·rot·id b.
in·ter·me·di·ate b. of Flemming
in·ter·re·nal b.'s
b. of is·chi·um
Jaworski's b.'s
Joest b.'s
Jolly b.'s
jux·ta·glo·mer·u·lar b.
jux·ta·res·ti·form b.
ke·tone b.
Koch's blue b.'s
Kurloff's b.'s
Lafora b.
Lallemand's b.'s
Landolt's b.'s
lat·er·al ge·nic·u·late b.
L-D b.
L.E. b.
Leishman-Donovan b.
Lewy b.'s
Lieutaud's b.
Lindner's b.'s
loose b.
Luse b.'s
Luys' b.
Mallory b.'s
mal·pi·ghi·an b.'s
mam·il·lary b.
b. of mam·ma·ry gland
b. of man·di·ble
b. of max·il·la
me·di·al ge·nic·u·late b.
mel·on-seed b.
met·a·chro·mat·ic b.'s
Michaelis-Gutmann b.
Miyagawa b.'s
mol·lus·cum b.
Mooser b.'s
mul·ti·lam·el·lar b.
mul·ti·ve·sic·u·lar b.'s
my·e·lin b.
b. of nail
Negri b.'s
nerve cell b.
neu·ro·ep·i·the·li·al b.
Nissl b.'s
nod·u·lar b.
nu·cle·ar in·clu·sion b.'s
Odland b.
ol·i·vary b.

on·ion b.'s
pac·chi·o·ni·an b.'s
pam·pin·i·form b.
b. of pan·cre·as
Pappenheimer b.'s
para-aor·tic b.'s
par·a·ba·sal b.
par·a·neph·ric b.
par·a·nu·cle·ar b.
par·a·ter·mi·nal b.
Paschen b.'s
b. of pe·nis
per·i·ne·al b.
b. of pha·lanx
Pick's b.'s
pin·e·al b.
Plimmer's b.'s
po·lar b.
Prowazek b.'s
Prowazek-Greeff b.'s
psam·mo·ma b.'s
psit·ta·co·sis in·clu·sion b.'s
pu·bic b.
b. of pu·bic bone
pu·rine b.'s
quad·ri·gem·i·nal b.'s
re·sid·u·al b.
re·sid·u·al b. of Regaud
rest b.
res·ti·form b.
b. of rib
rice b.
Russell b.'s
sand b.'s
Sandström's b.'s
Savage's per·i·ne·al b.
Schaumann b.'s
scle·rot·ic b.'s
seg·ment·ing b.
b. of sphe·noid bone
spongy b. of pe·nis
b. of ster·num
b. of stom·ach
stri·ate b.
su·pra·re·nal b.
b. of sweat gland
Symington's ano·coc·cyg·e·al b.
b. of ta·lus
b. of thigh bone
thresh·old b.
thy·roid b.
b. of tib·ia
ti·groid b.'s
b. of tongue
tra·cho·ma b.'s
trap·e·zoid b.
Trousseau-Lallemand b.'s

tuff·stone b.
tur·bi·nat·ed b.
tym·pan·ic b.
b. of ul·na
ul·ti·mo·bran·chi·al b.
b. of uri·nary blad·der
b. of uter·us
vac·cine b.'s
Verocay b.'s
b. of ver·te·bra
Virchow-Hassall b.'s
vit·re·ous b.
Weibel-Palade b.'s
wolff·i·an b.
Wolf-Orton b.'s
X b.
Y b.
yel·low b.
ze·bra b.
Zuckerkandl's b.'s
body
cav·i·ty
im·age
lan·guage
me·chan·ics
ple·thys·mo·graph
sche·ma
stalk
body bur·den
body mass
in·dex
body right·ing
re·flex·es
body-weight
ra·tio
Boeck's
dis·ease
sar·coid
Boehmer's
he·ma·tox·y·lin
Boerhaave's
glands
syn·drome
bog
spav·in
bog·bean
Bogros'
space
Bogros' se·rous
mem·brane
Bohn's
nod·ules
Bohr
ef·fect
mag·ne·ton
Bohr's
at·om

equa·tion
the·o·ry
boil
Alep·po b.
Bag·dad b.
blind b.
date b.
Del·hi b.
Jer·i·cho b.
Ma·du·ra b.
Or·i·en·tal b.
salt wa·ter b.'s
shoe b.
trop·i·cal b.
boil·er·mak·er's
deaf·ness
boil·ing
point
bol·de·none
bol·din
bol·dine
bol·do
bol·do·glu·cin
bol·dus
bol·et·ic ac·id
Boley
gauge
Bo·liv·i·an hem·or·rhag·ic
fe·ver
Bollinger
bod·ies
gran·ules
Boll's
cells
Bolognini's
symp·tom
bo·lom·e·ter
bol·ster
fin·ger
Bolton
plane
point
Bolton-Broadbent
plane
Bolton-na·si·on
line
plane
bo·lus
dress·ing
bo·lus
in·tra·ve·nous b.
bomb
cal·o·rim·e·ter
bom·bard
Bom·bay
phe·nom·e·non
trait
bom·be·sin

131

bond

ac·yl·mer·cap·tan b.
con·ju·gat·ed dou·ble b.'s
co·or·di·nate b.
di·sul·fide b.
dou·ble b.
high en·er·gy phos·phate b.
hy·dro·gen b.
pep·tide b.
sem·i·po·lar b.
sin·gle b.
tri·ple b.

bone

Albrecht's b.
al·ve·o·lar b.
al·ve·o·lar sup·port·ing b.
an·kle b.
ba·sal b.
bas·i·lar b.
ba·si·oc·cip·i·tal b.
ba·si·sphe·noid b.
Bertin's b.'s
blade b.
breast b.
Breschet's b.'s
brit·tle b.'s
bun·dle b.
cal·ca·ne·al b.
calf b.
can·cel·lous b.
can·non b.
cap·i·tate b.
car·pal b.'s
car·ti·lage b.
cav·al·ry b.
cen·tral b.
cen·tral b. of an·kle
cheek b.
coc·cyg·eal b.
col·lar b.
com·pact b.
con·vo·lut·ed b.
cor·ti·cal b.
cox·al b.
cra·ni·al b.'s
cu·bi·tal b.
cu·boid b.
cu·ne·i·form b.
der·mal b.
b.'s of dig·its
dor·sal ta·lo·na·vic·u·lar b.
ear b.'s
el·bow b.
en·do·chon·dral b.
epac·tal b.'s
ep·i·hy·al b.
ep·i·pter·ic b.
ep·i·ster·nal b.

eth·moid b.
ex·er·cise b.
ex·oc·cip·i·tal b.
fa·cial b.'s
first cu·ne·i·form b.
flank b.
flat b.
Flower's b.
fourth tur·bi·nat·ed b.
fron·tal b.
Goethe's b.
great·er mult·ang·u·lar b.
ha·mate b.
heel b.
het·er·o·top·ic b.'s
high·est tur·bi·nat·ed b.
hip b.
hol·low b.
hooked b.
hy·oid b.
il·i·ac b.
in·ca·ri·al b.
in·ci·sive b.
b.'s of in·fe·ri·or limb
in·fe·ri·or tur·bi·nat·ed b.
in·nom·i·nate b.
in·ter·max·il·lary b.
in·ter·me·di·ate cu·ne·i·form b.
in·ter·pa·ri·e·tal b.
ir·reg·u·lar b.
is·chi·al b.
jaw b.
ju·gal b.
Krause's b.
lac·ri·mal b.
lam·el·lar b.
lat·er·al cu·ne·i·form b.
len·tic·u·lar b.
len·ti·form b.
less·er mult·ang·u·lar b.
lin·gual b.
long b.
lu·nate b.
ma·lar b.
mar·ble b.'s
mas·toid b.
me·di·al cu·ne·i·form b.
med ul·lary b.
mem·brane b.
mes·eth·moid b.
mid·dle cu·ne·i·form b.
mid·dle tur·bi·nat·ed b.
mult·ang·u·lar b.
na·sal b.
na·vic·u·lar b.
na·vic·u·lar b. of hand
non·la·mel·lar b.

oc·cip·i·tal b.
or·bic·u·lar b.
pal·a·tine b.
pa·ri·e·tal b.
pe·nis b.
per·i·chon·dral b.
per·i·os·te·al b.
per·i·o·tic b.
per·o·ne·al b.
pe·tro·sal b.
pet·rous b.
ping-pong b.
pipe b.
Pirie's b.
pis·i·form b.
pneu·mat·ic b.
post·sphe·noid b.
pre·in·ter·pa·ri·e·tal b.
pre·max·il·lary b.
pre·sphe·noid b.
pu·bic b.
py·ram·i·dal b.
re·place·ment b.
re·tic·u·lated b.
rid·er's b.
Riolan's b.'s
sa·cred b.
scaph·oid b.
scroll b.'s
sec·ond cu·ne·i·form b.
sem·i·lu·nar b.
sep·tal b.
ses·a·moid b.
shank b.
shin b.
short b.
sieve b.
sphe·noid b.
sphe·noi·dal tur·bi·nat·ed
 b.'s
splint b.
spongy b.
sti·fle b.
b.'s of su·pe·ri·or limb
su·pe·ri·or tur·bi·nat·ed b.
su·pra·in·ter·pa·ri·e·tal b.
su·pra·ster·nal b.
su·preme tur·bi·nat·ed b.
su·tur·al b.'s
tail b.
tar·sal b.'s
tem·po·ral b.
thigh b.
third cu·ne·i·form b.
three-cor·nered b.
tongue b.
tra·bec·u·lar b.
tra·pe·zi·um b.

trap·e·zoid b.
tri·an·gu·lar b.
tri·que·tral b.
tur·bi·nat·ed b.'s
tym·pan·ic b.
tym·pa·no·hy·al b.
un·ci·form b.
up·per jaw b.
Vesalius' b.
b.'s of vis·cer·al cra·ni·um
wedge b.
wor·mi·an b.'s
wo·ven b.
yoke b.
zy·go·mat·ic b.
bone
ab·scess
ache
age
block
can·a·lic·u·lus
cell
char·coal
chips
con·duc·tion
cor·pus·cle
cyst
flap
for·ceps
graft
in·farct
is·land
mar·row
ma·trix
phos·phate
plate
re·flex
re·sorp·tion
salt
scle·ro·sis
sen·si·bil·i·ty
spav·in
tis·sue
wax
bone ar·chi·tec·ture
bone ash
bone black
bone·let
bone mar·row
trans·plan·ta·tion
bone-salt
Bonhoeffer's
sign
Bonnet's
cap·sule
op·er·a·tion
Bonnevie-Ullrich
syn·drome

Bonnier's
  syn·drome
Bonwill
  tri·an·gle
bony
  an·ky·lo·sis
  crep·i·tus
  heart
  lab·y·rinth
  pal·ate
  part of au·di·to·ry tube
  part of na·sal sep·tum
bony na·sal
  sep·tum
bony sem·i·cir·cu·lar
  ca·nals
Böök
  syn·drome
Bo·oph·i·lus
  B. an·nu·la·tus
  B. de·col·or·a·tus
  B. mi·cro·pus
boost·er
  dose
boot
  Junod's b.
bo·rac·ic ac·id
bo·rate
bo·rat·ed
bo·rax
bor·bo·ryg·mi
bor·bo·ryg·mus
Bordeau
  the·o·ry
Bordeaux
  mix·ture
bor·der
  cells
  mold·ing
  move·ments
  seal
bor·der
  al·ve·o·lar b.
  an·te·ri·or b.
  brush b.
  den·ture b.
  b.'s of eye·lids
  in·fe·ri·or b.
  oc·cult b. of nail
  pos·te·ri·or b. of pet·rous
    part of tem·po·ral bone
  ra·di·al b.
  sag·it·tal b.
  sphe·noi·dal b.
  stri·at·ed b.
  su·pe·ri·or b. of pet·rous
    part of tem·po·ral bone
  tib·i·al b.

  b. of uter·us
  ver·mil·ion b.
bor·der·line
  lep·ro·sy
  per·son·al·i·ty
  rays
bor·der·line per·son·al·i·ty
  dis·or·der
bor·der tis·sue
  move·ments
Bor·de·tel·la
  B. bron·chi·sep·ti·ca
  B. par·a·per·tus·sis
  B. per·tus·sis
Bordet-Gengou
  ba·cil·lus
  phe·nom·e·non
Bordet-Gengou po·ta·to blood
  agar
Bordeu
  the·o·ry
bo·ric ac·id
bor·ism
Börjeson-Forssman-Lehmann
  syn·drome
Born
  meth·od of wax plate re·
    con·struc·tion
Bor·na
  dis·ease
Bor·na dis·ease
  vi·rus
bor·nane
Bornholm dis·ease
  vi·rus
bo·ro·glyc·er·in
bo·ro·glyc·er·ol
bo·ron
Borrel
  bod·ies
Bor·rel·ia
  B. an·se·ri·na
  B. burg·dor·feri
  B. cau·ca·si·ca
  B. croc·i·du·rae
  B. dut·to·nii
  B. herm·sii
  B. his·pa·ni·ca
  B. ko·chii
  B. la·ty·sche·wii
  B. maz·zot·tii
  B. par·keri
  B. per·si·ca
  B. re·cur·ren·tis
  B. thei·leri
  B. tu·ri·ca·tae
  B. ve·ne·zu·e·len·sis

bor·re·li·o·sis
  bo·vine b.
  ca·nine b.
Borrel's blue
  stain
Borst-Jadassohn type in·tra·ep·i·der·mal
  ep·i·the·li·o·ma
bosch
  yaws
boss
bos·se·lat·ed
bos·se·la·tion
Bos·ton
  ex·an·the·ma
  opi·um
Boston's
  sign
Botallo's
  duct
  fo·ra·men
  lig·a·ment
bot·fly
  head b.'s
  hu·man b.
  skin b.'s
  war·ble b.
both·ria
both·ri·o·ceph·a·li·a·sis
Both·ri·o·ceph·a·lus
  B. cor·da·tus
  B. la·tus
  B. man·so·ni
  B. man·so·noi·des
both·ri·um
bo·throp·ic
  an·ti·tox·in
Bo·throps
  an·ti·tox·in
bot·ry·oid
  sar·co·ma
Bot·ry·o·my·ces
bot·ry·o·my·co·sis
bot·ry·o·my·cot·ic
bots
  ox b.
  sheep b.
Böttcher's
  ca·nal
  cells
  crys·tals
  gan·gli·on
  space
bot·tle
  Mariotte b.
  wash-b.
  Woulfe's b.
bot·u·lin

bot·u·lin·o·gen·ic
bot·u·li·num
  an·ti·tox·in
bot·u·li·nus
  tox·in
bot·u·lism
  an·ti·tox·in
bot·u·lis·mo·tox·in
bot·u·lo·gen·ic
bou·bas
Bouchard's
  dis·ease
bouche de ta·pir
Bouchut's
  tube
Bouffardi's black
  my·ce·to·ma
Bouffardi's my·ce·to·mas
Bouffardi's white
  my·ce·to·ma
bou·gie
  b. à boule
  bul·bous b.
  elas·tic b.
  el·bowed b.
  fi·li·form b.
  fol·low·ing b.
  Hurst b.'s
  Maloney b.'s
  ta·pered b.
  wax-tipped b.
  whip b.
bou·gie·nage
Bouillaud's
  dis·ease
bouil·lon
Bouin's
  fix·a·tive
bou·lim·i·a
bound
  wa·ter
bound·ing
  pu·pil
bou·quet
  fe·ver
bou·quet
  Riolan's b.
Bourdon
  tube
Bourgery's
  lig·a·ment
Bourneville-Pringle
  dis·ease
Bourneville's
  dis·ease
bou·ton
  ax·o·nal ter·mi·nal b.'s
  b. de Bag·dad

bou·ton *(continued)*
    b. de Bis·kra
    b. d'O·ri·ent
    b. en che·mise
    b.'s en pas·sage
    syn·ap·tic b.'s
    ter·mi·nal b.'s
    b. ter·mi·naux
bou·ton·neuse
    fe·ver
bou·ton·nière
    de·for·mi·ty
Bovero's
    mus·cle
Bo·vic·o·la
bo·vine
    ac·e·ton·e·mia
    achon·dro·pla·sia
    ad·e·no·vi·rus·es
    an·ti·tox·in
    ba·be·si·o·sis
    bor·re·li·o·sis
    bru·cel·lo·sis
    col·loid
    he·mo·glo·bi·nu·ria
    hy·per·ker·a·to·sis
    ke·to·sis
    lym·pho·sar·co·ma
    mas·ti·tis
    por·phyr·ia
    rhi·no·vi·rus·es
    trich·o·mo·ni·a·sis
bo·vine can·cer
    eye
bo·vine con·gen·i·tal
    atax·ia
bo·vine ephem·er·al
    fe·ver
bo·vine her·pes
    mam·mil·li·tis
bo·vine in·fec·tious
    abor·tion
bo·vine leu·ke·mia
    vi·rus
bo·vine leu·ko·sis
    vi·rus
bo·vine pap·u·lar
    sto·ma·ti·tis
bo·vine pap·u·lar sto·ma·ti·tis
    vi·rus
bo·vine se·rum
    al·bu·min
bo·vine spo·rad·ic
    en·ceph·a·lo·my·e·li·tis
bo·vine ul·cer·a·tive
    mam·mil·li·tis
bo·vine vac·cin·ia
    mam·mil·li·tis

bo·vine vi·rus
    di·ar·rhea
bo·vine vi·rus di·ar·rhea
    vi·rus
bow
    Logan's b.
bow-leg
Bowditch's
    law
bowed
    ten·don
bow·el
    by·pass
    sounds
bow·el
bow·el by·pass
    syn·drome
bow·en·oid
    pa·pu·lo·sis
Bowen's
    dis·ease
Bowen's pre·can·cer·ous
    der·ma·to·sis
Bowie's
    stain
bow·leg
Bowles type
    steth·o·scope
Bowman's
    cap·sule
    disks
    gland
    mem·brane
    mus·cle
    op·er·a·tion
    probe
    space
    the·o·ry
box
    frac·ture b.
    Hogness b.
    Pribnow b.
    Skinner b.
    TATA b.
box·er's
    ear
    frac·ture
box·ing
    wax
Boyden
    meal
Boyden's
    sphinc·ter
Boyer's
    bur·sa
    cyst
Boyle's
    law

Bozeman-Fritsch
cath·e·ter
Bozeman's
op·er·a·tion
po·si·tion
Bozzolo's
sign
Braasch
cath·e·ter
brace
Taylor's back b.
brace·let
Nussbaum's b.
brac·es
bra·chia
brach·i·al
an·es·the·sia
ar·tery
fas·cia
gland
mus·cle
neu·ri·tis
plex·us
veins
brach·i·al birth
pal·sy
bra·chi·al·gia
b. sta·ti·ca pa·res·the·ti·ca
brach·i·al lymph
nodes
brach·i·al plex·us
neu·rop·a·thy
bra·chi·o·ce·phal·ic
mus·cle
trunk
veins
bra·chi·o·cru·ral
bra·chi·o·cu·bi·tal
bra·chi·o·gram
bra·chi·o·ra·di·al
mus·cle
re·flex
bra·chi·um
b. con·junc·ti·vum ce·re·bel·li
b. of the in·fe·ri·or col·lic·u·lus
in·fe·ri·or quad·ri·gem·i·nal b.
b. pon·tis
b. quad·ri·ge·mi·num in·fe·ri·us
b. quad·ri·ge·mi·num su·pe·ri·us
b. of su·pe·ri·or col·lic·u·lus
su·pe·ri·or quad·ri·gem·i·nal b.

Bracht
ma·neu·ver
Bracht-Wachter
le·sion
brach·y·ba·sia
brach·y·ba·so·camp·to·dac·ty·ly
brach·y·ba·so·pha·lan·gia
brach·y·car·dia
brach·y·ce·pha·lia
brach·y·ce·phal·ic
brach·y·ceph·a·lism
brach·y·ceph·a·lous
brach·y·ceph·a·ly
brach·y·chei·lia
brach·y·chi·lia
brach·y·cne·mic
brach·y·cra·nic
brach·y·dac·tyl·ia
brach·y·dac·tyl·ic
brach·y·dac·ty·ly
brach·y·e·soph·a·gus
brach·y·fa·cial
brach·y·glos·sal
bra·chyg·na·thia
bra·chyg·na·thous
brach·y·ker·kic
brach·y·me·lia
brach·y·me·so·pha·lan·gia
brach·y·met·a·car·pa·lia
brach·y·met·a·car·pa·lism
brach·y·met·a·car·pia
brach·y·me·tap·o·dy
brach·y·met·a·tar·sia
brach·y·mor·phic
brach·y·o·dont
brach·y·pel·lic
pel·vis
brach·y·pel·vic
brach·y·pha·lan·gia
bra·chyp·o·dous
brach·y·pro·sop·ic
brach·y·rhi·nia
brach·y·rhyn·chus
brach·y·skel·ic
brach·y·staph·y·line
brach·y·syn·dac·ty·ly
brach·y·te·le·pha·lan·gia
brach·y·ther·a·py
brach·y·type
brach·y·u·ran·ic
brac·ing
brack·en
poi·son·ing
stag·gers
brack·et
Bradford
frame
bra·dy·ar·rhyth·mia

bra·dy·arth·ria
bra·dy·car·dia
  car·di·o·mus·cu·lar b.
  cen·tral b.
  es·sen·tial b.
  fe·tal b.
  id·i·o·path·ic b.
  no·dal b.
  post·in·fec·tious b.
  si·nus b.
  ven·tric·u·lar b.
brad·y·car·di·ac
bra·dy·car·dic
bra·dy·ci·ne·sia
bra·dy·crot·ic
bra·dy·di·as·to·le
bra·dy·es·the·sia
bra·dy·glos·sia
bra·dy·ki·ne·sia
bra·dy·ki·net·ic
  anal·y·sis
bra·dy·ki·nin
bra·dy·ki·nin·o·gen
brad·y·ki·nin-po·ten·ti·at·ing
  pep·tide
bra·dy·ki·nin po·ten·ti·a·tor B
bra·dy·la·lia
bra·dy·lex·ia
bra·dy·lo·gia
bra·dy·men·or·rhea
bra·dy·pep·sia
bra·dy·pha·gia
bra·dy·pha·sia
bra·dy·phe·mia
bra·dyp·nea
bra·dy·pra·gia
bra·dy·psy·chia
bra·dy·rhyth·mia
bra·dy·sper·ma·tism
bra·dy·sphyg·mia
bra·dy·stal·sis
bra·dy·tel·e·o·ci·ne·sia
bra·dy·tel·e·o·ki·ne·sis
bra·dy·to·cia
bra·dy·u·ria
bra·dy·zo·ite
braille
Brailsford-Morquio
  dis·ease
brain
  cic·a·trix
  con·cus·sion
  con·ges·tion
  con·tu·sion
  death
  ede·ma
  lac·er·a·tion
  lip·id

  man·tle
  mur·mur
  po·ten·tial
  sand
  stem
  sug·ar
  swell·ing
  wave
brain
  ab·dom·i·nal b.
  res·pi·ra·tor b.
  split b.
  vis·cer·al b.
brain·case
brain-heart in·fu·sion
  agar
Brain's
  re·flex
brain·stem
  hem·or·rhage
brain·stem evoked re·sponse
  au·di·om·e·try
brain·wash·ing
brain wave
  com·plex
  cy·cle
bran
branch
branched
  cal·cu·lus
branched chain
  ke·to·ac·i·du·ria
  ke·ton·u·ria
bran·chia
bran·chi·ae
bran·chi·al
  ap·pa·ra·tus
  arch·es
  car·ti·lag·es
  cells
  clefts
  cyst
  duct
  fis·sure
  fis·tu·la
  groove
  mes·o·derm
  pouch·es
bran·chi·al cleft
  cyst
bran·chi·al ef·fer·ent
  col·umn
branch·ing
  en·zyme
  fac·tor
branch·ing
  false b.

branch·ing de·fi·cien·cy
am·y·lo·pec·tin·o·sis
bran·chi·o·gen·ic
bran·chi·og·en·ous
bran·chi·o·ma
bran·chi·o·mere
bran·chi·o·mer·ic
mus·cles
bran·chi·om·er·ism
bran·chi·o·mo·tor
nu·clei
Brandt-Andrews
ma·neu·ver
bran·dy
nose
Bran·ha·mel·la
B. ca·tar·rha·lis
Branham's
sign
bran·ny
des·qua·ma·tion
tet·ter
Brasdor's
meth·od
brassy
body
cough
Braune's
ca·nal
mus·cle
valve
Braun's
anas·to·mo·sis
brawny
arm
scle·ri·tis
Braxton-Hicks
con·trac·tion
sign
ver·sion
braxy
Ger·man b.
Bra·zil
wax
bra·zil·ein
Bra·zil·ian
oph·thal·mia
pem·phi·gus
braz·i·lin
braz·ing
BrDu-
band·ing
bread
pill
bread-and-but·ter
per·i·car·di·um
break
shock

break·a·way
phe·nom·e·non
break·bone
fe·ver
break·off
phe·nom·e·non
break·through
breast
ac·ces·so·ry b.
caked b.
chick·en b.
fun·nel b.
ir·ri·ta·ble b.
male b.
pi·geon b.
breast
bone
pang
pump
breath
ure·mic b.
breath anal·y·sis
test
breath-hold·ing
test
breath·ing
bag
re·serve
breath·ing
ap·neus·tic b.
Biot's b.
bron·chi·al b.
con·tin·u·ous pos·i·tive
pres·sure b.
glos·so·pha·ryn·ge·al b.
in·ter·mit·tent pos·i·tive
pres·sure b.
mouth b.
pos·i·tive-neg·a·tive pres·
sure b.
pursed lips b.
shal·low b.
Breda's
dis·ease
bre·douille·ment
breech
de·liv·ery
ex·trac·tion
pre·sen·ta·tion
breed·ing
breg·ma
breg·mat·ic
fon·ta·nel
breg·ma·to·lamb·doid
arc
breg·mo·car·di·ac
re·flex
brei

brems·strah·lung
Brenner
  tu·mor
breph·o·plas·tic
  graft
Breschet's
  bones
  ca·nals
  hi·a·tus
  si·nus
  vein
Brescia-Cimino
  fis·tu·la
Breslow's
  thick·ness
bre·tyl·i·um tos·yl·ate
Breus
  mole
brev·i·col·lis
Brewer's
  in·farcts
brew·ers'
  yeast
brick·dust
  de·pos·it
Bricker
  op·er·a·tion
brick·mak·er's
  ane·mia
bridge
  cor·pus·cle
bridge
  ar·te·ri·o·lo·ven·u·lar b.
  cell b.'s
  cy·to·plas·mic b.'s
  Gaskell's b.
  in·ter·cel·lu·lar b.'s
  my·o·car·di·al b.
  re·mov·a·ble b.
  Wheatstone's b.
bridge·work
bridg·ing he·pa·tic
  ne·cro·sis
bri·dle
  stric·ture
  su·ture
bri·dle
  b. of clit·o·ris
bright·ness dif·fer·ence
  thresh·old
Bright's
  dis·ease
bril·liant cres·yl blue
bril·liant green
bril·liant green bile salt
  agar
bril·liant vi·tal red
bril·liant yel·low

Brill's
  dis·ease
Brill-Symmers
  dis·ease
Brill-Zinsser
  dis·ease
brim
  pel·vic b.
brim·stone
brin·dle
Brinell hard·ness
  num·ber
Briquet's
  atax·ia
  syn·drome
brise·ment forcé
bris·ket
  dis·ease
bris·ket
Brissaud-Marie
  syn·drome
Brissaud's
  dis·ease
  in·fan·ti·lism
  re·flex
bris·tle
  cell
Brit·ish
  gum
Brit·ish an·ti-Lew·is·ite
Brit·ish Phar·ma·co·poe·ia
Brit·ish ther·mal
  unit
brit·tle
  bones
  di·a·be·tes
broach
  barbed b.
  smooth b.
broad
  fas·cia
  lig·a·ment of the uter·us
  spec·trum
Broadbent's
  law
  sign
broad·est
  mus·cle of back
broad mar·gi·nal con·fron·ta·tion
  meth·od
broad spec·trum
  an·ti·bi·ot·ic
Broca's
  an·gles
  apha·sia
  ar·ea
  cen·ter

field
fis·sure
for·mu·la
pouch
Broca's bas·i·lar
an·gle
Broca's di·ag·o·nal
band
Broca's fa·cial
an·gle
Broca's par·ol·fac·to·ry
ar·ea
Broca's vi·su·al
plane
Brock
op·er·a·tion
Brockenbrough
sign
Brock's
syn·drome
Brocq's
dis·ease
bro·cre·sine
Brödel's blood·less
line
Brodie
flu·id
Brodie's
ab·scess
bur·sa
dis·ease
knee
lig·a·ment
Brodmann's
ar·e·as
Broesike's
fos·sa
bro·mate
bro·mat·ed
bro·ma·ze·pam
bro·ma·zine hy·dro·chlo·ride
brom·cre·sol green
brom·cre·sol pur·ple
bro·me·lain
bro·me·lin
brom·hex·ine hy·dro·chlo·ride
brom·hi·dro·sis
bro·mic
bro·mide
ac·ne
bro·mi·dro·si·pho·bia
bro·mi·dro·sis
bro·min·at·ed
bro·min·di·one
bro·mine
wa·ter
bro·min·ism
bro·mism

brom·i·so·val·um
bro·mo·cre·sol green
bro·mo·crip·tine
bro·mo·de·ox·y·ur·i·dine
bro·mo·der·ma
bro·mo·di·phen·hy·dra·mine
hy·dro·chlo·ride
bro·mo·hy·per·hi·dro·sis
bro·mo·hy·per·i·dro·sis
bro·mo·phe·nol blue
bro·mop·nea
bro·mo·sul·fo·phtha·lein
brom·phen·ir·a·mine ma·le·ate
brom·phe·nol
test
brom·phe·nol blue
Bromp·ton
cock·tail
brom·sul·fo·phtha·lein
brom·sul·pha·lein
test
brom·thy·mol blue
bro·mum
bron·ca·tar
bron·chi
bron·chia
bron·chi·al
ad·e·no·ma
ar·ter·ies
asth·ma
breath·ing
bud
cal·cu·lus
frem·i·tus
glands
pneu·mo·nia
pol·yp
res·pi·ra·tion
tubes
veins
voice
bron·chic
cells
bron·chi·ec·ta·sia
b. sic·ca
bron·chi·ec·ta·sic
bron·chi·ec·ta·sis
cy·lin·dri·cal b.
dry b.
sac·cu·lar b.
bron·chi·ec·tat·ic
bron·chil·o·quy
bron·chi·o·cele
bron·chi·o·gen·ic
bron·chi·o·lar
ad·e·no·car·ci·no·ma
car·ci·no·ma

bron·chi·ole
  res·pi·ra·to·ry b.'s
  ter·mi·nal b.
bron·chi·o·lec·ta·sia
bron·chi·o·lec·ta·sis
bron·chi·o·li
bron·chi·ol·i·tis
  ex·ud·a·tive b.
  b. fi·bro·sa ob·li·te·r·ans
  pro·lif·er·a·tive b.
bron·chi·o·lo-al·ve·o·lar
  car·ci·no·ma
bron·chi·o·lo·pul·mo·nary
bron·chi·o·lus
  b. ter·mi·na·lis
bron·chi·o·ste·no·sis
bron·chit·ic
  asth·ma
bron·chi·tis
  asth·mat·ic b.
  Castellani's b.
  chron·ic b.
  croup·ous b.
  fi·brin·ous b.
  hem·or·rhag·ic b.
  in·fec·tious avi·an b.
  b. ob·li·te·r·ans
  oblit·er·a·tive b.
  plas·tic b.
  pseu·do·mem·bra·nous b.
  pu·trid b.
  ver·min·ous b.
bron·chi·um
bron·cho·al·ve·o·lar
bron·cho·cav·ern·ous
bron·cho·cele
bron·cho·cen·tric
  gran·u·lo·ma·to·sis
bron·cho·con·stric·tion
bron·cho·con·stric·tor
bron·cho·di·la·ta·tion
bron·cho·di·la·tion
bron·cho·di·la·tor
bron·cho·e·de·ma
bron·cho·e·soph·a·ge·al
  fis·tu·la
  mus·cle
bron·cho·e·soph·a·gol·o·gy
bron·cho·e·soph·a·gos·co·py
bron·cho·fi·ber·scope
bron·cho·gen·ic
  car·ci·no·ma
  cyst
bron·cho·gram
bron·chog·ra·phy
bron·cho·lith
bron·cho·li·thi·a·sis
bron·cho·ma·la·cia

bron·cho·me·di·as·ti·nal
  trunk
bron·cho·mo·tor
bron·cho·my·co·sis
bron·choph·o·ny
  whis·pered b.
bron·cho·plas·ty
bron·cho·pleu·ral
  fis·tu·la
bron·cho·pneu·mo·nia
  tu·ber·cu·lous b.
bron·cho·pul·mo·nary
  as·per·gil·lo·sis
  dys·pla·sia
  seg·ment
  se·ques·tra·tion
  spi·ro·che·to·sis
bron·cho·pul·mo·nary lymph
  nodes
bron·chor·rha·phy
bron·chor·rhea
bron·cho·scope
bron·cho·scop·ic
  brush
  smear
  sponge
bron·chos·co·py
bron·cho·spasm
bron·cho·spi·ro·che·to·sis
bron·cho·spi·rog·ra·phy
bron·cho·spi·rom·e·ter
bron·cho·spi·rom·e·try
bron·cho·stax·is
bron·cho·ste·no·sis
bron·chos·to·my
bron·cho·tome
bron·chot·o·my
bron·cho·tra·che·al
bron·cho·ve·sic·u·lar
  res·pi·ra·tion
bron·chus
  ep·ar·te·ri·al b.
  hyp·ar·te·ri·al bron·chi
  in·ter·me·di·ate b.
  b. in·ter·me·di·us
  left main b.
  lo·bar bron·chi
  pri·mary b.
  right main b.
  seg·men·tal b.
  stem b.
Brønsted
  base
  the·o·ry
bron·to·pho·bia
bronze
  di·a·be·tes

bronzed
dis·ease
skin
brood
cap·sules
cell
Brooke
il·e·os·to·my
Brooke's
dis·ease
tu·mor
broom
broth·er
com·plex
brow
pre·sen·ta·tion
brow·lift
brown
at·ro·phy
ede·ma
fat
in·du·ra·tion of the lung
lay·er
pel·li·cle
stri·ae
tu·mor
Brown-Adson
for·ceps
Brown-Brenn
stain
brown·i·an
mo·tion
move·ment
brown·i·an-Zsigmondy
move·ment
Browning's
vein
Brown's
syn·drome
Brown-Séquard's
pa·ral·y·sis
syn·drome
Bru·cel·la
B. abor·tus
B. ca·nis
B. mel·i·ten·sis
B. su·is
Bru·cel·la·ce·ae
bru·cel·ler·gin
bru·cel·lin
bru·cel·lo·sis
bo·vine b.
Bruch's
glands
mem·brane
bru·cine
Brücke-Bartley
phe·nom·e·non

Brücke's
mus·cle
tu·nic
Bruck's
dis·ease
Brudzinski's
sign
Bru·gi·a
B. ma·la·yi
Brugsch's
syn·drome
bruise
bruisse·ment
bru·it
an·eu·rys·mal b.
ca·rot·id b.
b. de can·on
b. de di·a·ble
b. de gal·op
b. de lime
b. de mou·lin
b. de rap·pel
b. de Roger
b. de scie ou de rape
b. de souf·flet
b. de ta·bour·ka
b. de tri·o·let
thy·roid b.
Traube's b.
Brumpt's white
my·ce·to·ma
Brunn
re·ac·tion
brun·ner·o·ma
brun·ner·o·sis
Brunner's
glands
Brunn's
mem·brane
nests
Bruns
atax·ia
Brunschwig's
op·er·a·tion
brush
bi·op·sy
bor·der
burn
cath·e·ter
brush
Ayre b.
bron·cho·scop·ic b.
den·ture b.
Haidinger's b.'s
Kruse's b.
pol·ish·ing b.
brush burn
abra·sion

Brushfield's
  spots
Brushfield-Wyatt
  dis·ease
brush heap
  struc·ture
brush·ite
Bruton's
  dis·ease
Bruton type
  agam·ma·glob·u·lin·e·mia
brux·ism
Bryant's
  am·pul·la
  sign
  trac·tion
  tri·an·gle
BSER
  au·di·om·e·try
BSP
  test
bu·aki
bu·ba mad·re
bu·bas
  b. bra·zi·li·a·na
bub·ble gum
  der·ma·ti·tis
bub·bling
  rale
bu·bo
  bul·let b.
  chan·croi·dal b.
  cli·mat·ic b.
  in·do·lent b.
  ma·lig·nant b.
  pa·rot·id b.
  pri·mary b.
  trop·i·cal b.
  ve·ne·re·al b.
  vir·u·lent b.
bu·bon·al·gia
bu·bon·ic
  plague
bu·bon·u·lus
bu·car·dia
buc·ca
buc·cae
buc·cal
  an·gles
  ar·tery
  car·ies
  cav·i·ty
  curve
  em·bra·sure
  flange
  gin·gi·va
  glands
  nerve

  node
  oc·clu·sion
  pit
  re·gion
  smear
  sur·face
  tab·let
  ves·ti·bule
buc·ci·na·tor
  ar·tery
  crest
  nerve
  node
buc·co·ax·i·al
buc·co·ax·i·o·cer·vi·cal
buc·co·ax·i·o·gin·gi·val
buc·co·cer·vi·cal
  ridge
buc·co·clu·sal
buc·co·dis·tal
buc·co·gin·gi·val
  ridge
buc·co·la·bi·al
buc·co·lin·gual
  di·am·e·ter
  di·men·sion
  re·la·tion
buc·co·me·si·al
buc·co·na·sal
  mem·brane
buc·co·neu·ral
  duct
buc·co-oc·clu·sal
  an·gle
buc·co·pha·ryn·ge·al
  fas·cia
  mem·brane
  part
buc·co·pul·pal
buc·co·ver·sion
buc·cu·la
Buchner
  ex·tract
  fun·nel
bu·chu
Buchwald's
  at·ro·phy
buck
  tooth
buck·bean
buck·et-han·dle
  in·ci·sion
  tear
buck·led
  aor·ta
Buck's
  ex·ten·sion

fas·cia
trac·tion
buck·thorn
  pol·y·neu·rop·a·thy
Bucky
  di·a·phragm
Bucky's
  rays
bu·cli·zine hy·dro·chlo·ride
buc·lo·sa·mide
bu·cry·late
bud
  bron·chi·al b.
  end b.
  gus·ta·to·ry b.
  limb b.
  liv·er b.
  lung b.
  me·di·an tongue b.
  met·a·neph·ric b.
  per·i·os·te·al b.
  syn·cy·tial b.
  tail b.
  taste b.
  tooth b.
  ure·ter·ic b.
  vas·cu·lar b.
bud
  fis·sion
Budd-Chiari
  syn·drome
Budde
  pro·cess
bud·de·ized
  milk
bud·ding
Budd's
  cir·rho·sis
  syn·drome
Budge's
  cen·ter
Budin's ob·stet·ri·cal
  joint
Buerger's
  dis·ease
bu·fa·di·en·o·lide
bu·fa·di·en·o·lides
bu·fa·gen·ins
bu·fa·gins
bu·fan·o·lide
bu·fa·tri·en·o·lide
bu·fen·o·lide
buf·fa·lo
  neck
buff·er
  ca·pac·i·ty
  in·dex
  pair

val·ue
val·ue of the blood
buff·er
  sec·on·dary b.
buff·ered crys·tal·line
  pen·i·cil·lin G
buffy
  coat
Bu·fon·i·dae
bu·for·min
bu·fo·ten·ine
bu·fo·tox·ins
bug·gery
bulb
  aor·tic b.
  ar·te·ri·al b.
  ca·rot·id b.
  b. of cor·pus spon·gi·o·sum
  den·tal b.
  du·o·de·nal b.
  end b.
  b. of eye
  hair b.
  b. of jug·u·lar vein
  Krause's end b.'s
  b. of lat·er·al ven·tri·cle
  ol·fac·to·ry b.
  b. of pe·nis
  b. of pos·te·ri·or horn of
    lat·er·al ven·tri·cle of
    brain
  Rouget's b.
  speech b.
  taste b.
  b. of ure·thra
  b. of ves·ti·bule
bul·bar
  ap·o·plexy
  con·junc·ti·va
  my·e·li·tis
  pal·sy
  pa·ral·y·sis
  pulse
  ridge
  sep·tum
bul·bi
bul·bi·tis
bul·bo·cav·er·no·sus
  re·flex
bul·boid
  cor·pus·cles
bul·bo·mim·ic
  re·flex
bul·bo·nu·cle·ar
bul·bo·pon·tine
bul·bo·sa·cral
  sys·tem
bul·bo·spi·nal

bul·bo·u·re·thral
  gland
bul·bous
  bou·gie
bul·bo·ven·tric·u·lar
  loop
  ridge
bul·bus
  b. cor·dis
  b. ure·thrae
bu·le·sis
bulg·ing eye
  dis·ease
bu·lim·ia
  b. ner·vo·sa
bu·lim·ic
Bu·li·nus
bulk
  mo·du·lus
bulk·age
bull
  neck
bul·la
  eth·moi·dal b.
  pul·mo·nary b.
  b. tym·pa·ni·ca
bul·lae
bull·dog
  calf
  for·ceps
  head
bul·let
  bu·bo
  for·ceps
bull·nose
bul·lous
  ede·ma
  ede·ma ve·si·cae
  fe·ver
  im·pe·ti·go of new·born
  ker·a·top·a·thy
  myr·in·gi·tis
  pem·phi·goid
  syph·i·lid
bull's-eye
  mac·u·lop·a·thy
bu·met·a·nide
Bumke's
  pu·pil
bun·am·i·dine hy·dro·chlo·ride
bun·dle
  ab·er·rant b.'s
  an·te·ri·or ground b.
  Arnold's b.
  atri·o·ven·tric·u·lar b.
  Bachmann's b.
  com·ma b. of Schultze
  Flechsig's ground b.'s

  Gantzer's ac·ces·so·ry b.
  Gierke's res·pi·ra·to·ry b.
  ground b.'s
  Held's b.
  Helie's b.
  Helweg's b.
  b. of His
  His' b.
  Hoche's b.
  hooked b. of Russell
  Keith's b.
  Kent-His b.
  Kent's b.
  Killian's b.
  Krause's res·pi·ra·to·ry b.
  lat·er·al ground b.
  Lissauer's b.
  Loewenthal's b.
  lon·gi·tu·di·nal pon·tine b.'s
  me·di·al fore·brain b.
  me·di·al lon·gi·tu·di·nal b.
  Meynert's ret·ro·flex b.
  Monakow's b.
  mus·cle b.
  ob·lique b. of pons
  ol·fac·to·ry b.
  ol·i·vo·co·chle·ar b.
  Pick's b.
  pos·te·ri·or lon·gi·tu·di·nal b.
  pre·com·mis·sur·al b.
  pre·dor·sal b.
  Rathke's b.'s
  Schütz' b.
  sol·i·tary b.
  ten·don b.
  Türck's b.
  un·ci·nate b. of Russell
  Vicq d'Azyr's b.
bun·dle
  bone
bun·dle-branch
  block
bung·pag·ga
bun·ion
bun·ion·ec·to·my
  Keller b.
  Mayo b.
Bunnell's
  su·ture
bu·no·dont
bu·no·lol hy·dro·chlo·ride
bu·no·loph·o·dont
bu·no·se·le·no·dont
Bu·nos·to·mum
  B. phle·bo·to·mum
  B. trig·o·no·ceph·a·lum
Bunsen burn·er

Bunsen-Roscoe
law
Bunsen's sol·u·bil·i·ty
co·ef·fi·cient
Bun·yam·we·ra
fe·ver
vi·rus
Bun·ya·vir·i·dae
Bun·ya·vi·rus
bun·ya·vi·rus
en·ceph·a·li·tis
buph·thal·mia
buph·thal·mos
buph·thal·mus
bu·piv·a·caine
bu·pre·nor·phine hy·dro·chlo·ride
bu·pro·pi·on hy·dro·chlo·ride
bur
cross-cut b.
end-cut·ting b.
fin·ish·ing b.
fis·sure b.
in·vert·ed cone b.
round b.
bur
drill
Burchard-Liebermann
re·ac·tion
Burdach's
col·umn
fas·cic·u·lus
nu·cle·us
tract
bur·den
Burdwan
fe·ver
bu·ret
bu·rette
Bürger-Grütz
syn·drome
Bur·gun·dy
pitch
bur·ied
flap
su·ture
Burkitt's
lym·pho·ma
Burlew
disk
wheel
burn
brush b.
chem·i·cal b.
first de·gree b.
flash b.
full-thick·ness b.
mat b.

par·tial-thick·ness b.
ra·di·a·tion b.
rope b.
sec·ond de·gree b.
su·per·fi·cial b.
ther·mal b.
third de·gree b.
Burnett's
syn·drome
burn·ing drops
sign
bur·nish·er
burn·out
Burn and Rand
the·o·ry
Burns'
lig·a·ment
space
Burns' fal·ci·form
pro·cess
burnt
al·um
Burow's
op·er·a·tion
so·lu·tion
tri·an·gle
vein
burr
cell
bur·row
bur·row·ing
hairs
bur·sa
Achilles b.
b. of acro·mi·on
ad·ven·ti·tious b.
an·ser·ine b.
an·te·ri·or tib·i·al b.
bi·cip·i·to·ra·di·al b.
Boyer's b.
Brodie's b.
Calori's b.
cor·a·co·brach·i·al b.
deep in·fra·pa·tel·lar b.
b. of ex·ten·sor car·pi ra·di·a·lis bre·vis
b. fa·bri·cii
Fleischmann's b.
b. of gas·troc·ne·mi·us
glu·te·o·fem·o·ral b.
glu·te·us me·di·us bur·sas
glu·te·us mi·ni·mus b.
b. of great toe
b. of hy·oid
il·i·ac b.
il·i·o·pec·tin·e·al b.
in·fe·ri·or b. of bi·ceps fe·mo·ris

bur·sa *(continued)*
in·fra·car·di·ac b.
in·fra·hy·oid b.
in·fra·spi·na·tus b.
in·ter·mus·cu·lar glu·te·al b.
in·ter·os·se·ous b. of el·bow
in·tra·ten·di·nous b. of el·bow
is·chi·al b.
la·ryn·ge·al b.
lat·er·al mal·le·o·lus b.
b. of la·tis·si·mus dor·si
Luschka's b.
me·di·al mal·le·o·lar b.
b. of Monro
b. mu·co·sa
b. of ob·tu·ra·tor in·ter·nus
b. of olec·ra·non
omen·tal b.
b. ova·ri·ca
pha·ryn·ge·al b.
b. of the pi·ri·for·mis
b. of pop·li··te·us
pre·pa·tel·lar b.
b. quad·ra·tus fe·mo·ris
quad·ra·tus fe·mo·ris b.
ra·di·al b.
ret·ro·hy·oid b.
rid·er's b.
sar·to·ri·us bur·sas
b. of sem·i·mem·bra·no·sus
sub·a·cro·mi·al b.
sub·cu·ta·ne·ous cal·ca·ne·al b.
sub·cu·ta·ne·ous in·fra·pa·tel·lar b.
sub·cu·ta·ne·ous b. of tib·i·al tu·ber·os·i·ty
sub·del·toid b.
sub·fas·cial pre·pa·tel·lar b.
sub·hy·oid b.
b. sub·lin·gua·lis
sub·scap·u·lar b.
sub·ten·di·nous b. of gas·troc·ne·mi·us
sub·ten·di·nous il·i·ac b.
sub·ten·di·nous pre·pa·tel·lar b.
su·pe·ri·or b. of bi·ceps fe·mo·ris
su·pra·pa·tel·lar b.
syn·o·vi·al b.
syn·o·vi·al troch·le·ar b.
b. of ten·do cal·ca·ne·us
b. of ten·sor ve·li pa·la·ti·ni mus·cle

b. of te·res ma·jor
tib·i·al in·ter·ten·di·nous b.
b. of tra·pe·zi·us
tri·ceps b.
tro·chan·ter·ic b.
troch·le·ar syn·o·vi·al b.
ul·nar b.
bur·sae
bur·sal
ab·scess
cyst
syn·o·vi·tis
bur·sec·to·my
bur·si·tis
an·ser·ine b.
bi·cip·i·tal b.
cal·ca·ne·al b.
in·ter·tu·ber·cu·lar b.
olec·ra·non b.
pre·pa·tel·lar b.
shoul·der b.
sub·a·cro·mi·al b.
sub·del·toid b.
tro·chan·ter·ic b.
bur·so·lith
bur·sop·a·thy
bur·sot·o·my
burst
res·pi·ra·to·ry b.
bur·su·la
b. tes·ti·um
Burton's
line
Bu·ru·li
ul·cer
Bury's
dis·ease
Buschke-Löwenstein
tu·mor
Buschke-Ollendorf
syn·drome
Buschke's
dis·ease
bush
sick·ness
yaws
bu·spi·rone hy·dro·chlo·ride
Busquet's
dis·ease
Buss
dis·ease
Busse-Buschke
dis·ease
bu·sul·fan
bu·sul·phan
bu·ta·bar·bi·tal
bu·ta·caine sul·fate
bu·tal·bi·tal

bu·tam·ben
bu·tane
bu·ta·nil·i·caine
bu·ta·no·ic ac·id
bu·ta·nol
bu·ta·nol-ex·tract·a·ble
io·dine
bu·ta·nol-ex·tract·a·ble io·dine
test
bu·tan·o·yl
bu·ta·per·a·zine
bu·tav·er·ine
bu·te·thal
bu·teth·a·mate
bu·teth·a·mine hy·dro·chlo·ride
bu·thal·i·tal
bu·thi·a·zide
bu·to·con·a·zole ni·trate
bu·to·py·ro·nox·yl
bu·tor·pha·nol tar·trate
bu·tox·a·mine hy·dro·chlo·ride
t-bu·tox·y·car·bon·yl
bu·trip·ty·line hy·dro·chlo·ride
butt
but·ter
   b. of an·ti·mo·ny
   b. of bis·muth
   ca·cao b.
   co·coa b.
   b. of tin
   b. of zinc
but·ter
   stools
but·ter·fly
   ad·re·nal
   erup·tion
   frag·ment
   lung
   patch
   rash
   ver·te·bra
but·ter·milk
but·ter yel·low
but·tocks
but·ton
   Am·boy·na b.
   Bis·kra b.
   Murphy's b.
   Or·i·en·tal b.
   per·i·to·ne·al b.
but·ton
   su·ture
but·ton·hole
   ir·i·dec·to·my
   ste·no·sis

but·tress
   foot
   plate
bu·tyl
   b. al·co·hol
   b. ami·no·ben·zo·ate
   iso·bu·tyl al·co·hol
   pri·mary b. al·co·hol
   sec·on·dary b. al·co·hol
   ter·ti·ary b. al·co·hol
tert-bu·tyl·ox·y·car·bon·yl
bu·tyl·par·a·ben
bu·ty·ra·ce·ous
bu·ty·rate
bu·ty·rate-CoA li·gase
bu·tyr·ic
bu·tyr·ic ac·id
bu·tyr·o·cho·lin·es·ter·ase
bu·ty·roid
bu·tyr·om·e·ter
bu·ty·ro·phe·none
bu·tyr·ous
bu·tyr·yl
bu·tyr·yl·cho·line es·ter·ase
bu·tyr·yl-CoA syn·the·tase
bu·yo cheek
   can·cer
Buzzard's
   ma·neu·ver
Bwam·ba
   fe·ver
   vi·rus
By
   an·ti·gen
Byler
   dis·ease
by·pass
   aor·to·cor·o·nary b.
   aor·to·il·i·ac b.
   aor·to·re·nal b.
   bow·el b.
   car·di·o·pul·mo·nary b.
   cor·o·nary b.
   ex·tra·in·tra·cra·ni·al b.
   fem·o·ro·pop·lit·e·al b.
   gas·tric b.
   je·ju·no·il·e·al b.
   par·tial il·e·al b.
bys·si·no·sis
By·zan·tine arch
   pal·ate

C
bile
cell
chain
fac·tors
fi·bers
wave
C-
band·ing
ter·mi·nus
CA
vi·rus
c-a
in·ter·val
caa·pi
cab·bage
goi·ter
cab·bage tree
cab·i·net
pneu·mat·ic c.
Sauerbruch's c.
ca·ble
graft
Cabot-Locke
mur·mur
Cabot's ring
bod·ies
ca·cao
but·ter
ca·cao
c. oil
ca·ché
ca·chec·tic
ede·ma
en·do·car·di·tis
fe·ver
pal·lor
cac·hec·tin
ca·chet
ca·chex·ia
c. aph·tho·sa
c. aquo·sa
c. hy·po·phys·e·o·pri·va
hy·po·phy·si·al c.
ma·lar·i·al c.
pi·tu·i·tary c.
c. stru·mi·pri·va
c. thy·roi·dea
c. thy·ro·pri·va

cach·in·na·tion
cac·o·cho·lia
cac·o·de·mon·o·ma·nia
cac·o·dyl
cac·o·dyl·ate
cac·o·dyl·ic
cac·o·dyl·ic ac·id
cac·o·gen·e·sis
cac·o·gen·ic
cac·o·gen·ics
cac·o·geu·sia
cac·o·me·lia
cac·o·plas·tic
ca·cos·mia
cac·ti·no·my·cin
cac·u·men
cac·u·mi·na
cac·u·mi·nal
ca·dav·er
ca·dav·er·ic
ri·gid·i·ty
spasm
ca·dav·er·ine
ca·dav·er·ous
cad·dis
worm
cade oil
cad·mi·um
ca·du·ca
ca·fe
cor·o·nary
ca·fé au lait
spots
caf·fe·a·rine
caf·feine
c. cit·rate
c. hy·drate
c. and so·di·um ben·zo·ate
c. and so·di·um sa·lic·y·
late
caf·fein·ism
Caffey's
dis·ease
syn·drome
Caffey-Silverman
syn·drome
cage
tho·rac·ic c.

Cagot
ear
Cain
com·plex
cais·son
dis·ease
Cajal's
cell
Cajal's as·tro·cyte
stain
caj·e·put oil
caj·e·put·ol
caj·u·put oil
caj·u·put·ol
cake
al·um
kid·ney
caked
breast
Cal·a·bar
swell·ing
Cal·a·bar bean
cal·a·mine
cal·a·mus
c. scrip·to·ri·us
cal·ca·ne·al
ar·ter·ies
bone
bur·si·tis
gait
pro·cess of cu·boid bone
re·gion
sul·cus
tu·ber
tu·ber·cle
tu·ber·os·i·ty
cal·ca·ne·al ar·tic·u·lar
sur·face of ta·lus
cal·ca·ne·an
ten·don
cal·ca·nei
cal·ca·ne·o·a·poph·y·si·tis
cal·ca·ne·o·as·trag·a·loid
cal·ca·ne·o·cu·boid
joint
lig·a·ment
cal·can·e·o·dyn·ia
cal·ca·ne·o·fib·u·lar
lig·a·ment
cal·ca·ne·o·na·vic·u·lar
lig·a·ment
cal·ca·ne·o·scaph·oid
cal·ca·ne·o·tib·i·al
lig·a·ment
cal·ca·ne·o·val·gus
cal·ca·ne·o·var·us
cal·ca·ne·um
cal·ca·ne·us

cal·car
c. fe·mo·ra·le
c. pe·dis
cal·car·e·ous
con·junc·ti·vi·tis
de·gen·er·a·tion
in·fil·tra·tion
me·tas·ta·sis
cal·ca·rine
ar·tery
fas·cic·u·lus
fis·sure
sul·cus
cal·car·i·u·ria
cal·cer·gy
cal·ces
cal·cic
wa·ter
cal·ci·co·sis
cal·ci·di·ol
cal·ci·fe·di·ol
cal·cif·er·ol
cal·cif·er·ous
cal·ci·fi·ca·tion
dys·tro·phic c.
met·a·stat·ic c.
Mönckeberg's c.
path·o·log·ic c.
pulp c.
cal·ci·fi·ca·tion
lines of Retzius
cal·cif·ic nod·u·lar aor·tic
ste·no·sis
cal·ci·fied
car·ti·lage
cal·ci·fy
cal·ci·fy·ing ep·i·the·li·al
odon·to·gen·ic
tu·mor
cal·ci·fy·ing and ker·a·tin·iz·
ing odon·to·gen·ic
cyst
cal·ci·fy·ing odon·to·gen·ic
cyst
cal·cii
cal·ci·na·tion
cal·cine
cal·cined
mag·ne·sia
cal·ci·no·sis
c. cir·cum·scrip·ta
c. cu·tis
dys·tro·phic c.
c. in·ter·ver·te·bra·lis
re·vers·i·ble c.
tu·mor·al c.
c. uni·ver·sa·lis

cal·ci·nu·ric
  di·a·be·tes
cal·ci·ol
cal·ci·o·stat
cal·ci·o·trau·mat·ic
cal·ci·pe·nia
cal·ci·pe·nic
cal·ci·pex·ic
cal·ci·pex·is
cal·ci·pexy
cal·ci·phil·ia
cal·ci·phy·lax·is
cal·ci·priv·ia
cal·ci·priv·ic
cal·cis
cal·cite
cal·ci·tet·rol
cal·ci·to·nin
cal·ci·tri·ol
cal·ci·tro·ic ac·id
cal·ci·um
  c. al·gi·nate
  c. ami·no·sa·lic·y·late
  c. ben·zo·yl·pas
  c. bro·mide
  c. carb·as·pi·rin
  c. car·bide
  c. car·bi·mide
  c. car·bon·ate
  c. ca·sein·ate
  c. chlo·ride
  cit·rat·ed c. car·bi·mide
  crude c. sul·fide
  c. cy·an·a·mide
  di·ba·sic c. phos·phate
  c. di·so·di·um ed·e·tate
  c. di·so·di·um eth·yl·ene·
    di·a·mine·tet·ra·ac·e·tate
  c. fo·li·nate
  c. glu·bi·o·nate
  c. glu·cep·tate
  c. glu·co·hep·to·nate
  c. glu·co·nate
  c. glyc·er·o·phos·phate
  c. hip·pu·rate
  c. hy·drox·ide
  c. hy·po·phos·phite
  c. io·date
  c. io·do·be·hen·ate
  c. ipo·date
  c. lac·tate
  c. lac·to·phos·phate
  c. leu·co·vo·rin
  c. lev·u·li·nate
  c. man·del·ate
  c. mon·o·hy·dro·gen phos·
    phate
  c. ox·a·late

  c. ox·ide
  c. pan·to·then·ate
  pre·cip·i·tat·ed c. car·bon·
    ate
  c. pro·pi·o·nate
  ra·ce·mic c. pan·to·then·ate
  c. sac·cha·rate
  sec·on·dary c. phos·phate
  c. ste·a·rate
  c. sul·fate
  c. sul·fite
  ter·ti·ary c. phos·phate
  tri·ba·sic c. phos·phate
  c. tri·so·di·um pen·te·tate
cal·ci·um
  an·tag·o·nist
  gout
  rig·or
  time
cal·ci·um chan·nel-block·ing
  agent
cal·ci·um group
cal·ci·u·ria
cal·co·dyn·ia
cal·coph·or·ous
cal·co·sphe·rite
calc·spar
cal·cu·lat·ed mean
  or·ga·nism
cal·cu·lat·ed se·rum
  os·mo·lal·i·ty
cal·cu·li
cal·cu·lo·sis
cal·cu·lus
  ap·a·tite c.
  ar·thrit·ic c.
  bil·i·ary c.
  blood c.
  branched c.
  bron·chi·al c.
  car·di·ac c.
  ce·re·bral c.
  com·bi·na·tion c.
  cor·al c.
  cys·tine c.
  de·cu·bi·tus c.
  den·drit·ic c.
  den·tal c.
  en·cyst·ed c.
  fi·brin c.
  fu·si·ble c.
  gas·tric c.
  he·ma·to·ge·net·ic c.
  he·mic c.
  in·di·go c.
  in·tes·ti·nal c.
  lac·ri·mal c.
  mam·ma·ry c.

cal·cu·lus *(continued)*
  ma·trix c.
  mul·ber·ry c.
  na·sal c.
  ne·phrit·ic c.
  ox·a·late c.
  pan·cre·at·ic c.
  pha·ryn·ge·al c.
  pleu·ral c.
  pock·et·ed c.
  pre·pu·ti·al c.
  pri·mary re·nal c.
  pros·tat·ic c.
  pulp c.
  re·nal c.
  sal·i·vary c.
  sec·on·dary re·nal c.
  se·rum·al c.
  stag·horn c.
  stru·vite c.
  sub·gin·gi·val c.
  su·pra·gin·gi·val c.
  ton·sil·lar c.
  uri·nary c.
  uter·ine c.
  ves·i·cal c.
  wed·del·lite c.
  whe·wel·lite c.
Cal·cu·lus Sur·face In·dex
Caldani's
  lig·a·ment
Caldwell
  pro·jec·tion
  view
Caldwell-Luc
  op·er·a·tion
Caldwell-Moloy
  clas·si·fi·ca·tion
cal·e·fa·cient
calf
  bull-dog c.
  foot·ball c.
  gnome's c.
calf
  bone
  diph·the·ria
calf-bone
cal·i·ber
cal·i·brate
cal·i·bra·tion
cal·i·bra·tor
cal·i·ce·al
cal·i·cec·ta·sis
cal·i·cec·to·my
ca·li·ces
ca·lic·i·form
  cell
  end·ing

cal·i·cine
Ca·lic·i·vi·rus
ca·li·co·plas·ty
cal·i·cot·o·my
ca·lic·u·li
ca·lic·u·lus
  c. oph·thal·mi·cus
ca·li·ec·ta·sis
ca·li·ec·to·my
Cal·i·for·nia
  en·ceph·a·li·tis
  vi·rus
Cal·i·for·nia psy·cho·log·i·cal
  in·ven·to·ry
  test
cal·i·for·ni·um
cal·i·ga·tion
ca·li·go
ca·li·o·plas·ty
ca·li·or·rha·phy
ca·li·ot·o·my
cal·i·per
  mi·cro·me·ter
cal·i·pers
cal·is·then·ics
ca·lix
  ma·jor ca·li·ces
  mi·nor ca·li·ces
Calkins'
  sign
Callahan's
  meth·od
Callander's
  am·pu·ta·tion
Call-Exner
  bod·ies
Cal·liph·o·ra
Callison's
  flu·id
Cal·li·tro·ga
cal·lo·sal
  con·vo·lu·tion
  gy·rus
  sul·cus
cal·lose
cal·los·i·tas
cal·los·i·ty
cal·lo·so·mar·gin·al
  ar·tery
  fis·sure
cal·lous
cal·lus
  cen·tral c.
  de·fin·i·tive c.
  en·sheath·ing c.
  med·ul·lary c.
  per·ma·nent c.

pro·vi·sion·al c.
tem·po·rary c.
calm·a·tive
Calmette
test
Calmette-Guérin
ba·cil·lus
vac·cine
cal·mod·u·lin
cal·o·mel
veg·e·ta·ble c.
cal·o·mel
elec·trode
ca·lor
ca·lor·ic
nys·tag·mus
test
val·ue
cal·o·rie
gram c.
kil·o·gram c.
large c.
mean c.
small c.
cal·o·rif·ic
ca·lor·i·gen·ic
ac·tion
cal·o·rim·e·ter
Benedict-Roth c.
bomb c.
cal·o·ri·met·ric
cal·o·rim·e·try
di·rect c.
in·di·rect c.
Calori's
bur·sa
ca·lor·i·tro·pic
cal·o·ry
Calot's
tri·an·gle
ca·lum·ba
ca·lum·bin
cal·u·ster·one
cal·var·ia
cal·var·i·ae
cal·var·i·al
hook
cal·var·i·um
Calvé-Perthes
dis·ease
calves
cal·vi·ti·es
calx
cal·y·ce·al
cal·y·cec·ta·sis
cal·y·cec·to·my
ca·ly·ces

ca·lyc·i·form
end·ing
ca·ly·cine
ca·ly·cle
ca·ly·co·plas·ty
cal·y·cot·o·my
ca·lyc·u·lus
ca·ly·ec·ta·sis
Ca·lym·ma·to·bac·te·ri·um
C. gran·u·lo·ma·tis
ca·ly·o·plas·ty
ca·ly·or·rha·phy
ca·ly·ot·o·my
ca·lyx
cam·ben·da·zole
cam·bi·um
lay·er
cam·el·oid
ane·mia
cell
cam·el·pox
cam·era
Anger c.
gam·ma c.
c. oc·u·li an·te·ri·or
c. oc·u·li ma·jor
c. oc·u·li mi·nor
c. oc·u·li pos·te·ri·or
ret·i·nal c.
vit·re·ous c.
cam·er·ae
cam·er·as
cam·er·o·stome
cam·i·sole
cam·o·mile
CAMP
test
camp
fe·ver
Campbell
sound
Campbell's
lig·a·ment
Camper's
chi·asm
fas·cia
lig·a·ment
line
plane
cam·phane
cam·phene
cam·phet·a·mide
cam·phor
can·tha·ris c.
c. lin·i·ment
mon·o·bro·mat·ed c.
pep·per·mint c.

cam·phor *(continued)*
    tar c.
    thyme c.
cam·pho·ra·ceous
cam·phor·at·ed
    men·thol
    phe·nol
cam·phor·at·ed oil
cam·pho·ta·mide
cam·phra·mine
cam·pi fo·reli
cam·pim·e·ter
cAMP re·cep·tor
    pro·tein
camp·to·cor·mia
camp·to·dac·tyl·ia
camp·to·dac·ty·ly
camp·to·me·lia
camp·to·mel·ic
    dwarf·ism
camp·to·spasm
Cam·py·lo·bac·ter
    C. fe·tus
    C. fe·tus subsp. *je·ju·ni*
    C. spu·to·rum
cam·py·lo·bac·ter·i·o·sis
camp·y·lo·dac·ty·ly
ca·myl·o·fine
Can·a·da
    bal·sam
    snake·root
    tur·pen·tine
can·a·dine
ca·nal
    ab·dom·i·nal c.
    ac·ces·so·ry c.
    ad·duc·tor c.
    Alcock's c.
    al·i·men·ta·ry c.
    al·ve·o·lar c.'s
    al·ve·o·lo·den·tal c.'s
    anal c.
    an·te·ri·or con·dy·loid c. of
      oc·cip·i·tal bone
    an·te·ri·or sem·i·cir·cu·lar
      c.'s
    arch·en·ter·ic c.
    Arnold's c.
    ar·te·ri·al c.
    atri·o·ven·tric·u·lar c.
    au·di·to·ry c.
    ba·si·pha·ryn·ge·al c.
    Bernard's c.
    Bichat's c.
    birth c.
    blas·to·por·ic c.
    bony sem·i·cir·cu·lar c.'s
    Böttcher's c.

    Braune's c.
    Breschet's c.'s
    ca·rot·id c.
    car·pal c.
    cau·dal c.
    cen·tral c.
    cen·tral c.'s of co·chlea
    cer·vi·cal c.
    cil·i·ary c.'s
    Civinini's c.
    Cloquet's c.
    co·chle·ar c.
    con·dy·lar c.
    con·dy·loid c.
    Corti's c.
    Cotunnius' c.
    cra·ni·o·pha·ryn·ge·al c.
    cru·ral c.
    def·er·ent c.
    den·tal c.'s
    den·ti·nal c.'s
    di·plo·ic c.'s
    Dorello's c.
    Dupuytren's c.
    en·do·der·mal c.
    fa·cial c.
    fal·lo·pi·an c.
    fem·o·ral c.
    Ferrein's c.
    Fontana's c.
    gal·ac·toph·o·rous c.'s
    Gartner's c.
    gas·tric c.
    great·er pal·a·tine c.
    gu·ber·nac·u·lar c.
    gy·ne·co·phor·ic c.
    Hannover's c.
    ha·ver·si·an c.'s
    Hensen's c.
    c. of Hering
    Hirschfeld's c.'s
    Holmgrén-Golgi c.'s
    c. of Hovius
    Hoyer's c.'s
    Huguier's c.
    Hunter's c.
    hy·a·loid c.
    hy·po·glos·sal c.
    in·ci·sive c.
    in·ci·sor c.
    in·fe·ri·or den·tal c.
    in·fra·or·bit·al c.
    in·gui·nal c.
    in·ter·den·tal c.'s
    in·ter·fa·cial c.'s
    ir·rup·tion c.
    Jacobson's c.
    Kuersteiner's c.'s

Kürsteiner's c.'s
lat·er·al c.
lat·er·al sem·i·cir·cu·lar c.'s
Laurer's c.
Lauth's c.
Leeuwenhoek's c.'s
c.'s for less·er pal·a·tine nerves
lon·gi·tu·di·nal c.'s of mo·di·o·lus
Löwenberg's c.
man·dib·u·lar c.
mar·row c.
men·tal c.
mus·cu·lo·tu·bal c.
na·so·lac·ri·mal c.
neu·ral c.
neur·en·ter·ic c.
no·to·chor·dal c.
c. of Nuck
nu·tri·ent c.
ob·tu·ra·tor c.
op·tic c.
pal·a·to·vag·i·nal c.
par·tu·ri·ent c.
pel·vic c.
per·i·car·di·o·per·i·to·ne·al c.
per·sis·tent atri·o·ven·tric·u·lar c.
Petit's c.'s
pha·ryn·ge·al c.
pleu·ro·per·i·car·di·al c.'s
pleu·ro·per·i·to·ne·al c.
por·tal c.'s
pos·te·ri·or sem·i·cir·cu·lar c.'s
pter·y·goid c.
pter·y·go·pal·a·tine c.
pu·den·dal c.
pulp c.
py·lor·ic c.
Rivinus' c.'s
root c. of tooth
Rosenthal's c.
sa·cral c.
Santorini's c.
Schlemm's c.
sem·i·cir·cu·lar c.'s
small c. of chor·da tym·pa·ni
Sondermann's c.
spi·nal c.
spi·ral c. of co·chlea
spi·ral c. of mo·di·o·lus
Stilling's c.
sub·sar·to·ri·al c.

Sucquet-Hoyer c.'s
Sucquet's c.'s
tar·sal c.
tem·po·ral c.
Theile's c.
tu·bo·tym·pan·ic c.
tym·pan·ic c.
unit·ing c.
uro·gen·i·tal c.
uter·o·vag·i·nal c.
van Horne's c.
Velpeau's c.
ver·te·bral c.
ves·i·co·u·re·thral c.
ves·tib·u·lar c.
vid·i·an c.
Volkmann's c.'s
vo·mer·ine c.
vom·er·o·bas·i·lar c.
vom·er·o·ros·tral c.
vom·e·ro·vag·i·nal c.
Walther's c.'s
Wirsung's c.
ca·na·les
can·a·lic·u·lar
  ducts
  sphinc·ter
can·a·lic·u·li
can·a·lic·u·li·tis
can·a·lic·u·li·za·tion
can·a·lic·u·lus
  au·ric·u·lar c.
  bil·i·ary c.
  bone c.
  co·chle·ar c.
  c. in·no·mi·na·tus
  in·ter·cel·lu·lar c.
  in·tra·cel·lu·lar c.
  lac·ri·mal c.
  mas·toid c.
  c. re·u·ni·ens
  se·cre·to·ry c.
  Thiersch's can·a·lic·u·li
ca·na·lis
  c. ner·vi pe·tro·si su·per·fi·ci·a·lis min·or·ris
  c. re·u·ni·ens
  c. um·bil·i·cus
can·a·li·za·tion
ca·nar·y·pox
  vi·rus
can·av·a·nase
Canavan's
  dis·ease
  scle·ro·sis
can·cel·lat·ed
can·cel·li

can·cel·lous
　bone
　tis·sue
can·cel·lus
can·cer
　be·tel c.
　bu·yo cheek c.
　chim·ney sweep's c.
　col·loid c.
　con·ju·gal c.
　c. à deux
　en·ceph·a·loid c.
　c. en cui·rasse
　ep·i·der·moid c.
　ep·i·the·li·al c.
　fa·mil·i·al c.
　glan·du·lar c.
　green c.
　kang c.
　kan·gri c.
　mouse c.
　mule-spin·ner's c.
　par·af·fin c.
　pipe-smok·er's c.
　pitch-work·er's c.
　scar c.
　spi·der c.
　stump c.
　tel·an·gi·ec·tat·ic c.
　wa·ter c.
can·cer
　bod·ies
　fam·i·ly
　juice
can·cer·a·tion
can·cer·i·ci·dal
can·cer·i·gen·ic
can·cer·o·ci·dal
can·cer·o·pho·bia
can·cer·ous
can·cra
can·cri·form
can·croid
can·crum
　c. na·si
　c. oris
can·de·la
can·di·cans
can·di·ci·din
Can·di·da
　C. al·bi·cans
can·di·de·mia
can·di·di·a·sis
can·di·do·sis
can·dle
can·dle-me·ter
can·dle-pow·er

cane
　sug·ar
cane·field
　fe·ver
ca·nic·o·la
　fe·ver
Can·i·dae
ca·nine
　am·e·bi·a·sis
　ba·be·si·o·sis
　bor·re·li·o·sis
　ehr·lich·i·o·sis
　em·i·nence
　fos·sa
　her·pe·to·vi·rus
　hys·te·ria
　leish·man·i·a·sis
　prom·i·nence
　spasm
　tooth
Ca·nine dis·tem·per
ca·nine dis·tem·per
　vi·rus
ca·nine he·red·i·tary
　blind·ness
ca·nine oral
　pap·il·lo·ma
ca·nine par·vo·vi·rus
　dis·ease
ca·nine ve·ne·re·al
　gran·u·lo·ma
ca·ni·ni·form
can·is·ter
ca·ni·ti·es
　c. cir·cum·scrip·ta
　rap·id c.
　c. un·gui·um
can·ker
　wa·ter c.
can·ker
　sores
can·na·bi·di·ol
can·nab·i·noids
can·na·bi·nol
can·na·bis
can·na·bism
Cannizzaro's
　re·ac·tion
can·non
　bone
　sound
　wave
can·non·ball
　pulse
Cannon-Bard
　the·o·ry

Cannon's
ring
the·o·ry
can·nu·la
Karmen c.
Lindemann's c.
per·fu·sion c.
wash·out c.
can·nu·la·tion
can·nu·li·za·tion
can·ren·one
Cantelli's
sign
can·ter·ing
rhythm
can·thal
hy·per·tel·or·ism
can·thar·i·dal
col·lo·di·on
can·thar·i·date
can·thar·i·des
can·thar·i·dic ac·id
can·thar·i·din
can·thar·i·dis
can·tha·ris
cam·phor
can·thec·to·my
can·thi
can·thi·tis
can·thol·y·sis
can·tho·me·a·tal
plane
can·tho·plas·ty
can·thor·rha·phy
can·thot·o·my
can·thus
ex·ter·nal c.
in·ter·nal c.
lat·er·al c.
me·di·al c.
can·ti·le·ver
beam
Cantor
tube
caou·tchouc
pel·vis
cap
splint
stage
cap
ac·ro·so·mal c.
c. of the am·pul·la·ry crest
chin c.
cra·dle c.
den·tal c.'s
du·o·de·nal c.
Dutch c.
enam·el c.

head c.
met·a·neph·ric c.
phryg·i·an c.
py·lor·ic c.
x-ray c. of Zinn
ca·pac·i·tance
ca·pac·i·ta·tion
ca·pac·i·tor
ca·pac·i·ty
buff·er c.
cra·ni·al c.
dif·fus·ing c.
forced vi·tal c.
func·tion·al re·sid·u·al c.
heat c.
in·spi·ra·to·ry c.
iron-bind·ing c.
max·i·mum breath·ing c.
ox·y·gen c.
re·sid·u·al c.
res·pi·ra·to·ry c.
ther·mal c.
to·tal lung c.
vi·tal c.
cap·ac·tins
cap·e·line
ban·dage
Capgras'
phe·nom·e·non
syn·drome
cap·il·lar·ec·ta·sia
Ca·pil·la·ria
C. aer·o·phi·la
C. bo·vis
C. bre·vi·pes
C. he·pat·i·ca
C. phi·lip·pi·nen·sis
C. pli·ca
ca·pil·la·ri·a·sis
in·tes·ti·nal c.
cap·il·lar·i·o·mo·tor
cap·il·lar·i·os·co·py
cap·il·lar·i·tis
cap·il·lar·i·ty
cap·il·la·ron
cap·il·la·rop·a·thy
cap·il·lar·os·co·py
cap·il·lary
ar·te·ri·al c.
bile c.
blood c.
con·tin·u·ous c.
fen·es·trat·ed c.
lymph c.
si·nus·oi·dal c.
ve·nous c.
cap·il·lary
an·gi·o·ma

cap·il·lary *(continued)*
  ar·te·ri·ole
  at·trac·tion
  bed
  cir·cu·la·tion
  drain·age
  frac·ture
  he·man·gi·o·ma
  lake
  loops
  ne·vus
  per·i·cyte
  pulse
  vein
  ves·sel
cap·il·lary fra·gil·i·ty
  test
cap·il·lary per·me·a·bil·i·ty
  fac·tor
cap·il·lary re·sis·tance
  test
ca·pil·li
ca·pil·lus
Ca·pim
  vi·rus·es
cap·i·stra·tion
ca·pi·ta
cap·i·tal
  op·er·a·tion
cap·i·tate
  bone
cap·i·tel·lum
ca·pi·tis
ca·pit·i·um
cap·i·ton·nage
cap·i·to·ped·al
ca·pit·u·la
ca·pit·u·lar
  joint
ca·pit·u·lum
Caplan's
  nod·ules
  syn·drome
cap·no·gram
cap·no·graph
ca·pon-comb-growth
  test
capped
  el·bow
  hock
  knee
  uter·us
cap·ping
  di·rect pulp c.
  in·di·rect pulp c.
Capps'
  re·flex
Cap·ra

cap·rate
cap·re·o·my·cin sul·fate
n-cap·ric ac·id
ca·pril·o·quism
cap·rin
cap·rine
  her·pe·to·vi·rus
Cap·ri·pox·vi·rus
cap·ri·zant
cap·ro·ate
n-ca·pro·ic ac·id
cap·ro·yl
cap·ro·y·late
cap·ry·late
ca·pryl·ic ac·id
cap·sa·i·cin
cap·si·cin
cap·si·cum
cap·sid
cap·so·mer
cap·so·mere
cap·su·la
  c. bul·bi
  c. cor·dis
  c. ex·tre·ma
  c. li·e·nis
  c. vas·cu·lo·sa len·tis
cap·su·lae
cap·su·lar
  ad·vance·ment
  an·ti·gen
  cat·a·ract
  cir·rho·sis of liv·er
  glau·co·ma
  lig·a·ment
  space
cap·su·lar flap
  py·e·lo·plas·ty
cap·su·la·tion
cap·sule
  ad·i·pose c.
  ad·re·nal c.
  ar·tic·u·lar c.
  at·ra·bil·i·ary c.
  au·di·to·ry c.
  bac·te·ri·al c.
  Bonnet's c.
  Bowman's c.
  brood c.'s
  car·ti·lage c.
  cri·co·ar·y·te·noid ar·tic·u·lar c.
  cri·co·thy·roid ar·tic·u·lar c.
  Crosby c.
  crys·tal·line c.
  ex·ter·nal c.
  ex·treme c.

eye c.
fi·brous c.
fi·brous ar·tic·u·lar c.
fi·brous c. of kid·ney
Gerota's c.
Glisson's c.
in·ter·nal c.
joint c.
len·tic·u·lar c.
mal·pi·ghi·an c.
Müller's c.
na·sal c.
op·tic c.
otic c.
per·i·vas·cu·lar fi·brous c.
ra·di·o·tel·e·me·ter·ing c.
sem·i·nal c.
su·pra·re·nal c.
Tenon's c.
cap·sule
cell
for·ceps
cap·su·li·tis
ad·he·sive c.
he·pa·tic c.
cap·su·lo·len·tic·u·lar
cat·a·ract
cap·su·lo·plas·ty
cap·su·lor·rha·phy
cap·su·lo·tome
cap·su·lot·o·my
re·nal c.
cap·to·di·a·mine
cap·to·dra·min
cap·to·pril
cap·ture
atri·al c.
elec·tron c.
ven·tric·u·lar c.
cap·ture
beat
cap·u·ride
Capuron's
points
ca·put
c. an·gu·la·re qua·dra·ti la·
bii su·pe·ri·o·ris
c. cor·nus
c. fe·mo·ris
c. gal·li·na·gi·nis
c. in·fra·or·bi·ta·le qua·
dra·ti la·bii su·pe·ri·o·ris
c. me·du·sae
c. qua·dra·tum
c. suc·ce·da·ne·um
c. zy·go·ma·ti·cum qua·dra·
ti la·bii su·pe·ri·o·ris

car
sick·ness
Carabelli
tu·ber·cle
car·a·mel
ca·ram·i·phen eth·ane·di·sul·
fo·nate
ca·ram·i·phen hy·dro·chlo·ride
Caraparu
vi·rus
ca·ra·te
car·ba·chol
car·ba·cryl·a·mine
res·ins
car·ba·dox
car·ba·mate
c. ki·nase
car·bam·az·e·pine
car·bam·ic ac·id
car·bam·ide
carb·a·mi·no
com·pound
carb·a·mi·no·he·mo·glo·bin
car·ba·mo·ate
car·bam·o·yl
car·bam·o·yl·as·par·tate de·hy·
drase
N-**car·bam·o·yl·as·par·tic**
car·bam·o·yl·a·tion
car·bam·o·yl·car·bam·ic ac·id
car·bam·o·yl·glu·tam·ic ac·id
car·bam·o·yl phos·phate
car·bam·o·yl-phos·phate syn·
thase
car·bam·o·yl·trans·fer·as·es
car·bam·o·yl·u·rea
car·ba·myl
car·ba·myl·a·tion
carb·an·i·on
car·bar·sone
car·ba·zides
car·baz·o·chrome sa·lic·y·late
car·ba·zole
carb·a·zot·ic ac·id
car·ben·i·cil·lin di·so·di·um
car·be·ni·um
car·ben·ox·o·lone di·so·di·um
car·be·ta·pen·tane cit·rate
carb·he·mo·glo·bin
car·bide
car·bi·do·pa
car·bi·ma·zole
car·bi·nol
car·bi·nox·a·mine ma·le·ate
car·bo
car·bo·ben·zoxy
car·bo·cat·i·on

car·bo·chro·mene hy·dro·chlo·ride
car·bo·cy·clic
  com·pound
car·bo·he·mo·glo·bin
car·bo·hy·dras·es
car·bo·hy·drate
  me·tab·o·lism
car·bo·hy·drate-in·duced
  hy·per·li·pe·mia
car·bo·hy·drates
car·bo·hy·drate uti·li·za·tion
  test
car·bo·hy·drat·u·ria
car·bo·hy·dra·zides
car·bol
  fuch·sin
car·bo·late
car·bo·lat·ed
car·bol-fuch·sin
  paint
car·bol·ic ac·id
car·bo·lize
car·bol-thi·o·nin
  stain
car·bo·lu·ria
car·bo·mer
car·bom·e·try
car·bon
  ac·tive c. di·ox·ide
  an·o·mer·ic c.
  c. bi·sul·fide
  c. di·chlo·ride
  c. di·ox·ide
  c. di·ox·ide snow
  c. di·sul·fide
  c. mon·ox·ide
  c. tet·ra·chlo·ride
car·bon
  cy·cle
car·bon·ate
  c. de·hy·dra·tase
  c. hy·dro-ly·ase
car·bon·at·ed
  wa·ter
car·bon·ate de·hy·dra·tase
  in·hib·i·tor
car·bon di·ox·ide
  ac·i·do·sis
  con·tent
  cy·cle
  elec·trode
  elim·i·na·tion
car·bon di·ox·ide-free
  wa·ter
car·bon di·sul·fide
  poi·son·ing

car·bon·ic
  an·hy·drase
  wa·ter
car·bon·ic ac·id
  gas
car·bon·ic an·hy·drase
  in·hib·i·tor
car·bon·ic an·hy·dride
car·bo·ni·um
car·bon mon·ox·ide
  he·mo·glo·bin
  poi·son·ing
car·bo·nom·e·ter
car·bo·nom·e·try
car·bo·nu·ria
car·bon·yl
car·bo·prost tro·meth·a·mine
car·box·am·ide
car·box·im·ide
N-car·box·y·an·hy·drides
car·box·y·ca·thep·sin
car·box·y·dis·mu·tase
car·box·y·he·mo·glo·bin
car·box·y·he·mo·glo·bi·ne·mia
car·box·yl
car·box·yl·ase
car·box·yl·a·tion
car·box·yl·trans·fer·as·es
car·box·y·meth·yl
  cel·lu·lose
car·box·y·pep·ti·dase
  ac·id c.
  ser·ine c.
car·box·y·pep·ti·dase A
car·box·y·pep·ti·dase B
car·box·y·pep·ti·dase C
car·box·y·pep·ti·dase G
car·box·y·pol·y·pep·ti·dase
N-car·box·y·u·rea
car·bun·cle
  kid·ney c.
  re·nal c.
car·bun·cu·lar
car·bun·cu·lo·sis
car·bu·ret
car·bu·ta·mide
car·bu·te·rol hy·dro·chlo·ride
car·cass
car·ci·no·em·bry·on·ic
  an·ti·gen
car·cin·o·gen
  com·plete c.
car·ci·no·gen·e·sis
car·ci·no·gen·ic
car·ci·noid
  syn·drome
  tu·mor
car·ci·no·lyt·ic

car·ci·no·ma
ac·i·nar c.
acin·ic cell c.
ac·i·nose c.
ac·i·nous c.
ad·e·noid cys·tic c.
ad·e·noid squa·mous cell c.
ad·nex·al c.
ad·re·nal cor·ti·cal car·ci·no·mas
al·ve·o·lar cell c.
an·a·plas·tic c.
ap·o·crine c.
ba·sal cell c.
ba·sa·loid c.
ba·sal squa·mous cell c.
ba·si·squa·mous c.
ba·so·squa·mous c.
bron·chi·o·lar c.
bron·chi·o·lo-al·ve·o·lar c.
bron·cho·gen·ic c.
clear cell c. of kid·ney
col·loid c.
c. cu·ta·ne·um
cyl·in·drom·a·tous c.
cys·tic c.
duct c.
duc·tal c.
em·bry·o·nal c.
en·do·me·tri·oid c.
ep·i·der·moid c.
fi·bro·la·mel·lar liv·er cell c.
fol·lic·u·lar car·ci·no·mas
gi·ant cell c.
gi·ant cell c. of thy·roid gland
glan·du·lar c.
he·pa·to·cel·lu·lar c.
Hürthle cell c.
in·flam·ma·to·ry c.
in·ter·me·di·ate c.
in·tra·duc·tal c.
in·tra·ep·i·der·mal c.
in·tra·ep·i·the·li·al c.
in·va·sive c.
ju·ve·nile c.
kan·gri burn c.
large cell c.
la·tent c.
lat·er·al ab·er·rant thy·roid c.
lep·to·me·nin·ge·al c.
liv·er cell c.
lob·u·lar c.
lob·u·lar c. in si·tu
Lucké c.
med·ul·lary c.

mel·a·not·ic c.
me·nin·ge·al c.
mes·o·met·a·neph·ric c.
met·a·plas·tic c.
met·a·stat·ic c.
met·a·typ·i·cal c.
mi·cro·in·va·sive c.
mu·ci·nous c.
mu·co·ep·i·der·moid c.
c. myx·o·ma·to·des
non·in·fil·trat·ing lob·u·lar c.
oat cell c.
oc·cult c.
on·co·plas·tic c.
pap·il·lary c.
pri·mary c.
re·nal cell c.
sar·co·ma·toid c.
scar c.
scir·rhous c.
sec·on·dary c.
se·cre·to·ry c.
sig·net ring cell c.
c. sim·plex
c. in si·tu
small cell c.
spin·dle cell c.
squa·mous cell c.
sweat gland c.
tra·bec·u·lar c.
tran·si·tion·al cell c.
tu·bu·lar c.
ver·ru·cous c.
vil·lous c.
Walker c.
wolff·i·an duct c.
car·ci·no·ma ex ple·o·mor·phic ad·e·no·ma
car·ci·no·mas
car·ci·no·ma·ta
car·ci·no·ma·to·sis
lep·to·me·nin·ge·al c.
me·nin·ge·al c.
car·ci·nom·a·tous
en·ceph·a·lo·my·e·lop·a·thy
im·plants
my·e·lop·a·thy
my·op·a·thy
neu·ro·my·op·a·thy
car·ci·no·pho·bia
car·ci·no·sar·co·ma
em·bry·o·nal c.
re·nal c.
Walker c.
car·ci·no·sis
car·ci·no·stat·ic
car·co·ma

Carden's
am·pu·ta·tion
car·dia
car·di·ac
ac·ci·dent
al·bu·min·ur·ia
an·eu·rysm
ar·rest
ar·rhyth·mia
asth·ma
cal·cu·lus
cath·e·ter
cir·rho·sis
com·pe·tence
cy·cle
de·com·pres·sion
di·as·to·le
di·u·ret·ic
dys·rhyth·mia
ede·ma
fail·ure
gan·glia
gland
glands of esoph·a·gus
he·mop·ty·sis
het·er·o·tax·ia
his·ti·o·cyte
hor·mone
im·pres·sion of liv·er
im·pres·sion of lung
im·pulse
in·com·pe·tence
in·dex
in·farc·tion
in·suf·fi·cien·cy
jel·ly
liv·er
lung
mas·sage
mon·i·tor
mur·mur
mus·cle
neu·ro·sis
notch
notch of left lung
open·ing
out·put
part of stom·ach
plex·us
pol·yp
prom·i·nence
re·serve
seg·ment
skel·e·ton
souf·fle
sound
stand·still
sym·phy·sis

tam·pon·ade
te·lem·e·try
tube
veins
car·di·ac bal·let
car·di·ac de·pres·sor
re·flex
car·di·ac lym·phat·ic
ring
car·di·ac mus·cle
tis·sue
car·di·ac valve
pros·the·sis
car·di·al·gia
car·di·a·tax·ia
car·di·a·te·lia
car·di·ec·ta·sia
car·di·ec·to·my
car·di·ec·to·pia
car·di·nal
lig·a·ment
points
symp·tom
veins
car·di·nal oc·u·lar
move·ments
card·ing
car·di·o·ac·cel·er·a·tor
car·di·o·ac·tive
car·di·o·an·gi·og·ra·phy
car·di·o·a·or·tic
car·di·o·ar·te·ri·al
in·ter·val
car·di·o·cai·ro·graph
car·di·o·cele
car·di·o·cen·te·sis
car·di·o·cha·la·sia
car·di·o·cla·sia
car·di·o·di·o·sis
car·di·o·dy·nam·ics
car·di·o·dyn·ia
car·di·o·e·soph·a·ge·al
re·lax·a·tion
car·di·o·gen·e·sis
car·di·o·gen·ic
plate
shock
car·di·o·gram
esoph·a·ge·al c.
car·di·o·graph
car·di·og·ra·phy
ul·tra·sound c.
car·di·o·he·mo·throm·bus
car·di·o·he·pat·ic
an·gle
tri·an·gle
car·di·o·he·pa·to·meg·a·ly

car·di·oid
  con·dens·er
car·di·o·in·hib·i·to·ry
car·di·o·ki·net·ic
car·di·o·ky·mo·gram
car·di·o·ky·mo·graph
car·di·o·ky·mog·ra·phy
car·di·o·lip·in
car·di·o·lith
car·di·ol·o·gist
car·di·ol·o·gy
car·di·ol·y·sis
car·di·o·ma·la·cia
car·di·o·meg·a·ly
  gly·co·gen c.
car·di·om·e·try
car·di·o·mo·til·i·ty
car·di·o·mus·cu·lar
  bra·dy·car·dia
car·di·o·my·o·li·po·sis
car·di·o·my·op·a·thy
  al·co·hol·ic c.
  beer-drink·er's c.
  di·lat·ed c.
  hy·per·tro·phic c.
  id·i·o·path·ic c.
  post·par·tum c.
  pri·mary c.
  re·stric·tive c.
  sec·on·dary c.
car·di·o·my·ot·o·my
car·di·o·ne·cro·sis
car·di·o·nec·tor
car·di·o·neph·ric
car·di·o·neu·ral
car·di·o·neu·ro·sis
car·di·o-o·men·to·pexy
car·di·o·pal·u·dism
car·di·o·path
car·di·o·path·ia nig·ra
car·di·op·a·thy
car·di·o·per·i·car·di·o·pexy
car·di·o·pho·bia
car·di·o·phone
car·di·oph·o·ny
car·di·o·phre·nia
car·di·o·plas·ty
car·di·o·ple·gia
car·di·o·ple·gic
car·di·op·to·sia
car·di·o·pul·mo·nary
  by·pass
  mur·mur
  re·sus·ci·ta·tion
car·di·o·py·lo·ric
car·di·o·re·nal
car·di·o·res·pi·ra·to·ry
  mur·mur

car·di·or·rha·phy
car·di·or·rhex·is
car·di·os·chi·sis
car·di·o·scope
car·di·o·se·lec·tive
car·di·o·se·lec·tiv·i·ty
car·di·o·spasm
car·di·o·sphyg·mo·graph
car·di·o·ta·chom·e·ter
car·di·o·tho·rac·ic
  in·dex
  ra·tio
car·di·o·throm·bus
car·di·o·thy·ro·tox·i·co·sis
car·di·ot·o·my
car·di·o·ton·ic
car·di·o·tox·ic
  my·ol·y·sis
car·di·o·val·vot·o·my
car·di·o·val·vu·li·tis
car·di·o·val·vu·lot·o·my
car·di·o·vas·cu·lar
  sys·tem
car·di·o·vas·cu·lo·re·nal
car·di·o·ver·sion
car·di·o·ver·ter
car·di·tis
  rheu·mat·ic c.
care
  com·pre·hen·sive med·i·cal
    c.
  health c.
  in·ten·sive c.
  med·i·cal c.
  pri·mary med·i·cal c.
  sec·on·dary med·i·cal c.
  ter·ti·ary med·i·cal c.
car·e·ba·ria
Carey Coombs
  mur·mur
ca·ri·bi
car·i·ca
car·ies
  ac·tive c.
  ar·rest·ed den·tal c.
  buc·cal c.
  ce·ment·al c.
  com·pound c.
  den·tal c.
  dis·tal c.
  fis·sure c.
  in·cip·i·ent c.
  in·ter·den·tal c.
  me·si·al c.
  oc·clu·sal c.
  pit c.
  pit and fis·sure c.
  pri·mary c.

car·ies *(continued)*
    prox·i·mal c.
    ra·di·a·tion c.
    re·cur·rent c.
    root c.
    sec·on·dary c.
    se·nile den·tal c.
    smooth sur·face c.
ca·ri·na
    c. for·ni·cis
    c. va·gi·nae
ca·ri·nae
car·i·nate
    ab·do·men
car·i·o·gen·e·sis
car·i·o·gen·ic
car·i·o·ge·nic·i·ty
car·i·ol·o·gy
car·i·o·stat·ic
car·i·ous
car·i·so·pro·date
car·i·so·pro·dol
ca·ris·sin
Carlen's
    tube
carm·al·um
car·mi·nate
car·min·a·tive
car·mine
    Schneider's c.
car·min·ic ac·id
car·min·o·phil
car·min·o·phile
car·mi·noph·i·lous
Carmody-Batson
    op·er·a·tion
car·mus·tine
car·nas·si·al
    tooth
car·nau·ba
    wax
car·ne·ous
    de·gen·er·a·tion
    mole
car·nes
Carnett's
    sign
car·ni·fi·ca·tion
car·nis
car·ni·tine
Car·niv·o·ra
car·ni·vore
car·niv·o·rous
car·no·sine
car·nos·i·ty
Carnoy's
    fix·a·tive

ca·ro
    c. qua·dra·ta syl·vii
car·ob flour
Caroli's
    dis·ease
car·o·ten·ase
car·o·tene
    c. ox·i·dase
car·o·ten·e·mia
ca·rot·e·noid
ca·rot·e·noids
car·o·te·no·sis cu·tis
ca·rot·ic
ca·rot·i·co·cli·noid
    lig·a·ment
ca·rot·i·co·tym·pan·ic
    ar·ter·ies
    nerve
ca·rot·id
    ar·ter·ies
    body
    bru·it
    bulb
    ca·nal
    duct
    end·ar·ter·ec·to·my
    fo·ra·men
    gan·gli·on
    groove
    sheath
    shud·der
    si·nus
    sul·cus
    tri·an·gles
    tu·ber·cle
    wall of mid·dle ear
ca·rot·id body
    tu·mor
ca·rot·id-cav·ern·ous
    fis·tu·la
ca·rot·id si·nus
    nerve
    re·flex
    syn·co·pe
    syn·drome
ca·rot·i·dyn·ia
car·o·tin
car·o·ti·nase
car·o·tin·e·mia
ca·rot·i·noid
ca·rot·i·no·sis cu·tis
ca·rot·o·dyn·ia
carp
    mouth
car·pal
    arch·es
    ar·tery
    ar·tic·u·la·tion

bones
ca·nal
groove
joints
tun·nel
car·pal ar·tic·u·lar
sur·face of ra·di·us
car·pal tun·nel
syn·drome
car·pec·to·my
Carpenter's
syn·drome
car·phen·a·zine ma·le·ate
car·pho·lo·gia
car·phol·o·gy
car·pi
car·pi·tis
car·po·car·pal
Car·po·glyp·tus
car·po·met·a·car·pal
joints
joint of thumb
lig·a·ments
car·po·ped·al
con·trac·tion
spasm
car·pop·to·sia
car·pop·to·sis
Carpue's
meth·od
car·pus
c. cur·vus
car·ra·geen
car·ra·gee·nan
car·ra·gee·nin
car·ra·gheen
car·re·four sen·si·tif
Carrel-Lindbergh
pump
Carrel's
treat·ment
car·ri·er
cell
screen·ing
state
strain
car·ri·er
amal·gam c.
con·va·les·cent c.
ge·net·ic c.
hy·dro·gen c.
in·cu·ba·to·ry c.
man·i·fest·ing c.
trans·lo·ca·tion c.
Carrión's
dis·ease
Carr-Price
re·ac·tion

car·ry·ing
an·gle
Carter's
fe·ver
Carter's black
my·ce·to·ma
car·te·sian
nom·o·gram
car·tha·mus
car·ti·lage
ac·ces·so·ry c.
ac·ces·so·ry na·sal c.'s
ac·ces·so·ry quad·rate c.
c. of acous·tic me·a·tus
al·i·sphe·noid c.
an·nu·lar c.
ar·thro·di·al c.
ar·tic·u·lar c.
ar·y·te·noid c.
au·di·to·ry c.
c. of au·di·to·ry tube
au·ric·u·lar c.
bas·i·lar c.
bran·chi·al c.'s
cal·ci·fied c.
cel·lu·lar c.
cil·i·ary c.
cir·cum·fer·en·tial c.
con·chal c.
con·nect·ing c.
cor·nic·u·late c.
cos·tal c.
cri·coid c.
cu·ne·i·form c.
di·ar·thro·di·al c.
c. of ear
elas·tic c.
en·si·form c.
en·sis·ter·num c.
ep·i·glot·tic c.
ep·i·phys·i·al c.
fal·ci·form c.
float·ing c.
great·er alar c.
Huschke's c.'s
hy·a·line c.
hyp·si·loid c.
in·nom·i·nate c.
in·ter·os·se·ous c.
in·ter·ver·te·bral c.
in·tra-ar·tic·u·lar c.
in·tra·thy·roid c.
in·vest·ing c.
Jacobson's c.
c.'s of lar·ynx
lat·er·al c.
lat·er·al c. of nose
less·er alar c.'s

car·ti·lage *(continued)*
  loose c.
  Luschka's c.
  man·dib·u·lar c.
  me·a·tal c.
  Meckel's c.
  Meyer's c.'s
  Morgagni's c.
  c. of na·sal sep·tum
  or·bi·to·sphe·noid c.
  par·a·chor·dal c.
  par·a·sep·tal c.
  per·i·o·tic c.
  per·ma·nent c.
  c. of pha·ryn·go·tym·pan·ic tube
  pre·cur·so·ry c.
  pri·mor·di·al c.
  qua·dran·gu·lar c.
  Reichert's c.
  re·tic·u·lar c.
  ret·i·form c.
  Santorini's c.
  sec·on·dary c.
  Seiler's c.
  sem·i·lu·nar c.
  sep·tal c.
  ses·a·moid c. of lar·ynx
  ses·a·moid c.'s of nose
  slip·ping rib c.
  ster·nal c.
  su·pra-ar·y·te·noid c.
  tar·sal c.
  tem·po·rary c.
  thy·roid c.
  tra·che·al c.'s
  tri·an·gu·lar c.
  tri·que·trous c.
  tub·al c.
  unit·ing c.
  vo·mer·ine c.
  vom·er·o·na·sal c.
  Weitbrecht's c.
  Wrisberg's c.
  xi·phoid c.
  Y c.
  yel·low c.
  Y-shaped c.
car·ti·lage
  bone
  cap·sule
  cell
  knife
  la·cu·na
  ma·trix
  space
car·ti·lage-hair
  hy·po·pla·sia

car·ti·la·gi·nes
car·ti·lag·i·noid
car·ti·lag·i·nous
  joint
  neu·ro·cra·ni·um
  part of au·di·to·ry tube
  part of skel·e·tal sys·tem
  sep·tum
  tis·sue
  vis·cer·o·cra·ni·um
car·ti·la·go
ca·ru·bin·ose
ca·run·cle
  Morgagni's c.
  Santorini's ma·jor c.
  Santorini's mi·nor c.
  ure·thral c.
ca·run·cu·la
  ca·run·cu·lae myr·ti·for·mes
  c. myr·ti·for·mis
  c. sa·li·va·ris
ca·run·cu·lae
Carus'
  cir·cle
  curve
car·va·crol
Carvallo's
  sign
carv·er
car·y·o·phyl·lum
car·y·o·phyl·lus
car·y·o·the·ca
Casal's
  neck·lace
cas·a·mi·no ac·ids
cas·cade
  stom·ach
cas·cara
  c. am·a·ra
  c. sa·gra·da
case
  in·dex c.
  tri·al c.
ca·se·a·tion
  ne·cro·sis
case-con·trol
  study
case fa·tal·i·ty
  rate
ca·sein
  io·di·nat·ed c.
  c. io·dine
  plant c.
ca·sein·ate
ca·sein·o·gen
ca·seo·io·dine
ca·se·ose

ca·se·ous
  ab·scess
  de·gen·er·a·tion
  lym·phad·e·ni·tis
  ne·cro·sis
  os·te·i·tis
  pneu·mo·nia
  rhi·ni·tis
  tu·ber·cle
Caslick's
  op·er·a·tion
Casoni in·tra·der·mal
  test
Casoni skin
  test
cas·sa·va starch
Casselberry
  po·si·tion
Casser's
  fon·ta·nel
Casser's per·fo·rat·ed
  mus·cle
cas·sette
cas·sia
  cin·na·mon
cas·sia bark
cas·sia fis·tu·la
cas·sia oil
cast
  blood c.
  co·ma c.
  de·cid·u·al c.
  den·tal c.
  di·ag·nos·tic c.
  ep·i·the·li·al c.
  false c.
  fat·ty c.
  fi·brin·ous c.
  gran·u·lar c.
  hair c.
  ha·lo c.
  hy·a·line c.
  in·vest·ment c.
  mas·ter c.
  mu·cous c.
  re·frac·to·ry c.
  re·nal c.
  spu·ri·ous c.
  tube c.
  uri·nary c.'s
  waxy c.
cast brace
Castellani-Low
  sign
Castellani's
  bron·chi·tis
  paint

Cas·tile
  soap
cast·ing
  flask
  ring
  wax
cast·ing
  cen·trif·u·gal c.
  cer·a·mo·met·al c.
  gold c.
  vac·u·um c.
Castleman's
  dis·ease
Castle's in·trin·sic
  fac·tor
cas·tor bean
cas·tor oil
  ar·o·mat·ic c. o.
cas·trate
  cells
cas·tra·tion
  anx·i·e·ty
  cells
  com·plex
cas·tra·tion
  func·tion·al c.
ca·su·al·ty
cat
  unit
cat·a·ba·si·al
cat·a·bi·ot·ic
cat·a·bol·ic
ca·tab·o·lism
ca·tab·o·lite
ca·tab·o·lite gene
  ac·ti·va·tor
ca·tab·o·lite (gene) ac·ti·va·tor
  pro·tein
cat·a·chron·o·bi·ol·o·gy
cat·a·crot·ic
  pulse
ca·tac·ro·tism
cat·a·di·crot·ic
  pulse
cat·a·di·cro·tism
cat·a·did·y·mus
cat·a·di·op·tric
cat·a·gen
cat·a·gen·e·sis
cat·a·lase
cat·a·lat·ic
  re·ac·tion
cat·a·lep·sy
cat·a·lep·tic
cat·a·lep·toid
cat·a·lo·gia

ca·tal·y·sis
  con·tact c.
  sur·face c.
cat·a·lyst
  in·or·gan·ic c.
  neg·a·tive c.
  or·gan·ic c.
  pos·i·tive c.
  Raney c.
cat·a·lyt·ic
cat·a·lyze
cat·a·lyz·er
cat·a·me·nia
cat·a·me·ni·al
cat·a·men·o·gen·ic
cat·am·ne·sis
cat·am·nes·tic
cat·a·pasm
cat·a·pha·sia
ca·taph·o·ra
cat·a·pho·re·sis
cat·a·pho·ret·ic
cat·a·phy·lax·is
cat·a·pla·sia
cat·a·pla·sis
cat·a·plasm
cat·a·plec·tic
cat·a·plexy
cat·a·ract
  an·nu·lar c.
  ar·bo·res·cent c.
  atop·ic c.
  ax·i·al c.
  ax·il·lary c.
  black c.
  blue c.
  cap·su·lar c.
  cap·su·lo·len·tic·u·lar c.
  cen·tral c.
  com·plete c.
  com·pli·cat·ed c.
  con·cus·sion c.
  con·gen·i·tal c.
  cop·per c.
  cor·al·li·form c.
  cor·o·nary c.
  cor·ti·cal c.
  crys·tal·line c.
  cu·ne·i·form c.
  cu·pu·li·form c.
  den·drit·ic c.
  di·a·bet·ic c.
  disk-shaped c.
  elec·tric c.
  em·bry·on·ic c.
  fi·brin·ous c.
  fi·broid c.
  flo·ri·form c.

fur·nace·men's c.
fu·si·form c.
ga·lac·tose c.
glass·work·er's c.
glau·co·ma·tous c.
gray c.
hard c.
hook-shaped c.
hy·per·ma·ture c.
hy·po·cal·ce·mic c.
im·ma·ture c.
in·fan·tile c.
in·fra·red c.
in·tu·mes·cent c.
ju·ve·nile c.
lam·el·lar c.
life-belt c.
ma·ture c.
mem·bra·nous c.
Morgagni's c.
my·o·ton·ic c.
nu·cle·ar c.
over·ripe c.
per·i·nu·cle·ar c.
pe·riph·e·ral c.
pis·ci·form c.
po·lar c.
pos·te·ri·or sub·cap·su·lar
  c.
pro·gress·ive c.
punc·tate c.
py·ram·i·dal c.
ra·di·a·tion c.
re·du·pli·cat·ed c.
ripe c.
ru·bel·la c.
sau·cer-shaped c.
sec·on·dary c.
sed·i·men·ta·ry c.
se·nile c.
sid·er·a·tic c.
si·lic·u·lose c.
sil·i·quose c.
soft c.
spin·dle c.
sta·tion·ary c.
stel·late c.
sub·cap·su·lar c.
sug·ar c.
su·tur·al c.
syn·der·ma·tot·ic c.
tet·a·ny c.
to·tal c.
tox·ic c.
trau·mat·ic c.
um·bil·i·cat·ed c.
vas·cu·lar c.
zo·nu·lar c.

cat·a·ract
  lens
  nee·dle
  spoon
cat·a·rac·ta
  c. adi·po·sa
  c. bru·nes·cens
  c. ce·ru·lea
  c. der·mat·o·genes
  c. elec·tri·ca
  c. fi·bro·sa
  c. mem·bra·na·cea ac·cre·ta
  c. neu·ro·der·ma·ti·ca
  c. nig·ra
  c. no·di·for·mis
  c. os·sea
cat·a·rac·to·gen·e·sis
cat·a·rac·to·gen·ic
cat·a·ract-ol·i·go·phre·nia
  syn·drome
cat·a·rac·tous
ca·tar·ia
ca·tarrh
  au·tum·nal c.
  ma·lig·nant c. of cat·tle
  na·sal c.
  ver·nal c.
ca·tarrh·al
  asth·ma
  fe·ver
  gas·tri·tis
  in·flam·ma·tion
  jaun·dice
  oph·thal·mia
Cat·ar·rhi·na
cat·ar·rhine
cat·a·stal·sis
cat·a·stal·tic
ca·tas·ta·sis
cat·a·stroph·ic
  re·ac·tion
cat·a·to·nia
  ex·cit·ed c.
  pe·ri·od·ic c.
  stu·por·ous c.
cat·a·to·ni·ac
cat·a·ton·ic
  de·men·tia
  ex·cite·ment
  pu·pil
  ri·gid·i·ty
  schiz·o·phre·nia
  stu·por
cat·a·tor·u·lin
  test
cat·a·tri·chy
cat·a·tri·crot·ic
cat·a·tri·cro·tism

cat·a·tro·pic
  im·age
cat-bite
  dis·ease
  fe·ver
cat-cry
  syn·drome
cat dis·tem·per
  vi·rus
cat·e·chase
cat·e·chin
cat·e·chin·ic ac·id
cat·e·chol
  c. meth·yl·trans·fer·ase
  c. ox·i·dase
  c. ox·i·dase(di·mer·iz·ing)
cat·e·chol·a·mines
cat·e·chu
  c. ni·grum
cat·e·chu·ic ac·id
cat·e·gor·i·cal
  trait
cat·e·lec·trot·o·nus
Ca·te·na·bac·te·ri·um
  C. ca·te·na·for·me
  C. con·tor·tum
  C. fil·a·men·to·sum
  C. hel·min·thoi·des
cat·e·nat·ing
cat·e·noid
ca·ten·u·late
cat·er·pil·lar
  cell
  der·ma·ti·tis
  flap
  rash
cat·er·pil·lar-hair
  oph·thal·mia
cat·gut
  su·ture
cat·gut
  chro·mic c.
  IKI c.
  sil·ver·ized c.
Catha ed·u·lis
ca·thar·sis
ca·thar·tic
ca·thec·tic
ca·them·o·glo·bin
ca·thep·sin
cath·e·ter
  acorn-tipped c.
  bal·loon-tip c.
  bi·cou·date c.
  c. bi·cou·dé
  Bozeman-Fritsch c.
  Braasch c.
  brush c.

cath·e·ter *(continued)*
  car·di·ac c.
  cen·tral ve·nous c.
  con·i·cal c.
  c. cou·dé
  c. à de·meure
  de Pezzer c.
  dou·ble-chan·nel c.
  Drew-Smythe c.
  el·bowed c.
  eu·sta·chi·an c.
  fe·male c.
  Fogarty c.
  Foley c.
  Gouley's c.
  in·dwell·ing c.
  in·tra·car·di·ac c.
  Malecot c.
  Nélaton's c.
  ol·ive-tipped c.
  pac·ing c.
  Pezzer c.
  Phillips' c.
  pros·tat·ic c.
  Robinson c.
  self-re·tain·ing c.
  spi·ral tip c.
  Swan-Ganz c.
  two-way c.
  ver·te·brat·ed c.
  whis·tle-tip c.
  winged c.
cath·e·ter
  em·bo·lus
  fe·ver
  gauge
  guide
cath·e·ter·i·za·tion
cath·e·ter·ize
cath·e·ter·o·stat
ca·thex·is
cath·o·dal
cath·o·dal clo·sure
  con·trac·tion
  tet·a·nus
cath·o·dal du·ra·tion
  tet·a·nus
cath·o·dal open·ing
  clo·nus
  con·trac·tion
  tet·a·nus
cath·ode
  rays
cath·ode ray
  os·cil·lo·scope
  tube
ca·thod·ic
cath·ol·y·sis

cat·i·on
cat·i·on-an·i·on
  dif·fer·ence
cat·i·on-ex·change
  res·in
cat·i·on ex·change
cat·i·on ex·chang·er
cat·i·on·ic
  de·ter·gents
cat·i·on·o·gen
cat·lin
cat·ling
cat·mint
cat·nep
cat·nip
cat·o·chus
ca·top·tric
cat-scratch
  dis·ease
  fe·ver
cat's-eye
  pu·pil
  syn·drome
cat·tle
  plague
  warts
cat·tle plague
  vi·rus
Ca·tu
  vi·rus
cau·da
  c. fas·ci·ae den·ta·tae
  c. stri·a·ti
cau·dad
cau·dae
cau·da equi·na
  syn·drome
cau·dal
  an·es·the·sia
  ca·nal
  flex·ure
  lig·a·ment
  neu·ro·pore
  ret·i·nac·u·lum
  sheath
  ver·te·brae
cau·da·lis
cau·dal neu·ro·se·cre·to·ry
  sys·tem
cau·dal pan·cre·at·ic
  ar·tery
cau·dal pha·ryn·ge·al
  com·plex
cau·dal trans·ten·to·ri·al
  her·ni·a·tion
cau·dal trans·verse
  fis·sure

cau·date
  lobe
  nu·cle·us
  pro·cess
cau·da·to·len·tic·u·lar
cau·da·tum
cau·do·ceph·a·lad
cau·do·len·tic·u·lar
caul
  fat
cau·li·flow·er
  ear
cau·mes·the·sia
caus·al
  ad·di·tiv·i·ty
cau·sal·gia
caus·al in·di·ca·tion
cause
  con·sti·tu·tion·al c.
  ex·cit·ing c.
  pre·dis·pos·ing c.
  prox·i·mate c.
  spe·cif·ic c.
caus·tic
  al·ka·li
  pot·ash
  so·da
cau·ter·ant
cau·ter·i·za·tion
cau·ter·ize
cau·tery
  ac·tu·al c.
  bi·po·lar c.
  chem·i·cal c.
  cold c.
  elec·tric c.
  gal·van·ic c.
  gas c.
  mon·o·po·lar c.
cau·tery
  con·i·za·tion
  knife
ca·va
ca·va·gram
ca·val
  fold
  valve
cav·al·ry
  bone
cav·a·scope
cave
cav·e·o·la
cav·e·o·lae
cav·ern
ca·ver·na
ca·ver·nae
cav·er·nil·o·quy

cav·er·ni·tis
  fi·brous c.
cav·er·no·scope
cav·er·nos·copy
cav·er·no·si·tis
cav·er·nos·to·my
cav·ern·ous
  an·gi·o·ma
  ar·ter·ies
  body of clit·o·ris
  body of pe·nis
  groove
  he·man·gi·o·ma
  lym·phan·gi·ec·ta·sis
  nerves of clit·o·ris
  nerves of pe·nis
  part of in·ter·nal ca·rot·id
   ar·tery
  plex·us
  plex·us of clit·o·ris
  plex·us of con·chae
  plex·us of pe·nis
  rale
  res·o·nance
  res·pi·ra·tion
  rhon·chus
  si·nus
  tis·sue
  voice
cav·ern·ous-ca·rot·id
  an·eu·rysm
cav·ern·ous si·nus
  syn·drome
cav·ern·ous voice
  sound
Ca·via
  C. por·cel·lus
cav·i·ar
  le·sion
cav·i·tary
cav·i·tas
  c. oris pro·pria
cav·i·ta·tes
cav·i·ta·tion
ca·vi·tis
cav·i·ty
  ab·dom·i·nal c.
  al·lan·to·ic c.
  am·ni·ot·ic c.
  ax·il·lary c.
  body c.
  buc·cal c.
  cleav·age c.
  c. of con·cha
  c.'s of cor·po·ra ca·ver·no·
   sa
  c.'s of cor·pus spon·gi·o·
   sum

cav·i·ty *(continued)*
  cot·y·loid c.
  cra·ni·al c.
  crown c.
  ec·to·pla·cen·tal c.
  ec·to·troph·o·blas·tic c.
  ep·am·ni·ot·ic c.
  ep·i·du·ral c.
  gle·noid c.
  great·er per·i·to·ne·al c.
  head c.
  in·tra·cra·ni·al c.
  c. of lar·ynx
  less·er per·i·to·ne·al c.
  Meckel's c.
  med·ul·lary c.
  c. of mid·dle ear
  na·sal c.
  neph·ro·tom·ic c.
  oral c.
  oral c. prop·er
  or·bi·tal c.
  pel·vic c.
  per·i·car·di·al c.
  per·i·to·ne·al c.
  per·i·vis·cer·al c.
  pha·ryn·go·na·sal c.
  c. of phar·ynx
  pleu·ral c.
  pleu·ro·per·i·to·ne·al c.
  prim·i·tive per·i·vis·cer·al
    c.
  pulp c.
  Retzius' c.
  seg·men·ta·tion c.
  c. of sep·tum pel·lu·ci·dum
  so·mite c.
  splanch·nic c.
  sub·a·rach·noid c.
  sub·du·ral c.
  sub·ger·mi·nal c.
  ten·sion c.
  tho·rac·ic c.
  c. of tooth
  tri·gem·i·nal c.
  tym·pan·ic c.
  uter·ine c.
  c. of uter·us
  vis·cer·al c.
cav·i·ty
  li·ner
  mar·gin
  prep·a·ra·tion
  wall
cav·i·ty line
  an·gle

cav·i·ty prep·a·ra·tion
  base
  form
ca·vo·gram
ca·vog·ra·phy
ca·vo·sur·face
  an·gle
  bev·el
ca·vum
  c. ab·do·mi·nis
  c. ar·tic·u·la·re
  c. cor·o·na·le
  c. den·tis
  c. doug·lasi
  c. in·fra·glot·ti·cum
  c. la·ryn·gis
  c. me·di·a·sti·na·le
  c. me·dul·la·re
  c. na·si
  c. oris
  c. pel·vis
  c. pe·ri·car·dii
  c. pe·ri·to·nei
  c. pha·ryn·gis
  c. pleu·rae
  c. psal·te·rii
  c. ret·zii
  c. sub·du·ra·le
  c. tho·ra·cis
  c. tym·pa·ni
  c. uteri
  c. ver·gae
  c. ve·si·co·u·te·ri·num
ca·vy
Cazenave's
  vit·i·li·go
CB
  lead
C-band·ing
  stain
C car·bo·hy·drate
  an·ti·gen
CDE
  an·ti·gens
CDE blood group
ce·as·mic
  ter·a·to·sis
ce·bo·ceph·a·ly
ce·ca
ce·cal
  ar·ter·ies
  folds
  fo·ra·men of fron·tal bone
  fo·ra·men of the tongue
  her·nia
  re·cess
ce·cec·to·my
ce·ci·tis

ce·co·cen·tral
  sco·to·ma
ce·co·co·los·to·my
ce·co·fix·a·tion
ce·co·il·e·os·to·my
ce·co·pexy
ce·co·pli·ca·tion
ce·cor·rha·phy
ce·co·sig·moid·os·to·my
ce·cos·to·my
ce·cot·o·my
ce·cum
ce·dar leaf oil
ce·dar wood oil
Ceelen-Gellerstadt
  syn·drome
cef·a·clor
cef·a·drox·il
cef·a·man·dole nafate
ce·faz·o·lin
ce·fon·i·cid di·so·di·um
ce·fo·per·a·zone so·di·um
ce·for·a·nide
ce·fo·tax·ime so·di·um
cef·o·te·tan di·so·di·um
ce·fox·i·tin so·di·um
cef·taz·i·dime so·di·um
cef·ti·zox·ime so·di·um
cef·tri·ax·one di·so·di·um
ce·lec·tome
ce·len·ter·on
cel·ery seed
Celestin
  tube
ce·les·tine blue B
ce·li·ac
  ar·tery
  ax·is
  dis·ease
  gan·glia
  glands
  plex·us
  rick·ets
  trunk
ce·li·ac lymph
  nodes
ce·li·ac plex·us
  re·flex
ce·li·ag·ra
ce·li·ec·to·my
ce·li·o·cen·te·sis
ce·li·o·en·ter·ot·o·my
ce·li·o·gas·tros·to·my
ce·li·o·gas·trot·o·my
ce·li·o·hys·ter·ec·to·my
ce·li·o·hys·ter·ot·o·my
ce·li·o·my·al·gia
ce·li·o·my·o·mec·to·my

ce·li·o·my·o·mot·o·my
ce·li·o·my·o·si·tis
ce·li·o·par·a·cen·te·sis
ce·li·op·a·thy
ce·li·or·rha·phy
ce·li·o·sal·pin·gec·to·my
ce·li·o·sal·pin·got·o·my
ce·li·os·co·py
ce·li·ot·o·my
  vag·i·nal c.
ce·li·ot·o·my
  in·ci·sion
ce·li·tis
cell
  A c.'s
  ab·sorp·tion c.
  ab·sorp·tive c.'s of in·tes·
    tine
  ac·id c.
  ac·i·do·phil c.
  ac·i·nar c.
  ac·i·nous c.
  acous·tic c.
  ad·i·pose c.
  ad·ven·ti·tial c.
  air c.'s
  al·bu·min·ous c.
  al·goid c.
  al·pha c.'s of an·te·ri·or
    lobe of hy·poph·y·sis
  al·pha c.'s of pan·cre·as
  al·ve·o·lar c.
  am·a·crine c.
  ame·boid c.
  am·ni·o·gen·ic c.'s
  an·a·bi·ot·ic c.'s
  an·a·plas·tic c.
  an·gi·o·blas·tic c.'s
  Anitschkow c.
  an·te·ri·or c.'s
  an·ti·gen-pre·sent·ing c.
  an·ti·gen-re·spon·sive c.
  an·ti·gen-sen·si·tive c.
  apo·lar c.
  APUD c.'s
  ar·gen·taf·fin c.'s
  ar·gyr·o·phil·ic c.'s
  Askanazy c.
  as·trog·lia c.
  au·di·to·ry re·cep·tor c.'s
  B c.
  bal·loon c.
  band c.
  ba·sal c.
  ba·sa·loid c.
  bas·i·lar c.
  bas·ket c.

cell *(continued)*
  ba·so·phil c. of an·te·ri·or lobe of hy·poph·y·sis
  beak·er c.
  Beale's c.
  Berger c.'s
  ber·ry c.
  be·ta c. of an·te·ri·or lobe of hy·poph·y·sis
  be·ta c. of pan·cre·as
  Betz c.'s
  Bevan-Lewis c.'s
  bi·po·lar c.
  Bizzozero's red c.'s
  blast c.
  blood c.
  Boll's c.'s
  bone c.
  bor·der c.'s
  Böttcher's c.'s
  bran·chi·al c.'s
  bris·tle c.
  bron·chic c.'s
  brood c.
  burr c.
  C c.
  Cajal's c.
  ca·lic·i·form c.
  cam·el·oid c.
  cap·sule c.
  car·ri·er c.
  car·ti·lage c.
  cas·trate c.'s
  cas·tra·tion c.'s
  cat·er·pil·lar c.
  cen·tro·ac·i·nar c.
  chal·ice c.
  chief c.
  chief c. of cor·pus pi·ne·a·le
  chief c. of par·a·thy·roid gland
  chief c. of stom·ach
  chro·maf·fin c.
  chro·mo·phobe c.'s of an·te·ri·or lobe of hy·poph·y·sis
  Clara c.
  Claudius' c.'s
  clear c.
  cleav·age c.
  cleaved c.
  clo·no·gen·ic c.
  co·chle·ar hair c.'s
  col·umn c.'s
  com·mis·sur·al c.
  com·pound gran·ule c.
  cone c. of ret·i·na

  con·nec·tive tis·sue c.
  Corti's c.'s
  cres·cent c.
  cy·to·me·ga·lic c.'s
  cy·to·tox·ic c.
  cy·to·tro·pho·blas·tic c.'s
  D c.
  dark c.'s
  daugh·ter c.
  Davidoff's c.'s
  de·cid·u·al c.
  de·coy c.'s
  deep c.
  Deiters' c.'s
  del·ta c. of an·te·ri·or lobe of hy·poph·y·sis
  del·ta c. of pan·cre·as
  den·drit·ic c.'s
  Dogiel's c.'s
  dome c.
  Downey c.
  dust c.
  ef·fec·tor c.
  egg c.
  enam·el c.
  en·do·der·mal c.'s
  en·do·the·li·al c.
  en·ter·o·chro·maf·fin c.'s
  en·ter·o·en·do·crine c.'s
  en·to·der·mal c.'s
  ep·en·dy·mal c.
  ep·i·der·mic c.
  ep·i·the·li·al c.
  ep·i·the·li·al re·tic·u·lar c.
  ep·i·the·li·oid c.
  er·y·throid c.
  eth·moi·dal c.'s
  ex·ter·nal pil·lar c.'s
  ex·u·da·tion c.
  Fañanás c.
  fas·ci·cu·la·ta c.
  fat c.
  fat-stor·ing c.
  floor c.
  foam c.'s
  fol·lic·u·lar ep·i·the·li·al c.
  fol·lic·u·lar ovar·i·an c.'s
  for·eign body gi·ant c.
  form·a·tive c.'s
  fo·ve·o·lar c.'s of stom·ach
  fuch·sin·o·phil c.
  fu·si·form c.'s of ce·re·bral cor·tex
  G c.'s
  gam·ma c. of pan·cre·as
  gan·gli·on c.
  gan·gli·on c.'s of dor·sal spi·nal root

gan·gli·on c.'s of ret·i·na
Gaucher c.'s
ge·mäs·te·te c.
ge·mis·to·cyt·ic c.
germ c.
ger·mi·nal c.
ghost c.
Giannuzzi's c.'s
gi·ant c.
git·ter c.
glia c.'s
glit·ter c.'s
glo·boid c.
glo·mer·u·lo·sa c.
gob·let c.
Golgi ep·i·the·li·al c.
Golgi's c.'s
Goormaghtigh's c.'s
gran·ule c.'s
gran·ule c. of con·nec·tive
  tis·sue
gran·u·lo·sa c.
gran·u·lo·sa lu·te·in c.'s
great al·ve·o·lar c.'s
gua·nine c.
gus·ta·to·ry c.'s
gy·ro·chrome c.
hair c.'s
hairy c.'s
heart fail·ure c.
HeLa c.'s
hel·met c.
help·er c.
HEMPAS c.'s
Hensen's c.
het·er·o·mer·ic c.
hi·lus c.'s
hob·nail c.'s
Hofbauer c.
hor·i·zon·tal c. of Cajal
hor·i·zon·tal c.'s of ret·i·na
Hortega c.'s
Hürthle c.
I c.
im·mu·no·log·i·cal·ly ac·ti·
  vat·ed c.
im·mu·no·log·i·cal·ly com·
  pe·tent c.
in·clu·sion c.
in·dif·fer·ent c.
in·duc·er c.
in·ter·cap·il·lary c.
in·ter·nal pil·lar c.'s
in·ter·sti·tial c.'s
ir·ri·ta·tion c.
is·let c.
Ito c.'s
ju·ve·nile c.

jux·ta·glo·mer·u·lar c.'s
K c.'s
kar·y·o·chrome c.
kill·er c.'s
Kulchitsky c.'s
Kupffer c.'s
la·cis c.
Langerhans' c.'s
Langhans' c.'s
Langhans'-type gi·ant c.'s
LE c.
Leishman's chrome c.'s
lep·ra c.'s
Leydig's c.'s
light c.'s of thy·roid
lin·ing c.
Lipschütz c.
lit·to·ral c.
Loevit's c.'s
lu·pus er·y·the·ma·to·sus c.
lu·te·al c.
lu·te·in c.
lymph c.
lym·phoid c.
ma·crog·lia c.
mal·pi·ghi·an c.
Marchand's wan·der·ing c.
mar·row c.
Martinotti's c.
mast c.
mas·toid c.'s
Mauthner's c.
Merkel's tac·tile c.
mes·an·gi·al c.
me·sen·chy·mal c.'s
me·sog·li·al c.'s
mes·o·the·li·al c.
Mex·i·can hat c.
Meynert's c.'s
mi·crog·lia c.'s
mi·crog·li·al c.'s
mid·dle c.'s
midg·et bi·po·lar c.'s
Mikulicz' c.'s
mir·ror-im·age c.
mi·tral c.'s
mon·o·cy·toid c.
mossy c.
moth·er c.
mo·tor c.
mu·co·al·bu·mi·nous c.'s
mu·co·se·rous c.'s
mu·cous c.
mu·cous neck c.
Müller's ra·di·al c.'s
mul·ti·po·lar c.
mu·ral c.
my·e·loid c.

cell *(continued)*

my·o·ep·i·the·li·al c.
my·oid c.'s
Nageotte c.'s
nat·u·ral kill·er c.'s
nerve c.
Neumann's c.'s
neu·ri·lem·ma c.'s
neu·ro·en·do·crine c.
neu·ro·en·do·crine trans·
  duc·er c.
neu·ro·ep·i·the·li·al c.'s
neu·rog·lia c.'s
neu·ro·lem·ma c.'s
neu·ro·mus·cu·lar c.
neu·ro·se·cre·to·ry c.'s
ne·vus c.
Niemann-Pick c.
NK c.'s
no·ble c.'s
non·clo·no·gen·ic c.
null c.'s
nurse c.'s
oat c.
OKT c.'s
ol·fac·to·ry re·cep·tor c.'s
ol·i·go·den·drog·lia c.'s
Opalski c.
os·se·ous c.
os·te·o·chon·dro·gen·ic c.
os·te·o·gen·ic c.
os·te·o·pro·gen·i·tor c.
ox·yn·tic c.
ox·y·phil c.'s
P c.
packed hu·man blood c.'s
pag·et·oid c.'s
Paget's c.'s
Paneth's gran·u·lar c.'s
par·a·fol·lic·u·lar c.'s
par·a·gan·gli·on·ic c.'s
par·a·lu·te·al c.
pa·ren·chy·mal c.
par·en·chym·a·tous c. of
  cor·pus pi·ne·a·le
par·ent c.
pa·ri·e·tal c.
pep·tic c.
per·i·cap·il·lary c.
per·i·po·lar c.
per·i·the·li·al c.
per·i·tu·bu·lar con·trac·tile
  c.'s
pes·sa·ry c.
pha·lan·ge·al c.'s
phe·o·chrome c.
pho·to·re·cep·tor c.'s
phys·a·liph·or·ous c.

Pick c.
pig·ment c.
pig·ment c.'s of iris
pig·ment c.'s of ret·i·na
pig·ment c. of skin
pil·lar c.'s
pil·lar c.'s of Corti
pin·e·al c.'s
plas·ma c.
plu·rip·o·tent c.'s
po·lar c.
pol·y·chro·mat·ic c.
pol·y·chro·ma·to·phil c.
pos·te·ri·or c.'s
preg·nan·cy c.'s
pre·gra·nu·lo·sa c.'s
prick·le c.
pri·mary em·bry·on·ic c.
prim·i·tive re·tic·u·lar c.
pri·mor·di·al c.
pri·mor·di·al germ c.
pro·lac·tin c.
pseu·do-Gaucher c.
pseu·do·u·ni·po·lar c.
pseu·do·xan·tho·ma c.
pulp·ar c.
Purkinje's c.'s
pus c.
py·ram·i·dal c.'s
pyr·rhol c.
pyr·rol c.
Raji c.
re·ac·tive c.
red blood c.
Reed c.'s
Reed-Sternberg c.'s
Renshaw c.'s
rest·ing c.
rest·ing wan·der·ing c.
re·struc·tured c.
re·tic·u·lar c.
re·tic·u·la·ris c.
re·tic·u·lo·en·do·the·li·al c.
rha·gi·o·crine c.
Rieder c.'s
Rindfleisch's c.'s
rod nu·cle·ar c.
rod c. of ret·i·na
Rolando's c.'s
ro·sette-form·ing c.'s
Rouget c.
sar·co·gen·ic c.
sat·el·lite c.'s
sat·el·lite c. of skel·e·tal
  mus·cle
scav·eng·er c.
Schilling's band c.
Schultze's c.'s

Schwann c.'s
seg·ment·ed c.
sen·si·tized c.
sep·tal c.
se·ro·mu·cous c.'s
se·rous c.
Sertoli's c.'s
sex c.
Sézary c.
shad·ow c.'s
sick·le c.
sig·net ring c.'s
sil·ver c.
skein c.
small cleaved c.
smudge c.'s
so·mat·ic c.'s
sperm c.
spi·der c.
spin·dle c.
spine c.
splen·ic c.'s
squa·mous c.
squa·mous al·ve·o·lar c.'s
stab c.
staff c.
stan·dard c.
stel·late c.'s of ce·re·bral
  cor·tex
stel·late c.'s of liv·er
stem c.
Sternberg c.'s
Sternberg-Reed c.'s
stich·o·chrome c.
strap c.
sup·port·ing c.
sup·pres·sor c.
sur·face mu·cous c.'s of
  stom·ach
sus·ten·tac·u·lar c.
sym·pa·thet·ic form·a·tive
  c.
sym·path·i·co·tro·pic c.'s
sym·pa·tho·chro·maf·fin c.
syn·o·vi·al c.
T c.
tac·tile c.
tanned red c.'s
tar·get c.
tart c.
taste c.'s
ten·don c.'s
the·ca lu·te·in c.
the·ca c.'s of stom·ach
Tiselius elec·tro·pho·re·sis c.
to·tip·o·tent c.
touch c.
Touton gi·ant c.

trans·duc·er c.
tran·si·tion·al c.
tub·al air c.'s
tufted c.
tun·nel c.'s
Türk c.
tym·pan·ic c.'s
type II c.'s
Tzanck c.'s
un·dif·fer·en·ti·at·ed c.
uni·po·lar c.
va·so·for·ma·tive c.
veil c.
ves·tib·u·lar hair c.'s
Virchow's c.'s
vi·rus-trans·formed c.
vi·su·al re·cep·tor c.'s
vit·re·ous c.
wan·der·ing c.
Warthin-Finkeldey c.'s
was·ser·hel·le c.
wa·ter-clear c. of par·a·thy·
  roid
white blood c.
wing c.
yolk c.'s
zy·mo·gen·ic c.

cell
  body
  bridg·es
  cen·ter
  cul·ture
  cy·cle
  fu·sion
  hy·brid·i·za·tion
  in·clu·sions
  line
  mark·er
  ma·trix
  mem·brane
  nests
  or·gan·elle
  strain
  trans·for·ma·tion
  wall
cel·la
  c. me·dia
cel·lae
cell-bound
  an·ti·body
cel·lic·o·lous
cell-me·di·at·ed
  im·mu·ni·ty
  re·ac·tion
cel·lo·bi·ase
cel·lo·bi·ose
cel·lo·hex·ose
cel·loi·din

cel·lon
cel·lo·na
cel·lose
cel·lu·la
   cel·lu·lae an·te·ri·o·res
   cel·lu·lae co·li
   cel·lu·lae me·di·ae
   cel·lu·lae pos·te·ri·o·res
cel·lu·lae
cel·lu·lar
   bi·ol·o·gy
   car·ti·lage
   em·bo·lism
   im·mu·ni·ty
   im·mu·no·de·fi·cien·cy with
    ab·nor·mal im·mu·no·
    glob·u·lin syn·the·sis
   in·fil·tra·tion
   mo·sa·i·cism
   pa·thol·o·gy
   pol·yp
   spill
   te·nac·i·ty
   tu·mor
cel·lu·lar blue
   ne·vus
cel·lu·lar im·mu·ni·ty de·fi·
  cien·cy
   syn·drome
cel·lu·lar·i·ty
cel·lu·lase
cel·lule
cel·lu·li·ci·dal
cel·lu·lif·u·gal
cel·lu·lin
cel·lu·lip·e·tal
cel·lu·lite
cel·lu·lit·ic
   phleg·ma·sia
cel·lu·li·tis
   acute scalp c.
   dis·sect·ing c.
   eo·sin·o·phil·ic c.
   ep·i·zo·ot·ic c.
   pel·vic c.
   phleg·mon·ous c.
cel·lu·lo·cu·ta·ne·ous
   flap
cel·lu·loid
   strip
cel·lu·los·an
cel·lu·lose
   c. ac·e·tate
   c. ac·e·tate phthal·ate
   car·box·y·meth·yl c.
   di·eth·yl·a·mi·no·eth·yl c.
   mi·cro·crys·tal·line c.
   ox·i·dized c.

cel·lu·los·ic ac·id
CELO
   vi·rus
ce·lom
   ex·tra·em·bry·on·ic c.
ce·lo·ma
ce·lom·ic
   bays
   pouch·es
ce·lom·ic met·a·pla·sia
   the·o·ry of en·do·me·tri·o·
   sis
ce·lo·nych·ia
ce·lo·phle·bi·tis
ce·los·chi·sis
ce·lo·scope
ce·los·co·py
ce·lo·so·mia
ce·lo·the·li·um
ce·lot·o·my
ce·lo·zo·ic
Cel·si·us
   scale
Celsus'
   al·o·pe·cia
   ar·ea
   ke·ri·on
   pap·ules
   vit·i·li·go
ce·ment
   base
   cor·pus·cle
   line
ce·ment
   com·pos·ite den·tal c.
   cop·per phos·phate c.
   den·tal c.
   in·or·gan·ic den·tal c.
   in·ter·cel·lu·lar c.
   mod·i·fied zinc ox·ide-eu·
   ge·nol c.
   or·gan·ic den·tal c.
   pol·y·car·box·y·late c.
   sil·i·cate c.
   tooth c.
   un·mod·i·fied zinc ox·ide-
   eu·ge·nol c.
   zinc phos·phate c.
ce·ment·al
   car·ies
   dys·pla·sia
ce·men·ta·tion
ce·ment·i·cle
ce·ment·i·fi·ca·tion
ce·ment·i·fy·ing
   fi·bro·ma
ce·ment·o·blast

ce·ment·o·blas·to·ma
be·nign c.
ce·ment·o·cla·sia
ce·ment·o·clast
ce·ment·o·cyte
ce·ment·o·den·tin·al
junc·tion
ce·men·to·e·nam·el
junc·tion
ce·men·to·ma
gi·gan·ti·form c.
true c.
ce·men·tum
afi·bril·lar c.
pri·mary c.
sec·on·dary c.
ce·men·tum
hy·per·pla·sia
ce·nes·the·sia
ce·nes·the·sic
ce·nes·thet·ic
ce·nes·thop·a·thy
ce·no·cyte
ce·no·cyt·ic
ce·no·gen·e·sis
cen·o·site
ce·no·trope
cen·sor
cen·ter
ano·spi·nal c.
Broca's c.
Budge's c.
cell c.
chon·dri·fi·ca·tion c.
cil·i·o·spi·nal c.
den·ta·ry c.
di·a·phys·i·al c.
ep·i·ot·ic c.
ex·pi·ra·to·ry c.
feed·ing c.
ger·mi·nal c. of Flemming
in·spi·ra·to·ry c.
Kerckring's c.
med·ul·lary c.
mo·tor speech c.
os·sif·ic c.
c. of os·si·fi·ca·tion
pri·mary c. of os·si·fi·ca·tion
re·ac·tion c.
res·pi·ra·to·ry c.
c. of ridge
ro·ta·tion c.
sa·ti·e·ty c.
sec·on·dary c. of os·si·fi·ca·tion
sem·i·o·val c.
sen·so·ry speech c.

speech c.'s
sphe·not·ic c.
vi·tal c.
Wernicke's c.
cen·te·sis
cen·ti·bar
cen·ti·grade
scale
cen·ti·gram
cen·ti·li·ter
cen·ti·me·ter
cu·bic c.
cen·ti·me·ter-gram-sec·ond
sys·tem
unit
cen·ti·mor·gan
cen·ti·nor·mal
cen·ti·pede
cen·ti·poise
cen·tra
cen·trad
cen·trage
cen·tral
am·pu·ta·tion
ap·nea
ap·pa·ra·tus
ar·tery
ar·tery of ret·i·na
bear·ing
body
bone
bone of an·kle
bra·dy·car·dia
cal·lus
ca·nal
ca·nals of co·chlea
cat·a·ract
chro·ma·tol·y·sis
deaf·ness
gan·glio·neu·ro·ma
gy·ri
il·lu·mi·na·tion
im·plan·ta·tion
in·ci·sor
in·hi·bi·tion
lac·te·al
lob·ule
ne·cro·sis
neu·ri·tis
nys·tag·mus
os·te·i·tis
pa·ral·y·sis
pit
pla·cen·ta pre·via
pneu·mo·nia
sco·to·ma
spin·dle
sul·cus

cen·tral *(continued)*
   ten·don of di·a·phragm
   ten·don of per·i·ne·um
   vein of ret·i·na
   veins of liv·er
   vein of su·pra·re·nal gland
   vi·sion
cen·tral an·gi·o·spas·tic
   ret·i·ni·tis
   ret·i·nop·a·thy
cen·tral are·o·lar cho·roi·dal
   at·ro·phy
   scle·ro·sis
cen·tral-bear·ing
   de·vice
   point
cen·tral-bear·ing trac·ing
   de·vice
cen·tral ce·ment·i·fy·ing
   fi·bro·ma
cen·tral cord
   syn·drome
cen·tral core
   dis·ease
Cen·tral Eu·ro·pe·an tick-borne
   fe·ver
Cen·tral Eu·ro·pe·an tick-borne
   en·ceph·a·li·tis
   vi·rus
cen·tral ex·cit·a·to·ry
   state
cen·tral gray
   sub·stance
cen·tra·lis
cen·tral lymph
   nodes
cen·tral ner·vous
   sys·tem
cen·tral os·si·fy·ing
   fi·bro·ma
cen·tral pon·tine
   my·e·li·nol·y·sis
cen·tral se·rous
   cho·roi·dop·a·thy
   ret·i·nop·a·thy
cen·tral teg·men·tal
   fas·cic·u·lus
   tract
cen·tral ter·mi·nal
   elec·trode
cen·tral trans·ac·tion·al
   core
cen·tral ve·nous
   cath·e·ter
   pres·sure
cen·tre mé·di·an de Luys
cen·tren·ce·phal·ic
   ep·i·lep·sy

cen·tri-ac·i·nar
   em·phy·se·ma
cen·tric
   con·tact
   fu·sion
   oc·clu·sion
   po·si·tion
   re·la·tion
cen·tric in·ter·oc·clu·sal
   rec·ord
cen·tric·i·put
cen·tric jaw
   re·la·tion
cen·trif·u·gal
   cast·ing
   cur·rent
   nerve
cen·trif·u·gal fast
   an·a·lyz·er
cen·trif·u·gal·i·za·tion
cen·trif·u·gal·ize
cen·trif·u·ga·tion
   den·si·ty gra·di·ent c.
cen·tri·fuge
cen·tri·lob·u·lar
   em·phy·se·ma
cen·tri·ole
   dis·tal c.
   prox·i·mal c.
cen·trip·e·tal
   cur·rent
   nerve
cen·tro·ac·i·nar
   cell
cen·tro·blast
Cen·tro·ces·tus
cen·tro·cyte
cen·tro·fa·cial
   len·tig·i·no·sis
cen·tro·ki·ne·sia
cen·tro·ki·net·ic
cen·tro·lec·i·thal
   egg
   ovum
cen·tro·me·di·an
   nu·cle·us
cen·tro·mere
cen·tro·mere band·ing
   stain
cen·tro·mer·ic
   in·dex
cen·tro·nu·cle·ar
   my·op·a·thy
cen·tro·plasm
cen·tro·some
cen·tro·sphere
cen·tro·stal·tic

cen·trum
    c. me·di·a·num
    c. me·dul·la·re
    c. ova·le
    c. sem·i·o·va·le
    c. of a ver·te·bra
    Vicq d'Azyr's c. sem·i·o·va·le
    Vieussens' c.
    Willis' c. ner·vo·sum
Cen·tru·roi·des
ce·nu·ri·a·sis
cen·u·ris
cen·u·ro·sis
ce·pha·e·line
Ceph·a·e·lis
ceph·a·lad
ceph·a·lal·gia
    his·ta·min·ic c.
    Horton's c.
ceph·a·lea
    c. agi·ta·ta
    c. at·to·ni·ta
ceph·al·e·de·ma
ceph·a·le·mia
ceph·a·lex·in
ceph·al·he·ma·to·cele
ceph·al·he·ma·to·ma
ceph·al·hy·dro·cele
ce·phal·ic
    an·gle
    flex·ure
    in·dex
    pole
    pre·sen·ta·tion
    re·flex·es
    tet·a·nus
    tri·an·gle
    vein
    ver·sion
ceph·a·lin
ceph·a·line
ceph·a·li·tis
ceph·a·li·za·tion
ceph·a·lo·cau·dal
    ax·is
ceph·a·lo·cele
ceph·a·lo·cen·te·sis
ceph·a·lo·cer·cal
ceph·a·lo·chord
ceph·a·lo·did·y·mus
ceph·a·lo·di·pro·so·pus
ceph·a·lo·dyn·ia
ceph·a·lo·gen·e·sis
ceph·a·lo·gly·cin
ceph·a·lo·gram
ceph·a·lo·gy·ric
ceph·a·lo·he·ma·to·cele

ceph·a·lo·he·ma·to·ma
ceph·a·lo·he·mom·e·ter
ceph·a·lo·med·ul·lary
    an·gle
ceph·a·lo·meg·a·ly
ceph·a·lom·e·lus
ceph·a·lo·men·in·gi·tis
ceph·a·lom·e·ter
ceph·a·lo·met·ric
    anal·y·sis
    roent·gen·o·gram
    trac·ing
ceph·a·lo·met·rics
ceph·a·lom·e·try
    ul·tra·son·ic c.
ceph·a·lo·mo·tor
Ceph·a·lo·my·ia
ceph·a·lont
ceph·a·lo·oc·u·lo·cu·ta·ne·ous
    tel·an·gi·ec·ta·sia
ceph·a·lo·or·bit·al
    in·dex
ceph·a·lop·a·gus
ceph·a·lo·pal·pe·bral
    re·flex
ceph·a·lop·a·thy
ceph·a·lo·pel·vic
ceph·a·lo·pel·vim·e·try
ceph·a·lo·pha·ryn·ge·us
ceph·a·lor·i·dine
ceph·a·lor·rha·chid·i·an
    in·dex
ceph·a·lo·spor·an·ic ac·id
ceph·a·lo·spo·rin
    c. C
    c. N
    c. P
ceph·a·lo·spor·i·nase
Ceph·a·lo·spo·ri·um
ceph·a·lo·stat
ceph·a·lo·thin
ceph·a·lo·tho·rac·ic
ceph·a·lo·tho·ra·co·il·i·op·a·gus
ceph·a·lo·tho·ra·cop·a·gus
    c. asym·me·tros
    c. di·sym·me·tros
    c. mon·o·sym·met·ros
ceph·a·lo·tome
ceph·a·lot·o·my
ceph·a·lo·tox·in
ceph·a·lo·tribe
ceph·a·lo·tri·gem·i·nal
    an·gi·o·ma·to·sis
ceph·a·pi·rin so·di·um
ceph·ra·dine
cep·tor
    chem·i·cal c.

cep·tor *(continued)*
  con·tact c.
  dis·tance c.
ce·ra
ce·ra·ceous
cer·am·i·dase
cer·a·mide
  c. di·hex·o·side
  c. sac·cha·ride
cer·a·mo-met·al
  cast·ing
cer·a·sin
ce·rate
cer·a·tin
cer·a·to·cri·coid
  lig·a·ment
cer·a·to·glos·sus
cer·a·to·hy·al
cer·a·to·pha·ryn·ge·al
  part
Cer·a·to·phyl·li·dae
Cer·a·to·phyl·lus
  C. pun·ja·ten·sis
cer·car·ia
cer·car·i·ae
cer·ci
cer·clage
cer·co·cys·tis
cer·co·mer
cer·co·mo·nad
Cer·co·mo·nas
Cer·co·pi·the·coi·dea
Cer·co·pi·the·cus
cer·cus
ce·rea flex·i·bil·i·tas
ce·re·bel·la
cer·e·bel·lar
  ar·ter·ies
  atax·ia
  at·ro·phy
  cor·tex
  cyst
  fis·sures
  gait
  hem·i·sphere
  pyr·a·mid
  ri·gid·i·ty
  speech
  sul·ci
  syn·drome
  ton·sil
  veins
cer·e·bel·lin
cer·e·bel·li·tis
cer·e·bel·lo·len·tal
cer·e·bel·lo·med·ul·lary
  cis·tern

cer·e·bel·lo·med·ul·lary mal·
  for·ma·tion
  syn·drome
cer·e·bel·lo-ol·i·vary
cer·e·bel·lo·pon·tile
  an·gle
cer·e·bel·lo·pon·tine
  an·gle
  cis·tern·og·ra·phy
  re·cess
cer·e·bel·lo·pon·tine an·gle
  syn·drome
  tu·mor
cer·e·bel·lo·ru·bral
  tract
cer·e·bel·lo·tha·lam·ic
  tract
cer·e·bel·lum
ce·re·bra
ce·re·bral
  agraph·ia
  an·gi·og·ra·phy
  an·thrax
  ar·ter·ies
  ar·te·ri·og·ra·phy
  cal·cu·lus
  clad·o·spo·ri·o·sis
  clau·di·ca·tion
  com·pres·sion
  cor·tex
  cra·ni·um
  death
  de·com·pres·sion
  de·cor·ti·ca·tion
  di·a·tax·ia
  dys·pla·sia
  ede·ma
  fis·sures
  flex·ure
  gi·gan·tism
  hem·i·sphere
  hem·or·rhage
  her·nia
  hy·per·es·the·sia
  in·dex
  lay·er of ret·i·na
  lip·i·do·sis
  lo·cal·i·za·tion
  ma·lar·ia
  pal·sy
  part of in·ter·nal ca·rot·id
    ar·tery
  pe·dun·cle
  po·ro·sis
  si·nus·es
  sphin·go·lip·i·do·sis
  sul·ci
  sur·face

tet·a·nus
throm·bo·sis
tu·ber·cu·lo·sis
veins
ven·tri·cles
ves·i·cle
ce·re·bral am·y·loid
an·gi·op·a·thy
cer·e·bral·gia
cer·e·bra·tion
cer·e·bri·form
cer·e·bri·tis
sup·pu·ra·tive c.
cer·e·bro·a·troph·ic
hy·per·am·mo·ne·mia
cer·e·bro·cu·pre·in
cer·e·bro·ga·lac·tose
cer·e·bro·ga·lac·to·side
cer·e·bro·hep·a·to·re·nal
syn·drome
cer·e·bro·ma
cer·e·bro·ma·la·cia
cer·e·bro·men·in·gi·tis
cer·e·bron
cer·e·bron·ic ac·id
cer·e·bro·path·ia
cer·e·brop·a·thy
cer·e·bro·phys·i·ol·o·gy
cer·e·bro·pu·pil·lary
re·flex
cer·e·bro·scle·ro·sis
cer·e·brose
cer·e·bro·side
c.-sul·fa·tase
c. sul·fa·ti·dase
cer·e·bro·side
lip·i·do·sis
cer·e·bro·si·do·sis
cer·e·bro·sis
cer·e·bro·spi·nal
ax·is
fe·ver
flu·id
in·dex
men·in·gi·tis
nem·a·to·di·a·sis
pres·sure
sys·tem
cer·e·bro·spi·nal flu·id
otor·rhea
rhi·nor·rhea
cer·e·bro·spi·nant
cer·e·bro·ste·rol
cer·e·bro·ten·di·nous
cho·les·ter·in·o·sis
xan·tho·ma·to·sis
cer·e·brot·o·my
cer·e·bro·to·nia

cer·e·bro·vas·cu·lar
ac·ci·dent
dis·ease
cer·e·brum
c. ab·do·mi·na·le
cer·e·brums
cere·cloth
Cerenkov
ra·di·a·tion
cer·e·sin
ce·rin
Cer·i·thid·ea
ce·ri·um
c. ox·a·late
ce·roid
lip·o·fus·ci·no·sis
ce·ro·plas·ty
cer·o·sin
cer·ti·fi·a·ble
cer·ti·fi·ca·tion
cer·ti·fied
milk
cer·ti·fied pas·teur·ized
milk
cer·ti·fy
ce·ru·le·an
ce·ru·le·in
ce·ru·lo·plas·min
ce·ru·men
in·spis·sat·ed c.
c. in·spis·sa·tum
ce·ru·mi·nal
ce·ru·mi·no·lyt·ic
ce·ru·mi·no·ma
ce·ru·mi·no·sis
ce·ru·mi·nous
glands
ce·ruse
cer·veau iso·lé
cer·vi·cal
am·pu·ta·tion
an·chor·age
an·es·the·sia
au·ri·cle
ca·nal
di·ver·tic·u·lum
duct
dys·pla·sia
en·large·ment of spi·nal
cord
fas·cia
fi·bro·si·tis
fis·tu·la
flex·ure
fringe
glands
glands of uter·us
hy·dro·cele

cer·vi·cal *(continued)*
  hy·gro·ma
  hy·per·es·the·sia
  lig·a·ment of uter·us
  line
  loop
  mar·gin
  my·o·si·tis
  my·o·spasm
  nerves
  nys·tag·mus
  part
  part of esoph·a·gus
  part of in·ter·nal ca·rot·id
    ar·tery
  part of spi·nal cord
  part of tho·rac·ic duct
  pa·ta·gi·um
  pleu·ra
  plex·us
  preg·nan·cy
  rib
  si·nus
  smear
  spon·dy·lo·sis
  tri·an·gle
  vein
  ver·te·brae
  ves·i·cle
  zone
  zone of tooth
cer·vi·cal aor·tic
  knuck·le
cer·vi·cal com·pres·sion
  syn·drome
cer·vi·cal disc
  syn·drome
cer·vi·cal fu·sion
  syn·drome
cer·vi·cal il·i·o·cos·tal
  mus·cle
cer·vi·cal in·ter·spi·nal
  mus·cle
cer·vi·cal in·tra·ep·i·the·li·al
  ne·o·pla·sia
cer·vi·ca·lis
  c. as·cen·dens
cer·vi·cal lon·gis·si·mus
  mus·cle
cer·vi·cal par·a·tra·che·al
  lymph
  nodes
cer·vi·cal rib
  syn·drome
cer·vi·cal ro·ta·tor
  mus·cles
cer·vi·cal ten·sion
  syn·drome

cer·vi·cec·to·my
cer·vi·ces
cer·vi·cis
cer·vi·ci·tis
cer·vi·co·brach·i·al
cer·vi·co·buc·cal
cer·vi·co·dyn·ia
cer·vi·co·fa·cial
cer·vi·cog·ra·phy
cer·vi·co·la·bi·al
cer·vi·co·lin·gual
cer·vi·co·lin·guo·ax·i·al
cer·vi·co·lum·bar
  phe·nom·e·non
cer·vi·co-oc·cip·i·tal
cer·vi·co-oc·u·lo-a·cous·tic
  syn·drome
cer·vi·co·plas·ty
cer·vi·co·tho·rac·ic
  gan·gli·on
  tran·si·tion
cer·vi·cot·o·my
cer·vi·co·vag·i·nal
  ar·tery
cer·vi·co·ves·i·cal
cer·vix
  c. of the ax·on
  c. co·lum·nae pos·te·ri·o·ris
ce·ryl
ce·sar·e·an
  hys·ter·ec·to·my
  op·er·a·tion
  sec·tion
ce·si·um
Cestan-Chenais
  syn·drome
Ces·to·da
Ces·to·dar·ia
ces·tode
ces·to·di·a·sis
ces·toid
Ces·toi·dea
ce·ta·ce·um
cet·al·ko·ni·um chlo·ride
cet·hex·o·ni·um bro·mide
ce·to·ste·a·ryl al·co·hol
ce·trar·ia
ce·tri·mo·ni·um bro·mide
ce·tyl
  c. al·co·hol
  c. pal·mi·tate
ce·tyl·pyr·i·din·i·um chlo·ride
ce·tyl·tri·meth·yl·am·mo·ni·um
  bro·mide
cev·a·dil·la
cev·a·dine
ce·vi·tam·ic ac·id

Cey·lon
  cin·na·mon
  moss
CF
  an·ti·body
  lead
C group
  vi·rus·es
CGS
  unit
cgs
  unit
Cha·ber·tia
Chaddock
  re·flex
  sign
Chadwick's
  sign
chae·ta
chafe
Chagas'
  dis·ease
Chagas-Cruz
  dis·ease
cha·go·ma
Chagres
  vi·rus
chain
  re·ac·tion
  re·flex
chain
  A c.
  B c.
  be·hav·ior c.
  C c.
  gly·cyl c.
  H c.
  heavy c.
  he·mo·lyt·ic c.
  J c.
  L c.
  light c.
  long c.
  os·sic·u·lar c.
  phen·yl·al·a·nyl c.
  res·pi·ra·to·ry c.
  short c.
  side c.
chain-com·pen·sat·ed
  spi·rom·e·ter
chain·ing
chair
  form
cha·la·sia
cha·la·sis
cha·la·za
cha·la·zia

cha·la·zi·on
  acute c.
  col·lar-stud c.
chal·cone
chal·co·sis
  c. len·tis
chal·ice
  cell
chal·i·co·sis
chal·in·o·plas·ty
chalk
  French c.
  pre·pared c.
chal·ki·tis
chal·lenge
  di·et
cha·lone
cha·ly·be·ate
  wa·ter
cha·maz·u·lene
cham·ber
  Abbé-Zeiss count·ing c.
  al·ti·tude c.
  an·e·cho·ic c.
  an·te·ri·or c. of eye
  aque·ous c.'s
  de·com·pres·sion c.
  Haldane c.
  high al·ti·tude c.
  hy·per·bar·ic c.
  ion·i·za·tion c.
  pos·te·ri·or c. of eye
  pulp c.
  re·lief c.
  Sandison-Clark c.
  si·nu·a·tri·al c.
  Thoma's count·ing c.
  vit·re·ous c. of eye
  Zappert count·ing c.
Chamberlain's
  line
Chamberlen
  for·ceps
cham·e·ce·phal·ic
cham·e·ceph·a·lous
cham·e·pro·sop·ic
cham·fer
cham·o·mile
Champy's
  fix·a·tive
Chance
  frac·ture
chan·cre
  hard c.
  mixed c.
  mon·o·rec·i·dive c.
  c. re·dux
  soft c.

chan·cre *(continued)*
spo·ro·tri·cho·sit·ic c.
tu·la·re·mic c.
chan·cri·form
py·o·der·ma
syn·drome
chan·croid
chan·croi·dal
bu·bo
chan·crous
Chandler
syn·drome
change
Armanni-Ebstein c.
Baggenstoss c.
Crooke's hy·a·line c.
fat·ty c.
c. of life
tro·phic c.
chan·nel
ion c.
lig·and-gat·ed c.
trans·nex·us c.
volt·age-gat·ed c.
Chantemesse
re·ac·tion
cha·o·tro·pic
cha·o·tro·pism
chap·pa
chapped
char·ac·ter
ac·quired c.
com·pound c.
dom·i·nant c.
in·her·it·ed c.
men·de·li·an c.
pri·mary sex c.'s
re·ces·sive c.
sec·on·dary sex c.'s
sex-linked c.
unit c.
char·ac·ter
anal·y·sis
dis·or·der
neu·ro·sis
char·ac·ter ar·mor
char·ac·ter·is·tic
char·ac·ter·i·za·tion
den·ture c.
char·ac·ter·iz·ing
group
cha·ras
char·bon
char·coal
ac·ti·vat·ed c.
an·i·mal c.
bone c.
me·dic·i·nal c.

veg·e·ta·ble c.
wood c.
Charcot-Böttcher
crys·tal·loids
Charcot-Leyden
crys·tals
Charcot-Marie-Tooth
dis·ease
Charcot-Neumann
crys·tals
Charcot-Robin
crys·tals
Charcot's
ar·tery
dis·ease
gait
joint
syn·drome
tri·ad
ver·ti·go
Charcot's in·ter·mit·tent
fe·ver
Charcot-Weiss-Baker
syn·drome
charge
num·ber
nurse
charge trans·fer
com·plex
char·la·tan
char·la·tan·ism
Charles
law
char·ley horse
Charlin's
syn·drome
Charlouis'
dis·ease
Charnley hip
ar·thro·plas·ty
Charrière
scale
chart
Amsler's c.
col·or c.
qual·i·ty con·trol c.
Tanner growth c.
Walker's c.
Charters'
meth·od
chart·ing
Chassaignac's
space
tu·ber·cle
Chastek
pa·ral·y·sis
Chauffard's
syn·drome

chaul·moo·gra oil
Chaussier's
  are·o·la
  line
  sign
Chauveau's
  bac·te·ri·um
Chayes'
  meth·od
Cheadle's
  dis·ease
Cheatle
  slit
check
  lig·a·ments of eye·ball, me·
    di·al and lat·er·al
  lig·a·ments of odon·toid
check·bite
check·er·ber·ry oil
Chédiak-Higashi
  dis·ease
Chédiak-Steinbrinck-Higashi
  anom·a·ly
  syn·drome
cheek
  bone
  mus·cle
  tooth
cheese
  mag·got
cheese work·er's
  lung
cheesy
  pus
chei·lal·gia
chei·lec·to·my
cheil·ec·tro·pi·on
chei·li·on
chei·li·tis
  ac·tin·ic c.
  an·gu·lar c.
  com·mis·sur·al c.
  con·tact c.
  c. ex·fo·li·a·ti·va
  c. glan·du·la·ris
  c. gran·u·lo·ma·to·sa
  im·pe·tig·i·nous c.
  so·lar c.
  c. ve·ne·na·ta
  Volkmann's c.
chei·lo·al·ve·o·los·chi·sis
chei·lo·gnath·o·glos·sos·chi·sis
chei·lo·gnath·o·pal·a·tos·chi·sis
chei·lo·gnath·o·pros·o·pos·chi·
  sis
chei·lo·gna·thos·chi·sis
chei·lo·gnath·o·u·ra·nos·chi·sis
chei·lo·pha·gia

chei·lo·plas·ty
chei·lor·rha·phy
chei·los·chi·sis
chei·lo·sis
chei·lo·sto·ma·to·plas·ty
chei·lot·o·my
chei·rar·thri·tis
chei·ro·bra·chi·al·gia
chei·ro·cin·es·the·sia
chei·rog·nos·tic
chei·ro·kin·es·the·sia
chei·ro·kin·es·thet·ic
chei·rol·o·gy
chei·ro·meg·a·ly
chei·ro·plas·ty
chei·ro·po·dal·gia
chei·ro·pom·pho·lyx
chei·ro·spasm
che·late
che·la·tion
che·lic·era
che·lic·er·ae
chel·i·don
che·loid
Che·lo·nia
che·lo·ni·an
chem·ex·fo·li·a·tion
chem·i·cal
  an·ti·dote
  at·trac·tion
  burn
  cau·tery
  cep·tor
  con·junc·ti·vi·tis
  der·ma·ti·tis
  di·a·be·tes
  en·er·gy
  equa·tion
  for·mu·la
  ki·net·ics
  knife
  per·i·to·ni·tis
  pneu·mo·nia
  pro·phy·lax·is
  ray
  re·pair
  so·lu·tion
  sym·pa·thec·to·my
  thy·roid·ec·to·my
chem·i·co·cau·tery
chem·i·o·tax·is
che·mise
chem·ist
chem·is·try
  an·a·lyt·ic c.
  ap·plied c.
  bi·o·log·i·cal c.
  clin·i·cal c.

chem·is·try *(continued)*
ep·i·ther·mal c.
in·or·gan·ic c.
mac·ro·mo·lec·u·lar c.
med·i·cal c.
me·dic·i·nal c.
nu·cle·ar c.
or·gan·ic c.
phar·ma·ceu·ti·cal c.
phys·i·o·log·i·cal c.
ra·di·a·tion c.
syn·thet·ic c.
che·mo·au·to·troph
che·mo·au·to·tro·phic
che·mo·bi·o·dy·nam·ics
che·mo·bi·ot·ic
che·mo·cau·tery
che·mo·cep·tor
che·mo·dec·to·ma
che·mo·dec·to·ma·to·sis
che·mo·dif·fer·en·ti·a·tion
che·mo·het·er·o·troph
che·mo·het·er·o·troph·ic
che·mo·im·mu·nol·o·gy
che·mo·ki·ne·sis
che·mo·ki·net·ic
che·mo·lith·o·troph
che·mo·lith·o·tro·phic
che·mo·lu·mi·nes·cence
chem·ol·y·sis
che·mo·nu·cle·ol·y·sis
che·mo·or·ga·no·troph
che·mo·or·ga·no·tro·phic
che·mo·pal·li·dec·to·my
che·mo·pal·li·do·thal·a·mec·to·my
che·mo·pal·li·dot·o·my
che·mo·pro·phy·lax·is
che·mo·re·cep·tor
med·ul·lary c.
pe·riph·e·ral c.
che·mo·re·cep·tor
tu·mor
che·mo·re·flex
che·mo·re·sis·tance
che·mo·sen·si·tive
che·mo·se·ro·ther·a·py
che·mo·sis
chem·os·mo·sis
che·mo·sur·gery
che·mo·tac·tic
che·mo·tax·is
che·mo·thal·a·mec·to·my
che·mo·thal·a·mot·o·my
che·mo·ther·a·peu·tic
in·dex
che·mo·ther·a·peu·tics

che·mo·ther·a·py
con·sol·i·da·tion c.
in·duc·tion c.
in·ten·si·fi·ca·tion c.
sal·vage c.
che·mot·ic
che·mo·trans·mit·ter
che·mot·ro·pism
Cheney
syn·drome
che·no·de·ox·y·cho·lic ac·id
che·no·di·ol
che·no·po·di·um
cher·ry
an·gi·o·ma
cher·ry juice
cher·ry-red
spot
cher·ry-red spot my·oc·lo·nus
syn·drome
che·rub·ic
fa·ci·es
che·rub·ism
chess·board
grafts
chest
in·dex
leads
wall
chest
alar c.
bar·rel c.
blast c.
flail c.
flat c.
fo·ve·at·ed c.
fun·nel c.
keeled c.
phthin·oid c.
pter·y·goid c.
chest·nut
chev·ron
in·ci·sion
chew·ing
cy·cle
force
louse
Cheyne's
nys·tag·mus
Cheyne-Stokes
psy·cho·sis
res·pi·ra·tion
Chi·an
tur·pen·tine
Chiari-Budd
syn·drome
Chiari-Frommel
syn·drome

Chiari II
  syn·drome
Chiari's
  dis·ease
  net
  syn·drome
chi·asm
  Camper's c.
  op·tic c.
chi·as·ma
  syn·drome
chi·as·ma·pexy
chi·as·ma·ta
chi·as·mat·ic
  sul·cus
chi·as·mom·e·ter
chick·en
  breast
chick·en em·bryo le·thal or·
  phan
  vi·rus
chick·en fat
  clot
chick·en·pox
  im·mu·no·glob·u·lin
  vi·rus
chick·en·pox im·mune
  glob·u·lin (hu·man)
Chick-Martin
  test
chick nu·trit·ion·al
  der·ma·to·sis
chi·cle·ro's
  ul·cer
chief
  ag·glu·ti·nin
  ar·tery of thumb
  cell
  cell of cor·pus pi·ne·a·le
  cell of par·a·thy·roid gland
  cell of stom·ach
Chievitz'
  lay·er
  or·gan
chig·ger
chig·oe
chi·kun·gun·ya
  vi·rus
Chilaiditi's
  syn·drome
chi·lal·gia
chil·blain
CHILD
  syn·drome
child·bear·ing
  age
child·bed
  fe·ver

child·birth
child·hood
child·hood mus·cu·lar
  dys·tro·phy
child·hood type
  tu·ber·cu·lo·sis
Chil·e·an
  salt·pe·ter
chi·lec·to·my
chil·ec·tro·pi·on
chi·li·tis
chill
chi·lo·al·ve·o·los·chi·sis
chi·lo·gnath·o·glos·sos·chi·sis
chi·lo·gnath·o·pal·a·tos·chi·sis
chi·lo·gnath·o·pros·o·pos·chi·
  sis
chi·lo·gnath·os·chi·sis
chi·lo·gnath·o·u·ra·nos·chi·sis
chi·lo·mas·ti·gi·a·sis
Chi·lo·mas·tix
chi·lo·mas·to·sis
chi·lo·pha·gia
chi·lo·plas·ty
Chi·lo·po·da
chi·lo·po·di·a·sis
chi·lor·rha·phy
chi·los·chi·sis
chi·lo·sis
chi·lo·sto·ma·to·plas·ty
chi·lot·o·my
chi·me·ra
  ra·di·a·tion c.
chi·mer·ic
chi·me·rism
chim·ney sweep's
  can·cer
chim·pan·zee
chim·pan·zee co·ry·za
  agent
chin
  cap
  jerk
  mus·cle
  re·flex
chin
  dou·ble c.
  ga·lo·che c.
chin·chil·la
  gi·ar·di·a·sis
Chi·nese
  cin·na·mon
  gin·ger
  wax
Chi·nese res·tau·rant
  syn·drome
chin·ic ac·id
chi·ni·o·fon

chin·o·le·ine
chip
  bone c.'s
chip
  graft
  sy·ringe
chip-blow·er
chi·ral
  crys·tal
chi·ral·i·ty
chi·rar·thri·tis
chi·ro·bra·chi·al·gia
chi·ro·cin·es·the·sia
chi·rog·nos·tic
chi·ro·kin·es·the·sia
chi·rol·o·gy
chi·ro·meg·a·ly
chi·ro·plas·ty
chi·ro·po·dal·gia
chi·rop·o·dist
chi·rop·o·dy
chi·ro·pom·pho·lyx
chi·ro·prac·tic
chi·ro·prac·tor
Chi·rop·te·ra
chi·ro·scope
chi·ro·spasm
chi·rur·geon
chi·rur·gery
chi·rur·gi·cal
chis·el
  bin·an·gle c.
chi square
  test
chi·tin
chi·ti·nase
chi·tin·ous
chi·to·bi·ose
chi·to·dex·tri·nase
chi·to·neure
chi·to·sa·mine
chi·u·fa
Chla·myd·ia
  C. o·cu·lo·ge·ni·ta·lis
  C. psit·ta·ci
  C. tra·cho·ma·tis
chla·myd·ia
Chlam·y·di·a·ce·ae
chla·myd·i·ae
chla·myd·i·al
  ar·thri·tis
chla·myd·i·o·sis
Chlam·y·do·co·nid·i·um
Chlam·y·do·phrys
Chlam·y·do·zo·a·ce·ae
Chlam·y·do·zo·on
chlo·as·ma
  c. bron·zi·num

chlo·phe·di·a·nol hy·dro·chlo·ride
chlor·a·ce·tic ac·id
chlor·ac·ne
chlo·ral
  an·hy·drous c.
  c. be·ta·ine
  c. hy·drate
m-chlo·ral
p-chlo·ral
chlo·ral·ism
chlor·am·bu·cil
chlo·ra·mine B
chlo·ra·mine T
chlor·am·i·no·phene
chlor·am·i·phene
chlor·am·phen·i·col
  c. pal·mi·tate
  c. so·di·um suc·ci·nate
chlo·rate
chlo·raz·a·nil
chlor·a·zene
chlo·ra·zol black E
chlor·ben·zox·a·mine
chlor·ben·zox·y·eth·a·mine
chlor·bet·a·mide
chlor·bu·tol
chlor·cy·cli·zine hy·dro·chlo·ride
chlor·dane
chlor·dan·to·in
chlor·di·az·e·pox·ide hy·dro·chlo·ride
chlor·e·mia
chlor·eth·ene ho·mo·pol·y·mer
chlor·eth·yl
chlor·gua·nide hy·dro·chlo·ride
chlor·hex·a·dol
chlor·hex·i·dine hy·dro·chlo·ride
chlor·hy·dria
chlo·ric ac·id
chlo·ride
  de·ple·tion
  shift
chlor·i·dim·e·try
chlor·i·dom·e·ter
chlor·i·du·ria
chlo·rin
chlo·ri·nat·ed
  lime
  par·af·fin
chlor·in·da·nol
chlo·rine
  ac·ne
  wa·ter
chlo·rine group
chlor·i·o·dized

chlor·i·o·dized oil
chlor·i·o·do·quin
chlor·i·son·da·mine chlo·ride
chlo·rite
chlor·mad·i·none ac·e·tate
chlor·mer·od·rin
chlor·mez·a·none
chlo·ro·a·ce·tic ac·id
chlo·ro·ac·e·to·phe·none
chlo·ro·am·bu·cil
chlo·ro·a·ne·mia
chlo·ro·az·o·din
chlo·ro·bu·ta·nol
chlo·ro·cre·sol
chlo·ro·cru·o·rin
chlo·ro·eth·ane
chlo·ro·eth·yl·ene
chlo·ro·form
   ac·e·tone c.
chlo·ro·form·ism
chlo·ro·gua·nide hy·dro·chlo·ride
chlo·ro·he·min
chlo·ro·leu·ke·mia
chlo·ro·ma
p-chlo·ro·mer·cu·ri·ben·zo·ate
chlo·ro·meth·ane
chlo·rom·e·try
chlo·ro·my·e·lo·ma
chlo·ro·pe·nia
chlo·ro·per·cha
   meth·od
chlo·ro·phe·nol
o-chlo·ro·phe·nol
p-chlo·ro·phe·nol
chlo·ro·phen·o·thane
chlo·ro·phyll
   c. *a*
   c. *b*
   c. *c*
   c. *d*
   c. es·ter·ase
   wa·ter-sol·u·ble c. de·riv·a·tives
chlo·ro·phyll
   unit
chlo·ro·phyl·lase
chlo·ro·phyl·lid
chlo·ro·phyl·lide
chlo·ro·pic·rin
chlo·ro·plast
chlo·ro·pred·ni·sone
chlo·ro·pro·caine
   pen·i·cil·lin O
chlo·ro·pro·caine hy·dro·chlo·ride
chlo·rop·sia
chlo·ro·pyr·a·mine

chlo·ro·quine
chlo·ro·sis
chlo·ro·then cit·rate
chlo·ro·thi·a·zide
   c. so·di·um
chlo·ro·thy·mol
chlo·rot·ic
   ane·mia
chlo·ro·tri·an·i·sene
chlo·rous
chlo·rous ac·id
chlor·phen·e·sin
   c. car·ba·mate
chlor·phen·in·di·one
chlor·phen·ir·a·mine ma·le·ate
chlor·phe·nol red
chlor·phen·ox·a·mine
chlor·phen·ter·mine hy·dro·chlo·ride
chlor·pro·eth·a·zine hy·dro·chlo·ride
chlor·pro·guan·il hy·dro·chlo·ride
chlor·prom·a·zine
   c. hy·dro·chlo·ride
chlor·prop·a·mide
chlor·pro·thix·ene
chlor·quin·al·dol
chlor·tet·ra·cy·cline
chlor·thal·i·done
chlor·then·ox·a·zin
chlor·thy·mol
chlor·u·re·sis
chlor·u·ret·ic
chlor·u·ria
chlor·zox·a·zone
cho·a·na
   pri·mary c.
   prim·i·tive c.
   sec·on·dary c.
cho·a·nae
cho·a·nal
   atre·sia
   pol·yp
cho·a·nate
cho·a·no·flag·el·late
cho·a·noid
cho·a·no·mas·ti·gote
Cho·a·no·tae·nia in·fun·dib·u·lum
choc·o·late
   agar
   cyst
Chodzko's
   re·flex
choke
   tho·rac·ic c.

choked
   disk
chokes
cho·la·gog·ic
cho·la·gogue
cho·la·ic ac·id
cho·lal·ic ac·id
cho·lane
5β-cho·lane
chol·a·ner·e·sis
cho·lan·ge·i·tis
chol·an·gi·ec·ta·sis
chol·an·gi·o·car·ci·no·ma
chol·an·gi·o·en·ter·os·to·my
chol·an·gi·o·fi·bro·sis
chol·an·gi·o·gas·tros·to·my
chol·an·gi·o·gram
chol·an·gi·og·ra·phy
   cys·tic duct c.
   per·cu·ta·ne·ous c.
chol·an·gi·ole
chol·an·gi·o·lit·ic
   cir·rho·sis
   hep·a·ti·tis
chol·an·gi·o·li·tis
chol·an·gi·o·ma
chol·an·gi·o·pan·cre·a·tog·ra·
   phy
   en·do·scop·ic ret·ro·grade c.
chol·an·gi·os·co·py
chol·an·gi·os·to·my
chol·an·gi·ot·o·my
chol·an·gi·tis
   pri·mary scle·ros·ing c.
cho·lan·ic ac·id
cho·lan·o·poi·e·sis
cho·lan·o·poi·et·ic
chol·an·threne
cho·las·cos
cho·late
   c. li·gase
   c. syn·the·tase
   c. thi·o·ki·nase
cho·le·cal·cif·er·ol
cho·le·chro·mo·poi·e·sis
cho·le·cyst
cho·le·cys·ta·gog·ic
cho·le·cys·ta·gogue
cho·le·cys·tat·o·ny
cho·le·cys·tec·ta·sia
cho·le·cys·tec·to·my
cho·le·cys·ten·dy·sis
cho·le·cyst·en·ter·os·to·my
cho·le·cyst·en·ter·ot·o·my
cho·le·cys·tic
cho·le·cys·tis
cho·le·cys·ti·tis
   acute c.

chron·ic c.
em·phy·sem·a·tous c.
xan·tho·gran·u·lo·ma·tous c.
cho·le·cys·to·co·los·to·my
cho·le·cys·to·du·o·de·nal
   fis·tu·la
cho·le·cys·to·du·o·de·nos·to·my
cho·le·cys·to·gas·tros·to·my
cho·le·cys·to·gram
cho·le·cys·tog·ra·phy
cho·le·cys·to·il·e·os·to·my
cho·le·cys·to·je·ju·nos·to·my
cho·le·cys·to·ki·nase
cho·le·cys·to·ki·net·ic
cho·le·cys·to·ki·nin
cho·le·cys·to·li·thi·a·sis
cho·le·cys·to·lith·o·trip·sy
cho·le·cys·to·my
cho·le·cys·top·a·thy
cho·le·cys·to·pexy
cho·le·cys·tor·rha·phy
cho·le·cys·to·so·nog·ra·phy
cho·le·cys·tos·to·my
cho·le·cys·tot·o·my
cho·le·doch
   duct
cho·le·doch·al
   cyst
   sphinc·ter
cho·led·o·chec·to·my
cho·led·o·chen·dy·sis
cho·led·o·chi·arc·tia
cho·led·o·chi·tis
cho·led·o·cho·cho·led·o·chos·
   to·my
cho·led·o·cho·du·o·de·nal
   junc·tion
cho·led·o·cho·du·o·de·nos·to·
   my
cho·led·o·cho·en·ter·os·tomy
cho·led·o·chog·ra·phy
cho·led·o·cho·je·ju·nos·to·my
cho·led·o·cho·lith
cho·led·o·cho·li·thi·a·sis
cho·led·o·cho·li·thot·o·my
cho·led·o·cho·lith·o·trip·sy
cho·led·o·cho·li·thot·ri·ty
cho·led·o·cho·plas·ty
cho·led·o·chor·rha·phy
cho·led·o·chos·to·my
cho·led·o·chot·o·my
cho·led·o·chous
cho·led·o·chus
cho·le·glo·bin
cho·le·he·ma·tin
cho·le·he·mia
cho·le·ic
cho·le·ic ac·ids

cho·le·lith
cho·le·li·thi·a·sis
cho·le·li·thot·o·my
cho·le·lith·o·trip·sy
cho·le·li·thot·ri·ty
cho·lem·e·sis
cho·le·mia
cho·le·mic
   ne·phro·sis
cho·le·path·ia
   c. spas·ti·ca
cho·le·per·i·to·ne·um
cho·le·per·i·to·ni·tis
cho·le·poi·e·sis
cho·le·poi·et·ic
chol·era
   Asi·at·ic c.
   fowl c.
   hog c.
   c. in·fan·tum
   c. mor·bus
   pan·cre·at·ic c.
   c. sic·ca
   ty·phoid c.
chol·era
   agar
   ba·cil·lus
   tox·in
   vac·cine
chol·er·a·gen
chol·er·a·ic
   di·ar·rhea
chol·er·a·phage
chol·era-red
   re·ac·tion
cho·le·re·sis
cho·le·ret·ic
chol·e·rhe·ic
chol·er·ic
chol·er·i·form
chol·er·i·gen·ic
chol·er·ig·en·ous
chol·er·ine
chol·er·oid
cho·ler·rha·gia
cho·ler·rha·gic
cho·les·tane
cho·les·ta·nol
cho·les·tan·one
cho·le·sta·sia
cho·le·sta·sis
cho·le·stat·ic
   hep·a·ti·tis
   jaun·dice
cho·les·te·a·to·ma
cho·les·ten·one
cho·les·ter·e·mia
cho·les·ter·ide

cho·les·ter·in
cho·les·ter·in·e·mia
cho·les·ter·in·ized
   an·ti·gen
cho·les·ter·in·o·sis
   cer·e·bro·ten·di·nous c.
cho·les·ter·i·nu·ria
cho·les·ter·o·der·ma
cho·les·ter·ol
   cleft
   em·bo·lism
cho·les·ter·ol·e·mia
cho·les·ter·ol es·ter stor·age
   dis·ease
cho·les·ter·ol·o·gen·e·sis
cho·les·ter·ol·o·sis
   ex·tra·cel·lu·lar c.
cho·les·ter·ol·u·ria
cho·les·ter·o·sis
   c. cu·tis
cho·le·styr·a·mine
   res·in
cho·le·u·ria
cho·le·ver·din
cho·lic
cho·lic ac·id
cho·li·cele
cho·line
   c. acet·y·lase
   c. ace·tyl·trans·fer·ase
   c. chlo·ride
   c. di·hy·dro·gen cit·rate
   c. es·ter·ase I
   c. es·ter·ase II
   c. ki·nase
   c. phos·pha·tase
   c. phos·pho·ki·nase
   c. sa·lic·y·late
   c. the·o·phyl·li·nate
cho·line·phos·pho·trans·fer·ase
cho·lin·er·gic
   agent
   block·ade
   fi·bers
   re·cep·tors
   ur·ti·car·ia
cho·lin·es·ter
cho·lin·es·ter·ase
   "e"-type c.
   non·spe·cif·ic c.
   spe·cif·ic c.
   "s"-type c.
   true c.
cho·lin·es·ter·ase
   in·hib·i·tor
cho·lin·es·ter·ase re·ac·ti·va·tor
cho·lin·o·cep·tive
cho·li·no·lyt·ic

chol·i·no·mi·met·ic
cho·lin·o·re·ac·tive
chol·i·no·re·cep·tors
cho·lis·tine sul·pho·meth·ate
  so·di·um
chol·o·lith
chol·o·li·thi·a·sis
chol·o·lith·ic
chol·o·pla·nia
chol·o·poi·e·sis
chol·or·rhea
cho·los·co·py
chol·o·tho·rax
cho·lo·yl
chol·ur·ia
cho·lyl·co·en·zyme A
chon·dral
chon·dral·gia
chon·dral·lo·pla·sia
chon·drec·to·my
Chon·drich·thyes
chon·dri·fi·ca·tion
  cen·ter
chon·dri·fy
chon·drin
  ball
chon·dri·tis
  cos·tal c.
chon·dro·blast
chon·dro·blas·to·ma
chon·dro·cal·ci·no·sis
  ar·tic·u·lar c.
chon·dro·clast
chon·dro·cos·tal
chon·dro·cra·ni·um
chon·dro·cyte
  isog·e·nous c.'s
chon·dro·der·ma·ti·tis no·du·
  la·ris, chron·i·ca he·li·cis
chon·dro·dyn·ia
chon·dro·dys·pla·sia
  he·red·i·tary de·form·ing c.
  c. punc·ta·ta
chon·dro·dys·tro·phia
  c. cal·ci·fi·cans con·gen·i·ta
  c. con·gen·i·ta punc·ta·ta
chon·dro·dys·tro·phic
  dwarf·ism
chon·dro·dys·tro·phy
  as·phyx·i·at·ing tho·rac·ic
  c.
  asym·met·ri·cal c.
  he·red·i·tary de·form·ing c.
chon·dro·ec·to·der·mal
  dys·pla·sia
chon·dro·fi·bro·ma
chon·dro·gen·e·sis
chon·dro·glos·sus

chon·dro·hy·po·pla·sia
chon·droid
  sy·rin·go·ma
  tis·sue
chon·dro·i·tin
  c. sul·fate A
  c. sul·fate B
  c. sul·fate C
chon·drol·o·gy
chon·drol·y·sis
chon·dro·ma
  ex·tra·ske·le·tal c.
  jux·ta·cor·ti·cal c.
  per·i·os·te·al c.
chon·dro·ma·la·cia
  c. fe·ta·lis
  gen·er·al·ized c.
  c. of lar·ynx
  sys·tem·ic c.
chon·dro·ma·to·sis
  syn·o·vi·al c.
chon·dro·ma·tous
chon·dro·mere
chon·dro·mu·cin
chon·dro·mu·coid
chon·dro·myx·oid
  fi·bro·ma
chon·dro·myx·o·ma
chon·dro-os·se·ous
chon·dro-os·te·o·dys·tro·phy
chon·drop·a·thy
chon·dro·pha·ryn·ge·al
  part
chon·dro·pha·ryn·ge·us
chon·dro·phyte
chon·dro·plast
chon·dro·plas·ty
chon·dro·po·ro·sis
chon·dro·pro·tein
chon·dro·sa·mine
chon·dro·sar·co·ma
chon·dro·sin
chon·dro·sine
chon·dro·sis
chon·dro·skel·e·ton
chon·dro·some
chon·dro·ster·nal
chon·dro·ster·no·plas·ty
chon·dro·tome
chon·drot·o·my
chon·dro·tro·phic
chon·dro·xi·phoid
  lig·a·ment
chon·drus
cho·ne·chon·dro·ster·non
Chopart's
  am·pu·ta·tion
  joint

chor·da
sa·li·va
chor·da
c. dor·sa·lis
c. mag·na
c. sper·ma·ti·ca
c. um·bi·li·ca·lis
c. ver·te·bra·lis
chor·dae vo·ca·les
c. vo·ca·lis
chor·dae wil·li·sii
chor·dae
chord·al
chor·da-me·so·derm
Chor·da·ta
chor·date
chor·dee
chor·di·tis
c. fi·bri·no·sa
c. no·do·sa
c. tu·be·ro·sa
c. vo·ca·lis
c. vo·ca·lis in·fe·ri·or
chor·do·ma
chor·do·skel·e·ton
chor·dot·o·my
cho·rea
au·to·mat·ic c.
chron·ic pro·gress·ive c.
c. cor·dis
danc·ing c.
de·gen·er·a·tive c.
c. di·mi·di·a·ta
elec·tric c.
c. fes·ti·nans
fi·bril·lary c.
c. grav·i·dar·um
hab·it c.
hem·i·lat·er·al c.
Henoch's c.
he·red·i·tary c.
Huntington's c.
hys·ter·i·cal c.
ju·ve·nile c.
la·ryn·ge·al c.
c. ma·jor
me·thod·i·cal c.
mi·met·ic c.
c. mi·nor
Morvan's c.
c. nu·tans
par·a·lyt·ic c.
post·hem·i·ple·gic c.
pro·cur·sive c.
rheu·mat·ic c.
rhyth·mic c.
c. ro·ta·to·ria
sal·ta·to·ry c.

se·nile c.
Sydenham's c.
tet·a·noid c.
cho·re·a-a·can·tho·cy·to·sis
cho·re·al
cho·re·ic
aba·si·a
move·ment
cho·re·i·form
cho·re·o·ath·e·toid
cho·re·o·ath·e·to·sis
cho·re·oid
cho·re·o·phra·sia
cho·ri·o·ad·e·no·ma
c. des·tru·ens
cho·ri·o·al·lan·to·ic
graft
mem·brane
pla·cen·ta
cho·ri·o·al·lan·to·is
cho·ri·o·am·ni·on·ic
pla·cen·ta
cho·ri·o·am·ni·o·ni·tis
cho·ri·o·an·gi·o·ma
cho·ri·o·an·gi·o·ma·to·sis
cho·ri·o·an·gi·o·sis
cho·ri·o·cap·il·la·ris
cho·ri·o·cap·il·la·ry
lay·er
cho·ri·o·car·ci·no·ma
cho·ri·o·cele
cho·ri·o·ep·i·the·li·o·ma
cho·ri·o·go·nad·o·tro·pin
cho·ri·o·ma
cho·ri·o·mam·mo·tro·pin
cho·ri·o·men·in·gi·tis
lym·pho·cyt·ic c.
cho·ri·on
c. fron·do·sum
c. lae·ve
pre·vil·lous c.
prim·i·tive c.
shag·gy c.
smooth c.
cho·ri·on·ic
ep·i·the·li·o·ma
go·nad·o·tro·pin
plate
sac
vil·li
cho·ri·on·ic go·nad·o·tro·phic
hor·mone
cho·ri·on·ic go·nad·o·tro·pic
hor·mone
cho·ri·on·ic go·nad·o·tro·pin
unit
Cho·ri·op·tes

cho·ri·op·tic
mange
cho·ri·o·ret·i·nal
cho·ri·o·ret·i·ni·tis
c. sclo·pe·ta·ria
cho·ri·o·ret·i·nop·a·thy
cho·ri·o·vi·tel·line
pla·cen·ta
cho·ris·ta
cho·ris·to·blas·to·ma
cho·ris·to·ma
cho·roid
fis·sure
glo·mus
plex·us
plex·us of fourth ven·tri·cle
plex·us of lat·er·al ven·tri·cle
plex·us of third ven·tri·cle
skein
te·la of fourth ven·tri·cle
te·la of third ven·tri·cle
vein
veins of eye
cho·roi·dal
ring
cho·roi·dal vas·cu·lar
at·ro·phy
cho·roi·dea
cho·roi·der·e·mia
cho·roid·i·tis
an·te·ri·or c.
are·o·lar c.
dif·fuse c.
dis·sem·i·nat·ed c.
ex·ud·a·tive c.
jux·ta·pu·pil·lary c.
met·a·stat·ic c.
mul·ti·fo·cal c.
pos·te·ri·or c.
pro·lif·er·a·tive c.
sup·pu·ra·tive c.
cho·roid·o·cy·cli·tis
cho·roi·dop·a·thy
are·o·lar c.
cen·tral se·rous c.
Doyne's hon·ey·comb c.
ge·o·graph·ic c.
gut·tate c.
hel·i·coid c.
my·o·pic c.
se·nile gut·tate c.
ser·pig·i·nous c.
cho·roid·o·ret·i·ni·tis
cho·roi·do·sis
Chotzen
syn·drome

Chr^a
an·ti·gens
Christ·church
chro·mo·some
Christensen-Krabbe
dis·ease
Christian's
dis·ease
syn·drome
Christison's
for·mu·la
Christmas
dis·ease
fac·tor
Christ-Siemens
syn·drome
chro·maf·fin
body
cell
re·ac·tion
sys·tem
tis·sue
tu·mor
chro·maf·fin·o·ma
chro·maf·fin·op·a·thy
chro·man
chro·mane
chro·man·ol
chro·ma·phil
chro·mate
stain for lead
chro·mat·ic
ab·er·ra·tion
ap·pa·ra·tus
au·di·tion
fi·ber
gran·ule
spec·trum
vi·sion
chro·ma·tid
chro·ma·tin
het·er·o·pyk·not·ic c.
ox·y·phil c.
sex c.
chro·ma·tin
body
net·work
nu·cle·o·lus
par·ti·cles
chro·ma·ti·nol·y·sis
chro·mat·i·nor·rhex·is
chro·ma·tism
chro·ma·tog·e·nous
chro·mat·o·gram
chro·mat·o·graph
chro·mat·o·graph·ic
chro·ma·tog·ra·phy
ab·sorp·tion c.

chron·ic fa·mil·i·al
  ic·ter·us
  jaun·dice
  pol·y·neu·ri·tis
chron·ic fol·lic·u·lar
  con·junc·ti·vi·tis
chron·ic gran·u·lom·a·tous
  dis·ease
chron·ic hem·or·rhag·ic vil·lous
  syn·o·vi·tis
chron·ic hy·per·ten·sive
  dis·ease
chron·ic hy·per·tro·phic
  vul·vi·tis
chron·ic hy·per·ven·ti·la·tion
  syn·drome
chron·ic id·i·o·path·ic
  jaun·dice
chron·ic in·ter·sti·tial
  hep·a·ti·tis
  sal·pin·gi·tis
chro·nic·i·ty
chron·ic lead
  poi·son·ing
chron·ic mer·cu·ry
  poi·son·ing
chron·ic moun·tain
  sick·ness
chron·ic non·leu·ke·mic
  my·e·lo·sis
chron·ic ob·struc·tive pul·mo·
  nary
  dis·ease
chron·ic pro·gress·ive
  cho·rea
chron·ic res·pi·ra·to·ry
  dis·ease
chron·ic sub·glot·tic
  lar·yn·gi·tis
chron·ic ul·cer·a·tive
  proc·ti·tis
chro·no·bi·ol·o·gy
chron·og·no·sis
chro·no·graph
chro·no·log·ic
  age
chro·nom·e·try
  men·tal c.
chron·o-on·col·o·gy
chro·no·phar·ma·col·o·gy
chro·no·pho·bia
chro·no·pho·to·graph
chro·no·ta·rax·is
chro·no·tro·pic
chro·not·ro·pism
  neg·a·tive c.
  pos·i·tive c.

chry·san·the·mum-car·box·yl·ic
  ac·ids
chrys·a·ro·bin
chrys·a·zine
chry·si·a·sis
chrys·o·cy·a·no·sis
chrys·o·der·ma
chrys·oi·din
Chrys·o·my·ia
Chrys·ops
Chrys·o·spo·ri·um par·vum
chrys·o·ther·a·py
chthon·o·pha·gia
chthon·oph·a·gy
chunk·ing
Churg-Strauss
  syn·drome
chut·ta
Chvostek's
  sign
chy·lan·gi·o·ma
chy·la·que·ous
chyle
  cis·tern
  cor·pus·cle
  cyst
  per·i·to·ni·tis
  ves·sel
chy·le·mia
chy·li·dro·sis
chy·li·fac·tion
chy·li·fac·tive
chy·lif·er·ous
chy·li·fi·ca·tion
chy·li·form
  as·ci·tes
chy·lo·cele
  par·a·sit·ic c.
chy·lo·cyst
chy·lo·der·ma
chy·lo·me·di·as·ti·num
chy·lo·mi·cra
chy·lo·mi·cron
chy·lo·mi·cro·ne·mia
chy·lo·mi·crons
chy·lo·per·i·car·di·tis
chy·lo·per·i·car·di·um
chy·lo·per·i·to·ne·um
chy·lo·phor·ic
chy·lo·pleu·ra
chy·lo·pneu·mo·tho·rax
chy·lo·poi·e·sis
chy·lo·poi·et·ic
chy·lor·rhea
chy·lo·sis
chy·lo·tho·rax
chy·lous
  ar·thri·tis

chy·lous *(continued)*
  as·ci·tes
  hy·dro·tho·rax
  urine
chy·lu·ria
chy·mase
chyme
chy·mi·fi·ca·tion
chy·mo·pa·pa·in
chy·mo·poi·e·sis
chy·mor·rhea
chy·mo·sin
chy·mo·sin·o·gen
chy·mo·tryp·sin
chy·mo·tryp·sin·o·gen
chy·mous
Ciaccio's
  glands
  stain
ci·bo·pho·bia
cic·a·trec·to·my
cic·a·tri·ces
cic·a·tri·cial
  al·o·pe·cia
  con·junc·ti·vi·tis
  ec·tro·pi·on
  en·tro·pi·on
  horn
  pem·phi·goid
cic·a·tri·cot·o·my
cic·a·tri·sot·o·my
cic·a·trix
  brain c.
  fil·ter·ing c.
  me·nin·go·ce·re·bral c.
  vi·cious c.
cic·a·tri·zant
cic·a·tri·za·tion
ci·clo·pir·ox ol·a·mine
cic·u·tox·in
cig·a·rette
  drain
cig·a·rette-pa·per
  scars
ci·gua·te·ra
ci·gua·tox·in
ci·la·stat·in so·di·um
cil·ia
cil·i·a·rot·o·my
cil·i·ary
  bleph·a·ri·tis
  body
  ca·nals
  car·ti·lage
  crown
  disk
  folds
  gan·gli·on

glands
lig·a·ment
mar·gin
move·ment
mus·cle
part of ret·i·na
pro·cess
ring
staph·y·lo·ma
veins
wreath
zone
zon·ule
cil·i·ary gan·gli·on·ic
  plex·us
cil·i·a·stat·ic
Ci·li·a·ta
cil·i·at·ed
  ep·i·the·li·um
cil·i·ates
cil·i·ec·to·my
cil·i·o·gen·e·sis
Ci·li·oph·o·ra
cil·i·o·ret·i·nal
cil·i·o·scle·ral
cil·i·o·spi·nal
  cen·ter
  re·flex
cil·i·ot·o·my
cil·i·o·tox·ic·i·ty
cil·i·um
cil·lo
Cil·lo·bac·te·ri·um
cil·lo·sis
ci·met·i·dine
Ci·mex lec·tu·lar·i·us
cim·i·co·sis
cin·an·es·the·sia
ci·nan·ser·in hy·dro·chlo·ride
cin·chol
cin·cho·na
  bark
cin·chon·ic
cin·cho·nine
cin·cho·nism
cin·cho·phen
cin·cli·sis
cinc·ture
  sen·sa·tion
cin·e·an·gi·o·car·di·og·ra·phy
cin·e·an·gi·og·ra·phy
cin·e·flu·o·rog·ra·phy
cin·e·flu·o·ros·co·py
cin·e·gas·tros·co·py
cin·e·mat·ic
  am·pu·ta·tion
cin·e·mat·ics
cin·e·mat·i·za·tion

cin·e·ol
cin·e·ole
cin·e·pho·to·mi·crog·ra·phy
cin·e·plas·tic
   am·pu·ta·tion
cin·e·plas·tics
cin·e·ra·di·og·ra·phy
ci·ne·rea
ci·ne·re·al
ci·ner·i·tious
cin·e·roent·gen·og·ra·phy
cin·e·seis·mog·ra·phy
ci·ne·to·plasm
ci·ne·to·plas·ma
cin·e·u·rog·ra·phy
cin·gu·la
cin·gu·late
   con·vo·lu·tion
   gy·rus
   her·ni·a·tion
cin·gu·lec·to·my
cin·gu·li
cin·gu·lot·o·my
cin·gu·lum
   c. of tooth
cin·gu·lum
   rest
cin·na·bar
cin·na·mal·de·hyde
cin·na·mate
cin·nam·e·drine
cin·nam·e·in
cin·na·mene
cin·nam·ic
cin·nam·ic ac·id
cin·nam·ic al·co·hol
cin·nam·ic al·de·hyde
cin·na·mon
   cas·sia c.
   Cey·lon c.
   Chi·nese c.
   Sai·gon c.
cin·na·mon oil
cin·na·myl·ic ac·id
cin·nar·i·zine
cin·nip·i·rine
cin·o·cen·trum
ci·nox·a·cin
ci·nox·ate
ci·on
cip·ro·flox·a·cin hy·dro·chlo·ride
cir·an·tin
cir·ca·di·an
   rhythm
cir·cel·lus
   c. ve·no·sus hy·po·glos·si
cir·cho·ral

cir·ci·nate
   ret·i·ni·tis
   ret·i·nop·a·thy
cir·cle
   ar·te·ri·al c. of cer·e·brum
   ar·tic·u·lar vas·cu·lar c.
   Baudelocque's uter·ine c.
   Carus' c.
   closed c.
   de·fen·sive c.
   great·er ar·te·ri·al c. of iris
   Haller's c.
   Huguier's c.
   least dif·fu·sion c.
   less·er ar·te·ri·al c. of iris
   Pagenstecher's c.
   Ridley's c.
   semi-closed c.
   vas·cu·lar c.
   vas·cu·lar c. of op·tic nerve
   ve·nous c. of mam·ma·ry gland
   vi·cious c.
   c. of Willis
   Zinn's vas·cu·lar c.
cir·cle ab·sorp·tion
   an·es·the·sia
cir·cling
   dis·ease
cir·cuit
   an·es·thet·ic c.
   Papez c.
   re·ver·ber·at·ing c.
cir·cu·lar
   am·pu·ta·tion
   anas·to·mo·sis
   ban·dage
   di·chro·ism
   fi·bers
   folds
   lay·ers of mus·cu·lar tu·nics
   lay·er of tym·pan·ic mem·brane
   re·ac·tion
   si·nus
   sul·cus of Reil
cir·cu·la·tion
   time
cir·cu·la·tion
   blood c.
   cap·il·lary c.
   col·lat·er·al c.
   com·pen·sa·to·ry c.
   cross c.
   em·bry·on·ic c.
   en·ter·o·he·pat·ic c.
   ex·tra·cor·po·re·al c.
   fe·tal c.

cir·cu·la·tion *(continued)*
  great·er c.
  less·er c.
  lymph c.
  pla·cen·tal c.
  por·tal c.
  pul·mo·nary c.
  Servetus' c.
  sys·tem·ic c.
cir·cu·la·to·ry
  ar·rest
  col·lapse
  sys·tem
cir·cu·li
cir·cu·lus
  c. ar·te·ri·o·sus hal·leri
  c. ve·no·sus hal·leri
  c. ve·no·sus rid·leyi
  c. zinn·ii
cir·cum·al·ve·o·lar
  fix·a·tion
cir·cum·a·nal
  glands
cir·cum·ar·tic·u·lar
cir·cum·ax·il·lary
cir·cum·bul·bar
cir·cum·cise
cir·cum·ci·sion
cir·cum·cor·ne·al
cir·cum·duc·tion
cir·cum·fer·ence
  ar·tic·u·lar c. of ra·di·us
  ar·tic·u·lar c. of ul·na
cir·cum·fer·en·tia
cir·cum·fer·en·tial
  car·ti·lage
  clasp
  fi·bro·car·ti·lage
  im·plan·ta·tion
  la·mel·la
  wir·ing
cir·cum·fer·en·tial clasp
  arm
cir·cum·flex
  nerve
  veins
cir·cum·flex fib·u·lar
  ar·tery
cir·cum·flex scap·u·lar
  ar·tery
cir·cum·gem·mal
cir·cum·in·tes·ti·nal
cir·cum·len·tal
cir·cum·man·dib·u·lar
  fix·a·tion
cir·cum·ne·vic
  vit·i·li·go
cir·cum·nu·cle·ar

cir·cum·oc·u·lar
cir·cum·o·ral
cir·cum·or·bit·al
cir·cum·re·nal
cir·cum·scribed
  cra·ni·o·ma·la·cia
  ede·ma
  myx·e·de·ma
  per·i·to·ni·tis
  py·o·ceph·a·lus
cir·cum·scrip·tus
cir·cum·stan·ti·al·i·ty
cir·cum·val·late
  pa·pil·la
cir·cum·vas·cu·lar
cir·cum·ven·tric·u·lar
  or·gans
cir·cum·vo·lute
cir·cum·zy·go·mat·ic
  fix·a·tion
cir·cus
  move·ment
  rhythm
cir·rho·gen·ic
cir·rhog·e·nous
cir·rhon·o·sus
cir·rho·sis
  al·co·hol·ic c.
  bil·i·ary c.
  Budd's c.
  cap·su·lar c. of liv·er
  car·di·ac c.
  chol·an·gi·o·lit·ic c.
  con·ges·tive c.
  cryp·to·gen·ic c.
  fat·ty c.
  Glisson's c.
  Hanot's c.
  ju·ve·nile c.
  Laënnec's c.
  ne·crot·ic c.
  nu·trit·ion·al c.
  pig·men·tary c.
  por·tal c.
  post·hep·a·tit·ic c.
  post·ne·crot·ic c.
  pri·mary bil·i·ary c.
  sta·sis c.
  tox·ic c.
cir·rhot·ic
cir·ri
cir·rose
cir·rous
cir·rus
cir·sec·to·my
cir·so·cele
cir·sod·e·sis

cir·soid
  an·eu·rysm
  var·ix
cir·som·pha·los
cir·soph·thal·mia
cir·so·tome
cir·sot·o·my
cis
  phase
cis·plat·in
cis·sa
cis·tern
  cer·e·bel·lo·med·ul·lary c.
  c. of chi·asm
  chyle c.
  c. of cy·to·plas·mic re·tic·u·lum
  c. of great vein of cer·e·brum
  in·ter·pe·dun·cu·lar c.
  c. of lat·er·al fos·sa of cer·e·brum
  c. of nu·cle·ar en·ve·lope
  Pecquet's c.
  pon·tine c.
  sub·ar·ach·noi·dal c.'s
cis·ter·na
  c. am·bi·ens
  am·bi·ent c.
  c. ba·sa·lis
  c. car·y·o·the·cae
  c. cru·ra·lis
  c. mag·na
  c. pe·ri·lym·phat·i·ca
  c. pon·tis
  sub·sur·face c.
  c. su·pe·ri·o·ris
  ter·mi·nal cis·ter·nae
  c. ve·nae mag·nae ce·re·bri
cis·ter·nae
cis·ter·nal
  punc·ture
cis·tern·og·ra·phy
  cer·e·bel·lo·pon·tine c.
  ra·di·o·nu·clide c.
cis·tron
cis·ves·tism
cis·ves·ti·tism
Ci·tel·lus
cit·ral
cit·rase
cit·ra·tase
cit·rate
  c. al·dol·ase
  c. ly·ase
  c. syn·thase
cit·rate
  in·tox·i·ca·tion

cit·rat·ed
  cal·ci·um car·bi·mide
cit·ric ac·id
  cy·cle
cit·ri·des·mo·lase
cit·rin
Cit·ro·bac·ter
  C. ama·lo·na·ti·ca
  C. di·ver·sus
  C. freun·dii
  C. ko·seri
ci·trog·en·ase
cit·ro·nel·la
ci·trov·o·rum
  fac·tor
ci·trul·line
cit·rul·li·ne·mia
cit·rul·li·nu·ria
cit·ta
cit·to·sis
Civatte
  bod·ies
Civatte's
  dis·ease
Civinini's
  ca·nal
  lig·a·ment
  pro·cess
CL
  lead
clad·i·o·sis
Cla·dor·chis wat·soni
Clado's
  anas·to·mo·sis
  band
  lig·a·ment
  point
clad·o·spo·ri·o·sis
  ce·re·bral c.
Clad·o·spo·ri·um
  C. ban·ti·a·num
  C. car·rion·ii
  C. wer·nec·kii
clair·voy·ance
clam·ox·y·quin hy·dro·chlo·ride
clamp
  Cope's c.
  Crafoord c.
  Crile's c.
  Fogarty c.
  Gant's c.
  Gaskell's c.
  gin·gi·val c.
  Goldblatt's c.
  Kelly c.
  Kocher c.
  Mikulicz c.
  mo·gen c.

clamp *(continued)*
mos·qui·to c.
Ochsner c.
Payr's c.
Potts' c.
Rankin's c.
rub·ber dam c.
Willett's c.
clamp
for·ceps
clamp con·nec·tion
clang
as·so·ci·a·tion
cla·po·tage
cla·pote·ment
Clapton's
line
Clara
cell
cla·rif·i·cant
clar·i·fi·ca·tion
Clark
elec·trode
Clarke-Hadfield
syn·drome
Clarke's
col·umn
nu·cle·us
Clark's
lev·el
Clark's weight
rule
clas·mat·o·cyte
clas·ma·to·sis
clasp
bar c.
cir·cum·fer·en·tial c.
con·tin·u·ous c.
ex·tend·ed c.
Roach c.
clasp
arm
bar
guide·line
clasp·ing
re·flex
clasp-knife
ef·fect
ri·gid·i·ty
spas·tic·i·ty
class
clas·sic
mi·graine
clas·si·cal
con·di·tion·ing
clas·si·cal ce·sar·e·an
sec·tion

clas·si·fi·ca·tion
ad·an·so·ni·an c.
Angle's c. of mal·oc·clu·sion
Arneth c.
Black's c.
Caldwell-Moloy c.
Cummer's c.
Denver c.
Dukes c.
Galton's sys·tem of c. of
fin·ger·prints
Jansky's c.
Kennedy c.
Kiel c.
Lancefield c.
Lennert c.
Lukes-Collins c.
mul·ti·ax·i·al c.
Rappaport c.
Rye c.
Salter-Harris c. of ep·i·
phys·i·al frac·tures
clas·tic
anat·o·my
clas·to·gen
clas·to·gen·ic
clas·to·thrix
clath·rate
crys·tal
clath·rin
Clauberg
test
unit
Claude's
syn·drome
clau·di·ca·tion
ce·re·bral c.
in·ter·mit·tent c.
clau·di·ca·tory
Claudius'
cells
fos·sa
claus·tra
claus·tral
lay·er
claus·tro·pho·bia
claus·tro·pho·bic
claus·trum
c. gut·tu·ris
c. oris
c. vir·gi·na·le
clau·su·ra
cla·va
cla·val
cla·vate
pa·pil·lae
cla·vi
Clav·i·ceps pur·pu·rea

clav·i·cle
clav·i·cot·o·my
cla·vic·u·la
cla·vic·u·lae
cla·vic·u·lar
  fac·et
  notch
  part
  per·cus·sion
cla·vic·u·li
cla·vic·u·lus
cla·vi·pec·to·ral
  fas·cia
clav·u·lan·ic ac·id
cla·vus
claw
  dew c.
  grif·fin c.
claw
  foot
  hand
claw·foot
claw·hand
Claybrook's
  sign
clay pi·geon
  poi·son·ing
clean·ing
  ul·tra·son·ic c.
cleans·ing
  cream
clear
  cell
  lay·er of ep·i·der·mis
clear·ance
  p-ami·no·hip·pu·rate c.
  cre·at·i·nine c.
  en·dog·e·nous cre·at·i·nine
    c.
  ex·og·e·nous cre·at·i·nine c.
  free wa·ter c.
  in·ter·oc·clu·sal c.
  in·u·lin c.
  iso·tope c.
  max·i·mum urea c.
  oc·clu·sal c.
  os·mo·lal c.
  stan·dard urea c.
  urea c.
clear cell
  ac·an·tho·ma
  ad·e·no·car·ci·no·ma
  car·ci·no·ma of kid·ney
  hi·drad·e·no·ma
clear·er
clear·ing
  fac·tors
  me·di·um

clear liq·uid
  di·et
cleav·age
  cav·i·ty
  cell
  di·vi·sion
  lines
  pro·duct
  site
  spin·dle
cleav·age
  ab·nor·mal c. of car·di·ac
    valve
  ad·e·qual c.
  com·plete c.
  de·ter·mi·nate c.
  dis·coi·dal c.
  enam·el c.
  equal c.
  equa·to·ri·al c.
  hol·o·blas·tic c.
  hy·dro·lyt·ic c.
  in·com·plete c.
  in·de·ter·mi·nate c.
  me·rid·i·o·nal c.
  mer·o·blas·tic c.
  phos·phor·o·clas·tic c.
  pro·gress·ive c.
  pu·den·dal c.
  su·per·fi·cial c.
  thi·o·clas·tic c.
  un·e·qual c.
  yolk c.
cleaved
  cell
cleav·er
  enam·el c.
Cleemann's
  sign
cleft
  hand
  lip
  nose
  pal·ate
  spine
  tongue
cleft
  anal c.
  bran·chi·al c.'s
  cho·les·ter·ol c.
  fa·cial c.
  first vis·cer·al c.
  gill c.'s
  gin·gi·val c.
  glu·te·al c.
  hy·o·bran·chi·al c.
  hy·o·man·dib·u·lar c.
  in·ter·neu·ro·mer·ic c.'s

cleft *(continued)*
  Larrey's c.
  Maurer's c.'s
  na·tal c.
  ob·lique fa·cial c.
  re·sid·u·al c.
  Schmidt-Lanterman c.'s
  syn·ap·tic c.
  uro·gen·i·tal c.
  vis·cer·al c.
clei·dag·ra
clei·dal
clei·do·cos·tal
clei·do·cra·ni·al
  dys·os·to·sis
  dys·pla·sia
cleis·to·the·ci·um
Cleland's
  re·a·gent
clem·as·tine
clem·i·zole
clenched fist
  sign
cle·oid
clep·to·par·a·site
cler·i·cal
  spec·ta·cles
Clevenger's
  fis·sure
click
  ejec·tion c.
  mi·tral c.
  sys·tol·ic c.
click·ing
  rale
  tin·ni·tus
cli·dag·ra
cli·dal
cli·din·i·um bro·mide
cli·do·cos·tal
cli·do·cra·ni·al
  dys·os·to·sis
  dys·pla·sia
cli·do·ic
cli·ent-cen·tered
  ther·a·py
cli·ma·co·pho·bia
cli·mac·ter·ic
  grand c.
cli·mac·ter·ic
  psy·cho·sis
  syn·drome
cli·mac·ter·i·um
cli·mat·ic
  bu·bo
  ker·a·top·a·thy
cli·ma·tol·o·gy
cli·ma·to·ther·a·py

cli·max
climb·ing
  fi·bers
cli·mo·graph
clin·da·my·cin
cline
clin·ic
clin·i·cal
  chem·is·try
  crown
  di·ag·no·sis
  erup·tion
  fit·ness
  ge·net·ics
  le·thal
  med·i·cine
  nurse spe·cial·ist
  pa·thol·o·gy
  phar·ma·col·o·gist
  phar·ma·col·o·gy
  phar·ma·cy
  psy·chol·o·gy
  re·cord·ing
  root
  spec·trom·e·try
  spec·tros·co·py
  ther·mom·e·ter
cli·ni·cian
clin·i·co·path·o·log·ic
cli·no·ce·phal·ic
cli·no·ceph·a·lous
cli·no·ceph·a·ly
cli·no·dac·ty·ly
cli·nog·ra·phy
cli·noid
  pro·cess
cli·no·scope
  ex·og·e·nous cre·at·i·nine c.
cli·o·quin·ol
cli·ox·a·nide
clip
  wound c.
clip
  for·ceps
clipped
  speech
clith·ro·pho·bia
clit·i·on
clit·o·rid·e·an
clit·o·ri·dec·to·my
cli·to·ri·des
clit·o·ri·di·tis
clit·o·ris
clit·o·rism
clit·o·ri·tis
clit·or·o·meg·a·ly
cli·val
cli·vi

cli·vus
Blumenbach's c.
c. o·cu·la·ris
clo·a·ca
ec·to·der·mal c.
en·do·der·mal c.
per·sis·tent c.
clo·a·cal
mem·brane
plate
the·o·ry
clo·a·ci·tis
clo·be·ta·sol pro·pi·o·nate
clo·cor·to·lone
clo·faz·i·mine
clo·fen·a·mide
clo·fi·brate
clo·ges·tone ac·e·tate
clo·ma·cran phos·phate
clo·me·ges·tone ac·e·tate
clo·mi·phene
test
clo·mi·phene cit·rate
clo·mip·ra·mine hy·dro·chlo·ride
clo·nal
ag·ing
clo·nal se·lec·tion
the·o·ry
clo·na·ze·pam
clone
clo·nic
con·vul·sion
spasm
clon·ic·i·ty
clon·i·co·ton·ic
clo·ni·dine hy·dro·chlo·ride
clon·ing
vec·tor
clo·nism
clo·nix·in
clo·no·gen·ic
as·say
cell
clon·o·graph
clo·nor·chi·a·sis
clo·nor·chi·o·sis
Clo·nor·chis si·nen·sis
clon·o·spasm
clo·nus
an·kle c.
cath·o·dal open·ing c.
toe c.
wrist c.
clo·pam·ide
Cloquet's
ca·nal
her·nia

sep·tum
space
clor·az·e·pate
clor·pren·a·line hy·dro·chlo·ride
close
bite
closed
an·es·the·sia
an·gi·og·ra·phy
bite
cir·cle
com·e·do
dis·lo·ca·tion
drain·age
frac·ture
hos·pi·tal
re·duc·tion of frac·tures
sur·gery
closed-an·gle
glau·co·ma
closed chain
com·pound
closed chest
mas·sage
closed cir·cuit
meth·od
closed head
in·ju·ry
closed-loop
ob·struc·tion
closed skull
frac·ture
clos·ing
con·trac·tion
mem·branes
snap
vol·ume
clo·sir·a·mine acet·u·rate
clos·trid·ia
clos·trid·i·al
my·o·ne·cro·sis
clos·trid·i·o·pep·ti·dase A
clos·trid·i·o·pep·ti·dase B
Clos·trid·i·um
C. aer·o·foe·ti·dum
C. bi·fer·men·tans
C. bot·u·li·num
C. bu·ty·ri·cum
C. ca·da·ve·ris
C. ca·pi·to·va·le
C. car·nis
C. chau·voei
C. chro·mo·genes
C. co·chle·a·ri·um
C. dif·fi·cile
C. fal·lax
C. fe·seri
C. gum·mo·sum

Clos·trid·i·um *(continued)*
  C. hae·mo·ly·ti·cum
  C. his·to·lyt·i·cum
  C. in·no·mi·na·tum
  C. mi·cros·po·rum
  C. mul·ti·fer·men·tans
  C. ni·gri·fi·cans
  C. nov·yi
  C. oe·de·ma·tiens
  C. par·a·bot·u·lin·um
  C. par·a·pu·trif·i·cum
  C. per·frin·gens
  C. ra·mo·sum
  C. sep·ti·cum
  C. sphe·noi·des
  C. spo·ro·genes
  C. tale
  C. ter·ti·um
  C. te·ta·ni
  C. tet·a·noi·des
  C. tet·a·no·mor·phum
  C. ther·mo·sac·cha·ro·ly·ti·cum
  C. welch·ii
clos·trid·i·um
Clos·trid·i·um his·to·lyt·i·cum col·la·gen·ase
Clos·trid·i·um his·to·lyt·i·cum pro·tein·ase B
clos·tri·pain
clo·sure
  flask c.
  vel·o·pha·ryn·ge·al c.
clo·sure
  prin·ci·ple
clo·sy·late
clot
  ag·o·ny c.
  an·te·mor·tem c.
  blood c.
  chick·en fat c.
  cur·rant jel·ly c.
  lam·i·nat·ed c.
  pas·sive c.
  post·mor·tem c.
  Schede's c.
clot re·trac·tion
  time
clo·trim·a·zole
clot·tage
clot·ting
  fac·tor
  time
cloud·ing of
  con·scious·ness
Cloudman
  mel·a·no·ma

cloudy
  swell·ing
  urine
clove oil
clo·ver
  dis·ease
clo·ver·leaf
  skull
clo·ver·leaf skull
  syn·drome
clox·a·cil·lin so·di·um
clo·za·pine
club
  foot
  hair
  hand
  moss
clubbed
  dig·its
  fin·gers
  pe·nis
club·bing
club·foot
club·hand
clump
clump·ing
clu·ne·al
clu·nes
clus·ter
  anal·y·sis
  head·ache
clut·ter·ing
Clutton's
  joints
cly·sis
clys·ter
CM-cel·lu·lose
cne·mi·al
cne·mis
cni·da
cni·dae
cni·do·cyst
cni·do·sis
Cnid·o·spora
Cni·do·spo·rid·ia
co·ac·er·vate
co·ac·er·va·tion
co·ad·ap·ta·tion
co·ag·glu·ti·nin
co·ag·u·la
co·ag·u·la·ble
co·ag·u·lant
co·ag·u·late
co·ag·u·la·tion
  dis·sem·i·nat·ed in·tra·vas·cu·lar c.
co·ag·u·la·tion
  fac·tor

ne·cro·sis
time
co·ag·u·la·tive
co·ag·u·lop·a·thy
   con·sump·tion c.
co·ag·u·lum
co·a·les·cence
coal oil
coal tar
   naph·tha
co·apt
co·ap·ta·tion
   splint
   su·ture
co·arct
co·arc·tate
   ret·i·na
co·arc·ta·tion
   re·versed c.
co·arc·tot·o·my
coarse
   dis·per·sion
   trem·or
coast·al
   er·y·sip·e·las
coat
   buffy c.
   scle·rot·ic c.
   se·rous c.
coat·ed
   tongue
coat·ing
   an·ti·re·flec·tion c.
CoA trans·fer·as·es
Coats'
   dis·ease
co·bal·a·min
   c. con·cen·trate
co·balt
co·bal·tous chlo·ride
co·bam·ic ac·id
co·bam·ide
Cobb
   syn·drome
cob·bler's
   su·ture
co·bin·am·ide
co·bin·ic ac·id
co·bra
   he·mo·tox·in
co·bra ven·om
   co·fac·tor
   fac·tor
co·bro·tox·in
co·byr·ic ac·id
co·byr·in·a·mide
co·byr·in·ic ac·id
co·byr·in·ic hex·a-am·ide

co·ca
co·caine
co·cain·i·za·tion
co·car·box·yl·ase
co·car·cin·o·gen
co·carde
   re·ac·tion
Coc·ca·ce·ae
coc·cal
coc·ci
Coc·cid·ia
coc·cid·ia
coc·cid·i·al
Coc·ci·di·as·i·na
coc·cid·i·oi·dal
   gran·u·lo·ma
Coc·cid·i·oi·des
coc·cid·i·oi·din
   test
coc·cid·i·oi·do·ma
coc·cid·i·oi·do·my·co·sis
   asymp·tom·at·ic c.
   dis·sem·i·nate c.
   la·tent c.
   pri·mary c.
   pri·mary ex·tra·pul·mo·nary
     c.
   sec·on·dary c.
coc·cid·i·o·sis
coc·cid·i·o·stat
coc·cid·i·um
coc·ci·nel·la
coc·ci·nel·lin
coc·co·bac·il·lary
coc·co·ba·cil·lus
coc·coid
coc·cu·lin
coc·cus
   Neisser's c.
   Weichselbaum's c.
coc·cy·al·gia
coc·cy·ceph·a·ly
coc·cy·dyn·ia
coc·cy·gal·gia
coc·cyg·eal
   body
   bone
   dim·ple
   fis·tu·la
   fo·ve·o·la
   gan·gli·on
   gland
   horn
   joint
   mus·cle
   nerve
   part of spi·nal cord
   plex·us

coc·cyg·eal *(continued)*
  si·nus
  ver·te·brae
  whorl
coc·cy·gec·to·my
coc·cy·ges
coc·cyg·e·us
coc·cy·gis
coc·cy·go·dyn·ia
coc·cy·got·o·my
coc·cy·o·dyn·ia
coc·cyx
Co·chin Chi·na
  di·ar·rhea
coch·i·neal
co·chlea
  mem·bra·nous c.
co·chle·ae
co·chle·ar
  aq·ue·duct
  ar·ea
  ca·nal
  can·a·lic·u·lus
  duct
  im·plant
  joint
  lab·y·rinth
  nerve
  nu·clei
  part of ves·tib·u·lo·co·chle·
   ar nerve
  pros·the·sis
  re·cess
  root of ves·tib·u·lo·co·chle·
   ar nerve
  win·dow
co·chle·a·re
co·chle·ar hair
  cells
co·chle·ar·i·form
  pro·cess
co·chle·ate
co·chle·i·tis
co·chle·o-or·bic·u·lar
  re·flex
co·chle·o·pal·pe·bral
  re·flex
co·chle·o·pu·pil·lary
  re·flex
co·chle·o·sac·cu·lot·o·my
co·chle·o·sta·pe·di·al
  re·flex
co·chle·o·ves·tib·u·lar
Co·chli·o·my·ia
  C. amer·i·cana
  C. hom·i·niv·o·rax
  C. ma·cel·la·ria
co·chli·tis

co·cil·la·na
cock·ade
  re·ac·tion
Cockayne's
  dis·ease
  syn·drome
cocks·comb
  ul·cer
cocks comb
cock·tail
  Bromp·ton c.
  lyt·ic c.
  Phil·a·del·phia c.
  Rivers' c.
co·coa
  but·ter
co·con·scious·ness
co·co·nut
  sound
coc·to·la·bile
coc·to·sta·bile
coc·to·sta·ble
code
  ge·net·ic c.
co·de·car·box·yl·ase
co·de·hy·dro·gen·ase I
co·de·hy·dro·gen·ase II
co·deine
Co·dex med·i·ca·men·tar·i·us
cod·fish
  ver·te·brae
cod·ing
  se·quence
cod liv·er oil
Codman's
  sign
  tri·an·gle
  tu·mor
co·dom·i·nant
  al·lele
  in·her·i·tance
  trait
co·don
  in·i·ti·a·ting c.
  ter·mi·na·tion c.
Coe
  vi·rus
co·ef·fi·cient
  ab·sorp·tion c.
  ac·tiv·i·ty c.
  bi·o·log·i·cal c.
  Bunsen's sol·u·bil·i·ty c.
  c. of con·san·guin·i·ty
  cor·re·la·tion c.'s
  cre·at·i·nine c.
  dif·fu·sion c.
  dis·tri·bu·tion c.
  ex·tinc·tion c.

ex·trac·tion c.
fil·tra·tion c.
hy·gien·ic lab·o·ra·tory c.
c. of in·breed·ing
iso·ton·ic c.
c. of kin·ship
le·thal c.
lin·e·ar ab·sorp·tion c.
Long's c.
mo·lar ab·sorp·tion c.
mo·lar ex·tinc·tion c.
Ostwald's sol·u·bil·i·ty c.
ox·y·gen uti·li·za·tion c.
par·ti·tion c.
phe·nol c.
Poiseuille's vis·cos·i·ty c.
re·flec·tion c.
c. of re·la·tion·ship
re·li·a·bil·i·ty c.
res·pi·ra·to·ry c.
Rideal-Walker c.
se·lec·tion c.
spe·cif·ic ab·sorp·tion c.
tem·per·a·ture c.
ul·tra·fil·tra·tion c.
c. of var·i·a·tion
ve·loc·i·ty c.
c. of vis·cos·i·ty
Coe·len·ter·a·ta
coe·len·ter·ate
coe·lom
coe·nes·the·sia
coe·no·cyte
coe·no·cyt·ic
coe·nu·ro·sis
Coe·nu·rus
C. ce·re·bra·lis
C. se·ri·a·lis
co·en·zyme
fac·tor
co·en·zyme A
trans·fer·as·es
co·en·zyme I
co·en·zyme II
co·en·zyme Q
co·en·zyme R
coeur
c. en sa·bot
co·fac·tor
co·bra ven·om c.
plate·let c.
plate·let c. II
c. of throm·bo·plas·tin
c. V
co·fer·ment
cof·fee-ground
vom·it

Coffey
sus·pen·sion
cof·fin
joint
Coffin-Lowry
syn·drome
Coffin-Siris
syn·drome
Cogan-Reese
syn·drome
Cogan's
syn·drome
cog·ni·tion
cog·ni·tive
psy·chol·o·gy
ther·a·py
cog·ni·tive dis·so·nance
the·o·ry
cog·ni·tive lat·er·al·i·ty
quo·tient
cog·wheel
phe·nom·e·non
pu·pil
res·pi·ra·tion
ri·gid·i·ty
cog·wheel oc·u·lar
move·ments
co·he·sion
co·he·sive
gold
Cohnheim's
ar·ea
field
the·o·ry
co·ho·ba
co·hort
study
coil
gland
coiled
ar·tery of the uter·us
coin
le·sions of lungs
test
coin-count·ing
coin·o·site
co·i·tal
Coiter's
mus·cle
co·i·tion
co·i·to·pho·bia
co·i·tus
c. in·ter·rup·tus
c. re·ser·va·tus
co·la
col·chi·cine

cold
 c. in the head
 rose c.
cold
 ab·scess
 ag·glu·ti·na·tion
 ag·glu·ti·nin
 al·ler·gy
 au·to·ag·glu·ti·nin
 au·to·an·ti·body
 cau·tery
 con·i·za·tion
 cream
 gan·grene
 he·mo·ly·sin
 light
 nod·ule
 pack
 snare
 sore
 stage
 ul·cer
 ur·ti·car·ia
 vi·rus
cold bend
 test
cold-blood·ed
 an·i·mal
cold cure
 res·in
cold-cur·ing
 res·in
cold he·mag·glu·ti·nin
 dis·ease
cold-rig·or
 point
Cole-Cecil
 mur·mur
co·lec·ta·sia
col·ec·to·my
col·e·i·tis
co·le·o·cele
Co·le·op·te·ra
co·le·op·to·sis
co·le·ot·o·my
co·les
co·les·ti·pol
co·li
 gran·u·lo·ma
co·li·ba·cil·li
co·li·bac·il·lo·sis
co·li·ba·cil·lus
col·ic
 im·pres·sion
 in·tus·sus·cep·tion
 sphinc·ter
 sur·face of spleen

 te·ni·ae
 veins
col·ic
 ap·pen·dic·u·lar c.
 bil·i·ary c.
 cop·per c.
 Dev·on·shire c.
 gall·stone c.
 gas·tric c.
 he·pa·tic c.
 lead c.
 me·co·ni·al c.
 men·stru·al c.
 milk c.
 ovar·i·an c.
 paint·er's c.
 pan·cre·at·ic c.
 re·nal c.
 sal·i·vary c.
 sat·ur·nine c.
 tub·al c.
 uter·ine c.
 ver·mic·u·lar c.
 zinc c.
col·i·ca
col·i·cin
col·i·ci·nog·e·ny
col·icky
col·i·co·ple·gia
col·i·form
co·li·my·cin
co·li·pase
co·li·phage
co·li·pli·ca·tion
co·li·punc·ture
co·lis·ti·meth·ate so·di·um
co·lis·tin
 c. sul·fate
 c. sul·fo·meth·ate so·di·um
co·li·tis
 ame·bic c.
 col·lag·e·nous c.
 c. cys·ti·ca pro·fun·da
 c. cys·ti·ca su·per·fi·ci·a·lis
 gran·u·lom·a·tous c.
 c. gra·vis
 hem·or·rhag·ic c.
 mu·cous c.
 myx·o·mem·bra·nous c.
 pseu·do·mem·bra·nous c.
 ul·cer·a·tive c.
 ure·mic c.
col·i·tose
col·la
col·la·cin
col·la·gen
 type I c.
 type II c.

type III c.
type IV c.
col·la·gen
dis·eas·es
fi·ber
fi·brils
col·la·gen·ase A
col·la·gen·ase I
col·la·ge·na·tion
col·la·gen·ic
col·lag·e·ni·za·tion
col·lag·e·no·lyt·ic
col·lag·e·no·sis
re·ac·tive per·fo·rat·ing c.
col·lag·e·nous
co·li·tis
fi·ber
col·la·gen-vas·cu·lar
dis·eas·es
col·lapse
de·lir·i·um
ther·a·py
col·lapse
ab·sorp·tion c.
cir·cu·la·to·ry c.
c. of den·tal arch
mas·sive c.
pres·sure c.
pul·mo·nary c.
col·laps·ing
pulse
col·lar
bone
col·lar
re·nal c.
c. of Ve·nus
col·lar-but·ton
ab·scess
col·lared
flag·el·late
col·lar·ette
col·lar-stud
cha·la·zi·on
col·las·tin
col·lat·er·al
ar·tery
cir·cu·la·tion
em·i·nence
fis·sure
hy·per·e·mia
in·her·i·tance
lig·a·ment
sul·cus
tri·gone
ves·sel
col·lat·er·al dig·i·tal
ar·tery

col·lect·ing
tu·bule
col·lec·tive
un·con·scious
Colles'
fas·cia
frac·ture
lig·a·ment
space
Collet-Sicard
syn·drome
col·lic·u·lec·to·my
col·lic·u·li
col·lic·u·li·tis
col·lic·u·lus
fa·cial c.
in·fe·ri·or c.
sem·i·nal c.
su·pe·ri·or c.
c. ure·thra·lis
Collier's
tract
col·lier's
lung
col·li·ga·tion
col·li·ga·tive
col·li·ma·tion
col·li·ma·tor
col·lin·e·ar·i·ty
col·li·ot·o·my
col·li·qua·tion
bal·loon·ing c.
re·tic·u·lat·ing c.
col·liq·ua·tive
al·bu·min·ur·ia
de·gen·er·a·tion
di·ar·rhea
ne·cro·sis
sweat
Collis
gas·tro·plas·ty
col·li·sion
tu·mor
col·lo·di·on
ba·by
col·lo·di·on
blis·ter·ing c.
can·thar·i·dal c.
flex·i·ble c.
he·mo·stat·ic c.
iodized c.
sal·i·cyl·ic ac·id c.
styp·tic c.
c. ve·si·cans
col·lo·di·um
col·loid
bo·vine c.
dis·per·sion c.

col·loid *(continued)*
  emul·sion c.
  hy·dro·phil c.
  hy·dro·phil·ic c.
  hy·dro·pho·bic c.
  ir·re·vers·i·ble c.
  ly·o·phil·ic c.
  ly·o·pho·bic c.
  pro·tec·tive c.
  re·vers·i·ble c.
  sta·ble c.
  styp·tic c.
  sus·pen·sion c.
  thy·roid c.
  un·sta·ble c.
col·loid
  ac·ne
  ad·e·no·ma
  bath
  bod·ies
  can·cer
  car·ci·no·ma
  cor·pus·cle
  cyst
  de·gen·er·a·tion
  goi·ter
  mil·i·um
  sys·tem
  the·o·ry of nar·co·sis
col·loi·dal
  dis·per·sion
  gel
  met·al
  sil·i·con di·ox·ide
  sil·ver io·dide
  so·lu·tion
col·loi·dal ra·di·o·ac·tive
  gold
col·loi·din
col·loi·do·cla·sia
col·loi·do·cla·sis
col·loi·do·clas·tic
col·loi·do·gen
col·lox·y·lin
col·lum
  c. den·tis
  c. dis·tor·tum
  c. fe·mo·ris
  c. fol·lic·u·li pi·li
  c. hu·meri
  c. ve·si·cae bil·i·ar·is
col·lu·nar·i·um
col·lu·to·ri·um
col·lu·tory
Col·lyr·i·clum
col·lyr·i·um
col·o·bo·ma
  c. of cho·roid

  Fuchs' c.
  c. ir·i·dis
  c. len·tis
  c. lob·u·li
  mac·u·lar c.
  c. of op·tic nerve
  c. pal·pe·bra·le
  c. of vit·re·ous
co·lo·cen·te·sis
co·lo·cho·le·cys·tos·to·my
co·lo·col·ic
co·lo·co·los·to·my
co·lo·cu·ta·ne·ous
  fis·tu·la
col·o·cynth
co·lo·cys·to·plas·ty
co·lo·en·ter·i·tis
co·lo·hep·a·to·pexy
co·lo·il·e·al
  fis·tu·la
co·lol·y·sis
co·lom·ba
col·o·min·ic ac·id
co·lon
  as·cend·ing c.
  de·scend·ing c.
  gi·ant c.
  il·i·ac c.
  ir·ri·ta·ble c.
  lead-pipe c.
  c. pel·vi·num
  sig·moid c.
  trans·verse c.
co·lon
  ba·cil·lus
co·lon·al·gia
co·lon·ic
  fis·tu·la
  smear
col·o·ni·za·tion
  ge·net·ic c.
co·lon·o·gram
co·lo·nom·e·ter
co·lon·op·a·thy
co·lon·or·rha·gia
co·lon·or·rhea
co·lon·o·scope
co·lon·os·co·py
col·o·ny
  daugh·ter c.
  fil·a·men·tous c.
  Gheel c.
  H c.
  len·tic·u·lar c.
  moth·er c.
  mu·coid c.
  O c.
  rough c.

smooth c.
sphe·roid c.
co·lop·a·thy
co·lo·pex·os·to·my
co·lo·pex·ot·o·my
col·o·pexy
co·lo·pho·ny
co·lo·pli·ca·tion
co·lo·proc·tia
co·lo·proc·ti·tis
co·lo·proc·tos·to·my
co·lop·to·sia
co·lop·to·sis
co·lo·punc·ture
col·or
    com·ple·men·ta·ry c.'s
    con·fu·sion c.'s
    ex·trin·sic c.
    in·ci·den·tal c.
    in·trin·sic c.
    op·po·nent c.
    pri·mary c.
    pure c.
    re·flect·ed c.'s
    sat·u·rat·ed c.
    sim·ple c.
    tone c.
col·or
    ab·er·ra·tion
    blind·ness
    chart
    con·stan·cy
    hear·ing
    in·dex
    rad·i·cal
    sco·to·ma
    sense
    spec·trum
    taste
    vi·sion
Col·o·ra·do tick
    fe·ver
Col·o·ra·do tick fe·ver
    vi·rus
col·or-con·trast
    mi·cro·scope
co·lo·rec·tal
co·lo·rec·ti·tis
co·lo·rec·tos·to·my
col·or·im·e·ter
    Duboscq's c.
col·or·i·met·ric
    ti·tra·tion
col·or·i·met·ric car·ies sus·cep·
  ti·bil·i·ty
    test
col·or·im·e·try
col·or match

co·lor·rha·gia
co·lor·rha·phy
co·lor·rhea
col·or sol·id
co·los·co·py
co·lo·sig·moi·dos·to·my
co·los·to·my
    bag
co·los·tra·tion
co·los·tric
co·los·tror·rhea
co·los·trous
co·los·trum
    cor·pus·cle
co·lot·o·my
co·lo·vag·i·nal
    fis·tu·la
co·lo·ves·i·cal
    fis·tu·la
col·pa·tre·sia
col·pec·ta·sia
col·pec·ta·sis
col·pec·to·my
col·pi·tis
    c. my·co·ti·ca
col·po·cele
col·po·clei·sis
col·po·cys·ti·tis
col·po·cys·to·cele
col·po·cys·to·plas·ty
col·po·cys·tot·o·my
col·po·cys·to·u·re·ter·ot·o·my
col·po·dyn·ia
col·po·hy·per·pla·sia
    c. cys·ti·ca
    c. em·phy·se·ma·to·sa
col·po·hys·ter·ec·to·my
col·po·hys·ter·o·pexy
col·po·hys·ter·ot·o·my
col·po·mi·cro·scope
col·po·mi·cros·co·py
col·po·my·co·sis
col·po·my·o·mec·to·my
col·pop·a·thy
col·po·per·i·ne·o·plas·ty
col·po·per·i·ne·or·rha·phy
col·po·pexy
col·po·plas·ty
col·po·poi·e·sis
col·po·pto·sia
col·po·pto·sis
col·po·rec·to·pexy
col·por·rha·gia
col·por·rha·phy
col·por·rhex·is
col·po·scope
col·pos·co·py
col·po·spasm

col·po·stat
col·po·ste·no·sis
col·po·ste·not·o·my
col·pot·o·my
col·po·u·re·ter·ot·o·my
col·po·xe·ro·sis
Co·lu·bri·dae
Co·lum·bia Men·tal Ma·tu·ri·ty
  Scale
Co·lum·bia S. K.
  vi·rus
co·lum·bin
co·lum·bi·um
co·lum·bo
col·u·mel·la
  c. au·ris
  c. co·chle·ae
  c. na·si
col·u·mel·lae
col·umn
  af·fin·i·ty c.
  anal c.'s
  an·te·ri·or c. of me·dul·la ob·lon·ga·ta
  an·te·ri·or c. of spi·nal cord
  an·ter·o·lat·er·al c. of spi·nal cord
  Bertin's c.'s
  bran·chi·al ef·fer·ent c.
  Burdach's c.
  Clarke's c.
  dor·sal c. of spi·nal cord
  c. of for·nix
  gen·er·al so·mat·ic af·fer·ent c.
  gen·er·al so·mat·ic ef·fer·ent c.
  gen·er·al vis·cer·al c.
  Goll's c.
  Gowers' c.
  gray c.'s
  in·ter·me·di·o·lat·er·al cell c. of spi·nal cord
  lat·er·al c. of spi·nal cord
  Morgagni's c.'s
  pos·te·ri·or c. of spi·nal cord
  rec·tal c.'s
  re·nal c.'s
  Rolando's c.
  Sertoli's c.'s
  spe·cial so·mat·ic af·fer·ent c.
  spe·cial vis·cer·al c.
  spi·nal c.
  splanch·nic af·fer·ent c.

  splanch·nic ef·fer·ent c.
  Stilling's c.
  Türck's c.
  vag·i·nal c.'s
  ven·tral c. of spi·nal cord
  ver·te·bral c.
col·umn
  cells
  chro·ma·tog·ra·phy
co·lum·na
  co·lum·nae car·ne·ae
  c. na·si
co·lum·nae
co·lum·nar
  ep·i·the·li·um
  lay·er
co·lum·nel·la
col·um·nel·lae
co·ly·pep·tic
co·ma
  c. car·ci·no·ma·to·sum
  di·a·bet·ic c.
  he·pa·tic c.
  hy·per·os·mo·lar hy·per·gly·ce·mic non·ke·ton·ic c.
  Kussmaul's c.
  met·a·bol·ic c.
  thy·ro·tox·ic c.
  trance c.
co·ma
  ab·er·ra·tion
  cast
  scale
  vig·il
co·ma·tose
comb-growth
  test
com·bi·na·tion
  beat
  cal·cu·lus
  res·to·ra·tion
com·bi·na·tion
  bi·na·ry c.
  new c.
com·bi·na·tion oral
  con·tra·cep·tive
com·bined
  glau·co·ma
  im·mu·no·de·fi·cien·cy
  preg·nan·cy
  scle·ro·sis
  ver·sion
com·bined fat- and car·bo·hy·drate-in·duced
  hy·per·li·pe·mia
com·bined sys·tem
  dis·ease

com·bin·ing
  weight
comb·like
  sep·tum
com·bus·ti·ble
com·bus·tion
  slow c.
  spon·ta·ne·ous c.
com·bus·tion
  equiv·a·lent
Comby's
  sign
com·e·do
  ne·vus
com·e·do
  closed c.
  open c.
com·e·do·car·ci·no·ma
com·e·do·gen·ic
com·e·do·nes
com·e·dos
co·mes
com·fort
  zone
com·i·tance
com·i·tes
com·ma
  ba·cil·lus
  bun·dle of Schultze
  tract of Schultze
com·man·do
  op·er·a·tion
  pro·ce·dure
com·mem·o·ra·tive
  sign
com·men·sal
  par·a·site
com·men·sal·ism
  ep·i·zo·ic c.
com·mi·nut·ed
  frac·ture
com·mi·nut·ed skull
  frac·ture
com·mi·nu·tion
com·mis·sura
  c. an·te·ri·or gri·sea
  c. bul·bo·rum
  c. ci·ne·rea
  c. gri·sea
  c. hip·po·cam·pi
  c. pos·te·ri·or gri·sea
  c. ven·tra·lis al·ba
com·mis·sur·ae
com·mis·sur·al
  cell
  chei·li·tis
  fi·bers
  my·e·lot·o·my

com·mis·sure
  an·te·ri·or c.
  an·te·ri·or la·bi·al c.
  an·te·ri·or white c.
  c. of bulb
  c. of ce·re·bral hem·i·
    spheres
  c. of for·nix
  Ganser's c.'s
  Gudden's c.'s
  c. of ha·ben·u·lae
  ha·ben·u·lar c.
  hip·po·cam·pal c.
  lat·er·al pal·pe·bral c.
  c. of lips
  me·di·al pal·pe·bral c.
  Meynert's c.'s
  pos·te·ri·or ce·re·bral c.
  pos·te·ri·or la·bi·al c.
  su·pra·op·tic c.'s
  Wernekinck's c.
  white c.
com·mis·sur·ot·o·my
  mi·tral c.
com·mit·ment
com·mon
  an·ti·gen
  limb of mem·bra·nous sem·
    i·cir·cu·lar ducts
  mi·graine
  op·so·nin
  salt
  wart
com·mon ba·sal
  vein
com·mon bile
  duct
com·mon car·di·nal
  veins
com·mon ca·rot·id
  ar·tery
  plex·us
com·mon cold
  vi·rus
com·mon fa·cial
  vein
com·mon fib·u·lar
  nerve
com·mon flex·or
  sheath
com·mon he·pa·tic
  ar·tery
  duct
com·mon il·i·ac
  ar·tery
  vein
com·mon il·i·ac lymph
  nodes

com·mon in·ter·os·se·ous
 ar·tery
com·mon pal·mar dig·i·tal
 ar·tery
 nerves
com·mon per·o·ne·al
 nerve
com·mon plan·tar dig·i·tal
 ar·tery
 nerves
com·mon ten·di·nous
 ring
com·mon var·i·a·ble
 im·mu·no·de·fi·cien·cy
com·mo·tio
 c. ce·re·bri
 c. spi·na·lis
com·mu·ni·ca·ble
 dis·ease
com·mu·ni·cans
com·mu·ni·can·tes
com·mu·ni·cat·ing
 ar·tery
 hy·dro·ceph·a·lus
com·mu·ni·ca·tion
com·mu·ni·ty
 bi·ot·ic c.
 ther·a·peu·tic c.
com·mu·ni·ty
 den·tis·try
 psy·chi·a·try
 psy·chol·o·gy
com·mu·ni·ty health
 nurse
Comolli's
 sign
co·mor·bid·i·ty
com·pact
 bone
 sub·stance
com·pac·ta
com·pa·ges tho·ra·cis
com·pan·ion
 ar·tery to sci·at·ic nerve
 vein
 veins
com·pan·ion lymph
 nodes of ac·ces·so·ry nerve
com·par·a·scope
com·par·a·tive
 anat·o·my
 pa·thol·o·gy
 phys·i·ol·o·gy
 psy·chol·o·gy
com·par·a·tor
 mi·cro·scope
com·part·men·tal
 syn·drome

com·pat·i·bil·i·ty
com·pat·i·ble
com·pen·sat·ed
 ac·i·do·sis
 al·ka·lo·sis
 glau·co·ma
com·pen·sat·ing
 curve
 em·phy·se·ma
 oc·u·lar
com·pen·sa·tion
 neu·ro·sis
com·pen·sa·tion
 depth c.
 gene dos·age c.
com·pen·sa·to·ry
 at·ro·phy
 cir·cu·la·tion
 em·phy·se·ma
 hy·per·tro·phy
 hy·per·tro·phy of the heart
 pause
 pol·y·cy·the·mia
com·pe·tence
 car·di·ac c.
 im·mu·no·log·i·cal c.
com·pe·ti·tion
 an·ti·gen·ic c.
com·pet·i·tive
 an·tag·o·nist
 in·hi·bi·tion
com·pet·i·tive bind·ing
 as·say
com·pet·i·tor
 DNA
com·plaint
com·ple·ment
 fix·a·tion
 unit
com·ple·men·tal
 air
com·ple·men·tar·i·ty
com·ple·men·ta·ry
 air
 col·ors
 DNA
 hy·per·tro·phy
 role
 strand
com·ple·men·ta·tion
 in·ter·gen·ic c.
 in·tra·gen·ic c.
com·ple·ment bind·ing
 as·say
com·ple·ment che·mo·tac·tic
 fac·tor

com·ple·ment-fix·a·tion
  re·ac·tion
  test
com·ple·ment-fix·ing
  an·ti·body
com·plete
  abor·tion
  achro·ma·top·sia
  an·ti·body
  an·ti·gen
  as·cer·tain·ment
  blood count
  car·cin·o·gen
  cat·a·ract
  cleav·age
  den·ture
  dis·in·fec·tant
  fis·tu·la
  hem·i·a·nop·sia
  her·nia
  ir·i·do·ple·gia
  me·di·um
  met·a·mor·pho·sis
  tet·a·nus
  trans·duc·tion
com·plete atri·o·ven·tric·u·lar
  dis·so·ci·a·tion
com·plete A-V
  block
  dis·so·ci·a·tion
com·plete den·ture
  im·pres·sion
com·plex
  ab·sence
  lo·cus
  odon·to·ma
com·plex
  ab·er·rant c.
  AIDS-re·lat·ed c.
  amyg·da·loid c.
  anom·a·lous c.
  an·ti·gen·ic c.
  ap·i·cal c.
  atri·al c.
  au·ric·u·lar c.
  avi·an leu·ke·mia-sar·co·ma
    c.
  avi·an leu·ko·sis-sar·co·ma
    c.
  brain wave c.
  broth·er c.
  Cain c.
  cas·tra·tion c.
  cau·dal pha·ryn·ge·al c.
  charge trans·fer c.
  Di·ana c.
  di·pha·sic c.

Eisenmenger's c.
Elec·tra c.
elec·tro·car·di·o·graph·ic c.
equi·pha·sic c.
fa·ther c.
fe·line leu·ke·mia-sar·co·ma
  vi·rus c.
fem·i·nin·i·ty c.
Golgi c.
HLA c.
im·mune c.
in·fe·ri·or·i·ty c.
iron-dex·tran c.
iso·di·pha·sic c.
j-g c.
Jocasta c.
junc·tion·al c.
jux·ta·glo·mer·u·lar c.
K c.
Lear c.
ma·jor his·to·com·pat·i·bil·
  i·ty c.
mem·brane at·tack c.
Meyenburg's c.
mon·o·pha·sic c.
moth·er su·pe·ri·or c.
Oedipus c.
per·se·cu·tion c.
pri·mary c.
QRS c.
ri·bo·some-la·mel·la c.
sic·ca c.
spike and wave c.
Steidele's c.
su·pe·ri·or·i·ty c.
symp·tom c.
syn·ap·ti·ne·mal c.
Tac·a·ribe c. of vi·rus·es
ter·na·ry c.
tri·ple symp·tom c.
VATER c.
ven·tric·u·lar c.
com·plex·ion
com·plex learn·ing
  pro·cess·es
com·plex par·tial
  sei·zure
com·plex pre·cip·i·tat·ed
  ep·i·lep·sy
com·plex·us
com·pli·ance
  dy·nam·ic c. of lung
  c. of heart
  spe·cif·ic c.
  stat·ic c.
  tho·rac·ic c.
  ven·ti·la·to·ry c.

com·pli·cat·ed
  cat·a·ract
  frac·ture
com·pli·ca·tion
com·po·nent
  an·te·ri·or c. of force
  c. A of pro·throm·bin
  c. of com·ple·ment
  c. of force
  c.'s of mas·ti·ca·tion
  c.'s of oc·clu·sion
  plas·ma throm·bo·plas·tin c.
  throm·bo·plas·tic plas·ma c.
com·pos·ite
  flap
  graft
  res·in
com·pos·ite den·tal
  ce·ment
com·po·si·tion
  base c.
  mod·el·ing c.
com·pos men·tis
com·pound
  ac·e·tone c.
  acy·clic c.
  ad·di·tion c.
  al·i·cy·clic c.'s
  al·i·phat·ic c.
  ar·o·mat·ic c.
  carb·a·mi·no c.
  car·bo·cy·clic c.
  closed chain c.
  con·den·sa·tion c.
  con·ju·gat·ed c.
  cy·clic c.
  ge·net·ic c.
  gly·co·syl c.
  het·er·o·cy·clic c.
  high en·er·gy c.'s
  ho·mo·cy·clic c.
  im·pres·sion c.
  in·clu·sion c.
  in·or·gan·ic c.
  iso·cy·clic c.
  meso c.'s
  me·tho·ni·um c.'s
  mod·el·ing c.
  non·po·lar c.
  open chain c.
  or·gan·ic c.
  po·lar c.
  ring c.
com·pound
  an·eu·rysm
  car·ies
  char·ac·ter
  cyst

dis·lo·ca·tion
  eye
  flap
  frac·ture
  gland
  het·er·o·zy·gote
  joint
  lens
  lip·ids
  mi·cro·scope
  ne·vus
  odon·to·ma
  preg·nan·cy
  pro·tein
  res·to·ra·tion
com·pound gran·ule
  cell
com·pound hy·per·o·pic
  astig·ma·tism
com·pound my·o·pic
  astig·ma·tism
com·pound skull
  frac·ture
com·pre·hen·sion
com·pre·hen·sive med·i·cal
  care
com·press
  grad·u·at·ed c.
  wet c.
com·pressed
  sponge
  tab·let
  yeast
com·press·i·ble cav·ern·ous
  bod·ies
com·pres·sion
  an·es·the·sia
  cy·a·no·sis
  mold·ing
  pa·ral·y·sis
  plat·ing
  ret·i·nop·a·thy
  syn·drome
  throm·bo·sis
com·pres·sion
  c. of brain
  ce·re·bral c.
  c. of tis·sue
com·pres·sive
  my·e·lop·a·thy
  nys·tag·mus
  strength
com·pres·sor
  mus·cle of lips
com·pres·sor
  c. ve·nae dor·sa·lis pe·nis
com·pres·sor·i·um

Compton
  ef·fect
com·pul·sion
com·pul·sive
  idea
  neu·ro·sis
  per·son·al·i·ty
com·put·ed
  pe·rim·e·try
  to·mog·ra·phy
com·put·er
  mod·el
  sim·u·la·tion
com·put·er·ized ax·i·al
  to·mog·ra·phy
con·al·bu·min
con·a·nine
co·nar·i·um
co·na·tion
co·na·tive
co·na·tus
con·cam·er·a·tion
con·ca·nav·a·lin A
con·cat·e·nate
Concato's
  dis·ease
con·cave
  lens
  mir·ror
con·cav·i·ty
con·ca·vo·con·cave
  lens
con·ca·vo·con·vex
  lens
con·cealed
  con·duc·tion
  hem·or·rhage
  her·nia
con·cen·trat·ed hu·man red
  blood
  cor·pus·cle
con·cen·tra·tion
  gra·di·ent
con·cen·tra·tion
  M c.
  mean cell he·mo·glo·bin c.
  min·i·mal al·ve·o·lar c.
  min·i·mal al·ve·o·lar an·es·
    thet·ic c.
  min·i·mal in·hib·i·to·ry c.
  mo·lar c.
  nor·mal c.
con·cen·tric
  fi·bro·ma
  hy·per·tro·phy
  la·mel·la
con·cept
  for·ma·tion

con·cept
  no-thresh·old c.
  self c.
con·cep·ti
con·cep·tion
  im·per·a·tive c.
con·cep·tu·al
con·cep·tus
con·cha
  c. of ear
  high·est c.
  in·fe·ri·or c.
  mid·dle c.
  Morgagni's c.
  na·sal c.
  c. san·to·ri·ni
  Santorini's c.
  sphe·noi·dal con·chae
  su·pe·ri·or c.
  su·preme c.
con·chae
con·chal
  car·ti·lage
  crest
con·chi·tis
con·choi·dal
  bod·ies
con·cho·scope
con·com·i·tance
con·com·i·tant
  im·mu·ni·ty
  stra·bis·mus
  symp·tom
con·cor·dance
  rate
con·cor·dant
  al·ter·nans
  al·ter·na·tion
con·cre·ment
con·cres·cence
con·crete
  op·er·a·tions
  seb·or·rhea
  think·ing
con·cre·tio cor·dis
con·cre·tion
con·cret·i·za·tion
con·cur·rent
  va·lid·i·ty
con·cus·sion
  cat·a·ract
  my·e·li·tis
con·cus·sion
  brain c.
  spi·nal c.
con·cus·sor
con·den·sa·tion
  com·pound

con·dense
con·densed
  milk
con·dens·er
  Abbé's c.
  au·to·mat·ic c.
  car·di·oid c.
  dark-field c.
  pa·rab·o·loid c.
con·dens·ing
  en·zyme
  os·te·i·tis
con·di·tion
con·di·tion·al-le·thal
  mu·tant
con·di·tion·al·ly le·thal
  mu·tant
con·di·tioned
  avi·ta·min·o·sis
  he·mol·y·sis
  re·flex
  re·sponse
  stim·u·lus
con·di·tion·ing
  as·ser·tive c.
  aver·sive c.
  avoid·ance c.
  clas·si·cal c.
  es·cape c.
  high·er or·der c.
  in·stru·men·tal c.
  op·er·ant c.
  pav·lov·i·an c.
  re·spon·dent c.
  sec·ond-or·der c.
  skin·ner·i·an c.
  trace c.
con·dom
con·dom·i·nant
  gene
con·duct
  dis·or·der
con·duc·tance
con·duct·ing
  air·way
  sys·tem of heart
con·duc·tion
  an·al·ge·sia
  an·es·the·sia
  apha·sia
con·duc·tion
  ab·er·rant ven·tric·u·lar c.
  ac·cel·er·at·ed c.
  air c.
  an·ter·o·grade c.
  atri·o·ven·tric·u·lar c.
  A-V c.
  av·a·lanche c.

  bone c.
  con·cealed c.
  dec·re·men·tal c.
  de·layed c.
  for·ward c.
  in·tra-a·tri·al c.
  in·tra·ven·tric·u·lar c.
  nerve c.
  Purkinje c.
  ret·ro·grade c.
  sal·ta·to·ry c.
  su·pra·nor·mal c.
  syn·ap·tic c.
  V-A c.
  ven·tric·u·lar c.
  ven·tric·u·lo·a·tri·al c.
con·duc·tive
  deaf·ness
  heat
con·duc·tiv·i·ty
  hy·drau·lic c.
con·duc·tor
con·duit
  il·e·al c.
con·du·pli·cate
con·du·pli·ca·to cor·pore
con·du·ran·go
con·dy·lar
  ar·tic·u·la·tion
  ax·is
  ca·nal
  fos·sa
  guid·ance
  guide
  joint
  pro·cess
con·dy·lar em·is·sary
  vein
con·dy·lar guid·ance
  in·cli·na·tion
con·dy·lar hinge
  po·si·tion
con·dy·lar·thro·sis
con·dyle
  c. of hu·mer·us
  lat·er·al c.
  lat·er·al c. of fe·mur
  lat·er·al c. of tib·ia
  man·dib·u·lar c.
  me·di·al c.
  me·di·al c. of fe·mur
  me·di·al c. of tib·ia
  oc·cip·i·tal c.
  work·ing side c.
con·dyle
  cord
  path
con·dy·lec·to·my

con·dyl·i·on
con·dy·loid
  ca·nal
  pro·cess
con·dy·lo·ma
  c. acu·mi·na·tum
  flat c.
  gi·ant c.
  c. la·tum
  poin·ted c.
con·dy·lo·ma·ta
con·dy·lom·a·tous
con·dy·lot·o·my
con·dy·lus
cone
  an·tip·o·dal c.
  ar·te·ri·al c.
  elas·tic c.
  ether c.
  fer·til·i·za·tion c.
  gut·ta-per·cha c.
  Haller's c.'s
  im·plan·ta·tion c.
  ker·a·to·sic c.'s
  c. of light
  med·ul·lary c.
  oc·u·lar c.
  Politzer's lu·mi·nous c.
  pul·mo·nary c.
  ret·i·nal c.'s
  sil·ver c.
  the·ca in·ter·na c.
  twin c.
  vas·cu·lar c.'s
cone
  achro·ma·top·sia
  cell of ret·i·na
  de·gen·er·a·tion
  disks
  fi·ber
  gran·ule
  vi·sion
con·e·nine
co·nes·si
co·nes·sine
co·nex·us
con·fab·u·la·tion
con·fec·tio
con·fec·tion
con·fec·ti·o·nes
con·fec·ti·o·nis
con·fer·tus
con·fi·den·ti·al·i·ty
con·fig·u·ra·tion
con·fine·ment
con·flict
  ap·proach-ap·proach c.
  ap·proach-avoid·ance c.

  avoid·ance-avoid·ance c.
  role c.
con·flu·ence
  c. of si·nus·es
con·flu·ens
con·flu·ent
  ar·tic·u·la·tion
  small·pox
con·flu·ent and re·tic·u·late
  pap·il·lo·ma·to·sis
con·for·ma·tion
  boat c.
  en·ve·lope c.
con·form·er
con·fron·ta·tion
  meth·od
con·fu·sion
  col·ors
con·fu·sion·al
con·ge·la·tion
  ur·ti·car·ia
con·ge·ner
con·ge·ner·ous
con·gen·ic
  strain
con·gen·i·tal
  afi·brin·o·gen·e·mia
  agam·ma·glob·u·lin·e·mia
  al·o·pe·cia
  am·pu·ta·tion
  ane·mia
  apla·sia of thy·mus
  bald·ness
  cat·a·ract
  co·nus
  dys·pha·go·cy·to·sis
  el·e·phan·ti·a·sis
  epu·lis of new·born
  glau·co·ma
  hy·dro·cele
  hy·dro·ceph·a·lus
  hy·po·phos·pha·ta·sia
  leu·ko·der·ma
  leu·ko·path·ia
  lymph·e·de·ma
  meg·a·co·lon
  met·he·mo·glo·bi·ne·mia
  myx·e·de·ma
  ne·vus
  nys·tag·mus
  pan·cy·to·pe·nia
  par·a·my·o·to·nia
  pneu·mo·nia
  stri·dor
  syph·i·lis
  tor·ti·col·lis
  tox·o·plas·mo·sis
  valve

con·gen·i·tal ad·re·nal
  hy·per·pla·sia
con·gen·i·tal aplas·tic
  ane·mia
con·gen·i·tal are·gen·er·a·tive
  ane·mia
con·gen·i·tal aton·ic
  pseu·do·pa·ral·y·sis
con·gen·i·tal ce·re·bral
  an·eu·rysm
con·gen·i·tal di·a·phrag·mat·ic
  her·nia
con·gen·i·tal dys·e·ryth·ro·poi·
  et·ic
  ane·mia
con·gen·i·tal dys·plas·tic
  an·gi·ec·ta·sia
  an·gi·o·ma·to·sis
  an·gi·op·a·thy
con·gen·i·tal ec·to·der·mal
  de·fect
  dys·pla·sia
con·gen·i·tal eryth·ro·poi·et·ic
  por·phyr·ia
con·gen·i·tal fa·cial
  di·ple·gia
con·gen·i·tal gen·er·al·ized
  fi·bro·ma·to·sis
con·gen·i·tal he·mo·lyt·ic
  ane·mia
  ic·ter·us
  jaun·dice
con·gen·i·tal hy·po·plas·tic
  ane·mia
con·gen·i·tal ich·thy·o·si·form
  eryth·ro·der·ma
con·gen·i·tal py·lor·ic
  ste·no·sis
con·gen·i·tal se·ba·ceous
  hy·per·pla·sia
con·gen·i·tal spas·tic
  par·a·ple·gia
con·gen·i·tal su·tur·al
  al·o·pe·cia
con·gen·i·tal to·tal
  lip·o·dys·tro·phy
con·gen·i·tus
con·gest·ed
con·ges·tion
  ac·tive c.
  brain c.
  func·tion·al c.
  hy·po·stat·ic c.
  pas·sive c.
  phys·i·o·log·ic c.
  ve·nous c.

con·ges·tive
  cir·rho·sis
  sple·no·meg·a·ly
con·ges·tive heart
  fail·ure
con·glo·bate
con·glo·ba·tion
con·glom·er·ate
con·glu·ti·nant
con·glu·ti·na·tion
con·glu·ti·nin
Con·go·li·an red
  fe·ver
con·go·phil·ic
  an·gi·op·a·thy
Con·go red
  pa·per
con·gru·ent
  points
con·gru·ous
  hem·i·a·nop·sia
co·ni
con·ic
  pa·pil·lae
con·i·cal
  cath·e·ter
  cor·nea
co·nid·ia
co·nid·i·al
co·nid·i·o·bo·lus
co·nid·i·og·e·nous
co·nid·i·o·phore
  Phi·a·lo·phore-type c.
co·nid·i·um
co·ni·ine
co·ni·o·fi·bro·sis
co·ni·o·lymph·sta·sis
co·ni·om·e·ter
co·ni·o·phage
co·ni·o·sis
co·ni·ot·o·my
co·ni·um
con·i·za·tion
  cau·tery c.
  cold c.
con·joined
  anas·to·mo·sis
  ten·don
  twins
con·joined asym·met·ri·cal
  twins
con·joined equal
  twins
con·joined nerve
  root
con·joined sym·met·ri·cal
  twins

con·joined un·e·qual
  twins
con·joint
  ten·don
  ther·a·py
con·ju·gal
  can·cer
con·ju·gant
con·ju·gase
con·ju·ga·ta
  c. di·ag·o·na·lis
con·ju·gate
  di·ag·o·nal c.
  ef·fec·tive c.
  ex·ter·nal c.
  false c.
  fo·lic ac·id c.
  c. of in·let
  in·ter·nal c.
  ob·stet·ric c.
  ob·stet·ric c. of out·let
  c. of out·let
  true c.
con·ju·gate
  ax·is
  de·vi·a·tion of the eyes
  di·am·e·ter of the pel·vic
   in·let
  dis·par·i·ty
  di·vi·sion
  fo·ci
  fo·ra·men
  gaze
  lig·a·ment
  move·ment of eyes
  nys·tag·mus
  pa·ral·y·sis
  point
con·ju·gate ac·id-base
  pair
con·ju·gat·ed
  an·ti·gen
  bil·i·ru·bin
  com·pound
  es·tro·gen
  hap·ten
  pro·tein
con·ju·gat·ed dou·ble
  bonds
con·ju·ga·tion
con·ju·ga·tive
  plas·mid
con·junc·ti·va
  bul·bar c.
  pal·pe·bral c.
con·junc·ti·vae
con·junc·ti·val
  ar·ter·ies

cul-de-sac
glands
lay·er of bulb
lay·er of eye·lids
re·flex
ring
sac
var·ix
veins
con·junc·tive
con·junc·ti·vi·plas·ty
con·junc·ti·vi·tis
  ac·tin·ic c.
  acute ca·tarrh·al c.
  acute con·ta·gious c.
  acute ep·i·dem·ic c.
  acute fol·lic·u·lar c.
  acute hem·or·rhag·ic c.
  al·ler·gic c.
  an·gu·lar c.
  arc-flash c.
  c. ar·i·da
  atop·ic c.
  Béal's c.
  blen·nor·rhe·al c.
  cal·car·e·ous c.
  chem·i·cal c.
  chron·ic c.
  chron·ic fol·lic·u·lar c.
  cic·a·tri·cial c.
  con·ta·gious gran·u·lar c.
  croup·ous c.
  diph·the·rit·ic c.
  dip·lo·ba·cil·la·ry c.
  fol·lic·u·lar c.
  gon·o·coc·cal c.
  gran·u·lar c.
  in·clu·sion c.
  in·fan·tile pu·ru·lent c.
  Koch-Weeks c.
  lac·ri·mal c.
  lar·val c.
  lig·ne·ous c.
  li·thi·a·sis c.
  c. me·di·ca·men·to·sa
  mei·bo·mi·an c.
  mem·bra·nous c.
  mol·lus·cum c.
  Morax-Axenfeld c.
  mu·co·pu·ru·lent c.
  ne·crot·ic in·fec·tious c.
  Parinaud's c.
  Pascheff's c.
  c. pet·ri·fi·cans
  phlyc·ten·u·lar c.
  prai·rie c.
  pseu·do·mem·bra·nous c.
  pu·ru·lent c.

con·junc·ti·vi·tis *(continued)*
  sim·ple c.
  snow c.
  spring c.
  squir·rel plague c.
  swim·ming pool c.
  tox·i·co·gen·ic c.
  tra·chom·a·tous c.
  tu·la·re·mic c.
  c. tu·la·ren·sis
  ver·nal c.
  weld·er's c.
con·junc·ti·vo·dac·ry·o·cys·to·
rhi·nos·to·my
con·junc·ti·vo·dac·ry·o·cys·tos·
to·my
con·junc·ti·vo·ma
con·junc·ti·vo·plas·ty
con·junc·ti·vo·rhi·nos·to·my
con·nect·ing
  car·ti·lage
  stalk
  tu·bule
con·nec·tins
con·nec·tion
  in·ter·ten·di·ne·us c.'s
con·nec·tive
  tis·sue
  tu·mor
con·nec·tive-tis·sue
  dis·eas·es
con·nec·tive tis·sue
  cell
  group
con·nec·tor
  bar
con·nec·tor
  ma·jor c.
  mi·nor c.
Connell's
  su·ture
con·nex·on
con·nex·us
Conn's
  syn·drome
co·noid
  lig·a·ment
  pro·cess
  tu·ber·cle
co·noid
  Sturm's c.
co·no·my·oi·din
con·qui·nine
Conradi-Drigalski
  agar
Conradi's
  dis·ease
  line

con·san·guin·e·ous
con·san·guin·i·ty
con·scious
  per·cep·tion
con·scious·ness
  cloud·ing of c.
  dou·ble c.
  field of c.
con·sec·u·tive
  am·pu·ta·tion
  an·eu·rysm
  an·gi·i·tis
  an·oph·thal·mia
  es·o·tro·pia
con·sen·su·al
  re·ac·tion
  val·i·da·tion
con·sen·su·al light
  re·flex
con·ser·va·tion
  c. of en·er·gy
con·ser·va·tive
con·serve
con·sis·ten·cy
  prin·ci·ple
con·sol·i·dant
con·sol·i·da·tion
  che·mo·ther·a·py
con·so·nat·ing
  rale
con·spe·cif·ic
con·stan·cy
  col·or c.
  ob·ject c.
con·stan·cy
  phe·nom·e·non
con·stant
  cou·pling
  re·gion
con·stant
  Ambard's c.
  as·so·ci·a·tion c.
  Avogadro's c.
  de·cay c.
  dif·fu·sion c.
  dis·in·te·gra·tion c.
  dis·so·ci·a·tion c.
  dis·so·ci·a·tion c. of an
   ac·id
  dis·so·ci·a·tion c. of a base
  dis·so·ci·a·tion c. of wa·ter
  equi·lib·ri·um c.
  Far·a·day's c.
  flo·ta·tion c.
  Michaelis c.
  Michaelis-Menten c.
  new·to·ni·an c. of grav·i·
   ta·tion

Planck's c.
ra·di·o·ac·tive c.
rate c.'s
sed·i·men·ta·tion c.
time c.
ve·loc·i·ty c.'s
con·stant field
equa·tion
con·stant in·fu·sion
pump
con·stel·la·tion
con·sti·pate
con·sti·pat·ed
con·sti·pa·tion
con·sti·tu·tion
con·sti·tu·tion·al
cause
dis·ease
for·mu·la
hir·sut·ism
psy·chol·o·gy
re·ac·tion
symp·tom
throm·bop·a·thy
ul·cer
con·sti·tu·tion·al he·pa·tic
dys·func·tion
con·sti·tu·tive
het·er·o·chro·ma·tin
con·stric·tion
hy·per·e·mia
ring
con·stric·tion
pri·mary c.
sec·on·dary c.
con·stric·tive
en·do·car·di·tis
con·stric·tor
con·struct
va·lid·i·ty
con·sul·tand
dum·my c.
con·sul·tant
con·sul·ta·tion
con·sult·ing
staff
con·sump·tion
co·ag·u·lop·a·thy
con·sump·tion
ox·y·gen c.
con·sump·tive
con·tact
bal·anc·ing c.
cen·tric c.
de·flec·tive oc·clu·sal c.
in·i·tial c.
in·ter·cep·tive oc·clu·sal c.

pre·ma·ture c.
prox·i·mal c.
prox·i·mate c.
c. with re·al·i·ty
work·ing c.'s
con·tact
al·ler·gy
ar·ea
ca·tal·y·sis
cep·tor
chei·li·tis
der·ma·ti·tis
il·lu·mi·na·tion
in·hi·bi·tion
lens
point
splint
sur·face of tooth
con·tac·tant
con·tact-type
der·ma·ti·tis
con·ta·gion
im·me·di·ate c.
me·di·ate c.
psy·chic c.
con·ta·gious
abor·tion
ag·a·lac·tia
aph·thae
dis·ease
ec·thy·ma
con·ta·gious bo·vine
pleu·ro·pneu·mo·nia
py·e·lo·ne·phri·tis
con·ta·gious cap·rine
pleu·ro·pneu·mo·nia
con·ta·gious ec·thy·ma
(pus·tu·lar der·ma·ti·tis)
vi·rus of sheep
con·ta·gious equine
me·tri·tis
con·ta·gious gran·u·lar
con·junc·ti·vi·tis
con·ta·gious·ness
con·ta·gious pus·tu·lar
der·ma·ti·tis
con·ta·gious pus·tu·lar sto·ma·
ti·tis
vi·rus
con·ta·gium
con·tam·i·nant
con·tam·i·nate
con·tam·i·na·tion
con·tent
car·bon di·ox·ide c.
la·tent c.
man·i·fest c.

con·tent
  anal·y·sis
  va·lid·i·ty
con·ti·gu·i·ty
con·tig·u·ous
con·ti·nence
con·ti·nent
con·tin·ued
  fe·ver
con·ti·nu·i·ty
con·tin·u·ous
  beam
  cap·il·lary
  clasp
  erup·tion
  mur·mur
  phase
  spec·trum
  su·ture
  trem·or
  var·i·a·tion
con·tin·u·ous bar
  re·tain·er
con·tin·u·ous ep·i·du·ral
  an·es·the·sia
con·tin·u·ous loop
  wir·ing
con·tin·u·ous pas·sive
  mo·tion
con·tin·u·ous pos·i·tive air·way
  pres·sure
con·tin·u·ous pos·i·tive pres·sure
  breath·ing
  ven·ti·la·tion
con·tin·u·ous re·in·force·ment
  sched·ule
con·tin·u·ous spi·nal
  an·es·the·sia
con·tour
  lines of Owen
con·tour
  flange c.
  gin·gi·val c.
  gum c.
  height of c.
con·tra-an·gle
con·tra-ap·er·ture
con·tra·bev·el
con·tra·cep·tion
con·tra·cep·tive
  com·bi·na·tion oral c.
  in·tra·u·ter·ine c. de·vice
  oral c.
  se·quen·tial oral c.
con·tra·cep·tive
  de·vice
  sponge

con·tract
con·tract·ed
  foot
  heel
  kid·ney
  pel·vis
  ten·don
con·trac·tile
  stric·ture
  vac·u·ole
con·trac·til·i·ty
con·trac·tion
  af·ter-c.
  anod·al clo·sure c.
  anod·al open·ing c.
  au·to·mat·ic c.
  Brax·ton-Hicks c.
  car·po·ped·al c.
  cath·o·dal clo·sure c.
  cath·o·dal open·ing c.
  clos·ing c.
  es·caped c.
  es·caped ven·tric·u·lar c.
  fi·bril·lary c.'s
  front-tap c.
  Gowers' c.
  hour·glass c.
  hun·ger c.'s
  id·i·o·mus·cu·lar c.
  my·o·tat·ic c.
  open·ing c.
  par·a·dox·i·cal c.
  pos·tur·al c.
  pre·ma·ture c.
  te·tan·ic c.
  ton·ic c.
  uter·ine c.
con·trac·tion
  band
con·trac·tu·al
  psy·chi·a·try
  psy·cho·ther·a·py
con·trac·tu·ral
  di·ath·e·sis
con·trac·ture
  de·for·mi·ty
con·trac·ture
  Dupuytren's c.
  func·tion·al c.
  is·che·mic c. of the left
    ven·tri·cle
  or·gan·ic c.
  Volkmann's c.
con·tra·fis·sura
con·tra·in·di·cant
con·tra·in·di·ca·tion
con·tra·lat·er·al
  hem·i·ple·gia

re·flex
sign
con·trary
  sex·u·al
con·trast
  bath
  en·e·ma
  en·hance·ment
  me·di·um
  sen·si·tiv·i·ty
  stain
con·trast
  si·mul·ta·ne·ous c.
  suc·ces·sive c.
con·tra·stim·u·lant
con·tre·coup
  in·ju·ry of brain
con·trec·ta·tion
con·trol
  bi·o·log·i·cal c.
  birth c.
  id·i·o·dy·nam·ic c.
  own c.'s
  qual·i·ty c.
  re·flex c.
  so·cial c.
  stim·u·lus c.
  syn·er·gic c.
  time-var·ied gain c.
  ton·ic c.
  ves·tib·u·lo-e·quil·i·bra·to·ry
    c.
con·trol
  an·i·mal
  ex·per·i·ment
  gene
  group
  sy·ringe
con·trolled
  hy·po·ten·sion
  res·pi·ra·tion
  sub·stance
  ven·ti·la·tion
con·trolled me·chan·i·cal
  ven·ti·la·tion
con·tu·sion
  pneu·mo·nia
con·tu·sion
  brain c.
  scalp c.
  wind c.
con·u·lar
Co·nus
co·nus
  con·gen·i·tal c.
  dis·trac·tion c.
  my·o·pic c.
  pul·mo·nary c.

su·per·trac·tion c.
co·ni vas·cu·lo·si
con·va·les·cence
con·va·les·cent
  car·ri·er
  se·rum
con·val·lar·ia
con·vec·tion
con·vec·tive
  heat
con·ve·nience
  form
con·ven·tion·al
  an·i·mal
  signs
  tho·ra·co·plas·ty
con·ver·gence
  ex·cess
  in·suf·fi·cien·cy
  nu·cle·us of Perlia
con·ver·gence
  ac·com·mo·da·tive c.
  am·pli·tude of c.
  an·gle of c.
  far point of c.
  near point of c.
  neg·a·tive c.
  pos·i·tive c.
  range of c.
  unit of c.
con·ver·gent
  ev·o·lu·tion
  squint
  stra·bis·mus
con·verg·ing
  me·nis·cus
con·ver·sion
  dis·or·der
  elec·tron
  hys·te·ria
  re·ac·tion
con·ver·sion hys·te·ria
  neu·ro·sis
con·ver·sive
  heat
con·ver·tase
con·ver·tin
con·vex
  high c.
  low c.
con·vex
  lens
  mir·ror
con·vex·i·ty
  cor·ti·cal c.
con·vex·o·ba·sia
con·vex·o·con·cave
  lens

con·vex·o·con·vex
  lens
con·vo·lute
con·vo·lut·ed
  bone
  gland
  part of kid·ney lob·ule
  tu·bule of kid·ney
con·vo·lut·ed sem·i·nif·er·ous
  tu·bule
con·vo·lu·tion
  an·gu·lar c.
  an·te·ri·or cen·tral c.
  as·cend·ing fron·tal c.
  as·cend·ing pa·ri·e·tal c.
  cal·lo·sal c.
  cin·gu·late c.
  first tem·po·ral c.
  hip·po·cam·pal c.
  in·fe·ri·or fron·tal c.
  in·fe·ri·or tem·po·ral c.
  mid·dle fron·tal c.
  mid·dle tem·po·ral c.
  pos·te·ri·or cen·tral c.
  sec·ond tem·po·ral c.
  su·pe·ri·or fron·tal c.
  su·pe·ri·or tem·po·ral c.
  su·pra·mar·gin·al c.
  third tem·po·ral c.
  tran·si·tion·al c.
  trans·verse tem·po·ral c.'s
  Zuckerkandl's c.
con·vul·sant
  thresh·old
con·vul·sion
  clo·nic c.
  co·or·di·nate c.
  ether c.
  feb·rile c.
  hys·ter·i·cal c.
  hys·ter·oid c.
  im·me·di·ate post·trau·mat·
   ic c.
  in·fan·tile c.
  mim·ic c.
  pu·er·per·al c.'s
  sa·laam c.'s
  stat·ic c.
  te·tan·ic c.
  ton·ic c.
con·vul·sive
  re·flex
  state
  tic
Cooke's
  spec·u·lum
cooled-knife
  meth·od

Cooley's
  ane·mia
Coolidge
  tube
coo·lie
  itch
Coombs
  mur·mur
Coombs'
  se·rum
  test
Coo·pe·ria
  C. bis·o·nis
  C. cur·ti·cei
  C. field·ingi
  C. on·co·pho·ra
  C. pec·ti·na·ta
  C. punc·ta·ta
  C. spa·tu·la·ta
Coopernail's
  sign
Cooper's
  fas·cia
  her·nia
  her·ni·o·tome
  lig·a·ments
co·or·di·nate
  bond
  con·vul·sion
co·or·di·nat·ed
  re·flex
co·or·di·na·tion
co-os·si·fi·ca·tion
co-os·si·fy
co·pai·ba
co·par·af·fi·nate
cope
co·pe·pod
Co·pep·o·da
Cope's
  clamp
cop·ing
  trans·fer c.
co·pol·y·mer
  res·in
cop·per
  cat·a·ract
  col·ic
  nose
cop·per
  c. ar·se·nite
  c. bi·chlo·ride
  c. chlo·ride
  c. cit·rate
  c. di·chlo·ride
  c. sul·fate
  c. sul·phate
cop·per·as

cop·per·head
Cop·per Ket·tle
   va·por·iz·er
cop·per pen·nies
cop·per phos·phate
   ce·ment
cop·per sul·fate
   meth·od
Coppet's
   law
co·pra
   itch
co·pre·cip·i·ta·tion
cop·rem·e·sis
cop·ro·an·ti·bod·ies
cop·ro·lag·nia
cop·ro·la·lia
cop·ro·lith
co·prol·o·gy
cop·ro·ma
co·proph·a·gous
co·proph·a·gy
cop·ro·phil
cop·ro·phil·ia
cop·ro·phil·ic
cop·ro·pho·bia
cop·ro·phra·sia
cop·ro·plan·e·sia
cop·ro·por·phyr·ia
cop·ro·por·phy·rin
cop·ro·por·phy·rin·o·gen
cop·ro·stane
epi-co·pros·ta·nol
cop·ros·tan·one
cop·ro·sta·sis
cop·ros·ten·ol
cop·ros·ter·in
co·pros·ter·ol
epi-co·pros·ter·ol
cop·ro·stig·mas·tane
cop·ro·zoa
cop·ro·zo·ic
cop·to·sis
cop·u·la
   His' c.
   c. lin·guae
cop·u·la·tion
co·quille
cor
   c. adi·po·sum
   c. bi·lo·cu·la·re
   c. bo·vi·num
   c. mo·bile
   c. pen·du·lum
   c. pul·mo·na·le
   c. tri·at·ri·a·tum
   c. tri·lo·cu·la·re

   c. tri·lo·cu·la·re bi·a·tri·a·tum
   c. tri·lo·cu·la·re bi·ven·tri·cu·la·re
cor·a·cid·i·um
cor·a·co·a·cro·mi·al
   lig·a·ment
cor·a·co·brach·i·al
   bur·sa
   mus·cle
cor·a·co·bra·chi·a·lis
cor·a·co·cla·vic·u·lar
   lig·a·ment
cor·a·co·hu·mer·al
   lig·a·ment
cor·a·coid
   pro·cess
   tu·ber·os·i·ty
cor·al
   cal·cu·lus
cor·al·li·form
   cat·a·ract
cor·al·lin
   yel·low c.
cord
   Bergmann's c.'s
   Billroth's c.'s
   con·dyle c.
   den·tal c.
   false vo·cal c.
   Ferrein's c.'s
   gan·gli·at·ed c.
   gen·i·tal c.
   ger·mi·nal c.'s
   go·nad·al c.'s
   gu·ber·nac·u·lar c.
   he·pa·tic c.'s
   lat·er·al c. of brach·i·al
     plex·us
   me·di·al c. of brach·i·al
     plex·us
   med·ul·lary c.'s
   neph·ro·gen·ic c.
   ob·lique c.
   pos·te·ri·or c. of brach·i·al
     plex·us
   psal·ter·i·al c.
   red pulp c.'s
   re·te c.'s
   sex c.'s
   sper·mat·ic c.
   spi·nal c.
   splen·ic c.'s
   ten·di·nous c.'s
   tes·tic·u·lar c.
   tes·tis c.'s
   true vo·cal c.
   um·bil·i·cal c.

cord *(continued)*
vi·tel·line c.
vo·cal c.
Weitbrecht's c.
Wilde's c.'s
Willis' c.'s
cord
blad·der
blood
cord·a·bra·sion
cor·date
pel·vis
cor·dec·to·my
cor·dial
cor·di·a·nine
cor·di·form
pel·vis
uter·us
cor·dis
cor·do·pexy
cor·dot·o·my
an·ter·o·lat·er·al c.
open c.
pos·te·ri·or col·umn c.
spi·no·tha·lam·ic c.
ster·e·o·tac·tic c.
cordy
pulse
Cor·dy·lo·bia
C. an·thro·poph·a·ga
cor·dy·lo·bi·a·sis
core
atom·ic c.
cen·tral trans·ac·tion·al c.
core
pneu·mo·nia
cor·e·clei·sis
cor·e·cli·sis
cor·ec·ta·sia
cor·ec·ta·sis
cor·ec·to·me·di·al·y·sis
cor·ec·to·pia
cor·e·di·as·ta·sis
co·rel·y·sis
co·re·mi·um
cor·e·o·plas·ty
cor·e·pexy
cor·e·praxy
co·re·pres·sor
cor·e·ste·no·ma
c. con·ge·ni·tum
Co·ri
cy·cle
es·ter
co·ria
co·ri·an·der
Co·ri's
dis·ease

co·ri·um
c. co·ro·nae
c. lim·bi
c. pa·ri·e·tis
c. so·le·ae
c. un·gu·lae
corn
as·bes·tos c.
hard c.
seed c.
soft c.
corn
er·got
sug·ar
cor·nea
con·i·cal c.
c. fa·ri·na·ta
floury c.
c. pla·na con·gen·i·ta fa·
mi·li·a·res
c. uri·ca
c. ver·ti·cil·la·ta
cor·ne·al
astig·ma·tism
cor·pus·cles
de·com·pen·sa·tion
dys·tro·phy
ec·ta·sia
fac·et
graft
lay·er of ep·i·der·mis
lens
mar·gin
pan·nus
re·flex
space
spot
staph·y·lo·ma
trans·plan·ta·tion
trep·a·na·tion
Cornelia de Lange
syn·drome
cor·ne·o·bleph·a·ron
cor·ne·o·cyte
en·ve·lope
cor·ne·o·sclera
cor·ne·o·scler·al
part
cor·ne·ous
Corner-Allen
test
unit
Corner's
tam·pon
cor·ne·um
cor·nic·u·late
car·ti·lage
tu·ber·cle

cor·nic·u·lo·pha·ryn·ge·al
   lig·a·ment
cor·nic·u·lum
   c. la·ryn·gis
cor·ni·fi·ca·tion
cor·ni·fied
   lay·er of nail
corn·meal
   agar
   dis·ease
cor·noid
   la·mel·la
corn oil
corn·silk
corn-smut
cor·nu
   c. am·mo·nis
   c. cu·ta·ne·um
   cor·nua of hy·oid bone
   cor·nua of lat·er·al ven·tri·cle
   cor·nua of sa·phe·nous open·ing
   cor·nua of spi·nal cord
   sty·loid c.
   cor·nua of thy·roid car·ti·lage
cor·nua
cor·nu·al
   preg·nan·cy
cor·nus
co·ro·na
   c. ca·pi·tis
   c. ra·di·a·ta
   c. seb·or·rhe·i·ca
   c. ve·ne·ris
   Zinn's c.
cor·o·nad
co·ro·nae
cor·o·nal
   plane
   pulp
   sec·tion
   su·ture
cor·o·na·le
cor·o·na·lis
cor·o·na·ria
cor·o·nar·ism
cor·o·na·ri·tis
cor·o·nary
   ca·fe c.
cor·o·nary
   ar·tery
   band
   by·pass
   cat·a·ract
   end·ar·ter·ec·to·my
   fail·ure

in·suf·fi·cien·cy
   lig·a·ment of knee
   lig·a·ment of liv·er
   node
   oc·clu·sion
   plex·us
   si·nus
   sul·cus
   ten·don
   throm·bo·sis
   valve
   vein
cor·o·nary care
   unit
cor·o·nary no·dal
   rhythm
cor·o·nary os·ti·al
   ste·no·sis
cor·o·nary si·nus
   rhythm
Co·ro·na·vir·i·dae
co·ro·na·vi·rus
cor·o·ner
cor·o·net
co·ro·ni·on
cor·o·ni·tis
cor·o·noid
   fos·sa
   pro·cess
cor·o·noi·dec·to·my
co·ro·par·el·cy·sis
cor·o·plas·ty
co·rot·o·my
cor·po·ra
cor·po·ra lu·tea
   cysts
cor·po·re·al
cor·po·rin
cor·po·ris
corpse
corps ronds
cor·pu·lence
cor·pu·len·cy
cor·pu·lent
cor·pus
   cor·po·ra al·la·ta
   cor·po·ra am·y·la·cea
   c. am·y·la·ce·um
   c. aor·ti·cum
   c. aran·tii
   cor·po·ra ar·e·na·cea
   atret·ic c. lu·te·um
   c. atre·ti·cum
   cor·po·ra bi·gem·i·na
   c. can·di·cans
   c. ca·ver·no·sum con·chae
   c. ca·ver·no·sum ure·thrae
   c. den·ta·tum

cor·pus *(continued)*
c. fe·mo·ris
c. fi·bro·sum
c. fim·bri·a·tum
c. ge·ni·cu·la·tum ex·ter·num
c. ge·ni·cu·la·tum in·ter·num
c. glan·du·lae su·do·ri·fe·rae
c. he·mor·rha·gi·cum
c. high·mori
c. high·mor·i·a·num
c. luy·sii
c. oli·va·re
c. pam·pi·ni·for·me
c. pa·pil·la·re
c. pa·ra·ter·mi·na·le
c. pon·to·bul·ba·re
cor·po·ra quad·ri·gem·i·na
c. quad·ri·ge·mi·num an·te·ri·us
c. quad·ri·ge·mi·num pos·te·ri·us
c. res·ti·for·me
c. spon·gi·o·sum ure·thrae mu·li·e·bris
c. tri·tic·e·um

cor·pus·cle
am·ni·ot·ic c.
am·y·la·ceous c.
am·y·loid c.
ar·tic·u·lar c.'s
ax·ile c.
ax·is c.
ba·sal c.
Bizzozero's c.
blood c.
bone c.
bridge c.
bul·boid c.'s
ce·ment c.
chyle c.
col·loid c.
co·los·trum c.
con·cen·trat·ed hu·man red blood c.
cor·ne·al c.'s
Dogiel's c.
Donné's c.
dust c.'s
Eichhorst's c.'s
ex·u·da·tion c.
gen·i·tal c.'s
ghost c.
Gluge's c.'s
Golgi-Mazzoni c.
Grandry's c.'s

Hassall's con·cen·tric c.'s
Herbst's c.'s
in·flam·ma·to·ry c.
Key-Retzius c.'s
lam·el·lat·ed c.'s
lymph c.
lym·phat·ic c.
lym·phoid c.
mal·pi·ghi·an c.'s
Mazzoni's c.
Meissner's c.
Merkel's c.
Mex·i·can hat c.
milk c.
mol·lus·cum c.
Negri c.'s
Norris' c.'s
oval c.
pac·chi·o·ni·an c.'s
pa·ci·ni·an c.'s
pes·sa·ry c.
phan·tom c.
plas·tic c.
Purkinje's c.'s
pus c.
Rainey's c.'s
red c.
re·nal c.
re·tic·u·lated c.
Ruffini's c.'s
sal·i·vary c.
Schwalbe's c.
shad·ow c.
splen·ic c.'s
tac·tile c.
taste c.
ter·mi·nal nerve c.'s
third c.
thy·mic c.
touch c.
Toynbee's c.'s
Traube's c.
Tröltsch's c.'s
Valentin's c.'s
Vater-Pacini c.'s
Vater's c.'s
Virchow's c.'s
white c.
Zimmermann's c.

cor·pus·cu·la
cor·pus·cu·lar
lymph
ra·di·a·tion
cor·pus·cu·lum
cor·pus lu·te·um
he·ma·to·ma
hor·mone

cor·pus lu·te·um de·fi·cien·cy
  syn·drome
cor·pus lu·te·um hor·mone
  unit
cor·rect·ed
  dex·tro·car·dia
cor·rec·tion
  oc·clu·sal c.
  spon·ta·ne·ous c. of pla·
    cen·ta pre·via
cor·rec·tive
cor·rec·tive emo·tion·al
  ex·pe·ri·ence
cor·re·la·tion
  co·ef·fi·cients
cor·re·la·tion
  pro·duct-mo·ment c.
  rank-dif·fer·ence c.
cor·re·la·tion·al
  meth·od
cor·rel·a·tive
  dif·fer·en·ti·a·tion
Correra's
  line
cor·re·spon·dence
  ab·nor·mal c.
  anom·a·lous c.
  dys·har·mo·ni·ous c.
  har·mo·ni·ous c.
cor·ri·dor
  dis·ease
Corrigan's
  dis·ease
  pulse
cor·ri·gent
cor·rin
cor·rode
cor·ro·sion
  prep·a·ra·tion
cor·ro·sive
  mer·cu·ry chlo·ride
  sub·li·mate
  ul·cer
cor·ru·ga·tor
  mus·cle
cor·tex
  ad·re·nal c.
  agran·u·lar c.
  as·so·ci·a·tion c.
  au·di·to·ry c.
  cer·e·bel·lar c.
  ce·re·bral c.
  deep c.
  dys·gran·u·lar c.
  fe·tal c.
  fe·tal ad·re·nal c.
  fron·tal c.

gran·u·lar c.
c. of hair shaft
het·er·o·typ·ic c.
ho·mo·typ·ic c.
in·su·lar c.
lam·i·nat·ed c.
c. of lens
c. of lymph node
mo·tor c.
ol·fac·to·ry c.
or·bi·to·fron·tal c.
c. of ova·ry
par·a·stri·ate c.
per·i·stri·ate c.
pir·i·form c.
pre·fron·tal c.
pre·mo·tor c.
pri·mary vi·su·al c.
pro·vi·sion·al c.
re·nal c.
sec·on·dary sen·so·ry c.
sec·on·dary vi·su·al c.
sen·so·ry c.
so·mat·ic sen·so·ry c.
so·ma·to·sen·so·ry c.
stri·ate c.
sup·ple·men·tary mo·tor c.
su·pra·re·nal c.
tem·po·ral c.
ter·ti·ary c.
c. of thy·mus
vi·su·al c.
cor·ti·cal
  aprax·ia
  arch·es of kid·ney
  ar·ter·ies
  au·di·om·e·try
  blind·ness
  bone
  cat·a·ract
  con·vex·i·ty
  deaf·ness
  ep·i·lep·sy
  hor·mones
  im·plan·ta·tion
  os·te·i·tis
  part
  sen·si·bil·i·ty
  sub·stance
cor·ti·cal·i·za·tion
cor·ti·cal·os·te·ot·o·my
cor·ti·cec·to·my
cor·ti·ces
cor·ti·cif·u·gal
cor·ti·cip·e·tal
cor·ti·cis
cor·ti·co·af·fer·ent

cor·ti·co·bul·bar
  fi·bers
  tract
cor·ti·co·cer·e·bel·lum
cor·ti·co·ef·fer·ent
cor·ti·cof·u·gal
cor·ti·coid
cor·ti·co·lib·er·in
cor·ti·co·me·di·al
cor·ti·co·nu·cle·ar
  fi·bers
cor·ti·co·pon·tine
  fi·bers
  tract
cor·ti·co·pu·pil·lary
  re·flex
cor·ti·co·re·tic·u·lar
  fi·bers
cor·ti·co·spi·nal
  fi·bers
  tract
cor·ti·co·ste·roid
cor·ti·co·ste·roid-bind·ing
  glob·u·lin
  pro·tein
cor·ti·co·ste·roid-in·duced
  glau·co·ma
cor·ti·cos·ter·one
cor·ti·co·tha·lam·ic
cor·ti·co·troph
cor·ti·co·tro·pic
  hor·mone
cor·ti·co·tro·pin
  c.-zinc hy·drox·ide
cor·ti·co·tro·pin-re·leas·ing
  fac·tor
  hor·mone
Cor·ti·co·vir·i·dae
Corti's
  arch
  ca·nal
  cells
  gan·gli·on
  mem·brane
  or·gan
  pil·lars
  rods
  tun·nel
Corti's au·di·to·ry
  teeth
cor·ti·sol
  c. ac·e·tate
cor·ti·sone
co·run·dum
cor·us·ca·tion
Corvisart's
  fa·ci·es
cor·yl·o·phy·line

co·rym·bi·form
cor·ym·bose
  syph·i·lid
cor·y·ne·bac·te·ria
cor·y·ne·bac·te·ri·o·phage
Cor·y·ne·bac·te·ri·um
  C. ac·nes
  C. bo·vis
  C. diph·the·ri·ae
  C. en·zy·mi·cum
  C. equi
  C. hof·man·nii
  C. kut·scheri
  C. mi·nu·tis·si·mum
  C. mu·ri·sep·ti·cum
  C. ovis
  C. par·vum
  C. pho·cae
  C. pseu·do·diph·the·ri·ti·cum
  C. pseu·do·tu·ber·cu·lo·sis
  C. py·og·e·nes
  C. re·na·le
  C. stri·a·tum
  C. ul·ce·rans
  C. xe·ro·sis
cor·y·ne·bac·te·ri·um
co·ry·za
  al·ler·gic c.
co·ry·za·vi·rus
cos·me·sis
cos·met·ic
  der·ma·ti·tis
  sur·gery
cos·met·ics
cos·mic
  rays
cos·mid
cos·mo·pol·i·tan
cos·ta
  cos·tae fluc·tu·an·tes
cos·tae
cos·tal
  an·gle
  arch
  car·ti·lage
  chon·dri·tis
  fringe
  groove
  notch
  part of di·a·phragm
  pit of trans·verse pro·cess
  pleu·ri·sy
  pro·cess
  res·pi·ra·tion
  sur·face
  sur·face of lung

sur·face of scap·u·la
tu·ber·os·i·ty
cos·tal arch
  re·flex
cos·tal·gia
cos·tec·to·my
Costen's
  syn·drome
cos·ti·car·ti·lage
cos·ti·form
cos·tive
cos·tive·ness
cos·to·ax·il·lary
  vein
cos·to·cen·tral
cos·to·cer·vi·cal
  ar·tery
  trunk
cos·to·chon·dral
  joint
  syn·drome
cos·to·chon·dri·tis
cos·to·cla·vic·u·lar
  lig·a·ment
  line
  syn·drome
cos·to·col·ic
  lig·a·ment
cos·to·cor·a·coid
cos·to·di·a·phrag·mat·ic
  re·cess
cos·to·gen·ic
cos·to·in·fe·ri·or
cos·to·me·di·as·ti·nal
  re·cess
  si·nus
cos·to·pec·to·ral
  re·flex
cos·to·phren·ic sep·tal
  lines
cos·to·scap·u·lar
cos·to·sca·pu·la·ris
cos·to·ster·nal
cos·to·ster·no·plas·ty
cos·to·su·pe·ri·or
cos·to·tome
cos·tot·o·my
cos·to·trans·verse
  fo·ra·men
  joint
  lig·a·ment
cos·to·trans·ver·sec·to·my
cos·to·ver·te·bral
  joints
cos·to·xi·phoid
  lig·a·ment
co·syn·tro·pin

Cotard's
  syn·drome
co·tar·nine
co·throm·bo·plas·tin
co·ti·nine
co·trans·port
Cotte's
  op·er·a·tion
Cotton
  ef·fect
cot·ton
  ab·sor·bent c.
  pu·ri·fied c.
  sol·u·ble gun c.
  styp·tic c.
cot·ton-fi·ber
  em·bo·lism
cot·ton-mill
  fe·ver
cot·ton·seed oil
cot·ton-wool
  patch·es
  spots
Cotunnius
  dis·ease
Cotunnius'
  aq·ue·duct
  ca·nal
  liq·uid
  space
cot·y·le
cot·y·le·don
  fe·tal c.
  ma·ter·nal c.
cot·y·le·don·ary
  pla·cen·ta
Cot·y·lo·gon·i·mus
cot·y·loid
  cav·i·ty
  joint
  lig·a·ment
  notch
couch·ing
  nee·dle
cough
  frac·ture
  re·flex
cough
  brassy c.
  ear c.
  he·bet·ic c.
  ken·nel c.
  priv·et c.
  re·flex c.
  stom·ach c.
  tooth c.
  tri·gem·i·nal c.

cough *(continued)*
  weav·er's c.
  whoop·ing c.
cou·lomb
cou·mar·a·none
cou·ma·ric an·hy·dride
cou·ma·rin
cou·met·a·rol
Councilman
  body
Councilman hy·a·line
  body
Coun·cil·ma·nia
Councilman's
  le·sion
coun·sel·ing
  psy·chol·o·gy
coun·sel·ing
  ge·net·ic c.
  mar·i·tal c.
  pas·to·ral c.
count
  Addis c.
  Arneth c.
  blood c.
  ep·i·der·mal ridge c.
  fil·a·ment-non·fil·a·ment c.
count
  den·si·ty
count·er
  au·to·mat·ed dif·fer·en·tial
    leu·ko·cyte c.
  elec·tron·ic cell c.
  Geiger-Müller c.
  pro·por·tion·al c.
  scin·til·la·tion c.
  whole-body c.
counter-
  shock
count·er·bal·anc·ing
count·er·con·di·tion·ing
count·er·cur·rent
  dis·tri·bu·tion
  mech·a·nism
count·er·cur·rent ex·chang·er
count·er·cur·rent mul·ti·pli·er
count·er·de·pres·sant
count·er·die
count·er·ex·ten·sion
count·er·im·mu·no·e·lec·tro·
  pho·re·sis
count·er·in·ci·sion
count·er·in·vest·ment
count·er·ir·ri·tant
count·er·ir·ri·ta·tion
count·er·o·pen·ing
count·er·pho·bic
count·er·pul·sa·tion

count·er·punc·ture
count·er·shock
count·er·stain
count·er·trac·tion
count·er·trans·fer·ence
count·er·trans·port
coup
  in·ju·ry of brain
coup de sa·bre
cou·ple
cou·pled
  beats
  pulse
  rhythm
cou·pling
  de·fect
  fac·tors
  in·ter·val
  phase
cou·pling
  con·stant c.
  fixed c.
  var·i·a·ble c.
Couranand's
  dip
Courvoisier's
  law
  sign
cou·vade
Couvelaire
  uter·us
cou·ver·cle
co·va·lent
cov·er
  glass
  test
cov·er·slip
cov·ert
  sen·si·ti·za·tion
cov·er-un·cov·er
  test
cow
  face
  kid·ney
Cowden's
  dis·ease
Cow·dria ru·mi·nan·ti·um
cow·dri·o·sis
Cowdry's type A in·clu·sion
  bod·ies
Cowdry's type B in·clu·sion
  bod·ies
cowl
  mus·cle
Cowling's
  rule
cow·per·i·tis

Cowper's
  cyst
  gland
  lig·a·ment
cow·pox
  vi·rus
coxa
  c. ad·duc·ta
  false c. va·ra
  c. flexa
  c. mag·na
  c. pla·na
  c. val·ga
  c. va·ra
  c. va·ra lux·ans
cox·ae
cox·al
  bone
cox·al·gia
  c. fu·gax
Cox·i·el·la
  C. bur·ne·tii
cox·it·ic
  sco·li·o·sis
cox·o·dyn·ia
cox·o·fem·o·ral
cox·ot·o·my
cox·o·tu·ber·cu·lo·sis
Cox·sack·ie
  en·ceph·a·li·tis
  vi·rus
Cox·sack·ie·vi·rus
co·zy·mase
C-pep·tide
CR
  lead
crab
  hand
  yaws
Crabtree
  ef·fect
cracked
  heel
cracked-pot
  res·o·nance
  sound
crack·ling
  jaw
cra·dle
  cap
Crafoord
  clamp
craft
  pal·sy
Craig·ia
Cramer wire
  splint

cramp
  ac·ces·so·ry c.
  heat c.'s
  in·ter·mit·tent c.
  min·er's c.'s
  mu·si·cian's c.
  pi·a·nist's c.
  pi·a·no-play·er's c.
  seam·stress's c.
  shav·ing c.
  stok·er's c.'s
  tai·lor's c.
  typ·ist's c.
  vi·o·lin·ist's c.
  wait·er's c.
  watch·mak·er's c.
  writ·er's c.
Crampton
  test
Crampton's
  line
  mus·cle
Crandall's
  syn·drome
cra·nia
cra·ni·ad
cra·ni·al
  ar·te·ri·tis
  base
  bones
  ca·pac·i·ty
  cav·i·ty
  flex·ure
  fon·ta·nels
  in·dex
  nerves
  roots
  si·nus·es
  su·tures
  syn·chon·dro·ses
  ver·te·bra
cra·ni·a·lis
cra·ni·am·phit·o·my
Cra·ni·a·ta
cra·ni·ec·to·my
  lin·e·ar c.
cra·ni·o-au·ral
cra·ni·o·car·di·ac
  re·flex
cra·ni·o·car·po·tar·sal
  dys·pla·sia
  dys·tro·phy
cra·ni·o·cele
cra·ni·o·ce·re·bral
cra·ni·o·cla·sia
cra·ni·o·cla·sis
cra·ni·o·clast
cra·ni·o·clei·do·dys·os·to·sis

cra·ni·o·di·a·phys·i·al
  dys·pla·sia
cra·ni·o·did·y·mus
cra·ni·o·fa·cial
  an·gle
  ap·pli·ance
  ax·is
  dys·os·to·sis
  fix·a·tion
  notch
  sur·gery
cra·ni·o·fa·cial dys·junc·tion
  frac·ture
cra·ni·o·fa·cial sus·pen·sion
  wir·ing
cra·ni·o·fe·nes·tria
cra·ni·og·no·my
cra·ni·o·graph
cra·ni·og·ra·phy
cra·ni·o·la·cu·nia
cra·ni·ol·o·gy
  Gall's c.
cra·ni·o·ma·la·cia
  cir·cum·scribed c.
cra·ni·o·me·nin·go·cele
cra·ni·o·met·a·phys·si·al
  dys·pla·sia
cra·ni·om·e·ter
cra·ni·o·met·ric
  points
cra·ni·om·e·try
cra·ni·op·a·gus
  c. oc·ci·pi·ta·lis
  c. pa·ra·si·ti·cus
cra·ni·op·a·thy
  met·a·bol·ic c.
cra·ni·o·pha·ryn·ge·al
  ca·nal
  duct
cra·ni·o·pha·ryn·gi·o·ma
  cys·tic pap·il·lo·ma·tous c.
cra·ni·o·phore
cra·ni·o·plas·ty
cra·ni·o·punc·ture
cra·ni·or·rha·chid·i·an
cra·ni·or·rha·chis·chi·sis
cra·ni·o·sa·cral
  sys·tem
cra·ni·os·chi·sis
cra·ni·o·scle·ro·sis
cra·ni·os·co·py
cra·ni·o·si·nus
  fis·tu·la
cra·ni·o·spi·nal
cra·ni·o·ste·no·sis
cra·ni·os·to·sis
cra·ni·o·syn·os·to·sis
cra·ni·o·tabes

cra·ni·o·tome
cra·ni·ot·o·my
  at·tached c.
  de·tached c.
  os·te·o·plas·tic c.
cra·ni·o·to·nos·co·py
cra·ni·o·try·pe·sis
cra·ni·o·tym·pan·ic
cra·ni·um
  bi·fid c.
  c. bi·fi·dum
  ce·re·bral c.
  c. ce·re·bra·le
  vis·cer·al c.
  c. vis·ce·ra·le
crap·u·lent
crap·u·lous
cras·sa·men·tum
cra·ter
  arc
cra·ter·i·form
cra·ter·i·za·tion
cra·vat
  ban·dage
craw-craw
craz·ing
cra·zy chick
  dis·ease
C-re·ac·tive
  pro·tein
cream of
  tar·tar
cream
  cleans·ing c.
  cold c.
  grease·less c.
  leu·ko·cyte c.
  lu·bri·cat·ing c.
  van·ish·ing c.
crease
  flex·ion c.
  pal·mar c.
  sim·i·an c.
  Sydney c.
crease
  wound
cre·a·ti·nase
cre·a·tine
  c. ki·nase
  c. phos·phate
  c. phos·pho·ki·nase
cre·a·ti·ne·mia
cre·at·i·nin·ase
cre·at·i·nine
  clear·ance
  co·ef·fi·cient
cre·a·tin·u·ria

cre·a·tive
  think·ing
Credé's
  ma·neu·vers
  meth·ods
creep
  re·cov·ery
creep·ing
  erup·tion
  my·i·a·sis
  pal·sy
  throm·bo·sis
  ul·cer
cre·mas·ter
  mus·cle
crem·as·ter·ic
  ar·tery
  fas·cia
  re·flex
crem·no·cele
crem·no·pho·bia
cre·na
  c. clu·ni·um
  c. cor·dis
cre·nae
cre·nate
cre·nat·ed
cre·na·tion
creno·cyte
cre·no·cy·to·sis
Cren·o·so·ma vul·pis
cre·o·la
  bod·ies
cre·oph·a·gism
cre·oph·a·gy
cre·o·sol
cre·o·sote
crep·i·tant
  rale
crep·i·ta·tion
crep·i·tus
  ar·tic·u·lar c.
  bony c.
cre·pus·cu·lar
cre·scen·do
  an·gi·na
  mur·mur
  sleep
cres·cent
  cell
cres·cent
  ar·tic·u·lar c.
  Giannuzzi's c.'s
  glo·mer·u·lar c.
  Heidenhain's c.'s
  ma·lar·i·al c.
  my·o·pic c.
  sub·lin·gual c.

cres·cent cell
  ane·mia
cres·cen·tic
  lob·ules of the cer·e·bel·
  lum
cres·co·graph
cre·sol
m-cre·sol
cre·so·lase
cre·sol red
CREST
  syn·drome
crest
  acous·tic c.
  acous·ti·co·fa·cial c.
  al·ve·o·lar c.
  am·pul·la·ry c.
  an·te·ri·or lac·ri·mal c.
  arched c.
  ar·cu·ate c.
  ar·tic·u·lar c.'s
  bas·i·lar c. of co·chle·ar
    duct
  buc·ci·na·tor c.
  c. of co·chle·ar open·ing
  con·chal c.
  del·toid c.
  den·tal c.
  eth·moi·dal c.
  ex·ter·nal oc·cip·i·tal c.
  fal·ci·form c.
  fron·tal c.
  gan·gli·on·ic c.
  gin·gi·val c.
  glu·te·al c.
  c. of great·er tu·ber·cle
  c. of head of rib
  il·i·ac c.
  in·ci·sor c.
  in·fra·tem·po·ral c.
  in·gui·nal c.
  in·ter·me·di·ate sa·cral c.'s
  in·ter·nal oc·cip·i·tal c.
  in·ter·os·se·ous c.
  in·ter·tro·chan·ter·ic c.
  lat·er·al ep·i·con·dy·lar c.
  lat·er·al sa·cral c.'s
  lat·er·al su·pra·con·dy·lar c.
  c. of less·er tu·ber·cle
  mar·gi·nal c.
  me·di·al c.
  me·di·al ep·i·con·dy·lar c.
  me·di·al su·pra·con·dy·lar
    c.
  me·di·an sa·cral c.
  c.'s of nail bed
  na·sal c.
  c. of neck of rib

crest *(continued)*
 neu·ral c.
 ob·tu·ra·tor c.
 pal·a·tine c.
 c. of pal·a·tine bone
 pos·te·ri·or lac·ri·mal c.
 pu·bic c.
 c. of ridge
 sa·cral c.
 sag·it·tal c.
 c. of scap·u·lar spine
 sphe·noid c.
 spi·ral c.
 su·pi·na·tor c.
 c. of su·pi·na·tor mus·cle
 su·pra·mas·toid c.
 su·pra·ven·tric·u·lar c.
 ter·mi·nal c.
 tib·i·al c.
 trans·verse c.
 tri·an·gu·lar c.
 tri·gem·i·nal c.
 tro·chan·ter·ic c.
 tur·bi·nat·ed c.
 tym·pan·ic c.
 ure·thral c.
 ves·tib·u·lar c.
 c. of ves·ti·bule
cres·ta
cres·yl·ate
cres·yl blue
cres·yl blue bril·liant
cres·yl echt
cres·yl fast vi·o·let
cres·yl vi·o·let ac·e·tate
cre·ta
cre·tin
cre·tin·ism
cre·tin·is·tic
cre·tin·oid
cre·tin·ous
Creutzfeldt-Jakob
 dis·ease
crev·ice
 gin·gi·val c.
cre·vic·u·lar
 ep·i·the·li·um
 flu·id
crib
 death
cri·bra
crib·rate
cri·bra·tion
crib·ri·form
 ar·ea
 fas·cia
 hy·men
 plate of eth·moid bone

cri·brum
Cri·cet·i·nae
Cri·ce·tu·lus
Cri·ce·tus
Crichton-Browne's
 sign
cri·co·ar·y·te·noid
 ar·tic·u·la·tion
 joint
cri·co·ar·y·te·noid ar·tic·u·lar
 cap·sule
cri·co·ar·y·te·noi·de·us
cri·co·e·soph·a·ge·al
 ten·don
cri·coid
 car·ti·lage
cri·coi·dec·to·my
cri·coi·dyn·ia
cri·co·pha·ryn·ge·al
 lig·a·ment
 part
cri·co·san·to·ri·ni·an
 lig·a·ment
cri·co·thy·roid
 ar·tery
 ar·tic·u·la·tion
 joint
 lig·a·ment
 mem·brane
 mus·cle
cri·co·thy·roid ar·tic·u·lar
 cap·sule
cri·co·thy·roi·de·us
cri·co·thy·roi·dot·o·my
cri·co·thy·rot·o·my
cri·cot·o·my
cri·co·tra·che·al
 lig·a·ment
 mem·brane
cri·co·vo·cal
 mem·brane
cri-du-chat
 syn·drome
Crigler-Najjar
 dis·ease
 syn·drome
Crile's
 clamp
Cri·me·an-Con·go hem·or·rhag·ic
 fe·ver
Cri·me·an-Con·go hem·or·rhag·ic fe·ver
 vi·rus
crim·i·nal
 abor·tion
 an·thro·pol·o·gy
 hy·giene

in·san·i·ty
ir·re·spon·si·bil·i·ty
psy·chol·o·gy
crim·i·nol·o·gy
cri·nes
crin·in
cri·nis
crin·o·gen·ic
crin·oph·a·gy
crip·pled
cri·ses
cri·sis
  ad·di·so·ni·an c.
  ad·o·les·cent c.
  ad·re·nal c.
  an·a·phy·lac·toid c.
  blast c.
  blood c.
  Dietl's c.
  feb·rile c.
  gas·tric c.
  glau·co·ma·to·cy·clit·ic c.
  iden·ti·ty c.
  la·ryn·ge·al c.
  mid·life c.
  my·e·lo·cyt·ic c.
  oc·u·lar c.
  oc·u·lo·gy·ric cri·ses
  sick·le cell c.
  ta·bet·ic c.
  ther·a·peu·tic c.
  thy·roid c.
  thy·ro·tox·ic c.
cri·sis
  in·ter·ven·tion
cris·pa·tion
cris·ta
  c. buc·ci·na·to·ria
  c. den·ta·lis
  c. di·vi·dens
  c. glu·tea
  c. he·li·cis
  cris·tae of mi·to·chon·dria
  cris·tae mi·to·chon·dri·a·les
  c. phal·li·ca
  c. quar·ta
  c. tym·pa·ni·ca
cris·tae
cri·te·ria
cri·te·ri·on
  Spiegelberg's cri·te·ria
cri·te·ri·on-re·lat·ed
  va·lid·i·ty
Cri·thid·ia
cri·thid·ia
crit·i·cal
  an·gle
  il·lu·mi·na·tion

or·gan
pe·ri·od
pH
point
pres·sure
rate
tem·per·a·ture
crit·i·cal care
  unit
crit·i·cal flick·er fu·sion
  fre·quen·cy
croc·i·dis·mus
croc·o·dile
  tears
croc·o·dile tears
  syn·drome
Crocq's
  dis·ease
cro·cus
Crohn's
  dis·ease
cro·mo·lyn so·di·um
Cronkhite-Canada
  syn·drome
Crookes'
  glass
Crooke's
  gran·ules
Crooke's hy·a·line
  change
  de·gen·er·a·tion
crop
  gland
  milk
Crosby
  cap·sule
cross
  ag·glu·ti·na·tion
  birth
  cir·cu·la·tion
  flap
  hy·brid·i·za·tion
  in·fec·tion
  mat·ing
  re·ac·tion
  tol·er·ance
cross
  back c.
  dou·ble back c.
  hair c.'s
  Ranvier's c.'s
  test c.
cross-bite
  teeth
cross·breed
cross·breed·ing
cross-cut
  bur

crossed
an·es·the·sia
cyl·in·ders
di·plo·pia
em·bo·lism
eyes
fix·a·tion
hem·i·an·es·the·sia
hem·i·a·nop·sia
hem·i·ple·gia
im·mu·no·e·lec·tro·pho·re·
sis
jerk
lat·er·al·i·ty
pa·ral·y·sis
re·flex
re·flex of pel·vis
crossed ad·duc·tor
jerk
re·flex
crossed ex·ten·sion
re·flex
crossed knee
jerk
re·flex
crossed phren·ic
phe·nom·e·non
crossed py·ram·i·dal
tract
crossed spi·no-ad·duc·tor
re·flex
cross-eye
cross·ing-over
so·mat·ic c.
un·e·qual c.
un·e·ven c.
cross-linked
pol·y·mer
res·in
cross-match·ing
cross·over
cross-re·act·ing
ag·glu·ti·nin
an·ti·body
ma·te·ri·al
cross-sec·tion·al
ech·o·car·di·og·ra·phy
meth·od
study
cross·way
sen·so·ry c.
cro·ta·lar·ia
poi·son·ing
cro·ta·lid
Cro·tal·i·dae
cro·ta·lin
cro·ta·line
cro·tal·ism

Cro·ta·lus
an·ti·tox·in
cro·tam·i·ton
cro·taph·i·on
cro·ton·ase
cro·ton oil
cro·to·nyl-ACP re·duc·tase
croup
croup-as·so·ci·at·ed
vi·rus
croup·ous
bron·chi·tis
con·junc·ti·vi·tis
in·flam·ma·tion
lar·yn·gi·tis
lymph
mem·brane
phar·yn·gi·tis
rhi·ni·tis
croupy
Crouzon's
dis·ease
syn·drome
crowd·ing
crow·ing
in·spi·ra·tion
crown
cav·i·ty
flask
glass
tu·ber·cle
crown
an·a·tom·i·cal c.
ar·ti·fi·cial c.
bell-shaped c.
cil·i·ary c.
clin·i·cal c.
c. of head
jack·et c.
ra·di·ate c.
c. of tooth
crown-heel
length
crown·ing
crown-rump
length
CRST
syn·drome
cru·ces
cru·cial
anas·to·mo·sis
ban·dage
lig·a·ment
cru·ci·ate
anas·to·mo·sis
em·i·nence
lig·a·ment of the at·las
lig·a·ment of leg

lig·a·ments of knee
mus·cle
cru·ci·ble
cru·ci·form
  em·i·nence
  lig·a·ment of at·las
  part of fi·brous sheath
crude
  cal·ci·um sul·fide
  drug
  urine
cru·fo·mate
cruor
cru·ra
cru·ral
  arch
  ar·tery
  ca·nal
  fos·sa
  her·nia
  ring
  sep·tum
  sheath
  tri·an·gle
cru·re·us
cru·ris
crus
  c. of clit·o·ris
  c. cor·po·ris ca·ver·no·si
   pe·nis
  c. of for·nix
  left c. of atri·o·ven·tric·u·
   lar trunk
  left c. of di·a·phragm
  long c. of in·cus
  right c. of atri·o·ven·tric·u·
   lar trunk
  right c. of di·a·phragm
  short c. of in·cus
crush
  kid·ney
  syn·drome
crus I
crus II
crus·ot·o·my
crust
  milk c.
crus·ta
  c. in·flam·ma·to·ria
  c. lac·tea
  c. phlo·gis·ti·ca
Crus·ta·cea
crus·tae
crust·ed
  ring·worm
  tet·ter

crutch
  pal·sy
  pa·ral·y·sis
Cruveilhier-Baumgarten
  dis·ease
  mur·mur
  sign
  syn·drome
Cruveilhier's
  dis·ease
  fas·cia
  fos·sa
  joint
  lig·a·ments
  plex·us
crux
  c. of heart
Cruz
  try·pan·o·so·mi·a·sis
cry
  re·flex
cry·al·ge·sia
cry·an·es·the·sia
cry·es·the·sia
cry for help
cry·mo·dyn·ia
cry·mo·phil·ic
cry·mo·phy·lac·tic
cry·mo·ther·a·py
cry·o·an·es·the·sia
cry·o·bi·ol·o·gy
cry·o·cau·tery
cry·o·con·i·za·tion
cry·o·ex·trac·tion
cry·o·ex·trac·tor
cry·o·fi·brin·o·gen
cry·o·fi·brin·o·gen·e·mia
cry·o·flu·o·rane
cry·o·gen
cry·o·gen·ic
cry·o·gen·ics
cry·o·glob·u·lin·e·mia
  crys·tal c.
cry·o·glob·u·lins
cry·o·hy·drate
cry·o·hy·poph·y·sec·to·my
cry·ol·y·sis
cry·om·e·ter
cry·o·pal·li·dec·to·my
cry·op·a·thy
cry·o·pexy
cry·o·phil·ic
cry·o·phy·lac·tic
cry·o·pre·cip·i·tate
cry·o·pre·cip·i·ta·tion
cry·o·pres·er·va·tion
cry·o·probe
cry·o·pros·ta·tec·to·my

cry·o·pro·tein
cry·o·pul·vi·nec·to·my
cry·o·scope
cry·os·co·py
cry·o·spasm
cry·o·stat
cry·o·sty·let
cry·o·sty·lette
cry·o·sur·gery
cry·o·thal·a·mec·to·my
cry·o·ther·a·py
cry·o·tol·er·ant
cry·o·u·nit
crypt
 den·tal c.
 enam·el c.
 c.'s of iris
 Lieberkühn's c.'s
 lin·gual c.
 Morgagni's c.'s
 syn·o·vi·al c.
 ton·sil·lar c.
crypt
 abscesses
cryp·ta
cryp·tae
cryp·tec·to·my
cryp·ten·a·mine ac·e·tates
cryp·ten·a·mine tan·nates
cryp·tic
cryp·ti·tis
cryp·to·coc·co·ma
cryp·to·coc·co·sis
Cryp·to·coc·cus
 C. ne·o·for·mans
cryp·to·crys·tal·line
Cryp·to·cys·tis trich·o·dec·tis
cryp·to·did·y·mus
Cryp·to·gam·ia
cryp·to·gen·ic
 cir·rho·sis
 in·fec·tion
 py·e·mia
 sep·ti·ce·mia
cryp·to·lith
cryp·to·men·or·rhea
cryp·toph·thal·mia
cryp·toph·thal·mus
 syn·drome
cryp·to·po·dia
cryp·to·pyr·role
cryp·tor·chid
 tes·tis
cryp·tor·chi·dec·to·my
cryp·tor·chi·dism
cryp·tor·chi·do·pexy
cryp·tor·chism
cryp·to·spo·rid·i·o·sis

Cryp·to·spo·rid·i·um
Cryp·to·stro·ma cor·ti·ca·le
cryp·to·tia
cryp·to·xan·thin
cryp·to·zo·ite
cryp·to·zy·gous
crys·tal
 asth·ma c.'s
 blood c.'s
 Böttcher's c.'s
 Charcot-Leyden c.'s
 Charcot-Neumann c.'s
 Charcot-Robin c.'s
 chi·ral c.
 clath·rate c.
 ear c.'s
 Florence's c.'s
 he·ma·toi·din c.'s
 hy·drate c.
 knife-rest c.
 Leyden's c.'s
 Lubarsch's c.'s
 sperm c.
 sperm·in c.
 Teichmann's c.'s
 thorn ap·ple c.'s
 twin c.
 Virchow's c.'s
 whet·stone c.'s
crys·tal
 cry·o·glob·u·lin·e·mia
 rash
 struc·ture
crys·tal·lin
 gam·ma c.
crys·tal·line
 cap·sule
 cat·a·ract
 dig·i·tal·in
 in·ter·face
 lens
crys·tal·line in·su·lin zinc
 sus·pen·sion
crys·tal·li·za·tion
crys·tal·lized
 tryp·sin
crys·tal·lo·gram
crys·tal·log·ra·phy
crys·tal·loid
 Charcot-Böttcher c.'s
 Reinke c.'s
crys·tal·lo·pho·bia
crys·tal·lu·ria
crys·tal vi·o·let
 vac·cine
C-sec·tion
Csillag's
 dis·ease

"C" slid·ing
os·te·ot·o·my
CT
num·ber
unit
Cteno·ce·phal·i·des
Cu·ban
itch
cu·beb
cu·bic
cen·ti·me·ter
ni·ter
cu·bi·tal
bone
fos·sa
joint
nerve
cu·bi·tal lymph
nodes
cu·bi·ti
cu·bi·tus
c. val·gus
c. var·us
cu·boid
bone
cu·boi·dal
ep·i·the·li·um
cu·boi·dal ar·tic·u·lar
sur·face of cal·ca·ne·us
cu·boi·de·o·na·vic·u·lar
joint
lig·a·ment
cu·boi·do·dig·i·tal
re·flex
cue
re·sponse-pro·duced c.'s
cuff
mus·cu·lo·ten·di·nous c.
per·i·vas·cu·lar c.'s
ro·ta·tor c. of shoul·der
cuff·ing
cui·rass
an·al·ge·sic c.
ta·bet·ic c.
cui·rass
res·pi·ra·tor
cul-de-sac
smear
cul-de-sac
con·junc·ti·val c.
Douglas' c.
great·er c.
Gruber's c.
less·er c.
cul·do·cen·te·sis
cul·do·plas·ty
cul·do·scope
cul·dos·co·py

cul·dot·o·my
Cu·lex
C. pi·pi·ens
C. tar·sa·lis
Cu·lic·i·dae
cu·li·ci·dal
cu·li·cide
cu·lic·i·fuge
Cu·li·coi·des
C. aus·te·ni
C. fu·rens
C. mil·nei
C. var·i·i·pen·nis
cu·li·co·sis
Cu·li·se·ta melanura
Cullen's
sign
cul·men
cul·mi·na
Culp
py·e·lo·plas·ty
culs-de-sac
cult
cul·ti·vat·ed
yeast
cul·ti·va·tion
cul·tur·al
an·thro·pol·o·gy
shock
cul·ture
me·di·um
cul·ture
cell c.
elec·tive c.
hang·ing-block c.
mixed lym·pho·cyte c.
nee·dle c.
ne·o·type c.
or·gan c.
pure c.
roll-tube c.
sen·si·tized c.
shake c.
slant c.
slope c.
smear c.
stab c.
stock c.
streak c.
tis·sue c.
type c.
cu·ma·rin
cu·meth·a·rol
cu·me·thox·a·eth·ane
Cummer's
clas·si·fi·ca·tion
guide·line

cu·mu·la·tive
  ac·tion
  dose
  ef·fect
cu·mu·li
cu·mu·lus
  c. ooph·or·us
  c. ova·ri·cus
cu·ne·ate
  fas·cic·u·lus
  fu·nic·u·lus
  nu·cle·us
cu·nei
cu·ne·i·form
  bone
  car·ti·lage
  cat·a·ract
  lobe
  tu·ber·cle
cu·ne·o·cer·e·bel·lar
  tract
cu·ne·o·cu·boid
  joint
  lig·a·ment
cu·ne·o·met·a·tar·sal
  joints
cu·ne·o·na·vic·u·lar
  ar·tic·u·la·tion
  joint
  lig·a·ments
cu·ne·o·scaph·oid
cu·ne·us
cu·nic·u·li
cu·nic·u·lus
cun·ni·linc·tion
cun·ni·linc·tus
cun·ni·lin·gus
Cun·ning·ham·el·la el·e·gans
cun·nus
cup
  Diogenes c.
  dry c.
  eye c.
  glau·co·ma·tous c.
  oc·u·lar c.
  op·tic c.
  per·i·lim·bal suc·tion c.
  phys·i·o·log·ic c.
  suc·tion c.
  wet c.
cup bi·op·sy
  for·ceps
cu·po·la
cupped
cup·ping
  glass
cu·pric
cu·pric ac·e·tate

cu·pric ac·e·tate nor·mal
cu·pric ar·se·nite
cu·pric chlo·ride
cu·pric cit·rate
cu·pric sul·fate
cu·pri·u·re·sis
cu·pu·la
cu·pu·lae
cu·pu·lar
  part
cu·pu·lar blind
  sac
cu·pu·late
  part
cu·pu·li·form
  cat·a·ract
cu·pu·lo·gram
cu·rage
cu·ra·re
cu·ra·ri·form
cu·rar·i·mi·met·ic
cu·ra·rine
cu·ra·ri·za·tion
cur·a·tive
  dose
curb
  te·not·o·my
curby
  hock
curd
  soap
curdy
  pus
cure
cu·ret
cu·ret·ment
cu·ret·tage
  per·i·ap·i·cal c.
  sub·gin·gi·val c.
cu·rette
  Hartmann's c.
cu·rette·ment
cu·rie
cur·ing
  den·tal c.
cu·ri·um
cur·li·cue
  ure·ter
Curling's
  ul·cer
cur·rant jel·ly
  clot
cur·rent of
  in·ju·ry
cur·rent
  ac·tion c.
  af·ter-c.
  al·ter·nat·ing c.

anod·al c.
as·cend·ing c.
ax·i·al c.
cen·trif·u·gal c.
cen·trip·e·tal c.
d'Arsonval c.
de·mar·ca·tion c.
de·scend·ing c.
di·rect c.
elec·tro·ton·ic c.
gal·van·ic c.
high fre·quen·cy c.
c. of in·ju·ry
la·bile c.
Tesla c.
Curschmann's
dis·ease
spi·rals
curse
Ondine's c.
cur·va·tu·ra
cur·va·tu·rae
cur·va·ture
an·gu·lar c.
an·te·ri·or c.
back·ward c.
gin·gi·val c.
great·er c. of stom·ach
lat·er·al c.
less·er c. of stom·ach
oc·clu·sal c.
Pott's c.
spi·nal c.
cur·va·ture
ab·er·ra·tion
hy·per·o·pia
my·o·pia
curve
re·sponse
curve
align·ment c.
an·ti-Monson c.
Barnes' c.
buc·cal c.
Carus' c.
com·pen·sat·ing c.
dis·tri·bu·tion c.
dose-re·sponse c.
dye-di·lu·tion c.
ep·i·dem·ic c.
flow-vol·ume c.
Frank-Starling c.
fre·quen·cy c.
Friedman c.
gaus·si·an c.
growth c.
in·di·ca·tor-di·lu·tion c.
in·tra·car·di·ac pres·sure c.

iso·vol·ume pres·sure-flow c.
lo·gis·tic c.
milled-in c.'s
Monson c.
mus·cle c.
c. of oc·clu·sion
Pleasure c.
Price-Jones c.
prob·a·bil·i·ty c.
pulse c.
re·verse c.
c. of Spee
Starling's c.
strength-du·ra·tion c.
stress-strain c.
ten·sion c.
Traube-Hering c.'s
von Spee's c.
whole-body ti·tra·tion c.
Cur·vu·la·ria
Cushing
ef·fect
phe·nom·e·non
re·sponse
cush·ing·oid
Cushing's
ba·soph·i·lism
dis·ease
su·ture
syn·drome
syn·drome med·i·ca·men·to·
sus
cush·ion
atri·o·ven·tric·u·lar ca·nal
c.'s
en·do·car·di·al c.'s
c. of ep·i·glot·tis
eu·sta·chi·an c.
le·va·tor c.
Passavant's c.
pha·ryn·go·e·soph·a·ge·al
c.'s
plan·tar c.
suck·ing c.
cusp
an·te·ri·or c.
c. of Carabelli
pos·te·ri·or c.
sep·tal c.
c. of tooth
cusp
an·gle
height
cus·pad
cus·pal
in·ter·fer·ence
cus·par·ia bark

251

cus·pid
  tooth
cus·pi·date
  tooth
cus·pi·des
cus·pis
cusp·less
  tooth
cu·ta·ne·o·man·dib·u·lar
  pol·y·on·co·sis
cu·ta·ne·o·me·nin·go·spi·nal
  an·gi·o·ma·to·sis
cu·ta·ne·o·mu·co·sal
cu·ta·ne·o·mu·cous
  mus·cle
cu·ta·ne·o·mu·cou·veal
  syn·drome
cu·ta·ne·ous
  ab·sorp·tion
  al·bi·nism
  an·cy·lo·sto·mi·a·sis
  an·thrax
  ap·o·plexy
  diph·the·ria
  em·phy·se·ma
  gan·grene
  hab·ro·ne·mi·a·sis
  hem·or·rhoids
  horn
  lar·va mi·grans
  lay·er of tym·pan·ic mem·
    brane
  leish·man·i·a·sis
  lep·ro·sy
  me·nin·gi·o·ma
  mus·cle
  nerve
  re·ac·tion
  re·flex
  test
  tu·ber·cu·lo·sis
  vas·cu·li·tis
  vein
cu·ta·ne·ous cer·vi·cal
  nerve
cu·ta·ne·ous pu·pil
  re·flex
cu·ta·ne·ous-pu·pil·lary
  re·flex
cu·ta·ne·ous sys·tem·ic
  an·gi·i·tis
cu·ta·ne·ous tu·ber·cu·lin
  test
cutch
cut·down
Cu·te·reb·ra
cu·ti·cle
  ac·quired c.

ac·quired enam·el c.
den·tal c.
enam·el c.
c. of hair
Nasmyth's c.
post·e·rup·tion c.
c. of root sheath
cu·tic·u·la
  c. pi·li
  c. va·gi·nae fol·lic·u·li pi·li
cu·tic·u·lae
cu·tic·u·lar·i·za·tion
cu·tin
cu·ti·re·ac·tion
  test
cu·tis
  graft
  plate
cu·tis
  c. an·se·ri·na
  c. hy·per·e·las·ti·ca
  c. laxa
  c. mar·mo·ra·ta
  c. rhom·boi·da·lis nu·chae
  c. unc·tu·o·sa
  c. ve·ra
  c. ver·ti·cis gy·ra·ta
cu·ti·sec·tor
cu·ti·za·tion
cut·ting
  edge
  for·ceps
  teeth
cut·tle·fish
  disk
cu·vet
cu·vette
  ox·im·e·ter
Cuvier's
  ducts
  veins
cy·a·mem·a·zine
cy·an·al·co·hols
cy·an·a·mide
cy·a·nate
cy·a·ne·mia
cy·a·nide
  c. met·he·mo·glo·bin
cy·a·nide
  poi·son·ing
cy·an·ide-ni·tro·prus·side
  test
cy·a·nid·e·non
cy·an·i·dol
cy·an·met·he·mo·glo·bin
Cy·a·no·bac·te·ria
cy·a·no·chro·ic
cy·an·och·rous

cy·a·no·co·bal·a·min
  ra·di·o·ac·tive c.
cy·an·o·gen
  c. chlo·ride
cy·a·no·gen·ic
cy·a·no·hy·drins
cy·an·o·phil
cy·an·o·phile
cy·a·noph·i·lous
Cy·a·no·phy·ce·ae
cy·a·no·pia
cy·a·nop·sia
  c. ret·i·nae
cy·a·nosed
cy·a·nose tar·dive
cy·a·no·sis
  com·pres·sion c.
  en·ter·og·e·nous c.
  false c.
  he·red·i·tary met·he·mo·
    glo·bi·ne·mic c.
  c. ret·i·nae
  tar·dive c.
  tox·ic c.
cy·a·not·ic
  as·phyx·ia
  at·ro·phy
  at·ro·phy of the liv·er
  in·du·ra·tion
cy·a·nu·ria
cy·a·nu·ric ac·id
Cy·a·tho·sto·ma
  C. bron·chi·a·lis
Cy·a·tho·sto·mum
cy·ber·net·ics
cy·brid
cy·cla·mate
cy·clam·ic ac·id
cy·cla·mide
cy·clan·de·late
cy·clar·ba·mate
cy·clar·thro·di·al
cy·clar·thro·sis
cy·clase
cy·cla·zo·cine
cy·cle
  an·ov·u·la·to·ry c.
  brain wave c.
  car·bon c.
  car·bon di·ox·ide c.
  car·di·ac c.
  cell c.
  chew·ing c.
  cit·ric ac·id c.
  Cori c.
  di·car·box·yl·ic ac·id c.
  en·dog·e·nous c.
  es·trous c.

ex·o·e·ryth·ro·cyt·ic c.
ex·og·e·nous c.
fat·ty ac·id ox·i·da·tion c.
forced c.
ge·ne·si·al c.
gly·cine suc·ci·nate c.
gly·ox·yl·ic ac·id c.
hair c.
Krebs c.
Krebs-Henseleit c.
Krebs or·ni·thine c.
Krebs urea c.
life c.
mas·ti·cat·ing c.'s
men·stru·al c.
ni·tro·gen c.
or·ni·thine c.
ovar·i·an c.
re·pro·duc·tive c.
re·stored c.
re·turn·ing c.
suc·cin·ic ac·id c.
tri·car·box·yl·ic ac·id c.
urea c.
vi·su·al c.
cy·clec·to·my
cy·clen·ce·pha·lia
cy·clen·ceph·a·ly
cy·cles per sec·ond
cy·clic
  ad·e·nyl·ic ac·id
  al·bu·min·ur·ia
  com·pound
  es·o·tro·pia
  neu·tro·pe·nia
  phos·phate
  phos·phor·ic ac·id
  stra·bis·mus
cy·clic AMP
cy·cli·cot·o·my
cy·cli·tis
  het·er·o·chro·mic c.
  plas·tic c.
  pu·ru·lent c.
cy·cli·zine hy·dro·chlo·ride
cy·cli·zine lac·tate
cy·clo·bar·bi·tal
cy·clo·ben·za·prine hy·dro·chlo·
  ride
cy·clo·ce·pha·lia
cy·clo·ceph·a·ly
cy·clo·cho·roid·i·tis
cy·clo·cry·o·ther·a·py
cy·clo·cu·ma·rol
cy·clo·di·al·y·sis
cy·clo·di·a·ther·my
cy·clo·duc·tion
cy·clo·e·lec·trol·y·sis

cy·clo·guan·il pam·o·ate
cy·clo·hex·ane·sul·fam·ic ac·id
cy·clo·hex·a·tri·ene
cy·clo·hex·i·mide
cy·clo·hex·i·tol
cy·clo·hex·yl·sul·fam·ic ac·id
cy·cloid
cy·clol
cy·clo·meth·y·caine sul·fate
cy·clo·na·mine
cy·clo·pea
cy·clo·pe·an
  eye
cy·clo·pent·a·mine hy·dro·chlo·ride
cy·clo·pen·tane
cy·clo·pen·ta *a*phen·an·threne
cy·clo·pen·ta·phene
cy·clo·pen·thi·a·zide
cy·clo·pen·to·late hy·dro·chlo·ride
cy·clo·pep·tide
cy·clo·phen·a·zine hy·dro·chlo·ride
cy·clo·pho·ras·es
cy·clo·pho·ria
cy·clo·phos·pha·mide
cy·clo·pho·to·co·ag·u·la·tion
cy·clo·phre·nia
Cy·clo·phyl·li·dae
cy·clo·pia
cy·clo·pi·an
  eye
cy·clo·ple·gia
cy·clo·ple·gic
cy·clo·pro·pane
cy·clops
cy·clo·ser·ine
cy·clo·sis
cy·clo·spor·in A
cy·clo·spor·ine
cy·clo·thi·a·zide
cy·clo·thy·mia
cy·clo·thy·mi·ac
cy·clo·thy·mic
  dis·or·der
  per·son·al·i·ty
cy·clo·tome
cy·clot·o·my
cy·clo·tron
cy·clo·tro·pia
cy·clo·zo·o·no·sis
cy·cri·mine hy·dro·chlo·ride
cy·e·sis
cy·hep·ta·mide
cyl·in·der
  ax·is c.
  Bence Jones c.'s

  crossed c.'s
  Külz's c.
cyl·in·der
  ret·i·nos·co·py
cyl·in·drax·is
cy·lin·dri·cal
  bron·chi·ec·ta·sis
  ep·i·the·li·um
  lens
cyl·in·dro·ad·e·no·ma
cyl·in·droid
  an·eu·rysm
cyl·in·dro·ma
cyl·in·drom·a·tous
  car·ci·no·ma
cyl·in·dro·sar·co·ma
cyl·in·dru·ria
cyl·lo·so·ma
cy·ma·rin
cym·ba con·chae
cym·bo·ce·phal·ic
cym·bo·ceph·a·lous
cym·bo·ceph·a·ly
cyn·an·che
cy·nan·thro·py
cyn·ic
  spasm
cyn·o·ceph·a·ly
cyn·o·dont
cy·no·pho·bia
Cyon's
  nerve
cy·pri·do·pho·bia
Cy·prin·i·dae
cy·pro·hep·ta·dine hy·dro·chlo·ride
cy·pro·ter·one ac·e·tate
cyr·tom·e·ter
cyst
  ad·ven·ti·tious c.
  al·lan·to·ic c.
  al·ve·o·lar hy·da·tid c.
  an·eu·rys·mal bone c.
  ap·i·cal per·i·o·don·tal c.
  ap·o·plec·tic c.
  arach·noid c.
  Baker's c.
  Bartholin's c.
  bile c.
  Blessig's c.'s
  blood c.
  blue dome c.
  bone c.
  Boyer's c.
  bran·chi·al c.
  bran·chi·al cleft c.
  bron·cho·gen·ic c.
  bur·sal c.

cal·ci·fy·ing and ker·a·tin·
  iz·ing odon·to·gen·ic c.
cal·ci·fy·ing odon·to·gen·ic
  c.
cer·e·bel·lar c.
choc·o·late c.
cho·le·doch·al c.
chyle c.
col·loid c.
com·pound c.
cor·po·ra lu·tea c.'s
Cowper's c.
daugh·ter c.
den·tig·er·ous c.
den·ti·nal lam·i·na c.
der·moid c.
der·moid c. of ova·ry
dis·ten·tion c.
du·pli·ca·tion c.
echi·no·coc·cus c.
en·do·me·tri·al c.
en·do·the·li·al c.
en·ter·og·e·nous c.'s
ep·en·dy·mal c.
ep·i·der·mal c.
ep·i·der·moid c.
ep·i·the·li·al c.
ex·trav·a·sa·tion c.
ex·u·da·tion c.
false c.
fis·sur·al c.
fol·lic·u·lar c.
Gartner's c.
gas c.
gin·gi·val c.
glo·mer·u·lar c.'s
Gorlin c.
grand·daugh·ter c.
hem·or·rhag·ic c.
he·pa·tic c.'s
hy·da·tid c.
im·plan·ta·tion c.
in·clu·sion c.
in·vo·lu·tion c.
io·dine c.'s
Iwanoff's c.'s
junc·tion·al c.
ke·rat·i·nous c.
lac·te·al c.
lat·er·al per·i·o·don·tal c.
mei·bo·mi·an c.
milk c.
mor·ga·gni·an c.
moth·er c.
mu·cous c.
mul·ti·loc·u·lar c.
mul·ti·loc·u·lar hy·da·tid c.

mul·ti·loc·u·late hy·da·tid
  c.
myx·oid c.
na·both·i·an c.
ne·crot·ic c.
neu·ral c.
odon·to·gen·ic c.
oil c.
ooph·or·it·ic c.
os·se·ous hy·da·tid c.
ovar·i·an c.
par·a·phys·i·al c.'s
par·a·sit·ic c.
par·ent c.
par·o·oph·o·rit·ic c.
par·vi·loc·u·lar c.
pearl c.
per·i·ap·i·cal c.
phae·o·my·cot·ic c.
pi·lar c.
pi·lif·er·ous c.
pi·lo·ni·dal c.
pin·e·al c.
post·trau·mat·ic lep·to·me·
  nin·ge·al c.
pri·mor·di·al c.
pro·lif·er·at·ing trich·o·lem·
  mal c.
pro·lif·er·a·tion c.
pro·lif·er·a·tive c.
pro·lif·er·ous c.
pro·to·zo·an c.
pseu·do·mu·ci·nous c.
ra·dic·u·lar c.
Rathke's cleft c.
re·ten·tion c.
re·te c. of ova·ry
root end c.
san·guin·e·ous c.
se·ba·ceous c.
se·cre·to·ry c.
se·ques·tra·tion c.
se·rous c.
sol·i·tary bone c.
Stafne bone c.
stat·ic bone c.
ster·ile c.
sub·lin·gual c.
su·pra·sel·lar c.
syn·o·vi·al c.
Tarlov's c.
tar·ry c.
tar·sal c.
ter·a·tom·a·tous c.
thy·ro·glos·sal duct c.
thy·ro·lin·gual c.
Tornwaldt's c.
trich·i·lem·mal c.

cyst *(continued)*
 tu·bu·lar c.
 um·bil·i·cal c.
 uni·cam·er·al c.
 uni·cam·er·al bone c.
 uni·loc·u·lar c.
 uni·loc·u·lar hy·da·tid c.
 ura·chal c.
 uri·nary c.
 vi·tel·lo·in·tes·tin·al c.
 wolff·i·an c.
cys·ta·canth
cyst·ad·e·no·car·ci·no·ma
cyst·ad·e·no·ma
 pap·il·lary c. lym·pho·ma·
  to·sum
cyst·al·gia
cys·ta·mine
cys·ta·thi·o·nase
cys·ta·thi·o·nine
cys·ta·thi·o·nin·u·ria
cys·tau·chen·i·tis
cys·tau·chen·ot·o·my
cys·tec·ta·sia
cys·tec·ta·sy
cys·tec·to·my
 Bartholin's c.
 par·tial c.
 rad·i·cal c.
 to·tal c.
 vul·vo·vag·i·nal c.
cys·te·ic ac·id
cys·te·ine
 c. de·sulf·hy·drase
 c. syn·thase
cys·te·ine·sul·fin·ic ac·id
cys·tein·yl
cys·ten·de·sis
cys·tic
 ac·ne
 ar·tery
 car·ci·no·ma
 di·ath·e·sis
 dis·ease of the breast
 dis·ease of re·nal me·dul·la
 duct
 fi·bro·sis
 fi·bro·sis of the pan·cre·as
 goi·ter
 hy·per·pla·sia
 hy·per·pla·sia of the breast
 kid·ney
 lym·phan·gi·ec·ta·sis
 mole
 node
 pol·yp
 vein

cys·tic duct
 chol·an·gi·og·ra·phy
cys·ti·cer·ci
cys·ti·cer·coid
cys·ti·cer·co·sis
Cys·ti·cer·cus
 C. bo·vis
 C. cel·lu·lo·sae
 C. fas·ci·o·la·ris
 C. pi·si·for·mis
 C. ten·u·i·col·lis
cys·ti·cer·cus
cys·tic gall
 duct
cys·tic me·di·al
 ne·cro·sis
cys·tic pap·il·lo·ma·tous
 cra·ni·o·pha·ryn·gi·o·ma
cys·ti·des
cys·ti·do·ce·li·ot·o·my
cys·ti·do·lap·a·rot·o·my
cys·ti·do·trach·e·lot·o·my
cys·ti·fel·le·ot·o·my
cys·ti·form
cys·tig·er·ous
cys·tine
 c. de·sulf·hy·drase
 c. ly·ase
cys·tine
 cal·cu·lus
meso-cys·tine
cys·ti·ne·mia
cys·tine stor·age
 dis·ease
cys·ti·no·sis
cys·ti·not·ic
 leu·ko·cyte
cys·ti·nu·ria
 fa·mil·i·al c.
cys·tin·yl
cys·tiph·or·ous
cys·tis
 c. fel·lea
 c. uri·na·ria
cys·ti·stax·is
cys·ti·tis
 c. col·li
 c. cys·ti·ca
 fol·lic·u·lar c.
 c. glan·du·la·ris
 in·ter·sti·tial c.
cys·to·ad·e·no·ma
cys·to·car·ci·no·ma
cys·to·cele
cys·to·chro·mos·co·py
cys·to·co·los·to·my
cys·to·di·aph·a·nos·co·py
cys·to·di·ver·tic·u·lum

cys·to·du·o·de·nal
 lig·a·ment
cys·to·du·o·de·nos·to·my
cys·to·en·ter·o·cele
cys·to·en·ter·os·to·my
cys·to·e·pip·lo·cele
cys·to·ep·i·the·li·o·ma
cys·to·fi·bro·ma
cys·to·gas·tros·to·my
cys·to·gram
 void·ing c.
cys·tog·ra·phy
 an·te·grade c.
cys·toid
 mac·u·lop·a·thy
cys·toid mac·u·lar
 de·gen·er·a·tion
 ede·ma
cys·to·je·ju·nos·to·my
cys·to·lith
cys·to·li·thec·to·my
cys·to·li·thi·a·sis
cys·to·lith·ic
cys·to·li·thot·o·my
cys·to·ma
cys·tom·e·ter
cys·to·met·ro·gram
cys·to·me·trog·ra·phy
cys·tom·e·try
cys·to·mor·phous
cys·to·my·o·ma
cys·to·myx·o·ad·e·no·ma
cys·to·myx·o·ma
cys·to·pan·en·dos·co·py
cys·to·pa·ral·y·sis
cys·to·pexy
cys·toph·er·ous
cys·to·pho·tog·ra·phy
cys·to·plas·ty
cys·to·ple·gia
cys·to·proc·tos·to·my
cys·to·pto·sia
cys·to·pto·sis
cys·to·py·e·li·tis
cys·to·py·e·lo·ne·phri·tis
cys·to·ra·di·og·ra·phy
cys·to·rec·tos·to·my
cys·tor·rha·gia
cys·tor·rha·phy
cys·tor·rhea
cys·to·sar·co·ma
 c. phyl·lodes
cys·to·scope
cys·to·scop·ic
 urog·ra·phy
cys·tos·co·py
cys·to·spasm
cys·to·stax·is

cys·tos·to·my
cys·to·tome
cys·tot·o·my
 su·pra·pu·bic c.
cys·to·trach·e·lot·o·my
cys·to·u·re·ter·i·tis
cys·to·u·re·ter·o·gram
cys·to·u·re·ter·og·ra·phy
cys·to·u·re·thri·tis
cys·to·u·re·thro·cele
cys·to·u·re·thro·gram
cys·to·u·re·throg·ra·phy
cys·to·u·re·thro·scope
cyst·ous
Cys·to·vir·i·dae
cys·tyl-a·mi·no·pep·ti·dase
cy·ta·pher·e·sis
cy·tar·a·bine
cy·tase
Cy·taux·zo·on
cy·taux·zo·on·o·sis
cy·the·mo·lyt·ic
 ic·ter·us
cyt·i·dine
 c. di·phos·phate cho·line
 c. phos·phate
cyt·i·dine·di·phos·pho·cho·line
cyt·i·dyl·ic ac·id
cy·to·an·a·lyz·er
cy·to·ar·chi·tec·ton·ics
cy·to·ar·chi·tec·tur·al
cy·to·ar·chi·tec·ture
cy·to·bi·ol·o·gy
cy·to·bi·o·tax·is
cy·to·cen·trum
cy·to·chal·a·sins
cy·to·chem·is·try
cy·to·chrome
 sys·tem
cy·to·chrome *cd*
cy·to·chrome *c* ox·i·dase
cy·to·chrome *c* re·duc·tase
cy·to·chrome ox·i·dase (*Pseu·do·mo·nas*)
cy·to·chrome per·ox·i·dase
cy·to·chrome re·duc·tase
cy·to·chy·le·ma
cy·toc·i·dal
cy·to·cide
cy·to·ci·ne·sis
cy·toc·la·sis
cy·to·clas·tic
cy·to·cle·sis
cy·to·crine
 se·cre·tion
cy·to·cu·pre·in
cy·to·cyst
cy·to·di·ag·no·sis

cy·to·di·er·e·sis
cy·to·gene
cy·to·gen·e·sis
cy·to·ge·net·i·cist
cy·to·ge·net·ics
cy·to·gen·ic
  re·pro·duc·tion
cy·tog·e·nous
cy·to·glu·co·pe·nia
cy·to·het
cy·to·hy·a·lo·plasm
cy·toid
  bod·ies
cy·to·ker·a·tin
  fil·a·ments
cy·to·kine
cy·to·ki·ne·sis
cy·to·lem·ma
cy·to·lip·in
cy·to·lip·in H
cy·to·lip·in K
cy·to·log·ic
  ex·am·i·na·tion
  screen·ing
  smear
  spec·i·men
cy·to·log·ic fil·ter
  prep·a·ra·tion
cy·tol·o·gist
cy·tol·o·gy
  ex·fo·li·a·tive c.
cy·to·lymph
cy·tol·y·sin
cy·tol·y·sis
cy·to·ly·so·some
cy·to·lyt·ic
cy·to·ma
cy·to·ma·trix
cy·to·me·ga·lic
  cells
cy·to·me·ga·lic in·clu·sion
  dis·ease
cy·to·meg·a·lo·vi·rus
  dis·ease
cy·to·mem·brane
cy·to·mere
cy·to·met·a·pla·sia
cy·tom·e·ter
cy·tom·e·try
cy·to·mi·cro·some
cy·to·mi·tome
cy·to·mor·phol·o·gy
cy·to·mor·pho·sis
cy·ton
cy·to·path·ic
  ef·fect
cy·to·path·o·gen·ic
  vi·rus

cy·to·path·o·log·ic
cy·to·path·o·log·i·cal
cy·to·pa·thol·o·gist
cy·to·pa·thol·o·gy
cy·top·a·thy
cy·to·pemp·sis
cy·to·pe·nia
cy·to·phag·ic
  pan·nic·u·li·tis
cy·toph·a·gous
cy·toph·a·gy
cy·to·phan·ere
cy·to·phar·ynx
cy·to·phil
  group
cy·to·phil·ic
  an·ti·body
cy·to·pho·tom·e·try
  flow c.
cy·to·phy·lac·tic
cy·to·phy·lax·is
cy·to·phy·let·ic
cy·to·pi·pette
cy·to·plasm
  ground-glass c.
cy·to·plas·mic
  bridg·es
  in·her·i·tance
  ma·trix
Cy·to·plas·mic in·clu·sion
  bod·ies
cy·to·plas·mic in·clu·sion
  bod·ies
cy·to·plast
cy·to·poi·e·sis
cy·to·prep·a·ra·tion
cy·to·py·ge
cy·to·re·duc·tive
  ther·a·py
cy·tor·rhyc·tes
cy·to·ryc·tes
cy·to·sides
cy·to·sine
  c. ar·a·bi·no·side
  c. ri·bo·nu·cle·o·side
cy·to·sis
cy·to·skel·e·ton
cy·to·smear
cy·to·sol
cy·to·sol·ic
cy·to·some
cy·tos·ta·sis
cy·to·stat·ic
cy·to·stome
cy·to·tac·tic
cy·to·tax·ia
cy·to·tax·is
cy·toth·e·sis

cy·to·ton·ic
  en·ter·o·tox·in
cy·to·tox·ic
  cell
  re·ac·tion
cy·to·tox·ic·i·ty
  lym·pho·cyte-me·di·at·ed c.
cy·to·tox·in
cy·to·tro·pho·blast
cy·to·tro·pho·blas·tic
  cells
  shell
cy·to·tro·pic
  an·ti·body
cy·to·tro·pic an·ti·body
  test

cy·tot·ro·pism
cy·to·zo·ic
cy·to·zo·on
cy·to·zyme
cy·tu·ria
Czapek-Dox
  me·di·um
Czapek's so·lu·tion
  agar
Czerny-Lembert
  su·ture
Czerny's
  su·ture

D
cell
en·zyme
wave
Daae's
dis·ease
da·boia
da·boya
da·car·ba·zine
DaCosta's
syn·drome
dac·ry·ad·e·ni·tis
dac·ry·a·gogue
dac·ry·o·ad·en·al·gia
dac·ry·o·ad·e·ni·tis
dac·ry·o·blen·nor·rhea
dac·ry·o·cele
dac·ry·o·cyst
dac·ry·o·cys·tal·gia
dac·ry·o·cys·tec·to·my
dac·ry·o·cys·ti·tis
dac·ry·o·cys·to·blen·nor·rhea
dac·ry·o·cys·to·cele
dac·ry·o·cys·to·eth·moid·os·to·my
dac·ry·o·cys·to·gram
dac·ry·o·cys·top·to·sia
dac·ry·o·cys·top·to·sis
dac·ry·o·cys·to·rhi·no·ste·no·sis
dac·ry·o·cys·to·rhi·nos·to·my
dac·ry·o·cys·to·tome
dac·ry·o·cys·tot·o·my
dac·ry·o·hem·or·rhea
dac·ry·o·lith
Desmarres' d.'s
dac·ry·o·li·thi·a·sis
dac·ry·o·ma
dac·ry·on
dac·ry·ops
dac·ry·o·py·or·rhea
dac·ry·o·py·o·sis
dac·ry·o·rhi·no·cys·tot·o·my
dac·ry·or·rhea
dac·ry·o·scin·tig·ra·phy
dac·ry·o·so·le·ni·tis
dac·ry·o·ste·no·sis
dac·ry·o·syr·inx
dac·ti·no·my·cin
dac·tyl

dac·ty·lag·ra
dac·ty·lal·gia
Dac·ty·la·ria
dac·tyl·e·de·ma
dac·ty·li
dac·tyl·ia
dac·ty·li·tis
sick·le cell d.
dac·tyl·i·um
dac·ty·lo·camp·sis
dac·ty·lo·camp·so·dyn·ia
dac·ty·lo·dyn·ia
dac·ty·lo·gry·po·sis
dac·ty·lol·o·gy
dac·ty·lol·y·sis spon·ta·nea
dac·tyl·o·meg·a·ly
dac·ty·los·co·py
dac·ty·lo·spasm
dac·ty·lus
dac·u·ro·ni·um
Da Fano's
stain
dag·ga
dah·lin
dahll·ite
dai·ly
dose
dai·sy
Da·kar
vac·cine
Dakin-Carrel
treat·ment
Dakin's
flu·id
so·lu·tion
Dale
re·ac·tion
Dale-Feldberg
law
Dalen-Fuchs
nod·ules
Dalrymple's
sign
dal·ton
Dalton-Henry
law
dal·to·ni·an
dal·ton·ism

Dalton's
law
Dam
unit
dam
post d.
rub·ber d.
Dam·a·lin·ia
dam·mar
damp
damp·ing
Dana's
op·er·a·tion
da·na·zol
dance
hi·lar d.
Saint Anthony's d.
Saint John's d.
Saint Vitus d.
Dance's
sign
danc·ing
cho·rea
dis·ease
spasm
dan·der
dan·druff
Dandy
op·er·a·tion
dan·dy
fe·ver
Dandy-Walker
syn·drome
Dane
par·ti·cles
Dane's
stain
Danforth's
sign
Danielssen-Boeck
dis·ease
Danielssen's
dis·ease
dan·syl
dan·thron
dan·tro·lene so·di·um
Da·nu·bi·an en·dem·ic fa·mil·i·al
ne·phrop·a·thy
Danysz
phe·nom·e·non
DAPI
stain
DA preg·nan·cy
test
dap·sone
d'Arcet's
met·al

Darier's
dis·ease
sign
dark
ad·ap·ta·tion
cells
re·ac·tion
dark-adapt·ed
eye
dark-field
con·dens·er
il·lu·mi·na·tion
mi·cro·scope
dark-ground
il·lu·mi·na·tion
Darling's
dis·ease
Darrow red
d'Arsonval
cur·rent
gal·va·nom·e·ter
dar·to·ic
tis·sue
dar·toid
dar·tos
d. mu·li·e·bris
dar·tos
mus·cle
dar·win·i·an
ear
re·flex
tu·ber·cle
Das·y·proc·ta
date
boil
fe·ver
da·tum
plane
Da·tu·ra
poi·son·ing
Da·tu·ra
D. me·tel
D. stra·mo·ni·um
da·tu·rine
Daubenton's
an·gle
line
plane
Dau·er·schlaf
daugh·ter
cell
col·o·ny
cyst
star
dau·no·my·cin
dau·no·ru·bi·cin
Davidoff's
cells

Davidson
  sy·ringe
Daviel's
  op·er·a·tion
  spoon
Davies'
  dis·ease
Davis
  grafts
Davis-Crowe mouth
  gag
Davis in·ter·lock·ing
  sound
Dawbarn's
  sign
dawn
  phe·nom·e·non
Dawson's
  en·ceph·a·li·tis
day
  blind·ness
  hos·pi·tal
  res·i·due
  sight
Day's
  test
daz·zling
  glare
daz·zling
de·a·cid·i·fi·ca·tion
de·ac·ti·va·tion
de·ac·yl·ase
dead
  fin·gers
  nerve
  pulp
  space
  tooth
  tracts
dead-end
  host
dead fe·tus
  syn·drome
dead·ly
  ag·a·ric
  night·shade
DEAE-cel·lu·lose
deaf
de·af·fer·en·ta·tion
deaf-mute
deaf·mut·ism
  en·dem·ic d.
deaf·ness
  acous·tic trau·ma d.
  Alexander's d.
  boil·er·mak·er's d.
  cen·tral d.
  con·duc·tive d.

  cor·ti·cal d.
  func·tion·al d.
  high fre·quen·cy d.
  hys·ter·i·cal d.
  in·dus·tri·al d.
  lab·y·rin·thine d.
  low tone d.
  mid·brain d.
  Mondini d.
  nerve d.
  neu·ral d.
  oc·cu·pa·tion·al d.
  or·gan·ic d.
  per·cep·tive d.
  post·lin·gual d.
  pre·lin·gual d.
  psy·cho·gen·ic d.
  ret·ro·co·chle·ar d.
  Scheibe's d.
  sen·so·ri·neu·ral d.
  word d.
de·al·ba·tion
de·al·co·hol·i·za·tion
de·al·ler·gize
de·am·i·das·es
de·am·i·da·tion
de·am·i·di·za·tion
de·am·i·dize
de·am·i·diz·ing
  en·zymes
de·am·i·nas·es
de·am·i·nat·ing
  en·zymes
de·am·i·na·tion
de·am·i·ni·za·tion
de·am·in·ize
de·a·nol ac·et·a·mi·do·ben·zo·
  ate
Dean's flu·o·ro·sis
  in·dex
de·ar·te·ri·al·i·za·tion
death
  black d.
  brain d.
  ce·re·bral d.
  crib d.
  di·rect ma·ter·nal d.
  ear·ly ne·o·na·tal d.
  fe·tal d.
  ge·net·ic d.
  in·di·rect ma·ter·nal d.
  in·fant d.
  late ne·o·na·tal d.
  lo·cal d.
  ma·ter·nal d.
  ne·o·na·tal d.
  per·i·na·tal d.

death *(continued)*
  so·mat·ic d.
  sys·tem·ic d.
death
  in·stinct
  rate
  trance
death-rat·tle
Deaver's
  in·ci·sion
de·band·ing
de·bil·i·tant
de·bil·i·tat·ing
de·bil·i·ty
de Bordeau
  the·o·ry
de·bouch
dé·bouche·ment
de·branch·ing
  en·zymes
  fac·tors
de·branch·ing de·fi·cien·cy lim·it
  dex·tri·no·sis
Debré
  phe·nom·e·non
dé·bride·ment
de·bris·o·quine sul·fate
debt
  alac·tic ox·y·gen d.
  lact·ac·id ox·y·gen d.
  ox·y·gen d.
de·bulk·ing
  op·er·a·tion
dec·a·gram
de·cal·ci·fi·ca·tion
de·cal·ci·fy
de·cal·ci·fy·ing
dec·a·li·ter
de·cal·vant
dec·a·me·ter
dec·a·me·tho·ni·um bro·mide
dec·a·mine
dec·ane
dec·a·no·ic ac·id
dec·a·no·in
dec·a·nor·mal
de·cant
de·can·ta·tion
de·ca·pac·i·ta·tion
  fac·tor
de·cap·i·tate
de·cap·i·ta·tion
de·cap·su·la·tion
  d. of kid·ney
de·car·bo·ni·za·tion
de·car·box·yl·ase

de·car·box·yl·at·ed
  do·pa
de·car·box·yl·a·tion
de·cay
  con·stant
  the·o·ry
de·cel·er·a·tion
  ear·ly d.
  late d.
  var·i·a·ble d.
de·cen·tered
  lens
de·cen·tra·tion
de·cer·e·brate
  ri·gid·i·ty
de·cer·e·bra·tion
  blood·less d.
de·cer·e·brize
de·chlo·ri·da·tion
de·chlo·ri·na·tion
de·chlo·ru·ra·tion
de·cho·les·ter·ol·i·za·tion
dec·i·bel
de·cid·ua
  ec·top·ic d.
  d. men·stru·a·lis
  d. po·ly·po·sa
  d. re·flexa
  d. ser·o·ti·na
  d. spon·gi·o·sa
  d. ve·ra
de·cid·u·al
  cast
  cell
  en·do·me·tri·tis
  fis·sure
  re·ac·tion
de·cid·u·ate
  pla·cen·ta
de·cid·u·a·tion
de·cid·u·i·tis
de·cid·u·o·ma
  Loeb's d.
de·cid·u·ous
  den·ti·tion
  mem·brane
  skin
  tooth
dec·i·gram
dec·i·li·ter
dec·i·me·ter
dec·i·mor·gan
dec·i·nor·mal
de·clamp·ing
  phe·nom·e·non
  shock
de Clerambault
  syn·drome

dec·li·na·tion
dec·lin·a·tor
de·clive
de·cli·vis
de·coc·tion
dé·colle·ment
de·com·pen·sa·tion
  cor·ne·al d.
de·com·pose
de·com·po·si·tion
de·com·po·si·tion of
  move·ment
de·com·pres·sion
  cham·ber
  dis·ease
  op·er·a·tions
  sick·ness
de·com·pres·sion
  car·di·ac d.
  ce·re·bral d.
  ex·plo·sive d.
  in·ter·nal d.
  nerve d.
  or·bi·tal d.
  per·i·car·di·al d.
  rap·id d.
  spi·nal d.
  sub·oc·cip·i·tal d.
  sub·tem·po·ral d.
  tri·gem·i·nal d.
de·con·ges·tant
de·con·ges·tive
de·con·tam·i·na·tion
de·cor·ti·ca·tion
  ce·re·bral d.
  re·vers·i·ble d.
de·cor·ti·za·tion
de·coy
  cells
dec·re·ment
dec·re·men·tal
  con·duc·tion
de·crep·i·ta·tion
de·cru·des·cence
de·cu·ba·tion
de·cu·bi·tal
  gan·grene
de·cu·bi·tus
  cal·cu·lus
  pa·ral·y·sis
  ul·cer
de·cu·bi·tus
  Andral's d.
de·cur·rent
de·cus·sate
de·cus·sa·tio
  d. bra·chii con·junc·ti·vi
  d. fon·ti·na·lis

de·cus·sa·tion
  d. of bra·chia con·junc·ti·
    va
  dor·sal teg·men·tal d.
  d. of the fil·let
  Forel's d.
  foun·tain d.
  Held's d.
  d. of me·di·al lem·nis·cus
  Meynert's d.
  mo·tor d.
  op·tic d.
  py·ram·i·dal d.
  ru·bro·spi·nal d.
  sen·so·ry d. of me·dul·la
    ob·lon·ga·ta
  d. of su·pe·ri·or cer·e·bel·
    lar pe·dun·cles
  tec·to·spi·nal d.
  teg·men·tal d.'s
  d. of troch·le·ar nerves
  ven·tral teg·men·tal d.
  Wernekinck's d.
de·cus·sa·ti·o·nes
de·den·ti·tion
de·dif·fer·en·ti·a·tion
de·do·la·tion
de-ef·fer·en·ta·tion
de-e·met·in·ized
  ip·e·cac·u·a·nha
deep
  ar·tery of clit·o·ris
  ar·tery of pe·nis
  ar·tery of thigh
  ar·tery of tongue
  bite
  cell
  cor·tex
  fas·cia
  fas·cia of arm
  fas·cia of fore·arm
  fas·cia of leg
  head
  lay·er
  part
  per·cus·sion
  re·flex
  scle·ri·tis
  sen·si·bil·i·ty
  vein of pe·nis
  veins of clit·o·ris
deep ab·dom·i·nal
  re·flex·es
deep an·te·ri·or cer·vi·cal
lymph
  nodes
deep au·ric·u·lar
  ar·tery

deep brach·i·al
   ar·tery
deep car·di·ac
   plex·us
deep cer·e·bel·lar
   nu·clei
deep ce·re·bral
   veins
deep cer·vi·cal
   ar·tery
   vein
deep cir·cum·flex il·i·ac
   ar·tery
   vein
deep dor·sal
   vein of clit·o·ris
   vein of pe·nis
deep dor·sal sa·cro·coc·cyg·e·al
   lig·a·ment
deep ep·i·gas·tric
   ar·tery
   vein
deep fa·cial
   vein
deep fem·o·ral
   vein
deep fib·u·lar
   nerve
deep flex·or
   mus·cle of fin·gers
de-ep·i·car·di·al·i·za·tion
deep in·fra·pa·tel·lar
   bur·sa
deep in·gui·nal
   ring
deep in·gui·nal lymph
   nodes
deep lat·er·al cer·vi·cal lymph
   nodes
deep lin·gual
   vein
deep lym·phat·ic
   ves·sel
deep mid·dle ce·re·bral
   vein
deep or·i·gin
deep pal·mar
   arch
deep pal·mar ve·nous
   arch
deep pa·rot·id lymph
   nodes
deep per·i·ne·al
   space
deep per·o·ne·al
   nerve
deep pe·tro·sal
   nerve

deep pos·te·ri·or sa·cro·coc·
   cyg·e·al
   lig·a·ment
deep punc·tate
   ker·a·ti·tis
deep tem·po·ral
   ar·tery
   nerves
   veins
deep tran·si·tion·al
   gy·rus
deep trans·verse
   mus·cle of per·i·ne·um
deep trans·verse met·a·car·pal
   lig·a·ment
deep trans·verse met·a·tar·sal
   lig·a·ment
deer-fly
   dis·ease
   fe·ver
deer hem·or·rhag·ic
   fe·ver
deer hem·or·rhag·ic fe·ver
   vi·rus
Deetjen's
   bod·ies
de·fat·i·ga·tion
DEF car·ies
   in·dex
def car·ies
   in·dex
def·e·cate
def·e·ca·tion
de·fect
   aor·ti·co·pul·mo·nary sep·
      tal d.
   aor·tic sep·tal d.
   atri·al sep·tal d.
   con·gen·i·tal ec·to·der·mal
      d.
   cou·pling d.
   en·do·car·di·al cush·ion d.
   fi·brous cor·ti·cal d.
   fill·ing d.
   io·dide trans·port d.
   io·do·ty·ro·sine de·i·o·di·
      nase d.
   lu·te·al phase d.
   met·a·phy·si·al fi·brous
      cor·ti·cal d.
   or·gan·i·fi·ca·tion d.
   ven·tric·u·lar sep·tal d.
de·fec·tive
   bac·te·ri·o·phage
   phage
   pro·bac·te·ri·o·phage
   pro·phage
   vi·rus

de·fem·i·na·tion
de·fense
    screen d.
    ur-d.'s
de·fense
    mech·a·nism
    re·flex
de·fen·sive
    cir·cle
    med·i·cine
def·er·ent
    ca·nal
    duct
def·er·en·tec·to·my
def·er·en·tial
    plex·us
def·er·en·ti·tis
de·fer·ox·a·mine mes·y·late
de·ferred
    shock
de·fer·ves·cence
de·fer·ves·cent
    stage
de·fi·bril·la·tion
de·fi·bril·la·tor
    ex·ter·nal d.
de·fi·bri·na·tion
de·fi·cien·cy
    an·ti·tryp·sin d.
    arch length d.
    fa·mil·i·al high den·si·ty
      lip·o·pro·tein d.
    ga·lac·to·ki·nase d.
    glu·cose·phos·phate isom·er·
      ase d.
    im·mune d.
    im·mu·ni·ty d.
    im·mu·no·log·i·cal d.
    LCAT d.
    lu·te·al phase d.
    men·tal d.
    phos·pho·hex·ose isom·er·
      ase d.
    pla·cen·tal sul·fa·tase d.
    prox·i·mal fem·o·ral fo·cal
      d.
    pseu·do·cho·lin·es·ter·ase d.
    py·ru·vate ki·nase d.
    ri·bo·fla·vin d.
    sec·on·dary an·ti·body d.
    taste d.
de·fi·cien·cy
    ane·mia
    dis·ease
    symp·tom
def·i·cit
    base d.

ox·y·gen d.
    pulse d.
def·i·ni·tion
de·fin·i·tive
    cal·lus
    host
    ly·so·somes
    meth·od
    pros·the·sis
de·flec·tion
    in·trin·sic d.
    in·trin·si·coid d.
de·flec·tive oc·clu·sal
    con·tact
def·lo·ra·tion
def·lo·res·cence
de·flu·o·ri·da·tion
de·flu·vi·um
    d. ca·pil·lo·rum
    d. un·gui·um
de·flux·ion
de·for·ma·tion
de·form·ing
de·for·mi·ty
    Åkerlund d.
    Arnold-Chia·ri d.
    bou·ton·nière d.
    con·trac·ture d.
    Erlenmeyer flask d.
    gun·stock d.
    Haglund's d.
    J-sel·la d.
    key·hole d.
    lob·ster-claw d.
    Madelung's d.
    mer·maid d.
    par·a·chute d.
    pseu·do·lob·ster-claw d.
    re·duc·tion d.
    seal-fin d.
    sil·ver-fork d.
    Sprengel's d.
    swan-neck d.
    tor·sion·al d.
    whis·tling d.
    Whitehead d.
de·fur·fur·a·tion
de·gan·gli·on·ate
de·gen·er·a·cy
de·gen·er·ate
de·gen·er·a·tio
    d. hy·a·loi·dea gran·u·li·
      for·mis
    d. sphe·ru·la·ris elai·oi·des
de·gen·er·a·tion
    ad·i·pose d.
    ad·i·po·so·gen·i·tal d.
    al·bu·mi·noid d.

de·gen·er·a·tion *(continued)*
al·bu·min·ous d.
am·y·loid d.
an·gi·o·lith·ic d.
as·cend·ing d.
ath·er·om·a·tous d.
bal·loon·ing d.
ba·so·phil·ic d.
cal·car·e·ous d.
car·ne·ous d.
ca·se·ous d.
col·liq·ua·tive d.
col·loid d.
cone d.
Crooke's hy·a·line d.
cys·toid mac·u·lar d.
de·scend·ing d.
dis·ci·form d.
ec·tat·ic mar·gi·nal d. of
cor·nea
elas·toid d.
elas·tot·ic d.
fa·mil·i·al pseu·do·in·flam·
ma·to·ry mac·u·lar d.
fas·cic·u·lar d.
fat·ty d.
fi·brin·oid d.
fi·brin·ous d.
fi·brous d.
gran·u·lar d.
gran·u·lo·vac·u·o·lar d.
gray d.
he·pa·to·len·tic·u·lar d.
her·e·do·mac·u·lar d.
hy·a·line d.
hy·a·loi·de·o·ret·i·nal d.
hy·drop·ic d.
in·fan·tile neu·ro·nal d.
Kuhnt-Junius d.
len·tic·u·lar pro·gress·ive d.
liq·ue·fac·tion d.
mac·u·lar d.
mar·gi·nal cor·ne·al d.
Mönckeberg's d.
mu·ci·noid d.
mu·coid d.
mu·coid me·di·al d.
my·e·lin·ic d.
my·o·pic d.
myx·oid d.
myx·o·ma·tous d.
neu·ro·fi·bril·la·ry d.
Nissl d.
ol·i·vo·pon·to·cer·e·bel·lar
d.
or·tho·grade d.
par·en·chym·a·tous d.
pri·mary neu·ro·nal d.

pri·mary pig·men·tary d. of
ret·i·na
pri·mary pro·gress·ive cer·e·
bel·lar d.
pseu·do·tu·bu·lar d.
red d.
re·tic·u·lar d.
ret·ro·grade d.
Salzmann's nod·u·lar cor·
ne·al d.
sec·on·dary d.
se·nile d.
Sorsby's mac·u·lar d.
spongy d.
sub·a·cute com·bined d. of
the spi·nal cord
ta·pe·to·ret·i·nal d.
Terrien's mar·gi·nal d.
trans·syn·ap·tic d.
Türck's d.
vac·u·o·lar d.
vi·tel·li·form d.
vi·tel·li·rup·tive d.
wal·le·ri·an d.
waxy d.
xe·rot·ic d.
Zenker's d.
de·gen·er·a·tive
ar·thri·tis
cho·rea
in·dex
in·flam·ma·tion
my·o·pia
de·gen·er·a·tive joint
dis·ease
de·glov·ing
in·ju·ry
de·glu·ti·tion
ap·nea
pneu·mo·nia
re·flex
de·glu·ti·tive
Degos
syn·drome
Degos'
ac·an·tho·ma
dis·ease
deg·ra·da·tion
de·gran·u·la·tion
de·gree
d.'s of free·dom
de·gus·ta·tion
de·hal·o·gen·ase
Dehio's
test
de·his·cence
iris d.

root d.
wound d.
de·hu·man·i·za·tion
de·hy·drase
de·hy·dra·tase
de·hy·drate
de·hy·drat·ed
al·co·hol
de·hy·dra·tion
fe·ver
de·hy·dra·tion
ab·so·lute d.
rel·a·tive d.
vol·un·tary d.
de·hy·dro·a·ce·tic ac·id
de·hy·dro·a·scor·bic ac·id
de·hy·dro·bil·i·ru·bin
de·hy·dro·cho·late
test
de·hy·dro·cho·lic ac·id
de·hy·dro·em·e·tine
d. res·in·ate
de·hy·dro·gen·ase
aer·o·bic d.
an·aer·o·bic d.
Robison es·ter d.
de·hy·dro·gen·ate
de·hy·dro·gen·a·tion
de·hy·dro·i·so·an·dros·ter·one
de·hy·dro·pep·ti·dase II
de·hy·dro·ret·i·nal·de·hyde
de·hy·dro·ret·i·no·ic ac·id
de·hy·dro·ret·i·nol
de·hy·dro·sug·ars
de·hy·dro·tes·tos·ter·one
de·hyp·no·tize
de·im·i·nas·es
de·in·sti·tu·tion·al·i·za·tion
de·it·er·o·spi·nal
tract
Deiters'
cells
nu·cle·us
pro·cess
Deiters' ter·mi·nal
frames
dé·jà vu
phe·nom·e·non
de·jec·ta
de·jec·tion
Dejerine-Lichtheim
phe·nom·e·non
Dejerine-Roussy
syn·drome
Dejerine's
dis·ease
re·flex
sign

Dejerine's hand
phe·nom·e·non
Déjérine-Sottas
dis·ease
Dejerine's pe·riph·e·ral
neu·ro·ta·bes
de·lac·ri·ma·tion
Delafield's
he·ma·tox·y·lin
de·lam·i·na·tion
Delaney clause
de Lange
syn·drome
de·layed
al·ler·gy
con·duc·tion
den·ti·tion
erup·tion
flap
graft
hy·per·sen·si·tiv·i·ty
im·plan·ta·tion
re·ac·tion
re·flex
sen·sa·tion
shock
su·ture
de·layed re·ac·tion
ex·per·i·ment
Delbet's
sign
Del Castillo
syn·drome
de-lead
DeLee's
ma·neu·ver
del·e·te·ri·ous
de·le·tion
chro·mo·som·al d.
gene d.
in·ter·sti·tial d.
nu·cle·o·tide d.
point d.
ter·mi·nal d.
Del·hi
boil
del·i·cate
de·lim·i·ta·tion
de·lim·it·ing
ker·a·tot·o·my
del·i·quesce
del·i·ques·cence
del·i·ques·cent
de·lir·i·ant
de·lir·i·ous
shock
de·lir·i·um
acute d.

de·lir·i·um *(continued)*
anx·ious d.
col·lapse d.
d. cor·dis
low d.
d. mus·si·tans
mut·ter·ing d.
post·trau·mat·ic d.
se·nile d.
tox·ic d.
d. tre·mens
del·i·tes·cence
de·liv·er
de·liv·ery
as·sist·ed ce·phal·ic d.
breech d.
for·ceps d.
high for·ceps d.
low for·ceps d.
mid·for·ceps d.
post·mor·tem d.
pre·ma·ture d.
spon·ta·ne·ous ce·phal·ic d.
del·le
del·len
d. of Fuchs
del·o·mor·phous
de·louse
del·phi·an
node
del·phi·nine
Del·phin·i·um aja·cis
del·ta
d. for·ni·cis
Galton's d.
d. mes·o·scap·u·lae
del·ta
agent
al·co·hol·ism
an·ti·gen
cell of an·te·ri·or lobe of
hy·poph·y·sis
cell of pan·cre·as
gran·ule
hep·a·ti·tis
rhythm
vi·rus
wave
del·toid
crest
em·i·nence
im·pres·sion
lig·a·ment
mus·cle
re·gion
tu·ber·os·i·ty

del·toi·de·o·pec·to·ral
tri·an·gle
tri·gone
del·to·pec·to·ral
flap
de·lu·sion
d. of be·ing con·trolled
d. of con·trol
ex·pan·sive d.
d. of gran·deur
d. of ne·ga·tion
ni·hil·is·tic d.
d. of pas·siv·i·ty
d. of per·se·cu·tion
per·se·cu·to·ry d.
d. of ref·er·ence
so·mat·ic d.
sys·tem·a·tized d.
un·sys·tem·a·tized d.
de·lu·sion·al
de·mand
pace·mak·er
de·mand pulse
gen·er·a·tor
de·mar·ca·tion
cur·rent
line of ret·i·na
po·ten·tial
Demarquay's
symp·tom
de·mas·cu·lin·iz·ing
De·mat·i·a·ce·ae
de·mat·i·a·ceous
deme
dem·e·car·i·um bro·mide
dem·e·clo·cy·cline
dem·e·col·cine
de·ment·ed
de·men·tia
Alzheimer's d.
cat·a·ton·ic d.
di·al·y·sis d.
ep·i·lep·tic d.
he·be·phren·ic d.
mul·ti·in·farct d.
par·a·lyt·ic d.
d. pa·ra·ly·ti·ca
d. pa·r·a·noi·des
post·trau·mat·ic d.
d. pre·cox
pre·se·nile d.
d. pre·se·ni·lis
pri·mary d.
pri·mary se·nile d.
sec·on·dary d.
se·nile d.
tox·ic d.
vas·cu·lar d.

de·meth·yl·ase
dem·i·gaunt·let
  ban·dage
dem·i·lune
  body
dem·i·lune
  Giannuzzi's d.'s
  Heidenhain's d.'s
  se·rous d.'s
de·min·er·al·i·za·tion
dem·i·pen·ni·form
dem·o·dec·tic
  ac·a·ri·a·sis
  bleph·a·ri·tis
  mange
Dem·o·dex
  D. bo·vis
  D. ca·nis
  D. cati
  D. fol·lic·u·lo·rum
de·mog·ra·phy
  dy·nam·ic d.
Demoivre's
  for·mu·la
de·mo·ni·ac
dem·on·stra·tion
  oph·thal·mo·scope
dem·on·stra·tor
De Morgan's
  spots
de·mor·phin·i·za·tion
de Morsier's
  syn·drome
de·mu·co·sa·tion
de·mul·cent
de·my·e·li·nat·ing
  dis·ease
  en·ceph·a·lop·a·thy
de·my·e·li·na·tion
de·my·e·lin·i·za·tion
de·nar·co·tize
de·nar·co·tized
  opi·um
de·na·to·ni·um ben·zo·ate
de·na·tur·a·tion
  tem·per·a·ture of DNA
de·na·tured
  al·co·hol
  pro·tein
den·drax·on
den·dri·form
  ker·a·ti·tis
den·drite
  ap·i·cal d.
den·drit·ic
  cal·cu·lus
  cat·a·ract
  cells

de·po·lar·i·za·tion
ker·a·ti·tis
pro·cess
spines
thorns
den·drit·ic cor·ne·al
  ul·cer
den·dro·gram
den·droid
den·dron
de·ner·vate
de·ner·va·tion
den·gue
  hem·or·rhag·ic d.
den·gue
  fe·ver
  vi·rus
den·gue hem·or·rhag·ic
  fe·ver
den·gue shock
  syn·drome
de·ni·al
den·i·da·tion
Denis Browne
  splint
Denis Browne's
  pouch
de·ni·tra·tion
de·ni·tri·fi·ca·tion
de·ni·tri·fy
de·ni·tro·gen·a·tion
Denman's spon·ta·ne·ous
  ev·o·lu·tion
Dennie's
  fold
  line
Dennie's in·fra·or·bit·al
  fold
Denonvilliers'
  ap·o·neu·ro·sis
  lig·a·ment
dens
  d. an·gu·la·ris
  den·tes bi·cus·pi·di
  d. bi·cus·pi·dus
  den·tes cus·pi·da·ti
  d. cus·pi·da·tus
  d. in dente
  d. lac·te·us
  d. sa·pi·en·ti·ae
  d. suc·ce·da·ne·us
dense-de·pos·it
  dis·ease
den·sim·e·ter
den·si·tom·e·ter
den·si·tom·e·try
den·si·ty
  count d.

271

den·si·ty *(continued)*
  flux d.
  op·ti·cal d.
  pho·ton d.
  va·por d.
den·si·ty
  gra·di·ent
den·si·ty gra·di·ent
  cen·trif·u·ga·tion
den·tal
  ab·scess
  anat·o·my
  an·es·the·sia
  an·ky·lo·sis
  ap·pa·ra·tus
  arch
  ar·tic·u·la·tion
  bi·o·me·chan·ics
  bi·o·phys·ics
  bulb
  cal·cu·lus
  ca·nals
  caps
  car·ies
  cast
  ce·ment
  cord
  crest
  crypt
  cur·ing
  cu·ti·cle
  drill \
  dys·func·tion
  en·gi·neer·ing
  fi·bers
  fis·tu·la
  floss
  fol·li·cle
  for·ceps
  for·mu·la
  fur·nace
  ger·i·at·rics
  germ
  gran·u·lo·ma
  groove
  hy·gien·ist
  im·pac·tion
  in·dex
  jur·is·pru·dence
  lam·i·na
  ledge
  le·ver
  lymph
  ma·te·ri·al
  neck
  nerve
  or·tho·pe·dics
  os·te·o·ma

  pa·thol·o·gy
  plaque
  pol·yp
  pro·cess
  pro·phy·lax·is
  pros·the·sis
  pros·thet·ics
  pulp
  pump
  ridge
  sac
  se·nes·cence
  shelf
  sur·geon
  sy·ringe
  tu·ber·cle
  tu·bules
  ul·cer
  wedge
den·tal en·gine
den·tal·gia
den·ta·ry
  cen·ter
den·tate
  fas·cia
  fis·sure
  frac·ture
  gy·rus
  line
  nu·cle·us of cer·e·bel·lum
  su·ture
den·ta·tec·to·my
den·ta·to·tha·lam·ic
  tract
den·ta·tum
den·tes
den·ti·cle
den·tic·u·late
  hy·men
  lig·a·ment
den·tic·u·lat·ed
den·ti·form
den·ti·frice
den·tig·er·ous
  cyst
den·ti·la·bi·al
den·ti·lin·gual
den·tin
  dys·pla·sia
  glob·ule
den·tin
  he·red·i·tary opal·es·cent d.
  hy·per·sen·si·tive d.
  ir·reg·u·lar d.
  ir·ri·ta·tion d.
  per·i·tu·bu·lar d.
  pri·mary d.
  re·par·a·tive d.

scle·rot·ic d.
sec·on·dary d.
ter·ti·ary d.
trans·par·ent d.
vas·cu·lar d.
den·ti·nal
  ca·nals
  fi·bers
  flu·id
  pa·pil·la
  pulp
  sheath
  tu·bules
den·ti·nal·gia
den·ti·nal lam·i·na
  cyst
den·tine
den·tin·o·ce·ment·al
  junc·tion
den·tin·o·e·nam·el
  junc·tion
den·tin·o·gen·e·sis
  d. im·per·fec·ta
den·ti·noid
den·ti·no·ma
den·ti·num
den·tip·a·rous
den·tist
den·tis·try
  com·mu·ni·ty d.
  fo·ren·sic d.
  le·gal d.
  op·er·a·tive d.
  pe·di·at·ric d.
  pre·ven·tive d.
  pros·thet·ic d.
  pub·lic health d.
  re·stor·a·tive d.
den·ti·tion
  ar·ti·fi·cial d.
  de·cid·u·ous d.
  de·layed d.
  first d.
  man·dib·u·lar d.
  max·il·lary d.
  nat·u·ral d.
  pri·mary d.
  re·tard·ed d.
  sec·on·dary d.
  suc·ce·da·ne·ous d.
den·to·al·ve·o·lar
  ab·scess
  joint
den·tode
den·to·gin·gi·val
  lam·i·na
den·toid

den·to·le·gal
den·to·li·va
den·tu·lous
den·ture
  bar joint d.
  com·plete d.
  de·sign d.
  fixed par·tial d.
  full d.
  im·me·di·ate d.
  im·me·di·ate in·ser·tion d.
  im·plant d.
  in·ter·im d.
  over·lay d.
  par·tial d.
  par·tial d., dis·tal ex·ten·
    sion
  pro·vi·sion·al d.
  re·mov·a·ble par·tial d.
  tel·e·scop·ic d.
  tem·po·rary d.
  tran·si·tion·al d.
  treat·ment d.
  tri·al d.
  wax mod·el d.
den·ture
  base
  bor·der
  brush
  char·ac·ter·i·za·tion
  edge
  es·thet·ics
  flange
  flask
  foun·da·tion
  hy·per·pla·sia
  pack·ing
  prog·no·sis
  re·ten·tion
  space
  sta·bil·i·ty
den·ture ba·sal
  sur·face
den·ture-bear·ing
  ar·ea
den·ture foun·da·tion
  ar·ea
  sur·face
den·ture im·pres·sion
  sur·face
den·ture oc·clu·sal
  sur·face
den·ture pol·ished
  sur·face
den·ture ser·vice
den·ture sore
  mouth

den·ture-sup·port·ing
 ar·ea
 struc·tures
den·tur·ist
Denucé's
 lig·a·ment
de·nu·cle·at·ed
de·nu·da·tion
de·nude
Denver
 clas·si·fi·ca·tion
 shunt
Denys-Leclef
 phe·nom·e·non
de·ob·stru·ent
de·o·dor·ant
de·o·dor·ize
de·o·dor·ized
 opi·um
de·o·dor·iz·er
de·on·tol·o·gy
de·op·pi·la·tive
de·or·sum·duc·tion
de·os·si·fi·ca·tion
de·ox·i·da·tion
de·ox·i·dize
de·oxy
 sug·ar
de·ox·y·a·den·o·sine
de·ox·y·ad·e·nyl·ic ac·id
de·ox·y·cho·late
de·ox·y·cho·lic ac·id
de·ox·y·cor·ti·cos·ter·one
 d. ac·e·tate
 d. piv·a·late
de·ox·y·cor·tone
de·ox·y·cyt·i·dine
de·ox·y·cyt·i·dyl·ic ac·id
de·ox·y·ep·i·neph·rine
de·ox·y·gua·no·sine
de·ox·y·gua·nyl·ic ac·id
de·ox·y·hex·ose
de·ox·y·pen·tose
de·ox·y·ri·bo·al·dol·ase
de·ox·y·ri·bo·di·py·rim·i·dine
 pho·to·ly·ase
de·ox·y·ri·bo·nu·cle·ase
 ac·id d.
 pan·cre·at·ic d.
 spleen d.
de·ox·y·ri·bo·nu·cle·ic ac·id
 an·ti·sense
 com·pet·i·tor
 com·ple·men·ta·ry
 li·gase
 nu·cle·o·ti·dyl·ex·o·trans·
  fer·ase
 pal·in·drom·ic pol·y·mer·ase

re·com·bi·nant
re·pet·i·tive
sat·el·lite
de·ox·y·ri·bo·nu·cle·o·pro·tein
de·ox·y·ri·bo·nu·cle·o·side
de·ox·y·ri·bo·nu·cle·o·tide
de·ox·y·ri·bose
de·ox·y·ri·bose·phos·phate al·
 dol·ase
de·ox·y·ri·bo·side
de·ox·y·ri·bo·syl
de·ox·y·ri·bo·tide
de·ox·y·thy·mi·dyl·ic ac·id
de·ox·y·vi·rus
de·o·zon·ize
de·pen·dence
de·pen·dent
 beat
 drain·age
 ede·ma
 per·son·al·i·ty
 var·i·a·ble
De·pen·do·vi·rus
de·per·son·al·i·za·tion
de Pezzer
 cath·e·ter
de·phos·pho·ryl·a·tion
de·pig·men·ta·tion
dep·i·late
dep·i·la·tion
de·pil·a·to·ry
de·ple·tion
 chlo·ride d.
 salt d.
 wa·ter d.
de·ple·tion
 re·sponse
de·po·lar·i·za·tion
 den·drit·ic d.
de·po·lar·ize
de·po·lar·iz·ing
 block
 re·lax·ant
de·pol·y·mer·ase
de·pop·u·la·tion
de·pos·it
 brick·dust d.
de·pot
 in·jec·tion
 re·ac·tion
 ther·a·py
dep·ra·va·tion
de·praved
de·prav·i·ty
de·pres·sant
de·pressed
 frac·ture

de·pressed skull
frac·ture
de·pres·sion
ag·i·tat·ed d.
an·a·clit·ic d.
en·do·ge·no·mor·phic d.
en·dog·e·nous d.
lin·gual sal·i·vary gland d.
pac·chi·o·ni·an d.'s
post·drive d.
pter·y·goid d.
re·ac·tive d.
spread·ing d.
de·pres·sive
stu·por
de·pres·so·mo·tor
de·pres·sor
tongue d.
de·pres·sor
fi·bers
mus·cle of ep·i·glot·tis
mus·cle of eye·brow
mus·cle of low·er lip
mus·cle of sep·tum
nerve of Ludwig
re·flex
dep·ri·va·tion
am·bly·o·pia
dep·ri·va·tion
emo·tion·al d.
sen·so·ry d.
depth
an·es·thet·ic d.
fo·cal d.
d. of fo·cus
depth
com·pen·sa·tion
dose
per·cep·tion
psy·chol·o·gy
re·cord·ing
dep·tro·pine cit·rate
de·pu·li·za·tion
dep·u·rant
dep·u·ra·tion
dep·u·ra·tive
de·qua·lin·i·um ac·e·tate
de·qua·lin·i·um chlo·ride
de Quervain's
dis·ease
frac·ture
thy·roid·i·tis
der·a·del·phus
de·rail·ment
der·an·en·ce·pha·lia
der·an·en·ceph·a·ly
de·range·ment
Hey's in·ter·nal d.

der·by hat
frac·ture
Dercum's
dis·ease
de·re·al·i·za·tion
de·re·ism
de·re·is·tic
der·en·ce·pha·lia
der·en·ceph·a·lo·cele
der·en·ceph·a·ly
de·re·pres·sion
der·ic
der·i·va·tion
de·riv·a·tive
chro·mo·some
de·rived
pro·tein
der·ma·brad·er
der·ma·bra·sion
Der·ma·cen·tor
D. al·bo·pic·tus
D. an·der·soni
D. ni·tens
D. oc·ci·den·ta·lis
D. re·ti·cu·la·tus
D. va·ri·a·bi·lis
der·mad
der·mag·ra·phy
der·ma·he·mia
der·mal
bone
graft
leish·man·oid
pa·pil·lae
si·nus
sys·tem
tu·ber·cu·lo·sis
der·ma·lax·ia
der·mal duct
tu·mor
der·mal-fat
graft
der·ma·met·rop·a·thism
der·ma·my·i·a·sis
Der·ma·nys·sus gal·li·nae
der·ma·tal·gia
der·ma·tan sul·fate
der·mat·ic
der·ma·tit·i·des
der·ma·ti·tis
ac·tin·ic d.
d. aes·ti·va·lis
d. am·bus·ti·o·nis
an·cy·lo·sto·mi·a·sis d.
d. ar·te·fac·ta
atop·ic d.
d. atroph·i·cans
d. au·to·phy·ti·ca

der·ma·ti·tis *(continued)*
  ber·lock d.
  ber·loque d.
  blas·to·my·ce·tic d.
  d. blas·to·my·co·ti·ca
  bub·ble gum d.
  d. ca·lo·ri·ca
  cat·er·pil·lar d.
  chem·i·cal d.
  d. com·bus·tio·nis
  d. con·ge·la·ti·o·nis
  con·tact d.
  con·tact-type d.
  con·ta·gious pus·tu·lar d.
  cos·met·ic d.
  dho·bie mark d.
  di·a·per d.
  d. ex·fo·li·a·ti·va
  d. ex·fo·li·a·ti·va in·fan·tum
  d. ex·fo·li·a·ti·va ne·o·na·to·rum
  ex·fo·li·a·tive d.
  ex·ud·a·tive dis·coid and li·chen·oid d.
  d. fac·ti·tia
  d. gan·gre·no·sa in·fan·tum
  d. her·pet·i·for·mis
  d. hi·e·ma·lis
  in·fec·tious ec·ze·ma·toid d.
  d. li·ne·a·ris mi·grans
  liv·e·doid d.
  man·go d.
  mead·ow d.
  mead·ow grass d.
  d. me·di·ca·men·to·sa
  d. mul·ti·for·mis
  nick·el d.
  d. no·do·sa
  d. no·du·la·ris ne·cro·ti·ca
  d. pa·pil·la·ris ca·pil·li·tii
  pap·u·lar d. of preg·nan·cy
  d. pe·dic·u·loi·des ven·tri·co·sus
  plant d.
  pri·mary ir·ri·tant d.
  pro·lif·er·a·tive d.
  rat mite d.
  d. re·pens
  rhus d.
  san·dal strap d.
  Schamberg's d.
  schis·to·some d.
  seb·or·rhe·ic d.
  d. seb·or·rhe·i·ca
  shoe dye d.
  d. sim·plex
  so·lar d.

  sta·sis d.
  sub·cor·ne·al pus·tu·lar d.
  trau·mat·ic d.
  tre·foil d.
  d. ve·ge·tans
  d. ve·ne·na·ta
  d. ver·ru·co·sa
der·mat·o·al·lo·plas·ty
der·mat·o·ar·thri·tis
  lip·oid d.
der·mat·o·au·to·plas·ty
Der·ma·to·bia
  D. cy·a·ni·ven·tris
  D. hom·i·nis
der·ma·to·bi·a·sis
der·mat·o·cele
der·mat·o·cel·lu·li·tis
der·mat·o·cha·la·sis
der·mat·o·co·ni·o·sis
der·mat·o·cyst
der·mat·o·dyn·ia
der·mat·o·fi·bro·ma
der·mat·o·fi·bro·sar·co·ma pro·tu·ber·ans
  pig·ment·ed d. p.
der·ma·to·fi·bro·sis len·tic·u·lar·is dis·sem·i·na·ta
der·mat·o·gen·ic
  tor·ti·col·lis
der·mat·o·glyph·ics
der·mat·o·graph
der·ma·tog·ra·phism
der·ma·tog·ra·phy
der·mat·o·het·er·o·plas·ty
der·mat·o·ho·mo·plas·ty
der·ma·toid
der·mat·o·log·ic
  paste
der·ma·tol·o·gist
der·ma·tol·o·gy
der·ma·tol·y·sis
  d. pal·pe·bra·rum
der·ma·to·ma
der·ma·tome
  elec·tric d.
der·mat·o·meg·a·ly
der·mat·o·mere
der·ma·tom·ic
  ar·ea
der·mat·o·my·co·sis
  d. pe·dis
der·mat·o·my·o·ma
der·mat·o·my·o·si·tis
der·mat·o·neu·ro·sis
der·mat·o·no·sol·o·gy
der·mat·o·path·ia
  d. pig·men·to·sa re·tic·u·la·ris

der·mat·o·path·ic
  lym·phad·e·ni·tis
  lym·phad·e·nop·a·thy
der·mat·o·pa·thol·o·gy
der·ma·top·a·thy
Der·ma·toph·a·goi·des pter·o·
  nys·si·nus
der·ma·to·phi·lo·sis
Der·ma·toph·i·lus con·go·len·
  sis
der·mat·o·pho·bia
der·mat·o·phone
der·mat·o·phy·lax·is
der·mat·o·phyte
der·mat·o·phy·tid
der·mat·o·phy·to·sis
der·mat·o·plas·tic
der·mat·o·plas·ty
der·mat·o·pol·y·neu·ri·tis
der·ma·tor·rha·gia
  d. pa·ra·sit·i·ca
der·ma·tor·rhea
der·ma·tor·rhex·is
der·mat·o·scle·ro·sis
der·ma·tos·co·py
der·ma·to·ses
der·ma·to·sis
  ac·a·rine d.
  acute neu·tro·phil·ic d.
  be·nign chron·ic bul·lous d.
   of child·hood
  Bowen's pre·can·cer·ous d.
  chick nu·trit·ion·al d.
  der·mo·ly·tic bul·lous d.
  fi·lar·i·al d.
  li·chen·oid d.
  d. me·di·ca·men·to·sa
  d. pa·pu·lo·sa nig·ra
  pig·ment·ed pur·pu·ric li·
   chen·oid d.
  pro·gress·ive pig·men·tary
   d.
  ra·di·a·tion d.
  seb·or·rhe·ic d.
  sub·cor·ne·al pus·tu·lar d.
  tran·sient acan·tho·lyt·ic d.
  ul·cer·a·tive d.
der·mat·o·skel·e·ton
der·mat·o·ther·a·py
der·mat·o·thla·si·a
der·mat·o·tro·pic
der·ma·to·xen·o·plas·ty
der·mat·o·zo·i·a·sis
der·mat·o·zo·on
der·mat·o·zo·o·no·sis
der·ma·tro·phia
der·mat·ro·phy
der·men·chy·sis

der·mic
der·mis
der·mo·blast
der·mo·cy·ma
der·mo·ep·i·der·mal
  in·ter·face
der·mo·graph·ia
der·mog·ra·phism
der·mog·ra·phy
der·moid
  im·plan·ta·tion d.
  in·clu·sion d.
  se·ques·tra·tion d.
der·moid
  cyst
  cyst of ova·ry
  sys·tem
  tu·mor
der·moi·dec·to·my
der·mol·y·sis
der·mo·ly·tic bul·lous
  der·ma·to·sis
der·mo·ne·crot·ic
der·mo·neu·ro·sis
der·mo·no·sol·o·gy
der·mop·a·thy
  di·a·bet·ic d.
der·mo·phle·bi·tis
der·mo·plas·ty
der·mo·skel·e·ton
der·mo·ste·no·sis
der·mos·to·sis
der·mo·syph·i·lop·a·thy
der·mo·tox·in
der·mo·tro·p·ic
der·mo·tu·ber·cu·lin
  re·ac·tion
der·mo·vas·cu·lar
der·o·did·y·mus
de·ro·ta·tion
des·am·i·dize
De Sanctis-Cacchione
  syn·drome
de·sat·u·rate
de·sat·u·ra·tion
Desault's
  ban·dage
  lig·a·ture
Descartes'
  law
des·ce·me·ti·tis
des·ce·met·o·cele
Descemet's
  mem·brane
de·scen·dens
  d. cer·vi·ca·lis
  d. hy·po·glos·si

de·scend·ing
 ar·tery of knee
 co·lon
 cur·rent
 de·gen·er·a·tion
 neu·ri·tis
 nu·cle·us of the tri·gem·i·
 nus
 part
 tract of tri·gem·i·nal nerve
de·scend·ing pal·a·tine
 ar·tery
de·scend·ing scap·u·lar
 ar·tery
de·scen·sus
 d. aber·rans tes·tis
 d. par·a·dox·us tes·tis
 d. uteri
 d. ven·tric·u·li
de·scent
Deschamps
 nee·dle
de·scrip·tive
 anat·o·my
 my·ol·o·gy
 sta·tis·tics
de·sen·si·tiz·a·tion
 het·er·ol·o·gous d.
 ho·mol·o·gous d.
 sys·tem·at·ic d.
de·sen·si·tize
de·sen·si·tiz·ing
 paste
de·ser·pi·dine
de·sert
 fe·ver
 sore
des·fer·ri·ox·a·mine mes·y·late
des·ic·cant
des·ic·cate
des·ic·cat·ed
 liv·er
 pi·tu·i·tary
des·ic·ca·tion
des·ic·ca·tive
des·ic·ca·tor
 vac·u·um d.
de·sign
 den·ture
de·si·pra·mine hy·dro·chlo·ride
des·lan·o·side
Desmarres'
 dac·ry·o·liths
des·mec·ta·sia
des·mec·ta·sis
des·mins
des·mi·tis
des·mo·cra·ni·um

Des·mo·dus
des·mo·dyn·ia
des·mog·e·nous
des·mog·ra·phy
des·moid
 ex·tra-ab·dom·i·nal d.
des·moid
 tu·mor
des·mo·las·es
des·mol·o·gy
des·mon
des·mop·a·thy
des·mo·pla·sia
des·mo·plas·tic
 fi·bro·ma
 trich·o·ep·i·the·li·o·ma
des·mo·pres·sin ac·e·tate
des·mo·some
des·mos·te·rol
des·o·mor·phine
des·o·nide
des·ose
des·ox·i·met·a·sone
des·ox·y·cor·tone
de·spe·ci·at·ed
 an·ti·tox·in
de·spe·ci·a·tion
D'Éspine's
 sign
des·pu·ma·tion
des·qua·mate
des·qua·ma·tion
 bran·ny d.
des·qua·ma·tive
des·qua·ma·tive in·flam·ma·to·
 ry
 vag·i·ni·tis
des·qua·ma·tive in·ter·sti·tial
 pneu·mo·nia
de·ster·nal·i·za·tion
des·thi·o·bi·o·tin
de·struc·tive
 dis·til·la·tion
de·stru·do
de·sulf·hy·dras·es
de·sul·fi·nase
de·sul·fu·ras·es
de·syn·chro·nous
de·tached
 cra·ni·ot·o·my
 ret·i·na
de·tached cra·ni·al
 sec·tion
de·tach·ment
 dis·ci·form d. of ret·i·na
 ex·ud·a·tive ret·i·nal d.
 d. of ret·i·na
 ret·i·nal d.

rheg·ma·tog·e·nous ret·i·nal
   d.
   vit·re·ous d.
de·tec·tor
de·ter·gent
   an·i·on·ic d.'s
   cat·i·on·ic d.'s
de·te·ri·o·ra·tion
   al·co·hol·ic d.
   se·nile d.
de·ter·mi·nant
   al·lo·typ·ic d.'s
   an·ti·gen·ic d.
   dis·ease d.'s
   ge·net·ic d.
   id·i·o·typ·ic an·ti·gen·ic d.
   iso·al·lo·typ·ic d.'s
de·ter·mi·nant
   group
de·ter·mi·nate
   cleav·age
de·ter·mi·na·tion
   sex d.
de·ter·mi·nism
   psy·chic d.
de·ter·sive
De Toni-Fanconi
   syn·drome
de·tox·i·cate
de·tox·i·ca·tion
de·tox·i·fi·ca·tion
de·tox·i·fy
de·tri·tion
de·tri·tus
de·tru·sor
   d. uri·nae
de·tru·sor
   pres·sure
de·tru·sor sphinc·ter
   dys·syn·er·gia
de·tu·mes·cence
de·tur·ges·cence
deu·ten·ceph·a·lon
deu·ter·a·nom·a·ly
deu·ter·an·ope
deu·ter·an·o·pia
deu·ter·an·o·pic
deu·te·ri·um
   d. ox·ide
Deu·te·ro·my·ce·tes
deu·ter·on
deu·ter·o·path·ic
deu·ter·op·a·thy
deu·ter·o·plasm
deu·ter·o·por·phy·rin
deu·ter·o·some
deu·ter·o·to·cia
deu·ter·ot·o·ky

deu·to·gen·ic
deu·tom·er·ite
deu·ton
deu·to·plasm
deu·to·plas·mic
deu·to·plas·mi·gen·on
deu·to·plas·mol·y·sis
Deutschländer's
   dis·ease
de·vas·cu·lar·i·za·tion
de·vel·op·ment
   life-span d.
   psy·cho·sex·u·al d.
de·vel·op·men·tal
   age
   anat·o·my
   anom·a·ly
   dis·a·bil·i·ty
   grooves
   lines
   phys·i·ol·o·gy
   psy·chol·o·gy
Deventer's
   pel·vis
de·vi·ance
de·vi·ant
de·vi·a·tion
   ax·is d.
   con·ju·gate d. of the eyes
   im·mune d.
   d. to the left
   left ax·is d.
   pri·mary d.
   d. to the right
   right ax·is d.
   sec·on·dary d.
   sex·u·al d.
   skew d.
   stan·dard d.
de·vi·a·tion·al
   nys·tag·mus
de·vice
   cen·tral-bear·ing d.
   cen·tral-bear·ing trac·ing d.
   con·tra·cep·tive d.
   in·tra-a·or·tic bal·loon d.
   in·tra·u·ter·ine d.'s
   in·tra·u·ter·ine con·tra·cep·tive d.'s
Devic's
   dis·ease
dev·il's
   grip
de Vincentiis
   op·er·a·tion
Devine
   ex·clu·sion
de·vi·om·e·ter

de·vi·tal·i·za·tion
de·vi·tal·ize
de·vi·tal·ized
    tooth
dev·o·lu·tion
Dev·on·shire
    col·ic
De Vries'
    the·o·ry
dew
    claw
    itch
    point
Dewar
    flask
de Wecker's
    scis·sors
dex·a·meth·a·sone
dex·a·meth·a·sone sup·pres·
    sion
    test
dex·am·phet·a·mine
    d. so·di·um phos·phate
dex·brom·phen·ir·a·mine ma·
    le·ate
dex·chlor·phen·ir·a·mine ma·le·
    ate
dex·i·o·car·dia
dex·pan·the·nol
dex·ter
dex·trad
dex·tral
dex·tral·i·ty
dex·tran
    an·i·mal d.
    d. sul·fate
dex·tran·ase
dex·tran·su·crase
dex·trase
dex·tri·fer·ron
dex·trin
    lim·it d.
dex·tri·nase
    lim·it d.
dex·trin dex·tran·ase
dex·trin → dex·tran trans·glu·
    co·si·dase
dex·trin gly·co·syl·trans·fer·ase
dex·trin lim·it
dex·trin·o·gen·ic
dex·tri·no·sis
    de·branch·ing de·fi·cien·cy
      lim·it d.
      lim·it d.
dex·trin trans·gly·co·syl·ase
dex·tri·nu·ria
dex·tro·am·phet·a·mine phos·
    phate

dex·tro·am·phet·a·mine sul·fate
dex·tro·car·dia
    cor·rect·ed d.
    false d.
    iso·lat·ed d.
    sec·on·dary d.
    d. with si·tus in·ver·sus
dex·tro·car·di·o·gram
dex·tro·ce·re·bral
dex·tro·cli·na·tion
dex·troc·u·lar
dex·tro·cy·clo·duc·tion
dex·tro·duc·tion
dex·tro·gas·tria
dex·tro·glu·cose
dex·tro·gram
dex·tro·gy·ra·tion
dex·tro·man·u·al
dex·tro·meth·or·phan hy·dro·
    bro·mide
dex·tro·mor·a·mide tar·trate
dex·trop·e·dal
dex·tro·po·si·tion
    d. of the heart
dex·tro·pro·pox·y·phene hy·
    dro·chlo·ride
dex·tro·pro·pox·y·phene nap·
    syl·ate
dex·tro·ro·ta·tion
dex·tro·ro·ta·to·ry
dex·trose
dex·tro·si·nis·tral
dex·tro·su·ria
dex·tro·thy·rox·ine so·di·um
dex·tro·tor·sion
dex·tro·tro·p·ic
dex·tro·ver·sion
    d. of the heart
DF car·ies
    in·dex
df car·ies
    in·dex
Dharmendra
    an·ti·gen
d'Herelle
    phe·nom·e·non
dho·bie
    itch
    mark
dho·bie mark
    der·ma·ti·tis
D-ho·mo·ster·oid
Di
    an·ti·gen
di·a·be·tes
    adult-on·set d.
    al·i·men·ta·ry d.
    al·lox·an d.

brit·tle d.
bronze d.
cal·ci·nu·ric d.
chem·i·cal d.
ga·lac·tose d.
growth-on·set d.
d. in·no·cens
d. in·sip·i·dus
in·su·lin-de·pen·dent d.
  mel·li·tus
in·su·lin-o·pe·nic d.
d. in·ter·mit·tens
ju·ve·nile-on·set d.
la·tent d.
lip·o·a·tro·phic d.
li·pog·e·nous d.
ma·tu·ri·ty-on·set d.
d. mel·li·tus
met·a·hy·po·phy·si·al d.
Mosler's d.
neph·ro·gen·ic d. in·sip·i·
  dus
non-in·su·lin de·pen·dent d.
  mel·li·tus
pan·cre·at·ic d.
phlo·rid·zin d.
phos·phate d.
pi·qûre d.
preg·nan·cy d.
punc·ture d.
re·nal d.
star·va·tion d.
ste·roid d.
sub·clin·i·cal d.
thi·a·zide d.
type I d.
type II d.
va·so·pres·sin-re·sis·tant d.
di·a·bet·ic
ac·i·do·sis
ar·throp·a·thy
cat·a·ract
co·ma
der·mop·a·thy
di·et
fe·top·a·thy
gan·grene
gin·gi·vi·tis
glo·mer·u·lo·scle·ro·sis
li·pe·mia
my·e·lop·a·thy
neu·rop·a·thy
punc·ture
ret·i·ni·tis
ret·i·nop·a·thy
di·a·be·to·gen·ic
fac·tor
di·a·be·tog·en·ous

di·a·be·tol·o·gy
di·a·cele
di·ac·e·tate
di·ac·e·te·mia
di·a·ce·tic ac·id
di·ac·e·ton·u·ria
di·ac·e·tu·ria
di·a·ce·tyl
di·a·ce·tyl·cho·line
di·a·ce·tyl·mon·ox·ime
di·a·ce·tyl·mor·phine
di·a·ce·tyl·tan·nic ac·id
di·a·chron·ic
study
di·ac·id
di·a·cla·sia
di·ac·la·sis
di·ac·ri·nous
di·ac·ri·sis
di·a·crit·ic
di·a·crit·i·cal
di·ac·tin·ic
di·ac·yl·glyc·er·ol li·pase
di·ad
di·a·der·mic
di·ad·o·cho·ci·ne·sia
di·ad·o·cho·ki·ne·sia
di·ad·o·cho·ki·ne·sis
di·ad·o·cho·ki·net·ic
di·ag·nose
di·ag·no·sis
an·te·na·tal d.
clin·i·cal d.
dif·fer·en·tial d.
d. by ex·clu·sion
lab·o·ra·tory d.
ne·o·na·tal d.
path·o·log·ic d.
phys·i·cal d.
pre·na·tal d.
di·ag·no·sis-re·lat·ed group
di·ag·nos·tic
an·es·the·sia
au·di·om·e·try
cast
sen·si·tiv·i·ty
spec·i·fic·i·ty
ul·tra·sound
di·ag·nos·tic diph·the·ria
tox·in
di·ag·nos·ti·cian
di·ag·o·nal
con·ju·gate
di·a·ki·ne·sis
di·al
as·tig·mat·ic d.
di·al
ma·nom·e·ter

Di·a·lis·ter
di·al·lyl
di·al·y·sance
di·al·y·sate
di·al·y·sis
  equi·lib·ri·um d.
  ex·tra·cor·po·re·al d.
  per·i·to·ne·al d.
  d. ret·i·nae
di·al·y·sis
  de·men·tia
  shunt
di·al·y·sis dis·e·qui·lib·ri·um
  syn·drome
di·al·y·sis en·ceph·a·lop·a·thy
  syn·drome
di·a·lyze
di·a·lyz·er
di·a·mag·net·ic
di·a·mag·net·ism
di-a·me·lia
di·am·e·ter
  an·ter·o·pos·te·ri·or d. of
    the pel·vic in·let
  Baudelocque's d.
  bi·pa·ri·e·tal d.
  buc·co·lin·gual d.
  con·ju·gate d. of the pel·vic
    in·let
  d. me·di·a·nus
  ob·lique d.
  oc·cip·i·to·fron·tal d.
  oc·cip·i·to·men·tal d.
  pos·te·ri·or sag·it·tal d.
  sub·oc·cip·i·to·breg·mat·ic
    d.
  to·tal end-di·a·stol·ic d.
  to·tal end-sys·tol·ic d.
  trach·e·lo·breg·mat·ic d.
  trans·verse d.
  zy·go·mat·ic d.
di·am·ide
di·am·i·dines
di·a·mine
  d. ox·i·dase
di·a·mi·no ox·y·hy·drase
di·am·ni·ot·ic
di·a·mond
  disk
  fuch·sin
  skin
Diamond-Blackfan
  ane·mia
  syn·drome
di·a·mond cut·ting
  in·stru·ments
di·a·mond-shaped
  mur·mur

di·a·mond skin
  dis·ease
di·am·tha·zole di·hy·dro·chlo·ride
Di·ana
  com·plex
di·an·dria
di·an·dry
di·a·no·et·ic
di·a·pause
  em·bry·on·ic d.
di·a·pe·de·sis
di·a·per
  der·ma·ti·tis
  rash
di·aph·a·nos·cope
di·aph·a·nos·co·py
di·a·phe·met·ric
di·a·phen hy·dro·chlo·ride
di·aph·o·rase
di·a·pho·re·sis
di·a·pho·ret·ic
di·a·phragm
  Bucky d.
  pel·vic d.
  d. of pel·vis
  d. of sel·la
  uro·gen·i·tal d.
di·a·phragm
  pes·sa·ry
  phe·nom·e·non
di·a·phrag·ma
di·a·phrag·mal·gia
di·a·phrag·ma·ta
di·a·phrag·mat·ic
  flut·ter
  her·nia
  lig·a·ment of the mes·o·
    neph·ros
  nodes
  per·i·to·ni·tis
  pleu·ra
  pleu·ri·sy
  sur·face
di·a·phrag·mat·ic my·o·car·di·al
  in·farc·tion
di·a·phrag·mat·o·cele
di·a·phrag·mo·dyn·ia
di·aph·y·se·al
di·a·phy·sec·to·my
di·aph·y·ses
di·a·phys·i·al
  ac·la·sis
  cen·ter
  dys·pla·sia

di·a·phys·i·al jux·ta·ep·i·phys·
    i·al
    ex·os·to·sis
di·aph·y·sis
di·aph·y·si·tis
di·a·pi·re·sis
di·a·pla·cen·tal
di·ap·la·sis
di·a·plas·tic
di·a·plex·us
di·ap·no·ic
di·ap·not·ic
di·a·poph·y·sis
Di·ap·to·mus
di·ar·rhea
    d. al·ba
    bo·vine vi·rus d.
    chol·er·a·ic d.
    Co·chin Chi·na d.
    col·liq·ua·tive d.
    dys·en·ter·ic d.
    fat·ty d.
    gas·trog·e·nous d.
    li·en·ter·ic d.
    morn·ing d.
    mu·cous d.
    noc·tur·nal d.
    pan·cre·a·tog·en·ous d.
    se·rous d.
    sum·mer d.
    trav·el·er's d.
    trop·i·cal d.
    white d.
di·ar·rhe·al
di·ar·rhe·ic
di·ar·thric
di·ar·thro·di·al
    car·ti·lage
    joint
di·ar·thro·ses
di·ar·thro·sis
di·ar·tic·u·lar
di·as·chi·sis
di·a·scope
di·as·co·py
di·a·stal·sis
di·a·stal·tic
di·a·stase
di·as·ta·sis
    d. rec·ti
di·as·tas·u·ria
di·a·stat·ic
di·a·stat·ic skull
    frac·ture
di·a·ste·ma
di·a·ste·ma·ta
di·a·ste·ma·to·cra·nia
di·a·ste·ma·to·my·e·lia

di·as·ter
di·a·ste·re·o·i·so·mers
di·as·to·le
    car·di·ac d.
    gas·tric d.
di·a·stol·ic
    af·ter·po·ten·tial
    mur·mur
    pres·sure
    shock
    thrill
di·a·stroph·ic
    dwarf·ism
di·as·tro·phism
di·a·tax·ia
    ce·re·bral d.
di·a·te·la
di·a·ther·mal
di·a·ther·man·cy
di·a·ther·ma·nous
di·a·ther·mic
    ther·a·py
di·a·ther·mo·co·ag·u·la·tion
di·a·ther·my
    med·i·cal d.
    short wave d.
    sur·gi·cal d.
di·ath·e·sis
    con·trac·tu·ral d.
    cys·tic d.
    gouty d.
    hem·or·rhag·ic d.
    spas·mod·ic d.
    spas·mo·phil·ic d.
di·a·thet·ic
di·a·tom
di·a·to·ma·ceous
    earth
di·a·tom·ic
di·a·tor·ic
di·a·tri·zo·ate so·di·um
di·az·e·pam
di·a·zines
di·a·zo
    re·ac·tion
    re·a·gent
    stain for ar·gen·taf·fin
        gran·ules
di·a·zo·ni·um
    salts
di·az·o·tize
di·az·ox·ide
di·ba·sic
    ac·id
    am·mo·ni·um phos·phate
    cal·ci·um phos·phate
    po·tas·si·um phos·phate
    so·di·um phos·phate

di·benz·e·pin hy·dro·chlo·ride
di·benz·hep·tro·pine cit·rate
di·ben·zo·pyr·i·dine
di·ben·zo·thi·a·zine
di·benz·thi·one
Di blood group
Di·both·ri·o·ceph·a·lus
   D. la·tus
di·bro·mo·pro·pam·i·dine is·e·
   thi·o·nate
di·brom·sa·lan
di·bu·caine hy·dro·chlo·ride
di·bu·caine num·ber
di·bu·to·line sul·fate
di·bu·tyl phthal·ate
di·cac·o·dyl
di·car·box·yl·ic ac·id
   cy·cle
di·ce·lous
di·cen·tric
   chro·mo·some
di·ceph·a·lous
di·ceph·a·lus
   d. di·auch·e·nos
   d. di·pus di·bra·chi·us
   d. di·pus tet·ra·bra·chi·us
   d. di·pus tri·bra·chi·us
   d. di·py·gus
   d. mon·au·che·nos
di·chei·lia
di·chei·ria
di·chi·lia
di·chi·ria
di·chlo·ral·phen·a·zone
di·chlo·ra·mine-T
di·chlo·ride
di·chlo·ri·sone
di·chlor·i·so·pro·ter·e·nol
di·chlo·ro·ben·zene
di·chlo·ro·di·flu·o·ro·meth·ane
p,p'-di·chlo·ro·di·phen·yl meth·
   yl car·bi·nol
di·chlo·ro·di·phen·yl·tri·chlo·
   ro·eth·ane
di·chlo·ro·hy·drin
di·chlo·ro·i·so·pro·pyl al·co·hol
di·chlo·ro·i·so·pro·ter·e·nol
di·chlo·ro·phen
di·chlo·ro·phen·ar·sine hy·dro·
   chlo·ride
di·chlo·ro·vos
di·chlor·phen·a·mide
di·chlor·vos
di·cho·ri·al
   twins
di·cho·ri·on·ic
di·cho·ri·on·ic di·am·ni·ot·ic
   pla·cen·ta

di·chot·ic
di·chot·o·mous
di·chot·o·my
di·chro·ic
di·chro·ism
   cir·cu·lar d.
di·chro·mat
di·chro·mate
di·chro·mat·ic
di·chro·ma·tism
di·chro·ma·top·sia
di·chro·mic
di·chro·mo·phil
di·chro·mo·phile
Dick
   meth·od
   test
Dickens
   shunt
Dick test
   tox·in
di·clox·a·cil·lin so·di·um
di·co·phane
di·co·ria
di·cro·coe·li·o·sis
Di·cro·coe·li·um
di·crot·ic
   notch
   pulse
   wave
di·cro·tism
Dic·ty·o·cau·lus
   D. arn·fieldi
   D. fi·lar·ia
   D. vi·vip·a·rus
dic·ty·o·ma
dic·ty·o·tene
di·cu·ma·rol
di·cy·clo·mine hy·dro·chlo·ride
di·cys·te·ine
di·dac·tic
   anal·y·sis
di·dac·ty·lism
di·del·phic
Di·del·phis
did·y·mal·gi·a
did·y·mi·tis
did·y·mus
di·e·cious
Dieffenbach's
   meth·od
Diego blood group
di·el
di·el·drin
di·e·lec·trog·ra·phy
di·e·lec·trol·y·sis
Diels
   hy·dro·car·bon

di·en·ceph·a·la
di·en·ce·phal·ic
  ep·i·lep·sy
  syn·drome of in·fan·cy
di·en·ceph·a·lo·hy·po·phy·si·al
di·en·ceph·a·lon
die·ner
di·en·es·trol
Di·ent·a·moe·ba frag·i·lis
di·er·e·sis
di·e·ret·ic
di·es·ter·ase
di·es·trous
di·es·trus
di·et
  ac·id-ash d.
  al·ka·line-ash d.
  ba·sal d.
  ba·sic d.
  bland d.
  chal·lenge d.
  clear liq·uid d.
  di·a·bet·ic d.
  elim·i·na·tion d.
  full liq·uid d.
  Giordano-Giovannetti d.
  gout d.
  high cal·o·rie d.
  high fat d.
  ke·to·gen·ic d.
  low cal·o·rie d.
  low fat d.
  mac·ro·bi·ot·ic d.
  pu·rine-re·strict·ed d.
  re·duc·ing d.
  Sippy d.
  smooth d.
  soft d.
di·e·tary
  amen·or·rhea
  fi·ber
Dieterle's
  stain
di·e·tet·ic
  al·bu·min·ur·ia
di·e·tet·ics
di·eth·a·di·one
di·eth·a·nol·a·mine
  d. ac·e·tate
di·eth·a·zine
di·eth·e·noid
  fat·ty ac·id
di·eth·yl
di·eth·yl·a·mi·no·eth·yl
  cel·lu·lose
di·eth·yl·car·bam·a·zine cit·rate
di·eth·yl·ene·di·a·mine

di·eth·yl·ene·tri·a·mine pen·ta·a·ce·tic ac·id
di·eth·yl ether
di·eth·yl·mal·o·nyl·u·re·a
di·eth·y·lol·a·mine
di·eth·yl·pro·pi·on hy·dro·chlo·ride
di·eth·yl·stil·bes·trol
di·eth·yl·tol·u·am·ide
di·eth·yl·tryp·ta·mine
di·e·ti·tian
Dietl's
  cri·sis
di·e·to·ge·net·ics
Dieulafoy's
  ero·sion
  the·o·ry
di·far·ne·syl group
di·fen·ox·in
di·fen·ox·y·lic ac·id
dif·fer·ence
  al·ve·o·lar-ar·te·ri·al ox·y·gen d.
  ar·te·ri·o·ve·nous car·bon di·ox·ide d.
  ar·te·ri·o·ve·nous ox·y·gen d.
  cat·i·on-an·i·on d.
  in·di·vid·u·al d.'s
  light d.
  stan·dard er·ror of d.
dif·fer·en·tial
  thresh·old d.
dif·fer·en·tial
  di·ag·no·sis
  growth
  ma·nom·e·ter
  stain
  steth·o·scope
  ther·mom·e·ter
  thresh·old
dif·fer·en·tial blood
  pres·sure
dif·fer·en·tial re·nal func·tion
  test
dif·fer·en·tial spi·nal
  an·es·the·sia
dif·fer·en·tial ure·ter·al cath·e·ter·i·za·tion
  test
dif·fer·en·tial white
  blood count
dif·fer·en·ti·at·ed
dif·fer·en·ti·a·tion
  cor·rel·a·tive d.
  ech·o·car·di·o·graph·ic d.
  in·vis·i·ble d.
dif·flu·ence

dif·frac·tion
dif·frac·tion grat·ing
dif·fu·sate
dif·fuse
  ab·scess
  an·eu·rysm
  cho·roid·i·tis
  em·phy·se·ma
  gan·gli·on
  glo·mer·u·lo·ne·phri·tis
  goi·ter
  leish·man·i·a·sis
  per·i·to·ni·tis
  phleg·mon
dif·fuse ar·te·ri·al
  ec·ta·sia
dif·fuse cu·ta·ne·ous
  leish·man·i·a·sis
dif·fused
  pso·ri·a·sis
  re·flex
dif·fuse deep
  ker·a·ti·tis
dif·fuse id·i·o·path·ic skel·e·tal
  hy·per·os·to·sis
dif·fuse in·fan·tile fa·mil·i·al
  scle·ro·sis
dif·fuse mes·an·gi·al
  pro·lif·er·a·tion
dif·fuse small cleaved cell
  lym·pho·ma
dif·fuse waxy
  spleen
dif·fus·i·ble
  stim·u·lant
dif·fus·ing
  ca·pac·i·ty
  fac·tor
dif·fu·sion
  an·ox·ia
  co·ef·fi·cient
  con·stant
  hy·pox·ia
  meth·od
  res·pi·ra·tion
  shell
dif·fu·sion
  gel d.
di·flor·a·sone di·ac·e·tate
di·flu·cor·to·lone
di·flu·ni·sal
di·ga·met·ic
di·gas·tric
  fos·sa
  groove
  mus·cle
  notch
  tri·an·gle

di·gas·tri·cus
Di·ge·nea
di·gen·e·sis
di·ge·net·ic
DiGeorge
  syn·drome
di·gest
di·ges·tant
di·ges·tion
  gas·tric d.
  in·ter·cel·lu·lar d.
  in·tes·ti·nal d.
  in·tra·cel·lu·lar d.
  pan·cre·at·ic d.
  pep·tic d.
  pri·mary d.
  sal·i·vary d.
  sec·on·dary d.
di·ges·tive
  al·bu·min·ur·ia
  ap·pa·ra·tus
  fe·ver
  gly·cos·ur·ia
  leu·ko·cy·to·sis
  sys·tem
  tract
  tube
dig·in
dig·it
  clubbed d.'s
dig·i·tal
  fos·sa
  fur·row
  joints
  pulp
  re·flex
  veins
  whorl
dig·i·tal col·lat·er·al
  ar·tery
dig·i·tal·gia pa·res·the·ti·ca
dig·i·tal·in
  crys·tal·line d.
Dig·i·tal·is
dig·i·tal·is
  unit
dig·i·tal·ism
dig·i·tal·i·za·tion
dig·i·tal sub·trac·tion
  an·gi·og·ra·phy
dig·i·tate
  im·pres·sions
  wart
dig·i·ta·tion
dig·i·ta·ti·o·nes hip·po·cam·pi
di·gi·ti
dig·i·ti·grade
dig·i·tin

dig·i·to·nin
  re·ac·tion
dig·i·tox·ic·i·ty
dig·i·tox·in
dig·i·tus
  d. au·ric·u·la·ris
  di·gi·ti hip·po·cra·ti·ci
  d. val·gus
  d. var·us
di·glos·sia
di·glyc·er·ide li·pase
di·gly·co·coll hy·dro·i·o·dide-
  io·dine
di·gna·thus
di·gox·in
Di Guglielmo's
  dis·ease
  syn·drome
di·gyn·ia
di·gy·ny
di·het·er·o·zy·gote
di·hy·brid
di·hy·dral·a·zine
di·hy·drate
di·hy·dra·zone
di·hy·dric
  al·co·hol
di·hy·dro·a·scor·bic ac·id
di·hy·dro·cho·les·ter·ol
di·hy·dro·co·deine tar·trate
di·hy·dro·co·de·i·none
di·hy·dro·cor·ti·sone
di·hy·dro·er·go·cor·nine
di·hy·dro·er·go·cris·tine
di·hy·dro·er·go·cryp·tine
di·hy·dro·er·got·a·mine
di·hy·dro·er·go·tox·ine mes·y·
  late
di·hy·dro·fo·late re·duc·tase
di·hy·dro·gen
  phos·phate
di·hy·dro·lip·o·am·ide ace·tyl·
  trans·fer·ase
di·hy·dro·lip·o·am·ide de·hy·
  dro·gen·ase
di·hy·dro·li·po·ic ac·id
di·hy·dro·mor·phi·none hy·dro·
  chlo·ride
di·hy·dro-or·o·tase
di·hy·dro-or·o·tate
di·hy·dro·pte·ro·ic ac·id
di·hy·dro·strep·to·my·cin
di·hy·dro·ta·chys·ter·ol
di·hy·dro·tes·tos·ter·one
di·hy·dro·ur·a·cil
di·hy·dro·ur·i·dine
di·hy·drox·y·ac·e·tone

di·hy·drox·y·a·lu·mi·num ami·
  no·ac·e·tate
di·hy·drox·y·a·lu·mi·num so·
  di·um car·bon·ate
di·i·o·dide
di·i·o·do·hy·drox·y·quin
di·i·o·do·pyr·a·mine
di·i·so·pro·mine
di·i·so·pro·pyl flu·o·ro·phos·
  phate
di·ke·tone
di·ke·to·pi·per·a·zines
di·lac·er·a·tion
di·la·tan·cy
dil·a·ta·tion
dil·a·ta·tor
di·late
di·lat·ed
  car·di·o·my·op·a·thy
  pore
di·lat·ing
  la·ryn·go·tome
di·la·tion
  throm·bo·sis
di·la·tion
  ure·thral d.
di·la·tion and cu·ret·tage
di·la·tion and evac·u·a·tion
di·la·tor
  Goodell's d.
  Hanks d.'s
  Hegar's d.'s
  hy·dro·stat·ic d.
  d. ir·i·dis
  Kollmann's d.
  Plummer's d.
  d. of pu·pil
  d. tu·bae
  Tubbs' d.
  Walther's d.
di·la·tor
  mus·cle
dil·do
dil·doe
dill oil
di·lox·a·nide fu·ro·ate
dil·ti·a·zem hy·dro·chlo·ride
dil·u·ent
di·lute
  al·co·hol
  phos·phor·ic ac·id
di·lut·ed
  ace·tic ac·id
  hy·dro·chlo·ric ac·id
di·lu·tion
  ane·mia
di·ma·zole di·hy·dro·chlo·ride
di·ma·zon

di·me·lia
di·men·hy·dri·nate
di·men·sion
  buc·co·lin·gual d.
  oc·clu·sal ver·ti·cal d.
  rest ver·ti·cal d.
  ver·ti·cal d.
di·men·sion·al
  sta·bil·i·ty
di·mer
  thy·mine d.
di·mer·cap·rol
di·mer·cur·i·on
di·mer·ic
dim·er·ous
di·met·a·crine tar·trate
di·meth·i·cone
di·meth·in·dene ma·le·ate
di·me·thi·so·quin hy·dro·chlo·ride
di·me·this·ter·one
di·meth·o·thi·a·zine mes·y·late
di·me·thox·a·nate hy·dro·chlo·ride
di·meth·yl·a·mi·no·az·o·ben·zene
di·meth·yl·ar·sin·ic ac·id
di·meth·yl·ben·zene
di·meth·yl·car·bi·nol
di·meth·yl·eth·yl·car·bi·nol
di·meth·yl·eth·yl·car·bi·nol·chlo·ral
di·meth·yl ke·tone
di·meth·yl·phe·nol
di·meth·yl·phen·yl·pi·per·a·zin·i·um
di·meth·yl phthal·ate
di·meth·yl·pi·per·a·zine tar·trate
di·meth·yl sulf·ox·ide
N,N-di·meth·yl·tryp·ta·mine
di·meth·yl *d*-tu·bo·cu·ra·rine
di·meth·yl tu·bo·cu·ra·rine chlo·ride
di·meth·yl tu·bo·cu·ra·rine io·dide
di·me·tria
di·mid·i·ate
  her·maph·ro·dit·ism
Dimmer's
  ker·a·ti·tis
di·mor·phic
  ane·mia
di·mor·phism
  sex·u·al d.
di·mor·phol·a·mine
di·mor·phous
  lep·ro·sy

dim·ple
  sign
dim·ple
  coc·cyg·eal d.
dimp·ling
di·ner·ic
di·ni·tro·cel·lu·lose
di·ni·tro·gen mon·ox·ide
di·ni·tro·phen·yl·hy·dra·zine
  test
din·ner
  pad
di·no·flag·el·late
  tox·in
di·no·prost
  d. tro·meth·a·mine
di·no·pros·tone
di·nor·mo·cy·to·sis
Di·oc·to·phy·ma
  D. re·na·le
di·oc·to·phy·mi·a·sis
di·oc·tyl cal·ci·um sul·fo·suc·ci·nate
di·oc·tyl so·di·um sul·fo·suc·ci·nate
Di·o·don
di·o·done
di·o·do·quin
Diogenes
  cup
di·ol·a·mine
di·op·ter
  prism d.
di·op·tric
  ab·er·ra·tion
di·op·trics
di·or·tho·sis
di·ose
di·os·gen·in
di·ov·u·lar
  twins
di·ov·u·la·to·ry
di·ox·ane
di·ox·ide
di·ox·y·ben·zone
di·ox·y·gen·ase
DIP
  joints
dip
  phe·nom·e·non
di·pep·ti·dase
  me·thi·o·nyl d.
di·pep·tide
di·pep·ti·dyl car·box·y·pep·ti·dase
di·pep·ti·dyl pep·ti·dase
di·pep·ti·dyl pep·ti·dase I
di·pep·ti·dyl pep·ti·dase II

di·pep·ti·dyl trans·fer·ase
di·per·o·don hy·dro·chlo·ride
Di·pet·a·lo·ne·ma
   D. re·con·di·tum
   D. strep·to·cer·ca
di·phal·lus
di·pha·sic
   com·plex
di·pha·sic milk
   fe·ver
di·phe·ma·nil meth·yl·sul·fate
di·phem·e·thox·i·dine
di·phen·a·di·one
di·phen·an
di·phen·hy·dra·mine hy·dro·chlo·ride
di·phen·i·dol
o-di·phe·no·lase
di·phe·nol ox·i·dase
di·phe·nox·y·late hy·dro·chlo·ride
di·phen·yl·chlor·ar·sine
di·phen·yl·en·i·mine
di·phen·yl·hy·dan·to·in
   gin·gi·vi·tis
di·phen·yl·meth·ane
   dyes
di·phen·yl·pyr·a·line hy·dro·chlo·ride
di·phos·gene
di·phos·pho·pyr·i·dine nu·cle·o·tide
di·phos·pho·thi·a·min
diph·the·ria
   avi·an d.
   calf d.
   cu·ta·ne·ous d.
   false d.
   fowl d.
diph·the·ria
   an·ti·tox·in
   tox·in
diph·the·ria an·ti·tox·in
   unit
diph·the·ri·al
diph·the·ria, tet·a·nus tox·oids, and per·tus·sis
   vac·cine
diph·the·rit·ic
   con·junc·ti·vi·tis
   en·ter·i·tis
   mem·brane
   neu·rop·a·thy
   pa·ral·y·sis
   ul·cer
diph·the·ri·tis
diph·the·roid
diph·the·ro·tox·in

di·phyl·lo·both·ri·a·sis
Di·phyl·lo·both·ri·um
   D. cor·da·tum
   D. la·tum
   D. lin·gu·loi·des
   D. man·so·ni
   D. man·so·noi·des
di·phyl·lo·both·ri·um
   ane·mia
di·phy·o·dont
di·pip·a·none
di·pi·pro·ver·ine
di·piv·e·frin hy·dro·chlo·ride
dip·la·cu·sis
   d. bin·au·ra·lis
   d. dys·har·mon·i·ca
   d. echo·i·ca
   d. mon·au·ra·lis
di·ple·gia
   con·gen·i·tal fa·cial d.
   fa·cial d.
   in·fan·tile d.
   mas·ti·ca·to·ry d.
   spas·tic d.
dip·lo·al·bu·mi·nu·ria
dip·lo·ba·cil·la·ry
   con·junc·ti·vi·tis
dip·lo·ba·cil·lus
   Morax-Axenfeld d.
dip·lo·bac·te·ria
dip·lo·blas·tic
dip·lo·car·dia
dip·lo·ceph·a·lus
dip·lo·chei·ria
dip·lo·chi·ria
dip·lo·coc·ce·mia
dip·lo·coc·ci
dip·lo·coc·cin
dip·lo·coc·coid
Dip·lo·coc·cus
dip·lo·coc·cus
dip·lo·co·ri·a
dip·loë
dip·lo·gen·e·sis
Dip·lo·go·nop·o·rus
di·plo·ic
   ca·nals
   vein
dip·loid
   nu·cle·us
dip·lo·kar·y·on
dip·lo·mel·i·tu·ria
dip·lo·my·e·lia
dip·lon
dip·lo·ne·ma
dip·lo·neu·ral
dip·lop·a·gus

di·plo·pia
  crossed d.
  di·rect d.
  het·er·on·y·mous d.
  ho·mon·y·mous d.
  mo·noc·u·lar d.
  sim·ple d.
dip·lo·po·dia
dip·lo·some
dip·lo·so·mia
dip·lo·tene
dip·lo·ter·a·tol·o·gy
di·po·dia
di·po·lar
  ions
di·pole
  the·o·ry
di·po·tas·si·um phos·phate
di·pro·pyl·tryp·ta·mine
di·pro·so·pus
dip·se·sis
dip·so·gen
dip·so·ma·nia
dip·so·sis
dip·so·ther·a·py
Dip·tera
dip·ter·an
dip·ter·ous
Di·pus sa·git·ta
di·py·gus
dip·y·li·di·a·sis
Dip·y·lid·i·um ca·ni·num
di·py·rid·am·ole
di·py·rim·i·dine pho·to·ly·ase
di·py·rine
di·py·rone
di·rect
  astig·ma·tism
  aus·cul·ta·tion
  cal·o·rim·e·try
  cur·rent
  di·plo·pia
  di·u·ret·ic
  em·bo·lism
  flap
  frac·ture
  il·lu·mi·na·tion
  im·age
  lead
  meth·od for mak·ing in·lays
  oph·thal·mo·scope
  oph·thal·mos·co·py
  ox·i·dase
  per·cus·sion
  rays
  re·tain·er
  re·ten·tion
  tech·nique

  trans·fu·sion
  vi·sion
  zo·o·no·sis
di·rect acryl·ic
  res·to·ra·tion
di·rect bone
  im·pres·sion
di·rect com·pos·ite res·in
  res·to·ra·tion
di·rect Coombs'
  test
di·rect fill·ing
  res·in
di·rect flu·o·res·cent an·ti·body
  test
di·rect ful·gu·ra·tion
di·rect in·gui·nal
  her·nia
di·rec·tive
  psy·cho·ther·a·py
di·rect lyt·ic
  fac·tor of co·bra ven·om
di·rect ma·ter·nal
  death
di·rect nu·cle·ar
  di·vi·sion
di·rec·tor
di·rect o·vu·lar
  trans·mi·gra·tion
di·rect pulp
  cap·ping
di·rect py·ram·i·dal
  tract
di·rect re·act·ing
  bil·i·ru·bin
di·rect res·in
  res·to·ra·tion
di·rect vi·sion
  spec·tro·scope
dir·i·ga·tion
dir·i·go·mo·tor
Di·ro·fil·a·ria
  D. con·junc·ti·vae
  D. im·mi·tis
di·ro·fil·a·ri·a·sis
dirt-eat·ing
dis·a·bil·i·ty
  de·vel·op·men·tal d.
  learn·ing d.
dis·sac·cha·ride
dis·ag·gre·ga·tion
dis·ap·pear·ing bone
  dis·ease
dis·ar·tic·u·la·tion
dis·as·sim·i·la·tion
dis·as·so·ci·a·tion
disc
  elec·tro·pho·re·sis

disc·ec·to·my
dis·charge
   af·ter-d.
dis·charg·ing
   tu·bule
Dische
   re·ac·tion
dis·chro·na·tion
dis·ci
dis·ci·form
   de·gen·er·a·tion
   de·tach·ment of ret·i·na
dis·cis·sion
dis·ci·tis
dis·cli·na·tion
dis·clos·ing
   so·lu·tion
dis·co·blas·tic
dis·co·blas·tu·la
dis·co·gas·tru·la
dis·co·gen·ic
dis·co·gram
dis·cog·ra·phy
dis·coid
   lu·pus er·y·the·ma·to·sus
dis·coi·dal
   cleav·age
dis·con·nec·tion
   syn·drome
dis·con·tin·u·a·tion
   test
dis·con·tin·u·ous
   phase
   ster·il·i·za·tion
dis·cop·a·thy
   trau·mat·ic cer·vi·cal d.
dis·co·pla·cen·ta
dis·cor·dance
dis·cor·dant
   al·ter·nans
   al·ter·na·tion
dis·co·ria
dis·cot·o·my
dis·crete
   small·pox
dis·crim·i·nant
   func·tion
   stim·u·lus
dis·crim·i·na·tion
dis·cus
   d. len·ti·for·mis
   d. pro·lig·er·us
dis·cus·sive
dis·cu·ti·ent
dis·di·a·clast
dis·ease
   ABO he·mo·lyt·ic d. of the
   new·born

Acosta's d.
Adams-Stokes d.
ad·ap·ta·tion d.'s
Addison-Biermer d.
Addison's d.
ad·e·noid d.
ak·a·mu·shi d.
Aku·rey·ri d.
Albers-Schönberg d.
Albert's d.
Albright's d.
Aleu·tian d. of mink
Alexander's d.
al·ka·li d.
Almeida's d.
Alpers d.
Alzheimer's d.
an·ar·thrit·ic rheu·ma·toid
   d.
Anders' d.
Andersen's d.
an·ti·body de·fi·cien·cy d.
aor·to·il·i·ac oc·clu·sive d.
Aran-Duchenne d.
Aujeszky's d.
Aus·tra·li·an X d.
au·to·im·mune d.
avi·a·tor's d.
Ayerza's d.
Azor·e·an d.
Baelz' d.
Ballet's d.
Baló's d.
Bamberger-Marie d.
Bamberger's d.
Bang's d.
Bannister's d.
Banti's d.
Barclay-Baron d.
Barlow's d.
Barraquer's d.
Basedow's d.
Batten-Mayou d.
Bayle's d.
Bazin's d.
Bechterew's d.
Becker's d.
Begbie's d.
Béguez César d.
Behçet's d.
Behr's d.
Benson's d.
Bernhardt's d.
Besnier-Boeck-Schaumann d.
Best's d.
Bielschowsky's d.
Biermer's d.
big liv·er d.

dis·ease *(continued)*
Binswanger's d.
bird-breed·er's d.
black d.
black-tongue d.
blind·ing d.
Bloch-Sulzberger d.
Blocq's d.
Blount-Barber d.
Blount's d.
blue d.
blue·comb d. of chick·ens
blue·comb d. of tur·keys
Boeck's d.
Bor·na d.
Bornholm d.
Bouchard's d.
Bouillaud's d.
Bourneville-Pringle d.
Bourneville's d.
Bowen's d.
Brailsford-Morquio d.
Breda's d.
Bright's d.
Brill's d.
Brill-Symmers d.
Brill-Zinsser d.
bris·ket d.
Brissaud's d.
Brocq's d.
Brodie's d.
bronzed d.
Brooke's d.
Bruck's d.
Brushfield-Wyatt d.
Bruton's d.
Buerger's d.
bulg·ing eye d.
Bury's d.
Buschke's d.
Busquet's d.
Buss d.
Busse-Buschke d.
Byler d.
Caffey's d.
cais·son d.
Calvé-Perthes d.
Canavan's d.
ca·nine par·vo·vi·rus d.
Caroli's d.
Carrión's d.
Castleman's d.
cat-bite d.
cat-scratch d.
ce·li·ac d.
cen·tral core d.
cer·e·bro·vas·cu·lar d.
Chagas' d.

Chagas-Cruz d.
Charcot-Marie-Tooth d.
Charcot's d.
Charlouis' d.
Cheadle's d.
Chédiak-Higashi d.
Chiari's d.
cho·les·ter·ol es·ter stor·age d.
Christensen-Krabbe d.
Christian's d.
Christmas d.
chron·ic ac·tive liv·er d.
chron·ic gran·u·lom·a·tous d.
chron·ic hy·per·ten·sive d.
chron·ic ob·struc·tive pul·mo·nary d.
chron·ic res·pi·ra·to·ry d.
cir·cling d.
Civatte's d.
clo·ver d.
Coats' d.
Cockayne's d.
cold he·mag·glu·ti·nin d.
col·la·gen d.'s
col·la·gen-vas·cu·lar d.'s
com·bined sys·tem d.
com·mu·ni·ca·ble d.
Concato's d.
con·nec·tive-tis·sue d.'s
Conradi's d.
con·sti·tu·tion·al d.
con·ta·gious d.
Cori's d.
corn·meal d.
cor·ri·dor d.
Corrigan's d.
Cotunnius' d.
Cowden's d.
cra·zy chick d.
Creutzfeldt-Jakob d.
Crigler-Najjar d.
Crocq's d.
Crohn's d.
Crouzon's d.
Cruveilhier-Baumgarten d.
Cruveilhier's d.
Csillag's d.
Curschmann's d.
Cushing's d.
cys·tic d. of the breast
cys·tic d. of re·nal me·dul·la
cys·tine stor·age d.
cy·to·me·ga·lic in·clu·sion d.
cy·to·meg·a·lo·vi·rus d.

Daae's d.
danc·ing d.
Danielssen-Boeck d.
Danielssen's d.
Darier's d.
Darling's d.
Davies' d.
de·com·pres·sion d.
deer-fly d.
de·fi·cien·cy d.
de·gen·er·a·tive joint d.
Degos' d.
Dejerine's d.
Déjérine-Sottas d.
de·my·e·li·nat·ing d.
dense-de·pos·it d.
de Quervain's d.
Dercum's d.
Deutschländer's d.
Devic's d.
di·a·mond skin d.
Di Guglielmo's d.
dis·ap·pear·ing bone d.
dog d.
dom·i·nant·ly in·her·it·ed
  Lévi's d.
Donohue's d.
drug-in·duced d.
Dubini's d.
Dubois' d.
Duchenne-Aran d.
Duchenne's d.
Duhring's d.
Dukes' d.
Duncan's d.
Duplay's d.
Dupuytren's d. of the foot
Duroziez' d.
Dutton's d.
dy·nam·ic d.
Eales' d.
Ebstein's d.
Eisenmenger's d.
emo·tion·al d.
Engelmann's d.
English d.
Epstein's d.
Erb-Charcot d.
Erb's d.
Erdheim d.
Eulenburg's d.
ex·an·them·a·tous d.
ex·tra·mam·ma·ry Paget d.
ex·tra·py·ram·i·dal d.
Fabry's d.
Fahr's d.
Farber's d.
Feer's d.

fem·o·ro·pop·lit·e·al oc·clu·
  sive d.
Fenwick's d.
fi·bro·cys·tic d. of the
  breast
fi·bro·cys·tic d. of the pan·
  cre·as
fifth d.
Filatov's d.
Flatau-Schilder d.
Flegel's d.
flint d.
Folling's d.
foot-and-mouth d.
Forbes' d.
Fordyce's d.
Forrestier's d.
Fothergill's d.
Fournier's d.
fourth d.
Fox-Fordyce d.
Franklin's d.
Freiberg's d.
Friedmann's d.
Friedreich's d.
Friend d.
Fuerstner's d.
func·tion·al d.
fu·so·spi·ro·chet·al d.
Gairdner's d.
Gamna's d.
Gandy-Nanta d.
ga·ra·pa·ta d.
Garré's d.
gasp·ing d.
Gaucher's d.
Gerhardt's d.
Gerlier's d.
Gierke's d.
Gilbert's d.
Gilchrist's d.
Gilles de la Tourette's d.
Glanzmann's d.
gly·co·gen-stor·age d.
Goldflam d.
Gorham's d.
Gougerot and Blum d.
Gougerot-Ruiter d.
Gougerot-Sjögren d.
Gowers d.
Graefe's d.
graft ver·sus host d.
gran·u·lom·a·tous d.
Graves' d.
greasy pig d.
Greenfield's d.
Greenhow's d.
Griesinger's d.

dis·ease *(continued)*
Grover's d.
Guinon's d.
Gum·boro d.
Günther's d.
GVH d.
H d.
Haff d.
Haglund's d.
Hailey and Hailey d.
Hallervorden-Spatz d.
Hallopeau's d.
Hamman's d.
Hammond's d.
hand-foot-and-mouth d.
Hand-Schüller-Christian d.
Hansen's d.
Harada's d.
hard pad d.
Hartnup d.
Hashimoto's d.
heavy chain d.
Hebra's d.
Heck's d.
Heerfordt's d.
he·mo·glo·bin C d.
he·mo·glo·bin H d.
he·mo·lyt·ic d. of new·born
hem·or·rhag·ic d. of deer
hem·or·rhag·ic d. of the
new·born
he·pa·to·len·tic·u·lar d.
her·ring-worm d.
Hers' d.
hide·bound d.
Hippel-Lindau d.
Hippel's d.
Hirschsprung's d.
Hjärre's d.
Hodgkin's d.
Hodgson's d.
hoof-and-mouth d.
hook·worm d.
Hoppe-Goldflam d.
Huntington's d.
Hurler's d.
Hutchinson-Gilford d.
hy·a·line mem·brane d. of
the new·born
hy·da·tid d.
Hyde's d.
Ice·land d.
I-cell d.
id·i·o·path·ic Bamberger-
Marie d.
im·mune com·plex d.
im·mu·no·pro·lif·er·a·tive
small in·tes·ti·nal d.

in·clu·sion body d.
in·clu·sion cell d.
in·dus·tri·al d.
in·fec·tious d.
in·fec·tious bur·sal d.
in·fec·tive d.
in·ter·sti·tial d.
iron-stor·age d.
is·land d.
Itai-Itai d.
Jaffe-Lichtenstein d.
Jakob-Creutzfeldt d.
Jansky-Bielschowsky d.
Jem·bra·na d.
Jensen's d.
Johne's d.
jump·er d.
jump·er d. of Maine
Jüngling's d.
Kashin-Bek d.
Katayama d.
Kawasaki d.
Kienböck's d.
Kimmelstiel-Wilson d.
Kimura's d.
kinky-hair d.
Klippel's d.
Köhler's d.
Köhlmeier-Degos d.
Krabbe's d.
Kufs d.
Kugelberg-Welander d.
Kuhnt-Junius d.
Kussmaul's d.
Ky·as·a·nur For·est d.
Kyrle's d.
Lafora body d.
Lafora's d.
Lane's d.
Larrey-Weil d.
Lasègue's d.
laugh·ing d.
L-chain d.
Legg-Calvé-Perthes d.
Legg-Perthes d.
Legg's d.
Le·gion·naires' d.
Leigh's d.
Leiner's d.
Lenègre's d.
Leri-Weill d.
Letterer-Siwe d.
Lev's d.
Lewandowski-Lutz d.
Lhermitte-Duclos d.
Lindau's d.
lin·e·ar IgA bul·lous d. in
chil·dren

Little's d.
Lobo's d.
lo·co·weed d.
Löffler's d.
Lorain's d.
Luft's d.
lumpy skin d.
Lutz-Splendore-Almeida d.
Lyell's d.
Lyme d.
ly·so·so·mal d.
Machado-Joseph d.
Madelung's d.
Majocchi's d.
Malherbe's d.
Manson's d.
ma·ple bark d.
ma·ple syr·up urine d.
mar·ble bone d.
Mar·burg vi·rus d.
Marchiafava-Bignami d.
Marek's d.
Marfan's d.
mar·ga·rine d.
Marie-Strümpell d.
Marion's d.
Martin's d.
McArdle's d.
McArdle-Schmid-Pearson d.
Med·i·ter·ra·ne·an-he·mo·
   glo·bin E d.
Meige's d.
Ménétrièr's d.
Ménière's d.
men·tal d.
Merzbacher-Pelizaeus d.
Meyenburg's d.
Meyer's d.
mi·an·eh d.
Mibelli's d.
mi·cro·cys·tic d. of re·nal
   me·dul·la
mi·cro·met·a·stat·ic d.
Mikulicz' d.
Milian's d.
Milroy's d.
Milton's d.
Mi·na·ma·ta d.
min·er's d.
min·i·mal-change d.
Mitchell's d.
mixed con·nec·tive-tis·sue d.
Möbius d.
mo·lec·u·lar d.
Mondor's d.
Monge's d.
Morgagni's d.
Morquio's d.

Morquio-Ullrich d.
Morvan's d.
Moschcowitz' d.
mo·tor neu·ron d.
moy·a·moya d.
Mucha-Habermann d.
mu·co·sal d.
mul·ti·core d.
Nai·ro·bi sheep d.
na·vic·u·lar d.
Neftel's d.
Neumann's d.
neu·tral lip·id stor·age d.
New·cas·tle d.
Nicolas-Favre d.
Niemann-Pick d.
nil d.
nod·u·lar d.
Nonne-Milroy d.
Norrie's d.
no·ti·fi·a·ble d.
oast·house urine d.
oc·cu·pa·tion·al d.
Oguchi's d.
Ollier's d.
Oppenheim's d.
or·gan·ic d.
Ormond's d.
Osgood-Schlatter d.
Osler's d.
Osler-Vaquez d.
Otto's d.
Owren's d.
Paas' d.
Paget's d.
Panner's d.
pa·per mill work·er's d.
par·a·sit·ic d.
Parkinson's d.
par·rot d.
Parrot's d.
Parry's d.
Pauzat's d.
Pavy's d.
Paxton's d.
pearl-work·er's d.
Pel-Ebstein d.
Pelizaeus-Merzbacher d.
Pellegrini's d.
Pellegrini-Stieda d.
pel·vic in·flam·ma·to·ry d.
pe·ri·od·ic d.
per·na d.
Perthes d.
Pette-Döring d.
Peyronie's d.
Pick's d.
pink d.

dis·ease *(continued)*
plas·ter of Par·is d.
Plummer's d.
pol·y·cys·tic d. of kid·neys
pol·y·cys·tic liv·er d.
Pompe's d.
Por·tu·guese-A·zor·e·an d.
Posadas d.
Potter's d.
Pott's d.
poul·try han·dler's d.
preg·nan·cy d. of sheep
pri·mary d.
Pringle's d.
Profichet's d.
pul·lo·rum d.
pulpy kid·ney d.
pulse·less d.
Purtscher's d.
qui·et hip d.
Quincke's d.
Quinquaud's d.
rag-sort·er's d.
Ranikhet d.
Rayer's d.
Raynaud's d.
Recklinghausen's d.
Recklinghausen's d. of bone
Refsum's d.
Reiter's d.
Rendu-Osler-Weber d.
re·port·a·ble d.
rhe·sus d.
rheu·mat·ic d.
rheu·mat·ic heart d.
rheu·ma·toid d.
Riedel's d.
Riga-Fede d.
Ritter's d.
Robinson's d.
Robles' d.
Roger's d.
Rokitansky's d.
Romberg's d.
Rosenbach's d.
Roth-Bernhardt d.
Roth's d.
Rougnon-Heberden d.
Roussy-Lévy d.
Rubarth's d.
runt d.
Rust's d.
sal·i·vary gland vi·rus d.
salm·on d.
Sandhoff's d.
sand·worm d.
Schamberg's d.
Schaumberg's d.

Schenck's d.
Scheuermann's d.
Schilder's d.
Schlatter-Osgood d.
Schlatter's d.
Scholz' d.
Schönlein's d.
Schottmüller's d.
Schüller's d.
scle·ro·cys·tic d. of the
  ova·ry
sea-blue his·ti·o·cyte d.
sec·on·dary d.
Seitelberger's d.
Selter's d.
Senear-Usher d.
se·nile hip d.
se·rum d.
sex·u·al·ly trans·mit·ted d.
Shaver's d.
shi·ma·mu·shi d.
sick·le cell d.
sick·le cell C d.
sick·le cell-thal·as·se·mia d.
Siemerling-Creutzfeldt d.
si·lo-fil·ler's d.
Simmonds' d.
Simons' d.
sixth d.
sixth ve·ne·re·al d.
Sjögren's d.
skin·bound d.
slipped ten·don d.
slow vi·rus d.
Sneddon-Wilkinson d.
so·cial d.'s
spe·cif·ic d.
Spielmeyer-Sjögren d.
Spielmeyer-Stock d.
Spielmeyer-Vogt d.
Stargardt's d.
Steele-Richardson-Olszewski
  d.
Steinert's d.
Sticker's d.
stiff lamb d.
Still's d.
Stokes-Adams d.
stone-ma·sons' d.
stor·age d.
Strümpell-Marie d.
Strümpell's d.
Strümpell-Westphal d.
Sturge's d.
Sturge-Weber d.
Stuttgart d.
Sulzberger-Garbe d.
Sutton's d.

Swediauer's d.
sweet clo·ver d.
Sweet's d.
Swift's d.
swine ede·ma d.
swine·herd's d.
swine ve·sic·u·lar d.
Sydenham's d.
Sylvest's d.
sys·tem·ic au·to·im·mune
  d.'s
sys·tem·ic feb·rile d.'s
Takahara's d.
Takayasu's d.
Talma's d.
Tan·gier d.
Taussig-Bing d.
Taylor's d.
Tay's d.
Tay-Sachs d.
Teschen d.
Theiler's d.
third d.
Thomsen's d.
Thornwaldt's d.
Thygeson's d.
thy·ro·car·di·ac d.
Tommaselli's d.
Tornwaldt's d.
Tourette's d.
tsu·tsu·ga·mu·shi d.
tun·nel d.
Underwood's d.
Unna's d.
Unverricht's d.
Urbach-Wiethe d.
vag·a·bond's d.
va·grant's d.
van Bogaert's d.
van Buren's d.
Vaquez' d.
ve·ne·re·al d.
ve·no-oc·clu·sive d. of the
  liv·er
Vidal's d.
Vincent's d.
Virchow's d.
vi·rus X d.
Vogt-Spielmeyer d.
Voltolini's d.
von Economo's d.
von Gierke's d.
von Hippel-Lindau d.
von Meyenburg's d.
von Recklinghausen's d.
von Willebrand's d.
Voorhoeve's d.
Wagner's d.

Wardrop's d.
wast·ing d.
Weber-Christian d.
Wegner's d.
Weil's d.
Werdnig-Hoffmann d.
Werlhof's d.
Wernicke's d.
Werther's d.
Wesselsbron d.
Westphal's d.
Whipple's d.
white mus·cle d.
white spot d.
Wilkie's d.
Wilson's d.
Winiwarter-Buerger d.
Winkelman's d.
Winkler's d.
Wohlfart-Kugelberg-Welander
  d.
Wolman's d.
wool-sor·ters' d.
Woringer-Kolopp d.
X d. of cat·tle
yel·low d.
Ziehen-Oppenheim d.
dis·ease
  de·ter·mi·nants
dis·en·gage·ment
dis·e·qui·lib·ri·um
  ge·net·ic d.
  link·age d.
dis·ger·mi·no·ma
dish
  Petri d.
  Stender d.
dish
  face
dis·har·mo·ny
  oc·clu·sal d.
dish·pan
  frac·ture
dis·im·pac·tion
dis·in·fect
dis·in·fec·tant
  com·plete d.
  in·com·plete d.
dis·in·fec·tion
dis·in·hi·bi·tion
dis·in·sec·tion
dis·in·sec·ti·za·tion
dis·in·te·gra·tion
  con·stant
dis·in·vag·i·na·tion
dis·joined
  py·e·lo·plas·ty

dis·ju·gate
  move·ment of eyes
dis·junc·tion
dis·junc·tive
  ab·sorp·tion
disk
  kid·ney
  syn·drome
disk
  A d.'s
  acro·mi·o·cla·vic·u·lar d.
  an·i·so·tro·pic d.'s
  ar·tic·u·lar d.
  blas·to·der·mic d.
  blood d.
  Bowman's d.'s
  Burlew d.
  choked d.
  cil·i·ary d.
  cone d.'s
  cut·tle·fish d.
  di·a·mond d.
  em·bry·on·ic d.
  em·ery d.'s
  germ d.
  ger·mi·nal d.
  H d.
  hair d.
  Hensen's d.
  her·ni·at·ed d.
  I d.
  in·ter·ca·lat·ed d.
  in·ter·me·di·ate d.
  in·ter·pu·bic d.
  in·ter·ver·te·bral d.
  iso·tro·pic d.
  man·dib·u·lar d.
  Merkel's tac·tile d.
  Newton's d.
  op·tic d.
  Placido's d.
  pro·lig·er·ous d.
  pro·trud·ed d.
  Q d.'s
  ra·di·o·ul·nar d.
  ra·di·o·ul·nar ar·tic·u·lar d.
  Ranvier's d.'s
  rod d.'s
  rup·tured d.
  sa·cro·coc·cyg·e·al d.
  sand·pa·per d.'s
  sten·o·pa·ic d.
  sten·o·pe·ic d.
  ster·no·cla·vic·u·lar d.
  ster·no·cla·vic·u·lar ar·tic·u·lar d.
  stro·bo·scop·ic d.
  tac·tile d.

tem·po·ro·man·dib·u·lar ar·tic·u·lar d.
  trans·verse d.
  tri·an·gu·lar d. of wrist
  Z d.
dis·ki·tis
disk sen·si·tiv·i·ty
  meth·od
disk-shaped
  cat·a·ract
dis·lo·cate
dis·lo·ca·tio
  d. erec·ta
dis·lo·ca·tion
  d. of ar·tic·u·lar pro·cess·es
  closed d.
  com·pound d.
  frac·ture d.
  Kienböck's d.
  Nélaton's d.
  open d.
  sim·ple d.
dis·lo·ca·tion
  frac·ture
dis·mem·ber
dis·mem·bered
  py·e·lo·plas·ty
dis·mu·tase
dis·mu·ta·tion
di·so·di·um
  phos·phate
di·so·mic
di·so·my
di·so·pro·mine
di·so·pyr·a·mide
dis·or·der
  ad·just·ment d.'s
  af·fec·tive d.'s
  an·ti·so·cial per·son·al·i·ty d.
  at·ten·tion def·i·cit d.
  au·to·nom·ic d.
  be·hav·ior d.
  bi·po·lar d.
  bor·der·line per·son·al·i·ty d.
  char·ac·ter d.
  con·duct d.
  con·ver·sion d.
  cy·clo·thy·mic d.
  dys·thy·mic d.
  emo·tion·al d.
  func·tion·al d.
  gen·er·al·ized anx·i·e·ty d.
  iden·ti·ty d.
  im·mune com·plex d.
  im·mu·no·pro·lif·er·a·tive d.'s

im·pulse con·trol d.
in·ter·mit·tent ex·plo·sive
   d.
iso·lat·ed ex·plo·sive d.
men·tal d.
neu·ro·psy·cho·log·ic d.
op·po·si·tion·al d.
or·gan·ic men·tal d.
over·anx·ious d.
pan·ic d.
per·son·al·i·ty d.
per·va·sive de·vel·op·men·
   tal d.
plas·ma io·do·pro·tein d.
post·trau·mat·ic stress d.
psy·cho·gen·ic pain d.
psy·cho·phys·i·o·log·ic d.
psy·cho·so·mat·ic d.
schiz·o·phren·i·form d.
so·ma·ti·za·tion d.
so·mat·o·form d.'s
sub·stance abuse d.'s
thought pro·cess d.
vis·cer·al d.
dis·or·ga·ni·za·tion
dis·or·ga·nized
schiz·o·phre·nia
dis·o·ri·en·ta·tion
dis·par·ate
dis·par·i·ty
con·ju·gate d.
fix·a·tion d.
ret·i·nal d.
dis·par·i·ty
an·gle
dis·pen·sa·ry
dis·pen·sa·to·ry
dis·pense
dis·pens·ing
tab·let
di·sperm·ia
di·sper·my
dis·per·sal
flash d.
dis·perse
pla·cen·ta
dis·persed
phase
dis·pers·ing
elec·trode
dis·per·sion
col·loid
me·di·um
phase
dis·per·sion
coarse d.
col·loi·dal d.
mo·lec·u·lar d.

op·ti·cal ro·ta·to·ry d.
tem·po·ral d.
dis·per·si·ty
dis·per·soid
di·spi·reme
dis·place·a·bil·i·ty
tis·sue d.
dis·place·ment
af·fect d.
me·si·al d.
tis·sue d.
dis·place·ment
anal·y·sis
thresh·old
dis·pro·por·tion·at·ing
en·zyme
dis·sect
dis·sect·ing
an·eu·rysm
cel·lu·li·tis
dis·sec·tion
tu·ber·cle
dis·sem·i·nate
coc·cid·i·oi·do·my·co·sis
dis·sem·i·nat·ed
as·per·gil·lo·sis
cho·roid·i·tis
lip·o·gran·u·lo·ma·to·sis
lu·pus er·y·the·ma·to·sus
scle·ro·sis
tu·ber·cu·lo·sis
dis·sem·i·nat·ed cu·ta·ne·ous
gan·grene
leish·man·i·a·sis
**dis·sem·i·nat·ed in·tra·vas·cu·
lar**
co·ag·u·la·tion
dis·sem·i·nat·ed re·cur·rent
in·fun·dib·u·lo·fol·lic·u·li·
tis
dis·sep·i·ment
Disse's
space
dis·sim·i·la·tion
dis·sim·u·la·tion
dis·so·ci·at·ed
an·es·the·sia
nys·tag·mus
dis·so·ci·a·tion
con·stant
con·stant of an ac·id
con·stant of a base
con·stant of wa·ter
sen·si·bil·i·ty
dis·so·ci·a·tion
al·bu·mi·no·cy·to·log·ic d.
atri·al d.
atri·o·ven·tric·u·lar d.

dis·so·ci·a·tion *(continued)*
    com·plete atri·o·ven·tric·u·
      lar d.
    com·plete A-V d.
    elec·tro·me·chan·i·cal d.
    in·com·plete atri·o·ven·tric·
      u·lar d.
    in·com·plete A-V d.
    in·ter·fer·ence d.
    iso·rhyth·mic d.
    lon·gi·tu·di·nal d.
    sleep d.
    sy·rin·go·my·el·ic d.
    ta·bet·ic d.
dis·so·ci·a·tive
    an·es·the·sia
    re·ac·tion
dis·solve
dis·so·nance
dis·sym·me·try
dis·tad
dis·tal
    car·ies
    cen·tri·ole
    end
    il·e·i·tis
    my·op·a·thy
    oc·clu·sion
    part of an·te·ri·or lobe of
      hy·poph·y·sis
    sep·tum
    sur·face of tooth
dis·tal in·ter·pha·lan·ge·al
    joints
dis·ta·lis
dis·tal ra·di·o·ul·nar
    ar·tic·u·la·tion
dis·tal sple·no·re·nal
    shunt
dis·tance
    cep·tor
dis·tance
    fo·cal d.
    in·fi·nite d.
    in·ter·arch d.
    in·ter·oc·clu·sal d.
    in·ter·ridge d.
    large in·ter·arch d.
    pu·pil·lary d.
    re·duced in·ter·arch d.
    small in·ter·arch d.
    so·ci·o·met·ric d.
dis·tant
    flap
dis·tem·per
    vi·rus
dis·ten·si·bil·i·ty
dis·ten·sion

dis·ten·tion
    cyst
    ul·cer
dis·tich·ia
    ac·quired d.
dis·ti·chi·a·sis
dis·till
dis·til·late
dis·til·la·tion
    de·struc·tive d.
    dry d.
    frac·tion·al d.
    mo·lec·u·lar d.
dis·tilled
    wa·ter
dis·to·buc·cal
dis·to·buc·co-oc·clu·sal
dis·to·buc·co·pul·pal
dis·to·cer·vi·cal
dis·to·clu·sal
dis·to·clu·sion
dis·to·gin·gi·val
dis·to·in·ci·sal
dis·to·la·bi·al
dis·to·la·bi·o·pul·pal
dis·to·lin·gual
dis·to·lin·guo-oc·clu·sal
Dis·to·ma
dis·to·ma·to·sis
dis·to·mi·a·sis
    he·mic d.
    pul·mo·nary d.
dis·to·mo·lar
Dis·to·mum
dis·to-oc·clu·sal
dis·to-oc·clu·sion
dis·to·place·ment
dis·to·pul·pal
dis·tor·tion
    par·a·tax·ic d.
dis·tor·tion
    ab·er·ra·tion
dis·to·ver·sion
dis·tract·i·bil·i·ty
dis·trac·tion
    co·nus
dis·tress
    fe·tal d.
dis·trib·ut·ed
    ef·fort
dis·trib·ut·ing
    ar·tery
dis·tri·bu·tion
    co·ef·fi·cient
    curve
    leu·ko·cy·to·sis
    vol·ume

dis·tri·bu·tion
  bi·no·mi·al d.
  count·er·cur·rent d.
  ep·i·de·mi·o·log·i·cal d.
  ex·po·nen·tial d.
  fre·quen·cy d.
  gaus·si·an d.
  nor·mal d.
  Poisson d.
dis·trib·u·tive
  anal·y·sis
dis·tri·chi·a·sis
dis·trix
dis·tur·bance
  emo·tion·al d.
  men·tal d.
  psy·cho·graph·ic d.'s
di·sulf·am·ide
di·sul·fate
di·sul·fide
  bond
di·sul·fi·ram
di·ter·penes
di·thi·az·a·nine io·dide
di·thra·nol
Dittrich's
  plugs
  ste·no·sis
di·u·re·sis
  al·co·hol d.
  os·mot·ic d.
  wa·ter d.
di·u·ret·ic
  car·di·ac d.
  di·rect d.
  in·di·rect d.
  loop d.
di·ur·nal
  per·i·o·dic·i·ty
  rhythm
di·ur·nule
di·va·ga·tion
di·va·lence
di·va·len·cy
di·va·lent
di·val·pro·ex so·di·um
di·var·i·ca·tion
di·ver·gence
  in·suf·fi·cien·cy
di·ver·gence ex·cess
  ex·o·tro·pia
di·ver·gence in·suf·fi·cien·cy
  ex·o·tro·pia
di·ver·gent
  squint
  stra·bis·mus
di·verg·ing
  me·nis·cus

div·ers'
  spec·ta·cles
div·er's
  pa·ral·y·sis
di·ver·tic·u·la
di·ver·tic·u·lar
di·ver·tic·u·lec·to·my
di·ver·tic·u·li·tis
di·ver·tic·u·lo·ma
di·ver·tic·u·lo·pexy
di·ver·tic·u·lo·sis
di·ver·tic·u·lum
  al·lan·to·en·ter·ic d.
  al·lan·to·ic d.
  cer·vi·cal d.
  du·o·de·nal d.
  ep·i·phren·ic d.
  false d.
  Heister's d.
  hy·po·pha·ryn·ge·al d.
  Meckel's d.
  met·a·neph·ric d.
  Nuck's d.
  pan·cre·at·ic di·ver·tic·u·la
  Pertik's d.
  pha·ryn·go·e·soph·a·ge·al d.
  pi·tu·i·tary d.
  pul·sion d.
  Rathke's d.
  thy·ro·glos·sal d.
  thy·roid d.
  trac·tion d.
  true d.
  ure·thral d.
  ven·tric·u·lar d.
  ves·i·cal d.
  Zenker's d.
di·vic·ine
di·vid·ed
  dose
  spec·ta·cles
div·ing
  goi·ter
  re·flex
di·vi·nyl ether
di·vi·sion
  an·te·ri·or pri·mary d.
  cleav·age d.
  con·ju·gate d.
  di·rect nu·cle·ar d.
  equa·tion d.
  in·di·rect nu·cle·ar d.
  mei·ot·ic d.
  mi·tot·ic d.
  mul·ti·pli·ca·tive d.
  pos·te·ri·or pri·mary d.
  re·duc·tion d.
  Remak's nu·cle·ar d.

di·vulse
di·vul·sion
di·vul·sor
di·xyr·a·zine
di·zy·got·ic
  twins
di·zy·gous
diz·zi·ness
djen·kol
  poi·son·ing
djen·kol·ic ac·id
DMF car·ies
  in·dex
dmf car·ies
  in·dex
DMFS car·ies
  in·dex
dmfs car·ies
  in·dex
DNA
  gap
  he·lix
  ho·mol·o·gy
  hy·brid·i·za·tion
  pol·y·mor·phism
  vi·rus
do·bu·ta·mine
d'Ocagne
  nom·o·gram
dock
doc·o·sa·no·ic ac·id
doc·tor
doc·trine
  Arrhenius d.
  hu·mor·al d.
  Monro-Kellie d.
  Monro's d.
doc·u·sate cal·ci·um
doc·u·sate so·di·um
do·de·cane
do·dec·a·no·ic ac·id
do·de·car·bo·ni·um chlo·ride
do·de·cyl
  d. gal·late
  d. sul·fate
Döderlein's
  ba·cil·lus
Doerfler-Stewart
  test
dog
  dis·ease
  nose
  unit
dog dis·tem·per
  vi·rus
Dogiel's
  cells
  cor·pus·cle

Döhle
  bod·ies
  in·clu·sions
dol·i·cho·ce·phal·ic
dol·i·cho·ceph·a·lism
dol·i·cho·ceph·a·lous
dol·i·cho·ceph·a·ly
dol·i·cho·co·lon
dol·i·cho·cra·ni·al
dol·i·cho·ec·tat·ic
  ar·tery
dol·i·cho·fa·cial
dol·i·chol
dol·i·cho·pel·lic
  pel·vis
dol·i·cho·pel·vic
dol·i·cho·pro·sop·ic
dol·i·cho·pro·so·pous
dol·i·cho·sten·o·me·lia
dol·i·cho·u·ran·ic
dol·i·chu·ran·ic
doll's eye
  sign
do·lor
  d. ca·pi·tis
do·lo·rif·ic
do·lo·rim·e·try
do·lo·ro·gen·ic
  zone
do·lor·ol·o·gy
do·mains
Dombrock blood group
dome
  cell
do·mes·tic
  soap
dom·i·cil·i·at·ed
dom·i·nance
  false d.
  d. of genes
  ge·net·ic d.
dom·i·nance
  hi·er·ar·chy
dom·i·nant
  char·ac·ter
  eye
  fre·quen·cy
  gene
  hem·i·sphere
  idea
  in·her·i·tance
  trait
dom·i·nant·ly in·her·it·ed
  Lévi's
  dis·ease
do·mi·phen bro·mide
Donath-Landsteiner
  phe·nom·e·non

Donath-Landsteiner cold
  au·to·an·ti·body
Donders'
  glau·co·ma
  law
  pres·sure
  rings
Don Juan
Donnan
  equi·lib·ri·um
Donné's
  cor·pus·cle
Donohue's
  dis·ease
do·nor
  hy·dro·gen d.
  uni·ver·sal d.
Donovan
  body
don·o·va·no·sis
Doose
  syn·drome
DOPA
Do·pa
do·pa
  re·ac·tion
L-dopa
do·pa·mine
  d. hy·dro·chlo·ride
do·pa·min·er·gic
dope
Doppler
  ech·o·car·di·og·ra·phy
  ef·fect
  phe·nom·e·non
  shift
  ul·tra·so·nog·ra·phy
do·ra·pho·bia
Dorello's
  ca·nal
Dorendorf's
  sign
Dorfman-Chanarin
  syn·drome
dor·nase
  pan·cre·at·ic d.
Dorno
  rays
do·ro·ma·ni·a
dor·sa
dor·sab·dom·i·nal
dor·sad
dor·sal
  ar·tery of clit·o·ris
  ar·tery of foot
  ar·tery of nose
  ar·tery of pe·nis
  col·umn of spi·nal cord

fas·cia of foot
fas·cia of hand
flex·ure
fu·nic·u·lus
horn
mes·o·car·di·um
mus·cles
nerve of clit·o·ris
nerve of pe·nis
nerve of scap·u·la
nerves of toes
nu·cle·us
nu·cle·us of va·gus
pan·cre·as
part of pons
plate of neu·ral tube
po·si·tion
re·flex
root
spine
sur·face of dig·it
sur·face of sa·crum
sur·face of scap·u·la
tu·ber·cle
vein of cor·pus cal·lo·sum
veins of clit·o·ris
veins of pe·nis
ver·te·brae
dor·sal ac·ces·so·ry ol·i·vary
  nu·cle·us
dor·sal cal·lo·sal
  vein
dor·sal car·pal
  lig·a·ment
  net·work
dor·sal car·po·met·a·car·pal
  lig·a·ments
dor·sal col·umn
  stim·u·la·tion
dor·sal cu·boi·de·o·na·vic·u·lar
  lig·a·ment
dor·sal cu·ne·o·cu·boid
  lig·a·ment
dor·sal cu·ne·o·na·vic·u·lar
  lig·a·ments
dor·sal dig·i·tal
  ar·tery
  nerves
  nerves of foot
  veins of toes
dor·sal·gia
dor·sal in·ter·os·se·ous
  ar·tery
  mus·cle of foot
  mus·cle of hand
  nerve
dor·sa·lis

dor·sal lat·er·al cu·ta·ne·ous
  nerve
dor·sal lin·gual
  vein
dor·sal lon·gi·tu·di·nal
  fas·cic·u·lus
dor·sal me·di·al cu·ta·ne·ous
  nerve
dor·sal met·a·car·pal
  ar·tery
  lig·a·ments
  veins
dor·sal met·a·tar·sal
  ar·tery
  lig·a·ments
  veins
dor·sal mo·tor
  nu·cle·us of va·gus
dor·sal pan·cre·at·ic
  ar·tery
dor·sal ra·di·o·car·pal
  lig·a·ment
dor·sal root
  gan·gli·on
dor·sal sa·cro·coc·cyg·e·al
  mus·cle
dor·sal sa·cro·il·i·ac
  lig·a·ments
dor·sal scap·u·lar
  ar·tery
  vein
dor·sal spi·no·cer·e·bel·lar
  tract
dor·sal ta·lo·na·vic·u·lar
  bone
dor·sal teg·men·tal
  de·cus·sa·tion
dor·sal tho·rac·ic
  ar·tery
dor·sal ve·nous
  arch of foot
  net·work of foot
  net·work of hand
dor·sam of foot
  re·flex
Dorset's cul·ture egg
  me·di·um
dor·si
dor·si·duct
dor·si·flex·ion
dor·si·scap·u·lar
dor·si·spi·nal
  veins
dor·so·ceph·a·lad
dor·so·dyn·ia
dor·so·lat·er·al
  fas·cic·u·lus
  tract

dor·so·lum·bar
dor·so·me·di·al
  nu·cle·us
dor·so·me·di·al hy·po·tha·lam·ic
  nu·cle·us
dor·so·sa·cral
  po·si·tion
dor·so·ven·trad
dor·sum
  d. ephi·pii
  d. scap·u·lae
dor·sum pe·dis
  re·flex
dos·age
dose
  ab·sorbed d.
  air d.
  boost·er d.
  cu·mu·la·tive d.
  cur·a·tive d.
  dai·ly d.
  depth d.
  di·vid·ed d.
  ef·fec·tive d.
  ep·i·la·tion d.
  equi·an·al·ge·sic d.
  er·y·the·ma d.
  ex·it d.
  frac·tion·al d.
  in·i·tial d.
  L d.'s
  L$^+$ d.
  L$_+$ d.
  L$_f$ d.
  L$_r$ d.
  L$_o$ d.
  le·thal d.
  Lf d.
  Lo d.
  load·ing d.
  Lr d.
  main·te·nance d.
  max·i·mal d.
  max·i·mal per·mis·si·ble d.
  min·i·mal d.
  min·i·mal in·fect·ing d.
  min·i·mal le·thal d.
  min·i·mal re·act·ing d.
  op·ti·mum d.
  pre·ven·tive d.
  sen·si·tiz·ing d.
  shock·ing d.
  skin d.
  tis·sue cul·ture in·fec·tious
    d.
  tol·er·ance d.

dose-re·sponse
  curve
do·sim·e·try
  ther·mo·lu·mi·nes·cence d.
  x-ray d.
dot
  Gunn's d.'s
  Horner-Trantas d.'s
  Maurer's d.'s
  Schüffner's d.'s
  Trantas' d.'s
  Ziemann's d.'s
dot·age
dot·ard·ness
dot·ted
  tongue
dou·ble
  ath·e·to·sis
  bind
  bond
  chin
  con·scious·ness
  en·ter·os·to·my
  frac·ture
  he·lix
  hem·i·ple·gia
  im·mu·no·dif·fu·sion
  in·tus·sus·cep·tion
  pe·nis
  pneu·mo·nia
  pro·duct
  pro·tru·sion
  quar·tan
  re·frac·tion
  salt
  stain
  tach·y·car·dia
  ter·tian
  vi·sion
dou·ble an·ti·body
  im·mu·no·as·say
  meth·od
  pre·cip·i·ta·tion
dou·ble an·ti·body sand·wich
  as·say
dou·ble aor·tic
  ste·no·sis
dou·ble back
  cross
dou·ble blind
  ex·per·i·ment
  study
dou·ble-chan·nel
  cath·e·ter
dou·ble com·part·ment
  hy·dro·ceph·a·lus
dou·ble con·cave
  lens

dou·ble con·gen·i·tal
  ath·e·to·sis
dou·ble con·trast
  en·e·ma
dou·ble con·vex
  lens
dou·ble flap
  am·pu·ta·tion
dou·ble (gel) dif·fu·sion pre·cip·i·tin
  test in one di·men·sion
  test in two di·men·sions
dou·ble loop
  her·nia
dou·ble-masked
  ex·per·i·ment
dou·ble-mouthed
  uter·us
dou·ble ped·i·cle
  flap
dou·ble-point
  thresh·old
dou·ble quo·tid·i·an
  fe·ver
dou·ble-shock
  sound
dou·blet
  Wollaston's d.
dou·ble ter·tian
  ma·lar·ia
dou·bly
  het·er·o·zy·gous
dou·bly armed
  su·ture
douche
  bath
Douglas
  ab·scess
  bag
  graft
  mech·a·nism
Douglas'
  cul-de-sac
  fold
  line
  pouch
Douglas' spon·ta·ne·ous
  ev·o·lu·tion
dou·rine
dous·ing
  bath
dove·tail
dow·el
down
  ma·lig·nant d.
down·beat
  nys·tag·mus

Downey
cell
down-reg·u·la·tion
Downs'
anal·y·sis
Down's
syn·drome
down·ward
drain·age
dox·a·pram hy·dro·chlo·ride
dox·e·pin hy·dro·chlo·ride
dox·o·ru·bi·cin
dox·y·cy·cline
dox·yl·a·mine suc·ci·nate
Doyère's
em·i·nence
Doyle's
op·er·a·tion
Doyne's gut·tate
iri·tis
Doyne's hon·ey·comb
cho·roi·dop·a·thy
DPNH → **al·de·hyde trans·hy·**
dro·gen·ase
drachm
drac·on·ti·a·sis
dra·cun·cu·li·a·sis
dra·cun·cu·lo·sis
Dra·cun·cu·lus
D. loa
D. me·di·nen·sis
D. oc·u·li
D. per·sa·rum
draft
drag
sol·vent d.
dra·gée
Dragendorff's
test
Dräger
res·pi·rom·e·ter
drain
cig·a·rette d.
Mikulicz' d.
Penrose d.
stab d.
sump d.
drain·age
cap·il·lary d.
closed d.
de·pen·dent d.
down·ward d.
in·fu·sion-as·pi·ra·tion d.
open d.
pos·tur·al d.
suc·tion d.
through d.

tid·al d.
Wangensteen d.
drain·age
tube
drain-trap
stom·ach
dram
drape
Draper's
law
drap·e·to·ma·nia
draught
draw·er
sign
test
draw-sheet
dream
anx·i·e·ty d.
wet d.
dream
as·so·ci·a·tions
pain
dream-work
dreamy
state
Drechs·lera
drench
drep·a·nid·i·um
drep·a·no·cyte
drep·a·no·cy·the·mia
drep·a·no·cyt·ic
drep·a·no·cy·to·sis
dress·er
dress·ing
ad·he·sive ab·sor·bent d.
an·ti·sep·tic d.
bo·lus d.
dry d.
fixed d.
Lister's d.
oc·clu·sive d.
pres·sure d.
tie-o·ver d.
wa·ter d.
dress·ing
for·ceps
Dressler
beat
Dressler's
syn·drome
Drew-Smythe
cath·e·ter
Dreyer's
for·mu·la
drib·ble
dried
al·um
fer·rous sul·fate

mag·ne·si·um sul·fate
yeast
dried hu·man
al·bu·min
se·rum
dried hu·man plas·ma pro·tein
frac·tion
drift
move·ments
drift
an·ti·gen·ic d.
ge·net·ic d.
drift·ing
drifts
Drigalski-Conradi
agar
drill
bur d.
den·tal d.
Drinker
res·pi·ra·tor
drip
phleb·o·cly·sis
trans·fu·sion
drip
al·ka·line milk d.
in·tra·ve·nous d.
Murphy d.
post·na·sal d.
drip-suck
ir·ri·ga·tion
drive
ac·quired d.'s
ex·plor·a·to·ry d.
ki·net·ic d.
learned d.
mei·ot·ic d.
phys·i·o·log·i·cal d.'s
pri·mary d.'s
sec·on·dary d.'s
driv·er's
thigh
driv·ing
pho·tic d.
drom·ic
drom·o·graph
drom·o·ma·nia
dro·mo·stan·o·lone pro·pi·o·nate
dro·mo·tro·pic
neg·a·tive·ly d.
pos·i·tive·ly d.
dro·nab·i·nol
drop
hang·ing d.
drop
at·tack
fin·ger

foot
hand
heart
drop·a·cism
dro·per·i·dol
drop·let
in·fec·tion
nu·clei
dropped
beat
drop·per
drops
eye d.
knock-out d.
stom·ach d.
drop·si·cal
drop·sy
ab·dom·i·nal d.
ep·i·dem·ic d.
drows·i·ness
drug
crude d.
or·phan d.'s
rec·re·a·tion·al d.
sched·uled d.
drug
abuse
al·ler·gy
erup·tion
path·o·gen·e·sis
psy·cho·sis
rash
tet·a·nus
drug-fast
drug·gist
drug-in·duced
dis·ease
hep·a·ti·tis
drug in·ter·ac·tions
drum
mem·brane
drum·head
Drummond's
sign
drum·stick
ap·pend·age
fin·gers
drunk·en·ness
sleep d.
dru·sen
gi·ant d.
d. of op·tic disk
op·tic nerve d.
dry
ab·scess
am·pu·ta·tion
ber·i·beri
bron·chi·ec·ta·sis

dry *(continued)*
  cup
  dis·til·la·tion
  dress·ing
  gan·grene
  her·nia
  la·bor
  lep·ro·sy
  pack
  pleu·ri·sy
  rale
  sock·et
  syn·o·vi·tis
  tet·ter
  vom·it·ing
dry cu·ta·ne·ous
  leish·man·i·a·sis
dry eye
  syn·drome
dry ice
D-S
  test
DT-di·aph·o·rase
du·al
  per·son·al·i·ty
du·al·ism
Duane's
  syn·drome
Dubini's
  dis·ease
Dubin-Johnson
  syn·drome
DuBois'
  for·mu·la
Dubois'
  ab·scess·es
  dis·ease
du·boi·sine
Du Bois-Reymond's
  law
Duboscq's
  col·or·im·e·ter
Dubowitz
  score
Dubreuil-Chambardel
  syn·drome
Duchenne-Aran
  dis·ease
Duchenne-Erb
  pa·ral·y·sis
Duchenne's
  dis·ease
  dys·tro·phy
  pa·ral·y·sis
  sign
  syn·drome
duck
  plague

duck·bill
  spec·u·lum
duck em·bryo or·i·gin
  vac·cine
duck hep·a·ti·tis
  vi·rus
duck in·flu·en·za
  vi·rus
duck plague
  vi·rus
Duckworth's
  phe·nom·e·non
Ducrey
  test
Ducrey's
  ba·cil·lus
duct
  car·ci·no·ma
  pap·il·lo·ma
duct
  ab·er·rant d.
  ab·er·rant bile d.'s
  ac·ces·so·ry pan·cre·at·ic d.
  al·ve·o·lar d.
  am·ni·ot·ic d.
  anal d.'s
  ar·te·ri·al d.
  Bartholin's d.
  Bellini's d.'s
  Bernard's d.
  bile d.
  bil·i·ary d.
  Blasius' d.
  Botallo's d.
  bran·chi·al d.
  buc·co·neu·ral d.
  d. of bul·bo·u·re·thral
    gland
  can·a·lic·u·lar d.'s
  ca·rot·id d.
  cer·vi·cal d.
  cho·le·doch d.
  co·chle·ar d.
  com·mon bile d.
  com·mon he·pa·tic d.
  cra·ni·o·pha·ryn·ge·al d.
  Cuvier's d.'s
  cys·tic d.
  cys·tic gall d.
  def·er·ent d.
  ef·fer·ent d.
  ejac·u·la·to·ry d.
  en·do·lym·phat·ic d.
  d. of ep·i·did·y·mis
  ex·cre·to·ry d.
  ex·cre·to·ry d. of sem·i·nal
    ves·i·cle
  fron·to·na·sal d.

gal·ac·toph·o·rous d.'s
gall d.
Gartner's d.
gen·i·tal d.
gut·tur·al d.
hem·i·tho·rac·ic d.
Hensen's d.
he·pa·tic d.
he·pa·to·cys·tic d.
Hoffmann's d.
hy·po·phy·si·al d.
in·ci·sive d.
in·ter·ca·lat·ed d.'s
in·ter·lo·bar d.
in·ter·lob·u·lar d.
in·tra·lob·u·lar d.
jug·u·lar d.
lac·ri·mal d.
lac·tif·er·ous d.'s
left d. of cau·date lobe
left he·pa·tic d.
lon·gi·tu·di·nal d. of ep·o·
  oph·o·ron
Luschka's d.'s
lym·phat·ic d.
ma·jor sub·lin·gual d.
mam·il·lary d.'s
mam·ma·ry d.'s
mes·o·neph·ric d.
met·a·neph·ric d.
milk d.'s
mi·nor sub·lin·gual d.'s
mül·le·ri·an d.
Müller's d.
na·sal d.
na·so·lac·ri·mal d.
neph·ric d.
om·pha·lo·mes·en·ter·ic d.
pan·cre·at·ic d.
pap·il·lary d.'s
par·a·mes·o·neph·ric d.
par·a·u·re·thral d.'s
pa·rot·id d.
Pecquet's d.
per·i·lym·phat·ic d.
pha·ryn·go·bran·chi·al d.'s
pro·neph·ric d.
pros·tat·ic d.'s
right d. of cau·date lobe
right he·pa·tic d.
right lym·phat·ic d.
Rivinus' d.'s
sal·i·vary d.
Santorini's d.
Schüller's d.'s
se·cre·to·ry d.
sem·i·cir·cu·lar d.'s
sem·i·nal d.

d.'s of Skene's glands
sper·mat·ic d.
Steno's d.
Stensen's d.
stri·at·ed d.
sub·cla·vi·an d.
sub·man·dib·u·lar d.
sub·max·il·lary d.
su·do·rif·er·ous d.
sweat d.
tes·tic·u·lar d.
tho·rac·ic d.
thy·ro·glos·sal d.
thy·ro·lin·gual d.
unit·ing d.
utric·u·lo·sac·cu·lar d.
vi·tel·line d.
vi·tel·lo·in·tes·tin·al d.
Walther's d.'s
Wharton's d.
Wirsung's d.
wolff·i·an d.
duc·tal
  car·ci·no·ma
  hy·per·pla·sia
duc·tile
duc·tion
  F d.
  forced d.
  pas·sive d.
duct·less
  glands
duc·tu·lar
duc·tule
  ab·er·rant d.
  bil·i·ary d.'s
  ex·cre·to·ry d.'s of lac·ri·
    mal gland
  in·ter·lob·u·lar d.'s
  pros·tat·ic d.'s
  trans·verse d.'s of ep·o·
    oph·o·ron
duc·tu·li
duc·tu·lus
  duc·tu·li pa·ro·o·pho·ri
duc·tus
  d. aber·rans
  d. bil·i·fe·ri
  d. ca·ro·ti·cus
  d. dor·so·pan·cre·a·ti·cus
  d. ex·cre·to·ri·us
  d. hem·i·tho·ra·ci·cus
  d. lin·gua·lis
  d. om·pha·lo·me·sen·te·ri·
    cus
  pa·tent d. ar·te·ri·o·sus
  d. pha·ryn·go·bran·chi·a·lis
    III

duc·tus *(continued)*
 d. pha·ryn·go·bran·chi·a·lis IV
 d. pros·ta·ti·ci
 d. sub·max·il·la·ris
 d. su·do·ri·fe·rus
 d. thy·ro·glos·sus
 d. ve·no·sus aran·tii
duc·tus
Duddell's
 mem·brane
Duffy
 an·ti·gens
Duffy blood group
Dugas'
 test
Duhring's
 dis·ease
Dührssen's
 in·ci·sions
Dukes
 clas·si·fi·ca·tion
Dukes'
 dis·ease
dul·cin
dul·cite
dul·ci·tol
dul·cose
dull
dull·ness
 shift·ing d.
dul·ness
Dulong-Petit
 law
du·mas
dumb
 ra·bies
dumb·bell
 gan·glio·neu·ro·ma
Dum·dum
 fe·ver
dum·my
 con·sul·tand
Dumontpallier's
 pes·sa·ry
dump·ing
 syn·drome
Duncan's
 dis·ease
 folds
 mech·a·nism
 ven·tri·cle
du·o·crin·in
du·o·de·na
du·o·de·nal
 am·pul·la
 bulb
 cap

di·ver·tic·u·lum
fis·tu·la
fos·sae
glands
im·pres·sion
smear
sphinc·ter
du·o·de·nec·to·my
du·o·de·ni
du·o·de·ni·tis
du·o·de·no·cho·lan·gi·tis
du·o·de·no·cho·le·cys·tos·to·my
du·o·de·no·cho·led·o·chot·o·my
du·o·de·no·cys·tos·to·my
du·o·de·no·en·ter·os·to·my
du·o·de·no·je·ju·nal
 an·gle
 flex·ure
 fold
 fos·sa
 her·nia
 re·cess
 sphinc·ter
du·o·de·no·je·ju·nos·to·my
du·o·de·nol·y·sis
du·o·de·no·mes·o·col·ic
 fold
du·o··de·no·re·nal
 lig·a·ment
du·o·de·nor·rha·phy
du·o·de·nos·co·py
du·o·de·nos·to·my
du·o·de·not·o·my
du·o·de·num
du·o·vi·rus
Duplay's
 dis·ease
du·plex
 kid·ney
 trans·mis·sion
 uter·us
du·pli·ca·tion
 cyst
du·pli·ca·tion
 d. of chro·mo·somes
du·plic·i·tas
 d. an·te·ri·or
 d. pos·te·ri·or
du·plic·i·ty
 the·o·ry of vi·sion
Dupré's
 mus·cle
Dupuy-Dutemps
 op·er·a·tion
Dupuytren's
 am·pu·ta·tion
 ca·nal
 con·trac·ture

dis·ease of the foot
fas·cia
frac·ture
hy·dro·cele
sign
su·ture
tour·ni·quet
du·ra
du·ral
sheath
si·nus·es
du·ral·u·min
du·ra mat·er
d. m. of the brain
d. m. of the spi·nal cord
du·ra·ma·tral
Duran-Reynals per·me·a·bil·i·ty
fac·tor
Duran-Reynals spread·ing
fac·tor
du·ra·plas·ty
du·ra·tion
half am·pli·tude pulse d.
pulse d.
du·ra·tion
tet·a·ny
Dürck's
nodes
Duret's
le·sion
Durham
rule
Durham's
tube
Duroziez'
dis·ease
mur·mur
symp·tom
dust
ball
cell
cor·pus·cles
Dutch
cap
Dutton's
dis·ease
Dutton's re·laps·ing
fe·ver
Duverney's
fis·sures
fo·ra·men
gland
mus·cle
dwarf
pel·vis
dwarfed
enam·el
dwarf·ish·ness

dwarf·ism
achon·dro·plas·tic d.
ac·ro·mel·ic d.
aor·tic d.
asex·u·al d.
atel·i·ot·ic d.
camp·to·mel·ic d.
chon·dro·dys·tro·phic d.
di·a·stroph·ic d.
Fröhlich's d.
hy·po·thy·roid d.
id·i·o·path·ic d.
in·fan·tile d.
Laron type d.
le·thal d.
Lorain-Lévi d.
mes·o·mel·ic d.
met·a·tro·pic d.
mi·cro·mel·ic d.
pho·co·me·lic d.
phys·i·o·log·ic d.
pi·tu·i·tary d.
pol·y·dys·tro·phic d.
pri·mor·di·al d.
Seckel d.
se·nile d.
sex·u·al d.
Silver-Russell d.
snub-nose d.
than·a·to·phor·ic d.
true d.
dy·ad
dy·ad·ic
psy·cho·ther·a·py
sym·bi·o·sis
dy·clo·nine hy·dro·chlo·ride
dy·dro·ges·ter·one
dye
aci·dic d.'s
ac·ri·dine d.'s
azin d.'s
azo d.'s
az·o·car·mine d.'s
ba·sic d.'s
di·phen·yl·meth·ane d.'s
ke·ton·i·mine d.'s
nat·u·ral d.'s
ni·tro d.'s
ox·a·zin d.'s
ros·an·i·lin d.'s
salt d.
syn·thet·ic d.'s
thi·a·zin d.'s
tri·phen·yl·meth·ane d.'s
xan·thene d.'s
dye-di·lu·tion
curve

dye ex·clu·sion
test
Dyggve-Melchior-Clausen
syn·drome
dy·nam·ic
aor·ta
com·pli·ance of lung
de·mog·ra·phy
dis·ease
equi·lib·ri·um
force
fric·tion
il·e·us
mur·mur
psy·chi·a·try
psy·chol·o·gy
psy·cho·ther·a·py
rays
re·frac·tion
re·la·tions
splint
vis·cos·i·ty
dy·nam·ics
group d.
dy·na·mo·gen·e·sis
dy·na·mo·gen·ic
dy·na·mog·e·ny
dy·nam·o·graph
dy·na·mom·e·ter
dy·nam·o·scope
dy·na·mos·co·py
dy·na·therm
dyne
dyn·ein
arm
dy·phyl·line
dys·a·cou·sia
dys·a·cu·sia
dys·a·cu·sis
dys·ad·ap·ta·tion
dys·an·ti·graph·ia
dys·a·phia
dys·a·phic
dys·ap·ta·tion
dys·ar·te·ri·ot·o·ny
dys·ar·thria
d. li·te·ra·lis
d. syl·la·ba·ris spas·mo·di·ca
dys·ar·thric
dys·ar·thro·sis
dys·au·to·no·mia
fa·mil·i·al d.
dys·ba·rism
dys·ba·sia
d. an·gi·o·scle·ro·ti·ca
d. an·gi·o·spas·ti·ca
d. lor·do·ti·ca pro·gres·si·va

dys·bo·lism
dys·bu·lia
dys·bu·lic
dys·cal·cu·lia
dys·ce·pha·lia
d. man·di·bu·lo-oc·u·lo·fa·ci·a·lis
dys·ceph·a·ly
dys·chei·ral
dys·chei·ria
dys·che·zia
dys·chi·ral
dys·chi·ria
dys·chon·dro·gen·e·sis
dys·chon·dro·pla·sia
d. with he·man·gi·o·mas
dys·chon·dros·te·o·sis
dys·chroa
dys·chroia
dys·chro·ma·top·sia
dys·chro·ma·to·sis
dys·chro·mia
dys·ci·ne·sia
dys·coi·me·sis
dys·con·ju·gate
gaze
dys·con·trol
dys·co·ria
dys·cra·sia
blood d.
dys·cra·sic
frac·ture
dys·crat·ic
dys·di·ad·o·cho·ci·ne·sia
dys·di·ad·o·cho·ki·ne·sia
dys·em·bry·o·ma
dys·em·bry·o·pla·sia
dys·e·mia
dys·en·ce·pha·lia splanch·no·cys·ti·ca
dys·e·neia
dys·en·ter·ic
di·ar·rhea
dys·en·ter·ic al·gid
ma·lar·ia
dys·en·tery
an·ti·tox·in
ba·cil·lus
dys·en·tery
ame·bic d.
bac·il·la·ry d.
bal·an·tid·i·al d.
bil·har·zi·al d.
chron·ic d. of cat·tle
ful·mi·nat·ing d.
hel·min·thic d.
Jap·a·nese d.
lamb d.

ma·lig·nant d.
Sonne d.
spi·ril·lar d.
swine d.
vi·ral d.
win·ter d. of cat·tle
dys·er·e·thism
dys·er·gia
dys·es·the·sia
dys·fi·brin·o·ge·ne·mia
dys·func·tion
con·sti·tu·tion·al he·pa·tic d.
den·tal d.
min·i·mal brain d.
pap·il·lary mus·cle d.
psy·cho·sex·u·al d.
sex·u·al d.
tem·po·ro·man·dib·u·lar joint d.
dys·func·tion·al uter·ine
bleed·ing
dys·gam·ma·glob·u·lin·e·mia
dys·gen·e·sis
go·nad·al d.
ir·i·do·cor·ne·al mes·o·der·mal d.
sem·i·nif·er·ous tu·bule d.
tes·tic·u·lar d.
XO go·nad·al d.
XX go·nad·al d.
XY go·nad·al d.
dys·gen·ic
dys·ger·mi·no·ma
dys·geu·sia
dys·gna·thia
dys·gnath·ic
dys·gno·sia
dys·gon·ic
dys·gran·u·lar
cor·tex
dys·graph·ia
dys·har·mo·ni·ous
cor·re·spon·dence
dys·hem·a·to·poi·e·sis
dys·hem·a·to·poi·et·ic
dys·he·mo·poi·e·sis
dys·he·mo·poi·et·ic
ane·mia
dys·hid·ria
dys·hi·dro·sis
dys·id·ria
dys·i·dro·sis
dys·junc·tive
nys·tag·mus
dys·kar·y·o·sis
dys·kar·y·ot·ic

dys·ker·a·to·ma
warty d.
dys·ker·a·to·sis
be·nign d.
d. con·gen·i·ta
in·tra·ep·i·the·li·al d.
iso·lat·ed d. fol·lic·u·la·ris
ma·lig·nant d.
dys·ker·a·tot·ic
dys·ki·ne·sia
d. al·ge·ra
bil·i·ary d.
ex·tra·py·ram·i·dal d.'s
d. in·ter·mit·tens
tar·dive oral d.
tra·che·o·bron·chi·al d.
dys·ki·net·ic
dys·la·lia
dys·lex·ia
dys·lex·ic
dys·lip·i·do·sis
dys·lo·gia
dys·ma·se·sis
dys·ma·ture
dys·ma·tu·ri·ty
dys·meg·a·lop·sia
dys·me·lia
dys·men·or·rhea
es·sen·tial d.
func·tion·al d.
in·trin·sic d.
me·chan·i·cal d.
mem·bra·nous d.
ob·struc·tive d.
ovar·i·an d.
pri·mary d.
sec·on·dary d.
spas·mod·ic d.
tub·al d.
ure·ter·ic d.
uter·ine d.
vag·i·nal d.
dys·men·or·rhe·al
mem·brane
dys·met·ria
oc·u·lar d.
dys·mim·ia
dys·mne·sia
dys·mne·sic
psy·cho·sis
syn·drome
dys·mor·phia
man·dib·u·lo·oc·u·lo·fa·cial d.
dys·mor·phism
dys·mor·pho·gen·e·sis
dys·mor·phol·o·gy
dys·mor·pho·pho·bia

dys·my·e·li·na·tion
dys·my·o·to·nia
dys·nys·tax·is
dys·o·don·ti·a·sis
dys·on·to·gen·e·sis
dys·on·to·ge·net·ic
dys·o·rex·ia
dys·or·ic
  ret·i·nop·a·thy
dys·os·mia
dys·os·te·o·gen·e·sis
dys·os·to·sis
  ac·ro·fa·cial d.
  clei·do·cra·ni·al d.
  cli·do·cra·ni·al d.
  cra·ni·o·fa·cial d.
  man·dib·u·lo·ac·ral d.
  man·dib·u·lo·fa·cial d.
  met·a·phy·si·al d.
  d. mul·ti·plex
  or·o·dig·i·to·fa·cial d.
  oto·man·dib·u·lar d.
  pe·riph·e·ral d.
dys·pal·lia
dys·pa·reu·nia
dys·pep·sia
  ac·id d.
  ad·he·sion d.
  aton·ic d.
  fer·ment·a·tive d.
  flat·u·lent d.
  func·tion·al d.
  ner·vous d.
  re·flex d.
dys·pep·tic
dys·pha·gia
  d. lu·so·ria
  d. ner·vo·sa
  ner·vous d.
  sid·er·o·pe·nic d.
  val·lec·u·lar d.
dys·pha·go·cy·to·sis
  con·gen·i·tal d.
dys·pha·gy
dys·pha·sia
dys·phe·mia
dys·pho·nia
  d. pli·cae ven·tric·u·lar·is
  d. pu·be·rum
  d. spas·ti·ca
dys·pho·ria
dys·phra·sia
dys·phy·lax·ia
dys·pig·men·ta·tion
dys·pin·e·al·ism
dys·pi·tu·i·tar·ism

dys·pla·sia
  an·hi·drot·ic ec·to·der·mal d.
  an·ter·o·fa·cial d.
  an·ter·o·pos·te·ri·or d.
  an·ter·o·pos·te·ri·or fa·cial d.
  as·phyx·i·at·ing tho·rac·ic d.
  atri·o·dig·i·tal d.
  bron·cho·pul·mo·nary d.
  ce·ment·al d.
  ce·re·bral d.
  cer·vi·cal d.
  chon·dro·ec·to·der·mal d.
  clei·do·cra·ni·al d.
  cli·do·cra·ni·al d.
  con·gen·i·tal ec·to·der·mal d.
  cra·ni·o·car·po·tar·sal d.
  cra·ni·o·di·a·phys·i·al d.
  cra·ni·o·met·a·phy·si·al d.
  den·tin d.
  di·a·phys·i·al d.
  ec·to·der·mal d.
  enam·el d.
  en·ceph·a·lo-oph·thal·mic d.
  d. ep·i·phys·i·a·lis hem·i·me·lia
  d. ep·i·phys·i·a·lis mul·ti·plex
  d. ep·i·phys·i·a·lis punc·ta·ta
  ep·i·the·li·al d.
  fa·ci·o·dig·i·to·gen·i·tal d.
  fa·mil·i·al fi·brous d. of jaws
  fa·mil·i·al white fold·ed d.
  fi·bro·mus·cu·lar d.
  fi·brous d.
  fi·brous d. of bone
  flor·id os·se·ous d.
  he·red·i·tary re·nal-ret·i·nal d.
  hi·drot·ic ec·to·der·mal d.
  hy·po·hi·drot·ic ec·to·der·mal d.
  lym·pho·pe·nic thy·mic d.
  mam·ma·ry d.
  man·dib·u·lo·fa·cial d.
  met·a·phy·si·al d.
  Mondini d.
  mon·o·stot·ic fi·brous d.
  mu·co·ep·i·the·li·al d.
  mul·ti·ple ep·i·phys·i·al d.
  OAV d.
  oc·u·lo·au·ric·u·lo·ver·te·bral d.

oc·u·lo·den·to·dig·i·tal d.
oc·u·lo·ver·te·bral d.
ODD d.
odon·to·gen·ic d.
OMM d.
oph·thal·mo·man·dib·u·lo·mel·ic d.
per·i·ap·i·cal ce·ment·al d.
pol·y·os·tot·ic fi·brous d.
pseu·do··a·chon·dro·plas·tic spon·dy·lo·ep·i·phys·i·al d.
ret·i·nal d.
sep·to-op·tic d.
spon·dy·lo·ep·i·phys·i·al d.
ven·tric·u·lo·ra·di·al d.
dys·plas·tic
ne·vus
dys·plas·tic ne·vus
syn·drome
dysp·nea
par·ox·ys·mal noc·tur·nal d.
Traube's d.
dysp·ne·ic
dys·prax·ia
dys·pro·si·um
dys·pro·tein·e·mia
dys·pro·tein·e·mic
ret·i·nop·a·thy
dys·raph·ia
dys·ra·phism
dys·rhyth·mia
car·di·ac d.
elec·tro·en·ceph·a·lo·graph·ic d.
par·ox·ys·mal ce·re·bral d.
dys·se·ba·cia
dys·som·nia
dys·sper·mat·o·gen·ic
ste·ril·i·ty
dys·spon·dy·lism
dys·sta·sia
dys·stat·ic
dys·syl·la·bia
dys·syn·er·gia
d. ce·re·bel·la·ris my·o·clo·ni·ca
d. ce·re·bel·la·ris pro·gres·si·va
de·tru·sor sphinc·ter d.
dys·tax·ia
dys·tel·e·pha·lan·gy
dys·thy·mia
dys·thy·mic
dis·or·der
dys·thy·roi·dal
in·fan·ti·lism

dys·to·cia
fe·tal d.
ma·ter·nal d.
pla·cen·tal d.
dys·to·nia
d. len·tic·u·lar·is
d. mus·cu·lo·rum de·for·mans
tor·sion d.
dys·ton·ic
re·ac·tion
tor·ti·col·lis
dys·to·pia
d. can·tho·rum
d. trans·ver·sa ex·ter·na tes·tis
d. trans·ver·sa in·ter·na tes·tis
dys·top·ic
dys·tro·phia
d. ad·i·po·so·ge·ni·ta·lis
d. brev·i·col·lis
d. my·o·to·ni·ca
d. un·gui·um
dys·tro·phic
cal·ci·fi·ca·tion
cal·ci·no·sis
dys·tro·pho·neu·ro·sis
dys·tro·phy
ad·i·po·so·gen·i·tal d.
adult pseu·do·hy·per·tro·phic mus·cu·lar d.
Barnes' d.
Becker type tar·dive mus·cu·lar d.
child·hood mus·cu·lar d.
cor·ne·al d.
cra·ni·o·car·po·tar·sal d.
Duchenne's d.
en·do·the·li·al d. of cor·nea
ep·i·the·li·al d.
fa·ci·o·scap·u·lo·hu·mer·al mus·cu·lar d.
Favre's d.
fin·ger·print d.
fleck d. of cor·nea
Fuchs' ep·i·the·li·al d.
Groenouw's cor·ne·al d.
gut·ter d. of cor·nea
in·fan·tile neu·ro·ax·o·nal d.
ju·ve·nile ep·i·the·li·al d.
Landouzy-Dejerine d.
lat·tice cor·ne·al d.
Leyden-Möbius mus·cu·lar d.
limb-gir·dle mus·cu·lar d.
map-dot-fin·ger·print d.

dys·tro·phy *(continued)*
Meesman d.
mi·cro·cys·tic ep·i·the·li·al
d.
mus·cu·lar d.
my·o·ton·ic d.
pel·vo·fem·oral mus·cu·lar
d.
pro·gress·ive mus·cu·lar d.
pro·gress·ive ta·pe·to·cho·
roi·dal d.
pseu·do·hy·per·tro·phic
mus·cu·lar d.

re·tic·u·lar d. of cor·nea
ring-like cor·ne·al d.
sym·pa·thet·ic re·flex d.
tho·rac·ic-pel·vic-pha·lan·ge·
al d.
twen·ty-nail d.
vit·re·o-ta·pe·to·ret·i·nal d.
dys·tro·py
dys·u·ria
dys·u·ric
dys·u·ry
dys·ver·sion

Eagle
syn·drome
Eagle's ba·sal
me·di·um
Eagle's min·i·mum es·sen·tial
me·di·um
Eales'
dis·ease
ear
bones
cough
crys·tals
lobe
mange
sign
wax
ear
avi·a·tor's e.
Az·tec e.
Blainville e.'s
box·er's e.
Cagot e.
cau·li·flow·er e.
dar·win·i·an e.
lop e.
Morel's e.
Mozart e.
scroll e.
Stahl's e.
Wildermuth's e.
ear·ache
ear·drum
Earle L
fi·bro·sar·co·ma
Earle's
so·lu·tion
ear·ly
de·cel·er·a·tion
re·ac·tion
ear·ly di·a·stol·ic
mur·mur
ear·ly ne·o·na·tal
death
ear·ly-phase
re·sponse
ear·ly post·trau·mat·ic
ep·i·lep·sy
ear·ly re·cep·tor
po·ten·tial

earth
wax
earth
al·ka·line e.'s
di·a·to·ma·ceous e.
ful·ler's e.
rare e.'s
earth-eat·ing
earthy
wa·ter
ear·wax
East Af·ri·can
try·pan·o·so·mi·a·sis
East Af·ri·can sleep·ing
sick·ness
East Coast
fe·ver
east·ern equine
en·ceph·a·lo·my·e·li·tis
east·ern equine en·ceph·a·lo·my·e·li·tis
vi·rus
eat·ing
ep·i·lep·sy
Eaton
agent
Eaton agent
pneu·mo·nia
Eaton-Lambert
syn·drome
EB
vi·rus
Ebbecke's
re·ac·tion
Ebbinghaus
test
E·ber·thel·la
Eberth's
ba·cil·lus
lines
per·i·the·li·um
Ebner's
glands
re·tic·u·lum
E·bo·la
vi·rus
E·bo·la hem·or·rhag·ic
fe·ver
e·bo·na·tion

317

ébran·le·ment
Ebstein's
  anom·a·ly
  dis·ease
  sign
eb·ul·lism
ebur
  e. den·tis
eb·ur·na·tion
  e. of den·tin
ebur·ne·ous
ebur·ni·tis
écar·teur
ecau·date
ECBO
  vi·rus
ec·bo·line
ec·cen·tric
  am·pu·ta·tion
  fix·a·tion
  hy·per·tro·phy
  im·plan·ta·tion
  oc·clu·sion
  po·si·tion
  re·la·tion
ec·cen·tric in·ter·oc·clu·sal
  rec·ord
ec·cen·tro·chon·dro·pla·sia
ec·cen·tro·pi·e·sis
ec·chon·dro·ma
ec·chon·dro·sis
  e. phy·sa·li·for·mis
  e. phy·sal·i·phora
ec·chon·dro·tome
ec·chy·mo·ma
ec·chy·mosed
ec·chy·mos·es
ec·chy·mo·sis
  Tardieu's ec·chy·mos·es
ec·chy·mot·ic
  mask
ec·crine
  ac·ro·spi·ro·ma
  gland
  po·ro·ma
  spi·rad·e·no·ma
ec·cri·nol·o·gy
ec·cri·sis
ec·crit·ic
ec·cy·e·sis
ec·dem·ic
ec·dys·i·al
  glands
ec·dys·i·asm
ec·dy·sis
ec·go·nine
ech·e·o·sis
Echid·noph·a·ga gal·li·na·cea

echi·nate
Echi·no·chas·mus
echi·no·coc·co·sis
Echi·no·coc·cus
  E. gran·u·lo·sus
  E. mul·ti·lo·cu·la·ris
echi·no·coc·cus
  cyst
echi·no·cyte
echi·no·derm
Echi·no·der·ma·ta
Echi·no·rhyn·chus
ech·i·no·sis
Echi·no·sto·ma
  E. il·o·ca·num
  E. ma·lay·a·num
echi·no·sto·mi·a·sis
echin·u·late
Ech·is
ECHO
  vi·rus
echo
  beat
  re·ac·tion
  speech
ech·o·a·cou·sia
ech·o·a·or·tog·ra·phy
ech·o·car·di·o·gram
ech·o·car·di·o·graph·ic
  dif·fer·en·ti·a·tion
ech·o·car·di·og·ra·phy
  cross-sec·tion·al e.
  Doppler e.
  two-di·men·sion·al e.
ech·o·en·ceph·a·log·ra·phy
echo-free
ech·o·gen·ic
ech·o·gram
ech·o·graph
echog·ra·pher
ech·o·graph·ia
echog·ra·phy
ech·o·ki·ne·sia
ech·o·ki·ne·sis
ech·o·la·lia
ech·o·lo·ca·tion
e·cho·ma·tism
ech·o·mim·ia
ech·o·mo·tism
e·chop·a·thy
ech·o·pho·nia
e·choph·o·ny
ech·o·phot·o·ny
ech·o·phra·sia
ech·o·prax·ia
ech·o·scope
ech·o·thi·o·phate io·dide
ech·o·vi·rus

Eck
  fis·tu·la
Ecker's
  fis·sure
ec·la·bi·um
ec·lamp·sia
  pu·er·per·al e.
  su·per·im·posed e.
ec·lamp·tic
  ret·i·nop·a·thy
ec·lamp·to·gen·ic
ec·lamp·tog·e·nous
ec·lec·tic
eclipse
  am·bly·o·pia
  blind·ness
  pe·ri·od
  phase
ec·mne·sia
ECMO
  vi·rus
ecoid
ec·o·log·i·cal
  ec·to·crine
  sys·tem
e·col·o·gy
  hu·man e.
eco·ma·ni·a
econ·a·zole
econ·o·my
eco·pho·bia
ec·o·spe·cies
ec·o·sys·tem
  par·a·site-host e.
ec·o·tax·is
ec·o·tro·pic
  vi·rus
écou·teur
écou·vil·lon
ec·pho·ria
ec·pho·rize
ec·phy·ma
écra·seur
ECSO
  vi·rus
ec·sta·sy
ec·stat·ic
ec·stro·phe
ec·ta·co·lia
ec·tad
ec·tal
ec·tal or·i·gin
ec·ta·sia
  e. cor·dis
  cor·ne·al e.
  dif·fuse ar·te·ri·al e.
  hy·po·stat·ic e.
  mam·ma·ry duct e.

  pap·il·lary e.
  scle·ral e.
  se·nile e.
  e. ven·tric·u·li par·a·doxa
ec·ta·sis
ec·tat·ic
  an·eu·rysm
ec·tat·ic mar·gi·nal
  de·gen·er·a·tion of cor·nea
ec·ten·tal
ECTEOLA-cel·lu·lose
ect·eth·moid
ec·thy·ma
  con·ta·gious e.
  e. gan·gre·no·sum
ec·thy·mat·i·form
ec·thym·a·tous
  syph·i·lid
ec·thy·mi·form
ec·ti·ris
ec·to·an·ti·gen
ec·to·blast
ec·to·car·dia
ec·to·car·di·ac
ec·to·car·di·al
ec·to·cer·vi·cal
  smear
ec·to·cho·roi·dea
ec·to·cor·nea
ec·to·crine
  ec·o·log·i·cal e.
ec·to·cyst
ec·to·derm
  ep·i·the·li·al e.
  su·per·fi·cial e.
ec·to·der·mal
  clo·a·ca
  dys·pla·sia
ec·to·der·ma·to·sis
ec·to·der·mic
ec·to·der·mo·sis
  e. ero·si·va plu·ri·o·ri·fi·ci·
    a·lis
ec·to·en·tad
ec·to·en·tal
ec·to·en·zyme
ec·to·eth·moid
ec·to·gen·ic
  ter·a·to·sis
ec·tog·e·nous
ec·to·glob·u·lar
ec·to·hor·mone
ec·to·me·ninx
ec·to·mere
ec·to·me·rog·o·ny
ec·to·mes·en·chyme
ec·to·morph
ec·to·mor·phic

ec·top·a·gus
ec·to·par·a·site
ec·to·par·a·sit·i·cide
ec·to·par·a·sit·ism
ec·to·per·i·to·ni·tis
ec·to·phyte
ec·to·pia
  e. clo·a·cae
  e. cor·dis
  e. len·tis
  e. mac·u·lae
  e. pu·pil·lae con·gen·i·ta
  e. re·nis
  e. tes·tis
  e. ve·si·cae
ec·top·ic
  beat
  de·cid·ua
  eye·lash
  hor·mone
  im·pulse
  pace·mak·er
  pin·e·a·lo·ma
  preg·nan·cy
  rhythm
  schis·to·so·mi·a·sis
  tach·y·car·dia
  ter·a·to·sis
  tes·tis
ec·top·ic ACTH
  syn·drome
ec·to·pla·cen·tal
  cav·i·ty
ec·to·plasm
ec·to·plas·mat·ic
ec·to·py
ec·to·ret·i·na
ec·to·sarc
ec·tos·co·py
ec·tos·te·al
ec·tos·to·sis
ec·to·thrix
ec·to·tox·in
ec·to·troph·o·blas·tic
  cav·i·ty
ec·to·zo·on
ec·tro·chei·ry
ec·tro·chi·ry
ec·tro·dac·tyl·ia
ec·tro·dac·tyl·ism
ec·tro·dac·ty·ly
ec·tro·gen·ic
ec·trog·e·ny
ec·tro·me·lia
  vi·rus
ec·tro·mel·ic
ec·tro·pi·on
  aton·ic e.

  cic·a·tri·cial e.
  flac·cid e.
  par·a·lyt·ic e.
  spas·tic e.
  e. uve·ae
ec·tro·pi·um
ec·trop·o·dy
ec·tro·syn·dac·ty·ly
ec·trot·ic
ec·tyl·u·rea
ec·type
ec·u·re·sis
ec·ze·ma
  al·ler·gic e.
  atop·ic e.
  bak·er's e.
  chron·ic e.
  e. cra·que·lé
  e. di·a·be·ti·co·rum
  e. ep·i·lans
  e. er·y·the·ma·to·sum
  fa·cial e.
  flex·ur·al e.
  hand e.
  e. her·pe·ti·cum
  e. hy·per·tro·phi·cum
  in·fan·tile e.
  e. in·ter·tri·go
  li·chen·oid e.
  e. ma·di·dans
  e. mar·gi·na·tum
  e. num·mu·la·re
  e. pa·pu·lo·sum
  e. pa·ra·si·ti·cum
  e. pus·tu·lo·sum
  e. ru·brum
  seb·or·rhe·ic e.
  e. squa·mo·sum
  sta·sis e.
  trop·i·cal e.
  e. ty·lo·ti·cum
  e. vac·ci·na·tum
  var·i·cose e.
  e. ver·ru·co·sum
  e. ve·si·cu·lo·sum
  weep·ing e.
  win·ter e.
ec·zem·a·ti·za·tion
ec·ze·ma·toid
  seb·or·rhea
ec·ze·ma·tous
edath·a·mil
ed·dy
  sounds
edea
ede·ma
  an·gi·o·neu·rot·ic e.
  Berlin's e.

blue e.
brain e.
brown e.
bul·lous e.
bul·lous e. ve·si·cae
ca·chec·tic e.
car·di·ac e.
ce·re·bral e.
cir·cum·scribed e.
cys·toid mac·u·lar e.
de·pen·dent e.
ges·ta·tion·al e.
e. glot·ti·dis
heat e.
he·red·i·tary an·gi·o·neu·rot·ic e.
hy·dre·mic e.
in·flam·ma·to·ry e.
lym·phat·ic e.
ma·lig·nant e.
ma·ran·tic e.
men·stru·al e.
e. ne·o·na·to·rum
non·in·flam·ma·to·ry e.
nu·trit·ion·al e.
e. of the op·tic disk
pe·ri·od·ic e.
pit·ting e.
pre·men·stru·al e.
pul·mo·nary e.
Quincke's e.
salt e.
sol·id e.
Yang·tze e.
edem·a·ti·za·tion
edem·a·tous
eden·tate
eden·tu·lous
edes·tin
ed·e·tate
edet·ic ac·id
edge
cut·ting e.
den·ture e.
in·ci·sal e.
lead·ing e.
shear·ing e.
edge-to-edge
bite
oc·clu·sion
edge·wise
ap·pli·ance
Edinger-Westphal
nu·cle·us
edis·y·late
Edlefsen's
re·a·gent

Edman
meth·od
Edman's
re·a·gent
Edridge-Green
lamp
ed·ro·pho·ni·um chlo·ride
ed·u·ca·tion·al
psy·chol·o·gy
educt
edul·co·rant
edul·co·rate
Edwards'
syn·drome
Ed·ward·si·el·la
EEE
vi·rus
EEG
ac·ti·va·tion
ef·fect
ab·sco·pal e.
ad·di·tive e.
af·ter-e.
Arias-Stella e.
au·to·ki·net·ic e.
Bernoulli e.
Bohr e.
clasp-knife e.
Compton e.
Cotton e.
Crabtree e.
cu·mu·la·tive e.
Cushing e.
cy·to·path·ic e.
Doppler e.
elec·tro·phon·ic e.
ex·per·i·ment·er e.'s
Fahraeus-Lindqvist e.
Fenn e.
found·er e.
gene dos·age e.
Haldane e.
Orbeli e.
ox·y·gen e.
Pasteur's e.
pho·tech·ic e.
pho·to·e·lec·tric e.
po·si·tion e.
Raman e.
Rivero-Carvallo e.
Russell e.
sec·ond gas e.
sig·ma e.
Somogyi e.
Staub-Traugott e.
Stiles-Crawford e.
Venturi e.
Vulpian's e.

ef·fect *(continued)*
  Wedensky e.
  Wolff-Chaikoff e.
  Zeeman e.
ef·fec·tive
  con·ju·gate
  dose
  half-life
  tem·per·a·ture
ef·fec·tive os·mot·ic
  pres·sure
ef·fec·tive re·frac·to·ry
  pe·ri·od
ef·fec·tive tem·per·a·ture
  in·dex
ef·fec·tor
  cell
ef·fem·i·na·tion
ef·fer·ent
  gam·ma e.
ef·fer·ent
  duct
  lym·phat·ic
  nerve
  ves·sel
ef·fer·ent glo·mer·u·lar
  ar·te·ri·ole
ef·fer·vesce
ef·fer·ves·cent
  lith·i·um cit·rate
  mag·ne·si·um cit·rate
  mag·ne·si·um sul·fate
  po·tas·si·um cit·rate
  salts
  so·di·um phos·phate
ef·fi·cien·cy
  vi·su·al e.
ef·fleu·rage
ef·flo·resce
ef·flo·res·cent
ef·flu·via
ef·flu·vi·um
  tel·o·gen e.
ef·fort
  dis·trib·ut·ed e.
ef·fort
  syn·drome
  throm·bo·sis
ef·fuse
ef·fu·sion
eflor·ni·thine hy·dro·chlo·ride
eger·sis
eges·ta
egg
  cen·tro·lec·i·thal e.
  ho·mo·lec·i·thal e.
  iso·lec·i·thal e.

mi·cro·lec·i·thal e.
tel·o·lec·i·thal e.
egg
  al·bu·min
  cell
  mem·brane
egg clus·ter
Egger's
  line
Eggleston
  meth·od
egg shell
  nail
egg·shell
egg-white
  in·ju·ry
  syn·drome
egi·lops
eglan·du·lous
Eglis'
  glands
ego
  anal·y·sis
  ide·al
  iden·ti·ty
  in·stincts
ego-al·ien
ego·bron·choph·o·ny
ego·cen·tric
ego·cen·tric·i·ty
ego-dys·ton·ic
  ho·mo·sex·u·al·i·ty
ego·ma·nia
ego·phon·ic
egoph·o·ny
ego-syn·ton·ic
ego·tro·pic
Egyp·tian
  he·ma·tu·ria
  oph·thal·mia
  sple·no·meg·a·ly
Ehlers-Danlos
  syn·drome
Ehrenritter's
  gan·gli·on
Ehret's
  phe·nom·e·non
Ehrlich
  re·ac·tion
Ehr·lich·ia
  E. ca·nis
  E. ris·ti·cii
  E. sen·net·su
ehr·lich·i·o·sis
  ca·nine e.
  equine mon·o·cyt·ic e.
Ehrlich's
  ane·mia

phe·nom·e·non
pos·tu·late
the·o·ry
Ehrlich's ac·id he·ma·tox·y·lin
stain
Ehrlich's an·i·line crys·tal vi·o·let
stain
Ehrlich's benz·al·de·hyde
re·ac·tion
Ehrlich's di·a·zo
re·ac·tion
re·a·gent
Ehrlich's in·ner
body
Ehrlich's side-chain
the·o·ry
Ehrlich's tri·ac·id
stain
Ehrlich's tri·ple
stain
Ehrlich-Türk
line
Eichhorst's
cor·pus·cles
neu·ri·tis
Eicken's
meth·od
ei·co·nom·e·ter
n-**ei·co·sa·no·ic ac·id**
ei·co·sa·noids
ei·det·ic
im·age
ei·dop·tom·e·try
eighth cra·ni·al
nerve
eighth nerve
tu·mor
Ei·ken·el·la cor·ro·dens
ei·ko·nom·e·ter
ei·loid
Ei·me·ria
E. of cat·tle
E. of chick·ens
coc·cid·ia of cat·tle
coc·cid·ia of chick·ens
coc·cid·ia of geese
coc·cid·ia of pheas·ants
coc·cid·ia of rab·bits
coc·cid·ia of sheep and goats
coc·cid·ia of swine
coc·cid·ia of tur·keys
E. of geese
E. of pheas·ants
E. of rab·bits
E. sar·di·nae
E. of sheep and goats

E. of swine
E. of tur·keys
Ei·me·ri·i·dae
Einarson's gal·lo·cy·a·nin-chrome al·um
stain
ein·stein
ein·stein·i·um
Einthoven's
equa·tion
law
tri·an·gle
Eisenlohr's
syn·drome
Eisenmenger
syn·drome
Eisenmenger's
com·plex
dis·ease
te·tral·o·gy
ei·sod·ic
ejac·u·late
ejac·u·la·tio
e. de·fi·ciens
e. pre·cox
e. re·tar·da·ta
ejac·u·la·tion
pre·ma·ture e.
ejac·u·la·to·ry
duct
ejec·ta
ejec·tion
click
frac·tion
frac·tion sys·tol·ic
mur·mur
pe·ri·od
sound
ejec·tor
sa·li·va e.
Ejrup
ma·neu·ver
Ekbom
syn·drome
eki·ri
ek·to·plas·mic
ek·to·plas·tic
elab·o·ra·tion
sec·on·dary e.
Elae·oph·o·ra schnei·deri
el·a·id·ic ac·id
elai·o·path·ia
el·a·pid
Elap·i·dae
elas·mo·branch
elas·tance
elas·tase

elas·tic
  in·ter·max·il·lary e.
  ver·ti·cal e.
elas·tic
  ar·tery
  ban·dage
  bou·gie
  car·ti·lage
  cone
  fi·bers
  la·mel·la
  lam·i·nae of ar·ter·ies
  lay·ers of ar·ter·ies
  lay·ers of cor·nea
  lig·a·ture
  lim·it
  mem·brane
  skin
  tis·sue
elas·ti·ca
elas·tic band
  fix·a·tion
elas·ti·cin
elas·tic·i·ty
  phys·i·cal e. of mus·cle
  phys·i·o·log·ic e. of mus·cle
  to·tal e. of mus·cle
elas·tin
elas·to·fi·bro·ma
elas·toid
  de·gen·er·a·tion
elas·toi·din
elas·to·ma
  ju·ve·nile e.
  Miescher's e.
elas·tom·e·ter
elas·to·mu·cin
elas·tor·rhex·is
elas·to·sis
  e. col·loi·da·lis con·glo·me·
    ra·ta
  e. dys·tro·phi·ca
  e. per·fo·rans ser·pi·gi·no·
    sa
  so·lar e.
elas·tot·ic
  de·gen·er·a·tion
ela·tion
Elaut's
  tri·an·gle
el·bow
  bone
  jerk
  joint
  re·flex
el·bow
  capped e.
  Little Leagu·er's e.

min·er's e.
nurse·maid's e.
ten·nis e.
el·bowed
  bou·gie
  cath·e·ter
elec·tive
  cul·ture
  mut·ism
Elec·tra
  com·plex
elec·tric
  an·es·the·sia
  bath
  cat·a·ract
  cau·tery
  cho·rea
  der·ma·tome
  ir·ri·ta·bil·i·ty
  oph·thal·mia
  ret·i·nop·a·thy
  shock
  sleep
elec·tri·cal
  al·ter·nans
  al·ter·na·tion of heart
  ax·is
  fail·ure
  for·mu·la
elec·tri·cal heart
  po·si·tion
elec·tric car·di·ac
  pace·mak·er
elec·tro·an·al·ge·sia
elec·tro·a·nal·y·sis
elec·tro·an·es·the·sia
elec·tro·ax·on·og·ra·phy
elec·tro·ba·so·graph
elec·tro·ba·sog·ra·phy
elec·tro·bi·os·co·py
elec·tro·car·di·o·gram
  uni·po·lar e.
elec·tro·car·di·o·graph
elec·tro·car·di·o·graph·ic
  com·plex
  wave
elec·tro·car·di·og·ra·phy
  fe·tal e.
elec·tro·car·di·o·pho·no·gram
elec·tro·car·di·o·pho·nog·ra·phy
elec·tro·cau·ter·i·za·tion
elec·tro·cau·tery
elec·tro·ce·re·bral si·lence
elec·tro·chem·i·cal
  gra·di·ent
elec·tro·cho·le·cys·tec·to·my
elec·tro·cho·le·cys·to·cau·sis
elec·tro·co·ag·u·la·tion

elec·tro·co·chle·o·gram
elec·tro·co·chle·og·ra·phy
elec·tro·con·trac·til·i·ty
elec·tro·con·vul·sive
   ther·a·py
elec·tro·cor·ti·co·gram
elec·tro·cor·ti·cog·ra·phy
elec·tro·cute
elec·tro·cu·tion
elec·tro·cys·tog·ra·phy
elec·trode
   ac·tive e.
   cal·o·mel e.
   car·bon di·ox·ide e.
   cen·tral ter·mi·nal e.
   Clark e.
   dis·pers·ing e.
   ex·cit·ing e.
   ex·plor·ing e.
   glass e.
   hy·dro·gen e.
   in·dif·fer·ent e.
   ion-se·lec·tive e.'s
   lo·cal·iz·ing e.
   neg·a·tive e.
   ox·i·da·tion-re·duc·tion e.
   ox·y·gen e.
   pos·i·tive e.
   quin·hy·drone e.
   re·dox e.
   ref·er·ence e.
   Severinghaus e.
   si·lent e.
   ther·a·peu·tic e.
elec·trode
   knife
elec·tro·der·mal
   au·di·om·e·try
e·lec·tro·der·ma·tome
elec·tro·des·ic·ca·tion
elec·tro·di·ag·no·sis
elec·tro·di·al·y·sis
elec·tro·en·ceph·a·lo·gram
   flat e.
   iso·e·lec·tric e.
elec·tro·en·ceph·a·lo·graph
elec·tro·en·ceph·a·lo·graph·ic
   dys·rhyth·mia
elec·tro·en·ceph·a·log·ra·phy
elec·tro·en·dos·mo·sis
elec·tro·gas·tro·gram
elec·tro·gas·tro·graph
elec·tro·gas·trog·ra·phy
elec·tro·gram
   His bun·dle e.
elec·tro·he·mo·sta·sis
elec·tro·hys·ter·o·graph
elec·tro·im·mu·no·dif·fu·sion

elec·tro·ky·mo·gram
elec·tro·ky·mo·graph
elec·tro·ky·mog·ra·phy
elec·trol·y·sis
elec·tro·lyte
   am·pho·ter·ic e.
elec·tro·lyte
   me·tab·o·lism
elec·tro·lyt·ic
elec·tro·lyze
elec·tro·lyz·er
elec·tro·mag·net
elec·tro·mag·net·ic
   flow·me·ter
   in·duc·tion
   ra·di·a·tion
   unit
elec·tro·mas·sage
elec·tro·me·chan·i·cal
   dis·so·ci·a·tion
   sys·to·le
elec·tro·mic·tu·ra·tion
e·lec·tro·morph
elec·tro·mo·tive
   force
elec·tro·mus·cu·lar
   sen·si·bil·i·ty
elec·tro·my·o·gram
elec·tro·my·o·graph
elec·tro·my·og·ra·phy
elec·tron
   Auger e.
   con·ver·sion e.
   emis·sion e.
   in·ter·nal con·ver·sion e.
   pos·i·tive e.
   va·lence e.
elec·tron
   cap·ture
   in·ter·fer·om·e·ter
   in·ter·fer·o·me·try
   mag·ne·ton
   mi·cro·graph
   mi·cro·scope
   mi·cros·co·py
   ra·di·og·ra·phy
elec·tro·nar·co·sis
elec·tro·neg·a·tive
   el·e·ment
elec·tro·neu·rog·ra·phy
elec·tro·neu·rol·y·sis
elec·tro·neu·ro·my·og·ra·phy
elec·tron·ic
   num·ber
elec·tron·ic cell
   count·er
elec·tron·ic fe·tal
   mon·i·tor

elec·tron·ic pace·mak·er
  load
elec·tron res·o·nance
  ab·sorp·tion
elec·tron spin
  res·o·nance
elec·tron-trans·port
  sys·tem
elec·tron-volt
elec·tro·nys·tag·mog·ra·phy
elec·tro-oc·u·lo·gram
elec·tro-oc·u·log·ra·phy
elec·tro-ol·fac·to·gram
elec·tro-os·mo·sis
elec·tro·pa·thol·o·gy
elec·tro·pher·o·gram
elec·tro·phil
elec·tro·phile
elec·tro·phil·ic
elec·tro·pho·bia
elec·tro·phon·ic
  ef·fect
elec·tro·pho·re·sis
  disc e.
  gel e.
  iso·en·zyme e.
  lip·o·pro·tein e.
  thin-lay·er e.
elec·tro·pho·ret·ic
elec·tro·pho·ret·o·gram
elec·tro·pho·to·ther·a·py
elec·tro·phren·ic
  res·pi·ra·tion
elec·tro·phys·i·o·log·ic
  au·di·om·e·try
elec·tro·phys·i·ol·o·gy
elec·tro·pneu·mo·graph
elec·tro·pos·i·tive
  el·e·ment
elec·tro·punc·ture
elec·tro·ra·di·ol·o·gy
elec·tro·ra·di·om·e·ter
elec·tro·ret·i·no·gram
elec·tro·ret·i·nog·ra·phy
elec·tro·scis·sion
elec·tro·scope
elec·tro·shock
  ther·a·py
elec·tro·sol
elec·tro·spec·trog·ra·phy
elec·tro·spi·no·gram
elec·tro·spi·nog·ra·phy
elec·tro·stat·ic
  unit
elec·tro·ste·nol·y·sis
elec·tro·steth·o·graph
elec·tro·stric·tion

elec·tro·sur·gery
elec·tro·tax·is
  neg·a·tive e.
  pos·i·tive e.
elec·tro·tha·na·sia
elec·tro·ther·a·peu·tic
  bath
  sleep
elec·tro·ther·a·peu·tics
elec·tro·ther·a·peu·tic sleep
  ther·a·py
elec·tro·ther·a·py
elec·tro·therm
elec·tro·tome
elec·trot·o·my
elec·tro·ton·ic
  cur·rent
  junc·tion
  syn·apse
elec·trot·o·nus
elec·trot·ro·pism
elec·tu·ar·y
el·e·doi·sin
ele·i·din
el·e·ment
  ac·tin·i·de e.'s
  al·ka·line earth e.'s
  am·pho·ter·ic e.
  an·a·tom·i·cal e.
  elec·tro·neg·a·tive e.
  elec·tro·pos·i·tive e.
  ex·tra·chro·mo·som·al e.
  ex·tra·chro·mo·som·al ge·
   net·ic e.
  la·bile e.'s
  mor·pho·log·ic e.
  neu·tral e.
  no·ble e.
  pic·ture e.
  rare earth e.'s
  trace e.'s
  trans·pos·a·ble e.
  vol·ume e.
el·e·men·ta·ry
  bod·ies
  gran·ule
  par·ti·cle
el·e·o·ma
el·e·om·e·ter
el·e·op·a·thy
el·e·o·stear·ic ac·id
el·e·o·ther·a·py
el·e·o·tho·rax
el·e·phant
  leg
el·e·phan·ti·ac
el·e·phan·ti·as·ic

el·e·phan·ti·a·sis
  e. con·gen·i·ta an·gi·o·ma·
    to·sa
  con·gen·i·tal e.
  gin·gi·val e.
  e. neu·ro·ma·to·sa
  ne·void e.
  e. nos·tras
  e. scro·ti
  e. tel·an·gi·ec·to·des
  e. vul·vae
el·e·phan·toid
  fe·ver
eleu·ther·o·ma·nia
el·e·va·tion
  fron·to·na·sal e.
  lat·er·al na·sal e.
  me·di·al na·sal e.
  tac·tile e.'s
el·e·va·tor
  per·i·os·te·al e.
  screw e.
el·e·va·tor
  mus·cle of anus
  mus·cle of pros·tate
  mus·cle of rib
  mus·cle of scap·u·la
  mus·cle of soft pal·ate
  mus·cle of thy·roid gland
  mus·cle of up·per eye·lid
  mus·cle of up·per lip
  mus·cle of up·per lip and
    wing of nose
elev·enth cra·ni·al
  nerve
elf·in
  fa·ci·es
elf·wort
elim·i·nant
elim·i·na·tion
  car·bon di·ox·ide e.
elim·i·na·tion
  di·et
elin·gua·tion
el·i·nin
elix·ir
Ellik
  evac·u·a·tor
Elliot's
  op·er·a·tion
  po·si·tion
Elliott's
  law
el·lip·sis
el·lip·soid
el·lip·soi·dal
  joint

el·lip·ti·cal
  am·pu·ta·tion
  anas·to·mo·sis
  re·cess
el·lip·to·cyte
el·lip·to·cyt·ic
  ane·mia
el·lip·to·cy·to·sis
Ellis-van Creveld
  syn·drome
Ellsworth-Howard
  test
Eloesser
  pro·ce·dure
elon·ga·tion
Elschnig
  pearls
Elschnig's
  spots
El Tor
  vib·rio
el·u·ant
el·u·ate
el·u·ent
elu·sive
  ul·cer
elute
elu·tion
elu·tri·ate
elu·tri·a·tion
ema·ci·a·tion
emac·u·la·tion
em·a·na·tion
  ac·tin·i·um e.
  ra·di·um e.
  tho·ri·um e.
em·a·na·tor·i·um
eman·ci·pa·tion
em·a·non
em·a·no·ther·a·py
emar·gi·nate
emar·gi·na·tion
emas·cu·la·tion
EMB
  agar
Em·ba·dom·o·nas
em·balm
Embden
  es·ter
Embden-Meyerhof
  path·way
Embden-Meyerhof-Parnas
  path·way
em·bed
em·bed·ding
  agents
em·be·lin
em·bo·la·lia

em·bo·le
em·bo·lec·to·my
em·bo·le·mia
em·bo·li
em·bo·lia
em·bol·ic
  ab·scess
  an·eu·rysm
  ap·o·plexy
  gan·grene
  in·farct
  pneu·mo·nia
em·bol·i·form
  nu·cle·us
em·bo·lism
  air e.
  am·ni·ot·ic flu·id e.
  ath·er·o·ma e.
  bland e.
  cel·lu·lar e.
  cho·les·ter·ol e.
  cot·ton-fi·ber e.
  crossed e.
  di·rect e.
  fat e.
  gas e.
  he·ma·tog·e·nous e.
  in·fec·tive e.
  lymph e.
  lym·phog·e·nous e.
  mil·i·a·ry e.
  mul·ti·ple e.
  ob·tu·rat·ing e.
  oil e.
  pan·ta·loon e.
  par·a·dox·i·cal e.
  pul·mo·nary e.
  py·e·mic e.
  ret·i·nal e.
  ret·ro·grade e.
  rid·ing e.
  sad·dle e.
  strad·dling e.
  tu·mor e.
  ve·nous e.
em·bo·li·za·tion
em·bo·lo·la·lia
em·bo·lo·my·cot·ic
  an·eu·rysm
em·bo·lo·pha·sia
em·bo·lo·phra·sia
em·bo·lus
  cath·e·ter e.
em·bo·ly
em·bouche·ment
em·bra·sure
  buc·cal e.
  gin·gi·val e.
  in·ci·sal e.
  la·bi·al e.
  lin·gual e.
  oc·clu·sal e.
em·bro·ca·tion
em·bry·at·rics
em·bryo
  het·er·o·ga·met·ic e.
  hex·a·canth e.
  ho·mo·ga·met·ic e.
  on·co·sphere e.
  pre·so·mite e.
  pre·vil·lous e.
em·bryo
  trans·fer
em·bry·o·blast
em·bry·o·car·dia
  jug·u·lar e.
em·bry·o·gen·e·sis
em·bry·o·ge·ne·tic
em·bry·o·gen·ic
em·bry·og·e·ny
em·bry·oid
em·bry·ol·o·gist
em·bry·ol·o·gy
em·bry·o·ma
  e. of the kid·ney
em·bry·o·mor·phous
em·bry·o·nal
  ad·e·no·ma
  ar·ea
  car·ci·no·ma
  car·ci·no·sar·co·ma
  leu·ke·mia
  me·dul·lo·ep·i·the·li·o·ma
  rhab·do·my·o·sar·co·mas
  tu·mor
  tu·mor of cil·i·ary body
em·bry·o·nate
em·bry·on·ic
  an·id·e·us
  ar·ea
  ax·is
  blas·to·derm
  cat·a·ract
  cir·cu·la·tion
  di·a·pause
  disk
  mem·brane
  shield
  tu·mor
em·bry·on·i·form
em·bry·on·i·za·tion
em·bry·o·noid
em·bry·o·ny
em·bry·op·a·thy
em·bry·o·phore
em·bry·o·plas·tic

em·bry·o·scope
em·bry·ot·o·my
em·bry·o·tox·ic·i·ty
em·bry·o·tox·on
  an·te·ri·or e.
  pos·te·ri·or e.
em·bry·o·troph
em·bry·o·tro·phic
em·bry·ot·ro·phy
EMC
  vi·rus
emed·ul·late
emei·o·cy·to·sis
emer·gence
emer·gen·cy
  the·o·ry
emer·gent
  ev·o·lu·tion
em·ery
  disks
em·e·sis
  ba·sin
emet·ic
em·e·tine
em·e·to·ca·thar·tic
EMG
  syn·drome
emic·tion
em·i·gra·tion
  the·o·ry
em·i·nence
  ar·cu·ate e.
  ar·tic·u·lar e.
  ca·nine e.
  col·lat·er·al e.
  e. of con·cha
  cru·ci·ate e.
  cru·ci·form e.
  del·toid e.
  Doyère's e.
  fa·cial e.
  fore·brain e.
  fron·tal e.
  gen·i·tal e.
  hy·po·bran·chi·al e.
  hy·po·glos·sal e.
  hy·po·the·nar e.
  il·e·o·ce·cal e.
  il·i·o·pec·tin·e·al e.
  il·i·o·pu·bic e.
  in·ter·con·dy·lar e.
  in·ter·con·dy·loid e.
  max·il·lary e.
  me·di·al e.
  me·di·an e.
  ol·i·vary e.
  or·bi·tal e.
  pa·ri·e·tal e.

  py·ram·i·dal e.
  ra·di·al e. of wrist
  res·ti·form e.
  round e.
  e. of sca·pha
  the·nar e.
  thy·roid e.
  e. of tri·an·gu·lar fos·sa
  ul·nar e. of wrist
em·i·nen·tia
  e. ab·du·cen·tis
  e. ar·ti·cu·la·ris
  e. car·pi ra·di·a·lis
  e. car·pi ul·na·ris
  e. fa·ci·a·lis
  e. hy·po·glos·si
  e. in·ter·con·dy·loi·dea
  e. me·di·a·na
  e. or·bi·ta·lis
  e. pa·ri·e·tal·is
  e. res·ti·for·mis
  e. sym·phy·sis
  e. te·res
  e. tri·an·gu·la·ris
em·i·nen·ti·ae
em·i·o·cy·to·sis
em·is·sar·i·um
  e. con·dy·loi·de·um
  e. mas·toi·de·um
  e. oc·ci·pi·ta·le
  e. pa·ri·e·ta·le
em·is·sary
  vein
em·is·sary sphe·noi·dal
  fo·ra·men
emis·sion
  elec·tron
emis·siv·i·ty
em·men·a·gog·ic
em·men·a·gogue
em·men·ia
em·men·ic
em·men·i·op·a·thy
em·me·nol·o·gy
Emmens' S/L
  test
em·me·tro·pia
em·me·tro·pic
em·me·trop·i·za·tion
Emmet's
  nee·dle
  op·er·a·tion
Em·mon·si·el·la cap·su·la·ta
em·o·din
emol·lient
emo·tion
emo·tion·al
  age

emo·tion·al *(continued)*
  amen·or·rhea
  at·ti·tudes
  dep·ri·va·tion
  dis·ease
  dis·or·der
  dis·tur·bance
  leu·ko·cy·to·sis
  over·lay
  tone
emo·ti·o·vas·cu·lar
em·pasm
em·pas·ma
em·path·ic
  in·dex
em·pa·thize
em·pa·thy
  gen·er·a·tive e.
em·per·i·po·le·sis
em·phly·sis
em·phrac·tic
em·phrax·is
em·phy·se·ma
  cen·tri-ac·i·nar e.
  cen·tri·lob·u·lar e.
  com·pen·sat·ing e.
  com·pen·sa·to·ry e.
  cu·ta·ne·ous e.
  dif·fuse e.
  fa·mil·i·al e.
  gan·gre·nous e.
  gen·er·al·ized e.
  in·ter·lob·u·lar e.
  in·ter·sti·tial e.
  in·tes·ti·nal e.
  me·di·as·ti·nal e.
  pan·ac·i·nar e.
  pan·lob·u·lar e.
  par·a·sep·tal e.
  pul·mo·nary e.
  se·nile e.
  sub·cu·ta·ne·ous e.
  sub·ga·le·al e.
  sur·gi·cal e.
em·phy·sem·a·tous
  cho·le·cys·ti·tis
  gan·grene
  phleg·mon
em·pir·ic
  risk
em·pir·i·cal
  for·mu·la
em·pir·i·cism
em·pros·thot·o·nos
emp·ty
  sel·la
em·py·e·ma
  tube

em·py·e·ma
  e. ar·tic·u·li
  e. be·nig·num
  la·tent e.
  loc·u·lat·ed e.
  mas·toid e.
  e. ne·ces·si·ta·tis
  e. of the per·i·car·di·um
  pul·sat·ing e.
em·py·e·mic
  sco·li·o·sis
em·py·e·sis
em·py·o·cele
em·py·reu·ma
emul·gent
emul·si·fi·er
emul·si·fy
emul·si·fy·ing
  wax
emul·sin
emul·sion
  col·loid
emul·sive
emul·soid
em·u·re·sis
emyl·ca·mate
enal·a·pril ma·le·ate
enam·el
  dwarfed e.
  mot·tled e.
  nan·oid e.
  whorled e.
enam·el
  cap
  cell
  cleav·age
  cleav·er
  crypt
  cu·ti·cle
  dys·pla·sia
  ep·i·the·li·um
  fi·bers
  fis·sure
  germ
  hy·po·cal·ci·fi·ca·tion
  hy·po·pla·sia
  la·mel·la
  lay·er
  ledge
  mem·brane
  niche
  nod·ule
  or·gan
  pearl
  prisms
  pro·jec·tion
  pulp
  rods

tuft
wall
enam·el·o·gen·e·sis
  e. im·per·fec·ta
enam·el·o·ma
enam·el rod
  in·cli·na·tion
  sheath
enam·e·lum
enan·thal
enan·thate
en·an·them
en·an·the·ma
en·an·them·a·tous
en·an·the·sis
en·an·ti·o·mer
en·an·ti·o·mer·ic
en·an·ti·om·er·ism
en·an·ti·o·morph
en·an·ti·o·mor·phic
en·an·ti·o·mor·phism
en·an·ti·o·mor·phous
en·ar·thro·di·al
  joint
en·ar·thro·sis
en·cai·nide hy·dro·chlo·ride
en·can·this
en·cap·su·lat·ed
en·cap·su·la·tion
en·cap·suled
en·car·di·tis
en·ca·tar·rha·phy
en·ce·li·i·tis
en·ce·li·tis
en·ceph·a·la
en·ceph·a·lal·gia
en·ceph·a·la·tro·phic
en·ceph·a·lat·ro·phy
en·ceph·a·lauxe
en·céph·ale iso·lé
en·ceph·a·le·mia
en·ce·phal·ic
  an·gi·o·ma
  ves·i·cle
en·ceph·a·lit·ic
en·ceph·a·lit·i·des
en·ceph·a·li·tis
  acute hem·or·rhag·ic e.
  acute nec·ro·tiz·ing e.
  Aus·tra·li·an X e.
  bun·ya·vi·rus e.
  Cal·i·for·nia e.
  Cox·sack·ie e.
  Dawson's e.
  ep·i·dem·ic e.
  equine e.
  ex·per·i·men·tal al·ler·gic e.
  Far East Rus·sian e.

fox e.
e. hem·or·rha·gi·ca
her·pes e.
hy·per·er·gic e.
Ilhé·us e.
in·clu·sion body e.
Jap·a·nese B e.
e. ja·pon·i·ca
lead e.
e. le·thar·gi·ca
Men·go e.
Murray Val·ley e.
nec·ro·tiz·ing e.
e. ne·o·na·to·rum
opos·sum e.
e. per·i·ax·i·a·lis con·cen·
  tri·ca
e. per·i·ax·i·a·lis dif·fu·sa
post·vac·ci·nal e.
Pow·as·san e.
pu·ru·lent e.
e. py·o·ge·ni·ca
Rus·sian au·tumn e.
Rus·sian spring-sum·mer e.
  (East·ern sub·type)
Rus·sian spring-sum·mer e.
  (West·ern sub·type)
Rus·sian tick-borne e.
sec·on·dary e.
sub·a·cute in·clu·sion
  body e.
e. sub·cor·ti·ca·lis
  chron·i·ca
sup·pu·ra·tive e.
tick-borne e. (Cen·tral Eu·
  ro·pe·an sub·type)
tick-borne e. (East·ern sub·
  type)
var·i·cel·la e.
ver·nal e.
wood·cut·ter's e.
en·ceph·a·li·tis
  vi·rus
en·ceph·a·li·to·gen
en·ceph·a·li·to·gen·ic
En·ceph·a·li·to·zo·on
en·ceph·a·li·za·tion
en·ceph·a·lo·cele
en·ceph·a·lo·clas·tic
  mi·cro·ceph·a·ly
en·ceph·a·lo·cra·ni·o·cu·ta·ne·
ous
  lip·o·ma·to·sis
en·ceph·a·lo·dyn·ia
en·ceph·a·lo·dys·pla·sia
en·ceph·a·lo·gram
en·ceph·a·log·ra·phy
  gam·ma e.

en·ceph·a·loid
  can·cer
en·ceph·a·lo·lith
en·ceph·a·lol·o·gy
en·ceph·a·lo·ma
en·ceph·a·lo·ma·la·cia
  nu·trit·ion·al e. of chicks
en·ceph·a·lo·men·in·gi·tis
en·ceph·a·lo·me·nin·go·cele
en·ceph·a·lo·men·in·gop·a·thy
en·ceph·a·lo·mere
en·ceph·a·lom·e·ter
en·ceph·a·lo·my·e·li·tis
  acute dis·sem·i·nat·ed e.
  avi·an in·fec·tious e.
  be·nign my·al·gic e.
  bo·vine spo·rad·ic e.
  east·ern equine e.
  en·zo·ot·ic e.
  ep·i·dem·ic my·al·gic e.
  equine e.
  ex·per·i·men·tal al·ler·gic e.
  gran·u·lom·a·tous e.
  in·fec·tious por·cine e.
  mouse e.
  Ven·e·zu·e·lan equine e.
  vi·rus e.
  west·ern equine e.
  zos·ter e.
en·ceph·a·lo·my·e·lo·cele
en·ceph·a·lo·my·e·lo·neu·rop·a·thy
  non·spe·cif·ic e.
en·ceph·a·lo·my·e·lon·ic
  ax·is
en·ceph·a·lo·my·e·lop·a·thy
  car·ci·nom·a·tous e.
  ep·i·dem·ic my·al·gic e.
  nec·ro·tiz·ing e.
  par·a·car·ci·nom·a·tous e.
en·ceph·a·lo·my·e·lo·ra·dic·u·li·tis
en·ceph·a·lo·my·e·lo·ra·dic·u·lop·a·thy
en·ceph·a·lo·my·o·car·di·tis
  vi·rus
en·ceph·a·lon
en·ceph·a·lo·nar·co·sis
en·ceph·a·lo-oph·thal·mic
  dys·pla·sia
en·ceph·a·lo·path·ia
  e. ad·di·so·nia
en·ceph·a·lop·a·thy
  bil·i·ru·bin e.
  Binswanger's e.
  de·my·e·li·nat·ing e.
  fa·mil·i·al e.
  he·pa·tic e.

hy·per·na·tre·mic e.
hy·per·ten·sive e.
lead e.
met·a·bol·ic e.
pal·in·drom·ic e.
pan·cre·at·ic e.
por·tal-sys·tem·ic e.
pro·gress·ive sub·cor·ti·cal e.
re·cur·rent e.
sat·ur·nine e.
spon·gi·form e.
sub·a·cute spon·gi·form e.
sub·cor·ti·cal ar·te·ri·o·scle·rot·ic e.
thy·ro·tox·ic e.
trans·mis·si·ble e. of mink
trau·mat·ic e.
trau·mat·ic pro·gress·ive e.
Wernicke-Korsakoff e.
Wernicke's e.
en·ceph·a·lop·sy
en·ceph·a·lo·py·o·sis
en·ceph·a·lor·rha·chid·i·an
en·ceph·a·lor·rha·gia
en·ceph·a·los·chi·sis
en·ceph·a·lo·scle·ro·sis
en·ceph·a·lo·scope
en·ceph·a·los·co·py
en·ceph·a·lo·sis
en·ceph·a·lo·spi·nal
en·ceph·a·lo·thlip·sis
en·ceph·a·lo·tome
en·ceph·a·lot·o·my
en·ceph·a·lo·tri·gem·i·nal
  an·gi·o·ma·to·sis
en·ceph·a·lo·tri·gem·i·nal vas·cu·lar
  syn·drome
en·chon·dral
en·chon·dro·ma
en·chon·dro·ma·to·sis
en·chon·drom·a·tous
en·chon·dro·sar·co·ma
en·clave
en·cod·ing
en·cop·re·sis
en·coun·ter
  group
en·cra·ni·al
en·cra·ni·us
en·cyst·ed
  cal·cu·lus
  pleu·ri·sy
en·cyst·ment
end
  dis·tal e.

end
ar·tery
bud
bulb
or·gan
piece
plate
point
stage
End·a·moe·ba
end·an·ge·i·tis
end·an·gi·i·tis
e. ob·li·te·r·ans
end·a·or·ti·tis
end·ar·ter·ec·to·my
ca·rot·id e.
cor·o·nary e.
end·ar·te·ri·tis
bac·te·ri·al e.
e. de·for·mans
e. ob·li·te·r·ans
ob·lit·er·at·ing e.
e. pro·li·fe·rans
pro·lif·er·at·ing e.
end·au·ral
in·ci·sion
end·brain
end-brush
end-bulb
end-cut·ting
bur
end-di·a·stol·ic
vol·ume
en·de·mia
en·dem·ic
deaf·mut·ism
fu·nic·u·li·tis
goi·ter
he·ma·tu·ria
he·mop·ty·sis
hy·per·tro·phy
in·dex
in·flu·en·za
neu·ri·tis
sta·bil·i·ty
ty·phus
en·dem·ic non·bac·te·ri·al in·
fan·tile
gas·tro·en·ter·i·tis
en·dem·ic par·a·lyt·ic
ver·ti·go
en·dem·o·ep·i·dem·ic
end·er·gon·ic
en·der·mat·ic
en·der·mic
en·der·mism
en·der·mo·sis
end-feet

end·gut
end·ing
an·nu·lo·spi·ral e.
ca·lic·i·form e.
ca·lyc·i·form e.
ep·i·lem·mal e.
flow·er-spray e.
free nerve e.'s
grape e.'s
hed·er·i·form e.
nerve e.
sole-plate e.
syn·ap·tic e.'s
Endo
agar
en·do·ab·dom·i·nal
en·do·an·eu·rys·mo·plas·ty
en·do·an·eu·rys·mor·rha·phy
en·do·an·gi·i·tis
en·do-a·or·ti·tis
en·do·ap·pen·di·ci·tis
en·do·ar·te·ri·tis
en·do·aus·cul·ta·tion
en·do·ba·si·on
en·do·bi·ot·ic
en·do·blast
en·do·bron·chi·al
tube
en·do·car·dia
en·do·car·di·ac
en·do·car·di·al
cush·ions
fi·bro·e·las·to·sis
mur·mur
scle·ro·sis
en·do·car·di·al cush·ion
de·fect
en·do·car·di·og·ra·phy
en·do·car·dit·ic
en·do·car·di·tis
abac·te·ri·al throm·bot·ic e.
acute b. e.
acute bac·te·ri·al e.
atyp·i·cal ver·ru·cous e.
bac·te·ria-free stage of bac·
te·ri·al e.
bac·te·ri·al e.
ca·chec·tic e.
e. chor·da·lis
con·stric·tive e.
in·fec·tious e.
in·fec·tive e.
iso·lat·ed pa·ri·e·tal e.
Libman-Sacks e.
Löffler's e.
Löffler's fi·bro·plas·tic e.
ma·lig·nant e.
ma·ran·tic e.

en·do·car·di·tis *(continued)*
  mu·ral e.
  non·bac·te·ri·al throm·bot·
    ic e.
  non·bac·te·ri·al ver·ru·cous
    e.
  pol·y·pous e.
  rheu·mat·ic e.
  sep·tic e.
  sub·a·cute b. e.
  sub·a·cute bac·te·ri·al e.
  ter·mi·nal e.
  val·vu·lar e.
  veg·e·ta·tive e.
  ver·ru·cous e.
en·do·car·di·um
en·do·ce·li·ac
en·do·cer·vi·cal
  smear
en·do·cer·vi·ci·tis
en·do·cer·vix
en·do·chon·dral
  bone
  os·si·fi·ca·tion
en·do·co·li·tis
en·do·col·pi·tis
en·do·cra·ni·al
en·do·cra·ni·um
en·do·crine
  ex·oph·thal·mos
  glands
  oph·thal·mop·a·thy
  sys·tem
en·do·crine pol·y·glan·du·lar
  syn·drome
en·do·cri·nol·o·gist
en·do·cri·nol·o·gy
en·do·cri·no·ma
  mul·ti·ple e.
en·do·crin·o·path·ic
en·do·cri·nop·a·thy
  mul·ti·ple e.
en·do·cri·no·ther·a·py
en·do·cy·clic
en·do·cy·ma
en·do·cyst
en·do·cys·ti·tis
en·do·cy·to·sis
en·do·derm
en·do·der·mal
  ca·nal
  cells
  clo·a·ca
  pouch·es
en·do·der·mal si·nus
  tu·mor
En·do·der·mo·phy·ton
en·do·di·a·scope

en·do·di·as·co·py
en·do·don·tia
en·do·don·tic
  sta·bi·liz·er
en·do·don·tics
en·do·don·tist
en·do·don·tol·o·gist
en·do·don·tol·o·gy
en·do·dy·o·cyte
en·do·dy·og·e·ny
en·do·en·ter·i·tis
en·do·en·zyme
en·do·e·soph·a·gi·tis
en·do·far·a·dism
en·do·gal·va·nism
en·dog·a·my
en·do·gas·tric
en·do·gas·tri·tis
en·do·gen·ic
  tox·i·co·sis
en·do·ge·no·mor·phic
  de·pres·sion
en·do·ge·note
en·dog·e·nous
  cy·cle
  de·pres·sion
  fi·bers
  hy·per·glyc·er·i·de·mia
  in·fec·tion
en·dog·e·nous cre·at·i·nine
  clear·ance
en·do·glo·bar
en·do·glob·u·lar
en·do·gnath·i·on
en·do·her·ni·ot·o·my
en·do·in·tox·i·ca·tion
en·do·la·ryn·ge·al
En·do·li·max
en·do·lith
en·do·lymph
en·do·lym·pha
en·do·lym·phat·ic
  duct
  hy·drops
  sac
en·do·lym·phic
en·do·me·ninx
en·do·me·rog·o·ny
en·do·me·tria
en·do·me·tri·al
  cyst
  im·plants
  smear
en·do·me·tri·al stro·mal
  sar·co·ma
en·do·me·tri·oid
  car·ci·no·ma
  tu·mor

en·do·me·tri·o·ma
en·do·me·tri·o·sis
en·do·me·tri·tis
   de·cid·u·al e.
   e. dis·se·cans
en·do·me·tri·um
   Swiss cheese e.
en·do·me·tro·pic
en·do·mi·to·sis
en·do·morph
en·do·mor·phic
en·do·mo·tor·sonde
En·do·my·ces ge·ot·ri·chum
En·do·my·ce·ta·les
en·do·my·o·car·di·al
   fi·bro·e·las·to·sis
   fi·bro·sis
en·do·my·o·car·di·tis
en·do·my·o·me·tri·tis
en·do·mys·i·um
en·do·neu·ri·tis
en·do·neu·ri·um
end-on mat·tress
   su·ture
en·do·nu·cle·ase
   mi·cro·coc·cal e.
   nu·cle·ate e.
   re·stric·tion e.
   sin·gle-strand·ed nu·cle·ate
     e.
   spleen e.
en·do·nu·cle·ase (Ser·ra·tia
   mar·ces·cens)
en·do·nu·cle·o·lus
en·do-os·se·ous
   im·plant
en·do·par·a·site
en·do·par·a·sit·ism
en·do·pel·vic
   fas·cia
en·do·pep·ti·dase
en·do·per·i·ar·te·ri·tis
en·do·per·i·car·di·ac
en·do·per·i·car·di·tis
en·do·per·i·my·o·car·di·tis
en·do·per·i·neu·ri·tis
en·do·per·i·to·ni·tis
en·do·per·ox·ide
en·do·phle·bi·tis
en·doph·thal·mi·tis
   gran·u·lom·a·tous e.
   e. oph·thal·mia no·do·sa
   e. pha·co·a·na·phy·lac·ti·ca
en·do·phyte
en·do·phyt·ic
en·do·plasm
en·do·plas·mic
   re·tic·u·lum

en·do·plast
en·do·plas·tic
en·do·po·lyg·e·ny
en·do·pol·y·ploid
en·do·pol·y·ploi·dy
en·do·ra·di·og·ra·phy
en·do·rec·tal pull-through
   pro·ce·dure
en·do·re·du·pli·ca·tion
en·dor·phin·er·gic
en·dor·phins
en·dor·rha·chis
Endo's
   me·di·um
en·do·sal·pin·gi·o·sis
en·do·sal·pin·gi·tis
en·do·sarc
en·do·scope
en·do·scop·ic
   bi·op·sy
en·do·scop·ic ret·ro·grade
   chol·an·gi·o·pan·cre·a·tog·
     ra·phy
en·dos·co·pist
en·dos·co·py
Endo's fuch·sin
   agar
en·do·skel·e·ton
en·dos·mo·sis
en·do·some
en·do·so·nos·co·py
en·do·spore
en·dos·te·al
   im·plant
en·dos·te·i·tis
en·dos·te·o·ma
en·do·steth·o·scope
en·dos·te·um
en·dos·ti·tis
en·dos·to·ma
en·do·ten·din·e·um
en·do·ter·ic
   bac·te·ri·um
en·do·the·li·a
en·do·the·li·al
   cell
   cyst
   dys·tro·phy of cor·nea
   leu·ko·cyte
   my·e·lo·ma
en·do·the·li·o·cho·ri·al
   pla·cen·ta
en·do·the·li·o·cyte
en·do·the·li·o-en·do·the·li·al
   pla·cen·ta
en·do·the·li·oid
en·do·the·li·o·ma
en·do·the·li·o·sis

en·do·the·li·um
   e. of an·te·ri·or cham·ber
en·do·ther·mic
en·do·tho·rac·ic
   fas·cia
en·do·thrix
en·do·tox·e·mia
en·do·tox·ic
en·do·tox·i·co·sis
en·do·tox·in
   shock
en·do·tra·che·al
   an·es·the·sia
   in·tu·ba·tion
   sty·let
   tube
en·do·tra·che·li·tis
en·do·vac·ci·na·tion
en·do·vas·cu·li·tis
   hem·or·rhag·ic e.
en·do·ve·nous
   sep·tum
end-piece
end·plate
   mo·tor e.
end-point
   mea·sure·ment
end-po·si·tion
   nys·tag·mus
end-sys·tol·ic
   vol·ume
end-tid·al
   sam·ple
end-to-end
   bite
   oc·clu·sion
en·dy·ma
ene·di·ol
en·e·ma
   an·a·lep·tic e.
   bar·i·um e.
   blind e.
   con·trast e.
   dou·ble con·trast e.
   fla·tus e.
   high e.
   nu·tri·ent e.
   oil re·ten·tion e.
   soap·suds e.
   tur·pen·tine e.
en·e·ma·tor
en·e·mi·a·sis
en·er·get·ics
en·er·gom·e·ter
en·er·gy
   e. of ac·ti·va·tion
   bind·ing e.
   chem·i·cal e.

free e.
fu·sion e.
Gibbs free e.
ki·net·ic e.
la·tent e.
nu·cle·ar e.
nu·trit·ion·al e.
e. of po·si·tion
po·ten·tial e.
psy·chic e.
ra·di·ant e.
so·lar e.
to·tal e.
en·er·gy-rich
   phos·phates
en·er·va·tion
en·flu·rane
en·gage·ment
en·gas·tri·us
Engelmann's
   dis·ease
Engelmann's ba·sal
   knobs
en·gine
   ream·er
en·gi·neer·ing
   bi·o·med·i·cal e.
   den·tal e.
   ge·net·ic e.
Englisch's
   si·nus
English
   dis·ease
   po·si·tion
   rhi·no·plas·ty
en·globe
en·globe·ment
en·gorged
en·gorge·ment
en·gram
en·graph·ia
en grappe
en·hance·ment
   con·trast e.
   im·mu·no·log·i·cal e.
en·he·ma·to·spore
en·he·mo·spore
en·keph·a·lin·er·gic
en·keph·a·lins
en·large·ment
   cer·vi·cal e. of spi·nal cord
   gin·gi·val e.
   lum·bar e. of spi·nal cord
enol
eno·lase
eno·li·za·tion
enol py·ru·vate
en·oph·thal·mia

en·oph·thal·mos
en·or·gan·ic
en·o·si·ma·nia
en·os·to·sis
en·o·yl
en·o·yl-ACP re·duc·tase
en·o·yl-ACP re·duc·tase
  (NADPH)
en·o·yl-CoA hy·dra·tase
en·o·yl hy·drase
Enroth's
  sign
en·sheath·ing
  cal·lus
en·si·form
  car·ti·lage
  pro·cess
en·sis·ter·num
  car·ti·lage
en·stro·phe
en·tad
en·tal
en·tal or·i·gin
ent·am·e·bi·a·sis
Ent·a·moe·ba
  E. buc·ca·lis
  E. co·li
  E. gin·gi·va·lis
  E. hart·manni
  E. his·to·lyt·i·ca
  E. mosh·kov·skii
en·ta·sia
en·ta·sis
en·tat·ic
en·ter·al
en·ter·al·gia
en·ter·a·mine
en·ter·ec·ta·sis
en·ter·ec·to·my
en·ter·el·co·sis
en·ter·ic
  fe·ver
  plex·us
  tu·ber·cu·lo·sis
  vi·rus·es
en·ter·ic coat·ed
  tab·let
en·ter·ic cy·to·path·o·gen·ic
  bo·vine or·phan
  vi·rus
en·ter·ic cy·to·path·o·gen·ic
  hu·man or·phan
  vi·rus
en·ter·ic cy·to·path·o·gen·ic
  mon·key or·phan
  vi·rus

en·ter·ic cy·to·path·o·gen·ic
  swine or·phan
  vi·rus
en·ter·i·coid
  fe·ver
en·ter·ic or·phan
  vi·rus·es
en·ter·i·tis
  e. an·a·phy·lac·ti·ca
  chron·ic cic·a·triz·ing e.
  diph·the·rit·ic e.
  fe·line in·fec·tious e.
  gran·u·lom·a·tous e.
  e. of mink
  mu·co·mem·bra·nous e.
  e. ne·cro·ti·cans
  phleg·mon·ous e.
  e. po·ly·po·sa
  pseu·do·mem·bra·nous e.
  re·gion·al e.
  trans·mis·si·ble e.
  tu·ber·cu·lous e.
en·ter·o·a·nas·to·mo·sis
en·ter·o·an·the·lone
en·ter·o·ap·o·clei·sis
En·ter·o·bac·ter
  E. aer·o·genes
  E. clo·a·cae
en·ter·o·bac·te·ria
En·ter·o·bac·te·ri·a·ce·ae
en·ter·o·bac·te·ri·um
en·ter·o·bi·a·sis
En·te·ro·bi·us
en·ter·o·bro·sia
en·ter·o·bro·sis
en·ter·o·cele
  par·tial e.
en·ter·o·cen·te·sis
en·ter·o·cho·le·cys·tos·to·my
en·ter·o·cho·le·cys·tot·o·my
en·ter·o·chro·maf·fin
  cells
en·ter·o·clei·sis
  omen·tal e.
en·ter·oc·ly·sis
en·ter·o·coc·ci
en·ter·o·coc·cus
en·ter·o·co·li·tis
  an·ti·bi·ot·ic e.
  nec·ro·tiz·ing e.
  pseu·do·mem·bra·nous e.
  re·gion·al e.
en·ter·o·co·los·to·my
en·ter·o·cu·ta·ne·ous
  fis·tu·la
en·ter·o·cyst
en·ter·o·cys·to·cele
en·ter·o·cys·to·ma

337

en·ter·o·dyn·ia
en·ter·o·en·do·crine
  cells
en·ter·o·en·ter·os·to·my
en·ter·o·gas·tric
  re·flex
en·ter·o·gas·tri·tis
en·ter·o·gas·trone
en·ter·og·e·nous
  cy·a·no·sis
  cysts
  met·he·mo·glo·bi·ne·mia
en·ter·o·graph
en·ter·og·ra·phy
en·ter·o·he·pat·ic
  cir·cu·la·tion
en·ter·o·hep·a·ti·tis
  in·fec·tious e.
en·ter·o·hep·a·to·cele
en·ter·oi·dea
en·ter·o·ki·nase
en·ter·o·ki·ne·sis
en·ter·o·ki·net·ic
  agent
en·ter·o·lith
en·ter·o·li·thi·a·sis
en·ter·ol·o·gy
en·ter·ol·y·sis
en·ter·o·me·ga·lia
en·ter·o·meg·a·ly
en·ter·o·me·nia
en·ter·o·mer·o·cele
en·ter·om·e·ter
En·te·ro·mo·nas
en·ter·o·my·co·sis
en·ter·o·ni·tis
en·ter·o·pa·re·sis
en·ter·o·path·ic
  ar·thri·tis
en·ter·o·path·o·gen
en·ter·o·path·o·gen·ic
en·ter·op·a·thy
  glu·ten e.
  pro·tein-los·ing e.
en·ter·o·pep·ti·dase
en·ter·o·pex·y
en·ter·o·plas·ty
en·ter·o·ple·gia
en·ter·o·plex
en·ter·o·plexy
en·ter·o·proc·tia
en·ter·op·to·sia
en·ter·op·to·sis
en·ter·op·tot·ic
en·ter·o·re·nal
en·ter·or·rha·gia
en·ter·or·rha·phy
en·ter·or·rhex·is

en·ter·o·scope
en·ter·o·sep·sis
en·ter·o·spasm
en·ter·o·sta·sis
en·ter·o·stax·is
en·ter·o·ste·no·sis
en·ter·os·to·my
  dou·ble e.
en·ter·o·tome
en·ter·ot·o·my
en·ter·o·tox·e·mia
en·ter·o·tox·i·ca·tion
en·ter·o·tox·i·gen·ic
en·ter·o·tox·in
  cy·to·ton·ic e.
  Esch·e·rich·ia co·li e.
  staph·y·lo·coc·cal e.
en·ter·o·tox·ism
en·ter·o·tro·pic
en·ter·o·vag·i·nal
  fis·tu·la
en·ter·o·ves·i·cal
  fis·tu·la
En·te·ro·vi·rus
en·ter·o·zo·ic
en·ter·o·zo·on
en·thal·py
en·the·sis
en·the·si·tis
en·the·so·path·ic
en·the·sop·a·thy
en·thet·ic
en·thla·sis
en thyrse
en·tire
en·ti·ty
en·to·blast
en·to·cele
en·to·cho·roi·dea
en·to·cone
en·to·co·nid
en·to·cor·nea
en·to·cra·ni·al
en·to·cra·ni·um
en·to·derm
en·to·der·mal
  cells
en·to·ec·tad
En·to·lo·ma si·nu·a·tum
en·to·mi·on
en·to·mol·o·gy
en·to·mo·pho·bia
En·to·moph·tho·ra
en·to·moph·tho·ra·my·co·sis
  e. ba·sid·i·o·bo·lae
  e. co·nid·i·o·bo·lae
En·to·mo·pox·vi·rus
en·top·ic

en·to·plasm
ent·op·tic
  pulse
en·to·ret·i·na
en·to·rhi·nal
  ar·ea
en·to·sarc
En·to·zoa
en·to·zoa
en·to·zo·al
en·to·zo·on
en·trails
en·trance
  block
en·trap·ment
  neu·rop·a·thy
en·tro·pi·on
  aton·ic e.
  cic·a·tri·cial e.
  spas·tic e.
en·tro·pi·on·ize
en·tro·pi·um
en·tro·py
en·try
  zone
en·ty·py
enu·cle·ate
enu·cle·a·tion
en·u·re·sis
  noc·tur·nal e.
en·u·ret·ic
  ab·sence
en·ve·lope
  con·for·ma·tion
  flap
en·ve·lope
  cor·ne·o·cyte e.
  nu·cle·ar e.
  vi·ral e.
en·ven·om·a·tion
en·vi·ron·ment
en·vi·ron·men·tal
  psy·chol·o·gy
en·vy
  pe·nis e.
en·zo·ot·ic
  abor·tion of ewes
  atax·ia
  en·ceph·a·lo·my·e·li·tis
  sta·bil·i·ty
en·zo·ot·ic bo·vine
  leu·ko·sis
en·zo·ot·ic en·ceph·a·lo·my·e·li·tis
  vi·rus
en·zy·got·ic
  twins

en·zy·mat·ic
  syn·the·sis
en·zyme
  an·tag·o·nist
en·zyme
  ace·tyl-ac·ti·vat·ing e.
  ac·yl-ac·ti·vat·ing e.
  adap·tive e.
  an·gi·o·ten·sin-con·vert·ing e.
  au·to·lyt·ic e.
  branch·ing e.
  con·dens·ing e.
  D e.
  de·am·i·diz·ing e.'s
  de·am·i·nat·ing e.'s
  de·branch·ing e.'s
  dis·pro·por·tion·at·ing e.
  ex·tra·cel·lu·lar e.
  hy·dro·lyz·ing e.'s
  in·duced e.
  in·duc·i·ble e.
  in·tra·cel·lu·lar e.
  ma·late-con·dens·ing e.
  mal·ic e.
  me·thi·o·nine-ac·ti·vat·ing e.
  new yel·low e.
  old yel·low e.
  P e.
  pan·to·ate-ac·ti·vat·ing e.
  phos·pho·ryl·ase-rup·tur·ing e.
  pho·to·re·ac·ti·vat·ing e.
  PR e.
  Q e.
  R e.
  re·duc·ing e.
  re·press·i·ble e.
  res·pi·ra·to·ry e.
  re·stric·tion e.
  Schardinger e.
  split·ting e.'s
  T e.
  ter·mi·nal ad·di·tion e.
  trans·fer·ring e.'s
  Warburg's old yel·low e.
  Warburg's res·pi·ra·to·ry e.
en·zyme in·hi·bi·tion
  the·o·ry of nar·co·sis
en·zyme-linked im·mu·no·sor·bent
  as·say
en·zyme-mul·ti·plied
  im·mu·no·as·say
en·zy·mic
en·zy·mol·o·gist
en·zy·mol·o·gy

en·zy·mol·y·sis
en·zy·mop·a·thy
en·zy·mo·sis
eo·sin
   al·co·hol-sol·u·ble e.
   e. B
   eth·yl e.
   e. I blu·ish
   e. y
   e. yel·low·ish
   e. Ys
eo·sin-meth·yl·ene blue
   agar
eo·sin·o·cyte
eo·sin·o·pe·nia
eo·sin·o·pe·nic
   re·ac·tion
eo·sin·o·phil
   ad·e·no·ma
   gran·ule
eo·sin·o·phil che·mo·tac·tic
   fac·tor of an·a·phy·lax·is
eo·sin·o·phile
eo·sin·o·phil·ia
   sim·ple pul·mo·nary e.
   trop·i·cal e.
eo·sin·o·phil·ic
   cel·lu·li·tis
   fas·ci·i·tis
   gran·u·lo·ma
   leu·ke·mia
   leu·ko·cyte
   leu·ko·cy·to·sis
   leu·ko·pe·nia
   men·in·gi·tis
   me·nin·go·en·ceph·a·li·tis
   pneu·mo·nia
eo·sin·o·phil·ic non·al·ler·gic
   rhi·ni·tis
eo·sin·o·phil·ic pus·tu·lar
   fol·lic·u·li·tis
eo·sin·o·phil·o·cyt·ic
   leu·ke·mia
eo·sin·o·phil·u·ria
eo·sin·o·tac·tic
eo·sin·o·tax·is
eo·so·pho·bia
epac·tal
   bones
   os·si·cles
ep·am·ni·ot·ic
   cav·i·ty
ep·ar·sal·gia
ep·ar·te·ri·al
   bron·chus
ep·ax·i·al
ep·en·dy·ma

ep·en·dy·mal
   cell
   cyst
   lay·er
   zone
ep·en·dy·mi·tis
ep·en·dy·mo·blast
ep·en·dy·mo·blas·to·ma
ep·en·dy·mo·cyte
ep·en·dy·mo·ma
   myx·o·pap·il·lary e.
ep·er·sal·gia
Ep·e·ryth·ro·zo·on
   E. coc·coi·des
   E. ovis
   E. su·is
   E. wen·yoni
ep·e·ryth·ro·zo·on·o·sis
eph·apse
eph·ap·tic
ephe·bi·at·rics
ephe·bic
eph·e·bol·o·gy
ephed·rine
ephe·li·des
ephe·lis
ephem·er·al
   fe·ver
   fe·ver of cat·tle
ephem·er·al fe·ver
   vi·rus
ep·i·an·dros·ter·one
ep·i·blast
ep·i·blas·tic
ep·i·bleph·a·ron
epib·o·le
epib·o·ly
ep·i·bran·chi·al
   plac·odes
ep·i·bul·bar
ep·i·can·thus
   e. in·ver·sus
   e. pal·pe·bra·lis
   e. su·pra·ci·li·a·ris
   e. tar·sa·lis
ep·i·car·dia
ep·i·car·di·al
ep·i·car·di·um
ep·i·chord·al
ep·i·co·mus
ep·i·con·dy·lal·gia
   e. ex·ter·na
ep·i·con·dyle
   lat·er·al e.
   lat·er·al e. of fe·mur
   lat·er·al e. of hu·mer·us
   me·di·al e.

me·di·al e. of fe·mur
me·di·al e. of hu·mer·us
ep·i·con·dy·li
ep·i·con·dyl·i·an
ep·i·con·dyl·ic
ep·i·con·dy·li·tis
  lat·er·al hu·mer·al e.
ep·i·con·dy·lus
ep·i·cor·a·coid
ep·i·cor·ne·a·scle·ri·tis
ep·i·cra·ni·al
  ap·o·neu·ro·sis
  mus·cle
ep·i·cra·ni·um
ep·i·cri·sis
ep·i·crit·ic
  sen·si·bil·i·ty
ep·i·cys·ti·tis
ep·i·cys·tot·o·my
ep·i·cyte
ep·i·dem·ic
  point e.
ep·i·dem·ic
  curve
  drop·sy
  en·ceph·a·li·tis
  ex·an·the·ma
  he·mo·glo·bi·nu·ria
  hep·a·ti·tis
  hic·cup
  hys·te·ria
  ker·a·to·con·junc·ti·vi·tis
  my·al·gia
  my·o·si·tis
  nau·sea
  neu·ro·my·as·the·nia
  pa·rot·i·di·tis
  pleu·ro·dyn·ia
  pol·y·ar·thri·tis
  ro·se·o·la
  tet·a·ny
  trem·or
  ty·phus
  ver·ti·go
  vom·it·ing
ep·i·dem·ic be·nign dry
  pleu·ri·sy
ep·i·dem·ic cer·e·bro·spi·nal
  men·in·gi·tis
ep·i·dem·ic di·a·phrag·mat·ic
  pleu·ri·sy
ep·i·dem·ic gan·gre·nous
  proc·ti·tis
ep·i·dem·ic gas·tro·en·ter·i·tis
  vi·rus
ep·i·dem·ic hem·or·rhag·ic
  fe·ver
ep·i·de·mic·i·ty

ep·i·dem·ic ker·a·to·con·junc·ti·vi·tis
  vi·rus
ep·i·dem·ic my·al·gia
  vi·rus
ep·i·dem·ic my·al·gic
  en·ceph·a·lo·my·e·li·tis
  en·ceph·a·lo·my·e·lop·a·thy
ep·i·dem·ic non·bac·te·ri·al
  gas·tro·en·ter·i·tis
ep·i·dem·ic par·o·ti·tis
  vi·rus
ep·i·dem·ic pleu·ro·dyn·ia
  vi·rus
ep·i·dem·ic tran·sient di·a·phrag·mat·ic
  spasm
ep·i·de·mi·og·ra·phy
ep·i·de·mi·o·log·i·cal
  dis·tri·bu·tion
ep·i·de·mi·ol·o·gist
ep·i·de·mi·ol·o·gy
ep·i·derm
ep·i·der·ma
ep·i·der·mal
  cyst
  ridg·es
ep·i·der·mal growth
  fac·tor
ep·i·der·mal·i·za·tion
ep·i·der·mal ridge
  count
ep·i·der·mat·ic
ep·i·der·mat·o·plas·ty
ep·i·der·mic
  cell
  graft
ep·i·der·mic-der·mic
  ne·vus
ep·i·derm·i·des
ep·i·der·mi·do·sis
ep·i·der·mis
ep·i·der·mi·tis
ep·i·der·mi·za·tion
ep·i·der·mo·dys·pla·sia
  e. ver·ru·ci·for·mis
ep·i·der·moid
  can·cer
  car·ci·no·ma
  cyst
ep·i·der·mol·y·sis
  e. bul·lo·sa
  e. bul·lo·sa dys·tro·phi·ca
  e. bul·lo·sa le·tha·lis
  e. bul·lo·sa sim·plex
ep·i·der·mo·lyt·ic
  hy·per·ker·a·to·sis
Ep·i·der·mo·phy·ton

ep·i·der·mo·sis
ep·i·der·mot·ro·pism
ep·i·di·al·y·sis
ep·i·di·a·scope
ep·i·did·y·mal
ep·i·did·y·mec·to·my
ep·i·did·y·mid·ec·to·my
ep·i·did·y·mi·des
ep·i·did·y·mi·dis
ep·i·did·y·mis
ep·i·did·y·mis·o·plas·ty
ep·i·did·y·mi·tis
ep·i·did·y·mo-or·chi·tis
ep·i·did·y·mo·plas·ty
ep·i·did·y·mot·o·my
ep·i·did·y·mo·vas·ec·to·my
ep·i·did·y·mo·va·sos·to·my
ep·i·du·ral
  an·es·the·sia
  block
  cav·i·ty
  he·ma·to·ma
  men·in·gi·tis
  space
ep·i·du·rog·ra·phy
ep·i·es·tri·ol
ep·i·fas·cial
ep·i·gas·tral·gia
ep·i·gas·tric
  an·gle
  fold
  fos·sa
  her·nia
  re·flex
  re·gion
  veins
  voice
ep·i·gas·tri·um
ep·i·gas·tri·us
ep·i·gas·tro·cele
ep·i·glot·tic
  car·ti·lage
  tu·ber·cle
ep·i·glot·tid·e·an
ep·i·glot·ti·dec·to·my
ep·i·glot·ti·di·tis
ep·i·glot·tis
ep·i·glot·ti·tis
epig·na·thus
ep·i·hy·al
  bone
  lig·a·ment
ep·i·hy·oid
ep·i·ker·a·to·phak·ia
ep·i·ker·a·to·phak·ic
  ker·a·to·plas·ty
ep·i·ker·a·to·pros·the·sis
ep·i·la·mel·lar

ep·i·late
ep·i·la·tion
  dose
epil·a·to·ry
ep·i·lem·ma
ep·i·lem·mal
  end·ing
ep·i·lep·i·do·ma
ep·i·lep·sia
  e. nu·tans
  e. par·ti·a·lis con·tin·ua
ep·i·lep·sy
  ac·ti·vat·ed e.
  aki·net·ic e.
  ano·sog·no·sic e.
  aton·ic e.
  au·di·o·gen·ic e.
  au·to·mat·ic e.
  au·to·nom·ic e.
  cen·tren·ce·phal·ic e.
  com·plex pre·cip·i·tat·ed e.
  cor·ti·cal e.
  di·en·ce·phal·ic e.
  ear·ly post·trau·mat·ic e.
  eat·ing e.
  fo·cal e.
  gen·er·al·ized ton·ic-clo·nic
   e.
  grand mal e.
  id·i·o·path·ic e.
  jack·so·ni·an e.
  ju·ve·nile my·o·clon·ic e.
  Kojewnikoff's e.
  la·ryn·ge·al e.
  late e.
  lo·cal e.
  ma·jor e.
  masked e.
  ma·tu·ti·nal e.
  my·o·clon·ic astat·ic e.
  my·oc·lo·nus e.
  noc·tur·nal e.
  par·tial e.
  pat·tern sen·si·tive e.
  pe·tit mal e.
  pho·to·gen·ic e.
  post·trau·mat·ic e.
  pri·mary gen·er·al·ized e.
  pro·cur·sive e.
  psy·cho·mo·tor e.
  re·flex e.
  ro·lan·dic e.
  sec·on·dary gen·er·al·ized e.
  sen·so·ry e.
  sen·so·ry pre·cip·i·tat·ed e.
  sleep e.
  som·nam·bu·lic e.
  star·tle e.

symp·to·mat·ic e.
tar·dy e.
tem·po·ral lobe e.
ton·ic e.
tor·na·do e.
un·ci·nate e.
va·so·mo·tor e.
va·so·va·gal e.
vis·cer·al e.
ep·i·lep·tic
ab·sence
de·men·tia
ep·i·lep·ti·form
neu·ral·gia
ep·i·lep·to·gen·ic
zone
ep·i·lep·tog·e·nous
ep·i·lep·toid
ep·i·loia
ep·i·man·dib·u·lar
ep·i·mas·ti·cal
fe·ver
ep·i·mas·ti·gote
ep·i·men·or·rha·gia
ep·i·men·or·rhea
ep·i·mer
ep·i·mer·ase
ep·i·mere
epim·er·ite
ep·i·mi·cro·scope
ep·i·mor·pho·sis
ep·i·mys·i·ot·o·my
ep·i·mys·i·um
ep·i·neph·rine
re·ver·sal
ep·i·neph·ros
ep·i·neu·ral
ep·i·neu·ri·al
ep·i·neu·ri·um
ep·i·no·sic
ep·i·no·sis
ep·i·o·nych·i·um
ep·i·ot·ic
cen·ter
ep·i·pap·il·lary
mem·brane
ep·i·pas·tic
ep·i·per·i·car·di·al
ridge
ep·i·phar·ynx
ep·i·phe·nom·e·non
epiph·o·ra
aton·ic e.
ep·i·phre·nal
ep·i·phren·ic
di·ver·tic·u·lum
epiph·y·se·al
epiph·y·ses

ep·i·phys·i·al
ar·rest
car·ti·lage
eye
frac·ture
line
plate
ep·i·phys·i·al asep·tic
ne·cro·sis
epiph·y·si·od·e·sis
epiph·y·si·ol·y·sis
ep·i·phys·i·op·a·thy
epiph·y·sis
at·a·vis·tic e.
e. ce·re·bri
pres·sure e.
stip·pled e.
trac·tion e.
epiph·y·si·tis
ep·i·pi·al
epip·lo·cele
ep·i·plo·ic
ap·pend·age
fo·ra·men
epip·lo·on
epip·lo·pexy
ep·i·pter·ic
bone
ep·i·py·gus
ep·i·ret·i·nal
mem·brane
ᴅ-ep·i·rham·nose
ep·i·scle·ra
ep·i·scle·ral
ar·tery
lam·i·na
space
veins
ep·i·scle·ri·tis
e. mul·ti·no·du·la·ris
nod·u·lar e.
e. pe·ri·o·di·ca fu·gax
ep·i·si·o·per·i·ne·or·rha·phy
ep·i·si·o·plas·ty
ep·i·si·or·rha·phy
ep·i·si·o·ste·no·sis
ep·i·si·ot·o·my
ep·i·some
re·sis·tance-trans·fer·ring e.'s
ep·i·spa·dia
ep·i·spa·di·al
ep·i·spa·di·as
ep·i·spas·tic
ep·i·spi·nal
ep·i·sple·ni·tis
epis·ta·sis
epis·ta·sy
ep·i·stat·ic

ep·i·stax·is
  re·nal e.
epis·te·mo·phil·ia
ep·i·ster·nal
  bone
ep·i·ster·num
ep·i·stro·phe·us
ep·i·tar·sus
ep·i·taxy
ep·i·ten·din·e·um
epit·e·non
ep·i·thal·a·mus
ep·i·tha·lax·i·a
ep·i·the·lia
ep·i·the·li·al
  at·tach·ment
  body
  can·cer
  cast
  cell
  cyst
  dys·pla·sia
  dys·tro·phy
  ec·to·derm
  in·lay
  lam·i·na
  lay·ers
  mi·gra·tion
  nest
  pearl
  plug
  tis·sue
ep·i·the·li·al cho·roid
  lay·er
ep·i·the·li·al·i·za·tion
ep·i·the·li·al re·tic·u·lar
  cell
ep·i·the·li·o·cho·ri·al
  pla·cen·ta
ep·i·the·li·o·cyte
ep·i·the·li·o·fi·bril
ep·i·the·li·o·glan·du·lar
ep·i·the·li·oid
  cell
ep·i·the·li·oid cell
  ne·vus
ep·i·the·li·o·lyt·ic
ep·i·the·li·o·ma
  e. ad·e·noi·des cys·ti·cum
  ba·sal cell e.
  Borst-Jadassohn type in·tra·
    ep·i·der·mal e.
  cho·ri·on·ic e.
  e. con·ta·gi·o·sum
  e. cu·ni·cu·la·tum
  Malherbe's cal·ci·fy·ing e.
  ma·lig·nant cil·i·ary e.

  mul·ti·ple self-heal·ing squa·
    mous e.
  se·ba·ceous e.
ep·i·the·li·om·a·tous
ep·i·the·li·op·a·thy
  pig·ment e.
ep·i·the·li·o·sis
ep·i·the·lite
ep·i·the·li·um
  an·te·ri·or e. of cor·nea
  Barrett's e.
  cil·i·at·ed e.
  co·lum·nar e.
  cre·vic·u·lar e.
  cu·boi·dal e.
  cy·lin·dri·cal e.
  enam·el e.
  ex·ter·nal den·tal e.
  ex·ter·nal enam·el e.
  ger·mi·nal e.
  gin·gi·val e.
  glan·du·lar e.
  in·ner den·tal e.
  in·ner enam·el e.
  junc·tion·al e.
  lam·i·nat·ed e.
  e. of lens
  me·sen·chy·mal e.
  mus·cle e.
  ol·fac·to·ry e.
  pave·ment e.
  pig·ment e.
  pseu·do·strat·i·fied e.
  re·duced enam·el e.
  res·pi·ra·to·ry e.
  sem·i·nif·er·ous e.
  sim·ple e.
  sim·ple squa·mous e.
  strat·i·fied e.
  strat·i·fied cil·i·at·ed co·
    lum·nar e.
  strat·i·fied squa·mous e.
  sul·cu·lar e.
  sur·face e.
  tran·si·tion·al e.
ep·i·the·li·za·tion
ep·i·them
ep·i·ther·mal
  chem·is·try
  neu·tron
epith·e·sis
ep·i·thet
  spe·cif·ic e.
ep·i·thi·a·zide
ep·i·tope
ep·i·tox·oid
ep·i·trich·i·al
  lay·er

ep·i·trich·i·um
ep·i·troch·lea
ep·i·troch·le·ar
  nodes
ep·i·tu·ber·cu·lo·sis
ep·i·tu·ber·cu·lous
  in·fil·tra·tion
ep·i·tym·pan·ic
  re·cess
  space
ep·i·tym·pa·num
ep·i·zoa
ep·i·zo·ic
  com·men·sal·ism
ep·i·zo·ol·o·gy
ep·i·zo·on
ep·i·zo·ot·ic
  cel·lu·li·tis
  lym·phan·gi·tis
ep·i·zo·ot·i·ol·o·gy
éplu·chage
ep·o·nych·ia
ep·o·nych·i·um
ep·o·oph·o·rec·to·my
ep·o·öph·o·ron
epo·prost·en·ol
epo·prost·en·ol so·di·um
ep·ox·y
  res·in
ep·si·lon
  al·co·hol·ism
Ep·som
  salts
Ep·som salt
Epstein-Barr
  vi·rus
Epstein's
  dis·ease
  pearls
  symp·tom
epu·lis
  con·gen·i·tal e. of new·born
  e. fis·su·ra·tum
  gi·ant cell e.
  e. grav·i·dar·um
  pig·ment·ed e.
ep·u·loid
equal
  cleav·age
equa·tion
  di·vi·sion
equa·tion
  al·ve·o·lar gas e.
  Arrhenius e.
  Bohr's e.
  chem·i·cal e.
  con·stant field e.
  Einthoven's e.

GHK e.
Gibbs-Helmholtz e.
Goldman e.
Goldman-Hodgkin-Katz e.
Hasselbalch's e.
Henderson-Hasselbalch e.
Hill's e.
Hufner's e.
Lineweaver-Burk e.
Michaelis-Menten e.
Nernst's e.
per·son·al e.
Rayleigh e.
equa·tor
  e. of eye·ball
  e. of lens
equa·to·ri·al
  cleav·age
  plane
  plate
  staph·y·lo·ma
equi·an·al·ge·sic
  dose
equi·ax·i·al
equi·ca·lor·ic
eq·ui·len·in
equil·i·bra·tion
equi·lib·ri·um
  ac·id-base e.
  Donnan e.
  dy·nam·ic e.
  ge·net·ic e.
  Gibbs-Donnan e.
  Hardy-Weinberg e.
  ho·me·o·stat·ic e.
  ni·trog·e·nous e.
  nu·tri·tive e.
  phys·i·o·log·ic e.
  ra·di·o·ac·tive e.
  ran·dom mat·ing e.
  sta·ble e.
  un·sta·ble e.
equi·lib·ri·um
  con·stant
  di·al·y·sis
eq·ui·lin
equi·mo·lar
equi·mo·lec·u·lar
equine
  ba·be·si·o·sis
  en·ceph·a·li·tis
  en·ceph·a·lo·my·e·li·tis
  gait
  go·nad·o·tro·pin
  in·flu·en·za
  rhi·no·pneu·mo·ni·tis
  rhi·no·vi·rus·es
  syph·i·lis

equine abor·tion
vi·rus
equine ar·te·ri·tis
vi·rus
equine bil·i·ary
fe·ver
equine co·i·tal ex·an·the·ma
vi·rus
equine go·nad·o·tro·pin
unit
equine in·fec·tious
ane·mia
equine in·fec·tious ane·mia
vi·rus
equine in·flu·en·za
vi·rus·es
equine mon·o·cyt·ic
ehr·lich·i·o·sis
equine rhi·no·pneu·mo·ni·tis
vi·rus
equine se·rum
hep·a·ti·tis
equine spi·nal
atax·ia
equine vi·ral
ar·te·ri·tis
equine vi·rus
abor·tion
equi·no·val·gus
equi·no·var·us
equi·pha·sic
com·plex
equi·se·to·sis
equi·tox·ic
equiv·a·lence
zone
equiv·a·len·cy
equiv·a·lent
com·bus·tion e.
gold e.
gram e.
Joule's e.
le·thal e.
met·a·bol·ic e.
ni·tro·gen e.
starch e.
tox·ic e.
equiv·a·lent
ex·tract
pow·er
tem·per·a·ture
weight
equiv·a·lent form
re·li·a·bil·i·ty
equiv·o·cal
symp·tom
Eranko's flu·o·res·cence
stain

era·sion
Erb–Charcot
dis·ease
er·bi·um
Erb's
at·ro·phy
dis·ease
pal·sy
pa·ral·y·sis
sign
Erb's spi·nal
pa·ral·y·sis
Erb–Westphal
sign
er·cal·cid·i·ol
er·cal·ci·ol
er·cal·cit·ri·ol
Erdheim
dis·ease
tu·mor
Erdmann's
re·a·gent
erect
il·lu·mi·na·tion
erec·tile
tis·sue
erec·tion
erec·tor
mus·cles of the hairs
mus·cle of spine
erec·tor-spi·nal
re·flex
er·e·mo·phil·ia
er·e·mo·pho·bia
er·e·thism
er·e·this·mic
er·e·this·tic
shock
er·e·thit·ic
er·eu·tho·pho·bi·a
er·ga·sia
er·ga·si·o·ma·nia
er·ga·si·o·pho·bia
er·gas·the·nia
er·gas·to·plasm
er·gin
erg·ine
er·go·ba·sine
er·go·cal·cif·er·ol
er·go·cor·nine
er·go·cris·tine
er·go·cryp·tine
er·go·dy·nam·o·graph
er·go·es·the·si·o·graph
er·go·gen·ic
er·go·graph
Mosso's e.
er·go·graph·ic

er·gom·e·ter
er·go·met·rine
  e. ma·le·ate
er·go·nom·ics
er·go·no·vine
  e. ma·le·ate
er·go·sine
er·go·stat
er·gos·ter·in
er·gos·ter·ol
er·go·stet·rine
er·got
  corn e.
er·got·a·mine
er·got·am·i·nine
er·go·ther·a·py
er·go·thi·o·ne·ine
er·got·ism
er·go·tox·ine
er·go·tro·pic
Erichsen's
  sign
er·i·o·dic·ty·on
eris·o·phake
Erlenmeyer
  flask
Erlenmeyer flask
  de·for·mi·ty
erode
erog·e·nous
  zone
eros
erose
E-ro·sette
  test
ero·sion
  Dieulafoy's e.
  re·cur·rent cor·ne·al e.
ero·sive
  ad·e·no·ma·to·sis of nip·ple
erot·ic
  zo·oph·i·lism
erot·i·cism
er·o·tism
  anal e.
er·o·ti·za·tion
ero·to·gen·e·sis
ero·to·gen·ic
  zone
ero·to·ma·nia
ero·to·path·ic
er·o·top·a·thy
ero·to·pho·bia
er·rat·ic
er·ro·ne·ous
  pro·jec·tion

er·ror
  in·born e.'s of me·tab·o·lism
er·ta·cal·ci·ol
er·u·bes·cence
er·u·bes·cent
eru·cic ac·id
eruc·ta·tion
erup·tion
  ac·cel·er·at·ed e.
  but·ter·fly e.
  clin·i·cal e.
  con·tin·u·ous e.
  creep·ing e.
  de·layed e.
  drug e.
  feigned e.
  fixed drug e.
  io·dine e.
  Kaposi's var·i·cel·li·form e.
  me·dic·i·nal e.
  pas·sive e.
  pol·y·mor·phic light e.
  se·rum e.
  sur·gi·cal e.
erup·tive
  fe·ver
  phase
  xan·tho·ma
er·y·sip·e·las
  am·bu·lant e.
  coast·al e.
  e. in·ter·num
  e. mi·grans
  e. per·stans fa·ci·ei
  phleg·mon·ous e.
  e. pus·tu·lo·sum
  sur·gi·cal e.
  swine e.
  e. ver·ru·co·sum
  wan·der·ing e.
er·y·si·pel·a·tous
er·y·sip·e·loid
Er·y·sip·e·lo·thrix
  E. in·si·di·o·sa
  E. rhu·si·o·path·i·ae
er·y·sip·e·lo·tox·in
er·y·the·ma
  e. ab ig·ne
  ac·ro·dyn·ic e.
  e. an·nu·la·re
  e. an·nu·la·re cen·tri·fu·gum
  e. an·nu·la·re rheu·ma·ti·cum
  e. ar·thri·ti·cum ep·i·de·mi·cum
  e. bul·lo·sum

er·y·the·ma *(continued)*
e. ca·lo·ri·cum
e. chro·ni·cum mi·grans
e. cir·ci·na·tum
e. dys·chro·mi·cum per·stans
e. el·e·va·tum di·u·ti·num
e. ex·fo·li·a·ti·va
e. fig·u·ra·tum per·stans
e. fu·gax
e. gy·ra·tum
hem·or·rhag·ic ex·ud·a·tive e.
e. in·du·ra·tum
e. in·fec·ti·o·sum
e. in·ter·tri·go
e. iris
Jacquet's e.
e. ke·ra·to·des
mac·u·lar e.
e. mar·gi·na·tum
e. mi·grans
e. mi·grans lin·guae
Milian's e.
e. mul·ti·for·me
e. mul·ti·for·me bul·lo·sum
e. mul·ti·for·me ex·u·da·ti·vum
nec·ro·lyt·ic mi·gra·to·ry e.
e. ne·o·na·to·rum
ninth-day e.
e. no·do·sum
e. no·do·sum le·pro·sum
e. no·do·sum mi·grans
e. pal·ma·re he·re·di·ta·ri·um
e. pa·pu·la·tum
e. par·a·trim·ma
e. per·nio
e. per·stans
e. po·ly·mor·phe
scar·la·ti·ni·form e.
e. scar·la·ti·no·i·des
e. sim·plex
e. so·la·re
symp·to·mat·ic e.
e. tox·i·cum
e. tox·i·cum ne·o·na·to·rum
e. tu·ber·cu·la·tum
er·y·the·ma
dose
thresh·old
er·y·them·a·tous
syph·i·lid
er·y·the·ma·to·ve·sic·u·lar
er·y·ther·mal·gia
er·y·thral·gia
ery·thras·ma

eryth·re·de·ma
pol·y·neu·ri·tis
er·y·thre·mia
al·ti·tude e.
er·y·threm·ic
my·e·lo·sis
er·y·thrism
er·y·thris·tic
er·y·thrite
eryth·ri·tol
eryth·ri·tyl tet·ra·ni·trate
eryth·ro·blast
eryth·ro·blas·te·mia
eryth·ro·blas·tic
ane·mia
eryth·ro·blas·to·pe·nia
eryth·ro·blas·to·sis
avi·an e.
fe·tal e.
e. fe·ta·lis
fowl e.
eryth·ro·blas·tot·ic
eryth·ro·ca·tal·y·sis
eryth·ro·chro·mia
eryth·ro·cla·sis
eryth·ro·clas·tic
eryth·ro·cu·pre·in
eryth·ro·cy·a·no·sis
eryth·ro·cyte
in·di·ces
eryth·ro·cyte ad·her·ence phe·nom·e·non test
eryth·ro·cyte fra·gil·i·ty test
eryth·ro·cyte mat·u·ra·tion fac·tor
eryth·ro·cyte sed·i·men·ta·tion rate
eryth·ro·cy·the·mia
eryth·ro·cyt·ic
se·ries
eryth·ro·cy·to·blast
eryth·ro·cy·tol·y·sin
eryth·ro·cy·tol·y·sis
eryth·ro·cy·tom·e·ter
eryth·ro·cy·to·pe·nia
eryth·ro·cy·to·poi·e·sis
eryth·ro·cy·tor·rhex·is
eryth·ro·cy·tos·chi·sis
eryth·ro·cy·to·sis
eryth·ro·cy·tu·ria
eryth·ro·de·gen·er·a·tive
eryth·ro·der·ma
con·gen·i·tal ich·thy·o·si·form e.
e. des·qua·ma·ti·vum
e. ex·fo·li·a·ti·va

ich·thy·o·si·form e.
mac·u·lo·pap·u·lar e.
e. pso·ri·a·ti·cum
Sézary e.
eryth·ro·der·ma·ti·tis
eryth·ro·don·tia
eryth·ro·dys·es·the·sia
syn·drome
eryth·ro·gen·e·sis im·per·fec·ta
eryth·ro·gen·ic
tox·in
eryth·ro·go·nia
eryth·ro·go·ni·um
eryth·ro·he·pat·ic
por·phyr·ia
er·y·throid
cell
eryth·ro·ker·a·to·der·ma
e. va·ri·a·bi·lis
eryth·ro·ki·net·ics
er·y·throl
e. tet·ra·ni·trate
eryth·ro·leu·ke·mia
eryth·ro·leu·ko·sis
er·y·throl·y·sin
er·y·throl·y·sis
eryth·ro·mel·al·gia
eryth·ro·me·lia
eryth·ro·my·cin
er·y·thron
eryth·ro·ne·o·cy·to·sis
eryth·ro·pe·nia
eryth·ro·pha·gia
eryth·ro·phag·o·cy·to·sis
eryth·ro·phil
eryth·ro·phil·ic
eryth·ro·phore
re·ac·tion
eryth·ro·pla·kia
eryth·ro·pla·sia
e. of Queyrat
Zoon's e.
eryth·ro·poi·e·sis
eryth·ro·poi·et·ic
hor·mone
por·phyr·ia
pro·to·por·phyr·ia
eryth·ro·poi·e·tin
eryth·ro·pros·o·pal·gia
eryth·rop·sia
eryth·ro·pyk·no·sis
er·y·thror·rhex·is
er·y·throse
eryth·ro·sin B
er·y·throx·y·line
eryth·ru·lose
er·y·thru·ria

Esbach's
re·a·gent
es·cape
beat
con·di·tion·ing
im·pulse
in·ter·val
phe·nom·e·non
rhythm
es·cape
no·dal e.
ven·tric·u·lar e.
es·cape-cap·ture
bi·gem·i·ny
es·caped
beat
con·trac·tion
es·caped ven·tric·u·lar
con·trac·tion
es·char
es·cha·rot·ic
es·cha·rot·o·my
Esch·e·rich·ia
E. au·res·cens
E. co·li
E. freun·dii
Esch·e·rich·ia co·li
en·ter·o·tox·in
RNase I
Escherich's
sign
es·cor·cin
es·cor·cin·ol
es·cu·lent
es·cu·lin
es·cutch·eon
es·er·i·dine
es·er·ine
e. am·i·nox·ide
e. ox·ide
e. sa·lic·y·late
Esmarch
tour·ni·quet
es·mo·lol hy·dro·chlo·ride
es·o·de·vi·a·tion
es·od·ic
nerve
es·o·eth·moi·di·tis
es·o·gas·tri·tis
esoph·a·gal·gia
esoph·a·ge·al
acha·la·sia
ar·ter·ies
atre·sia
car·di·o·gram
glands
im·pres·sion
lead

esoph·a·ge·al *(continued)*
  ma·nom·e·try
  open·ing
  plex·us
  re·flux
  smear
  speech
  va·ri·ces
  veins
  web
esoph·a·gec·ta·sia
esoph·a·gec·ta·sis
e·soph·a·gec·to·my
  trans·hi·a·tal e.
  trans·tho·rac·ic e.
esoph·a·gi
esoph·a·gism
esoph·a·gi·tis
  pep·tic e.
  re·flux e.
esoph·a·go·car·di·o·plas·ty
esoph·a·go·cele
esoph·a·go·dyn·ia
esoph·a·go·en·ter·os·to·my
esoph·a·go·fi·ber·scope
esoph·a·go·gas·trec·to·my
esoph·a·go·gas·tric
  junc·tion
  or·i·fice
  ves·ti·bule
esoph·a·go·gas·tro·a·nas·to·mo·sis
esoph·a·go·gas·tro·my·ot·o·my
esoph·a·go·gas·tro·plas·ty
esoph·a·go·gas·tros·to·my
esoph·a·go·gram
esoph·a·gog·ra·phy
esoph·a·go·ma·la·cia
esoph·a·go·my·co·sis
esoph·a·go·my·ot·o·my
esoph·a·go·plas·ty
esoph·a·go·pli·ca·tion
esoph·a·go·pto·sia
esoph·a·go·pto·sis
esoph·a·go·sal·i·vary
  re·flex
esoph·a·go·scope
esoph·a·gos·co·py
esoph·a·go·spasm
esoph·a·go·ste·no·sis
esoph·a·go·sto·mi·a·sis
esoph·a·gos·to·my
esoph·a·got·o·my
esoph·a·gus
  Barrett e.
es·o·pho·ria
es·o·phor·ic
es·o·phy·lax·is

es·o·sphe·noid·i·tis
es·o·tro·pia
  A-e.
  ba·sic e.
  con·sec·u·tive e.
  cy·clic e.
  mixed e.
  non·ac·com·mo·da·tive e.
  non·re·frac·tive ac·com·mo·da·tive e.
  re·frac·tive ac·com·mo·da·tive e.
  V-e.
  X-e.
es·o·tro·pic
es·pun·dia
es·qui·nan·cea
es·sence
es·sen·tial
  al·bu·min·ur·ia
  ami·no ac·ids
  bra·dy·car·dia
  dys·men·or·rhea
  fe·ver
  fruc·to·su·ria
  he·ma·tu·ria
  hy·per·ten·sion
  oils
  pen·to·su·ria
  phthi·sis bul·bi
  pru·ri·tus
  tach·y·car·dia
  tel·an·gi·ec·ta·sia
  throm·bo·cy·to·pe·nia
es·sen·tial food
  fac·tors
es·sen·tial pro·gress·ive
  at·ro·phy of iris
Esser
  graft
  op·er·a·tion
Essick's cell
  bands
Essig
  splint
es·tab·lished cell
  line
es·ter
  Cori e.
  Embden e.
  Harden-Young e.
  Robison e.
  Robison-Embden e.
es·ter·ase
es·ter·i·fi·ca·tion
es·ter·i·fied
  es·tro·gens

Estes
op·er·a·tion
es·the·ma·tol·o·gy
es·the·sia
es·the·sic
es·the·si·od·ic
sys·tem
es·the·si·o·gen·e·sis
es·the·si·o·gen·ic
es·the·si·og·ra·phy
es·the·si·ol·o·gy
es·the·si·om·e·ter
es·the·si·om·e·try
es·the·si·o·neu·ro·blas·to·ma
ol·fac·to·ry e.
es·the·si·o·neu·ro·cy·to·ma
es·the·si·o·neu·ro·sis
es·the·si·on·o·sus
es·the·si·o·phys·i·ol·o·gy
es·the·si·os·co·py
es·the·sod·ic
es·thet·ic
sur·gery
es·thet·ics
den·ture e.
es·thi·o·mene
es·thi·om·e·nous
es·ti·val
es·ti·va·tion
es·ti·vo·au·tum·nal
Estlander
flap
op·er·a·tion
es·tra·di·ol
e. ben·zo·ate
e. cyp·i·o·nate
e. di·pro·pi·on·ate
eth·i·nyl e.
ethy·nyl e.
e. un·de·cy·late
e. val·er·ate
es·tra·di·ol ben·zo·ate
unit
es·tra·gon oil
es·tra·mus·tine phos·phate so·di·um
es·trane
es·tra·tri·ene
es·trin
es·tri·ol
es·tro·die·nol
es·tro·gen
con·ju·gat·ed e.
es·ter·i·fied e.'s
es·tro·gen·ic
hor·mone
es·trone
unit

es·trous
cy·cle
es·tru·al
es·trus
post·par·tum e.
es·y·late
et·a·fed·rine hy·dro·chlo·ride
etaf·e·none
etam·sy·late
état
e. cri·blé
e. mam·e·lon·né
eth·ac·ri·dine lac·tate
eth·a·cry·nate so·di·um
eth·a·cryn·ic ac·id
eth·a·di·one
eth·al·de·hyde
eth·am·bu·tol hy·dro·chlo·ride
etha·mi·van
eth·a·mox·y·tri·phe·tol
etham·sy·late
eth·a·nal
eth·ane
eth·ane·di·al
eth·ane·di·a·mine
eth·ane·di·ni·trile
eth·a·no·ic ac·id
eth·a·nol
eth·a·nol·a·mine
eth·a·nol·a·mine·phos·pho·trans·fer·ase
eth·av·e·rine hy·dro·chlo·ride
eth·chlor·vy·nol
eth·ene
eth·en·yl
eth·en·yl·ben·zene
eth·en·yl·ene
ether
an·es·thet·ic e.
sol·vent e.
xy·lo·styp·tic e.
ether
cone
con·vul·sion
test
ethe·re·al
oil
so·lu·tion
tinc·ture
ether·i·fi·ca·tion
ether·i·za·tion
ethi·a·zide
eth·i·cal
eth·ics
med·i·cal e.
eth·i·dene
Ethid·i·um
ethid·i·um bro·mide

ethin·a·mate
ethin·drone
eth·i·nyl
    e. tri·chlo·ride
eth·i·nyl
    es·tra·di·ol
eth·i·nyl·es·tre·nol
eth·i·o·dized oil
eth·i·on·am·ide
ethi·o·nine
ethis·ter·one
eth·mo·cra·ni·al
eth·mo·fron·tal
eth·moid
    an·gle
    bone
    in·fun·dib·u·lum
eth·moi·dal
    bul·la
    cells
    crest
    fo·ra·men
    groove
    lab·y·rinth
    notch
    pro·cess
    si·nus·es
    veins
eth·moi·da·le
eth·moi·dal-lac·ri·mal
    fis·tu·la
eth·moi·dec·to·my
eth·moid·i·tis
eth·moi·do·lac·ri·mal
    su·ture
eth·moi·do·max·il·lary
    su·ture
eth·mo·lac·ri·mal
eth·mo·max·il·lary
eth·mo·na·sal
eth·mo·pal·a·tal
eth·mo·sphe·noid
eth·mo·tur·bi·nals
eth·mo·vo·mer·ine
    plate
eth·no·cen·trism
eth·o·hep·ta·zine cit·rate
eth·o·hex·a·di·ol
ethol·o·gist
ethol·o·gy
eth·o·mox·ane
eth·o·phar·ma·col·o·gy
eth·o·pro·pa·zine hy·dro·chlo·ride
eth·o·sux·i·mide
eth·o·to·in
eth·o·tri·mep·ra·zine
ethox·a·zene hy·dro·chlo·ride

eth·oxy
eth·ox·y·bu·ta·mox·ane
eth·ox·y·zol·a·mide
eth·yl
    e. al·co·hol
    e. ami·no·ben·zo·ate
    e. bis·cou·ma·cet·ate
    e. bu·ty·rate
    e. car·ba·mate
    e. chlo·ride
    e. eo·sin
    e. for·mate
    e. ole·ate
    e. ox·ide
    e. sa·lic·y·late
eth·yl
    eo·sin
eth·yl·ate
eth·yl·benz·tro·pine
eth·yl·cel·lu·lose
eth·yl·ene
    e. di·bro·mide
    e. ox·ide
    e. tet·ra·chlo·ride
eth·yl·ene·di·a·mine
eth·yl·ene·di·a·mine·tet·ra·a·ce·tic ac·id
eth·yl·ene gly·col
eth·yl·es·tre·nol
eth·yl ether
eth·yl green
eth·yl·i·dene
eth·yl·i·dyne
eth·yl·i·so·bu·tra·zine
eth·yl·mor·phine hy·dro·chlo·ride
eth·yl·nor·ep·i·neph·rine
eth·yl·pa·pav·er·ine hy·dro·chlo·ride
eth·yl·par·a·ben
eth·yl·phen·ac·e·mide
eth·yl·phen·yl·eph·rine hy·dro·chlo·ride
eth·yl·stib·a·mine
eth·yl·vi·nyl ether
ethy·no·di·ol
    e. di·ac·e·tate
ethy·nyl
    e. es·tra·di·ol
ethy·nyl
    es·tra·di·ol
eti·ane
eti·an·ic ac·ids
eti·do·caine
eti·dro·nate di·so·di·um
eti·dron·ic ac·id
et·il·ef·rine hy·dro·chlo·ride
eti·o·al·lo·cho·lane

eti·o·cho·lane
eti·o·cho·lan·o·lone
eti·o·gen·ic
eti·o·lat·ed
eti·o·la·tion
eti·o·log·ic
eti·ol·o·gy
eti·o·path·ic
eti·o·por·phy·rin
eti·o·tro·pic
etom·i·date
eto·po·side
etor·phine
et·o·zo·lin
etret·i·nate
et·y·mem·a·zine
"e"-type
    cho·lin·es·ter·ase
eu·al·leles
Eu·bac·te·ri·a·les
Eu·bac·te·ri·um
    E. aer·o·fa·ci·ens
    E. bi·for·me
    E. com·be·si
    E. con·tor·tum
    E. cris·pa·tum
    E. dis·ci·for·mans
    E. eth·yl·i·cum
    E. fil·a·men·to·sum
    E. foe·dans
    E. len·tum
    E. li·mo·sum
    E. mi·nu·tum
    E. mo·nil·i·for·me
    E. mul·ti·for·me
    E. ni·o·sii
    E. par·vum
    E. poe·ci·loi·des
    E. pseu·do·tor·tu·o·sum
    E. quar·tum
    E. quin·tum
    E. rec·ta·le
    E. te·nue
    E. tor·tu·o·sum
eu·bi·ot·ics
eu·bo·lism
eu·caine
eu·ca·lyp·tol
eu·ca·lyp·tus
    e. oil
eu·ca·lyp·tus
    gum
eu·cap·nia
eu·car·y·ote
eu·car·y·ot·ic
eu·ca·sin
eu·cat·ro·pine hy·dro·chlo·ride
Eu·ces·to·da

eu·chlor·hy·dria
eu·cho·lia
eu·chro·mat·ic
eu·chro·ma·tin
eu·chro·mo·some
eu·cor·ti·cal·ism
eu·cra·sia
eu·cu·pine
eu·de·mo·nia
eu·di·a·pho·re·sis
eu·dip·sia
Eu·flag·el·la·ta
eu·gen·ic
eu·gen·ic ac·id
eu·gen·ics
eu·gen·ism
eu·ge·nol
Eu·gle·na
    E. grac·i·lis
    E. vi·ri·dis
Eu·gle·ni·dae
eu·glob·u·lin
eu·glob·u·lin clot ly·sis
    time
eu·gly·ce·mia
eu·gly·ce·mic
eu·gna·thia
eu·gnath·ic
    anom·a·ly
eu·gno·sia
eu·gon·ic
Eu·gre·ga·rin·i·da
eu·hy·dra·tion
Eu·kar·y·o·tae
eu·kar·y·ote
eu·kar·y·ot·ic
eu·ker·a·tin
eu·ki·ne·sia
Eulenburg's
    dis·ease
eu·mel·a·nin
eu·mel·a·no·some
eu·me·tria
eu·mor·phism
eu·my·cetes
Eu·my·ce·to·zo·ea
eu·noia
eu·nuch
eu·nuch·ism
eu·nuch·oid
    gi·gan·tism
    state
    voice
eu·nuch·oid·ism
    hy·per·go·nad·o·tro·pic e.
    hy·po·go·nad·o·tro·pic e.
eu·os·mia
eu·pan·cre·a·tism

eu·pa·ral
Eu·pa·ryph·i·um
eu·pav·er·in
eu·pep·sia
eu·pep·tic
eu·phen·ics
Eu·phor·bia pi·lu·lif·e·ra
eu·pho·ret·ic
eu·pho·ria
eu·pho·ri·ant
eu·pla·sia
eu·plas·tic
  lymph
eu·ploid
eu·ploidy
eup·nea
eu·prax·ia
eu·pro·cin hy·dro·chlo·ride
Eu·proc·tis
eu·rhyth·mia
Eu·ro·pe·an
  snake·root
  ta·ran·tu·la
eu·ro·pi·um
eu·rox·e·nous
  par·a·site
eu·ry·ce·phal·ic
eu·ry·ceph·a·lous
eu·ryg·nath·ic
eu·ryg·na·thism
eu·ryg·na·thous
eu·ry·on
eu·ry·o·pia
eu·ry·so·mat·ic
eu·scope
Eu·sim·u·li·um
eu·sta·chi·an
  cath·e·ter
  cush·ion
  ton·sil
  tube
  tu·ber
  valve
eu·sta·chi·tis
eus·the·nia
Eu·stron·gy·lus
eu·sys·to·le
eu·sys·tol·ic
eu·tec·tic
  al·loy
  tem·per·a·ture
eu·tel·e·gen·e·sis
eu·tha·na·sia
eu·then·ics
eu·ther·a·peu·tic
Eu·the·ria
eu·ther·mic
eu·thy·mia

eu·thy·mic
eu·thy·roid
  hy·po·me·tab·o·lism
eu·thy·roid·ism
eu·thy·scope
eu·thys·co·py
eu·ton·ic
eu·tri·cho·sis
eu·tro·phia
eu·tro·phic
eu·tro·phy
eu·vo·lia
evac·u·ant
evac·u·ate
evac·u·a·tion
evac·u·a·tor
  Ellik e.
evag·i·na·tion
ev·a·nes·cent
Evans
  for·ceps
Evans'
  syn·drome
Evans blue
e·vap·o·rate
evap·o·ra·tion
eva·sion
  mac·u·lar e.
even·tra·tion
  e. of the di·a·phragm
ever·sion
evert
evide·ment
evil
  joint e.
  king's e.
  poll e.
  quar·ter e.
ev·i·ra·tion
evis·cer·a·tion
evis·cer·o·neu·rot·o·my
evo·ca·tion
evo·ca·tor
evoked
  po·ten·tial
  re·sponse
evoked re·sponse
  au·di·om·e·try
ev·o·lu·tion
  bath·mic e.
  bi·o·log·ic e.
  con·ver·gent e.
  Denman's spon·ta·ne·ous e.
  Douglas' spon·ta·ne·ous e.
  emer·gent e.
  or·gan·ic e.
  or·tho·gen·ic e.

sal·ta·to·ry e.
spon·ta·ne·ous e.
ev·o·lu·tion·ary
fit·ness
evul·sion
Ewart's
pro·ce·dure
sign
Ewing's
sar·co·ma
sign
tu·mor
ex·ac·er·ba·tion
ex·am·i·na·tion
cy·to·log·ic e.
Papanicolaou e.
phys·i·cal e.
post·mor·tem e.
ex·am·in·er
med·i·cal e.
ex·am·in·ing
ta·ble
ex·an·them
ex·an·the·ma
Bos·ton e.
ep·i·dem·ic e.
ker·a·toid e.
e. sub·i·tum
ve·sic·u·lar e.
ex·an·them·a·tous
dis·ease
fe·ver
ex·an·the·sis
e. ar·thro·sia
ex·an·thrope
ex·an·throp·ic
ex·ar·te·ri·tis
ex·ar·tic·u·la·tion
ex·cal·a·tion
ex·ca·va·tio
e. pa·pil·lae
ex·ca·va·tion
atroph·ic e.
glau·co·ma·tous e.
e. of op·tic disk
phys·i·o·log·ic e.
ex·ca·va·tor
hatch·et e.
hoe e.
ex·ce·men·to·sis
ex·cen·tric
am·pu·ta·tion
ex·cess
lac·tate
ex·cess
an·ti·body e.
an·ti·gen e.
base e.

con·ver·gence e.
neg·a·tive base e.
ex·change
sis·ter chro·ma·tid e.
ex·change
trans·fu·sion
ex·cip·i·ent
ex·cise
ex·ci·sion
bi·op·sy
ex·cit·a·bil·i·ty
su·pra·nor·mal e.
ex·cit·a·ble
ar·ea
ex·cit·ant
ex·ci·ta·tion
spec·trum
wave
ex·cit·a·to·ry
ex·cit·a·to·ry post·syn·ap·tic
po·ten·tial
ex·cit·ed
at·om
cat·a·to·nia
state
ex·cite·ment
cat·a·ton·ic e.
man·ic e.
ex·cit·ing
cause
elec·trode
eye
ex·ci·to·glan·du·lar
ex·ci·to·met·a·bol·ic
ex·ci·to·mo·tor
ex·ci·to·mus·cu·lar
ex·ci·tor
nerve
ex·ci·to·re·flex
nerve
ex·ci·to·se·cre·to·ry
ex·ci·to·vas·cu·lar
ex·cla·ma·tion point
hair
ex·clave
ex·clu·sion
al·le·lic e.
Devine e.
e. of pu·pil
ex·con·ju·gant
ex·co·ri·ate
ex·co·ri·a·tion
neu·rot·ic e.
ex·cre·ment
ex·cre·men·ti·tious
ex·cres·cence
ex·cre·ta
ex·crete

ex·cre·tion
ex·cre·to·ry
  duct
  duct of sem·i·nal ves·i·cle
  duc·tules of lac·ri·mal gland
  gland
  urog·ra·phy
ex·cur·sion
  lat·er·al e.
  pro·tru·sive e.
ex·cy·clo·duc·tion
ex·cy·clo·pho·ria
ex·cy·clo·ver·gence
ex·cys·ta·tion
ex·e·mia
ex·en·ce·pha·lia
ex·en·ce·phal·ic
ex·en·ceph·a·lo·cele
ex·en·ceph·a·lous
ex·en·ceph·a·ly
ex·en·ter·a·tion
  an·te·ri·or pel·vic e.
  or·bi·tal e.
  pel·vic e.
  pos·te·ri·or pel·vic e.
  to·tal pel·vic e.
ex·en·ter·i·tis
ex·er·cise
  iso·met·ric e.
  Kegel's e.'s
ex·er·cise
  bone
  test
ex·er·e·sis
ex·er·gon·ic
ex·er·tion·al
  rhab·do·my·ol·y·sis
ex·flag·el·la·tion
ex·fo·li·a·tion
  e. of lens
ex·fo·li·a·tive
  cy·tol·o·gy
  der·ma·ti·tis
  gas·tri·tis
ex·ha·la·tion
ex·hale
ex·haus·tion
  heat e.
ex·haus·tion
  at·ro·phy
  psy·cho·sis
ex·hi·bi·tion·ism
ex·hi·bi·tion·ist
ex·hil·a·rant
ex·is·ten·tial
  psy·chi·a·try
  psy·chol·o·gy
  psy·cho·ther·a·py

ex·it
  block
  dose
ex·i·tus
Exner's
  plex·us
ex·o·an·ti·gen
ex·o·car·dia
ex·o·car·di·al
  mur·mur
ex·oc·cip·i·tal
  bone
ex·o·ce·lom·ic
  mem·brane
ex·o·crine
  gland
ex·o·cy·clic
ex·o·cy·to·sis
ex·o·de·vi·a·tion
ex·od·ic
  nerve
ex·o·don·tia
ex·o·don·tist
ex·o·en·zyme
ex·o·e·ryth·ro·cyt·ic
  cy·cle
  stage
ex·og·a·my
ex·o·gas·tru·la
ex·o·ge·net·ic
ex·o·gen·ic
  tox·i·co·sis
ex·o·ge·note
ex·og·e·nous
  cy·cle
  fi·bers
  he·mo·chro·ma·to·sis
  hy·per·glyc·er·i·de·mia
  ochro·no·sis
  pig·men·ta·tion
ex·og·e·nous cre·at·i·nine
  clear·ance
  cli·no·scope
ex·o·lev·er
ex·om·e·ter
ex·om·pha·los
ex·on
ex·on shuf·fle
ex·o·nu·cle·ase
ex·o·pep·ti·dase
Ex·o·phi·a·la
  E. jean·selmei
  E. wer·nec·kii
ex·o·pho·ria
ex·o·phor·ic
ex·oph·thal·mic
  goi·ter
  oph·thal·mo·ple·gia

ex·oph·thal·mom·e·ter
ex·oph·thal·mos
  en·do·crine e.
  ma·lig·nant e.
ex·oph·thal·mos-pro·duc·ing
  sub·stance
ex·oph·thal·mus
ex·o·phyte
ex·o·phyt·ic
ex·o·plasm
ex·o·se·ro·sis
ex·o·skel·e·ton
ex·os·mo·sis
ex·o·spore
ex·o·spo·ri·um
ex·os·tec·to·my
ex·os·to·sec·to·my
ex·os·to·ses
ex·os·to·sis
  e. bur·sa·ta
  e. car·ti·la·gi·nea
  di·a·phys·i·al jux·ta·ep·i·
    phys·i·al e.
  he·red·i·tary mul·ti·ple ex·
    os·to·ses
  ivo·ry e.
  mul·ti·ple e.
  sol·i·tary os·te·o·car·ti·lag·
    i·nous e.
ex·o·ter·ic
  bac·te·ri·um
ex·o·ther·mic
ex·o·tox·ic
ex·o·tox·in
ex·o·tro·pia
  A-e.
  ba·sic e.
  di·ver·gence ex·cess e.
  di·ver·gence in·suf·fi·cien·cy
    e.
  V-e.
  X-e.
ex·pan·sion
  hy·gro·scop·ic e.
  per·cep·tu·al e.
  set·ting e.
  wax e.
ex·pan·sion
  arch
ex·pan·sive
  de·lu·sion
ex·pan·sive·ness
ex·pec·ta·tion
  neu·ro·sis
ex·pec·to·rant
ex·pec·to·rate
ex·pec·to·ra·tion
  prune-juice e.

ex·pe·ri·ence
  cor·rec·tive emo·tion·al e.
ex·per·i·ment
  con·trol e.
  de·layed re·ac·tion e.
  dou·ble blind e.
  dou·ble-masked e.
  fac·to·ri·al e.'s
  hertz·i·an e.'s
  Mariotte's e.
  Nussbaum's e.
  Scheiner's e.
  Stensen's e.
  Toynbee's e.
  Weber's e.
ex·per·i·men·tal
  group
  med·i·cine
  meth·od
  neu·ro·sis
  psy·chol·o·gy
ex·per·i·men·tal al·ler·gic
  en·ceph·a·li·tis
  en·ceph·a·lo·my·e·li·tis
ex·per·i·ment·er
  ef·fects
ex·pi·ra·tion
ex·pi·ra·to·ry
  cen·ter
  re·sis·tance
  stri·dor
ex·pi·ra·to·ry re·serve
  vol·ume
ex·pire
ex·pired
  gas
ex·plant
ex·plan·ta·tion
ex·plo·ra·tion
ex·plor·a·to·ry
  drive
ex·plor·er
ex·plor·ing
  elec·trode
  nee·dle
ex·plo·sion
ex·plo·sive
  de·com·pres·sion
  speech
ex·po·nen·tial
  dis·tri·bu·tion
ex·pose
ex·posed
  pulp
ex·po·sure
  ker·a·ti·tis
ex·press

ex·pressed
  mus·tard oil
ex·pressed skull
  frac·ture
ex·pres·sion
  vec·tor
ex·pres·sive
  apha·sia
ex·pres·siv·i·ty
ex·pul·sive
  pains
ex·qui·site
ex·san·gui·nate
ex·san·gui·na·tion
  trans·fu·sion
ex·san·guine
ex·sect
ex·sec·tion
ex·sic·cant
ex·sic·cate
ex·sic·cat·ed
  al·um
  so·di·um sul·fite
ex·sic·ca·tion
  fe·ver
ex·so·ma·tize
ex·sorp·tion
ex·stro·phy
  e. of the blad·der
  e. of the clo·a·ca
ex·tem·po·ra·ne·ous
  mix·ture
ex·tend
ex·tend·ed
  clasp
  py·e·lot·o·my
ex·tend·ed fam·i·ly
  ther·a·py
ex·tend·ed in·su·lin zinc
  sus·pen·sion
ex·tend·ed rad·i·cal
  mas·tec·to·my
ex·ten·sion
  form
ex·ten·sion
  Buck's e.
  nail e.
  ridge e.
  skel·e·tal e.
ex·ten·sor
  ap·o·neu·ro·sis
  mus·cle of fin·gers
  mus·cle of lit·tle fin·ger
  ret·i·nac·u·lum
  tet·a·nus
ex·te·ri·or
ex·te·ri·or·ize
ex·tern

ex·ter·nal
  ab·sorp·tion
  ar·tery of nose
  ax·is of eye
  can·thus
  cap·sule
  con·ju·gate
  de·fi·bril·la·tor
  fis·tu·la
  fix·a·tion
  gen·i·ta·lia
  hem·or·rhoids
  hy·dro·ceph·a·lus
  lip of il·i·ac crest
  mal·le·o·lus
  me·di·um
  men·in·gi·tis
  nose
  oph·thal·mop·a·thy
  pace·mak·er
  phase
  py·o·ceph·a·lus
  res·pi·ra·tion
  squint
  stra·bis·mus
  sur·face of fron·tal bone
  sur·face of pa·ri·e·tal bone
  trac·tion
  ure·throt·o·my
  ver·sion
  wall of co·chle·ar duct
ex·ter·nal acous·tic
  fo·ra·men
  me·a·tus
  pore
ex·ter·nal ar·cu·ate
  fi·bers
ex·ter·nal au·di·to·ry
  fo·ra·men
  me·a·tus
  pore
ex·ter·nal car·di·ac
  mas·sage
ex·ter·nal ca·rot·id
  ar·tery
  nerves
  plex·us
ex·ter·nal col·lat·er·al
  lig·a·ment of wrist
ex·ter·nal cu·ne·ate
  nu·cle·us
ex·ter·nal den·tal
  ep·i·the·li·um
ex·ter·nal ear
ex·ter·nal enam·el
  ep·i·the·li·um
ex·ter·nal ex·ud·a·tive
  ret·i·nop·a·thy

ex·ter·nal il·i·ac
  ar·tery
  plex·us
  vein
ex·ter·nal il·i·ac lymph
  nodes
ex·ter·nal in·gui·nal
  ring
ex·ter·nal in·ter·cos·tal
  mus·cle
ex·ter·nal jug·u·lar
  vein
ex·ter·nal mal·le·o·lar
  sign
ex·ter·nal mam·ma·ry
  ar·tery
ex·ter·nal max·il·lary
  ar·tery
  plex·us
ex·ter·nal na·sal
  veins
ex·ter·nal ob·lique
  re·flex
  ridge
ex·ter·nal ob·tu·ra·tor
  mus·cle
ex·ter·nal oc·cip·i·tal
  crest
  pro·tu·ber·ance
ex·ter·nal o·vu·lar
  trans·mi·gra·tion
ex·ter·nal pil·lar
  cells
ex·ter·nal pin
  fix·a·tion
  fix·a·tion, bi·phase
ex·ter·nal pter·y·goid
  mus·cle
ex·ter·nal pu·den·dal
  ar·ter·ies
  veins
ex·ter·nal res·pi·ra·to·ry
  nerve of Bell
ex·ter·nal root
  sheath
ex·ter·nal sal·i·vary
  gland
ex·ter·nal sa·phe·nous
  nerve
ex·ter·nal sem·i·lu·nar
  fi·bro·car·ti·lage
ex·ter·nal sper·mat·ic
  ar·tery
  fas·cia
ex·ter·nal sphinc·ter
  mus·cle of anus
ex·ter·nal spi·ral
  sul·cus

ex·ter·nal ure·thral
  open·ing
ex·ter·nus
ex·ter·o·cep·tive
ex·ter·o·cep·tor
ex·ter·o·fec·tive
  sys·tem
ex·ti·ma
ex·tinc·tion
  spe·cif·ic e.
  vi·su·al e.
ex·tinc·tion
  co·ef·fi·cient
ex·tin·guish
ex·tir·pa·tion
Exton
  re·a·gent
ex·tor·sion
ex·tor·tor
ex·tra-sys·to·le
ex·tra-ab·dom·i·nal
  des·moid
ex·tra·am·ni·ot·ic
  preg·nan·cy
ex·tra-ar·tic·u·lar
ex·tra·buc·cal
ex·tra·bul·bar
ex·tra·cal·i·ce·al
ex·tra·cap·su·lar
  an·ky·lo·sis
  frac·ture
  lig·a·ments
ex·tra·car·di·ac
  mur·mur
ex·tra·car·pal
ex·tra·cel·lu·lar
  cho·les·ter·ol·o·sis
  en·zyme
  flu·id
  tox·in
ex·tra·cho·ri·al
  preg·nan·cy
ex·tra·chro·mo·som·al
  el·e·ment
  in·her·i·tance
ex·tra·chro·mo·som·al ge·net·ic
  el·e·ment
ex·tra·cor·o·nal
  re·tain·er
ex·tra·cor·po·re·al
  cir·cu·la·tion
  di·al·y·sis
ex·tra·cor·pus·cu·lar
ex·tra·cra·ni·al
  pneu·ma·to·cele
  pneu·mo·cele
ex·tract
  al·co·hol·ic e.

ex·tract *(continued)*
al·ler·gen·ic e.
al·ler·gic e.
Buchner e.
equiv·a·lent e.
flu·id e.
hy·dro·al·co·hol·ic e.
liq·uid e.
pol·len e.
ex·tract·ant
ex·tract·ing
for·ceps
ex·trac·tion
co·ef·fi·cient
ra·tio
ex·trac·tion
Baker's pyr·i·dine e.
breech e.
po·dal·ic e.
se·ri·al e.
ex·trac·tives
ex·trac·tor
vac·u·um e.
ex·tra·cys·tic
ex·tra·du·ral
an·es·the·sia
he·ma·tor·rha·chis
hem·or·rhage
ex·tra·em·bry·on·ic
blas·to·derm
ce·lom
mes·o·derm
ex·tra·ep·i·phy·si·al
ex·tra·gen·i·tal
ex·tra·glo·mer·u·lar
mes·an·gi·um
ex·tra·he·pat·ic
ex·tra·in·tra·cra·ni·al
by·pass
ex·tra·jec·tion
ex·tra·lig·a·men·tous
ex·tra·mal·le·o·lus
ex·tra·mam·ma·ry Paget
dis·ease
ex·tra·med·ul·lary
ex·tra·mem·bra·nous
preg·nan·cy
ex·tra·mu·ral
prac·tice
ex·tra·ne·ous
ex·tra·nu·cle·ar
in·her·i·tance
ex·tra·oc·u·lar
ex·tra·o·ral
an·chor·age
ex·tra·o·ral frac·ture
ap·pli·ance
ex·tra·ov·u·lar

ex·tra·pap·il·lary
ex·tra·pa·ren·chy·mal
ex·tra·per·i·ne·al
ex·tra·per·i·os·te·al
ex·tra·per·i·to·ne·al
fas·cia
ex·tra·phys·i·o·log·ic
ex·tra·pin·e·al
pin·e·a·lo·ma
ex·tra·pla·cen·tal
ex·tra·pleu·ral
pneu·mo·thor·ax
ex·tra·pros·tat·ic
ex·tra·pros·ta·ti·tis
ex·tra·pul·mo·nary
ex·tra·py·ram·i·dal
dis·ease
dys·ki·ne·si·as
syn·drome
ex·tra·py·ram·i·dal mo·tor
sys·tem
ex·tra·sac·cu·lar
her·nia
ex·tra·sen·so·ry
per·cep·tion
ex·tra·sen·so·ry thought
trans·fer·ence
ex·tra·se·rous
ex·tra·ske·le·tal
chon·dro·ma
ex·tra·so·mat·ic
ex·tra·sys·to·le
atri·al e.
atri·o·ven·tric·u·lar e.
atri·o·ven·tric·u·lar no·dal e.
au·ric·u·lar e.
A-V e.
A-V no·dal e.
in·fra·nod·al e.
in·ter·po·lat·ed e.
junc·tion·al e.
low·er no·dal e.
mid·no·dal e.
no·dal e.
re·turn e.
su·pra·ven·tric·u·lar e.
up·per no·dal e.
ven·tric·u·lar e.
ex·tra·tar·sal
ex·tra·tra·che·al
ex·tra·tub·al
ex·tra·u·ter·ine
preg·nan·cy
ex·tra·vag·i·nal
ex·trav·a·sate
ex·trav·a·sa·tion
cyst

ex·tra·vas·cu·lar
  flu·id
ex·tra·ven·tric·u·lar
ex·tra·ver·sion
ex·tra·vi·su·al
ex·tra·vi·tal
  ul·tra·vi·o·let
ex·treme
  cap·sule
ex·treme so·ma·to·sen·so·ry evoked
  po·ten·tial
in ex·tre·mis
ex·trem·i·tal
ex·trem·i·tas
ex·trem·i·ty
  acro·mi·al e. of clav·i·cle
  an·te·ri·or e.
  an·te·ri·or e. of cau·date nu·cle·us
  in·fe·ri·or e.
  low·er e.
  pos·te·ri·or e.
  ster·nal e. of clav·i·cle
  su·pe·ri·or e.
  tub·al e.
  up·per e.
  up·per e. of fib·u·la
  uter·ine e.
ex·trin·sic
  asth·ma
  col·or
  fac·tor
  mo·ti·va·tion
  sphinc·ter
ex·trin·sic al·ler·gic
  al·ve·o·li·tis
ex·trin·sic in·cu·ba·tion
  pe·ri·od
ex·tro·gas·tru·la·tion
ex·tro·spec·tion
ex·tro·ver·sion
ex·tro·vert
ex·trude
ex·trud·ed
  teeth
ex·tru·sion
  e. of a tooth
ex·tu·bate
ex·tu·ba·tion
ex·u·ber·ant
ex·u·date
ex·u·da·tion
  cell
  cor·pus·cle
  cyst
ex·ud·a·tive
  bron·chi·ol·i·tis

cho·roid·i·tis
glo·mer·u·lo·ne·phri·tis
in·flam·ma·tion
ret·i·ni·tis
vit·re·o·ret·i·nop·a·thy
ex·ud·a·tive dis·coid and li·chen·oid
  der·ma·ti·tis
ex·ud·a·tive ret·i·nal
  de·tach·ment
ex·ude
ex·ul·cer·ans
ex·um·bil·i·ca·tion
ex·u·vi·ae
eye
  cap·sule
  cup
  drops
  lens
  oint·ment
  re·flex
  sock·et
  spec·u·lum
  tooth
eye
  am·au·rot·ic cat's e.
  apha·kic e.
  ar·ti·fi·cial e.
  black e.
  blear e.
  bo·vine can·cer e.
  com·pound e.
  crossed e.'s
  cy·clo·pe·an e.
  cy·clo·pi·an e.
  dark-adapt·ed e.
  dom·i·nant e.
  ep·i·phys·i·al e.
  ex·cit·ing e.
  fix·ing e.
  hare's e.
  heavy e.
  hot e.
  light-adapt·ed e.
  Listing's re·duced e.
  mas·ter e.
  mas·ter-dom·i·nant e.
  pa·ri·e·tal e.
  pha·kic e.
  pho·top·ic e.
  pin·e·al e.
  pink e.
  rac·coon e.'s
  re·duced e.
  sche·mat·ic e.
  sco·top·ic e.
  spec·ta·cle e.'s
  squint·ing e.

eye *(continued)*
  sym·pa·thiz·ing e.
  wa·tery e.
  web e.
eye·ball
eye bank
eye·brow
eye-clo·sure
  re·flex
eye-ear
  plane
eye·glass·es
eye·grounds
eye·lash
  sign

eye·lash
  ec·top·ic e.
  pie·bald e.
eye·lid
  low·er e.
  third e.
  up·per e.
eye·piece
eye·spot
eye·stone
eye·strain
eye·wash

F
  agent
  duc·tion
  fac·tor
  ge·note
  pi·li
  plas·mid
  thal·as·se·mia
  wave
F-
  ac·tin
  ge·note
f
  wave
FA
  vi·rus
Fab
  frag·ment
  piece
fa·bel·la
Faber's
  ane·mia
  syn·drome
fa·bism
fab·ri·ca·tion
Fabricius'
  ship
Fabry's
  dis·ease
fab·u·la·tion
face
  bird f.
  cow f.
  dish f.
  frog f.
  hip·po·crat·ic f.
  mask·like f.
  moon f.
face
  form
  pre·sen·ta·tion
  va·lid·i·ty
face-bow
  fork
  rec·ord
face-bow
  ad·just·a·ble ax·is f.-b.
  kin·e·mat·ic f.-b.
face-lift

fac·et
  cla·vic·u·lar f.
  cor·ne·al f.
  Lenoir's f.
  locked f.'s
fac·et
  rhi·zot·o·my
fac·e·tec·to·my
fa·cette
fa·cial
  an·gle
  ar·tery
  ax·is
  bones
  ca·nal
  cleft
  col·lic·u·lus
  di·ple·gia
  ec·ze·ma
  em·i·nence
  height
  hem·i·at·ro·phy
  hem·i·ple·gia
  hil·lock
  in·dex
  mus·cles
  nerve
  neu·ral·gia
  pal·sy
  pa·ral·y·sis
  per·cep·tion
  plane
  plex·us
  pro·file
  re·flex
  root
  spasm
  sur·face of tooth
  tic
  tri·an·gle
  troph·o·neu·ro·sis
  vein
  vi·sion
fa·ci·a·lis
  phe·nom·e·non
fa·cial lymph
  nodes
fa·cial mo·tor
  nu·cle·us

fa·ci·es
fa·ci·es
   acro·mi·al ar·tic·u·lar f. of
      clav·i·cle
   ad·e·noid f.
   f. an·to·ni·na
   aor·tic f.
   f. bo·vi·na
   f. buc·ca·lis
   f. ce·re·bra·lis
   che·rub·ic f.
   Corvisart's f.
   f. do·lo·ro·sa
   elf·in f.
   hip·po·crat·ic f.
   f. hip·po·cra·ti·ca
   hound-dog f.
   hur·loid f.
   Hutchinson's f.
   f. la·bi·a·lis
   le·o·nine f.
   f. mas·ti·ca·to·ria
   mi·tral f.
   my·as·then·ic f.
   my·o·path·ic f.
   Parkinson's f.
   Potter's f.
   f. sca·phoi·dea
fa·cil·i·ta·tion
   Wedensky f.
fac·ing
fa·ci·o·ceph·a·lal·gia
fa·ci·o·dig·i·to·gen·i·tal
   dys·pla·sia
fa·ci·o·lin·gual
fa·ci·o·plas·ty
fa·ci·o·ple·gia
fa·ci·o·scap·u·lo·hu·mer·al
   at·ro·phy
fa·ci·o·scap·u·lo·hu·mer·al
   mus·cu·lar
   dys·tro·phy
fac·ti·tious
   mel·a·nin
   pur·pu·ra
   ur·ti·car·ia
fac·tor
   f. A
   ABO f.'s
   ac·cel·er·a·tor f.
   ac·e·tate re·place·ment f.
   ad·re·nal weight f.
   an·gi·o·gen·e·sis f.
   an·i·mal pro·tein f.
   an·ti·al·o·pe·cia f.
   an·ti·ber·i·beri f.
   an·ti-black-tongue f.
   an·ti·com·ple·men·ta·ry f.

an·ti·he·mo·phil·ic f. A
an·ti·he·mo·phil·ic f. B
an·ti·hem·or·rhag·ic f.
an·ti·neu·rit·ic f.
an·ti·nu·cle·ar f.
an·ti·pel·la·gra f.
an·ti·per·ni·cious ane·mia f.
an·ti·ste·ril·i·ty f.
atri·al na·tri·u·ret·ic f.
f. B
B_T f.
bac·te·ri·o·cin f.'s
bif·i·dus f.
bi·ot·ic f.'s
Bittner's milk f.
blood f.
branch·ing f.
C f.'s
CAMP f.
cap·il·lary per·me·a·bil·i·ty
   f.
Castle's in·trin·sic f.
Christmas f.
ci·trov·o·rum f.
clear·ing f.'s
clot·ting f.
co·ag·u·la·tion f.
co·bra ven·om f.
co·en·zyme f.
com·ple·ment che·mo·tac·tic
   f.
cor·ti·co·tro·pin-re·leas·ing
   f.
cou·pling f.'s
f. D
de·branch·ing f.'s
de·ca·pac·i·ta·tion f.
di·a·be·to·gen·ic f.
dif·fus·ing f.
di·rect lyt·ic f. of co·bra
   ven·om
Duran-Reynals per·me·a·bil·
   i·ty f.
Duran-Reynals spread·ing f.
f. E
eo·sin·o·phil che·mo·tac·tic
   f. of an·a·phy·lax·is
ep·i·der·mal growth f.
eryth·ro·cyte mat·u·ra·tion
   f.
es·sen·tial food f.'s
ex·trin·sic f.
F f.
F f.
fer·men·ta·tion Lac·to·ba·
   cil·lus ca·sei f.
fer·til·i·ty f.
fi·brin-sta·bi·liz·ing f.

fil·trate f.
fol·li·cle-stim·u·lat·ing hor·
    mone-re·leas·ing f.
G f.
ga·lac·ta·gogue f.
ga·lac·to·poi·et·ic f.
glass f.
gly·co·tro·pic f.
f. Gm
go·nad·o·tro·pin-re·leas·ing
    f.
growth hor·mone-re·leas·ing
    f.
f. H
Hageman f.
HG f.
hu·man an·ti·he·mo·phil·ic
    f.
hy·per·gly·ce·mic-gly·co·gen·
    o·lyt·ic f.
f. I
f. II
f. III
in·hi·bi·tion f.
in·i·ti·a·tion f.
in·su·lin-an·tag·o·niz·ing f.
in·su·lin-like growth f.
in·trin·sic f.
f. Inv
f. IV
f. IX
la·bile f.
Lac·to·ba·cil·lus bul·gar·i·
    cus f.
Lac·to·ba·cil·lus ca·sei f.
lac·to·gen·ic f.
Laki-Lorand f.
LE f.'s
le·thal f.
leu·ko·cy·to·sis-pro·mot·ing
    f.
leu·ko·pe·nic f.
lip·o·tro·pic f.
liv·er fil·trate f.
liv·er Lac·to·ba·cil·lus ca·
    sei f.
L-L f.
lu·te·i·niz·ing hor·mone/fol·
    li·cle-stim·u·lat·ing hor·
    mone-re·leas·ing f.
lu·te·i·niz·ing hor·mone-re·
    leas·ing f.
lymph node per·me·a·bil·i·
    ty f.
mam·mo·tro·pic f.
mat·u·ra·tion f.
mi·gra·tion-in·hib·i·tory f.
milk f.

mouse an·ti·al·o·pe·cia f.
mül·le·ri·an duct in·hib·i·
    to·ry f.
mül·le·ri·an re·gres·sion f.
my·o·car·di·al de·pres·sant
    f.
ne·phrit·ic f.
nerve growth f.
os·te·o·clast ac·ti·vat·ing f.
f. P
P f.
pel·lag·ra-pre·vent·ing (P-P)
    f.
plas·ma la·bile f.
plas·ma throm·bo·plas·tin f.
plas·ma throm·bo·plas·tin f.
    B
plas·ma f. X
plas·min pro·throm·bins
    con·ver·sion f.
plate·let-ac·ti·vat·ing f.
plate·let-ag·gre·gat·ing f.
plate·let-de·rived growth f.
plate·let tis·sue f.
pro·lac·tin in·hib·it·ing f.
pro·lac·tin re·leas·ing f.
pro·per·din f. A
pro·per·din f. B
pro·per·din f. D
pro·per·din f. E
pro·tein f.
py·ru·vate ox·i·da·tion f.
R f.'s
rec·og·ni·tion f.'s
re·lax·a·tion f.
re·leas·ing f.
re·sis·tance f.'s
re·sis·tance-in·duc·ing f.
re·sis·tance-trans·fer f.
rheu·ma·toid f.'s
risk f.
S f.
se·cre·tor f.
sex f.
slow-re·act·ing f. of an·a·
    phy·lax·is
SLR f.
so·ma·to·tro·pin re·lease-in·
    hib·it·ing f.
so·ma·to·tro·pin-re·leas·ing
    f.
spread·ing f.
sta·ble f.
Strep·to·coc·cus lac·tis R f.
Stuart f.
Stuart-Prower f.
sul·fa·tion f.
sun pro·tec·tion f.

fac·tor *(continued)*
  thy·mic lym·pho·poi·et·ic f.
  thy·roid-stim·u·lat·ing hor·
    mone-re·leas·ing f.
  thy·ro·tox·ic com·ple·ment-
    fix·a·tion f.
  thy·rot·ro·pin-re·leas·ing f.
  trans·fer f.
  trans·form·ing f.
  trans·meth·yl·a·tion f.
  tu·mor an·gi·o·gen·ic f.
  tu·mor ne·cro·sis f.
  un·cou·pling f.'s
  f. V
  f. VII
  f. VIII
  F. VIII:C
  f. VIIIR
  von Willebrand f.
  W f.
  f. X
  f. X for Hae·moph·i·lus
  f. XI
  f. XII
  f. XIII
  Y f.
  yeast el·u·ate f.
fac·to·ri·al
  ex·per·i·ments
fac·ul·ta·tive
  an·aer·obe
  het·er·o·chro·ma·tin
  hy·per·o·pia
  par·a·site
  sap·ro·phyte
fac·ul·ty
Fa·den
  su·ture
fad·ing
  time
Faget's
  sign
fag·o·py·rism
Fahraeus-Lindqvist
  ef·fect
Fahr·en·heit
  scale
Fahr's
  dis·ease
fail·ure
  back·ward heart f.
  car·di·ac f.
  con·ges·tive heart f.
  cor·o·nary f.
  elec·tri·cal f.
  for·ward heart f.
  heart f.
  high out·put f.

  left ven·tric·u·lar f.
  low out·put f.
  pace·mak·er f.
  pow·er f.
  pump f.
  right ven·tric·u·lar f.
  sec·on·dary f.
faint
faith
  heal·ing
fal·cate
fal·ces
fal·cial
fal·ci·form
  car·ti·lage
  crest
  lig·a·ment
  lig·a·ment of liv·er
  lobe
  mar·gin
  pro·cess
fal·ci·form ret·i·nal
  fold
fal·cine
fal·cip·a·rum
  fe·ver
  ma·lar·ia
fal·cu·la
fal·cu·lar
fall·en
  arch·es
fall·ing of the
  womb
fall·ing
  pal·ate
  sick·ness
fal·lo·pi·an
  aq·ue·duct
  arch
  ca·nal
  hi·a·tus
  lig·a·ment
  neu·ri·tis
  preg·nan·cy
  tube
Fallot's
  tet·rad
  te·tral·o·gy
  tri·ad
false
  ag·glu·ti·na·tion
  al·bu·min·ur·ia
  ane·mia
  an·eu·rysm
  an·gi·na
  an·ky·lo·sis
  bleph·a·rop·to·sis
  branch·ing

cast
con·ju·gate
coxa va·ra
cy·a·no·sis
cyst
dex·tro·car·dia
diph·the·ria
di·ver·tic·u·lum
dom·i·nance
glot·tis
he·ma·tu·ria
her·maph·ro·dit·ism
hy·per·tro·phy
im·age
joint
knots
knots of um·bil·i·cal cord
mac·u·la
mas·tur·ba·tion
mem·brane
mole
neg·a·tive
neu·ro·ma
nu·cle·o·lus
pains
par·a·cu·sis
pel·vis
pos·i·tive
preg·nan·cy
pro·jec·tion
ribs
ring·bone
su·ture
thirst
ver·te·brae
wa·ters
false-neg·a·tive
re·ac·tion
false-pos·i·tive
re·ac·tion
false vo·cal
cord
fal·si·fi·ca·tion
ret·ro·spec·tive f.
falx
f. ap·o·neu·ro·ti·ca
fa·mil·i·al
ag·gre·ga·tion
am·y·loi·do·sis
can·cer
cys·ti·nu·ria
dys·au·to·no·mia
em·phy·se·ma
en·ceph·a·lop·a·thy
gly·ci·nu·ria
goi·ter
hy·per·be·ta·lip·o·pro·tein·
e·mia

hy·per·be·ta·lip·o·pro·tein·
e·mia and hy·per·pre·be·
ta·lip·o·pro·tein·e·mia
hy·per·cho·les·ter·ol·e·mia
hy·per·cho·les·ter·ol·e·mia
with hy·per·li·pe·mia
hy·per·chy·lo·mi·cro·ne·mia
hy·per·chy·lo·mi·cro·ne·mia
with hy·per·pre·be·ta·lip·
o·pro·tein·e·mia
hy·per·lip·o·pro·tein·e·mia
hy·per·pre·be·ta·lip·o·pro·
tein·e·mia
hy·per·tri·glyc·er·i·de·mia
hy·po·par·a·thy·roid·ism
ne·phro·sis
screen·ing
fa·mil·i·al am·y·loid
neu·rop·a·thy
fa·mil·i·al be·nign chron·ic
pem·phi·gus
fa·mil·i·al eryth·ro·blas·tic
ane·mia
fa·mil·i·al fat-in·duced
hy·per·li·pe·mia
fa·mil·i·al fi·brous
dys·pla·sia of jaws
**fa·mil·i·al high den·si·ty lip·
o·pro·tein**
de·fi·cien·cy
**fa·mil·i·al hy·per·cho·les·ter·e·
mic**
xan·tho·ma·to·sis
**fa·mil·i·al hy·po·go·nad·o·tro·
pic**
hy·po·go·nad·ism
fa·mil·i·al hy·po·plas·tic
ane·mia
fa·mil·i·al in·tes·ti·nal
pol·yp·o·sis
fa·mil·i·al ju·ve·nile
neph·roph·thi·sis
fa·mil·i·al Med·i·ter·ra·ne·an
fe·ver
fa·mil·i·al mi·cro·cyt·ic
ane·mia
fa·mil·i·al non·he·mo·lyt·ic
jaun·dice
fa·mil·i·al par·ox·ys·mal
pol·y·ser·o·si·tis
rhab·do·my·ol·y·sis
fa·mil·i·al pe·ri·od·ic
pa·ral·y·sis
**fa·mil·i·al pseu·do·in·flam·ma·
to·ry**
mac·u·lop·a·thy

367

fa·mil·i·al pseu·do·in·flam·ma·
to·ry mac·u·lar
de·gen·er·a·tion
fa·mil·i·al pyr·i·dox·ine-re·
spon·sive
ane·mia
fa·mil·i·al re·cur·rent
pol·y·ser·o·si·tis
fa·mil·i·al spi·nal mus·cu·lar
at·ro·phy
fa·mil·i·al splen·ic
ane·mia
fa·mil·i·al white fold·ed
dys·pla·sia
fam·i·ly
med·i·cine
ther·a·py
fam·i·ly
can·cer f.
nu·cle·ar f.
fam·ine
fe·ver
fa·mo·ti·dine
fam·o·tine hy·dro·chlo·ride
fan
sign
FANA
test
Fañanás
cell
Fanconi's
ane·mia
pan·cy·to·pe·nia
syn·drome
fang
fan·go
Fan·nia
fan·ta·sy
far
point
sight
Farabeuf's
am·pu·ta·tion
tri·an·gle
far·ad
far·a·da·ic
far·a·day
Faraday's
con·stant
laws
fa·rad·ic
far·a·dism
surg·ing f.
far·a·di·za·tion
fa·ra·do·con·trac·til·i·ty
fa·ra·do·mus·cu·lar
far·a·do·pal·pa·tion
far·a·do·ther·a·py

far-and-near
su·ture
Farber's
dis·ease
syn·drome
far·cy
far·del
Far East Rus·sian
en·ceph·a·li·tis
far·fa·ra
fa·ri·na
far·i·na·ceous
farm·er's
lung
skin
far·ne·sene al·co·hol
far·ne·sol
Farnsworth-Munsell col·or
test
far point of
con·ver·gence
Farrant's mount·ing
flu·id
Farre's
line
Farr's
law
far·sight·ed·ness
fas·cia
Abernethy's f.
f. ad·he·rens
anal f.
an·te·brach·i·al f.
ax·il·lary f.
bi·cip·i·tal f.
brach·i·al f.
broad f.
buc·co·pha·ryn·ge·al f.
Buck's f.
f. bul·bi
Camper's f.
cer·vi·cal f.
f. ci·ne·rea
cla·vi·pec·to·ral f.
f. of clit·o·ris
Colles' f.
Cooper's f.
crem·as·ter·ic f.
crib·ri·form f.
Cruveilhier's f.
deep f.
deep f. of arm
deep f. of fore·arm
deep f. of leg
f. den·ta·ta hip·po·cam·pi
den·tate f.
f. di·a·phrag·ma·tis uro·ge·
ni·ta·lis su·pe·ri·or

dor·sal f. of foot
dor·sal f. of hand
Dupuytren's f.
en·do·pel·vic f.
en·do·tho·rac·ic f.
ex·ter·nal sper·mat·ic f.
f. of ex·tra·oc·u·lar mus·cles
ex·tra·per·i·to·ne·al f.
f. of fore·arm
Gerota's f.
Godman's f.
Hesselbach's f.
il·i·ac f.
il·i·o·pec·tin·e·al f.
in·fe·ri·or f. of pel·vic di·a·phragm
in·fe·ri·or f. of uro·gen·i·tal di·a·phragm
f. in·fra·spi·na·ta
in·fra·spi·na·tus f.
in·fun·dib·u·li·form f.
in·ter·co·lum·nar fas·ci·ae
in·ter·nal sper·mat·ic f.
in·ter·os·se·ous f.
lac·ri·mal f.
f. of leg
lum·bo·dor·sal f.
mas·se·ter·ic f.
mid·dle cer·vi·cal f.
mus·cu·lar f. of ex·tra·oc·u·lar mus·cle
f. of neck
nu·chal f.
ob·tu·ra·tor f.
or·bi·tal fas·ci·ae
pal·mar f.
pa·rot·id f.
f. pa·ro·ti·de·o·mas·se·te·ri·ca
pec·to·ral f.
per·i·re·nal f.
pha·ryn·go·bas·i·lar f.
phren·i·co·pleur·al f.
plan·tar f.
pop·lit·e·al f.
Porter's f.
pre·tra·che·al f.
pre·ver·te·bral f.
f. of pros·tate
rec·to·ves·i·cal f.
re·nal f.
Scarpa's f.
sem·i·lu·nar f.
Sibson's f.
sub·per·i·to·ne·al f.
su·per·fi·cial f.

su·per·fi·cial f. of per·i·ne·um
su·pe·ri·or f. of pel·vic di·a·phragm
su·pe·ri·or f. of uro·gen·i·tal di·a·phragm
tem·po·ral f.
Toldt's f.
Treitz's f.
tri·an·gu·lar f.
f. tri·an·gu·la·ris ab·do·mi·nis
Tyrrell's f.
um·bil·i·cal pre·ves·i·cal f.
um·bil·i·co·ves·i·cal f.
Zuckerkandl's f.
fas·cia
graft
fas·ci·ae
fas·cial
her·nia
fas·ci·cle
mus·cle f.
nerve f.
fas·cic·u·lar
block
de·gen·er·a·tion
graft
ker·a·ti·tis
oph·thal·mo·ple·gia
sar·co·ma
ul·cer
fas·ci·cu·la·ta
cell
fas·cic·u·late
blad·der
fas·cic·u·lat·ed
fas·cic·u·la·tion
fas·cic·u·li
fas·cic·u·lus
f. an·te·ri·or pro·pri·us
ar·cu·ate f.
f. atri·o·ven·tric·u·la·ris
Burdach's f.
cal·ca·rine f.
cen·tral teg·men·tal f.
f. cir·cum·o·li·va·ris py·ra·mi·dis
f. cor·ti·co·spi·na·lis an·te·ri·or
f. cor·ti·co·spi·na·lis la·te·ra·lis
cu·ne·ate f.
dor·sal lon·gi·tu·di·nal f.
dor·so·lat·er·al f.
Flechsig's fas·cic·u·li
Foville's f.
fron·to·oc·cip·i·tal f.

fas·cic·u·lus *(continued)*
  hooked f.
  in·fe·ri·or lon·gi·tu·di·nal f.
  in·ter·fas·cic·u·lar f.
  in·ter·seg·men·tal fas·cic·u·li
  f. la·te·ra·lis pro·pri·us
  f. len·tic·u·lar·is
  Lissauer's f.
  fas·cic·u·li lon·gi·tu·di·na·les pon·tis
  f. ma·cu·la·ris
  ma·mil·lo·teg·men·tal f.
  mam·il·lo·tha·lam·ic f.
  f. mar·gi·na·lis
  me·di·al lon·gi·tu·di·nal f.
  Meynert's f.
  f. ob·li·qu·us pon·tis
  oc·cip·i·to·fron·tal f.
  f. oc·cip·i·to·fron·ta·lis
  oval f.
  f. pe·dun·cu·lo·ma·mil·la·ris
  per·pen·dic·u·lar f.
  prop·er fas·cic·u·li
  f. py·ra·mi·da·lis an·te·ri·or
  f. py·ra·mi·da·lis la·te·ra·lis
  ret·ro·flex f.
  f. ro·tun·dus
  sem·i·lu·nar f.
  sep·to·mar·gi·nal f.
  slen·der f.
  f. so·li·ta·ri·us
  sub·cal·lo·sal f.
  su·pe·ri·or lon·gi·tu·di·nal f.
  f. tha·la·mi·cus
  f. thal·a·mo·mam·il·la·ris
  trans·verse fas·cic·u·li
  un·ci·form f.
  un·ci·nate f.
  un·ci·nate f. of Russell
  wedge-shaped f.
fas·ci·ec·to·my
fas·ci·i·tis
  eo·sin·o·phil·ic f.
  nec·ro·tiz·ing f.
  nod·u·lar f.
  par·os·te·al f.
  pro·lif·er·a·tive f.
  pseu·do·sar·co·ma·tous f.
fas·ci·od·e·sis
Fas·ci·o·la
  F. gi·gan·ti·ca
  F. he·pat·i·ca
fas·ci·o·la
  f. ci·ne·rea

fas·ci·o·lae
fas·ci·o·lar
  gy·rus
fas·ci·o·li·a·sis
fas·ci·o·lid
Fas·ci·o·loi·des mag·na
fas·ci·o·lop·si·a·sis
Fas·ci·o·lop·sis
  F. bus·ki
  F. rat·hou·isi
fas·ci·o·plas·ty
fas·ci·or·rha·phy
fas·ci·ot·o·my
fas·ci·tis
fast
  rhythm
  smear
fast green FCF
fas·tid·i·ous
  or·ga·nism
fas·tid·i·um ci·bi
fas·ti·ga·tum
fas·tig·i·o·bul·bar
  tract
fas·tig·i·um
fast·ness
fat
  brown f.
  caul f.
  mul·ti·loc·u·lar f.
  neu·tral f.
  sat·u·rat·ed f.
  split f.
  uni·loc·u·lar f.
  un·sat·u·rat·ed f.
  white f.
fat
  body of cheek
  body of is·chi·o·rec·tal fos·sa
  body of or·bit
  cell
  em·bo·lism
  graft
  in·di·ges·tion
  me·tab·o·lism
  ne·cro·sis
  pad
  sol·vents
  tide
fa·tal
fa·tal·i·ty
  rate
fa·ther
  com·plex
fat·i·ga·bil·i·ty
fa·ti·ga·ble

fa·tigue
  au·di·to·ry f.
  bat·tle f.
  func·tion·al vo·cal f.
fa·tigue
  fe·ver
  frac·ture
  strength
fat-pad
  Bichat's f.-p.
  Imlach's f.-p.
fat-sol·u·ble
  vi·ta·mins
fat-stor·ing
  cell
fat·ty
  ac·id
  al·co·hol
  as·ci·tes
  at·ro·phy
  cast
  change
  cir·rho·sis
  de·gen·er·a·tion
  di·ar·rhea
  heart
  her·nia
  in·fil·tra·tion
  kid·ney
  liv·er
  met·a·mor·pho·sis
  oil
  phan·er·o·sis
  se·ries
  tis·sue
fat·ty ac·id
  di·eth·e·noid f. a.
  sat·u·rat·ed f. a.
  f. a. thi·o·ki·nase
  un·sat·u·rat·ed f. a.
fat·ty ac·id ox·i·da·tion
  cy·cle
fau·ces
fau·cial
  pa·ral·y·sis
  re·flex
  ton·sil
fau·ci·tis
fau·ci·um
faulty
  un·ion
fau·na
faun tail
  ne·vus
fa·ve·o·late
fa·ve·o·li
fa·ve·o·lus
fa·vic chan·de·liers

fa·vid
fa·vism
Favre's
  dys·tro·phy
fa·vus
Fc
  frag·ment
  piece
  re·cep·tor
fear
feath·er
  louse
fea·tur·al
  sur·gery
fea·tures
feb·ri·cant
fe·bric·u·la
feb·ri·fa·cient
fe·brif·er·ous
fe·brif·ic
fe·brif·u·gal
feb·ri·fuge
feb·rile
  al·bu·min·ur·ia
  con·vul·sion
  cri·sis
  psy·cho·sis
  urine
  ur·ti·car·ia
fe·bris
fe·cal
  ab·scess
  fis·tu·la
  im·pac·tion
  tu·mor
  vom·it·ing
fe·ca·lith
fe·cal·oid
fe·ca·lo·ma
fe·ca·lu·ria
fe·ces
Fechner-Weber
  law
fec·u·lent
fe·cund
fec·un·date
fec·un·da·tion
fe·cun·di·ty
feed·back
  neg·a·tive f.
  pos·i·tive f.
feed·back
  in·hi·bi·tion
  sys·tem
feed·ing
  cen·ter
  tube

feed·ing
  fic·ti·tious f.
  forced f.
  forc·i·ble f.
  gas·tric f.
  na·sal f.
  sham f.
feel·ing
  tone
Feer's
  dis·ease
Fehling's
  re·a·gent
  so·lu·tion
feigned
  erup·tion
Feiss
  line
Fe·li·dae
fe·line
  agran·u·lo·cy·to·sis
  leu·ke·mia
  pneu·mo·ni·tis
Fe·line dis·tem·per
fe·line in·fec·tious
  en·ter·i·tis
  per·i·to·ni·tis
fe·line leu·ke·mia
  vi·rus
fe·line leu·ke·mia-sar·co·ma vi·
  rus
  com·plex
fe·line pan·leu·ko·pe·nia
  vi·rus
fe·line rhi·no·tra·che·i·tis
  vi·rus
fe·line vi·ral
  rhi·no·tra·che·i·tis
fel·la·tio
fel·la·tion
fel·la·tor·ism
fel·la·trix
fel·on
felt·work
Felty's
  syn·drome
fel·y·pres·sin
fe·male
  ge·net·ic f.
  XO f.
  XXX f.
fe·male
  cath·e·ter
  go·nad
  her·maph·ro·dit·ism
  pros·tate
  pseu·do·her·maph·ro·dit·ism

ste·ril·i·ty
ure·thra
fe·male gen·i·tal tract cy·to·
  log·ic
  smear
fe·male pro·nu·cle·us
fem·i·nin·i·ty
  com·plex
fem·i·ni·za·tion
  tes·tic·u·lar f.
fem·o·ra
fem·o·ral
  arch
  ar·tery
  ca·nal
  fos·sa
  her·nia
  mus·cle
  nerve
  open·ing
  plex·us
  re·flex
  re·gion
  ring
  sep·tum
  sheath
  tri·an·gle
  vein
fe·mo·ris
fem·o·ro·ab·dom·i·nal
  re·flex
fem·o·ro·cele
fem·o·ro·pa·tel·lar
  joint
fem·o·ro·pop·lit·e·al
  by·pass
fem·o·ro·pop·lit·e·al oc·clu·sive
  dis·ease
fem·o·ro·tib·i·al
fe·mur
fen·ca·mine
fen·clo·nine
fe·nes·tra
  f. of the co·chlea
  f. nov·o·va·lis
  f. ova·lis
  f. ro·tun·da
  f. of the ves·ti·bule
fe·nes·trae
fen·es·trat·ed
  cap·il·lary
  mem·brane
  sheath
fen·es·tra·tion
  op·er·a·tion
fen·es·tra·tion
  tra·che·al f.
fen·eth·yl·line hy·dro·chlo·ride

fen·flur·a·mine hy·dro·chlo·ride
Fenn
  ef·fect
fen·nel
fen·o·pro·fen cal·ci·um
fen·pip·ra·mide
fen·ta·nyl cit·rate
fen·ti·clor
fen·u·greek
Fenwick-Hunner
  ul·cer
Fenwick's
  dis·ease
Féréol-Graux
  pal·sy
Fergusson's
  in·ci·sion
fer·ment
fer·ment·a·ble
fer·men·ta·tion
  ace·tic f.
  ace·tous f.
  am·yl·ic f.
  lac·tic ac·id f.
fer·men·ta·tion Lac·to·ba·cil·
  lus ca·sei
  fac·tor
fer·ment·a·tive
  dys·pep·sia
fer·mi·um
fern
  test
Fernandez
  re·ac·tion
Fernbach
  flask
fern·ing
fer·ra·tin
fer·re·dox·ins
Ferrein's
  ca·nal
  cords
  fo·ra·men
  lig·a·ment
  pyr·a·mid
  tube
  va·sa aber·ran·tia
fer·ric
  al·um
fer·ric am·mo·ni·um cit·rate
fer·ric am·mo·ni·um sul·fate
fer·ric chlo·ride
  re·ac·tion of ep·i·neph·rine
  test
fer·ric cit·rate
fer·ric fruc·tose
fer·ric glyc·er·o·phos·phate
fer·ric hy·drox·ide

fer·ric ox·ide
fer·ric phos·phate
  sol·u·ble f. p.
fer·ric sul·fate
fer·ri·cy·a·nide
fer·ri·cy·to·chrome
fer·ri·heme
  f. chlo·ride
fer·ri·he·mo·glo·bin
fer·ri·por·phy·rin
  f. chlo·ride
fer·ri·pro·to·por·phy·rin
fer·ri·tin
fer·ro·che·la·tase
fer·ro·cho·li·nate
fer·ro·cy·a·nide
fer·ro·cy·an·o·gen
fer·ro·cy·to·chrome
fer·ro·heme
fer·ro·ki·net·ics
fer·ro·por·phy·rin
fer·ro·pro·teins
fer·ro·pro·to·por·phy·rin
fer·ro·so·fer·ric
fer·ro·ther·a·py
fer·rous
fer·rous bro·mide
fer·rous cit·rate
fer·rous fu·ma·rate
fer·rous glu·co·nate
fer·rous lac·tate
fer·rous suc·ci·nate
fer·rous sul·fate
  dried f. s.
fer·ru·gi·na·tion
fer·ru·gi·nous
  bod·ies
fer·rule
Ferry-Porter
  law
fer·tile
  pe·ri·od
fer·til·i·ty
  agent
  fac·tor
  vi·ta·min
fer·til·i·za·tion
  cone
  mem·brane
fer·til·i·za·tion
  in vit·ro f.
  in vi·vo f.
fer·til·ized
  ovum
fer·til·i·zin
Fer·u·la
fer·ves·cence

fes·cue
  foot
  poi·son·ing
fes·ter
fes·ti·nant
fes·ti·nat·ing
  gait
fes·ti·na·tion
fes·toon
  gin·gi·val f.
fes·toon·ing
fe·tal
  ad·e·no·ma
  age
  at·ti·tude
  bra·dy·car·dia
  cir·cu·la·tion
  cor·tex
  cot·y·le·don
  death
  dis·tress
  dys·to·cia
  elec·tro·car·di·og·ra·phy
  eryth·ro·blas·to·sis
  frac·ture
  hab·i·tus
  he·mo·glo·bin
  hy·drops
  in·clu·sion
  med·i·cine
  mem·brane
  move·ment
  ovoid
  pla·cen·ta
  souf·fle
  tach·y·car·dia
  zone
fe·tal ad·re·nal
  cor·tex
fe·tal al·co·hol
  syn·drome
fe·tal as·pi·ra·tion
  syn·drome
fe·tal death
  rate
fe·tal face
  syn·drome
fe·tal heart
  rate
fe·tal hy·dan·to·in
  syn·drome
fe·tal·ism
fe·tal re·tic·u·la·ris
fe·tal tri·meth·a·di·one
  syn·drome
fe·tal war·fa·rin
  syn·drome
fe·ta·tion

fe·ti·cide
fet·id
fet·ish
fet·ish·ism
fet·lock
fe·to·glob·u·lins
fe·tog·ra·phy
fe·tol·o·gy
fe·tom·e·try
fe·top·a·thy
  di·a·bet·ic f.
fe·to·pla·cen·tal
  an·a·sar·ca
fe·to·pro·teins
α-fe·to·pro·teins
β-fe·to·pro·teins
γ-fe·to·pro·teins
fe·tor
  f. he·pat·i·cus
  f. oris
fe·to·scope
fe·tos·co·py
fe·to·tox·ic·i·ty
fe·tus
  f. in fe·tu
  har·le·quin f.
  im·pact·ed f.
  f. pap·y·ra·ceus
fe·tus·es
Feulgen
  re·ac·tion
  stain
fe·ver
  blis·ter
  ther·a·py
fe·ver
  ab·sorp·tion f.
  ac·cli·mat·ing f.
  Aden f.
  aes·ti·vo·au·tum·nal f.
  Af·ri·can hem·or·rhag·ic f.
  Af·ri·can swine f.
  al·gid per·ni·cious f.
  aph·thous f.
  ar·dent f.
  Ar·gen·tin·i·an hem·or·rhag·ic f.
  asep·tic f.
  As·sam f.
  au·tumn f.
  bil·i·ary f. of dogs
  bil·i·ary f. of hors·es
  bil·ious re·mit·tent f.
  black f.
  black·wa·ter f.
  blue f.
  Bo·liv·i·an hem·or·rhag·ic f.

bou·quet f.
bou·ton·neuse f.
bo·vine ephem·er·al f.
break·bone f.
bul·lous f.
Bun·yam·we·ra f.
Burdwan f.
Bwam·ba f.
ca·chec·tic f.
camp f.
cane·field f.
ca·nic·o·la f.
Carter's f.
ca·tarrh·al f.
cat-bite f.
cath·e·ter f.
cat-scratch f.
Cen·tral Eu·ro·pe·an tick-borne f.
cer·e·bro·spi·nal f.
Charcot's in·ter·mit·tent f.
child·bed f.
Col·o·ra·do tick f.
Con·go·li·an red f.
con·tin·ued f.
cot·ton-mill f.
Cri·me·an-Con·go hem·or·rhag·ic f.
dan·dy f.
date f.
deer-fly f.
deer hem·or·rhag·ic f.
de·hy·dra·tion f.
den·gue f.
den·gue hem·or·rhag·ic f.
de·sert f.
di·ges·tive f.
di·pha·sic milk f.
dou·ble quo·tid·i·an f.
Dum·dum f.
Dutton's re·laps·ing f.
East Coast f.
E·bo·la hem·or·rhag·ic f.
el·e·phan·toid f.
en·ter·ic f.
en·ter·i·coid f.
ephem·er·al f.
ephem·er·al f. of cat·tle
ep·i·dem·ic hem·or·rhag·ic f.
ep·i·mas·ti·cal f.
equine bil·i·ary f.
erup·tive f.
es·sen·tial f.
ex·an·them·a·tous f.
ex·sic·ca·tion f.
fal·cip·a·rum f.

fa·mil·i·al Med·i·ter·ra·ne·an f.
fam·ine f.
fa·tigue f.
field f.
five-day f.
flood f.
food f.
Fort Bragg f.
Gam·bi·an f.
glan·du·lar f.
Haverhill f.
hay f.
he·ma·tu·ric bil·ious f.
he·mo·glo·bi·nu·ric f.
hem·or·rhag·ic f.
hem·or·rhag·ic f. with re·nal syn·drome
he·pa·tic in·ter·mit·tent f.
her·pet·ic f.
hos·pi·tal f.
Ilhé·us f.
in·a·ni·tion f.
in·ter·mit·tent ma·lar·i·al f.
in·un·da·tion f.
is·land f.
jail f.
Jap·a·nese riv·er f.
jun·gle f.
jun·gle yel·low f.
ke·da·ni f.
Kew Gar·dens f.
Kin·ki·ang f.
Ko·re·an hem·or·rhag·ic f.
Lassa f.
Lassa hem·or·rhag·ic f.
lau·rel f.
low f.
ma·lar·i·al f.
ma·lig·nant ca·tarrh·al f.
ma·lig·nant ter·tian f.
Mal·ta f.
Man·chu·ri·an f.
Man·chu·ri·an hem·or·rhag·ic f.
Mar·seilles f.
marsh f.
Med·i·ter·ra·ne·an f.
Med·i·ter·ra·ne·an ex·an·them·a·tous f.
me·nin·go·ty·phoid f.
met·al fume f.
Mex·i·can spot·ted f.
mi·an·eh f.
mil·i·a·ry f.
milk f.
mill f.
min·i·a·ture scar·let f.

fe·ver *(continued)*
mon·o·lep·tic f.
Mossman f.
mud f.
mu·mu f.
na·nu·ka·ya·mi f.
no·dal f.
North Queens·land tick f.
Omsk hem·or·rhag·ic f.
O'ny·ong-ny·ong f.
Oro·ya f.
Pah·vant Val·ley f.
pal·u·dal f.
pap·pa·ta·ci f.
pap·u·lar f.
par·a·ty·phoid f.
par·en·ter·ic f.
par·rot f.
Pel-Ebstein f.
Per·sian re·laps·ing f.
pe·te·chi·al f.
pha·ryn·go·con·junc·ti·val f.
phle·bot·o·mus f.
pol·ka f.
pol·y·lep·tic f.
pol·y·mer fume f.
Po·to·mac horse f.
pre·tib·i·al f.
pro·tein f.
pu·er·per·al f.
Pym's f.
py·o·gen·ic f.
Q f.
quar·tan f.
quin·tan f.
quo·tid·i·an f.
rab·bit f.
rat-bite f.
re·cru·des·cent ty·phus f.
re·cur·rent f.
red f.
red f. of the Con·go
red·wa·ter f.
re·laps·ing f.
re·mit·tent ma·lar·i·al f.
rheu·mat·ic f.
rice·field f.
Rift Val·ley f.
Rocky Moun·tain spot·ted f.
Ro·man f.
Ross River f.
sa·ku·shu f.
salt f.
sand·fly f.
San Joaquin f.
São Pau·lo f.
scar·let f.
Sen·net·su f.

sep·tic f.
sev·en-day f.
ship f.
ship·ping f.
Sind·bis f.
slow f.
snail f.
so·lar f.
South Af·ri·can tick-bite f.
spi·ril·lum f.
spot·ted f.
ste·roid f.
swamp f.
swine f.
symp·to·mat·ic f.
syph·i·lit·ic f.
ter·tian f.
Tex·as f.
ther·a·peu·tic f.
ther·mic f.
thirst f.
three-day f.
tick f.
Tobia f.
trau·mat·ic f.
trench f.
try·pan·o·some f.
tsu·tsu·ga·mu·shi f.
ty·phoid f.
un·dif·fer·en·ti·at·ed type
  f.'s
un·du·lant f.
ure·thral f.
uri·nary f.
ur·ti·car·i·al f.
uve·o·pa·rot·id f.
Uz·bek·i·stan hem·or·rhag·
  ic f.
val·ley f.
vi·ral hem·or·rhag·ic f.
vi·vax f.
Wesselsbron f.
West Af·ri·can f.
West Nile f.
wound f.
Yang·tze Val·ley f.
yel·low f.
Zi·ka f.
fe·ver·ish
urine
Fevold
test
FF
waves
ff
waves
FGT cy·to·log·ic
smear

fi·ber
  A f.'s
  ac·cel·er·a·tor f.'s
  ad·re·ner·gic f.'s
  af·fer·ent f.'s
  al·pha f.'s
  anas·to·mos·ing f.'s
  anas·to·mot·ic f.'s
  ar·cu·ate f.'s
  ar·gyr·o·phil·ic f.'s
  as·so·ci·a·tion f.'s
  as·tral f.'s
  aug·men·tor f.'s
  B f.'s
  Bergmann's f.'s
  be·ta f.'s
  C f.'s
  cho·lin·er·gic f.'s
  chro·mat·ic f.
  cir·cu·lar f.'s
  climb·ing f.'s
  col·la·gen f.
  col·lag·e·nous f.
  com·mis·sur·al f.'s
  cone f.
  cor·ti·co·bul·bar f.'s
  cor·ti·co·nu·cle·ar f.'s
  cor·ti·co·pon·tine f.'s
  cor·ti·co·re·tic·u·lar f.'s
  cor·ti·co·spi·nal f.'s
  den·tal f.'s
  den·ti·nal f.'s
  de·pres·sor f.'s
  di·e·tary f.
  elas·tic f.'s
  enam·el f.'s
  en·dog·e·nous f.'s
  ex·og·e·nous f.'s
  ex·ter·nal ar·cu·ate f.'s
  gam·ma f.'s
  Gerdy's f.'s
  Gratiolet's f.'s
  gray f.'s
  in·hib·i·to·ry f.'s
  in·ner cone f.
  in·ter·co·lum·nar f.'s
  in·ter·cru·ral f.'s
  in·ter·nal ar·cu·ate f.'s
  in·tra·fu·sal f.'s
  in·trin·sic f.'s
  James f.'s
  Korff's f.'s
  Kühne's f.
  f.'s of lens
  Mahaim f.'s
  med·ul·lat·ed nerve f.
  me·rid·i·o·nal f.'s
  mossy f.'s

  mo·tor f.'s
  Müller's f.'s
  my·e·li·nat·ed nerve f.
  Nélaton's f.'s
  nerve f.
  non·med·ul·lat·ed f.'s
  nu·cle·ar bag f.
  nu·cle·ar chain f.
  ob·lique f.'s of stom·ach
  os·te·o·col·lag·e·nous f.'s
  os·te·o·ge·net·ic f.'s
  out·er cone f.
  pec·ti·nate f.'s
  per·fo·rat·ing f.'s
  per·i·o·don·tal lig·a·ment
    f.'s
  per·i·ven·tric·u·lar f.'s
  pi·lo·mo·tor f.'s
  pre·col·lag·e·nous f.'s
  pres·sor f.'s
  pro·jec·tion f.'s
  Prussak's f.'s
  Purkinje's f.'s
  py·ram·i·dal f.'s
  red f.'s
  Reissner's f.
  Remak's f.'s
  re·tic·u·lar f.'s
  Retzius' f.'s
  rod f.
  Rosenthal f.
  Sappey's f.'s
  Sharpey's f.'s
  skel·e·tal mus·cle f.'s
  spin·dle f.
  su·do·mo·tor f.'s
  sus·ten·tac·u·lar f.'s of ret·
    i·na
  tau·to·mer·ic f.s
  Tomes' f.'s
  trans·sep·tal f.'s
  trans·verse f.'s of pons
  un·my·e·li·nat·ed f.'s
  Weitbrecht's f.'s
  white f.
  yel·low f.'s
  zo·nu·lar f.'s
fi·ber·op·tic
fi·ber·op·tics
fi·ber·scope
fi·bra
  fi·brae cor·ti·co·pon·ti·nae
  fi·brae py·ra·mi·da·les
fi·brae
fi·bre
fi·bre·mia
fi·bril
  col·la·gen f.'s

fi·bril *(continued)*
  mus·cu·lar f.
  sub·pel·lic·u·lar f.
  unit f.'s
fi·bril·la
fi·bril·lae
fi·bril·lar
  bas·kets
fi·bril·lary
  as·tro·cyte
  cho·rea
  con·trac·tions
  my·o·clo·nia
  neu·ro·ma
  trem·or
  waves
fi·bril·late
fi·bril·lat·ed
fi·bril·la·tion
  atri·al f.
  au·ric·u·lar f.
  ven·tric·u·lar f.
fi·bril·la·tion
  thresh·old
fi·bril·lo·gen·e·sis
fi·brin
  cal·cu·lus
  throm·bus
fi·brin·ase
fi·brin/fi·brin·o·gen deg·ra·da·tion
  pro·ducts
fi·bri·no·cel·lu·lar
fi·brin·o·gen
  hu·man f.
fi·brin·og·e·nase
fi·brin·o·ge·ne·mia
fi·bri·no·gen·e·sis
fi·brin·o·gen-fi·brin con·ver·sion
  syn·drome
fi·bri·no·gen·ic
fi·brin·o·gen·ol·y·sis
fi·brin·o·gen·o·pe·nia
fi·bri·nog·e·nous
fi·brin·oid
  de·gen·er·a·tion
  ne·cro·sis
fi·bri·no·ki·nase
fi·bri·nol·y·sin
  strep·to·coc·cal f.
fi·bri·nol·y·sis
fi·bri·no·ly·so·ki·nase
fi·bri·no·lyt·ic
  pur·pu·ra
fi·brin·o·pep·tide
fi·bri·no·pu·ru·lent
  in·flam·ma·tion

fi·bri·nos·co·py
fi·brin·ous
  ad·he·sion
  bron·chi·tis
  cast
  cat·a·ract
  de·gen·er·a·tion
  in·flam·ma·tion
  iri·tis
  lymph
  per·i·car·di·tis
  pleu·ri·sy
  pol·yp
  rhi·ni·tis
fi·brin-sta·bi·liz·ing
  fac·tor
fi·bri·nu·ria
fi·bro·ad·e·no·ma
  gi·ant f.
  in·tra·can·a·lic·u·lar f.
  per·i·can·a·lic·u·lar f.
fi·bro·ad·i·pose
fi·bro·a·re·o·lar
fi·bro·blast
  in·ter·fer·on
fi·bro·blas·tic
fi·bro·car·ci·no·ma
fi·bro·car·ti·lage
  cir·cum·fer·en·tial f.
  ex·ter·nal sem·i·lu·nar f.
  in·ter·ar·tic·u·lar f.
  in·ter·nal sem·i·lu·nar f. of knee joint
  sem·i·lu·nar f.
  strat·i·form f.
fi·bro·car·ti·lag·i·nous
  ring
fi·bro·car·ti·la·go
  f. ba·sa·lis
  f. in·ter·ar·tic·u·la·ris
  f. in·ter·ver·te·bra·lis
fi·bro·ca·se·ous
  per·i·to·ni·tis
fi·bro·cel·lu·lar
fi·bro·chon·dri·tis
fi·bro·chon·dro·ma
fi·bro·con·ges·tive
fi·bro·cyst
fi·bro·cys·tic
  dis·ease of the breast
  dis·ease of the pan·cre·as
fi·bro·cys·to·ma
fi·bro·cyte
fi·bro·dys·pla·sia
  f. os·sif·i·cans pro·gres·si·va
fi·bro·e·las·tic

fi·bro·e·las·to·sis
  en·do·car·di·al f.
  en·do·my·o·car·di·al f.
fi·bro·en·chon·dro·ma
fi·bro·ep·i·the·li·al
  pap·il·lo·ma
fi·bro·ep·i·the·li·o·ma
fi·bro·fat·ty
fi·bro·fol·lic·u·lo·ma
fi·bro·gen·e·sis
fi·bro·gli·o·sis
fi·bro·hy·a·line
  tis·sue
fi·broid
  ad·e·no·ma
  cat·a·ract
  in·flam·ma·tion
  lung
  tu·mor
fi·broid·ec·to·my
fi·bro·in
fi·bro·ker·a·to·ma
fi·bro·la·mel·lar liv·er cell
  car·ci·no·ma
fi·bro·lei·o·my·o·ma
fi·bro·li·po·ma
fi·bro·ma
  am·e·lo·blas·tic f.
  ap·o·neu·rot·ic f.
  ce·ment·i·fy·ing f.
  cen·tral ce·ment·i·fy·ing f.
  cen·tral os·si·fy·ing f.
  chon·dro·myx·oid f.
  con·cen·tric f.
  des·mo·plas·tic f.
  gi·ant cell f.
  ir·ri·ta·tion f.
  f. mol·le
  f. mol·le grav·i·dar·um
  f. myx·o·ma·to·des
  non·os·si·fy·ing f.
  non·os·te·o·gen·ic f.
  odon·to·gen·ic f.
  pe·riph·e·ral os·si·fy·ing f.
  per·i·un·gual f.
  rab·bit f.
  re·cur·ring dig·i·tal f.'s of
    child·hood
  se·nile f.
  Shope f.
  tel·an·gi·ec·tat·ic f.
fi·bro·ma·toid
fi·bro·ma·to·sis
  ab·dom·i·nal f.
  ag·gres·sive in·fan·tile f.
  f. col·li
  con·gen·i·tal gen·er·al·ized
    f.

in·fan·tile dig·i·tal f.
ju·ve·nile hy·a·lin f.
ju·ve·nile pal·mo-plan·tar f.
pal·mar f.
pe·nile f.
plan·tar f.
fi·bro·ma·to·sis
  vi·rus of rab·bits
fi·bro·ma·tous
fi·bro·mec·to·my
fi·bro·mus·cu·lar
  dys·pla·sia
  hy·per·pla·sia
fi·bro·my·ec·to·my
fi·bro·my·o·ma
fi·bro·my·o·si·tis
fi·bro·myx·o·ma
fi·bro·nec·tin
  plas·ma f.
fi·bro·neu·ro·ma
fi·bro-os·te·o·ma
fi·bro·pap·il·lo·ma
fi·bro·pla·sia
  ret·ro·len·tal f.
fi·bro·plas·tic
fi·bro·plate
fi·bro·pol·y·pus
fi·bro·psam·mo·ma
fi·bro·re·tic·u·late
fi·bro·sar·co·ma
  am·e·lo·blas·tic f.
  Earle L f.
  in·fan·tile f.
fi·brose
fi·bro·se·rous
fi·bros·ing
  ad·e·no·ma·to·sis
  ad·e·no·sis
fi·bro·sis
  cys·tic f.
  cys·tic f. of the pan·cre·as
  en·do·my·o·car·di·al f.
  id·i·o·path·ic ret·ro·per·i·
    to·ne·al f.
  lep·to·me·nin·ge·al f.
  me·di·as·ti·nal f.
  nod·u·lar sub·ep·i·der·mal
    f.
  per·i·cen·tral f.
  per·i·mus·cu·lar f.
  pipe·stem f.
  re·place·ment f.
  ret·ro·per·i·to·ne·al f.
  sub·ad·ven·ti·tial f.
  Symmers' f.
  Symmers' clay pipe·stem f.
fi·bro·sit·ic
  head·ache

fi·bro·si·tis
    cer·vi·cal f.
fi·bro·tho·rax
fi·brot·ic
fi·brous
    ad·he·sion
    an·ky·lo·sis
    ap·pen·dix of liv·er
    as·tro·cyte
    cap·sule
    cap·sule of kid·ney
    cav·er·ni·tis
    de·gen·er·a·tion
    dys·pla·sia
    dys·pla·sia of bone
    goi·ter
    ham·ar·to·ma of in·fan·cy
    his·ti·o·cy·to·ma
    joint
    lay·er
    mem·brane
    pol·yp
    pro·tein
    ring
    sheaths
    tis·sue
    tri·gones of heart
    tu·ber·cle
    tu·nic of cor·pus spon·gi·o·
      sum
    tu·nic of eye
    un·ion
    xan·tho·ma
fi·brous ar·tic·u·lar
    cap·sule
fi·brous bac·te·ri·al
    vi·rus·es
fi·brous cor·ti·cal
    de·fect
fi·bro·xan·tho·ma
    atyp·i·cal f.
fib·u·la
fib·u·lar
    ar·tery
    mar·gin of foot
    node
    notch
    veins
fib·u·lar ar·tic·u·lar
    sur·face of tib·ia
fib·u·lar col·lat·er·al
    lig·a·ment
fib·u·la·ris
fib·u·lo·cal·ca·ne·al
fi·cin
Fick
    prin·ci·ple

Fi·coll-Hy·paque
    tech·nique
fi·co·sis
fic·ti·tious
    feed·ing
Fiedler's
    my·o·car·di·tis
field of
    con·scious·ness
field
    block
    fe·ver
    lens
field
    au·di·to·ry f.
    Broca's f.
    Cohnheim's f.
    f. of con·scious·ness
    f. of fix·a·tion
    f.'s of Forel
    free f.
    H f.'s
    in·di·vid·u·a·tion f.
    mag·net·ic f.
    mi·cro·scop·ic f.
    nerve f.
    pre·ru·bral f.
    teg·men·tal f.'s of Forel
    vi·su·al f.
    Wernicke's f.
field block
    an·es·the·sia
Fielding's
    mem·brane
Field's rap·id
    stain
field-vole
Fiessinger-Leroy-Reiter
    syn·drome
fifth
    dis·ease
    fin·ger
    ven·tri·cle
fifth cra·ni·al
    nerve
fig
    wart
Figueira's
    syn·drome
fig·u·ra·tus
fig·ure
    au·thor·i·ty f.
    flame f.
    for·ti·fi·ca·tion f.'s
    mi·tot·ic f.
    my·e·lin f.
    Purkinje's f.'s
fig·ure and ground

fig·ure-of-eight
  ab·nor·mal·i·ty
fi·la
fi·la·ceous
fil·ag·grin
fil·a·men
fil·a·ment
  ac·tin f.
  ax·i·al f.
  cy·to·ker·a·tin f.'s
  in·ter·me·di·ate f.'s
  ker·a·tin f.'s
  my·o·sin f.
  par·a·ba·sal f.
  root f.'s
  sper·mat·ic f.
  Z f.
fil·a·men·ta
fil·a·men·ta·ry
  ker·a·top·a·thy
fil·a·ment-non·fil·a·ment
  count
fil·a·men·tous
  bac·te·ri·o·phage
  col·o·ny
fil·a·men·tous bac·te·ri·al
  vi·rus·es
fil·a·ment pol·y·mor·pho·nu·cle·ar
  leu·ko·cyte
fil·a·men·tum
fi·lar
  mass
  mi·cro·me·ter
  sub·stance
Fi·lar·ia
fi·lar·ia
fi·lar·i·ae
fi·lar·i·al
  ar·thri·tis
  der·ma·to·sis
  fu·nic·u·li·tis
  hy·dro·cele
  per·i·o·dic·i·ty
  syn·o·vi·tis
fil·a·ri·a·sis
  ban·croft·i·an f.
  pe·ri·od·ic f.
fi·lar·i·ci·dal
fi·lar·i·cide
fi·lar·i·form
  lar·va
Fil·a·ri·i·cae
Fi·lar·i·oi·dea
Fi·lar·oi·des
Filatov
  flap

Filatov-Gillies
  flap
Filatov-Gillies tubed
  ped·i·cle
Filatov's
  dis·ease
  op·er·a·tion
  spots
file
  Hedström f.
  per·i·o·don·tal f.
  root ca·nal f.
fil·i·al
  gen·er·a·tion
fi·li·form
  bou·gie
  pa·pil·lae
  pulse
  wart
fil·i·o·pa·ren·tal
fi·li·punc·ture
fill·er
  graft
fil·let
  lay·er
fil·let
  lat·er·al f.
  me·di·al f.
fill·ing
  de·fect
film
  ab·sorb·a·ble gel·a·tin f.
  bite·wing f.
  pan·o·ram·ic x-ray f.
  plain f.
  pre·cor·ne·al f.
  tear f.
fil·o·po·dia
fil·o·po·di·um
fi·lo·pres·sure
fi·lo·var·i·co·sis
fil·ter
  pa·per
fil·ter·a·ble
fil·ter·ing
  cic·a·trix
  op·er·a·tion
fil·tra·ble
  vi·rus
fil·trate
  fac·tor
  ni·tro·gen
fil·tra·tion
  an·gle
  co·ef·fi·cient
  frac·tion
  slits
  space

fil·tra·tion
  gel f.
fil·trum
  Merkel's f. ven·tric·u·li
  f. ven·tric·u·li
fi·lum
  fi·la ol·fac·to·ria
  ter·mi·nal f.
fim·bria
  ovar·i·an f.
  fim·bri·ae of uter·ine tube
fim·bri·ae
fim·bri·ate
fim·bri·at·ed
  fold
fim·bri·ec·to·my
fim·bri·o·cele
fim·bri·o·den·tate
  sul·cus
fim·bri·o·plas·ty
fi·nal
  host
  im·pres·sion
Finckh
  test
fine
  struc·ture
  trem·or
fine·ness
fin·ger
  base·ball f.
  bol·ster f.
  clubbed f.'s
  dead f.'s
  drop f.
  drum·stick f.'s
  fifth f.
  first f.
  fourth f.
  ham·mer f.
  hip·po·crat·ic f.'s
  in·dex f.
  jerk f.
  lit·tle f.
  lock f.
  mal·let f.
  mid·dle f.
  ring f.
  sau·sage f.'s
  sec·ond f.
  snap f.
  spade f.'s
  spi·der f.
  spring f.
  stuck f.
  third f.
  trig·ger f.
  waxy f.'s

webbed f.'s
white f.'s
fin·ger
  ag·no·sia
  per·cus·sion
  phe·nom·e·non
fin·ger·nail
fin·ger-nose
  test
fin·ger·print
  dys·tro·phy
fin·ger·print
  Galton's sys·tem of clas·si·fi·ca·tion of f.'s
fin·ger-thumb
  re·flex
fin·ger-to-fin·ger
  test
fin·ish·ing
  bur
Fink-Heimer
  stain
Finney
  py·lo·ro·plas·ty
Finney's
  op·er·a·tion
Finsen
  light
fire
fire·damp
first
  den·ti·tion
  fin·ger
  mes·sen·ger
  mo·lar
first aid
first arch
  syn·drome
first cra·ni·al
  nerve
first cu·ne·i·form
  bone
first de·gree
  burn
  pro·lapse
first de·gree A-V
  block
first du·o·de·nal
  sphinc·ter
first heart
  sound
first-or·der
  re·ac·tion
first par·al·lel pel·vic
  plane
first per·ma·nent
  mo·lar

first rank
symp·toms
first stage
first tem·po·ral
con·vo·lu·tion
first vis·cer·al
cleft
Fischer pro·jec·tion for·mu·las of
sug·ars
Fischer's
sign
symp·tom
Fischer's pro·jec·tion for·mu·las
fish
poi·son
skin
test
Fishberg con·cen·tra·tion
test
Fisher's
syn·drome
Fishman-Lerner
unit
fish-mouth
me·a·tus
fish-mouth mi·tral
ste·no·sis
fish tape·worm
ane·mia
fis·sion
fun·gi
pro·duct
fis·sion
bi·na·ry f.
bud f.
mul·ti·ple f.
sim·ple f.
fis·si·par·i·ty
fis·sip·a·rous
Fis·si·pe·dia
fis·su·ra
f. cal·ca·ri·na
f. ce·re·bri la·te·ra·lis
f. cho·roi·dea
f. col·la·te·ra·lis
f. den·ta·ta
f. hip·po·cam·pi
f. pa·ri·e·to·oc·cip·i·ta·lis
f. pte·ry·goi·dea
f. pte·ry·go·pa·la·ti·na
f. pu·den·di
f. trans·ver·sa ce·re·bel·li
fis·su·rae
fis·sur·al
cyst
fis·su·ra·tion

fis·sure
ab·dom·i·nal f.
Ammon's f.
anal f.
an·te·ri·or me·di·an f. of me·dul·la ob·lon·ga·ta
an·te·ri·or me·di·an f. of spi·nal cord
an·ti·tra·go·hel·i·cine f.
ape f.
au·ric·u·lar f.
Bichat's f.
bran·chi·al f.
Broca's f.
cal·ca·rine f.
cal·lo·so·mar·gin·al f.
cau·dal trans·verse f.
cer·e·bel·lar f.'s
ce·re·bral f.'s
cho·roid f.
Clevenger's f.
col·lat·er·al f.
de·cid·u·al f.
den·tate f.
Duverney's f.'s
Ecker's f.
enam·el f.
gla·se·ri·an f.
great hor·i·zon·tal f.
great lon·gi·tu·di·nal f.
Henle's f.'s
hip·po·cam·pal f.
hor·i·zon·tal f. of cer·e·bel·lum
hor·i·zon·tal f. of right lung
in·fe·ri·or or·bi·tal f.
lat·er·al ce·re·bral f.
left sag·it·tal f.
f. for lig·a·men·tum te·res
lin·guo·gin·gi·val f.
f.'s of liv·er
lon·gi·tu·di·nal f. of cer·e·brum
lu·nate f.
f.'s of lung
ob·lique f.
op·tic f.
oral f.
pal·pe·bral f.
Pansch's f.
par·a·cen·tral f.
pa·ri·e·to·oc·cip·i·tal f.
pet·ro·oc·cip·i·tal f.
pet·ro·squa·mous f.
pet·ro·tym·pan·ic f.
por·tal f.
post·cen·tral f.

fis·sure *(continued)*
  pos·te·ri·or me·di·an f. of
    the me·dul·la ob·lon·ga·ta
  pos·te·ri·or me·di·an f. of
    spi·nal cord
  pos·ter·o·lat·er·al f.
  post·hip·po·cam·pal f.
  post·lin·gual f.
  post·lu·nate f.
  post·py·ram·i·dal f.
  post·rhi·nal f.
  pre·nod·u·lar f.
  pri·mary f. of the cer·e·
    bel·lum
  pter·y·goid f.
  pter·y·go·max·il·lary f.
  rhi·nal f.
  right sag·it·tal f.
  f. of Rolando
  f. of round lig·a·ment
  Santorini's f.'s
  sec·on·dary f. of the cer·e·
    bel·lum
  sim·i·an f.
  sphe·noi·dal f.
  sphe·no·max·il·lary f.
  sphe·no·pe·tro·sal f.
  squa·mo·tym·pan·ic f.
  su·pe·ri·or or·bi·tal f.
  su·pe·ri·or tem·po·ral f.
  syl·vi·an f.
  f. of Sylvius
  trans·verse f. of cer·e·bel·
    lum
  trans·verse f. of cer·e·brum
  trans·verse f. of the lung
  tym·pa·no·mas·toid f.
  tym·pa·no·squa·mous f.
  um·bil·i·cal f.
  f. of ve·nous lig·a·ment
  ves·tib·u·lar f. of co·chlea
  zy·gal f.
fis·sure
  bur
  car·ies
  seal·ant
fis·sured
  frac·ture
  tongue
fis·tu·la
  knife
  test
fis·tu·la
  ab·dom·i·nal f.
  am·phi·bol·ic f.
  am·phib·o·lous f.
  anal f.
  ar·te·ri·o·ve·nous f.

  f. au·ris con·gen·i·ta
  bil·i·ary f.
  f. bi·mu·co·sa
  blind f.
  bran·chi·al f.
  Brescia-Cimino f.
  bron·cho·e·soph·a·ge·al f.
  bron·cho·pleu·ral f.
  ca·rot·id-cav·ern·ous f.
  cer·vi·cal f.
  cho·le·cys·to·du·o·de·nal f.
  coc·cyg·eal f.
  f. col·li con·gen·i·ta
  co·lo·cu·ta·ne·ous f.
  co·lo·il·e·al f.
  co·lon·ic f.
  co·lo·vag·i·nal f.
  co·lo·ves·i·cal f.
  com·plete f.
  cra·ni·o·si·nus f.
  den·tal f.
  du·o·de·nal f.
  Eck f.
  en·ter·o·cu·ta·ne·ous f.
  en·ter·o·vag·i·nal f.
  en·ter·o·ves·i·cal f.
  eth·moi·dal-lac·ri·mal f.
  ex·ter·nal f.
  fe·cal f.
  gas·tric f.
  gas·tro·co·lic f.
  gas·tro·cu·ta·ne·ous f.
  gas·tro·du·o·de·nal f.
  gas·tro·in·tes·ti·nal f.
  gen·i·to·u·ri·nary f.
  gin·gi·val f.
  he·pa·tic f.
  he·pa·to·pleu·ral f.
  horse·shoe f.
  in·com·plete f.
  in·ter·nal f.
  in·ter·nal lac·ri·mal f.
  in·tes·ti·nal f.
  lac·ri·mal f.
  f. la·cri·ma·lis
  lac·te·al f.
  lym·phat·ic f.
  mam·ma·ry f.
  Mann-Bollman f.
  me·tro·per·i·to·ne·al f.
  or·o·an·tral f.
  or·o·fa·cial f.
  or·o·na·sal f.
  pa·ri·e·tal f.
  per·i·ne·o·vag·i·nal f.
  pha·ryn·ge·al f.
  pi·lo·ni·dal f.
  pul·mo·nary f.

rec·to·la·bi·al f.
rec·to·u·re·thral f.
rec·to·vag·i·nal f.
rec·to·ves·i·cal f.
rec·to·ves·tib·u·lar f.
rec·to·vul·var f.
re·verse Eck f.
sal·i·vary f.
sig·moi·do·ves·i·cal f.
sper·mat·ic f.
ster·co·ral f.
Thiry's f.
Thiry-Vella f.
tho·rac·ic f.
tra·che·al f.
tra·che·o·bil·i·ary f.
tra·che·o·e·soph·a·ge·al f.
um·bil·i·cal f.
ura·chal f.
ure·ter·o·cu·ta·ne·ous f.
ure·ter·o·vag·i·nal f.
ure·thro·vag·i·nal f.
uri·nary f.
uro·gen·i·tal f.
uter·o·per·i·to·ne·al f.
Vella's f.
ves·i·cal f.
ves·i·co·co·lic f.
ves·i·co·cu·ta·ne·ous f.
ves·i·co·in·tes·ti·nal f.
ves·i·co·u·ter·ine f.
ves·i·co·vag·i·nal f.
ves·i·co·vag·i·no·rec·tal f.
vi·tel·line f.
fis·tu·lae
fis·tu·las
fis·tu·la·tion
fis·tu·la·tome
fis·tu·lec·to·my
fis·tu·li·za·tion
fis·tu·lo·en·ter·os·to·my
fis·tu·lot·o·my
fis·tu·lous
with·ers
FIT
test
fit
un·ci·nate f.
fit·ness
clin·i·cal f.
ev·o·lu·tion·ary f.
ge·net·ic f.
phys·i·cal f.
Fitz-Hugh and Curtis
syn·drome
five-day
fe·ver

fix·a·tion
dis·par·i·ty
nys·tag·mus
re·ac·tion
fix·a·tion
bi·fo·ve·al f.
bin·oc·u·lar f.
cir·cum·al·ve·o·lar f.
cir·cum·man·dib·u·lar f.
cir·cum·zy·go·mat·ic f.
com·ple·ment f.
cra·ni·o·fa·cial f.
crossed f.
ec·cen·tric f.
elas·tic band f.
ex·ter·nal f.
ex·ter·nal pin f.
ex·ter·nal pin f., bi·phase
freud·i·an f.
ge·net·ic f.
in·ter·max·il·lary f.
in·ter·nal f.
in·tra·os·se·ous f.
man·dib·u·lo·max·il·lary f.
max·il·lo·man·dib·u·lar f.
na·so·man·dib·u·lar f.
fix·a·tion·al oc·u·lar
move·ment
fix·a·tive
ac·e·tone f.
Altmann's f.
Bouin's f.
Carnoy's f.
Champy's f.
Flemming's f.
form·al·de·hyde f.
for·mol-cal·ci·um f.
for·mol-Müller f.
for·mol-sa·line f.
for·mol-Zenker f.
glu·tar·al·de·hyde f.
Golgi's os·mi·o·bi·chro·mate
f.
Helly's f.
Hermann's f.
Kaiserling's f.
Luft's po·tas·si·um per·
man·ga·nate f.
Marchi's f.
meth·a·nol f.
Müller's f.
neu·tral buff·ered for·ma·lin
f.
Newcomer's f.
Orth's f.
os·mic ac·id f.
Park-Williams f.
pic·ro·for·mol f.

fix·a·tive *(continued)*
   Regaud's f.
   Schaudinn's f.
   Thoma's f.
   Zenker's f.
fix·a·tor
   mus·cle
fixed
   al·ka·li
   al·ka·loid
   cou·pling
   dress·ing
   idea
   mac·ro·phage
   oil
   pu·pil
   tor·ti·col·lis
   vi·rus
fixed drug
   erup·tion
fixed-in·ter·val re·in·force·ment
   sched·ule
fixed par·tial
   den·ture
fixed-rate
   pace·mak·er
fixed rate pulse
   gen·er·a·tor
fixed-ra·tio re·in·force·ment
   sched·ule
fix·ing
   eye
flac·cid
   ec·tro·pi·on
   mem·brane
   part of tym·pan·ic mem·
     brane
flac·cid·i·ty
Flack's
   node
flag
   flap
   sign
fla·gel·la
fla·gel·lar
   ag·glu·ti·nin
   an·ti·gen
Flag·el·la·ta
flag·el·late
   col·lared f.
flag·el·lat·ed
flag·el·la·tion
fla·gel·lin
flag·el·lo·sis
fla·gel·lum
flail
   chest
   joint

flame
   arc
   fig·ure
   ne·vus
   pho·tom·e·ter
   spots
flame emis·sion
   spec·tro·pho·tom·e·try
flam·ma·ble
   an·es·thet·ic
flange
   con·tour
flange
   buc·cal f.
   den·ture f.
   la·bi·al f.
   lin·gual f.
flank
   bone
   in·ci·sion
   po·si·tion
flap
   am·pu·ta·tion
   op·er·a·tion
flap
   Abbe f.
   ad·vance·ment f.
   ar·te·ri·al f.
   ax·i·al pat·tern f.
   bi·lobed f.
   bi·ped·i·cle f.
   bone f.
   bur·ied f.
   cat·er·pil·lar f.
   cel·lu·lo·cu·ta·ne·ous f.
   com·pos·ite f.
   com·pound f.
   cross f.
   de·layed f.
   del·to·pec·to·ral f.
   di·rect f.
   dis·tant f.
   dou·ble ped·i·cle f.
   en·ve·lope f.
   Estlander f.
   Filatov f.
   Filatov-Gillies f.
   flag f.
   flat f.
   free f.
   free bone f.
   French f.
   full-thick·ness f.
   gin·gi·val f.
   hinged f.
   im·me·di·ate f.
   is·land f.
   jump f.

lined f.
lin·gual f.
liv·er f.
lo·cal f.
mu·co·per·i·chon·dri·al f.
mu·co·per·i·os·te·al f.
mus·cu·lo·cu·ta·ne·ous f.
my·o·cu·ta·ne·ous f.
my·o·der·mal f.
neu·ro·vas·cu·lar f.
open f.
par·a·bi·ot·ic f.
par·tial-thick·ness f.
ped·i·cle f.
per·i·cor·o·nal f.
per·ma·nent ped·i·cle f.
pha·ryn·ge·al f.
ran·dom pat·tern f.
rope f.
ro·ta·tion f.
sick·le f.
skin f.
slid·ing f.
split-thick·ness f.
sub·cu·ta·ne·ous f.
tongue f.
tubed f.
tubed ped·i·cle f.
turn·o·ver f.
waltzed f.
flap·less
am·pu·ta·tion
flap·ping
trem·or
flare
aque·ous f.
fla·rim·e·ter
flash
hot f.
flash
blind·ness
burn
dis·per·sal
ker·a·to·con·junc·ti·vi·tis
meth·od
point
flash·back
flash·ing pain
syn·drome
flask
clo·sure
flask
cast·ing f.
crown f.
den·ture f.
Dewar f.
Erlenmeyer f.
Fernbach f.

Florence f.
in·jec·tion f.
re·frac·to·ry f.
vac·u·um f.
vol·u·met·ric f.
flask·ing
flat
af·fect
bone
chest
con·dy·lo·ma
elec·tro·en·ceph·a·lo·gram
flap
foot
hand
pel·vis
plate
wart
Flatau's
law
Flatau-Schilder
dis·ease
flat·foot
flat pap·u·lar
syph·i·lid
flat top
waves
flat·u·lence
flat·u·lent
dys·pep·sia
fla·tus
en·e·ma
fla·tus
f. va·gi·na·lis
flat·worm
fla·ve·do
fla·vi·an·ic ac·id
fla·vin
f. ad·e·nine di·nu·cle·o·tide
f. mon·o·nu·cle·o·tide
fla·vine
Fla·vi·vi·rus
Fla·vo·bac·te·ri·um
F. aq·ua·tile
F. bre·ve
F. pis·ci·ci·da
fla·vo·en·zyme
fla·vo·ki·nase
fla·vone
fla·vo·noids
fla·vo·nol
fla·vo·pro·tein
fla·vor
fla·vox·ate hy·dro·chlo·ride
fla·vus
flax·seed
f. oil
flea

flea-bit·ten
 kid·ney
flea-borne
 ty·phus
fle·cai·nide ac·e·tate
Flechsig's
 ar·e·as
 fas·cic·u·li
 tract
Flechsig's ground
 bun·dles
fleck
 dys·tro·phy of cor·nea
 ret·i·na
 ret·i·na of Kandori
flecked
 ret·i·na
flecked ret·i·na
 syn·drome
flec·tion
fleece
 worm
Flegel's
 dis·ease
Fleisch
 pneu·mo·tach·o·graph
Fleischer's
 ring
Fleischmann's
 bur·sa
Fleischner
 lines
Fleitmann's
 test
Flemming's
 fix·a·tive
Flemming's tri·ple
 stain
Flesch
 for·mu·la
flesh
 proud f.
flesh·flies
fleshy
 mole
 pol·yp
flex
flex·i·bil·i·tas ce·rea
flex·i·ble
 col·lo·di·on
flex·im·e·ter
flex·ion
 pal·mar f.
 plan·tar f.
flex·ion
 crease
Flexner's
 ba·cil·lus

flex·or
 re·flex
 ret·i·nac·u·lum
 tet·a·nus
flex·u·ra
 f. sig·moi·dea
flex·u·rae
flex·ur·al
 ec·ze·ma
flex·ure
 ba·si·cra·ni·al f.
 cau·dal f.
 ce·phal·ic f.
 ce·re·bral f.
 cer·vi·cal f.
 cra·ni·al f.
 dor·sal f.
 du·o·de·no·je·ju·nal f.
 he·pa·tic f.
 in·fe·ri·or f. of du·o·de·num
 left col·ic f.
 lum·bar f.
 mes·en·ce·phal·ic f.
 per·i·ne·al f. of rec·tum
 pon·tine f.
 right col·ic f.
 sa·cral f.
 sa·cral f. of rec·tum
 sig·moid f.
 splen·ic f.
 su·pe·ri·or f. of du·o·de·num
 tel·en·ce·phal·ic f.
 trans·verse rhomb·en·ce·phal·ic f.
flick
 move·ments
flick·er
 fu·sion
 pe·rim·e·try
 pho·tom·e·ter
flick·er
flick·er fu·sion fre·quen·cy
 tech·nique
flicks
Flieringa's
 ring
flight
 blind·ness
flight or fight
 re·sponse
flight in·to dis·ease
flight in·to health
flint
 dis·ease
 glass

Flint's
  ar·cade
  mur·mur
flip
flit·ter·ing
  sco·to·ma
float·er
float·ing
  car·ti·lage
  kid·ney
  or·gan
  pa·tel·la
  ribs
  spleen
  vil·lus
floc
floc·cil·la·tion
floc·cose
floc·cu·la·ble
floc·cu·lar
  fos·sa
floc·cu·late
floc·cu·la·tion
  re·ac·tion
  test
floc·cule
floc·cu·lence
floc·cu·lent
floc·cu·li
floc·cu·lo·nod·u·lar
  lobe
floc·cu·lus
  ac·ces·so·ry f.
flood
  fe·ver
flood·ing
Flood's
  lig·a·ment
floor
  cell
  plate
flop·py valve
  syn·drome
flo·ra
flor·an·ty·rone
Florence
  flask
Florence's
  crys·tals
Florey
  unit
flor·id
flor·id oral
  pap·il·lo·ma·to·sis
flor·id os·se·ous
  dys·pla·sia
flo·ri·form
  cat·a·ract

Florschütz'
  for·mu·la
floss
  silk
floss
  den·tal f.
flo·ta·tion
  con·stant
  meth·od
Flourens'
  the·o·ry
floury
  cor·nea
flow
  cy·to·pho·tom·e·try
flow·er bas·ket of Bochdalek
flow·er of par·a·dise
Flow·er's
  bone
Flow·er's den·tal
  in·dex
flow·ers
  f. of an·ti·mo·ny
  f. of ben·zo·in
  f. of sul·fur
  f. of zinc
flow·er-spray
  end·ing
  or·gan of Ruffini
flow·ing
  hy·per·os·to·sis
flow·me·ter
  elec·tro·mag·net·ic f.
flow-over
  va·por·iz·er
flow-vol·ume
  curve
flox·ur·i·dine
flu·an·i·sone
flu·cry·late
fluc·tu·ate
fluc·tu·a·tion
flu·cy·to·sine
flu·dro·cor·ti·sone ac·e·tate
flu·fen·am·ic ac·id
flu·id
  al·lan·to·ic f.
  am·ni·ot·ic f.
  Brodie f.
  Callison's f.
  cer·e·bro·spi·nal f.
  cre·vic·u·lar f.
  Dakin's f.
  den·ti·nal f.
  ex·tra·cel·lu·lar f.
  ex·tra·vas·cu·lar f.
  Farrant's mount·ing f.
  gin·gi·val f.

flu·id *(continued)*
  in·fra·na·tant f.
  in·ter·sti·tial f.
  in·tra·cel·lu·lar f.
  in·tra·oc·u·lar f.
  new·to·ni·an f.
  non-new·to·ni·an f.
  pleu·ral f.
  pros·tat·ic f.
  pseu·do·plas·tic f.
  Rees-Ecker f.
  Scarpa's f.
  sem·i·nal f.
  sul·cu·lar f.
  su·per·na·tant f.
  syn·o·vi·al f.
  thix·o·tro·pic f.
  tis·sue f.
  trans·cel·lu·lar f.'s
  ven·tric·u·lar f.
flu·id
  ex·tract
  wave
flu·id·ex·tract
flu·id·glyc·er·ates
flu·id·i·ty
flu·id·ounce
flu·i·drachm
flu·i·dram
fluke
flu·men
flu·meth·a·sone
flu·me·thi·a·zide
flu·mi·na
flu·nis·o·lide
flu·o·cin·o·lone ac·e·to·nide
flu·o·cin·o·nide
flu·o·cor·to·lone
  f. cap·ro·ate
  f. hex·a·no·ate
  f. piv·a·late
flu·or·ap·a·tite
flu·o·res·ce·in
  f. iso·thi·o·cy·a·nate
  f. so·di·um
flu·o·res·ce·in
  an·gi·og·ra·phy
flu·o·res·ce·in in·stil·la·tion
  test
flu·o·res·ce·in string
  test
flu·o·res·cence
  mi·cro·scope
  mi·cros·co·py
  quench·ing
  spec·trum
flu·o·res·cence plus Giemsa
  stain

flu·o·res·cent
  an·ti·body
  screen
  stain
flu·o·res·cent an·ti·body
  tech·nique
flu·o·res·cent an·ti·nu·cle·ar an·ti·body
  test
flu·o·res·cent trep·o·ne·mal an·ti·body-ab·sorp·tion
  test
flu·o·res·cin
flu·o·ri·dat·ed
  teeth
flu·o·ri·da·tion
flu·o·ride
flu·o·ride num·ber
flu·o·ri·di·za·tion
flu·o·rine
flu·o·ro·chrome
flu·or·o·chrom·ing
flu·o·ro·cyte
flu·o·rog·ra·phy
flu·o·rom·e·ter
flu·o·ro·meth·o·lone
flu·o·rom·e·try
flu·o·ro·pho·tom·e·try
flu·o·ro·roent·gen·og·ra·phy
flu·o·ro·scope
flu·o·ro·scop·ic
flu·o·ros·co·py
flu·o·ro·sis
  chron·ic en·dem·ic f.
flu·o·ro·u·ra·cil
flu·ox·e·tine hy·dro·chlo·ride
flu·ox·y·mes·ter·one
flu·pen·tix·ol
flu·per·o·lone ac·e·tate
flu·phen·a·zine
  f. enan·thate
  f. hy·dro·chlo·ride
flu·pred·nis·o·lone
flur·an·dren·o·lide
flur·az·e·pam hy·dro·chlo·ride
flur·bi·pro·fen
flur·o·ges·tone ac·e·tate
flur·oth·yl
flur·ox·ene
Flury strain
  vac·cine
Flury strain ra·bies
  vi·rus
flush
  tech·nique
flush
  hec·tic f.

hot f.
ma·lar f.

flut·ter
atri·al f.
au·ric·u·lar f.
di·a·phrag·mat·ic f.
im·pure f.
oc·u·lar f.
ven·tric·u·lar f.

flut·ter-fi·bril·la·tion
waves

flux
den·si·ty
ra·tio

flux
lu·mi·nous f.
net f.
uni·di·rec·tion·al f.

flux·ion·ary
hy·per·e·mia

fly
ag·a·ric
blis·ter

fly
heel f.
louse f.'s
man·grove f.
Rus·sian f.
Span·ish f.
war·ble f.

fly·ing
blis·ter

fly·ing spot
mi·cro·scope

Flynn-Aird
syn·drome

FMD
vi·rus

foam
cells

foam
hu·man fi·brin f.

foam sta·bil·i·ty
test

foamy
agents
vi·rus·es

fo·cal
am·y·loi·do·sis
ap·pen·di·ci·tis
depth
dis·tance
ep·i·lep·sy
glo·mer·u·lo·ne·phri·tis
il·lu·mi·na·tion
in·fec·tion
in·ter·val
ne·cro·sis

ne·phri·tis
point
re·ac·tion
scle·ro·sis

fo·cal der·mal
hy·po·pla·sia

fo·cal der·mal hy·po·pla·sia
syn·drome

fo·cal em·bol·ic
glo·mer·u·lo·ne·phri·tis

fo·cal ep·i·the·li·al
hy·per·pla·sia

fo·cal lym·pho·cyt·ic
thy·roid·i·tis

fo·cal scle·ros·ing
glo·mer·u·lop·a·thy

fo·cal seg·men·tal
glo·mer·u·lo·scle·ro·sis

fo·ci

fo·cim·e·ter

fo·cus
con·ju·gate fo·ci
Ghon's f.
nat·u·ral f. of in·fec·tion
prin·ci·pal f.
real f.
vir·tu·al f.

Fogarty
cath·e·ter
clamp

fog·ging
ret·i·nos·co·py

fo·go sel·va·gem

foil

Foix-Alajouanine
my·e·li·tis

Foix's
syn·drome

fo·la·cin

fo·late

fold
ad·i·pose f.'s of the pleu·ra
alar f.'s
am·ni·ot·ic f.
ar·y·ep·i·glot·tic f.
ar·y·te·no·ep·i·glot·tid·e·an f.
ax·il·lary f.
ca·val f.
ce·cal f.'s
f. of chor·da tym·pa·ni
cil·i·ary f.'s
cir·cu·lar f.'s
Dennie's in·fra·or·bit·al f.
Douglas' f.
Duncan's f.'s
du·o·de·no·je·ju·nal f.
du·o·de·no·mes·o·col·ic f.

fold *(continued)*
ep·i·gas·tric f.
fal·ci·form ret·i·nal f.
fim·bri·at·ed f.
gas·tric f.'s
gas·tro·pan·cre·at·ic f.'s
gen·i·tal f.
gi·ant gas·tric f.'s
glos·so·pal·a·tine f.
glu·te·al f.
Guérin's f.
Hasner's f.
head f.
Houston's f.'s
il·e·o·ce·cal f.
in·cu·dal f.
in·fe·ri·or du·o·de·nal f.
in·fra·pa·tel·lar syn·o·vi·al f.
in·gui·nal f.
in·gui·nal ap·o·neu·rot·ic f.
in·ter·u·re·ter·ic f.
f.'s of iris
Kerckring's f.'s
la·bi·o·scro·tal f.'s
lac·ri·mal f.
f. of la·ryn·ge·al nerve
lat·er·al f.'s
lat·er·al glos·so·ep·i·glot·tic f.
lat·er·al na·sal f.
lat·er·al um·bil·i·cal f.
f. of left ve·na ca·va
lon·gi·tu·di·nal f. of du·o·de·num
ma·lar f.
mal·le·ar f.
mam·ma·ry f.
Marshall's ves·tig·i·al f.
me·di·al na·sal f.
me·di·al um·bil·i·cal f.
mes·o·neph·ric f.
mid·dle glos·so·ep·i·glot·tic f.
mid·dle um·bil·i·cal f.
mon·go·li·an f.
Morgan's f.
mu·co·buc·cal f.
mu·co·sal f.'s of gall·blad·der
nail f.
na·so·ju·gal f.
neu·ral f.'s
oper·cu·lar f.
pal·mate f.'s
pal·pe·bro·na·sal f.
par·a·du·o·de·nal f.
per·i·car·di·o·pleur·al f.

pha·ryn·go·ep·i·glot·tic f.
pleu·ro·per·i·to·ne·al f.
pre·splen·ic f.
rec·tal f.'s
rec·to·u·ter·ine f.
rec·to·vag·i·nal f.
rec·to·ves·i·cal f.
ret·i·nal f.
ret·ro·tar·sal f.
Rindfleisch's f.'s
sa·cro·gen·i·tal f.'s
sal·pin·go·pal·a·tine f.
sal·pin·go·pha·ryn·ge·al f.
Schultze's f.
sem·i·lu·nar f.
sem·i·lu·nar f. of co·lon
sem·i·lu·nar con·junc·ti·val f.
spi·ral f. of cys·tic duct
sta·pe·di·al f.
sub·lin·gual f.
su·pe·ri·or du·o·de·nal f.
syn·o·vi·al f.
tail f.
tar·sal f.
trans·verse f.'s of rec·tum
trans·verse ves·i·cal f.
Treves' f.
tri·an·gu·lar f.
Tröltsch's f.
ura·chal f.
ure·ter·ic f.
uro·rec·tal f.
uter·o·ves·i·cal f.
vas·cu·lar f. of the ce·cum
Vater's f.
ven·tric·u·lar f.
ves·tib·u·lar f.
ves·tig·i·al f.
vo·cal f.
fold·ed-lung
syn·drome
fold·ing
frac·ture
Foley
cath·e·ter
op·er·a·tion
Foley Y-plas·ty
py·e·lo·plas·ty
fo·lia
fo·li·a·ceous
fo·li·ar
fo·li·ate
pa·pil·lae
fo·lic ac·id
an·tag·o·nists
con·ju·gate

fo·lie
f. de pour·quoi
f. à deux
f. du doute
f. gé·mel·laire
fo·li·nate
fo·lin·ic ac·id
Folin-Looney
test
Folin's
re·ac·tion
test
fo·li·ose
fo·li·um
fo·lia lin·guae
folk
med·i·cine
fol·li·an
pro·cess
fol·lib·er·in
fol·li·cle
ag·gre·gat·ed lym·phat·ic f.'s
an·ov·u·lar ovar·i·an f.
atret·ic ovar·i·an f.
den·tal f.
gas·tric f.'s
gas·tric lym·phat·ic f.
graaf·i·an f.
grow·ing ovar·i·an f.
hair f.
in·tes·ti·nal f.'s
Lieberkühn's f.'s
lin·gual f.'s
lymph f.
lym·phat·ic f.
lym·phat·ic f.'s of lar·ynx
lym·phat·ic f.'s of rec·tum
ma·ture ovar·i·an f.
Montgomery's f.'s
na·both·i·an f.
ovar·i·an f.
pol·y·ov·u·lar ovar·i·an f.
pri·mary ovar·i·an f.
pri·mor·di·al ovar·i·an f.
se·ba·ceous f.'s
sec·on·dary f.
sol·i·tary f.'s
splen·ic lymph f.'s
f.'s of thy·roid gland
ve·sic·u·lar ovar·i·an f.
fol·li·cle-stim·u·lat·ing
hor·mone
hor·mone-re·leas·ing hor·mone
prin·ci·ple
fol·li·cle-stim·u·lat·ing hor·mone-re·leas·ing
fac·tor
fol·li·clis
fol·lic·u·lar
ab·scess
ad·e·no·ma
an·trum
car·ci·no·mas
con·junc·ti·vi·tis
cyst
cys·ti·tis
gland
goi·ter
hor·mone
im·pe·ti·go
iri·tis
lym·pho·ma
mange
mu·ci·no·sis
pap·ule
phar·yn·gi·tis
stig·ma
syph·i·lid
tra·cho·ma
ure·thri·tis
vul·vi·tis
fol·lic·u·lar ep·i·the·li·al
cell
fol·lic·u·lar ovar·i·an
cells
fol·lic·u·lar pre·dom·i·nant·ly large cell
lym·pho·ma
fol·lic·u·lar pre·dom·i·nant·ly small cleaved cell
lym·pho·ma
fol·lic·u·li
fol·lic·u·lin
f. hy·drate
fol·lic·u·li·tis
f. ab·sce·dens et suf·fo·di·ens
f. bar·bae
f. de·cal·vans
eo·sin·o·phil·ic pus·tu·lar f.
f. ex·ter·na
f. in·ter·na
f. ke·loi·da·lis
f. na·res per·fo·rans
per·fo·rat·ing f.
f. uler·y·the·ma·to·sa re·ti·cu·la·ta
fol·lic·u·lo·ma
fol·lic·u·lo·sis
fol·lic·u·lus
fol·lic·u·li glan·du·lae thy·roi·de·ae

fol·lic·u·lus *(continued)*
  fol·lic·u·li lin·gua·les
  fol·lic·u·li lym·pha·ti·ci la·
    ryn·gei
  fol·lic·u·li lym·pha·ti·ci
    rec·ti
  f. lym·pha·ti·cus
  f. lym·pha·ti·cus gas·tri·cus
Folling's
  dis·ease
Folli's
  pro·cess
fol·li·tro·pin
fol·low·ing
  bou·gie
Foltz'
  val·vule
fo·men·ta·tion
fo·mes
fo·mite
fom·i·tes
fo·na·zine mes·y·late
Fonio's
  so·lu·tion
Fonsecaea
Fontan
  op·er·a·tion
  pro·ce·dure
Fontana-Masson sil·ver
  stain
Fontana's
  ca·nal
  spac·es
  stain
fon·ta·nel
  an·te·ri·or f.
  an·ter·o·lat·er·al f.
  breg·mat·ic f.
  Casser's f.
  cra·ni·al f.'s
  fron·tal f.
  Gerdy's f.
  mas·toid f.
  oc·cip·i·tal f.
  pos·te·ri·or f.
  pos·ter·o·lat·er·al f.
  sag·it·tal f.
  sphe·noi·dal f.
fon·ta·nelle
fon·tic·u·li
fon·tic·u·lus
food
  ball
  fe·ver
  im·pac·tion
  poi·son·ing
foot
  plate

  plug·ger
  pre·sen·ta·tion
  pro·cess
  rot
  yaws
foot
  ath·lete's f.
  but·tress f.
  claw f.
  club f.
  con·tract·ed f.
  drop f.
  fes·cue f.
  flat f.
  fun·gous f.
  f. of hip·po·cam·pus
  Hong Kong f.
  im·mer·sion f.
  Madura f.
  Morand's f.
  mossy f.
  pum·iced f.
  reel f.
  san·dal f.
  spas·tic flat f.
  trench f.
foot-and-mouth
  dis·ease
foot-and-mouth dis·ease
  vi·rus
foot-and-mouth dis·ease vi·rus
  vac·cines
foot·ball
  calf
foot·can·dle
foot-drop
foot·ling
  pre·sen·ta·tion
foot·plate
foot-pound
foot-pound·al
foot-pound-second
  sys·tem
  unit
Foot's re·tic·u·lin im·preg·na·
tion
  stain
for·age
fo·ra·men
  al·ve·o·lar fo·ram·i·na
  an·te·ri·or con·dy·loid f.
  an·te·ri·or pal·a·tine fo·
    ram·i·na
  aor·tic f.
  ap·i·cal den·tal f.
  arach·noid f.
  f. of Arnold
  Bichat's f.

blind f. of fron·tal bone
blind f. of the tongue
Bochdalek's f.
Botallo's f.
f. bur·sae omen·ta·lis ma·
    jo·ris
ca·rot·id f.
ce·cal f. of fron·tal bone
ce·cal f. of the tongue
f. ce·cum me·dul·lae ob·
    lon·ga·tae
f. ce·cum pos·te·ri·us
con·ju·gate f.
cos·to·trans·verse f.
f. di·a·phrag·ma·tis sel·lae
Duverney's f.
em·is·sary sphe·noi·dal f.
ep·i·plo·ic f.
eth·moi·dal f.
ex·ter·nal acous·tic f.
ex·ter·nal au·di·to·ry f.
Ferrein's f.
fron·tal f.
great f.
great·er pal·a·tine f.
Huschke's f.
Hyrtl's f.
in·ci·sive f.
in·ci·sor f.
in·fe·ri·or den·tal f.
in·fra·or·bit·al f.
in·ter·a·tri·al f. pri·mum
in·ter·a·tri·al f. se·cun·dum
in·ter·nal acous·tic f.
in·ter·nal au·di·to·ry f.
in·ter·ven·tric·u·lar f.
in·ter·ver·te·bral f.
jug·u·lar f.
f. of Key-Retzius
lac·er·at·ed f.
f. la·ce·rum an·te·ri·us
f. la·ce·rum me·di·um
f. la·ce·rum pos·te·ri·us
Lannelongue's fo·ram·i·na
f. la·te·ra·lis ven·tric·u·li
    quar·ti
less·er pal·a·tine fo·ram·i·
    na
f. of Luschka
Magendie's f.
ma·lar f.
man·dib·u·lar f.
mas·toid f.
men·tal f.
Monro's f.
Morgagni's f.
na·sal f.
nu·tri·ent f.

ob·tu·ra·tor f.
ol·fac·to·ry f.
op·tic f.
f. op·ti·cum
oval f.
f. ova·le
pap·il·lary fo·ram·i·na of
    kid·ney
pa·ri·e·tal f.
pe·tro·sal f.
pos·te·ri·or con·dy·loid f.
pos·te·ri·or pal·a·tine f.
post·gle·noid f.
pri·mary in·ter·a·tri·al f.
f. qua·dra·tum
Retzius' f.
root f.
round f.
sa·cral f.
Scarpa's fo·ram·i·na
sci·at·ic f.
sec·on·dary in·ter·a·tri·al f.
fo·ram·i·na of the small·est
    veins
sol·i·tary f.
sphe·no·pal·a·tine f.
sphe·not·ic f.
Stensen's f.
sty·lo·mas·toid f.
f. sub·sep·ta·le
su·pra·or·bit·al f.
the·be·si·an fo·ram·i·na
thy·roid f.
f. trans·ver·sa·ri·um
trans·verse f.
f. of trans·verse pro·cess
f. of ve·na ca·va
ver·te·bral f.
ver·te·bro·ar·te·ri·al f.
Vesalius' f.
Vicq d'Azyr's f.
Vieussens' fo·ram·i·na
Weitbrecht's f.
Winslow's f.
zy·go·mat·i·co·fa·cial f.
zy·go·mat·i·co·or·bit·al f.
zy·go·mat·i·co·tem·po·ral f.
fo·ram·i·na
fo·ram·i·nal
    her·ni·a·tion
    node
Fo·ram·i·nif·e·ra
fo·ram·i·nif·er·ous
for·am·i·not·o·my
fo·ra·min·u·la
fo·ra·min·u·lum
Forbes'
    dis·ease

Forbes-Albright
syn·drome
force
an·i·mal f.
chew·ing f.
dy·nam·ic f.
elec·tro·mo·tive f.
G f.
London f.'s
f. of mas·ti·ca·tion
mas·ti·ca·to·ry f.
nerve f.
ner·vous f.
oc·clu·sal f.
psy·chic f.
re·cip·ro·cal f.'s
re·serve f.
van der Waals' f.'s
vi·tal f.
forced
al·i·men·ta·tion
beat
cy·cle
duc·tion
feed·ing
res·pi·ra·tion
forced ex·pi·ra·to·ry
time
vol·ume
forced grasp·ing
re·flex
forced vi·tal
ca·pac·i·ty
for·ceps
de·liv·ery
for·ceps
Adson f.
al·li·ga·tor f.
Allis f.
f. an·te·ri·or
Arruga's f.
ar·te·ri·al f.
ax·is-trac·tion f.
Barton's f.
bone f.
Brown-Adson f.
bull·dog f.
bul·let f.
cap·sule f.
Chamberlen f.
clamp f.
clip f.
cup bi·op·sy f.
cut·ting f.
den·tal f.
dress·ing f.
Evans f.
ex·tract·ing f.

Graefe f.
he·mo·stat·ic f.
jew·el·ler's f.
Kjelland's f.
Lahey f.
Laplace's f.
Levret's f.
li·on-jaw bone-hold·ing f.
Löwenberg's f.
mos·qui·to f.
mouse-tooth f.
nee·dle f.
non·fen·es·trat·ed f.
ob·stet·ri·cal f.
O'Hara f.
Piper's f.
f. pos·te·ri·or
Randall stone f.
rub·ber dam clamp f.
Simpson's f.
spec·u·lum f.
Tarnier's f.
te·nac·u·lum f.
thumb f.
tu·bu·lar f.
Tucker-McLean f.
vul·sel·la f.
vul·sel·lum f.
Willett's f.
Forchheimer's
sign
forc·i·ble
feed·ing
for·ci·pate
for·ci·pres·sure
Fordyce's
an·gi·o·ker·a·to·ma
dis·ease
gran·ules
spots
fore·arm
fore·brain
em·i·nence
prom·i·nence
ves·i·cle
fore·con·scious
fore·fin·ger
fore·foot
fore·gut
fore·head
olym·pi·an f.
for·eign
body
pro·tein
se·rum
for·eign body
gran·u·lo·ma

sal·pin·gi·tis
tu·mor·i·gen·e·sis
for·eign body gi·ant
cell
for·eign pro·tein
ther·a·py
fore·kid·ney
Forel's
de·cus·sa·tion
fore·milk
fo·ren·sic
den·tis·try
med·i·cine
odon·tol·o·gy
psy·chi·a·try
psy·chol·o·gy
fore·play
fore·pleas·ure
fore·quar·ter
am·pu·ta·tion
fore·skin
for·est
yaws
fore·stom·ach
fore·wa·ters
for·get·ting
fork
bite f.
face-bow f.
tun·ing f.
form
ac·co·lé f.'s
ap·pli·qué f.'s
arch f.
boat f.
cav·i·ty prep·a·ra·tion f.
chair f.
con·ve·nience f.
ex·ten·sion f.
face f.
half-chair f.
in·vo·lu·tion f.
L f.
oc·clu·sal f.
out·line f.
pos·te·ri·or tooth f.
rep·li·ca·tive f.
re·sis·tance f.
re·ten·tion f.
sick·le f.
skew f.
tooth f.
twist f.
wave f.
wax f.
Formad's
kid·ney

for·mal
op·er·a·tions
form·al·de·hyde
fix·a·tive
For·ma·lin
for·ma·lin
pig·ment
for·ma·lin·ize
for·mam·i·dase
for·mate
for·ma·tio
f. hip·po·cam·pa·lis
for·ma·tion
con·cept f.
per·son·al·i·ty f.
re·ac·tion f.
re·tic·u·lar f.
rou·leaux f.
symp·tom f.
for·ma·ti·o·nes
form·a·tive
cells
form·a·zan
form·board
formed vi·su·al
hal·lu·ci·na·tion
forme fruste
formes frustes
for·mic
for·mic ac·id
for·mic al·de·hyde
for·mi·ca·tion
for·mim·i·no·glu·tam·ic ac·id
for·mo·cre·sol
for·mol
ti·tra·tion
for·mol-cal·ci·um
fix·a·tive
for·mol-Müller
fix·a·tive
for·mol-sa·line
fix·a·tive
for·mol-Zenker
fix·a·tive
for·mo·sul·fa·thi·a·zole
for·mu·la
Arneth f.
Bazett's f.
Bernhardt's f.
Black's f.
Broca's f.
chem·i·cal f.
Christison's f.
con·sti·tu·tion·al f.
Demoivre's f.
den·tal f.
Dreyer's f.
DuBois' f.

for·mu·la *(continued)*
  elec·tri·cal f.
  em·pir·i·cal f.
  Fischer's pro·jec·tion for·mu·las
  Flesch f.
  Florschütz' f.
  Gorlin f.
  graph·ic f.
  Häser's f.
  Haworth per·spec·tive and con·for·ma·tion·al for·mu·las
  Long's f.
  Mall's f.
  Meeh f.
  Meeh-Dubois f.
  mo·lec·u·lar f.
  of·fi·cial f.
  Pignet's f.
  Poisson-Pearson f.
  Ranke's f.
  ra·tion·al f.
  Reuss' f.
  Runeberg's f.
  spa·tial f.
  ster·e·o·chem·i·cal f.
  struc·tur·al f.
  Trapp-Häser f.
  Trapp's f.
  Van Slyke's f.
  ver·te·bral f.
for·mu·lae
for·mu·lary
  hos·pi·tal f.
for·mu·las
for·myl
  ac·tive f.
for·my·lase
for·myl·ky·nur·e·nine
for·myl·me·thi·o·nine
Forney's
  syn·drome
for·ni·cate
for·ni·ca·tion
for·ni·ces
for·ni·cis
for·nix
  trans·verse f.
  f. uter·i
Forrestier's
  dis·ease
Forssman
  an·ti·body
  an·ti·gen
  re·ac·tion
Forssman an·ti·gen-an·ti·body
  re·ac·tion

Förster's
  uve·i·tis
Fort Bragg
  fe·ver
for·ti·fi·ca·tion
  fig·ures
  spec·trum
for·ti·fied vi·ta·min D
  milk
for·ward
  con·duc·tion
for·ward heart
  fail·ure
fos·car·net
Fosdick-Hansen-Epple
  test
Foshay
  test
fos·sa
  ac·e·tab·u·lar f.
  ad·i·pose fos·sae
  amyg·da·loid f.
  an·co·nal f.
  an·te·ri·or cra·ni·al f.
  f. of ant·he·lix
  ar·tic·u·lar f. of tem·po·ral bone
  ax·il·lary f.
  Bichat's f.
  Biesiadecki's f.
  Broesike's f.
  ca·nine f.
  f. ca·ro·ti·ca
  Claudius' f.
  con·dy·lar f.
  cor·o·noid f.
  cru·ral f.
  Cruveilhier's f.
  cu·bi·tal f.
  di·gas·tric f.
  dig·i·tal f.
  f. duc·tus ve·no·si
  du·o·de·nal fos·sae
  du·o·de·no·je·ju·nal f.
  ep·i·gas·tric f.
  f. ep·i·gas·tri·ca
  fem·o·ral f.
  floc·cu·lar f.
  gall·blad·der f.
  Gerdy's hy·oid f.
  gle·noid f.
  great·er su·pra·cla·vic·u·lar f.
  Gruber-Landzert f.
  f. of he·lix
  hy·a·loid f.
  hy·po·phy·si·al f.
  il·i·ac f.

il·i·a·co·sub·fas·cial f.
f. il·i·a·co·sub·fas·cia·lis
il·i·o·pec·tin·e·al f.
in·ci·sive f.
in·cu·dal f.
f. for in·cus
in·fe·ri·or du·o·de·nal f.
in·fra·cla·vic·u·lar f.
in·fra·du·o·de·nal f.
in·fra·spi·nous f.
in·fra·tem·po·ral f.
in·gui·nal f.
f. in·no·mi·na·ta
in·nom·i·nate f.
in·ter·con·dy·lar f.
in·ter·con·dyl·ic f.
in·ter·con·dy·loid f.
f. in·ter·mes·o·co·li·ca
  trans·ver·sa
in·ter·pe·dun·cu·lar f.
in·tra·bul·bar f.
is·chi·o·rec·tal f.
Jobert de Lamballe's f.
Jonnesco's f.
jug·u·lar f.
f. ju·gu·la·ris
lac·ri·mal f.
f. of lac·ri·mal gland
f. of lac·ri·mal sac
Landzert's f.
lat·er·al f. of brain
lat·er·al ce·re·bral f.
lat·er·al in·gui·nal f.
f. of lat·er·al mal·le·o·lus
len·tic·u·lar f.
less·er su·pra·cla·vic·u·lar f.
lit·tle f. of the co·chle·ar
  win·dow
lit·tle f. of the ves·tib·u·lar
  round win·dow
lit·tle f. of the ves·tib·u·lar
  win·dow
Malgaigne's f.
f. mal·le·o·li fib·u·lae
man·dib·u·lar f.
mas·toid f.
f. mas·toi·dea
me·di·al in·gui·nal f.
Merkel's f.
mes·en·ter·i·co·pa·ri·e·tal f.
mid·dle cra·ni·al f.
Mohrenheim's f.
Morgagni's f.
my·lo·hy·oid f.
f. na·vi·cu·la·ris au·ric·u·
  lae
f. na·vi·cu·la·ris au·ris

f. na·vi·cu·la·ris cru·veil·
  hier
f. na·vi·cu·la·ris ves·tib·u·
  lae va·gi·nae
na·vic·u·lar f. of ure·thra
olec·ra·non f.
oval f.
f. ova·lis
ovar·i·an f.
par·a·du·o·de·nal f.
par·a·je·ju·nal f.
f. pa·ra·je·ju·na·lis
par·a·rec·tal f.
par·a·ves·i·cal f.
pa·tel·lar f. of vit·re·ous
per·i·to·ne·al fos·sas
pe·tro·sal f.
pir·i·form f.
pi·tu·i·tary f.
pop·lit·e·al f.
pos·te·ri·or cra·ni·al f.
f. pro·ve·si·ca·lis
pter·y·goid f.
pter·y·go·max·il·lary f.
pter·y·go·pal·a·tine f.
ra·di·al f.
ret·ro·du·o·de·nal f.
ret·ro·man·dib·u·lar f.
f. ret·ro·man·di·bu·la·ris
ret·ro·mo·lar f.
rhom·boid f.
Rosenmüller's f.
scaph·oid f.
f. scar·pae ma·jor
sig·moid f.
sphe·no·max·il·lary f.
sub·ar·cu·ate f.
sub·ce·cal f.
sub·in·gui·nal f.
sub·lin·gual f.
sub·man·dib·u·lar f.
f. sub·man·di·bu·la·ris
sub·max·il·lary f.
sub·scap·u·lar f.
su·pe·ri·or du·o·de·nal f.
su·pra·mas·toid f.
su·pra·spi·nous f.
su·pra·ton·sil·lar f.
su·pra·ves·i·cal f.
f. of Sylvius
tem·po·ral f.
f. ter·mi·na·lis ure·thrae
ton·sil·lar f.
Treitz's f.
tri·an·gu·lar f.
tro·chan·ter·ic f.
troch·le·ar f.
f. troch·le·ar·is

fos·sa *(continued)*
um·bil·i·cal f.
Velpeau's f.
f. ve·nae ca·vae
f. ve·nae um·bi·li·ca·lis
f. ve·no·sa
ver·mi·an f.
ves·tib·u·lar f.
f. of ves·ti·bule of va·gi·na
Waldeyer's fos·sae
zy·go·mat·ic f.
fos·sae
fos·sette
fos·su·la
f. ro·tun·da
ton·sil·lar fos·su·lae
fos·su·lae
fos·su·late
Foster
frame
Foster Kennedy's
syn·drome
Fothergill's
dis·ease
neu·ral·gia
op·er·a·tion
sign
Fouchet's
re·a·gent
stain
fou·droy·ant
fou·lage
foun·da·tion
den·ture f.
found·er
ef·fect
prin·ci·ple
foun·tain
de·cus·sa·tion
sy·ringe
four·chette
Fournier's
dis·ease
gan·grene
four-tailed
ban·dage
fourth
dis·ease
fin·ger
ven·tri·cle
fourth cra·ni·al
nerve
fourth heart
sound
fourth lum·bar
nerve
fourth par·al·lel pel·vic
plane

fourth tur·bi·nat·ed
bone
fo·vea
f. an·te·ri·or
f. ar·ti·cu·la·ris in·fe·ri·or
at·lan·tis
f. ar·ti·cu·la·ris su·pe·ri·or
at·lan·tis
f. car·di·a·ca
f. coc·cy·gis
f. el·lip·ti·ca
f. eth·moi·da·lis
f. fe·mo·ra·lis
f. hem·i·el·lip·ti·ca
f. hem·i·sphe·ri·ca
f. in·gui·na·lis in·ter·na
Morgagni's f.
f. sphe·ri·ca
f. sub·max·il·la·ris
f. su·pra·ves·i·ca·lis
fo·ve·ae
fo·ve·ate
fo·ve·at·ed
chest
fo·ve·a·tion
fo·ve·o·la
coc·cyg·eal f.
f. o·cu·la·ris
f. pa·pil·la·ris
fo·ve·o·lae
fo·ve·o·lar
cells of stom·ach
fo·ve·o·late
Foville's
fas·cic·u·lus
syn·drome
fowl
chol·era
diph·the·ria
eryth·ro·blas·to·sis
leu·ko·sis
lym·pho·ma·to·sis
my·e·lo·blas·to·sis
pa·ral·y·sis
pest
plague
ty·phoid
Fowler's
po·si·tion
fowl eryth·ro·blas·to·sis
vi·rus
fowl lym·pho·ma·to·sis
vi·rus
fowl my·e·lo·blas·to·sis
vi·rus
fowl neu·ro·lym·pho·ma·to·sis
vi·rus

fowl plague
vi·rus
fowl·pox
vi·rus
fox en·ceph·a·li·tis
vi·rus
Fox-Fordyce
dis·ease
fox·glove
FPS
unit
fps
unit
frac·tion
amor·phous f. of ad·re·nal
cor·tex
blood plas·ma f.'s
dried hu·man plas·ma pro·
tein f.
ejec·tion f.
ejec·tion f. (sys·tol·ic)
fil·tra·tion f.
hu·man an·ti·he·mo·
phil·ic f.
hu·man plas·ma pro·tein f.
mole f.
re·com·bi·na·tion f.
re·gur·gi·tant f.
frac·tion·al
dis·til·la·tion
dose
ster·il·i·za·tion
frac·tion·al ep·i·du·ral
an·es·the·sia
frac·tion·al spi·nal
an·es·the·sia
frac·tion·a·tion
frac·ture
ap·o·phys·i·al f.
ar·tic·u·lar f.
avul·sion f.
Barton's f.
ba·sal skull f.
bend·ing f.
Bennett's f.
birth f.
blow-out f.
box·er's f.
cap·il·lary f.
Chance f.
closed f.
closed skull f.
Colles' f.
com·mi·nut·ed f.
com·mi·nut·ed skull f.
com·pli·cat·ed f.
com·pound f.
com·pound skull f.

f. by con·tre·coup
cough f.
cra·ni·o·fa·cial dys·junc·
tion f.
den·tate f.
de·pressed f.
de·pressed skull f.
de Quervain's f.
der·by hat f.
di·a·stat·ic skull f.
di·rect f.
dish·pan f.
dis·lo·ca·tion f.
dou·ble f.
Dupuytren's f.
dys·cra·sic f.
ep·i·phys·i·al f.
ex·pressed skull f.
ex·tra·cap·su·lar f.
fa·tigue f.
fe·tal f.
fis·sured f.
fold·ing f.
Galeazzi's f.
Gosselin's f.
green·stick f.
grow·ing f.
Guérin's f.
gut·ter f.
hair·line f.
hang·man's f.
hor·i·zon·tal f.
im·pact·ed f.
in·com·plete f.
in·di·rect f.
in·tra·ar·tic·u·lar f.
in·tra·cap·su·lar f.
in·tra·per·i·os·te·al f.
in·tra·u·ter·ine f.
Le Fort I f.
Le Fort II f.
Le Fort III f.
lin·e·ar f.
lin·e·ar skull f.
lon·gi·tu·di·nal f.
march f.
Monteggia's f.
mul·ti·ple f.
neu·ro·gen·ic f.
ob·lique f.
oc·cult f.
open f.
open skull f.
par·ry f.
path·o·log·ic f.
per·tro·chan·ter·ic f.
pi·lon f.
ping-pong f.

frac·ture *(continued)*
  pond f.
  Pott's f.
  py·ram·i·dal f.
  seg·men·tal f.
  sen·ti·nel spi·nous pro·cess
   f.
  Shepherd's f.
  sil·ver-fork f.
  sim·ple f.
  sim·ple skull f.
  Skillern's f.
  skull f.
  Smith's f.
  spi·ral f.
  splin·tered f.
  spon·ta·ne·ous f.
  sprain f.
  sta·ble f.
  stel·late f.
  stel·late skull f.
  strain f.
  stress f.
  sub·cap·i·tal f.
  sub·per·i·os·te·al f.
  su·pra·con·dy·lar f.
  tor·sion f.
  to·rus f.
  trans·cer·vi·cal f.
  trans·con·dy·lar f.
  trans·verse f.
  trans·verse fa·cial f.
  tri·mal·le·o·lar f.
  un·sta·ble f.
  un·u·nit·ed f.
  Wagstaffe's f.
frac·ture
  bed
  box
  dis·lo·ca·tion
Fraenkel's
  pneu·mo·coc·cus
Fraenkel-Weichselbaum
  pneu·mo·coc·cus
frag·ile
  site
frag·ile X
  chro·mo·some
  syn·drome
fra·gil·i·tas
  f. cri·ni·um
  f. os·si·um
  f. san·gui·nis
fra·gil·i·ty
  f. of the blood
fra·gil·i·ty
  test

fra·gil·o·cyte
fra·gil·o·cy·to·sis
frag·ment
  but·ter·fly f.
  Fab f.
  Fc f.
  one-car·bon f.
  two-car·bon f.
frag·men·ta·tion
  f. of the my·o·car·di·um
frag·men·ta·tion
  my·o·car·di·tis
frag·ment length
  pol·y·mor·phism
fraise
Fraley
  syn·drome
fram·be·sia
fram·be·si·form
  syph·i·lid
fram·be·si·o·ma
frame
  Bal·kan f.
  Bradford f.
  Deiters' ter·mi·nal f.'s
  Foster f.
  oc·clud·ing f.
  read·ing f.
  Stryker f.
  tri·al f.
  Whitman's f.
frame-shift
  mu·ta·gen
  mu·ta·tion
frame·work
Franceschetti-Jadassohn
  syn·drome
Franceschetti's
  syn·drome
Francisella
  F. no·vi·ci·da
  F. tu·la·ren·sis
fran·ci·um
Francke's
  nee·dle
fran·gu·la
fran·gu·lic ac·id
fran·gu·lin
frank
frank breech
  pre·sen·ta·tion
Frankenhäuser's
  gan·gli·on
Frankfort
  plane
Frankfort hor·i·zon·tal
  plane

Frankfort-man·dib·u·lar in·ci·sor
   an·gle
frank·in·cense
Franklin
   spec·ta·cles
frank·lin·ic
   taste
Franklin's
   dis·ease
Frank-Starling
   curve
Fräntzel's
   mur·mur
Fraser-Lendrum
   stain for fi·brin
Fraser's
   syn·drome
fra·ter·nal
   twins
Fraunhofer's
   lines
Frazier's
   nee·dle
Frazier-Spiller
   op·er·a·tion
freck·le
   Hutchinson's f.
   iris f.'s
   mel·a·not·ic f.
Fredet-Ramstedt
   op·er·a·tion
free
   as·so·ci·a·tion
   en·er·gy
   field
   flap
   gin·gi·va
   graft
   mac·ro·phage
   mar·gin
   rad·i·cal
   vil·lus
   wa·ter
free bone
   flap
free-float·ing
   anx·i·e·ty
free-hand
   knife
free man·dib·u·lar
   move·ments
Freeman-Sheldon
   syn·drome
free·mar·tin
free nerve
   end·ings

free thy·rox·ine
   in·dex
free wa·ter
   clear·ance
free·way
   space
freeze-dry·ing
freez·ing
   gas·tric f.
freez·ing
   point
Frei
   test
Freiberg's
   dis·ease
Frei-Hoffman
   re·ac·tion
Frejka pil·low
   splint
frem·i·tus
   bron·chi·al f.
   hy·da·tid f.
   per·i·car·di·al f.
   pleu·ral f.
   rhon·chal f.
   sub·jec·tive f.
   tac·tile f.
   tus·sive f.
   vo·cal f.
fre·na
fre·nal
French
   chalk
   flap
   po·lio
   scale
French proof
   agar
fre·nec·to·my
Frenkel's
   symp·tom
Frenkel's an·te·ri·or oc·u·lar
   trau·mat·ic
   syn·drome
fre·no·plas·ty
fre·not·o·my
fren·u·la
fren·u·lum
   f. ce·re·bel·li
   f. of clit·o·ris
   f. ep·i·glot·ti·dis
   f. of Giacomini
   f. of il·e·o·ce·cal valve
   f. la·bi·o·rum mi·no·rum
   f. of low·er lip
   f. of M'Dowel
   f. of Morgagni
   f. of pre·puce

fren·u·lum *(continued)*
    f. pre·pu·tii cli·to·ri·dis
    f. of pu·den·dal lips
    f. pu·den·di
    f. of su·pe·ri·or med·ul·lary
      ve·lum
    syn·o·vi·al fren·u·la
    f. of tongue
    f. of up·per lip
fre·num
    Morgagni's f.
    syn·o·vi·al fre·na
fren·zy
fre·quen·cy
    crit·i·cal flick·er fu·sion f.
    dom·i·nant f.
    fun·da·men·tal f.
    gene f.
    f. of mic·tu·ri·tion
    res·pi·ra·to·ry f.
fre·quen·cy
    curve
    dis·tri·bu·tion
Frerich's
    the·o·ry
fresh·en·ing
fresh fro·zen
    plas·ma
Fresnel
    lens
    prism
fress·re·flex
fre·ta
fret·ting
fre·tum
freud·i·an
    fix·a·tion
    psy·cho·a·nal·y·sis
freud·i·an slip
Freud's
    the·o·ry
Freund's
    anom·a·ly
    op·er·a·tion
Freund's com·plete
    ad·ju·vant
Freund's in·com·plete
    ad·ju·vant
Frey's
    syn·drome
Frey's ir·ri·ta·tion
    hairs
fri·a·ble
fric·a·tive
fric·tion
    dy·nam·ic f.
    start·ing f.
    stat·ic f.

fric·tion
    rub
    sound
fric·tion·al
    at·tach·ment
Fridenberg's stig·o·met·ric card
    test
Friderichsen-Waterhouse
    syn·drome
Friedländer's
    ba·cil·lus
    pneu·mo·nia
    stain for cap·sules
Friedman
    curve
Friedmann's
    dis·ease
Friedreich's
    atax·ia
    dis·ease
    phe·nom·e·non
    sign
Friend
    dis·ease
    vi·rus
Friend leu·ke·mia
    vi·rus
fright
    re·ac·tion
frig·id
fri·gid·i·ty
frig·o·rif·ic
frig·o·rism
fringe
    cer·vi·cal f.
    cos·tal f.
    Richard's f.'s
    syn·o·vi·al f.
frit
Froehde's
    re·a·gent
frog
    face
Fröhlich's
    dwarf·ism
    syn·drome
Frohn's
    re·a·gent
Froin's
    syn·drome
frôle·ment
Froment's
    sign
frons
front·ad
fron·tal
    an·gle of pa·ri·e·tal
    ar·ea

ar·tery
ax·is
bel·ly
bone
cor·tex
crest
em·i·nence
fon·ta·nel
fo·ra·men
grooves
gy·rec·to·my
horn
lobe
mar·gin
nerve
notch
plane
plate
pole
pro·cess
re·gion of head
si·nus
si·nus·i·tis
su·ture
tri·an·gle
tu·ber
veins
fron·ta·lis
fron·tal si·nus
ap·er·ture
fron·tis
fron·to·an·te·ri·or
po·si·tion
fron·to·eth·moi·dal
su·ture
fron·to·lac·ri·mal
su·ture
fron·to·ma·lar
fron·to·max·il·lary
su·ture
fron·to·na·sal
duct
el·e·va·tion
pro·cess
su·ture
fron·to·oc·cip·i·tal
fas·cic·u·lus
fron·to·or·bit·al
ar·ea
fron·to·pa·ri·e·tal
fron·to·pon·tine
tract
fron·to·pos·te·ri·or
po·si·tion
fron·to·sphe·noi·dal
pro·cess
fron·to·tem·po·ral
tract

fron·to·tem·po·ra·le
fron·to·trans·verse
po·si·tion
fron·to·zy·go·mat·ic
su·ture
front-tap
con·trac·tion
re·flex
Froriep's
gan·gli·on
in·du·ra·tion
Frost
su·ture
frost
itch
frost·bite
frost·ed
heart
liv·er
Frost-Lang
op·er·a·tion
frot·tage
frot·teur
fro·zen
pel·vis
sec·tion
shoul·der
fruc·to·fu·ra·nose
fruc·to·ki·nase
fruc·to·san
fruc·tose
fruc·tose-bis·phos·pha·tase
fruc·tose-bis·phos·phate al·dol·ase
fruc·tose-di·phos·phate al·dol·ase
fruc·to·se·mia
fruc·to·side
fruc·to·su·ria
es·sen·tial f.
fruit
sug·ar
fru·se·mide
frus·tra·tion
tol·er·ance
frus·tra·tion-ag·gres·sion
hy·poth·e·sis
FTA-ABS
test
Fuchs'
ad·e·no·ma
col·o·bo·ma
spur
sto·mas
syn·drome
uve·i·tis
Fuchs' black
spot

Fuchs' ep·i·the·li·al
  dys·tro·phy
fuch·sin
  agar
  bod·ies
fuch·sin
  ac·id f.
  al·de·hyde f.
  an·i·line f.
  ba·sic f.
  car·bol f.
  di·a·mond f.
fuch·sin·o·phil
  cell
  gran·ule
  re·ac·tion
fuch·sin·o·phil·ia
fuch·sin·o·phil·ic
fu·cose
fu·co·si·do·sis
Fuerstner's
  dis·ease
fu·gac·i·ty
fu·gi·tive
  swell·ing
  wart
fu·gu
  poi·son
fugue
fu·gu·tox·in
ful·cra
ful·crum
  line
ful·crums
ful·gu·rant
ful·gu·rat·ing
  mi·graine
ful·gu·ra·tion
full
  den·ture
full breech
  pre·sen·ta·tion
ful·ler's
  earth
full liq·uid
  di·et
full-thick·ness
  burn
  flap
  graft
ful·mi·nant
  hy·per·py·rex·ia
ful·mi·nat·ing
  dys·en·tery
  small·pox
fu·ma·rase
fu·ma·rate hy·dra·tase
fu·ma·rate re·duc·tase

fu·mar·ic ac·id
fu·mar·ic am·i·nase
fu·mar·ic hy·dro·gen·ase
fu·mi·gant
fu·mi·gate
fu·mi·ga·tion
fum·ing
  ni·tric ac·id
  sul·fu·ric ac·id
func·tio la·e·sa
func·tion
  al·lom·er·ic f.
  arous·al f.
  atri·al trans·port f.
  dis·crim·i·nant f.
  iso·mer·ic f.
  mod·u·la·tion trans·fer f.
func·tion·al
  al·bu·min·ur·ia
  am·bly·o·pia
  anat·o·my
  apha·sia
  ap·o·plexy
  au·ton·o·my
  blind·ness
  cas·tra·tion
  con·ges·tion
  con·trac·ture
  deaf·ness
  dis·ease
  dis·or·der
  dys·men·or·rhea
  dys·pep·sia
  group
  hy·per·tro·phy
  ill·ness
  mur·mur
  neu·ro·sur·gery
  oc·clu·sion
  pa·thol·o·gy
  spasm
  sphinc·ter
  splint
  stric·ture
func·tion·al aer·o·bic
  im·pair·ment
func·tion·al chew-in
  rec·ord
func·tion·al·ism
func·tion·al jaw
  or·tho·pe·dics
func·tion·al man·dib·u·lar
  move·ments
func·tion·al oc·clu·sal
  har·mo·ny
func·tion·al or·tho·don·tic
  ther·a·py

func·tion·al pre·pu·ber·tal cas·
  tra·tion
  syn·drome
func·tion·al re·frac·to·ry
  pe·ri·od
func·tion·al re·sid·u·al
  air
  ca·pac·i·ty
func·tion·al ter·mi·nal in·ner·
  va·tion
  ra·ti·o
func·tion·al vo·cal
  fa·tigue
func·tion cor·rec·tor
fun·da·ment
fun·da·men·tal
  fre·quen·cy
  tone
fun·dec·to·my
fun·di
fun·dic
fun·di·form
  lig·a·ment of foot
  lig·a·ment of pe·nis
fun·do·pli·ca·tion
Fun·du·lus
fun·dus
  f. al·bi·punc·ta·tus
  f. di·a·be·ti·cus
  f. fla·vi·mac·u·la·tus
  f. of gall·blad·der
  f. of in·ter·nal acous·tic
    me·a·tus
  f. of in·ter·nal au·di·to·ry
    me·a·tus
  leop·ard f.
  f. oc·u·li
  pep·per and salt f.
  f. po·ly·cy·the·mi·cus
  f. of stom·ach
  tes·sel·lat·ed f.
  f. ti·gré
  ti·groid f.
  f. tym·pa·ni
  f. of uri·nary blad·der
  f. of uter·us
fun·dus
  glands
  re·flex
fun·du·scope
fun·dus·co·py
fun·du·sec·to·my
fun·gal
fun·gate
fun·gat·ing
  sore
fun·ge·mia
Fun·gi

fun·gi
fun·gi·ci·dal
fun·gi·cide
fun·gi·ci·din
fun·gi·form
  pa·pil·lae
Fun·gi Im·per·fec·ti
fun·gil·li·form
fun·gi·stat·ic
fun·gi·tox·ic
fun·gi·tox·ic·i·ty
fun·goid
fun·gos·i·ty
fun·gous
  foot
fun·gus
  ball
fun·gus
  f. ce·re·bri
  fis·sion fun·gi
  im·per·fect f.
  mo·sa·ic f.
  per·fect f.
  ray f.
  slime f.
  thrush f.
  um·bil·i·cal f.
  yeast f.
fu·nic
  souf·fle
fu·ni·cle
fu·nic·u·lar
  graft
  hy·dro·cele
  my·e·li·tis
  my·e·lo·sis
  pro·cess
  souf·fle
fu·nic·u·li
fu·nic·u·li·tis
  en·dem·ic f.
  fi·lar·i·al f.
fu·nic·u·lo·pexy
fu·nic·u·lus
  f. am·nii
  an·te·ri·or f.
  cu·ne·ate f.
  dor·sal f.
  f. dor·sa·lis
  f. grac·i·lis
  lat·er·al f. of spi·nal cord
  pos·te·ri·or f.
  f. se·pa·rans
  f. so·li·ta·ri·us
  f. te·res
fu·ni·form
fu·nis

fun·nel
  Buchner f.
  Martegiani's f.
  pi·al f.
fun·nel
  breast
  chest
fun·nel-shaped
  pel·vis
fu·ral·ta·done
fu·ran
fu·ra·nose
fu·ra·zol·i·done
fur·cal
  nerve
fur·ca·tion
fur·cu·la
fur·fur
fur·fu·ra·ceous
fur·fu·ral
fur·fu·res
fur·fu·rol
  re·ac·tion
fur·fu·ryl
  f. al·co·hol
fu·ri·ous
  ra·bies
fur·nace
  den·tal f.
  muf·fle f.
fur·nace·men's
  cat·a·ract
fu·ror ep·i·lep·ti·cus
fu·ro·se·mide
furred
  tongue
fur·row
  dig·i·tal f.
  gen·i·tal f.
  glu·te·al f.
  men·to·la·bi·al f.
  prim·i·tive f.
fu·run·cle
fu·run·cu·lar
fu·run·cu·li
fu·run·cu·loid
fu·run·cu·lo·sis
  f. or·i·en·ta·lis
fu·run·cu·lous
fu·run·cu·lus
Fu·sar·i·um
fused
  kid·ney

sil·ver ni·trate
  teeth
fu·sel oil
fu·si·ble
  cal·cu·lus
  met·al
fu·si·date so·di·um
fu·sid·ic ac·id
fu·si·form
  an·eu·rysm
  cat·a·ract
  cells of ce·re·bral cor·tex
  gy·rus
  lay·er
  mus·cle
Fu·si·for·mis
fu·si·mo·tor
fus·ing
  point
fu·sion
  ar·ea
  beat
  en·er·gy
  tem·per·a·ture
fu·sion
  cell f.
  cen·tric f.
  flick·er f.
  nu·cle·ar f.
  spi·nal f.
  spine f.
  ver·te·bral f.
fu·sion·al
  move·ment
fu·sion-in·ferred thresh·old
  test
Fu·so·bac·te·ri·um
  F. fu·si·for·me
  F. mor·ti·fer·um
  F. nec·ro·pho·rum
  F. nu·cle·a·tum
  F. plau·ti
fu·so·cel·lu·lar
fu·so·spi·ro·chet·al
  dis·ease
  gin·gi·vi·tis
fus·tic
fus·ti·ga·tion
Futcher's
  line
Fy
  an·ti·gens
Fy blood group

G
an·ti·gen
cells
fac·tor
force
syn·drome
unit of strep·to·my·cin
G-
ac·tin
band·ing
Ga·boon
ul·cer
G ac·id
Gaddum and Schild
test
gad·fly
gad·o·le·ic ac·id
gad·o·lin·i·um
Gaenslen's
sign
Gaffky
scale
ta·ble
gag
re·flex
gag
Davis-Crowe mouth g.
gage
gain
pri·mary g.
sec·on·dary g.
time com·pen·sa·tion g.
time-var·ied g.
Gairdner's
dis·ease
Gaisböck's
syn·drome
gait
ant·al·gic g.
atax·ic g.
cal·ca·ne·al g.
cer·e·bel·lar g.
Charcot's g.
equine g.
fes·ti·nat·ing g.
glu·te·us max·i·mus g.
glu·te·us me·di·us g.
hel·i·co·pod g.
hem·i·ple·gic g.

high step·page g.
scis·sor g.
spas·tic g.
step·page g.
GAL
vi·rus
ga·lac·ta·cra·sia
ga·lac·ta·gogue
fac·tor
ga·lac·tans
ga·lac·tic
ga·lac·ti·dro·sis
ga·lac·to·blast
ga·lac·to·bol·ic
ga·lac·to·cele
ga·lac·to·gen
ga·lac·to·ki·nase
de·fi·cien·cy
ga·lac·to·lip·id
ga·lac·to·lip·in
ga·lac·tom·e·ter
gal·ac·toph·a·gous
ga·lac·to·phore
ga·lac·to·pho·ri·tis
gal·ac·toph·o·rous
ca·nals
ducts
ga·lac·to·poi·e·sis
ga·lac·to·poi·et·ic
fac·tor
hor·mone
ga·lac·to·pyr·a·nose
ga·lac·tor·rhea
ga·lac·tos·a·mine
ga·lac·tos·am·i·no·gly·can
ga·lac·to·sans
ga·lac·to·scope
ga·lac·tose
cat·a·ract
di·a·be·tes
ga·lac·to·se·mia
ga·lac·tose tol·er·ance
test
ga·lac·to·side
ga·lac·to·sis
ga·lac·tos·u·ria
ga·lac·to·syl
ga·lac·to·ther·a·py
ga·lac·to·wal·den·ase

ga·lac·to·zy·mase
ga·lac·tur·o·nan
ga·lac·tu·ron·ic ac·id
ga·lac·tur·o·nose
ga·lan·ga
ga·lan·gal
Galant's
  re·flex
Galassi's pu·pil·lary
  phe·nom·e·non
ga·lea
Galeati's
  glands
ga·le·at·o·my
Galeazzi's
  frac·ture
ga·le·na
ga·len·i·cals
Galen's
  anas·to·mo·sis
  nerve
gall
  blad·der
  duct
gal·la
gal·la·mine tri·eth·i·o·dide
Gallavardin's
  phe·nom·e·non
gall·blad·der
  fos·sa
gall·blad·der
  sand·pa·per g.
  straw·ber·ry g.
Gallego's dif·fer·en·ti·at·ing
  so·lu·tion
gal·le·in
gal·lic ac·id
Gallie's
  trans·plant
Gal·li·for·mes
gal·li·na·ceous
gal·li·um
gal·lo·cy·a·nin
gal·lo·cy·a·nine
gal·lon
gal·lop
  rhythm
  sound
gal·lop
  atri·al g.
  pre·sys·tol·ic g.
  pro·to·di·a·stol·ic g.
  sum·ma·tion g.
  sys·tol·ic g.
Gall's
  cra·ni·ol·o·gy

gall·stone
  col·ic
  il·e·us
gall·stone
  opac·i·fy·ing g.'s
  si·lent g.'s
Gal·lus
gal·lus ad·e·no-like
  vi·rus
ga·lo·che
  chin
gal·to·ni·an
  ge·net·ics
  in·her·i·tance
Galton's
  del·ta
  law
  whis·tle
Galton's sys·tem of clas·si·fi·
  ca·tion of
  fin·ger·prints
gal·van·ic
  cau·tery
  cur·rent
  nys·tag·mus
  thresh·old
  ver·ti·go
gal·van·ic skin
  re·ac·tion
  re·flex
  re·sponse
gal·va·nism
gal·va·ni·za·tion
gal·va·no·caus·tic
  snare
gal·va·no·cau·tery
gal·va·no·con·trac·til·i·ty
gal·va·no·far·a·di·za·tion
gal·va·nom·e·ter
  d'Ar·son·val g.
gal·va·no·mus·cu·lar
gal·va·no·pal·pa·tion
gal·va·no·scope
gal·va·no·sur·gery
gal·va·no·tax·is
gal·va·no·ther·a·py
gal·va·not·o·nus
gal·va·not·ro·pism
gam·a·bu·fa·gin
gam·a·bu·fo·gen·in
gam·a·bu·fo·tal·in
Gam·bi·an
  fe·ver
  try·pan·o·so·mi·a·sis
gam·bir
game
  lan·guage g.
  mod·el g.

game·keep·er's
  thumb
gam·e·tan·gi·um
ga·mete
  joint g.
ga·met·ic
  nu·cle·us
ga·me·to·cide
ga·me·to·cyst
ga·me·to·cyte
ga·me·to·gen·e·sis
ga·me·to·go·nia
gam·e·tog·o·ny
gam·e·toid
  the·o·ry
ga·me·to·ki·net·ic
  hor·mone
gam·e·to·pha·gia
Gam·gee
  tis·sue
gam·ic
gam·ma
  al·co·hol·ism
  an·gle
  cam·era
  cell of pan·cre·as
  crys·tal·lin
  ef·fer·ent
  en·ceph·a·log·ra·phy
  fi·bers
  loop
  rays
gam·ma-ben·zene hex·a·chlo·ride
gam·ma·cism
gam·ma·gram
gam·ma mo·tor
  neu·rons
  sys·tem
gam·mop·a·thy
  bi·clo·nal g.
  mon·o·clo·nal g.
Gamna-Favre
  bod·ies
Gamna-Gandy
  bod·ies
  nod·ules
Gamna's
  dis·ease
gam·o·gen·e·sis
gam·og·o·ny
gam·ont
gam·o·pha·gia
gam·o·pho·bia
gan·ci·clo·vir
Gandy-Gamna
  bod·ies

Gandy-Nanta
  dis·ease
gan·ga
gan·glia
gan·gli·al
gan·gli·ate
gan·gli·at·ed
  cord
  nerve
gan·gli·ec·to·my
gan·gli·form
gan·gli·i·tis
gan·gli·o·blast
gan·gli·o·cyte
gan·gli·o·cy·to·ma
gan·gli·o·form
gan·gli·o·gli·o·ma
gan·gli·ol·y·sis
  per·cu·ta·ne·ous ra·di·o·fre·quen·cy g.
gan·gli·o·ma
gan·gli·on
  ab·er·rant g.
  acous·ti·co·fa·cial g.
  Acrel's g.
  Andersch's g.
  aor·ti·co·re·nal gan·glia
  Arnold's g.
  au·di·to·ry g.
  Auerbach's gan·glia
  au·ric·u·lar g.
  au·to·nom·ic gan·glia
  gan·glia of au·to·nom·ic plex·us·es
  ba·sal gan·glia
  Bezold's g.
  Bochdalek's g.
  Bock's g.
  Böttcher's g.
  car·di·ac gan·glia
  ca·rot·id g.
  ce·li·ac gan·glia
  g. cer·vi·ca·le in·fe·ri·us
  cer·vi·co·tho·rac·ic g.
  cil·i·ary g.
  coc·cyg·eal g.
  Corti's g.
  dif·fuse g.
  dor·sal root g.
  Ehrenritter's g.
  g. ex·tra·cra·ni·a·le
  g. of fa·cial nerve
  Frankenhäuser's g.
  Froriep's g.
  gas·ser·i·an g.
  ge·nic·u·late g.
  Gudden's g.
  g. ha·ben·u·lae

gan·gli·on *(continued)*
 hy·po·gas·tric gan·glia
 in·fe·ri·or cer·vi·cal g.
 in·fe·ri·or g. of glos·so·
   pha·ryn·ge·al nerve
 in·fe·ri·or mes·en·ter·ic g.
 in·fe·ri·or g. of va·gus
 in·ter·cru·ral g.
 in·ter·me·di·ate gan·glia
 g. of in·ter·me·di·ate nerve
 in·ter·pe·dun·cu·lar g.
 in·ter·ver·te·bral g.
 in·tra·cra·ni·al g.
 g. isth·mi
 jug·u·lar g.
 Laumonier's g.
 Lee's g.
 len·tic·u·lar g.
 Lobstein's g.
 Ludwig's g.
 lum·bar gan·glia
 Meckel's g.
 mid·dle cer·vi·cal g.
 na·sal g.
 nerve g.
 neu·ral g.
 no·dose g.
 otic g.
 par·a·sym·pa·thet·ic gan·glia
 par·a·ver·te·bral gan·glia
 pel·vic gan·glia
 per·i·os·te·al g.
 pe·tro·sal g.
 pet·rous g.
 phren·ic gan·glia
 pre·ver·te·bral gan·glia
 pter·y·go·pal·a·tine g.
 Remak's gan·glia
 re·nal gan·glia
 Ribes' g.
 sa·cral gan·glia
 Scarpa's g.
 Schacher's g.
 sem·i·lu·nar g.
 sen·so·ry g.
 Soemmering's g.
 so·lar gan·glia
 sphe·no·pal·a·tine g.
 spi·nal g.
 spi·ral g. of co·chlea
 splanch·nic g.
 stel·late g.
 sub·lin·gual g.
 g. sub·lin·gua·le
 sub·man·dib·u·lar g.
 sub·max·il·lary g.
 su·pe·ri·or cer·vi·cal g.
 su·pe·ri·or g. of glos·so·
   pha·ryn·ge·al nerve
 su·pe·ri·or mes·en·ter·ic g.
 su·pe·ri·or g. of the va·gus
   nerve
 sym·pa·thet·ic gan·glia
 gan·glia of sym·pa·thet·ic
   trunk
 ter·mi·nal g.
 g. ter·mi·na·le
 tho·rac·ic gan·glia
 tri·gem·i·nal g.
 Troisier's g.
 g. of trunk of va·gus
 tym·pan·ic g.
 Valentin's g.
 ver·te·bral g.
 ves·tib·u·lar g.
 Vieussens' g.
 Walther's g.
 Wrisberg's gan·glia
gan·gli·on
 cell
 cells of dor·sal spi·nal root
 cells of ret·i·na
 ridge
gan·gli·on·at·ed
gan·gli·on·ec·to·my
gan·glio·neu·ro·ma
 cen·tral g.
 dumb·bell g.
gan·glio·neu·ro·ma·to·sis
gan·gli·on·ic
 block·ade
 crest
 lay·er of cer·e·bel·lar cor·
   tex
 lay·er of ce·re·bral cor·tex
 lay·er of op·tic nerve
 lay·er of ret·i·na
 sa·li·va
gan·gli·on·ic block·ing
 agent
gan·gli·on·ic mo·tor
 neu·ron
gan·gli·on·i·tis
gan·gli·o·nos·to·my
gan·gli·ons
gan·gli·o·ple·gic
gan·gli·o·side
 lip·i·do·sis
gan·gli·o·si·do·sis
 gen·er·al·ized g.
gan·go·sa
gan·grene
 ar·te·ri·o·scle·rot·ic g.
 cold g.
 cu·ta·ne·ous g.

de·cu·bi·tal g.
di·a·bet·ic g.
dis·sem·i·nat·ed cu·ta·ne·
ous g.
dry g.
em·bol·ic g.
em·phy·sem·a·tous g.
Fournier's g.
gas g.
hem·or·rhag·ic g.
hos·pi·tal g.
hot g.
Meleney's g.
moist g.
nos·o·co·mi·al g.
Pott's g.
pre·se·nile spon·ta·ne·ous g.
pres·sure g.
pro·gress·ive bac·te·ri·al
syn·er·gis·tic g.
se·nile g.
spon·ta·ne·ous g. of new·
born
stat·ic g.
sym·met·ri·cal g.
throm·bot·ic g.
tro·phic g.
ve·nous g.
wet g.
white g.
gan·gre·nous
ap·pen·di·ci·tis
em·phy·se·ma
phar·yn·gi·tis
pneu·mo·nia
rhi·ni·tis
sto·ma·ti·tis
Ganser's
com·mis·sures
syn·drome
gan·try
Gant's
clamp
Gantzer's
mus·cle
Gantzer's ac·ces·so·ry
bun·dle
Ganz·feld
stim·u·la·tion
gap
ar·thro·plas·ty
junc·tion
phe·nom·e·non
gap
air-bone g.
an·i·on g.
aus·cul·ta·to·ry g.
Bochdalek's g.

chro·mo·som·al g.
DNA g.
in·ter·oc·clu·sal g.
si·lent g.
gapes
gape·worm
ga·ra·pa·ta
dis·ease
Gard·ner-Di·a·mond
syn·drome
Gardner's
syn·drome
gar·gan·tuan
mas·ti·tis
gar·gle
gar·goyl·ism
Gariel's
pes·sa·ry
Garland's
tri·an·gle
gar·lic
g. oil
Garré's
dis·ease
Gartner's
ca·nal
cyst
duct
Gärtner's
ba·cil·lus
meth·od
to·nom·e·ter
Gärtner's vein
phe·nom·e·non
gas
ab·scess
ba·cil·lus
cau·tery
chro·ma·tog·ra·phy
cyst
em·bo·lism
gan·grene
per·i·to·ni·tis
phleg·mon
ther·mom·e·ter
gas
al·ve·o·lar g.
an·es·thet·ic g.
blood g.'s
car·bon·ic ac·id g.
ex·pired g.
he·mo·lyt·ic g.
ide·al al·ve·o·lar g.
in·ert g.'s
in·spired g.
laugh·ing g.
marsh g.
mixed ex·pired g.

gas *(continued)*
  mus·tard g.
  no·ble g.'s
  ole·fi·ant g.
  sew·er g.
  sneez·ing g.
  suf·fo·cat·ing g.
  tear g.
  ves·i·cat·ing g.
  vom·it·ing g.
  wa·ter g.
gas·e·ous
  me·di·as·ti·nog·ra·phy
  pulse
gas gan·grene
  an·ti·tox·in
Gaskell's
  bridge
  clamp
  nerves
gas-liq·uid
  chro·ma·tog·ra·phy
gas·om·e·ter
gas·o·met·ric
gas·om·e·try
gasp·ing
  dis·ease
gas·ser·i·an
  gan·gli·on
gas·sing
gas·ter
Gas·ter·o·phil·i·dae
Gas·ter·oph·i·lus
gas·trad·e·ni·tis
gas·tral
  mes·o·derm
gas·tral·gia
gas·trea
  the·o·ry
gas·trec·ta·sia
gas·trec·ta·sis
gas·trec·to·my
  Pólya g.
gas·tric
  anal·y·sis
  by·pass
  cal·cu·lus
  ca·nal
  col·ic
  cri·sis
  di·as·to·le
  di·ges·tion
  feed·ing
  fis·tu·la
  folds
  fol·li·cles
  freez·ing
  glands

  hem·or·rhage
  im·pres·sion
  in·di·ges·tion
  juice
  mu·cin
  neur·as·the·nia
  pit
  plex·us·es of au·to·nom·ic
   sys·tem
  smear
  sta·pling
  sur·face of spleen
  tet·a·ny
  ul·cer
  veins
  ver·ti·go
  vol·vu·lus
gas·tric al·gid
  ma·lar·ia
gas·tric car·dia
gas·tric in·hib·i·to·ry
  pol·y·pep·tide
gas·tric lym·phat·ic
  fol·li·cle
gas·tric·sin
gas·tri·cus
gas·trin·o·ma
gas·trins
gas·tri·tis
  atroph·ic g.
  ca·tarrh·al g.
  g. cys·ti·ca po·ly·po·sa
  ex·fo·li·a·tive g.
  g. fi·bro·plas·ti·ca
  hy·per·tro·phic g.
  in·ter·sti·tial g.
  phleg·mon·ous g.
  pol·y·pous g.
  pseu·do·mem·bra·nous g.
  scle·rot·ic g.
  trau·mat·ic g.
gas·tro·a·ceph·a·lus
gas·tro·ad·e·ni·tis
gas·tro·al·bum·or·rhea
gas·tro·a·mor·phus
gas·tro·a·nas·to·mo·sis
gas·tro·a·to·nia
gas·tro·blen·nor·rhea
gas·tro·car·di·ac
  syn·drome
gas·tro·cele
gas·tro·chron·or·rhea
gas·troc·ne·mi·us
  mus·cle
gas·tro·co·lic
  fis·tu·la
  lig·a·ment

omen·tum
re·flex
gas·tro·co·li·tis
gas·tro·co·lop·to·sis
gas·tro·co·los·to·my
gas·tro·cu·ta·ne·ous
fis·tu·la
gas·tro·di·al·y·sis
gas·tro·di·a·phrag·mat·ic
lig·a·ment
Gas·tro·dis·coi·des hom·i·nis
Gas·tro·dis·cus hom·i·nis
gas·tro·du·o·de·nal
ar·tery
fis·tu·la
or·i·fice
gas·tro·du·o·de·nal lymph
nodes
gas·tro·du·o·de·ni·tis
gas·tro·du·o·de·nos·co·py
gas·tro·du·o·de·nos·to·my
gas·tro·dyn·ia
gas·tro·en·ter·ic
gas·tro·en·ter·i·tis
acute in·fec·tious non·bac·
te·ri·al g.
en·dem·ic non·bac·te·ri·al
in·fan·tile g.
ep·i·dem·ic non·bac·te·ri·al
g.
in·fan·tile g.
por·cine trans·mis·si·ble g.
trans·mis·si·ble g. of swine
vi·ral g.
gas·tro·en·ter·i·tis
vi·rus type A
vi·rus type B
gas·tro·en·ter·o·a·nas·to·mo·sis
gas·tro·en·ter·o·co·li·tis
gas·tro·en·ter·o·co·los·to·my
gas·tro·en·ter·ol·o·gist
gas·tro·en·ter·ol·o·gy
gas·tro·en·ter·op·a·thy
gas·tro·en·ter·o·plas·ty
gas·tro·en·ter·op·to·sis
gas·tro·en·ter·os·to·my
gas·tro·en·ter·ot·o·my
gas·tro·ep·i·plo·ic
veins
gas·tro·e·soph·a·ge·al
her·nia
re·flux
ves·ti·bule
gas·tro·e·soph·a·gi·tis
gas·tro·e·soph·a·gos·to·my
gas·tro·gas·tros·to·my
gas·tro·ga·vage
gas·tro·gen·ic

gas·trog·e·nous
di·ar·rhea
gas·tro·graph
gas·tro·he·pat·ic
omen·tum
gas·tro·hy·dror·rhea
gas·tro·il·e·ac
re·flex
gas·tro·il·e·i·tis
gas·tro·il·e·os·to·my
gas·tro·in·tes·ti·nal
fis·tu·la
hor·mone
tract
gas·tro·je·ju·nal loop ob·struc·
tion
syn·drome
gas·tro·je·ju·no·co·lic
gas·tro·je·ju·nos·to·my
gas·tro·ki·ne·so·graph
gas·tro·la·vage
gas·tro·li·e·nal
lig·a·ment
gas·tro·lith
gas·tro·li·thi·a·sis
gas·trol·o·gist
gas·trol·o·gy
gas·trol·y·sis
gas·tro·ma·la·cia
gas·tro·meg·a·ly
gas·trom·e·lus
gas·tro·myx·or·rhea
gas·tro·ne·ste·os·to·my
gas·trop·a·gus
gas·tro·pan·cre·at·ic
folds
gas·tro·pa·ral·y·sis
gas·tro·par·a·si·tus
gas·tro·pa·re·sis
g. di·a·be·ti·co·rum
gas·tro·path·ic
gas·trop·a·thy
hy·per·tro·phic hy·per·se·
cre·to·ry g.
gas·tro·pex·y
Gas·tro·phil·i·dae
Gas·troph·i·lus
gas·tro·phren·ic
lig·a·ment
gas·tro·plas·ty
Collis g.
ver·ti·cal band·ed g.
gas·tro·pli·ca·tion
gas·tro·pneu·mon·ic
gas·tro·pod
Gas·trop·o·da
gas·trop·to·sia
gas·trop·to·sis

gas·tro·ptyx·is
gas·tro·pul·mo·nary
gas·tro·py·lor·ec·to·my
gas·tro·py·lor·ic
gas·tror·rha·gia
gas·tror·rha·phy
gas·tror·rhea
gas·tror·rhex·is
gas·tros·chi·sis
gas·tro·scope
gas·tro·scop·ic
gas·tros·co·py
gas·tro·spasm
gas·tro·splen·ic
  lig·a·ment
  omen·tum
gas·tro·stax·is
gas·tro·ste·no·sis
gas·tros·to·ga·vage
gas·tros·to·la·vage
gas·tros·to·my
gas·tro·tho·ra·cop·a·gus
gas·tro·tome
gas·trot·o·my
gas·tro·to·nom·e·ter
gas·tro·to·nom·e·try
gas·tro·tox·ic
gas·tro·tox·in
gas·tro·tro·pic
gas·trox·ia
gas·trox·yn·sis
gas·tru·la
gas·tru·la·tion
Gatch
  bed
gate
gate-con·trol
  hy·poth·e·sis
  the·o·ry
gat·ing
  mech·a·nism
Gaucher
  cells
Gaucher's
  dis·ease
gauge
  pres·sure
gauge
  bite g.
  Boley g.
  cath·e·ter g.
  strain g.
  un·der·cut g.
Gaule's
  spots
gaul·the·ria oil
gaul·the·rin

gaunt·let
  ban·dage
Gauss'
  sign
gauss
gaus·si·an
  curve
  dis·tri·bu·tion
gauze
  ban·dage
ga·vage
Gavard's
  mus·cle
Gay-Lussac's
  law
Gay's
  glands
gaze
  nys·tag·mus
gaze
  con·ju·gate g.
  dys·con·ju·gate g.
  ping-pong g.
G-band·ing
  stain
GDPman·nose phos·pho·ryl·ase
Ge
  an·ti·gen
Ge·doel·stia
ge·doel·sti·o·sis
Geigel's
  re·flex
Geiger-Müller
  count·er
  tube
gel
  dif·fu·sion
  elec·tro·pho·re·sis
  fil·tra·tion
  struc·ture
gel
  col·loi·dal g.
  phar·ma·co·pe·ial g.
ge·las·mus
gel·ate
gel·a·tin
  glyc·er·in·at·ed g.
  Irish moss g.
  veg·e·ta·ble g.
  zinc g.
gel·a·tin
  sug·ar
ge·la·ti·nif·er·ous
ge·lat·i·ni·za·tion
ge·lat·i·nize
ge·lat·i·noid
ge·lat·i·nous
  as·ci·tes

in·fil·tra·tion
pol·yp
scle·ri·tis
sub·stance
tis·sue
var·ix
ge·la·tion
ge·la·tum
gel dif·fu·sion
re·ac·tions
gel dif·fu·sion pre·cip·i·tin
tests
tests in one di·men·sion
tests in two di·men·sions
Gélineau's
syn·drome
Gell and Coombs
re·ac·tions
Gellé
test
ge·lo·sis
gel·o·trip·sy
gel·se·mine
Gély's
su·ture
ge·mäs·te·te
cell
Ge·mel·la
gem·el·lip·a·ra
ge·mel·lol·o·gy
ge·mel·lus
gem·fi·bro·zil
gem·i·nate
gem·i·nat·ed
teeth
gem·i·na·tion
gem·i·nous
ge·mis·to·cyte
ge·mis·to·cyt·ic
as·tro·cyte
as·tro·cy·to·ma
cell
re·ac·tion
ge·mis·to·cy·to·ma
gem·ma
gem·ma·tion
gem·mule
Hoboken's g.'s
ge·na
ge·nal
glands
gen·der
iden·ti·ty
role
gene
de·le·tion
fre·quen·cy

mo·sa·i·cism
pool
gene
al·le·lic g.
au·to·so·mal g.
con·dom·i·nant g.
con·trol g.
dom·i·nant g.
H g.
his·to·com·pat·i·bil·i·ty g.
hol·an·dric g.
im·mune re·sponse g.'s
Ir g.'s
jump·ing g.
le·thal g.
mim·ic g.'s
mi·to·chon·dri·al g.
mod·i·fi·er g.
mu·tant g.
op·er·a·tor g.
pen·e·trant g.
plei·o·tro·pic g.
pol·y·phen·ic g.
re·ces·sive g.
reg·u·la·tor g.
re·pres·sor g.
sex-linked g.
split g.
struc·tur·al g.
sup·pres·sor g.
trans·fer g.'s
trans·form·ing g.
X-linked g.
Y-linked g.
ge·ne·al·o·gy
gene dos·age
com·pen·sa·tion
ef·fect
gene li·brary
gene map·ping
gen·era
gen·er·al
anat·o·my
an·es·the·sia
an·es·thet·ic
blood·let·ting
hos·pi·tal
im·mu·ni·ty
per·i·to·ni·tis
phys·i·ol·o·gy
sen·sa·tion
stim·u·lant
trans·duc·tion
tu·ber·cu·lo·sis
gen·er·al ad·ap·ta·tion
re·ac·tion
syn·drome
gen·er·al·ist

gen·er·al·i·za·tion
  stim·u·lus g.
gen·er·al·ized
  an·a·phy·lax·is
  chon·dro·ma·la·cia
  em·phy·se·ma
  gan·gli·o·si·do·sis
  gly·co·ge·no·sis
  len·tig·i·no·sis
  tet·a·nus
  vac·cin·ia
  xan·the·las·ma
gen·er·al·ized anx·i·e·ty
  dis·or·der
gen·er·al·ized cor·ti·cal
  hy·per·os·to·sis
gen·er·al·ized erup·tive
  his·ti·o·cy·to·ma
gen·er·al·ized pus·tu·lar
  pso·ri·a·sis of Zambusch
gen·er·al·ized Shwartzman
  phe·nom·e·non
gen·er·al·ized ton·ic-clo·nic
  ep·i·lep·sy
  sei·zure
gen·er·al so·mat·ic af·fer·ent
  col·umn
gen·er·al so·mat·ic ef·fer·ent
  col·umn
gen·er·al vis·cer·al
  col·umn
gen·er·ate
gen·er·at·ed oc·clu·sal
  path
gen·er·a·tion
  asex·u·al g.
  fil·i·al g.
  non·sex·u·al g.
  pa·ren·tal g.
  sex·u·al g.
  skipped g.
  vir·gin g.
gen·er·a·tive
  em·pa·thy
gen·er·a·tor
  po·ten·tial
gen·er·a·tor
  aer·o·sol g.
  asyn·chro·nous pulse g.
  atri·al syn·chro·nous pulse
    g.
  atri·al trig·gered pulse g.
  de·mand pulse g.
  fixed rate pulse g.
  pulse g.
  ra·di·o·nu·clide g.
  stand·by pulse g.

ven·tric·u·lar in·hib·it·ed
  pulse g.
ven·tric·u·lar syn·chro·nous
  pulse g.
ven·tric·u·lar trig·gered
  pulse g.
ge·ner·ic
ge·ner·ic name
ge·ne·si·al
  cy·cle
ge·ne·si·ol·o·gy
gen·e·sis
gene splic·ing
ge·net·ic
  am·pli·fi·ca·tion
  ane·mia
  as·so·ci·a·tion
  bur·den
  car·ri·er
  code
  col·o·ni·za·tion
  com·pound
  coun·sel·ing
  death
  de·ter·mi·nant
  dis·e·qui·lib·ri·um
  dom·i·nance
  drift
  en·gi·neer·ing
  equi·lib·ri·um
  fe·male
  fit·ness
  fix·a·tion
  het·er·o·ge·ne·i·ty
  ho·me·o·sta·sis
  im·mu·ni·ty
  iso·late
  le·thal
  link·age
  load
  lo·cus
  male
  map
  mark·er
  pol·y·mor·phism
  psy·chol·o·gy
  re·com·bi·na·tion
ge·net·i·cist
ge·net·ics
  be·hav·ior g.
  bi·o·chem·i·cal g.
  clin·i·cal g.
  gal·to·ni·an g.
  hu·man g.
  math·e·mat·i·cal g.
  med·i·cal g.
  men·de·li·an g.
  mi·cro·bi·al g.

mo·lec·u·lar g.
pop·u·la·tion g.
quan·ti·ta·tive g.
so·mat·ic cell g.
sta·tis·ti·cal g.
trans·plan·ta·tion g.
ge·net·o·tro·phic
Ge·ne·va lens mea·sure
Gengou
phe·nom·e·non
ge·ni·al
tu·ber·cle
ge·ni·an
gen·ic
bal·ance
ge·nic·u·la
ge·nic·u·lar
ge·nic·u·late
body
gan·gli·on
neu·ral·gia
otal·gia
ge·nic·u·lat·ed
ge·nic·u·lo·cal·ca·rine
ra·di·a·tion
tract
ge·nic·u·lum
g. of fa·cial ca·nal
g. of fa·cial nerve
ge·ni·o·glos·sal
mus·cle
ge·ni·o·glos·sus
ge·ni·o·hy·oid
mus·cle
ge·ni·o·hy·oi·de·us
ge·ni·on
ge·ni·o·plas·ty
gen·i·tal
cord
cor·pus·cles
duct
em·i·nence
fold
fur·row
gland
her·pes
lig·a·ment
or·gans
phase
pri·ma·cy
ridge
swell·ings
sys·tem
tract
tu·ber·cle
wart

gen·i·ta·lia
am·big·u·ous ex·ter·nal g.
ex·ter·nal g.
gen·i·tal·i·ty
gen·i·tals
gen·i·to·cru·ral
nerve
gen·i·to·fem·o·ral
nerve
gen·i·to·in·gui·nal
lig·a·ment
gen·i·to·u·ri·nary
ap·pa·ra·tus
fis·tu·la
sys·tem
Gennari's
band
stri·a
gen·o·copy
ge·no·der·ma·tol·o·gy
ge·no·der·ma·to·sis
ge·nome
ge·nom·ic
ge·no·spe·cies
ge·note
F g.
F-g.
ge·no·tox·ic
gen·o·type
gen·o·typ·i·cal
gen·ta·mi·cin
gen·ta·my·cin
gen·tian
gen·tian an·i·line
wa·ter
gen·tian·o·phil
gen·tian·o·phile
gen·tian·oph·i·lous
gen·tian·o·pho·bic
gen·tian vi·o·let
gen·ti·o·bi·ase
genu
g. of cor·pus cal·lo·sum
g. of fa·cial nerve
g. of in·ter·nal cap·sule
g. re·cur·va·tum
g. val·gum
g. va·rum
gen·ua
gen·u·al
gen·u·cu·bi·tal
po·si·tion
gen·u·pec·to·ral
po·si·tion
ge·nus
gen·y·an·trum
ge·ode

ge·o·graph·ic
    cho·roi·dop·a·thy
    ker·a·ti·tis
    stip·pling of nails
    tongue
ge·o·med·i·cine
ge·o·met·ric
    isom·er·ism
    mean
ge·o·pa·thol·o·gy
ge·o·pha·gia
ge·oph·a·gism
ge·oph·a·gy
ge·o·phil·ic
Ge·oph·i·lus
ge·o·tax·is
ge·ot·ri·cho·sis
Ge·ot·ri·chum
ge·ot·ro·pism
geph·y·ro·pho·bia
Geraghty's
    test
ger·a·tol·o·gy
ger·bil
Gerdy's
    fi·bers
    fon·ta·nel
    lig·a·ment
    tu·ber·cle
Gerdy's hy·oid
    fos·sa
Gerdy's in·ter·a·tri·al
    loop
Gerhardt's
    dis·ease
    re·ac·tion
    sign
    test for ac·e·to·a·ce·tic ac·id
    test for uro·bi·lin in the urine
Gerhardt-Semon
    law
ger·i·at·ric
    ther·a·py
ger·i·at·rics
    den·tal g.
Gerlach's
    ton·sil
    valve
    val·vu·la
Gerlach's an·nu·lar
    ten·don
Gerlier's
    dis·ease
germ
    cell
    disk

    lay·er
    line
    mem·brane
    nu·cle·us
    the·o·ry
    tube
germ
    den·tal g.
    enam·el g.
    re·serve tooth g.
    tooth g.
Ger·man
    braxy
    mea·sles
ger·ma·ni·um
Ger·man mea·sles
    vi·rus
ger·mi·ci·dal
ger·mi·cide
ger·mi·nal
    apla·sia
    ar·ea
    cell
    cen·ter of Flemming
    cords
    disk
    ep·i·the·li·um
    lo·cal·i·za·tion
    mem·brane
    mo·sa·i·cism
    pole
    rod
    spot
    ves·i·cle
ger·mi·na·tive
    lay·er
    lay·er of nail
ger·mi·no·ma
germ lay·er
    the·o·ry
germ tube
    test
ger·o·der·ma
ger·o·don·tics
ger·o·don·tol·o·gy
ger·o·ma·ras·mus
ger·o·mor·phism
ge·ron·tal
ger·on·tine
ger·on·tol·o·gist
ger·on·tol·o·gy
ge·ron·to·phil·ia
ge·ron·to·pho·bia
ge·ron·to·ther·a·peu·tics
ge·ron·to·ther·a·py
ger·on·tox·on
Ge·ro·ta's
    cap·sule

fas·cia
meth·od
Gerstmann
syn·drome
Gerstmann-Straüssler
syn·drome
ges·ta·gen
ges·ta·gen·ic
ge·stalt
phe·nom·e·non
psy·chol·o·gy
the·o·ry
ther·a·py
ge·stalt·ism
ges·ta·tion
ges·ta·tion·al
age
ede·ma
pro·tein·u·ria
psy·cho·sis
ges·to·ses
ges·to·sis
ges·ture
su·i·cide g.
Gey's
so·lu·tion
ghat·ti
gum
ghee
Gheel
col·o·ny
GHK
equa·tion
Ghon's
fo·cus
tu·ber·cle
Ghon-Sachs
ba·cil·lus
Ghon's pri·mary
le·sion
ghost
cell
cor·pus·cle
tooth
ghost cell
glau·co·ma
ghoul
hand
Giannuzzi's
cells
cres·cents
dem·i·lunes
Gianotti-Crosti
syn·drome
gi·ant
ba·by
cell
chro·mo·some

co·lon
con·dy·lo·ma
dru·sen
fi·bro·ad·e·no·ma
hives
hy·per·tro·phy of gas·tric
mu·co·sa
mel·a·no·some
ur·ti·car·ia
gi·ant ax·o·nal
neu·rop·a·thy
gi·ant cell
aor·ti·tis
ar·te·ri·tis
car·ci·no·ma
car·ci·no·ma of thy·roid
gland
epu·lis
fi·bro·ma
gran·u·lo·ma
hep·a·ti·tis
my·e·lo·ma
my·o·car·di·tis
pneu·mo·nia
sar·co·ma
thy·roid·i·tis
tu·mor of bone
tu·mor of ten·don sheath
gi·ant fol·lic·u·lar
lym·pho·blas·to·ma
gi·ant gas·tric
folds
gi·ant·ism
gi·ant os·te·oid
os·te·o·ma
gi·ant pig·ment·ed
ne·vus
Gi·ar·dia
G. lam·blia
gi·ar·di·a·sis
chin·chil·la g.
gib·bon
gib·bous
Gibbs'
the·o·rem
Gibbs-Donnan
equi·lib·ri·um
Gibbs free
en·er·gy
Gibbs-Helmholtz
equa·tion
gib·bus
Gibney's fix·a·tion
ban·dage
Gibson
mur·mur
Gibson's
ban·dage

Giemsa
stain
Giemsa chro·mo·some band·ing
stain
Gierke's
dis·ease
Gierke's res·pi·ra·to·ry
bun·dle
Gifford's
op·er·a·tion
re·flex
sign
gi·gan·ti·form
ce·men·to·ma
gi·gan·tism
ac·ro·me·gal·ic g.
ce·re·bral g.
eu·nuch·oid g.
pi·tu·i·tary g.
pri·mor·di·al g.
gi·gan·to·cel·lu·lar
gli·o·ma
gi·gan·to·mas·tia
Gi·gan·to·rhyn·chus
gi·gan·to·so·ma
Gigli's
op·er·a·tion
saw
Gi·la mon·ster
gil·bert
Gilbert's
dis·ease
syn·drome
Gilchrist's
dis·ease
my·co·sis
gill
clefts
gill arch
skel·e·ton
Gilles de la Tourette's
dis·ease
syn·drome
Gillette's sus·pen·so·ry
lig·a·ment
Gilliam's
op·er·a·tion
Gillies'
op·er·a·tion
Gillmore
nee·dle
Gilmer
wir·ing
Gil-Vernet
op·er·a·tion
Gimbernat's
lig·a·ment

gin·ger
pa·ral·y·sis
gin·ger
Chi·nese g.
In·di·an g.
g. ole·o·res·in
wild g.
gin·gi·li oil
gin·gi·va
al·ve·o·lar g.
at·tached g.
buc·cal g.
free g.
la·bi·al g.
lin·gual g.
sep·tal g.
gin·gi·vae
gin·gi·val
abra·sion
ab·scess
at·ro·phy
clamp
cleft
con·tour
crest
crev·ice
cur·va·ture
cyst
el·e·phan·ti·a·sis
em·bra·sure
en·large·ment
ep·i·the·li·um
fes·toon
fis·tu·la
flap
flu·id
hy·per·pla·sia
mar·gin
mas·sage
mu·co·sa
pock·et
pro·lif·er·a·tion
re·ces·sion
re·po·si·tion·ing
re·sorp·tion
re·trac·tion
sep·tum
space
sul·cus
tis·sues
trough
zone
Gin·gi·val In·dex
Gin·gi·val-Per·i·o·don·tal In·dex
gin·gi·vec·to·my
gin·gi·vi·tis
acute nec·ro·tiz·ing g.

chron·ic des·qua·ma·tive g.
di·a·bet·ic g.
di·phen·yl·hy·dan·to·in g.
fu·so·spi·ro·chet·al g.
hor·mo·nal g.
hy·per·plas·tic g.
leu·ke·mic hy·per·plas·tic g.
mar·gi·nal g.
nec·ro·tiz·ing ul·cer·a·tive
  g.
pro·lif·er·a·tive g.
sup·pu·ra·tive g.
ul·cer·o·mem·bra·nous g.
gin·gi·vo·ax·i·al
gin·gi·vo·buc·cal
  groove
  sul·cus
gin·gi·vo·den·tal
  lig·a·ment
gin·gi·vo·glos·si·tis
gin·gi·vo·la·bi·al
  groove
  sul·cus
gin·gi·vo·lin·gual
  groove
  sul·cus
gin·gi·vo·lin·guo·ax·i·al
gin·gi·vo-os·se·ous
gin·gi·vo·plas·ty
gin·gi·vo·sis
gin·gi·vo·sto·ma·ti·tis
gin·gly·form
gin·glym·o·ar·thro·di·al
gin·gly·moid
  joint
gin·gly·mus
  hel·i·coid g.
  lat·er·al g.
gin·seng
Giordano-Giovannetti
  di·et
Girard's
  re·a·gent
gir·dle
  an·es·the·sia
  pain
  sen·sa·tion
gir·dle
  Hitzig's g.
  Neptune's g.
  pel·vic g.
  shoul·der g.
  tho·rac·ic g.
Girdlestone
  pro·ce·dure
gi·tal·in
gith·a·gism
gi·tog·e·nin

gi·to·nin
gi·tox·in
git·ter
  cell
git·ter·zel·le
gla·bel·la
gla·bel·lad
gla·brate
gla·brous
  skin
gla·cial
  ace·tic ac·id
  phos·phor·ic ac·id
glad·i·ate
glad·i·o·lus
glairy
  mu·cus
glanc·ing
  wound
gland
  ac·ces·so·ry g.
  ac·ces·so·ry lac·ri·mal g.'s
  ac·ces·so·ry pa·rot·id g.
  ac·ces·so·ry su·pra·re·nal
    g.'s
  ac·ces·so·ry thy·roid g.
  ac·id g.
  ac·i·no·tu·bu·lar g.
  ac·i·nous g.
  ad·max·il·lary g.
  ad·re·nal g.
  ag·gre·gate g.'s
  ag·mi·nate g.'s
  ag·mi·nat·ed g.'s
  Albarran's g.'s
  al·bu·min·ous g.
  al·ve·o·lar g.
  anal g.
  an·te·ri·or lin·gual g.
  ap·i·cal g.
  ap·o·crine g.
  are·o·lar g.'s
  ar·te·ri·o·coc·cyg·e·al g.
  ar·y·te·noid g.'s
  Aselli's g.
  g.'s of au·di·to·ry tube
  ax·il·lary g.'s
  ax·il·lary sweat g.'s
  Bartholin's g.
  Bauhin's g.
  Baumgarten's g.'s
  g.'s of bil·i·ary mu·co·sa
  Blandin's g.
  Boerhaave's g.'s
  Bowman's g.
  brach·i·al g.
  bron·chi·al g.'s
  Bruch's g.'s

gland *(continued)*

Brunner's g.'s
buc·cal g.'s
bul·bo·u·re·thral g.
car·di·ac g.
car·di·ac g.'s of esoph·a·gus
ce·li·ac g.'s
ce·ru·mi·nous g.'s
cer·vi·cal g.'s
cer·vi·cal g.'s of uter·us
Ciaccio's g.'s
cil·i·ary g.'s
cir·cum·a·nal g.'s
coc·cyg·eal g.
coil g.
com·pound g.
con·junc·ti·val g.'s
con·vo·lut·ed g.
Cowper's g.
crop g.
duct·less g.'s
du·o·de·nal g.'s
Duverney's g.
Ebner's g.'s
ec·crine g.
ec·dys·i·al g.'s
Eglis' g.'s
en·do·crine g.'s
esoph·a·ge·al g.'s
g.'s of eu·sta·chi·an tube
ex·cre·to·ry g.
ex·o·crine g.
ex·ter·nal sal·i·vary g.
fol·lic·u·lar g.
fun·dus g.'s
Galeati's g.'s
gas·tric g.'s
Gay's g.'s
ge·nal g.'s
gen·i·tal g.
Gley's g.'s
great·er ves·tib·u·lar g.
Guérin's g.'s
har·de·ri·an g.
Harder's g.
Havers' g.'s
he·mal g.
he·ma·to·poi·et·ic g.
he·mo·lymph g.
Henle's g.'s
hi·ber·nat·ing g.
hol·o·crine g.
in·gui·nal g.'s
in·ter·nal sal·i·vary g.
g.'s of in·ter·nal se·cre·tion
in·ter·re·nal g.'s
in·ter·scap·u·lar g.
in·ter·sti·tial g.

in·tes·ti·nal g.'s
in·tra·ep·i·the·li·al g.'s
jug·u·lar g.
Knoll's g.'s
Krause's g.'s
la·bi·al g.'s
lac·ri·mal g.
lac·tif·er·ous g.
la·ryn·ge·al g.'s
less·er ves·tib·u·lar g.'s
Lieberkühn's g.'s
Littre's g.'s
Luschka's g.
Luschka's cys·tic g.'s
lymph g.
ma·jor sal·i·vary g.'s
mal·pi·ghi·an g.'s
mam·ma·ry g.
mar·row-lymph g.
mas·ter g.
max·il·lary g.
mei·bo·mi·an g.'s
mer·o·crine g.
Méry's g.
mes·en·ter·ic g.'s
me·tri·al g.
milk g.
mi·nor sal·i·vary g.'s
mixed g.
mo·lar g.'s
Moll's g.'s
Montgomery's g.'s
g.'s of mouth
mu·ci·lag·i·nous g.
mu·cip·a·rous g.
mu·cous g.
mu·cous g.'s of au·di·to·ry
  tube
na·sal g.'s
Nuhn's g.
odor·if·er·ous g.
oil g.'s
ol·fac·to·ry g.'s
ox·yn·tic g.
pac·chi·o·ni·an g.'s
pal·a·tine g.'s
pal·pe·bral g.'s
par·a·thy·roid g.
par·a·u·re·thral g.'s
pa·rot·id g.
pec·to·ral g.'s
pep·tic g.
per·i·a·nal odor·if·er·
  ous g.'s
per·i·tra·che·al g.'s
per·spi·ra·to·ry g.'s
Peyer's g.'s
pha·ryn·ge·al g.'s

Philip's g.'s
pi·le·ous g.
pin·e·al g.
pi·tu·i·tary g.
Poirier's g.
preen g.
pre·hy·oid g.
pre·pu·ti·al g.'s
pros·tate g.
pro·tho·rac·ic g.'s
py·lor·ic g.'s
rac·e·mose g.
Rivinus' g.
Rosenmüller's g.
sac·cu·lar g.
sal·i·vary g.
sal·i·vary g. of ab·do·men
scent g.'s
se·ba·ceous g.'s
sem·i·nal g.
sen·ti·nel g.
se·ro·mu·cous g.
se·rous g.
Serres' g.'s
sex·u·al g.
Skene's g.'s
sol·i·tary g.'s
sub·lin·gual g.
sub·man·dib·u·lar g.
sub·max·il·lary g.
su·do·rif·er·ous g.'s
su·pra·hy·oid g.
su·pra·re·nal g.
Suzanne's g.
sweat g.'s
syn·o·vi·al g.'s
tar·get g.
tar·sal g.'s
Terson's g.'s
Theile's g.'s
tho·rac·ic g.'s
thy·mus g.
thy·roid g.
Tiedemann's g.
tra·che·al g.'s
tra·cho·ma g.'s
tu·bu·lar g.
tu·bu·lo·ac·i·nar g.
tu·bu·lo·al·ve·o·lar g.
tym·pan·ic g.
Tyson's g.'s
uni·cel·lu·lar g.
ure·thral g.'s
uro·pyg·i·al g.
uter·ine g.'s
vag·i·nal g.
vas·cu·lar g.
ven·tral g.'s

ves·i·cal g.
ves·tib·u·lar g.'s
vul·vo·vag·i·nal g.
Waldeyer's g.'s
Wasmann's g.'s
Weber's g.'s
Wepfer's g.'s
Wölfler's g.
Wolfring's g.'s
Zeis' g.'s
glan·ders
ba·cil·lus
glan·des
glan·di·lem·ma
glan·du·la
g. at·ra·bi·li·a·ris
g. bas·i·la·ris
g. par·o·tis
g. par·o·tis ac·ces·so·ria
g. pros·ta·ti·ca
g. uro·pyg·i·us
glan·du·lae
glan·du·lar
can·cer
car·ci·no·ma
ep·i·the·li·um
fe·ver
mas·ti·tis
phar·yn·gi·tis
plague
sub·stance of pros·tate
sys·tem
glan·dule
glan·du·lo·pre·pu·tial
la·mel·la
glan·du·lous
glans
Glanzmann-Riniker
syn·drome
Glanzmann's
dis·ease
throm·bas·the·nia
gla·phen·ine
glare
blind·ing g.
daz·zling g.
pe·riph·e·ral g.
spec·u·lar g.
veil·ing g.
gla·rom·e·ter
gla·se·ri·an
ar·tery
fis·sure
Glasgow co·ma scale
Glasgow's
sign
glass
body

glass *(continued)*
  elec·trode
  fac·tor
  rays
glass
  cov·er g.
  Crookes' g.
  crown g.
  cup·ping g.
  flint g.
  ob·ject g.
  quartz g.
  sol·u·ble g.
  vi·ta g.
  wa·ter g.
  Wood's g.
glass bead
  ster·il·iz·er
glass·es
glass·work·er's
  cat·a·ract
glas·sy
  mem·brane
Glauber's
  salt
glau·co·ma
  ab·so·lute g.
  acute g.
  an·gle-clo·sure g.
  apha·kic g.
  cap·su·lar g.
  chron·ic g.
  closed-an·gle g.
  com·bined g.
  com·pen·sat·ed g.
  con·gen·i·tal g.
  cor·ti·co·ste·roid-in·duced g.
  Donders' g.
  g. ful·mi·nans
  ghost cell g.
  hem·or·rhag·ic g.
  hy·per·se·cre·tion g.
  low ten·sion g.
  ma·lig·nant g.
  nar·row-an·gle g.
  ne·o·vas·cu·lar g.
  open-an·gle g.
  phac·o·gen·ic g.
  pha·co·lyt·ic g.
  phac·o·mor·phic g.
  pig·men·tary g.
  pseu·do·ex·fo·li·a·tive cap·
   su·lar g.
  pu·pil·lary block g.
  sec·on·dary g.
  sim·ple g.
  g. sim·plex

glau·co·ma·to·cy·clit·ic
  cri·sis
glau·co·ma·tous
  cat·a·ract
  cup
  ex·ca·va·tion
  ha·lo
  ring
glau·co·ma·tous nerve-fi·ber
  bun·dle
  sco·to·ma
glau·co·su·ria
Gleason's
  score
Gleason's tu·mor
  grade
gleet
gleety
Glenner-Lillie
  stain for pi·tu·i·tary
Glenn's
  op·er·a·tion
gle·no·hu·mer·al
  lig·a·ments
gle·noid
  cav·i·ty
  fos·sa
  lig·a·ment
  sur·face
gle·noi·dal
  lip
Gley's
  glands
glia
  cells
gli·a·cyte
gli·a·din
gli·al
glide
  man·dib·u·lar g.
glid·ing
  joint
  oc·clu·sion
gli·o·blast
gli·o·blas·to·ma
gli·o·blas·to·sis ce·re·bri
gli·o·ma
  gi·gan·to·cel·lu·lar g.
  mixed g.
  na·sal g.
  g. of op·tic chi·asm
  g. of the spi·nal cord
  tel·an·gi·ec·tat·ic g.
  g. tel·an·gi·ec·to·des
gli·o·ma·to·sis
gli·o·ma·tous
gli·o·myx·o·ma
gli·o·neu·ro·ma

gli·o·sar·co·ma
gli·o·sis
  iso·mor·phous g.
  pi·loid g.
  g. uter·i
glip·i·zide
glis·so·ni·tis
Glisson's
  cap·sule
  cir·rho·sis
  sphinc·ter
glit·ter
  cells
glob·al
  apha·sia
  pa·ral·y·sis
globe
  g. of eye
  pale g.
globe cell
  ane·mia
glo·bi
glo·bin
glo·bin zinc
  in·su·lin
Glo·bo·ceph·a·lus
glo·boid
  cell
glo·boid cell
  leu·ko·dys·tro·phy
glo·bo·side
glob·u·lar
  leu·ko·cyte
  pro·cess
  pro·tein
  spu·tum
  throm·bus
  val·ue
glob·ule
  den·tin g.
  Morgagni's g.'s
  po·lar g.
glob·u·lif·er·ous
glob·u·lin
  ac·cel·er·a·tor g.
  an·ti·he·mo·phil·ic g.
  an·ti·he·mo·phil·ic g. A
  an·ti·he·mo·phil·ic g. B
  an·ti·hu·man g.
  chick·en·pox im·mune g.
    (hu·man)
  cor·ti·co·ste·roid-bind·ing g.
  hu·man gam·ma g.
  im·mune se·rum g.
  mea·sles im·mune g. (hu·man)
  per·tus·sis im·mune g.
  plas·ma ac·cel·er·a·tor g.

po·li·o·my·e·li·tis im·mune
  g. (hu·man)
ra·bies im·mune g.
  (hu·man)
$RH_o(D)$ im·mune g.
se·rum ac·cel·er·a·tor g.
spe·cif·ic im·mune g.
  (hu·man)
tet·a·nus im·mune g.
thy·rox·ine-bind·ing g.
zos·ter im·mune g.
glob·u·li·nu·ria
glob·u·lus
glo·bus
  g. hys·ter·i·cus
  g. ma·jor
  g. mi·nor
glo·mal
glo·man·gi·o·ma
glo·man·gi·o·ma·tous os·se·ous
  mal·for·ma·tion
  syn·drome
glo·man·gi·o·sis
  pul·mo·nary g.
glome
glo·mec·to·my
glom·era
glo·mer·u·lar
  cres·cent
  cysts
  lay·er of ol·fac·to·ry bulb
  ne·phri·tis
  scle·ro·sis
glo·mer·u·lar fil·tra·tion
  rate
glom·er·ule
glo·mer·u·li
glo·mer·u·li·tis
glo·mer·u·lo·ne·phri·tis
  acute g.
  acute cres·cen·tic g.
  acute hem·or·rhag·ic g.
  acute post-strep·to·coc·cal g.
  an·ti-base·ment mem·brane
    g.
  Berger's fo·cal g.
  chron·ic g.
  dif·fuse g.
  ex·ud·a·tive g.
  fo·cal g.
  fo·cal em·bol·ic g.
  hy·po·com·ple·men·te·mic
    g.
  lob·u·lar g.
  lo·cal g.
  mem·bra·no·pro·lif·er·a·tive
    g.
  mem·bra·nous g.

glo·mer·u·lo·ne·phri·tis
(continued)
 mes·an·gi·al pro·lif·er·a·tive
   g.
 mes·an·gi·o·cap·il·lary g.
 pro·lif·er·a·tive g.
 rap·id·ly pro·gress·ive g.
 seg·men·tal g.
 sub·a·cute g.
glo·mer·u·lop·a·thy
 fo·cal scle·ros·ing g.
glo·mer·u·lo·sa
 cell
glo·mer·u·lo·scle·ro·sis
 di·a·bet·ic g.
 fo·cal seg·men·tal g.
 in·ter·cap·il·lary g.
glo·mer·u·lose
glo·mer·u·lus
 mal·pi·ghi·an g.
 g. of mes·o·neph·ros
 ol·fac·to·ry g.
 g. of pro·neph·ros
glo·mus
 g. aor·ti·cum
 cho·roid g.
 g. coc·cyg·e·um
 g. in·tra·va·ga·le
 g. ju·gu·la·re
 g. pul·mo·na·le
glo·mus
 body
 tu·mor
glo·mus ju·gu·la·re
 tu·mor
glo·no·in
glos·sa
glos·sag·ra
glos·sal
glos·sal·gia
glos·sec·to·my
Glos·si·na
 G. mor·si·tans
 G. pal·li·di·pes
 G. pal·pal·is
glos·si·tis
 g. ar·e·a·ta ex·fo·li·a·ti·va
 atroph·ic g.
 be·nign mi·gra·to·ry g.
 g. de·sic·cans
 Hunter's g.
 me·di·an rhom·boid g.
 Moeller's g.
glos·so·cele
glos·so·cin·es·thet·ic
glos·so·don·to·tro·pism
glos·so·dy·na·mom·e·ter
glos·so·dyn·ia

glos·so·dyn·i·o·tro·pism
glos·so·ep·i·glot·tic
 lig·a·ment
glos·so·ep·i·glot·tid·e·an
glos·so·graph
glos·so·hy·al
glos·so·kin·es·thet·ic
glos·so·la·bi·o·la·ryn·ge·al
 pa·ral·y·sis
glos·so·la·bi·o·pha·ryn·ge·al
 pa·ral·y·sis
glos·so·la·lia
glos·sol·o·gy
glos·sol·y·sis
glos·son·cus
glos·so·pal·a·tine
 arch
 fold
glos·so·pal·a·ti·nus
glos·sop·a·thy
glos·so·pha·ryn·ge·al
 breath·ing
 nerve
 neu·ral·gia
 part
 tic
glos·so·pha·ryn·ge·us
glos·so·plas·ty
glos·so·ple·gia
glos·sop·to·sia
glos·sop·to·sis
glos·so·py·ro·sis
glos·sor·rha·phy
glos·sos·co·py
glos·so·spasm
glos·so·ste·re·sis
glos·sot·o·my
glos·so·trich·ia
glossy
 skin
glot·tal
glot·tic
glot·ti·des
glot·ti·do·spasm
glot·tis
 false g.
 g. res·pi·ra·tor·ia
 g. spu·ria
 true g.
 g. ve·ra
 g. vo·ca·lis
glot·ti·tis
glot·tol·o·gy
glove
 an·es·the·sia
glov·er's
 su·ture

glu·ca·gon
  gut g.
glu·ca·gon·o·ma
  syn·drome
glu·cal
glu·can
glu·cas·es
glu·ce·mia
glu·cep·tate
glu·cide
glu·cin·i·um
glu·ci·phore
glu·co·am·y·lase
glu·co·a·scor·bic ac·id
glu·co·cer·e·bro·side
glu·co·coid
glu·co·cor·ti·coid
glu·co·cor·ti·co·tro·phic
glu·co·cy·a·mine
glu·co·fu·ra·nose
glu·co·gen·e·sis
glu·co·gen·ic
glu·co·he·mia
glu·co·in·vert·ase
glu·co·ki·nase
glu·co·ki·net·ic
glu·co·lip·ids
glu·col·y·sis
glu·co·ne·o·gen·e·sis
glu·con·ic ac·id
glu·con·o·lac·to·nase
glu·co·pe·nia
glu·co·pro·tein
glu·co·pyr·a·nose
glu·co·sa·mine
glu·co·sans
glu·cose
  g. de·hy·dro·gen·ase
  liq·uid g.
  g. ox·i·dase
  g. ox·y·hy·drase
  g. phos·pho·mu·tase
glu·cose ox·i·dase
  meth·od
glu·cose ox·i·dase pa·per strip
  test
glu·cose·phos·phate isom·er·ase
  de·fi·cien·cy
glu·cose tol·er·ance
  test
glu·cose trans·port
  max·i·mum
glu·co·si·das·es
glu·co·side
glu·co·sone
glu·co·sul·fone so·di·um
glu·cos·u·ria
glu·co·syl

glu·co·syl·cer·a·mide
glu·co·syl·trans·fer·ase
glu·cu·ro·nate
glu·cu·rone
glu·cu·ron·ic ac·id
glu·cu·ro·nide
ᴅ-glu·cu·ron·o·lac·tone
glu·cu·ron·ose
glu·cu·ron·o·syl·trans·fer·ase
glue-sniff·ing
Gluge's
  cor·pus·cles
glu·sul·ase
glu·ta·mate
  g. ace·tyl·trans·fer·ase
  g. de·car·box·yl·ase
  g. de·hy·dro·gen·as·es
glu·tam·ic ac·id
  g. a. de·hy·dro·gen·as·es
  g. a. hy·dro·chlo·ride
glu·tam·ic-as·par·tic trans·am·i·nase
glu·tam·ic-ox·a·lo·ace·tic trans·am·i·nase
glu·tam·ic-py·ru·vic trans·am·i·nase
glu·ta·min·ase
glu·ta·mine
  g. syn·the·tase
glu·ta·min·ic ac·id
glu·tam·i·nyl
glu·tam·o·yl
glu·tam·yl
  g. trans·pep·ti·dase
glu·ta·ral
glu·tar·al·de·hyde
  fix·a·tive
glu·tar·ic ac·id
glu·ta·ryl-CoA syn·the·tase
glu·ta·thi·one
glu·ta·thi·one re·duc·tase
glu·te·al
  cleft
  crest
  fold
  fur·row
  her·nia
  line
  re·flex
  re·gion
  ridge
  sur·face of il·i·um
  tu·ber·os·i·ty
  veins
glu·te·al lymph
  nodes
glu·te·lins

glu·ten
 g. ca·sein
glu·ten
 en·ter·op·a·thy
glu·te·nin
glu·te·o·fem·o·ral
 bur·sa
glu·te·o·in·gui·nal
glu·teth·i·mide
glu·te·us
glu·te·us max·i·mus
 gait
 mus·cle
glu·te·us me·di·us
 bur·sas
 gait
 mus·cle
glu·te·us mi·ni·mus
 bur·sa
 mus·cle
glu·ti·noid
glu·ti·nous
glu·ti·tis
gly·bu·ride
gly·cal
gly·can
gly·can·o·hy·dro·las·es
gly·cate
gly·ca·tion
gly·ce·mia
glyc·er·al·de·hyde
gly·cer·ic ac·id
ʟ-gly·cer·ic ac·i·du·ria
gly·cer·ic al·de·hyde
glyc·er·i·das·es
glyc·er·ide
 mixed g.'s
glyc·er·in
 g. jel·ly
glyc·er·in·at·ed
 gel·a·tin
 tinc·ture
glyc·er·ite
 starch g.
 tan·nic ac·id g.
glyc·er·o·gel·a·tin
glyc·er·o·ke·tone
glyc·er·o·ki·nase
glyc·er·ol
 io·di·nat·ed g.
 g. ki·nase
 g. phos·phate
glyc·er·one
glyc·er·o·phos·phate
glyc·er·o·phos·pho·cho·line
glyc·er·o·phos·phor·ic ac·id
glyc·er·o·phos·pho·ryl·cho·line
glyc·er·ose

glyc·er·u·lose
glyc·er·yl
 g. al·co·hol
 g. bo·rate
 g. ether
 g. guai·a·co·late
 g. mon·o·ste·a·rate
 g. tri·ac·e·tate
 g. tri·bu·tyr·ate
 g. tri·cap·rate
 g. tri·ni·trate
gly·cin·ate
gly·cine
 g. am·i·di·no·trans·fer·ase
 g. be·ta·ine
 g. de·hy·dro·gen·as·es
 g. trans·am·i·di·nase
gly·cine·a·mide ri·bo·nu·cle·o·tide
gly·ci·ne·mia
gly·cine suc·ci·nate
 cy·cle
gly·ci·nu·ria
 fa·mil·i·al g.
gly·co·bi·ar·sol
gly·co·ca·lyx
gly·co·cho·late
 g. so·di·um
gly·co·cho·lic ac·id
gly·co·cin
gly·co·coll
gly·co·cor·ti·coid
gly·co·cy·a·mine
gly·co·gel·a·tin
gly·co·gen
 g. phos·pho·ryl·ase
 g. starch syn·thase
 g. syn·thase
gly·co·gen
 ac·an·tho·sis
 car·di·o·meg·a·ly
 gran·ule
gly·co·ge·nase
gly·co·gen·e·sis
gly·co·ge·net·ic
gly·co·gen·ol·y·sis
gly·co·ge·no·sis
 gen·er·al·ized g.
 he·pa·to·phos·phor·y·lase de·fi·cien·cy g.
 my·o·phos·phor·y·lase de·fi·cien·cy g.
gly·cog·e·nous
gly·co·gen-stor·age
 dis·ease
gly·co·geu·sia
gly·co·gly·ci·nu·ria
gly·col

gly·col·al·de·hyde
gly·col·al·de·hyde·trans·fer·ase
gly·co·leu·cine
gly·col·ic ac·id
gly·col·ic ac·i·du·ria
gly·co·lip·id
   lip·i·do·sis
gly·co·lyl
gly·co·lyl·u·rea
gly·col·y·sis
gly·co·lyt·ic
gly·co·ne·o·gen·e·sis
gly·con·ic ac·ids
gly·co·pe·nia
gly·co·pep·tide
Gly·co·pha·gus
gly·co·phil·ia
gly·co·pro·tein
gly·co·pty·a·lism
gly·co·pyr·ro·late
gly·cor·rha·chia
gly·cor·rhea
gly·cos·am·i·no·gly·can
gly·co·se·cre·to·ry
gly·co·si·a·lia
gly·co·si·a·lor·rhea
gly·co·side
N-gly·co·side
gly·co·sphin·go·lip·id
gly·co·stat·ic
gly·cos·ur·ia
   al·i·men·ta·ry g.
   be·nign g.
   di·ges·tive g.
   nor·mo·gly·ce·mic g.
   path·o·log·ic g.
   phlo·rid·zin g.
   phlo·ri·zin g.
   re·nal g.
gly·co·syl
   com·pound
gly·co·syl·at·ed
   he·mo·glo·bin
gly·co·sy·la·tion
gly·co·syl·trans·fer·ase
gly·co·tro·phic
gly·co·tro·pic
   fac·tor
glyc·u·re·sis
gly·cu·ron·ate
gly·cu·ron·ic ac·id
gly·cu·ron·i·dase
gly·cu·ro·nide
gly·cur·on·ose
gly·cu·ro·nu·ria
gly·cy·cla·mide
gly·cyl
   g. be·ta·ine

gly·cyl
   chain
glyc·yr·rhi·za
gly·ox·al
gly·ox·a·lase
gly·ox·a·line
gly·ox·y·late trans·a·cet·y·lase
gly·ox·yl·di·u·reide
gly·ox·yl·ic ac·id
   cy·cle
gly·so·bu·zole
Gmelin's
   test
GMS
   stain
gnash·ing
gnat
gnath·ic
   in·dex
gnath·i·on
gnath·o·ceph·a·lus
gnath·o·dy·nam·ics
gnath·o·dy·na·mom·e·ter
gnath·og·ra·phy
gnath·o·log·ic·al
gnath·ol·o·gy
gnath·o·pal·a·tos·chi·sis
gnath·o·plas·ty
gnath·os·chi·sis
gnath·o·stat·ics
Gna·thos·to·ma
   G. si·am·ense
   G. spi·ni·ge·rum
gna·thos·to·mi·a·sis
gnome's
   calf
gnos·co·pine
gno·sia
gno·to·bi·ol·o·gy
gno·to·bi·o·ta
gno·to·bi·ote
gno·to·bi·ot·ic
goal
goat·pox
   vi·rus
goat's milk
   ane·mia
gob·let
   cell
Godélier's
   law
Godman's
   fas·cia
Godwin
   tu·mor
Goeckerman
   treat·ment

Goethe's
bone
Gofman
test
Gog·gi·a's
sign
gog·gle
ple·thys·mo·graph·ic g.
goi·ter
ab·er·rant g.
acute g.
ad·e·nom·a·tous g.
cab·bage g.
col·loid g.
cys·tic g.
dif·fuse g.
div·ing g.
en·dem·ic g.
ex·oph·thal·mic g.
fa·mil·i·al g.
fi·brous g.
fol·lic·u·lar g.
lin·gual g.
lym·phad·e·noid g.
mi·cro·fol·lic·u·lar g.
mul·ti·nod·u·lar g.
non·tox·ic g.
par·en·chym·a·tous g.
sim·ple g.
sub·ster·nal g.
suf·fo·ca·tive g.
tho·rac·ic g.
tox·ic g.
wan·der·ing g.
goi·tro·gen
goi·tro·gen·ic
goi·trous
gold
co·he·sive g.
col·loi·dal ra·di·o·ac·tive g.
mat g.
non·co·he·sive g.
pow·dered g.
g. so·di·um thi·o·mal·ate
g. so·di·um thi·o·sul·fate
g. thi·o·glu·cose
gold
al·loy
cast·ing
equiv·a·lent
in·lay
num·ber
Goldberg-Maxwell
syn·drome
Goldblatt
kid·ney
phe·nom·e·non

Goldblatt's
clamp
hy·per·ten·sion
Goldenhar's
syn·drome
gold·en seal
Goldflam
dis·ease
gold foil
Goldman
equa·tion
Goldman-Fox
knives
Goldman-Hodgkin-Katz
equa·tion
Goldmann
pe·rim·e·ter
Goldmann's ap·pla·na·tion
to·nom·e·ter
Goldscheider's
test
gold sol
test
Goldstein's toe
sign
Goldthwait's
sign
golf-hole ure·ter·al
or·i·fice
Golgi
ap·pa·ra·tus
com·plex
zone
Golgi ep·i·the·li·al
cell
Golgi in·ter·nal
re·tic·u·lum
Golgi-Mazzoni
cor·pus·cle
gol·gi·o·ki·ne·sis
Golgi's
cells
stain
Golgi's os·mi·o·bi·chro·mate
fix·a·tive
Golgi ten·don
or·gan
Golgi type I
neu·ron
Golgi type II
neu·ron
Goll's
col·umn
Goltz
syn·drome
Gombault's
tri·an·gle
go·me·nol

gom·i·to·li
Gomori-Jones pe·ri·od·ic ac·id-
me·the·na·mine-sil·ver
stain
Gomori's al·de·hyde fuch·sin
stain
Gomori's chrome al·um he·ma·
tox·y·lin-phlox·ine
stain
Gomori's meth·en·a·mine-sil·ver
stain
Gomori's non·spe·cif·ic ac·id
phos·pha·tase
stain
Gomori's non·spe·cif·ic al·ka·
line phos·pha·tase
stain
Gomori's one-step tri·chrome
stain
Gomori's sil·ver im·preg·na·tion
stain
Gompertz'
hy·poth·e·sis
gom·phol·ic
joint
gom·pho·sis
go·nad
fe·male g.
in·dif·fer·ent g.
male g.
streaked g.
go·nad
nu·cle·us
go·nad·al
agen·e·sis
apla·sia
cords
dys·gen·e·sis
mo·sa·i·cism
ridge
streak
go·nad·ec·to·my
go·nad·o·crins
go·nad·o·lib·er·in
gon·a·dop·athy
go·nad·o·rel·in hy·dro·chlo·ride
go·nad·o·troph
go·nad·o·tro·phic
go·nad·o·tro·phin
go·nad·o·tro·pic
hor·mone
go·nad·o·tro·pin
an·te·ri·or pi·tu·i·tary g.
cho·ri·on·ic g.
equine g.
hu·man cho·ri·on·ic g.
hu·man men·o·pau·sal g.
preg·nant mare's se·rum g.

go·nad·o·tro·pin-pro·duc·ing
ad·e·no·ma
go·nad·o·tro·pin-re·leas·ing
fac·tor
hor·mone
gon·a·duct
go·nal·gia
gon·ane
gon·an·gi·ec·to·my
gon·ar·thri·tis
gon·ar·throt·o·my
gon·a·tag·ra
go·nat·o·cele
gon·e·cyst
gon·e·cys·tis
gon·e·cys·to·lith
Gon·gy·lo·ne·ma
G. in·glu·vi·co·la
G. ne·o·plas·ti·cum
G. pul·chrum
gon·gy·lo·ne·mi·a·sis
go·nia
go·ni·o·cra·ni·om·e·try
go·ni·o·dys·gen·e·sis
gon·i·o·ma
go·ni·om·e·ter
go·ni·on
go·ni·o·punc·ture
go·ni·o·scope
go·ni·os·co·py
go·ni·os·pa·sis
go·ni·o·syn·ech·ia
go·ni·ot·o·my
go·ni·tis
gon·o·blen·nor·rhea
gon·o·cele
gon·o·cho·rism
gon·o·cho·ris·mus
gon·o·cide
gon·o·coc·cal
con·junc·ti·vi·tis
sto·ma·ti·tis
ure·thri·tis
gon·o·coc·ce·mia
gon·o·coc·ci
gon·o·coc·cic
gon·o·coc·ci·cide
gon·o·coc·cus
gon·o·cyte
gon·o·he·mia
go·nom·ery
gon·o·op·so·nin
gon·o·phage
gon·o·phore
gon·oph·o·rus
gon·or·rhea
gon·or·rhe·al
oph·thal·mia

gon·or·rhe·al *(continued)*
rheu·ma·tism
sal·pin·gi·tis
gon·o·some
gon·o·tox·e·mia
gon·o·tox·in
gon·o·tyl
Go·ny·au·lax cat·a·nel·la
go·ny·camp·sis
Good
an·ti·gen
good
ob·ject
Goodell's
di·la·tor
sign
Goodpasture's
stain
syn·drome
Goormaghtigh's
cells
goose·flesh
Gopalan's
syn·drome
Goppert's
sign
Gordius
Gordon
re·flex
Gordon's
sign
symp·tom
Gordon and Sweet
stain
gor·get
probe g.
Gorham's
dis·ease
Goriaew's
rule
Gorlin
cyst
for·mu·la
Gorlin-Chaudhry-Moss
syn·drome
Gorlin's
sign
syn·drome
Gorman's
syn·drome
go·ron·dou
Gosselin's
frac·ture
gos·sy·pine
gos·sy·pol
gos·sy·pose

Goth·ic
arch
pal·ate
Goth·ic arch
trac·ing
Göthlin's
test
gouge
Gougerot and Blum
dis·ease
Gougerot-Carteaud
syn·drome
Gougerot-Ruiter
dis·ease
Gougerot-Sjögren
dis·ease
Gould's
su·ture
Gouley's
cath·e·ter
goun·dou
gout
ab·ar·tic·u·lar g.
ar·tic·u·lar g.
cal·ci·um g.
in·ter·val g.
la·tent g.
lead g.
masked g.
ret·ro·ced·ent g.
sat·ur·nine g.
sec·on·dary g.
to·pha·ceous g.
gout
di·et
gouty
ar·thri·tis
di·ath·e·sis
pearl
to·phus
urine
gov·ern·ment
hos·pi·tal
Gowers
dis·ease
Gowers'
col·umn
con·trac·tion
syn·drome
tract
Gr
an·ti·gen
graaf·i·an
fol·li·cle
grac·ile
hab·i·tus
tu·ber·cle

grac·i·lis
  mus·cle
  syn·drome
grade
  Gleason's tu·mor g.
grade I
  as·tro·cy·to·ma
grade II
  as·tro·cy·to·ma
grade III
  as·tro·cy·to·ma
grade IV
  as·tro·cy·to·ma
Gradenigo's
  syn·drome
gra·di·ent
  atri·o·ven·tric·u·lar g.
  con·cen·tra·tion g.
  den·si·ty g.
  elec·tro·chem·i·cal g.
  mi·tral g.
  sys·tol·ic g.
  ven·tric·u·lar g.
grad·u·ate
grad·u·at·ed
  com·press
  te·not·o·my
Graefe
  for·ceps
Graefenberg
  ring
Graefe's
  dis·ease
  knife
  op·er·a·tion
  sign
  spots
Graffi's
  vi·rus
graft
  ac·cor·di·on g.
  ad·i·po·der·mal g.
  al·lo·ge·ne·ic g.
  anas·to·mosed g.
  an·i·mal g.
  aug·men·ta·tion g.
  au·to·der·mic g.
  au·to·ge·ne·ic g.
  au·tol·o·gous g.
  au·to·plas·tic g.
  Blair-Brown g.
  bone g.
  breph·o·plas·tic g.
  ca·ble g.
  chess·board g.'s
  chip g.
  cho·ri·o·al·lan·to·ic g.
  com·pos·ite g.

  cor·ne·al g.
  cu·tis g.
  Davis g.'s
  de·layed g.
  der·mal g.
  der·mal-fat g.
  Douglas g.
  ep·i·der·mic g.
  Esser g.
  fas·cia g.
  fas·cic·u·lar g.
  fat g.
  fill·er g.
  free g.
  full-thick·ness g.
  fu·nic·u·lar g.
  H g.
  het·er·ol·o·gous g.
  het·er·o·plas·tic g.
  het·er·o·spe·cif·ic g.
  het·er·o·top·ic g.
  ho·mol·o·gous g.
  ho·mo·plas·tic g.
  hy·per·plas·tic g.
  im·plan·ta·tion g.
  in·fu·sion g.
  in·lay g.
  in·ter·spe·cif·ic g.
  iso·ge·ne·ic g.
  isol·o·gous g.
  iso·plas·tic g.
  Krause g.
  mesh g.
  mu·co·sal g.
  nerve g.
  Ollier g.
  Ollier-Thiersch g.
  omen·tal g.
  on·lay g.
  or·tho·top·ic g.
  os·te·o·per·i·os·te·al g.
  par·tial-thick·ness g.
  ped·i·cle g.
  per·i·os·te·al g.
  Phemister g.
  pinch g.
  por·cine g.
  post·age stamp g.'s
  pri·mary skin g.
  punch g.'s
  Reverdin g.
  sieve g.
  skin g.
  sleeve g.
  split-skin g.
  split-thick·ness g.
  Stent g.
  syn·ge·ne·ic g.

graft *(continued)*
  ten·don g.
  Thiersch g.
  vas·cu·lar·ized g.
  white g.
  Wolfe g.
  Wolfe-Krause g.
  xen·o·gen·e·ic g.
  zo·o·plas·tic g.
graft·ing
graft ver·sus host
  dis·ease
  re·ac·tion
Gra·ha·mel·la
Graham Little
  syn·drome
Graham's
  law
Graham Steell's
  mur·mur
grain
  al·co·hol
  itch
grains
gram
  cal·o·rie
  equiv·a·lent
gram-ion
gram-atom·ic
  weight
gram-cen·ti·me·ter
gram·i·ci·din
gram-me·ter
gram-mo·lec·u·lar
  weight
gram-mol·e·cule
Gram-neg·a·tive
Gram-pos·i·tive
Gram's
  io·dine
  stain
gra·na
gra·na·tum
grand
  cli·mac·ter·ic
  mal
  mul·tip·a·ra
grand·daugh·ter
  cyst
gran·di·ose
grand mal
  ep·i·lep·sy
Grandry's
  cor·pus·cles
Granger's
  line
Granit's
  loop

gran·u·lar
  cast
  con·junc·ti·vi·tis
  cor·tex
  de·gen·er·a·tion
  kid·ney
  lay·er of cer·e·bel·lar cor·tex
  lay·er of ep·i·der·mis
  lay·ers of ce·re·bral cor·tex
  lay·ers of ret·i·na
  lay·er of a ve·sic·u·lar ovar·i·an fol·li·cle
  leu·ko·blast
  leu·ko·cyte
  lids
  oph·thal·mia
  phar·yn·gi·tis
  pits
  pneu·mo·no·cytes
  tra·cho·ma
  ure·thri·tis
  vag·i·ni·tis
gran·u·lar cell
  my·o·blas·to·ma
  tu·mor
gran·u·lar en·do·plas·mic
  re·tic·u·lum
gran·u·lat·ed
  opi·um
gra·nu·la·tio
gran·u·la·tion
  ar·ach·noi·dal g.'s
  pac·chi·o·ni·an g.'s
gran·u·la·tion
  tis·sue
gran·u·la·ti·o·nes
gran·ule
  ac·i·do·phil g.
  ac·ro·so·mal g.
  al·pha g.
  Altmann's g.
  am·pho·phil g.
  ar·gen·taf·fin g.'s
  az·u·ro·phil g.
  ba·sal g.
  ba·so·phil g.
  Bensley's spe·cif·ic g.'s
  be·ta g.
  Birbeck's g.
  Bollinger g.'s
  chro·mat·ic g.
  chro·mo·phil g.
  chro·mo·phobe g.'s
  cone g.
  Crooke's g.'s
  del·ta g.
  el·e·men·ta·ry g.

eo·sin·o·phil g.
Fordyce's g.'s
fuch·sin·o·phil g.
gly·co·gen g.
io·do·phil g.
jux·ta·glo·mer·u·lar g.'s
kap·pa g.
ker·a·to·hy·a·lin g.'s
lam·el·lar g.
Langerhans' g.
Langley's g.'s
mem·brane-coat·ing g.
met·a·chro·mat·ic g.'s
mu·cin·o·gen g.'s
Neusser's g.'s
neu·tro·phil g.
Nissl g.'s
ox·y·phil g.
Palade g.
pro·ac·ro·so·mal g.'s
pro·se·cre·tion g.'s
rod g.
Schüffner's g.'s
se·cre·to·ry g.
sem·i·nal g.
vol·u·tin g.'s
Zimmermann's g.
gran·ule
cell of con·nec·tive tis·sue
cells
gran·u·lo·blast
gran·u·lo·blas·to·sis
gran·u·lo·cyte
im·ma·ture g.
gran·u·lo·cyt·ic
leu·ke·mia
sar·co·ma
se·ries
gran·u·lo·cy·to·pe·nia
gran·u·lo·cy·to·poi·e·sis
gran·u·lo·cy·to·poi·et·ic
gran·u·lo·cy·to·sis
gran·u·lo·ma
ac·tin·ic g.
ame·bic g.
g. an·nu·la·re
ap·i·cal g.
be·ryl·li·um g.
bil·har·zi·al g.
ca·nine ve·ne·re·al g.
coc·cid·i·oi·dal g.
co·li g.
den·tal g.
g. en·de·mi·cum
eo·sin·o·phil·ic g.
g. fa·ci·a·le
for·eign body g.
g. gan·gre·nes·cens

gi·ant cell g.
g. grav·i·dar·um
in·fec·tious g.
g. in·gui·na·le
g. in·gui·na·le tro·pi·cum
la·ryn·ge·al g.
le·thal mid·line g.
lip·oid g.
lip·o·phag·ic g.
Majocchi g.'s
ma·lig·nant g.
g. mul·ti·for·me
oily g.
par·a·coc·cid·i·o·i·dal g.
par·a·sit·ic g.
per·i·ap·i·cal g.
g. pu·den·di
py·o·gen·ic g.
g. py·o·gen·i·cum
re·par·a·tive gi·ant cell g.
re·tic·u·lo·his·ti·o·cyt·ic g.
root end g.
sar·coid·al g.
schis·to·some g.
sea ur·chin g.
sil·i·con g.
swim·ming pool g.
g. tel·an·gi·ec·ta·ti·cum
g. tro·pi·cum
ul·cer·at·ing g. of pu·den·da
g. ve·ne·re·um
zir·co·ni·um g.
gran·u·lo·ma·to·sis
al·ler·gic g.
bron·cho·cen·tric g.
g. dis·ci·for·mis chron·i·ca et pro·gres·si·va
lip·id g.
lip·oid g.
lip·o·phag·ic in·tes·ti·nal g.
lym·pho·ma·toid g.
Miescher's g.
g. si·de·ro·ti·ca
Wegener's g.
gran·u·lom·a·tous
ar·te·ri·tis
co·li·tis
dis·ease
en·ceph·a·lo·my·e·li·tis
en·doph·thal·mi·tis
en·ter·i·tis
in·flam·ma·tion
mas·ti·tis
no·car·di·o·sis
gran·u·lo·mere
gran·u·lo·pe·nia
gran·u·lo·plasm

gran·u·lo·plas·tic
gran·u·lo·poi·e·sis
gran·u·lo·poi·et·ic
gran·u·lo·sa
   cell
gran·u·lo·sa cell
   tu·mor
gran·u·lo·sa lu·te·in
   cells
gran·u·lo·sis
   g. ru·bra na·si
gran·u·los·i·ty
gran·u·lo·vac·u·o·lar
   de·gen·er·a·tion
gra·num
grape
   end·ings
   mole
   sug·ar
graph
graph·an·es·the·sia
graph·es·the·sia
graph·ic
   apha·sia
   for·mu·la
graph·ite
gra·phol·o·gy
graph·o·ma·nia
graph·o·mo·tor
   apha·sia
graph·o·pa·thol·o·gy
graph·o·pho·bia
graph·or·rhea
graph·o·spasm
grasp
   palm g.
   pen g.
grasp
   re·flex
grasp·ing
   re·flex
grass
   ba·cil·lus
   tet·a·ny
Grasset-Gaussel
   phe·nom·e·non
Grasset's
   law
   phe·nom·e·non
   sign
Gratiolet's
   fi·bers
   ra·di·a·tion
grat·tage
Gräupner's
   meth·od
grave
   wax

grav·el
Graves'
   dis·ease
grav·id
   uter·us
grav·i·da
grav·i·da I
grav·i·da II
gra·vid·ic
   ret·i·ni·tis
   ret·i·nop·a·thy
grav·id·ism
gra·vid·i·tas
   g. ex·am·ni·a·lis
   g. ex·o·cho·ri·a·lis
gra·vid·i·ty
gra·vim·e·ter
grav·i·met·ric
grav·i·re·cep·tors
grav·i·ta·tion
   ab·scess
grav·i·ta·tion·al
   ul·cer
   units
grav·i·ty
   spe·cif·ic g.
   zero-g.
Grawitz'
   ba·so·phil·ia
   tu·mor
gray
   at·ro·phy
   cat·a·ract
   col·umns
   de·gen·er·a·tion
   fi·bers
   hep·a·ti·za·tion
   in·du·ra·tion
   in·fil·tra·tion
   lay·er of su·pe·ri·or col·lic·
     u·lus
   mat·ter
   scale
   sub·stance
   syn·drome
   tu·ber
   tu·ber·cle
   wing
gray ba·by
   syn·drome
gray-scale
   ul·tra·so·nog·ra·phy
grease
   heel
grease·less
   cream
greasy pig
   dis·ease

great
fo·ra·men
toe
vein of Galen
great ad·duc·tor
mus·cle
great al·ve·o·lar
cells
great anas·to·mot·ic
ar·tery
great au·ric·u·lar
nerve
great car·di·ac
vein
great ce·re·bral
vein
great·er
cir·cu·la·tion
cul-de-sac
cur·va·ture of stom·ach
horn
omen·tum
tro·chan·ter
tu·ber·cle of hu·mer·us
tu·ber·os·i·ty of hu·mer·us
wing of sphe·noid bone
great·er alar
car·ti·lage
great·er ar·te·ri·al
cir·cle of iris
great·er mult·ang·u·lar
bone
great·er oc·cip·i·tal
nerve
great·er pal·a·tine
ar·tery
ca·nal
fo·ra·men
groove
nerve
great·er pec·to·ral
mus·cle
great·er per·i·to·ne·al
cav·i·ty
great·er pe·tro·sal
nerve
great·er pos·te·ri·or rec·tus
mus·cle of head
great·er pso·as
mus·cle
great·er rhom·boid
mus·cle
great·er sci·at·ic
notch
great·er splanch·nic
nerve
great·er su·per·fi·cial pe·tro·sal
nerve

great·er su·pra·cla·vic·u·lar
fos·sa
great·er tym·pan·ic
spine
great·er ves·tib·u·lar
gland
great·er zy·go·mat·ic
mus·cle
great hor·i·zon·tal
fis·sure
great lon·gi·tu·di·nal
fis·sure
great pan·cre·at·ic
ar·tery
great sa·phe·nous
vein
great sci·at·ic
nerve
great su·pe·ri·or pan·cre·at·ic
ar·tery
great-toe
re·flex
green
can·cer
he·mo·glo·bin
pus
sick·ness
soap
spu·tum
stain
tooth
vi·sion
green
Scheele's g.
Greenfield's
dis·ease
Greenhow's
dis·ease
green mon·key
vi·rus
Greenough
mi·cro·scope
green·stick
frac·ture
gref·fo·tome
greg·a·loid
Greg·a·ri·na
greg·a·rine
Greg·a·ri·nia
greg·a·ri·no·sis
Greig's
syn·drome
grenz
ray
zone
gres·sion
Greville
bath

Grey Turner's
  sign
grid
  Wetzel g.
Gridley's
  stain
  stain for fun·gi
grief
Griesinger's
  dis·ease
  symp·tom
grif·fin
  claw
Griffith's
  sign
grin·de·lia
grind·ing
  se·lec·tive g.
grind·ing
  sur·face
grind·ing-in
grip
  dev·il's g.
grippe
gris·e·o·ful·vin
gris·e·us
Grisolle's
  sign
Gri·so·nel·la ra·tel·li·na
gris·tle
Gritti's
  op·er·a·tion
Gritti-Stokes
  am·pu·ta·tion
Grocco's
  sign
  tri·an·gle
gro·cer's
  itch
Grocott-Gomori meth·en·a·mine-sil·ver
  stain
Groenouw's cor·ne·al
  dys·tro·phy
groin
  ul·cer
Grönblad-Strandberg
  syn·drome
groove
  sign
groove
  al·ve·o·lo·buc·cal g.
  al·ve·o·lo·la·bi·al g.
  al·ve·o·lo·lin·gual g.
  an·te·ri·or au·ric·u·lar g.
  an·te·ri·or in·ter·me·di·ate
    g.

an·te·ri·or in·ter·ven·tric·u·
  lar g.
an·ter·o·lat·er·al g.
an·ter·o·me·di·an g.
ar·te·ri·al g.'s
atri·o·ven·tric·u·lar g.
g. for au·di·to·ry tube
au·ric·u·lo·ven·tric·u·lar g.
bi·cip·i·tal g.
bran·chi·al g.
ca·rot·id g.
car·pal g.
cav·ern·ous g.
cos·tal g.
g. of crus of the he·lix
den·tal g.
de·vel·op·men·tal g.'s
di·gas·tric g.
eth·moi·dal g.
fron·tal g.'s
gin·gi·vo·buc·cal g.
gin·gi·vo·la·bi·al g.
gin·gi·vo·lin·gual g.
great·er pal·a·tine g.
g. of great·er pe·tro·sal
  nerve
Harrison's g.
in·fe·ri·or pe·tro·sal g.
in·fra·or·bit·al g.
in·ter·os·se·ous g.
in·ter·tu·ber·cu·lar g.
in·ter·ven·tric·u·lar g.'s
lac·ri·mal g.
la·ryn·go·tra·che·al g.
lat·er·al bi·cip·i·tal g.
g. of less·er pe·tro·sal nerve
lin·guo·gin·gi·val g.
Lucas' g.
mas·toid g.
me·di·al bi·cip·i·tal g.
me·di·an g. of tongue
med·ul·lary g.
mus·cu·lo·spi·ral g.
my·lo·hy·oid g.
g. of nail ma·trix
na·so·la·bi·al g.
na·so·pal·a·tine g.
na·so·pha·ryn·ge·al g.
neu·ral g.
ob·tu·ra·tor g.
oc·cip·i·tal g.
ol·fac·to·ry g.
op·tic g.
pal·a·tine g.
pal·a·to·vag·i·nal g.
par·a·glen·oid g.
pha·ryn·ge·al g.'s
pha·ryn·go·tym·pan·ic g.

pon·to·med·ul·lary g.
pop·lit·e·al g.
pos·te·ri·or au·ric·u·lar g.
pos·te·ri·or in·ter·me·di·ate g.
pos·te·ri·or in·ter·ven·tric·u·lar g.
pos·ter·o·lat·er·al g.
pre·au·ric·u·lar g.
pri·mary la·bi·al g.
prim·i·tive g.
pter·y·go·pal·a·tine g.
g. for ra·di·al nerve
re·ten·tion g.
rhom·bic g.'s
sag·it·tal g.
Sibson's g.
sig·moid g.
skin g.'s
g. for spi·nal nerve
spi·ral g.
sub·cla·vi·an g.
g. for sub·cla·vi·an ar·tery
g. for sub·cla·vi·an vein
sub·cos·tal g.
g. for su·pe·ri·or sag·it·tal si·nus
sup·ple·men·tal g.
su·pra-ac·e·tab·u·lar g.
g. for ten·don of flex·or hal·lu·cis lon·gus
g. for ten·don of long per·o·ne·al mus·cle
tra·che·o·bron·chi·al g.
trans·verse na·sal g.
tym·pan·ic g.
g. for ul·nar nerve
ure·thral g.
ve·nous g.'s
ver·te·bral g.
vo·mer·al g.
vom·e·ro·vag·i·nal g.

grooved
tongue
Gross'
vi·rus
gross
anat·o·my
he·ma·tu·ria
le·sion
Gross' leu·ke·mia
vi·rus
ground
bun·dles
itch
la·mel·la
state
sub·stance

ground-glass
cy·to·plasm
ground itch
ane·mia
group
ag·glu·ti·na·tion
ag·glu·ti·nin
an·ti·gens
au·di·om·e·ter
au·di·om·e·try
dy·nam·ics
hos·pi·tal
im·mu·ni·ty
prac·tice
psy·cho·ther·a·py
re·ac·tion
test
group
blood g.
char·ac·ter·iz·ing g.
con·nec·tive tis·sue g.
con·trol g.
cy·to·phil g.
de·ter·mi·nant g.
en·coun·ter g.
ex·per·i·men·tal g.
func·tion·al g.
link·age g.
matched g.'s
par·tial g.'s
pros·thet·ic g.
sen·si·tiv·i·ty train·ing g.
symp·tom g.
T g.
task-o·ri·ent·ed g.
ther·a·peu·tic g.
train·ing g.
group I
my·co·bac·te·ria
group II
my·co·bac·te·ria
group III
my·co·bac·te·ria
group IV
my·co·bac·te·ria
Grover's
dis·ease
grow·ing
frac·ture
pains
grow·ing ovar·i·an
fol·li·cle
growth
curve
hor·mone
hor·mone-re·leas·ing hor·mone
lines

growth *(continued)*
quo·tient
rate
growth
ac·cre·tion·ary g.
ap·po·si·tion·al g.
aux·et·ic g.
dif·fer·en·tial g.
in·ter·sti·tial g.
in·tus·sus·cep·tive g.
mul·ti·pli·ca·tive g.
new g.
growth hor·mone-pro·duc·ing
ad·e·no·ma
growth hor·mone-re·leas·ing
fac·tor
growth-on·set
di·a·be·tes
grub
Gruber-Landzert
fos·sa
Gruber's
cul-de-sac
meth·od
re·ac·tion
syn·drome
Gruber-Widal
re·ac·tion
gru·el
gru·mous
Grunert's
spur
Grunstein-Hogness
as·say
Grynfeltt's
tri·an·gle
gry·o·chrome
gry·po·sis
g. un·gui·um
g-tol·er·ance
guai·ac
gum
test
guai·a·cin
guai·a·col
g. glyc·er·yl ether
g. phos·phate
guai·fen·e·sin
Gu·a·ma
vi·rus
guan·a·benz ac·e·tate
gua·na·cline sul·fate
gua·na·drel sul·fate
gua·nase
guanazolo
gua·neth·i·dine sul·fate
gua·ni·dine

gua·ni·di·no·ac·e·tate meth·yl·trans·fer·ase
gua·nine
g. am·i·nase
g. de·am·i·nase
g. de·ox·y·ri·bo·nu·cle·o·tide
g. ri·bo·nu·cle·o·tide
gua·nine
cell
gua·no·chlor sul·fate
gua·no·phores
gua·no·sine
guan·ox·an sul·fate
gua·nyl
g. cy·clase
guan·y·late cy·clase
gua·nyl·ic ac·id
gua·nyl·o·ri·bo·nu·cle·ase
gua·nyl·yl
g. cy·clase
guar
gum
gua·ra·na
gua·ra·nine
guard·ing
ab·dom·i·nal g.
Guarnieri
bod·ies
Guarnieri's gel·a·tin
agar
Gu·a·ro·a
vi·rus
gu·ber·nac·u·lar
ca·nal
cord
gu·ber·nac·u·lum
g. den·tis
Hunter's g.
Gubler's
hem·i·ple·gia
line
pa·ral·y·sis
syn·drome
tu·mor
Gudden's
com·mis·sures
gan·gli·on
Gudden's teg·men·tal
nu·clei
Guéneau de Mussy's
point
Guérin's
fold
frac·ture
glands
si·nus
valve

guid·ance
  con·dy·lar g.
  in·ci·sal g.
guide
  an·te·ri·or g.
  cath·e·ter g.
  con·dy·lar g.
  in·ci·sal g.
  mold g.
guide
  plane
guide·line
  clasp g.
  Cummer's g.
Guillain-Barré
  re·flex
  syn·drome
guil·lo·tine
  am·pu·ta·tion
guin·ea corn
  yaws
guin·ea green B
guin·ea pig
Guinon's
  dis·ease
Guldberg-Waage
  law
gul·let
L-gu·lon·ic ac·id
L-gu·lon·o·lac·tone
gu·lose
gum
  g. ar·a·bic
  Bas·so·ra g.
  g. ben·ja·min
  g. ben·zo·in
  Brit·ish g.
  eu·ca·lyp·tus g.
  ghat·ti g.
  guai·ac g.
  guar g.
  In·di·an g.
  ka·ra·ya g.
  lo·cust g.
  g. opi·um
  red g.
  sen·e·gal g.
  starch g.
  ster·cu·lia g.
  wheat g.
gum
  con·tour
  lan·cet
  line
  re·sec·tion
  res·in
gum·boil

Gum·boro
  dis·ease
gum·ma
gum·mas
gum·ma·ta
gum·ma·tous
  ab·scess
  syph·i·lid
  ul·cer
gum·my
Gumprecht's
  shad·ows
Gunn
  phe·nom·e·non
  pu·pil
Gunning
  splint
Günning's
  re·ac·tion
Gunn's
  dots
  sign
  syn·drome
gun·shot
  wound
gun·stock
  de·for·mi·ty
Günther's
  dis·ease
Günz'
  lig·a·ment
Günz·berg's
  re·a·gent
  test
gur·gling
  rale
gur·ney
Gussenbauer's
  su·ture
gus·ta·tion
gus·ta·to·ry
  an·es·the·sia
  au·di·tion
  bud
  cells
  hy·per·es·the·sia
  hy·per·hi·dro·sis
  lem·nis·cus
  nu·cle·us
  or·gan
  pore
  rhi·nor·rhea
gus·ta·to·ry-su·do·rif·ic
  re·flex
gus·ta·to·ry sweat·ing
  syn·drome
gut
  glu·ca·gon

gut
    blind g.
    post·a·nal g.
    post·clo·a·cal g.
    pre·o·ral g.
Guthrie
    test
Guthrie's
    mus·cle
gut·ta
    g. se·re·na
gut·tae
gut·ta-per·cha
    cone
    points
    spread·er
gut·tate
    cho·roi·dop·a·thy
gut·ter
    dys·tro·phy of cor·nea
    frac·ture
    wound
gut·tur·al
    duct
    pouch
    pulse
    rale
gut·tur·o·tet·a·ny
Gutzeit's
    test
Guyon's
    am·pu·ta·tion
    isth·mus
    sign
GVH
    dis·ease
Gym·na·moe·bi·da
gym·nas·tics
    Swed·ish g.
Gym·no·as·ca·ce·ae
gym·no·cyte
gym·no·pho·bia
gy·nan·drism
gy·nan·dro·blas·to·ma
gy·nan·droid
gy·nan·dro·mor·phism
gy·nan·dro·mor·phous
gy·na·tre·sia
gy·ne·cic
gy·ne·co·gen·ic
gy·ne·cog·ra·phy
gy·ne·coid
    pel·vis
gy·ne·co·log·ic
gy·ne·co·log·i·cal
gy·ne·col·o·gist
gy·ne·col·o·gy
gy·ne·co·ma·nia

gy·ne·co·ma·stia
gy·ne·co·mas·ty
gy·ne·co·phor·ic
    ca·nal
gy·ne·pho·bia
gy·ni·at·rics
gy·ni·at·ry
gy·no·car·dia oil
gy·no·gen·e·sis
gy·nop·a·thy
gy·no·plas·tics
gy·no·plas·ty
gyp·sum
gy·rate
    at·ro·phy of cho·roid and ret·i·na
gy·ra·tion
gy·rec·to·my
    fron·tal g.
gyr·en·ce·phal·ic
gy·ri
gy·ro·chrome
    cell
Gy·ro·mi·tra es·cu·len·ta
gy·ro·sa
gy·rose
gy·ro·spasm
gy·rus
    an·gu·lar g.
    an·nec·tent g.
    an·te·ri·or cen·tral g.
    an·te·ri·or pir·i·form g.
    as·cend·ing fron·tal g.
    as·cend·ing pa·ri·e·tal g.
    cal·lo·sal g.
    cen·tral gy·ri
    cin·gu·late g.
    deep tran·si·tion·al g.
    den·tate g.
    fas·ci·o·lar g.
    g. for·ni·ca·tus
    fu·si·form g.
    g. fu·si·for·mis
    Heschl's gy·ri
    hip·po·cam·pal g.
    in·fe·ri·or fron·tal g.
    in·fe·ri·or oc·cip·i·tal g.
    in·fe·ri·or pa·ri·e·tal g.
    in·fe·ri·or tem·po·ral g.
    in·ter·lock·ing gy·ri
    lat·er·al oc·cip·i·to·tem·po·ral g.
    lin·gual g.
    long g. of in·su·la
    mar·gi·nal g.
    me·di·al oc·cip·i·to·tem·po·ral g.
    mid·dle fron·tal g.

mid·dle tem·po·ral g.
oc·cip·i·tal gy·ri
or·bi·tal gy·ri
par·a·hip·po·cam·pal g.
par·a·ter·mi·nal g.
post·cen·tral g.
pos·te·ri·or cen·tral g.
pre·cen·tral g.
pre·pir·i·form g.
Retzius' g.
short gy·ri of the in·su·la
sple·ni·al g.

straight g.
sub·cal·lo·sal g.
su·pe·ri·or fron·tal g.
su·pe·ri·or oc·cip·i·tal g.
su·pe·ri·or pa·ri·e·tal g.
su·pe·ri·or tem·po·ral g.
su·pra·cal·lo·sal g.
su·pra·mar·gin·al g.
tran·si·tion·al g.
trans·verse tem·po·ral gy·ri
un·ci·nate g.

H
ag·glu·ti·nin
an·ti·gen
band
chain
col·o·ny
dis·ease
disk
fields
gene
graft
rays
re·flex
shunt
sub·stance
H-
mer·o·my·o·sin
Haab's
mag·net
re·flex
haar·scheibe
tu·mor
Haase's
rule
Habel
test
ha·be·na
ha·be·nae
hab·e·nal
ha·be·nar
ha·ben·u·la
h. of ce·cum
Haller's h.
ha·ben·u·lae per·fo·ra·ta
pin·e·al h.
Scarpa's h.
h. ure·thra·lis
ha·ben·u·lae
ha·ben·u·lar
com·mis·sure
nu·cle·us
ha·ben·u·lo·in·ter·pe·dun·cu·lar
tract
Haber's
syn·drome
hab·it
cho·rea
sco·li·o·sis

spasm
tic
hab·it
ha·bit·u·al
abor·tion
ha·bit·u·a·tion
hab·i·tus
fe·tal h.
grac·ile h.
hab·ro·ma·nia
Hab·ro·ne·ma
H. ma·jus
H. meg·a·sto·ma
H. mi·cro·sto·ma
H. mus·cae
hab·ro·ne·mi·a·sis
cu·ta·ne·ous h.
hack·ing
Ha·dru·rus
Haeckel's
law
Haeckel's gas·trea
the·o·ry
Hae·ma·dip·sa cey·lon·i·ca
Hae·ma·moe·ba
Hae·ma·phy·sa·lis
H. chor·dei·lis
H. cin·na·ba·ri·na
H. cin·na·ba·ri·na punc·ta·
ta
H. con·cin·na
H. lea·chi
H. le·po·ris-pa·lus·tris
H. spi·ni·ge·ra
Hae·ma·to·pi·nus
Hae·mo·bar·ton·el·la
H. mu·ris
Hae·mo·coc·cid·i·um
Hae·mo·dip·sus ven·tri·co·sus
Hae·mo·greg·a·ri·na
Hae·mon·chus
Hae·moph·i·lus
H. ae·gyp·ti·cus
H. aph·roph·i·lus
H. du·creyi
H. gal·li·na·rum
H. hae·mo·glo·bi·noph·i·lus
H. hae·mo·ly·ti·cus
H. in·flu·en·zae

Hae·moph·i·lus *(continued)*
   H. in·flu·en·zae-mu·ri·um
   H. ovis
   H. par·a·hae·mo·lyt·i·cus
   H. par·a·in·flu·en·zae
   H. per·tus·sis
   H. su·is
Hae·mo·pro·te·us
Hae·mo·spo·ri·na
Hae·mo·stron·gy·lus va·so·rum
Haenel's
   symp·tom
Haff
   dis·ease
Haffkine's
   vac·cine
haf·ni·um
ha·fussi
   bath
Hagedorn
   nee·dle
Hageman
   fac·tor
hag·i·o·ther·a·py
Haglund's
   de·for·mi·ty
   dis·ease
hahn·i·um
Hahn's ox·ine
   re·a·gent
Haidinger's
   brush·es
Hailey and Hailey
   dis·ease
hair
   ball
   bulb
   cast
   cells
   cross·es
   cy·cle
   disk
   fol·li·cle
   pa·pil·la
   root
   shaft
   streams
   whorls
hair
   au·di·to·ry h.'s
   bam·boo h.
   bay·o·net h.
   bead·ed h.
   bur·row·ing h.'s
   club h.
   ex·cla·ma·tion point h.
   Frey's ir·ri·ta·tion h.'s
   in·grown h.'s

   kinky h.
   la·nu·go h.
   mo·nil·i·form h.
   nett·ling h.'s
   ringed h.
   Schridde's can·cer h.'s
   stel·late h.
   tac·tile h.
   taste h.'s
   ter·mi·nal h.
   twist·ed h.'s
   vel·lus h.
   wool·ly h.
hair·line
   frac·ture
hair·worm
hairy
   cells
   heart
   leu·ko·pla·kia
   mole
   tongue
hairy cell
   leu·ke·mia
ha·la·tion
hal·az·e·pam
hal·a·zone
Halberstaedter-Prowazek
   bod·ies
hal·cin·o·nide
Haldane
   cham·ber
   ef·fect
   trans·for·ma·tion
   tube
Haldane-Priestley
   sam·ple
Haldane's
   ap·pa·ra·tus
Hales'
   pi·e·sim·e·ter
Hale's col·loi·dal iron
   stain
ha·leth·a·zole
half am·pli·tude pulse
   du·ra·tion
half-chair
   form
half-glass
   spec·ta·cles
half and half
   nail
half-life
   bi·o·log·i·cal h.-l.
   ef·fec·tive h.-l.
   phys·i·cal h.-l.
half-moon
   red h.-m.

half-val·ue
   lay·er
half·way house
hal·i·but liv·er oil
hal·ide
hal·i·pha·gia
hal·i·ste·re·sis
hal·i·ste·ret·ic
hal·i·to·sis
hal·i·tus
hal·la·chrome
Hallermann-Streiff
   syn·drome
Haller's
   an·nu·lus
   an·sa
   arch·es
   cir·cle
   cones
   ha·ben·u·la
   in·su·la
   line
   plex·us
   re·te
   tri·pod
   tu·ni·ca vas·cu·lo·sa
   un·guis
   vas aber·rans
Haller's vas·cu·lar
   tis·sue
Hallervorden
   syn·drome
Hallervorden-Spatz
   dis·ease
   syn·drome
Hallé's
   point
hal·lex
Hallgren's
   syn·drome
hal·li·ces
Hallion's
   test
Hallopeau's
   dis·ease
hal·lu·cal
hal·lu·ces
hal·lu·ci·na·tion
   formed vi·su·al h.
   hyp·na·gog·ic h.
   lil·li·pu·tian h.
   stump h.
   un·formed vi·su·al h.
hal·lu·ci·na·to·ry
   neu·ral·gia
hal·lu·ci·no·gen
hal·lu·ci·no·gen·ic
hal·lu·ci·no·sis

hal·lus
hal·lux
   h. do·lo·ro·sus
   h. ex·ten·sus
   h. flex·us
   h. mal·le·us
   h. ri·gi·dus
   h. val·gus
   h. var·us
ha·lo
   ane·mic h.
   glau·co·ma·tous h.
   se·nile h.
ha·lo
   cast
   mel·a·no·ma
   ne·vus
   sign
   sign of hy·drops
   trac·tion
   vi·sion
hal·o·an·i·sone
hal·o·der·mia
hal·o·gen
   ac·ne
hal·o·gen·a·tion
Hal·o·ge·ton
ha·lom·e·ter
hal·o·per·i·dol
hal·o·phil
hal·o·phile
hal·o·phil·ic
hal·o·pro·gin
hal·o·ste·re·sis
hal·o·thane
   hep·a·ti·tis
hal·o·thane-e·ther
   aze·o·trope
Halstead-Reitan
   bat·tery
Halsted's
   law
   op·er·a·tion
   su·ture
Hal·te·rid·i·um
hal·zoun
ham·a·me·lis
ha·mar·tia
ham·ar·to·blas·to·ma
ham·ar·to·chon·dro·ma·to·sis
ham·ar·to·ma
   fi·brous h. of in·fan·cy
   pul·mo·nary h.
ham·ar·tom·a·tous
ham·ar·to·pho·bia
ha·mate
   bone
ha·ma·tum

ha·max·o·pho·bia
Hamburger's
  law
  phe·nom·e·non
Hamilton's
  pseu·do·phleg·mon
Hamman-Rich
  syn·drome
Hamman's
  dis·ease
  sign
  syn·drome
Hammarsten's
  re·a·gent
ham·mer
  fin·ger
  nose
  toe
Hammerschlag's
  meth·od
ham·mock
  ban·dage
  lig·a·ment
Hammond's
  dis·ease
Hampson
  unit
Hampton
  hump
  line
  ma·neu·ver
  tech·nique
Ham's
  test
ham·ster
ham·string
  mus·cles
  ten·don
ham·string
ham·u·lar
  notch
  pro·cess of lac·ri·mal bone
  pro·cess of sphe·noid bone
ham·u·li
ham·u·lus
  h. co·chle·ae
  lac·ri·mal h.
  pter·y·goid h.
Hancock's
  am·pu·ta·tion
hand
  ec·ze·ma
  ra·ti·o
hand
  ac·cou·cheur's h.
  ape h.
  claw h.
  cleft h.

  club h.
  crab h.
  drop h.
  flat h.
  ghoul h.
  Marinesco's suc·cu·lent h.
  ob·stet·ri·cal h.
  op·e·ra-glass h.
  skel·e·ton h.
  spade h.
  split h.
  trench h.
  tri·dent h.
  writ·ing h.
hand-and-foot
  syn·drome
hand·ed·ness
hand-foot-and-mouth
  dis·ease
hand-foot-and-mouth dis·ease
  vi·rus
hand·i·cap
hand·piece
Hand-Schüller-Christian
  dis·ease
hang·ing
  drop
  heart
  sep·tum
hang·ing-block
  cul·ture
hang·man's
  frac·ture
hang·nail
Hanhart's
  syn·drome
Hanks
  di·la·tors
Hanks'
  so·lu·tion
Hannover's
  ca·nal
Hanot's
  cir·rho·sis
Hansemann
  mac·ro·phage
Hansen's
  ba·cil·lus
  dis·ease
Han·taan
  vi·rus
hap·a·lo·nych·ia
haph·al·ge·sia
haph·e·pho·bia
hap·lo·dont
hap·loid
hap·lol·o·gy
hap·lo·pro·tein

hap·lo·scope
  mir·ror h.
hap·lo·scop·ic
  vi·sion
Hap·lo·spo·rid·ia
hap·lo·type
hap·py pup·pet
  syn·drome
Hapsburg
  jaw and lip
  lip
hap·ten
  in·hi·bi·tion of pre·cip·i·ta·
  tion
hap·ten
  con·ju·gat·ed h.
hap·tics
hap·to·dys·pho·ria
hap·to·glo·bin
hap·tom·e·ter
Harada's
  dis·ease
  syn·drome
hard
  cat·a·ract
  chan·cre
  corn
  pal·ate
  pap·il·lo·ma
  par·af·fin
  pulse
  rays
  soap
  sore
  tis·sue
  tu·ber·cle
  ul·cer
  wa·ter
hard·ened
  pel·vis
Harden-Young
  es·ter
har·de·ri·an
  gland
Harder's
  gland
Harding-Passey
  mel·a·no·ma
hard·ness
  scale
hard·ness
  in·den·ta·tion h.
hard pad
  dis·ease
  vi·rus
Hardy-Rand-Ritter
  test

Hardy-Weinberg
  equi·lib·ri·um
  law
hare·lip
hare's
  eye
har·le·quin
  fe·tus
  re·ac·tion
har·ma·line
har·mi·dine
har·mine
har·mo·nia
har·mon·ic
  mean
  su·ture
har·mo·ni·ous
  cor·re·spon·dence
har·mo·ny
  func·tion·al oc·clu·sal h.
  oc·clu·sal h.
har·pax·o·pho·bia
har·poon
Harrington-Flocks
  test
Harris
  test
Harris'
  he·ma·tox·y·lin
  lines
  mi·graine
Harrison's
  groove
Harris and Ray
  test
Hartel
  tech·nique
Hart·man·nel·la
Hartmann's
  cu·rette
  op·er·a·tion
  pouch
  so·lu·tion
Hartman's
  so·lu·tion
Hartnup
  dis·ease
  syn·drome
harts·horn
har·vest bug
har·vest·er
  ant
has·a·mi·ya·mi
Häser's
  for·mu·la
Hashimoto's
  dis·ease

Hashimoto's *(continued)*
  stru·ma
  thy·roid·i·tis
hash·ish
Hasner's
  fold
  valve
Hassall-Henle
  bod·ies
Hassall's
  bod·ies
Hassall's con·cen·tric
  cor·pus·cles
Hasselbalch's
  equa·tion
hatch·et
  ex·ca·va·tor
hatch·et
Haubenfelder
Hauch
Haudek's
  niche
haus·to·ria
haus·to·ri·um
haus·tra
haus·tral
haus·tra·tion
haus·trum
haus·tus
Haverhill
  fe·ver
Ha·ver·hil·lia mul·ti·for·mis
Havers'
  glands
ha·ver·si·an
  ca·nals
  la·mel·la
  spac·es
  sys·tem
haw·kin·sin
haw·kin·si·nu·ria
Hawley
  ap·pli·ance
  re·tain·er
Haworth con·for·ma·tion·al for·
mu·las of cy·clic
  sug·ars
Haworth per·spec·tive and con·
for·ma·tion·al
  for·mu·las
Haworth per·spec·tive for·mu·
las of cy·clic
  sug·ars
hay
  asth·ma
  ba·cil·lus
  fe·ver

Hayem's
  he·ma·to·blast
  so·lu·tion
Hayem-Widal
  ane·mia
  syn·drome
Hayflick's
  lim·it
Haygarth's
  nodes
  no·dos·i·ties
ha·zel·wort
He
  an·ti·gens
head
  bot·flies
  cap
  cav·i·ty
  fold
  kid·ney
  mir·ror
  nurse
  pre·sen·ta·tion
  pro·cess
  tet·a·nus
  trem·ors
head
  bull·dog h.
  deep h.
  h. of ep·i·did·y·mis
  h. of fe·mur
  h. of fib·u·la
  hour·glass h.
  hu·mer·al h.
  hu·mer·o·ul·nar h.
  h. of hu·mer·us
  lat·er·al h.
  lit·tle h. of hu·mer·us
  long h.
  h. of mal·le·us
  h. of man·di·ble
  Medusa h.
  h. of met·a·car·pal bone
  h. of met·a·tar·sal bone
  ob·lique h.
  h. of pan·cre·as
  h. of pha·lanx
  ra·di·al h.
  h. of ra·di·us
  h. of rib
  sad·dle h.
  short h.
  h. of sta·pes
  su·per·fi·cial h.
  swelled h.
  h. of ta·lus
  h. of thigh bone
  trans·verse h.

h. of ul·na
ul·nar h.
head·ache
  bil·ious h.
  blind h.
  clus·ter h.
  fi·bro·sit·ic h.
  his·ta·min·ic h.
  Horton's h.
  mi·graine h.
  nod·u·lar h.
  or·gan·ic h.
  re·flex h.
  sick h.
  spi·nal h.
  symp·to·mat·ic h.
  ten·sion h.
  vac·u·um h.
  vas·cu·lar h.
head-bob·bing doll
  syn·drome
head-drop·ping
  test
head·gear
head·gut
head-nod·ding
Head's
  ar·e·as
  lines
  zones
head-tilt
heal
healed
  tu·ber·cu·lo·sis
  ul·cer
heal·er
heal·ing
  faith h.
  h. by first in·ten·tion
  h. by sec·ond in·ten·tion
  h. by third in·ten·tion
health
  men·tal h.
  pub·lic h.
health
  care
healthy
Heaney's
  op·er·a·tion
hear
hear·ing
  col·or h.
  nor·mal h.
hear·ing
  lev·el
hear·ing aid
hear·ing im·pair·ment

hear·ing loss
heart
  ar·mored h.
  ar·ti·fi·cial h.
  ath·let·ic h.
  beer h.
  bony h.
  drop h.
  fat·ty h.
  frost·ed h.
  hairy h.
  hang·ing h.
  hor·i·zon·tal h.
  hy·po·plas·tic h.
  ic·ing h.
  in·ter·me·di·ate h.
  ir·ri·ta·ble h.
  left h.
  lux·us h.
  mov·a·ble h.
  myx·e·de·ma h.
  parch·ment h.
  pen·du·lous h.
  pul·mo·nary h.
  right h.
  sa·bot h.
  sem·i·hor·i·zon·tal h.
  sem·i·ver·ti·cal h.
  skin h.
  sol·dier's h.
  stone h.
  sus·pend·ed h.
  sys·tem·ic h.
  tear·drop h.
  ti·ger h.
  to·bac·co h.
  ve·nous h.
  ver·ti·cal h.
  wood·en-shoe h.
heart
  an·ti·gen
  block
  fail·ure
  hor·mone
  po·si·tion
  rate
  re·flex
  sac
  sound
  stroke
  trans·plan·ta·tion
heart·beat
heart·burn
heart fail·ure
  cell
heart-hand
  syn·drome

heart-lung
  ma·chine
  prep·a·ra·tion
heart-shaped
  pel·vis
  uter·us
heart·wa·ter
heart·worm
heat
  atom·ic h.
  h. of com·bus·tion
  h. of com·pres·sion
  con·duc·tive h.
  con·vec·tive h.
  con·ver·sive h.
  h. of crys·tal·li·za·tion
  h. of dis·so·ci·a·tion
  h. of evap·o·ra·tion
  h. of for·ma·tion
  in·i·tial h.
  la·tent h.
  mo·lec·u·lar h.
  prick·ly h.
  ra·di·ant h.
  sen·si·ble h.
  h. of so·lu·tion
  spe·cif·ic h.
  h. of va·por·i·za·tion
heat
  ap·o·plexy
  ca·pac·i·ty
  cramps
  ede·ma
  ex·haus·tion
  hy·per·py·rex·ia
  lamp
  pros·tra·tion
  rash
  rig·or
  stroke
  treat·ment
  ur·ti·car·ia
heat co·ag·u·la·tion
  test
heat-cur·ing
  res·in
heat in·sta·bil·i·ty
  test
heat-la·bile
heat-ri·gor
  point
heat·stroke
heaves
heavy
  chain
  eye
  hy·dro·gen
  ni·tro·gen

  ox·y·gen
  wa·ter
heavy chain
  dis·ease
heavy liq·uid
  pe·tro·la·tum
Heb·e·lo·ma
he·be·phre·nia
he·be·phren·ic
  de·men·tia
  schiz·o·phre·nia
Heberden's
  an·gi·na
  nodes
  no·dos·i·ties
he·bet·ic
  cough
heb·e·tude
he·bi·at·rics
Hebra's
  dis·ease
  pru·ri·go
hec·a·ter·o·mer·ic
hec·a·tom·er·al
hec·a·to·mer·ic
Hecht's
  pneu·mo·nia
Heck's
  dis·ease
hec·tic
  flush
hec·to·gram
hec·to·li·ter
hed·e·o·ma
hed·er·i·form
  end·ing
he·do·no·pho·bia
hed·ro·cele
Hedström
  file
heel
  bone
  fly
  jar
  tap
  ten·don
heel
  con·tract·ed h.
  cracked h.
  grease h.
  pain·ful h.
  prom·i·nent h.
heel-tap
  re·ac·tion
  test
Heerfordt's
  dis·ease

Hegar's
di·la·tors
sign
Hegglin's
anom·a·ly
syn·drome
Hehner
num·ber
Heidenhain
pouch
Heidenhain's
cres·cents
dem·i·lunes
law
Heidenhain's azan
stain
Heidenhain's iron he·ma·tox·y·lin
stain
height of
con·tour
height
ver·ti·go
height
an·te·ri·or fa·cial h.
h. of con·tour
cusp h.
fa·cial h.
na·sal h.
or·bi·tal h.
height-length
in·dex
Heilbronner's
thigh
Heim-Kreysig
sign
Heimlich
ma·neu·ver
Heineke-Mikulicz
py·lo·ro·plas·ty
Heine's
op·er·a·tion
Heinz
bod·ies
Heinz body
test
Heinz-Ehrlich
body
Heister's
di·ver·tic·u·lum
valve
HeLa
cells
Helbings'
sign
hel·co·me·nia
hel·co·plas·ty

Held's
bun·dle
de·cus·sa·tion
he·li·an·thine
hel·i·cal
hel·i·ces
hel·i·cine
ar·tery
hel·i·coid
cho·roi·dop·a·thy
gin·gly·mus
hel·i·co·pod
gait
hel·i·co·po·dia
hel·i·co·tre·ma
he·li·en·ceph·a·li·tis
Helie's
bun·dle
he·li·o·aer·o·ther·a·py
he·li·op·a·thy
he·li·o·pho·bia
he·li·o·sis
he·li·o·tax·is
he·li·ot·ro·pism
He·li·o·zo·ea
he·li·um
speech
he·lix
DNA h.
dou·ble h.
Pauling-Corey h.
twin h.
Watson-Crick h.
hel·le·bore
hel·leb·o·rin
hel·le·bor·ism
hel·leb·o·rus
Heller
op·er·a·tion
Heller's
plex·us
Hellin's
law
Helly's
fix·a·tive
hel·met
cell
Helmholtz
the·o·ry of ac·com·mo·da·tion
the·o·ry of col·or vi·sion
the·o·ry of hear·ing
Helmholtz' ax·is
lig·a·ment
Helmholtz-Gibbs
the·o·ry
hel·minth
hel·min·tha·gogue

hel·min·them·e·sis
hel·min·thi·a·sis
hel·min·thic
   dys·en·tery
hel·min·thism
hel·min·thoid
hel·min·thol·o·gy
hel·min·tho·ma
hel·min·tho·pho·bia
Hel·min·tho·spo·ri·um
hel·min·tic
He·lo·der·ma
he·lo·ma
   h. du·rum
   h. mol·le
he·lo·sis
he·lot·o·my
help·er
   cell
   vi·rus
Hel·vel·la es·cu·len·ta
Helweg-Larssen
   syn·drome
Helweg's
   bun·dle
he·ma·chro·ma·to·sis
he·ma·chrome
he·ma·chro·sis
he·ma·cy·tom·e·ter
he·ma·cy·to·zo·on
he·ma·do·ste·no·sis
he·ma·drom·e·ter
he·ma·dro·mo·graph
he·ma·dro·mom·e·ter
he·mad·sorp·tion
he·mad·sorp·tion vi·rus
   test
he·ma·dy·na·mom·e·ter
he·ma·fa·ci·ent
he·mag·glu·ti·nat·ing cold
   au·to·an·ti·body
he·mag·glu·ti·na·tion
   in·hi·bi·tion
he·mag·glu·ti·na·tion
   pas·sive h.
   re·verse pas·sive h.
   vi·ral h.
he·mag·glu·ti·nin
he·ma·gog·ic
he·ma·gogue
he·mal
   arch·es
   gland
   node
   spine
he·mal·um
he·mam·e·bi·a·sis
he·ma·nal·y·sis

he·man·gi·ec·ta·sia
he·man·gi·ec·ta·sis
he·man·gi·ec·tat·ic
   hy·per·tro·phy
he·man·gi·o·blast
he·man·gi·o·blas·to·ma
he·man·gi·o·en·do·the·li·o·
   blas·to·ma
he·man·gi·o·en·do·the·li·o·ma
   h. tu·be·ro·sum mul·ti·plex
he·man·gi·o·fi·bro·ma
   ju·ve·nile h.
he·man·gi·o·ma
   ar·te·ri·al h.
   cap·il·lary h.
   cav·ern·ous h.
   h. con·ge·ni·tal·le
   h. pla·num ex·ten·sum
   rac·e·mose h.
   scle·ros·ing h.
   se·nile h.
   h. sim·plex
   ver·ru·cous h.
he·man·gi·o·ma-throm·bo·cy·to·
   pe·nia
   syn·drome
he·man·gi·o·ma·to·sis
he·man·gi·o·per·i·cy·to·ma
he·man·gi·o·sar·co·ma
he·ma·phe·ic
he·ma·phe·in
he·ma·phe·ism
he·mar·thron
he·mar·thros
he·mar·thro·sis
he·ma·stron·ti·um
he·ma·ta·chom·e·ter
he·mat·ap·os·te·ma
he·ma·te·in
   Ba·ker's ac·id h.
he·ma·tem·e·sis
he·mat·en·ceph·a·lon
he·ma·ther·a·py
he·ma·therm
he·ma·ther·mal
he·ma·ther·mous
he·mat·hi·dro·sis
he·ma·tho·rax
he·mat·ic
he·ma·tid
he·ma·ti·dro·sis
he·ma·tim·e·ter
hem·a·tin
   h. chlo·ride
   re·duced h.
he·ma·ti·ne·mia
hem·a·tin·ic
   prin·ci·ple

he·ma·to·bil·ia
he·ma·to·bi·um
he·ma·to·blast
   Hayem's h.
he·ma·to·cele
   pel·vic h.
   pu·den·dal h.
he·ma·to·ce·lia
hem·a·to·ceph·a·ly
he·ma·to·che·zia
he·ma·to·chlo·rin
he·ma·to·chy·lu·ria
he·ma·to·col·po·me·tra
he·ma·to·col·pos
he·mat·o·crit
he·ma·toc·ry·al
he·ma·to·cyst
he·ma·to·cys·tis
he·ma·to·cyte
he·ma·to·cy·to·blast
he·ma·to·cy·tol·y·sis
he·ma·to·cy·tom·e·ter
he·ma·to·cy·to·zo·on
he·ma·to·cy·tu·ria
he·ma·to·dys·cra·sia
he·ma·to·dys·tro·phy
he·ma·to·gen·e·sis
he·ma·to·ge·net·ic
   cal·cu·lus
he·ma·to·gen·ic
he·ma·tog·e·nous
   ab·scess
   em·bo·lism
   jaun·dice
   os·te·i·tis
   pig·ment
   the·o·ry of en·do·me·tri·o·sis
he·ma·tog·e·nous me·tas·ta·sis
he·ma·to·his·ti·o·blast
he·ma·to·his·ton
he·ma·toid
he·ma·toi·din
   crys·tals
he·ma·tol·o·gist
he·ma·tol·o·gy
he·ma·to·lymph·an·gi·o·ma
he·ma·tol·y·sis
he·ma·to·lyt·ic
he·ma·to·ma
   h. au·ris
   cor·pus lu·te·um h.
   ep·i·du·ral h.
   in·tra·cra·ni·al h.
   in·tra·mu·ral h.
   sub·du·ral h.
he·ma·to·ma·nom·e·ter
he·ma·to·me·tra

he·ma·tom·e·try
he·mat·om·pha·lo·cele
he·ma·to·my·e·lia
he·ma·to·my·e·lo·pore
he·ma·ton·ic
he·ma·to·pa·thol·o·gy
he·ma·top·a·thy
he·ma·to·pe·nia
he·ma·to·pha·gia
he·ma·toph·a·gous
he·ma·toph·a·gus
he·ma·to·phil·ia
he·ma·to·plas·tic
he·ma·to·poi·e·sis
he·ma·to·poi·et·ic
   gland
   sys·tem
he·ma·to·poi·e·tin
he·ma·to·por·phyr·ia
he·ma·to·por·phy·rin
he·ma·to·por·phy·ri·ne·mia
he·ma·to·por·phy·rin·u·ria
he·ma·top·sia
he·ma·tor·rha·chis
   h. ex·ter·na
   ex·tra·du·ral h.
   h. in·ter·na
   sub·du·ral h.
he·ma·to·sal·pinx
he·ma·to·sep·sis
he·ma·to·sin
he·ma·to·sis
he·ma·to·spec·tro·scope
he·ma·to·spec·tros·co·py
he·ma·to·sper·mat·o·cele
he·ma·to·sper·mia
he·ma·to·stat·ic
he·ma·to·stax·is
he·ma·tos·te·on
he·ma·to·ther·mal
he·ma·to·tox·ic
he·ma·to·tox·in
he·ma·to·trach·e·los
he·ma·to·tro·pic
he·ma·to·tym·pa·num
he·ma·tox·ic
he·ma·tox·in
he·ma·tox·y·lin
   Boehmer's h.
   Delafield's h.
   Harris' h.
   iron h.
   phos·pho·tung·stic ac·id h.
he·ma·tox·y·lin
   bod·ies
he·ma·tox·y·lin and eo·sin
   stain

he·ma·tox·y·lin-mal·a·chite
green-ba·sic fuch·sin
stain
he·ma·tox·y·lin-phlox·ine B
stain
he·ma·tox·y·phil
bod·ies
he·ma·to·zo·ic
he·ma·to·zo·on
he·ma·tu·re·sis
he·ma·tu·ria
an·gi·o·neu·rot·ic h.
Egyp·tian h.
en·dem·ic h.
es·sen·tial h.
false h.
gross h.
in·i·tial h.
mi·cro·scop·ic h.
pain·ful h.
pain·less h.
re·nal h.
ter·mi·nal h.
to·tal h.
ure·thral h.
ves·i·cal h.
he·ma·tu·ric bil·ious
fe·ver
heme
hem·el·y·tro·me·tra
he·men·do·the·li·o·ma
hem·er·a·lo·pia
hem·er·a·no·pia
he·me·ryth·rins
hem·i·a·car·di·us
hem·i·ac·e·tal
hem·i·ac·ro·so·mia
hem·i·a·geu·sia
hem·i·a·geus·tia
hem·i·al·gia
hem·i·a·my·os·the·nia
hem·i·an·al·ge·sia
hem·i·an·en·ceph·a·ly
hem·i·an·es·the·sia
al·ter·nate h.
crossed h.
hem·i·a·no·pia
hem·i·a·nop·ic
sco·to·ma
spec·ta·cles
hem·i·a·nop·sia
ab·so·lute h.
al·ti·tu·di·nal h.
bi·lat·er·al h.
bi·na·sal h.
bin·oc·u·lar h.
bi·tem·po·ral h.
com·plete h.

con·gru·ous h.
crossed h.
het·er·on·y·mous h.
ho·mon·y·mous h.
in·com·plete h.
in·con·gru·ous h.
pseudo-h.
quad·ran·tic h.
rel·a·tive h.
uni·lat·e·ral h.
uni·oc·u·lar h.
hem·i·a·nop·tic
hem·i·an·os·mia
hem·i·a·pla·sia
hem·i·a·prax·ia
hem·i-ar·thro·plas·ty
hem·i·a·sy·ner·gia
hem·i·a·tax·ia
hem·i·ath·e·to·sis
hem·i·at·ro·phy
fa·cial h.
pro·gress·ive lin·gual h.
hem·i·az·y·gos
vein
hem·i·bal·lism
hem·i·bal·lis·mus
hem·i·block
he·mic
cal·cu·lus
dis·to·mi·a·sis
mur·mur
hem·i·car·dia
h. dex·tra
h. si·nis·tra
hem·i·cel·lu·lose
hem·i·cen·trum
hem·i·ceph·a·lal·gia
hem·i·ce·pha·lia
hem·i·cer·e·brum
Hem·i·chor·da
Hem·i·chor·da·ta
hem·i·cho·rea
hem·i·chro·mo·some
hem·i·col·ec·to·my
hem·i·cor·po·rec·to·my
hem·i·cra·nia
hem·i·cra·ni·ec·to·my
hem·i·cra·ni·o·sis
hem·i·cra·ni·ot·o·my
hem·i·des·mo·somes
hem·i·di·a·pho·re·sis
hem·i·dro·sis
hem·i·dys·es·the·sia
hem·i·dys·tro·phy
hem·i·ec·tro·me·lia
hem·i·ep·i·lep·sy
hem·i·fa·cial
hem·i·gas·trec·to·my

hem·i·geu·sia
hem·i·glo·bin
hem·i·glos·sal
hem·i·glos·sec·to·my
hem·i·glos·si·tis
hem·i·gna·thia
hem·i·hep·a·tec·to·my
hem·i·hi·dro·sis
hem·i·hy·dran·en·ceph·a·ly
hem·i·hyp·al·ge·sia
hem·i·hy·per·es·the·sia
hem·i·hy·per·hi·dro·sis
hem·i·hy·per·i·dro·sis
hem·i·hy·per·to·nia
hem·i·hy·per·tro·phy
hem·i·hyp·es·the·sia
hem·i·hy·po·es·the·sia
hem·i·hy·po·to·nia
hem·i·kar·y·on
hem·i·ke·tal
hem·i·lam·i·nec·to·my
hem·i·lar·yn·gec·to·my
hem·i·lat·er·al
   cho·rea
hem·i·le·sion
hem·i·lin·gual
hem·i·mac·ro·glos·sia
hem·i·man·dib·u·lec·to·my
hem·i·me·tab·o·lous
he·min
hem·i·o·pal·gia
hem·ip·a·gus
hem·i·par·an·es·the·sia
hem·i·par·a·ple·gia
hem·i·pa·re·sis
hem·i·pel·vec·to·my
hem·i·ple·gia
   al·ter·nat·ing h.
   con·tra·lat·er·al h.
   crossed h.
   dou·ble h.
   fa·cial h.
   Gubler's h.
   in·fan·tile h.
   spas·tic h.
hem·i·ple·gic
   amy·ot·ro·phy
   gait
   mi·graine
He·mip·tera
hem·i·py·o·ne·phro·sis
hem·i·sec·tion
hem·i·sen·so·ry
hem·i·sep·tum
hem·i·spasm
hem·i·sphere
   cer·e·bel·lar h.

   ce·re·bral h.
   dom·i·nant h.
hem·i·spher·ec·to·my
hem·i·sphe·ri·um
   h. bul·bi ure·thrae
Hem·i·spo·ra
hem·i·stru·mec·to·my
hem·i·sul·fur
   mus·tard
hem·i·syn·drome
hem·i·sys·to·le
hem·i·ter·pene
hem·i·ther·mo·an·es·the·sia
hem·i·tho·rac·ic
   duct
hem·i·tho·rax
hem·i·to·nia
hem·i·trem·or
hem·i·ver·te·bra
hem·i·zy·gos·i·ty
hem·i·zy·gote
hem·i·zy·got·ic
hem·i·zy·gous
hem·lock
he·mo·ag·glu·ti·na·tion
he·mo·ag·glu·ti·nin
he·mo·an·ti·tox·in
He·mo·bar·ton·el·la
he·mo·bil·ia
he·mo·blast
   lym·phoid h. of Pappenheim
he·mo·blas·to·sis
he·mo·ca·thar·sis
he·mo·cath·e·re·sis
he·mo·cath·e·re·tic
he·moc·cult
   test
he·mo·cele
he·mo·cho·le·cyst
he·mo·cho·le·cys·ti·tis
he·mo·cho·ri·al
   pla·cen·ta
he·mo·chro·ma·to·sis
   ex·og·e·nous h.
   he·red·i·tary h.
   id·i·o·path·ic h.
   pri·mary h.
   sec·on·dary h.
he·mo·chrome
he·mo·chro·mo·gen
he·mo·cla·sia
he·moc·la·sis
he·mo·clas·tic
   re·ac·tion
he·mo·con·cen·tra·tion
he·mo·co·nia
he·mo·co·ni·o·sis
he·mo·cry·os·co·py

he·mo·cu·pre·in
he·mo·cy·a·nin
he·mo·cyte
he·mo·cy·to·blast
he·mo·cy·to·ca·ther·e·sis
he·mo·cy·tol·y·sis
he·mo·cy·tom·e·ter
he·mo·cy·tom·e·try
he·mo·cy·to·trip·sis
he·mo·cy·to·zo·on
he·mo·di·ag·no·sis
he·mo·di·al·y·sis
he·mo·di·a·lyz·er
   ul·tra·fil·tra·tion h.
he·mo·di·a·stase
he·mo·di·lu·tion
he·mo·drom·o·graph
he·mo·dro·mom·e·ter
he·mo·dy·nam·ic
he·mo·dy·nam·ics
he·mo·dy·na·mom·e·ter
he·mo·dys·cra·sia
he·mo·dys·tro·phy
he·mo·en·do·the·li·al
   pla·cen·ta
he·mo·fil·tra·tion
he·mo·flag·el·lates
he·mo·fus·cin
he·mo·gen·e·sis
he·mo·gen·ic
he·mo·glo·bin
   h. A
   h. A_{Ic}
   ab·er·rant h.
   h. Bart's
   bile pig·ment h.
   h. C
   h. $C_{George·town}$
   h. $C_{Har·lem}$
   car·bon mon·ox·ide h.
   h. Ches·a·peake
   h. $D_{Pun·jab}$
   h. E
   h. F
   fe·tal h.
   gly·co·syl·at·ed h.
   green h.
   h. H
   h. I
   h. $J_{Cape·town}$
   h. Kan·sas
   h. Le·pore
   h. M
   mean cell h.
   mus·cle h.
   ox·y·gen·at·ed h.
   h. Rai·nier
   re·duced h.

   h. S
   sick·le cell h.
   un·sta·ble h.'s
   var·i·ant h.
   h. Yak·i·ma
he·mo·glo·bin C
   dis·ease
he·mo·glo·bi·ne·mia
   h. pa·ra·ly·ti·ca
   pu·er·per·al h.
he·mo·glo·bin H
   dis·ease
he·mo·glo·bi·no·cho·lia
he·mo·glo·bi·nol·y·sis
he·mo·glo·bi·nop·a·thy
he·mo·glo·bi·no·pep·sia
he·mo·glo·bi·no·phil·ic
he·mo·glo·bi·nu·ria
   bo·vine h.
   ep·i·dem·ic h.
   ma·lar·i·al h.
   march h.
   par·ox·ys·mal noc·tur·nal h.
   post·par·tu·ri·ent h.
   pu·er·per·al h.
   tox·ic h.
he·mo·glo·bi·nu·ric
   fe·ver
   ne·phro·sis
he·mo·gram
he·mo·his·ti·o·blast
he·mo·la·mel·la
he·mo·leu·ko·cyte
he·mo·li·pase
he·mo·lith
he·mol·o·gy
he·mo·lymph
   gland
   node
he·mol·y·sate
he·mo·ly·sin
   bac·te·ri·al h.
   cold h.
   het·er·o·phil h.
   im·mune h.
   nat·u·ral h.
   spe·cif·ic h.
   warm-cold h.
he·mo·ly·sin
   unit
he·mo·ly·sin·o·gen
he·mol·y·sis
   bi·o·log·ic h.
   con·di·tioned h.
   im·mune h.
   ven·om h.
   vir·i·dans h.

he·mo·lyt·ic
  ane·mia
  ane·mia of new·born
  chain
  dis·ease of new·born
  gas
  jaun·dice
  sple·no·meg·a·ly
  strep·to·coc·ci
  unit
he·mo·lyt·ic ure·mic
  syn·drome
he·mo·ly·za·tion
he·mo·lyze
he·mo·ma·nom·e·ter
he·mo·me·di·as·ti·num
he·mo·me·tra
he·mom·e·try
he·mon·cho·sis
he·mo·ne·phro·sis
he·mo·pa·thol·o·gy
he·mop·a·thy
he·mo·per·fu·sion
he·mo·per·i·car·di·um
he·mo·per·i·to·ne·um
he·mo·pex·in
he·mo·pha·gia
he·mo·phag·o·cy·to·sis
he·mo·phil
he·mo·phile
he·mo·phil·ia
  h. A.
  h. B.
  re·nal h.
  vas·cu·lar h.
he·mo·phil·i·ac
he·mo·phil·ic
  ar·thri·tis
  joint
He·moph·i·lus
he·mo·pho·bia
he·mo·pho·re·sis
he·moph·thal·mia
he·moph·thal·mus
he·moph·thi·sis
he·mo·plas·tic
he·mo·plas·ty
he·mo·pneu·mo·per·i·car·di·um
he·mo·pneu·mo·tho·rax
he·mo·poi·e·sis
he·mo·poi·et·ic
  tis·sue
he·mo·poi·e·tin
he·mo·por·phy·rin
he·mo·pre·cip·i·tin
he·mo·pro·tein
he·mop·ty·sis
  car·di·ac h.

en·dem·ic h.
par·a·sit·ic h.
he·mo·py·el·ec·ta·sia
he·mo·py·el·ec·ta·sis
he·mo·re·pel·lant
he·mo·rhe·ol·o·gy
he·mor·rha·chis
hem·or·rhage
  brain·stem h.
  ce·re·bral h.
  con·cealed h.
  ex·tra·du·ral h.
  gas·tric h.
  in·ter·me·di·ate h.
  in·ter·nal h.
  in·tes·ti·nal h.
  in·tra·ce·re·bral h.
  in·tra·cra·ni·al h.
  in·tra·par·tum h.
  in·tra·ven·tric·u·lar h.
  na·sal h.
  par·en·chym·a·tous h.
  h. per rhex·is
  pe·te·chi·al h.
  pon·tine h.
  post·par·tum h.
  pri·mary h.
  punc·tate h.
  re·nal h.
  sec·on·dary h.
  se·rous h.
  splin·ter h.
  sub·a·rach·noid h.
  sub·du·ral h.
  sub·ga·le·al h.
  sy·rin·go·my·el·ic h.
  un·a·void·a·ble h.
hem·or·rha·gen·ic
hem·or·rhag·ic
  ane·mia
  as·ci·tes
  bron·chi·tis
  co·li·tis
  cyst
  den·gue
  di·ath·e·sis
  dis·ease of deer
  dis·ease of the new·born
  en·do·vas·cu·li·tis
  fe·ver
  fe·ver with re·nal syn·
    drome
  gan·grene
  glau·co·ma
  in·farct
  iri·tis
  mea·sles
  ne·phri·tis

hem·or·rhag·ic *(continued)*
  pach·y·men·in·gi·tis
  pi·an
  plague
  pleu·ri·sy
  rick·ets
  sep·ti·ce·mia
  shock
  small·pox
hem·or·rhag·ic ex·ud·a·tive
  er·y·the·ma
hem·or·rhag·ins
hem·or·rha·gip·a·rous
hem·or·rhea
hem·or·rhoid
hem·or·rhoi·dal
  nerves
  plex·us
  veins
hem·or·rhoid·ec·to·my
hem·or·rhoids
  cu·ta·ne·ous h.
  ex·ter·nal h.
  in·ter·nal h.
he·mo·sal·pinx
he·mo·si·al·em·e·sis
he·mo·sid·er·in
he·mo·sid·er·o·sis
  id·i·o·path·ic pul·mo·nary
    h.
  nu·trit·ion·al h.
  pul·mo·nary h.
he·mo·sper·mia
  h. spu·ria
  h. ve·ra
he·mo·spo·rid·i·um
he·mo·spo·rines
he·mo·sta·sia
he·mo·sta·sis
he·mo·stat
he·mo·stat·ic
  col·lo·di·on
  for·ceps
he·mo·styp·tic
he·mo·ta·chom·e·ter
he·mo·ther·a·peu·tics
he·mo·ther·a·py
he·mo·tho·rax
he·mo·thy·mia
he·mo·tox·ic
  ane·mia
he·mo·tox·in
  co·bra h.
he·mo·troph
he·mot·ro·phe
he·mo·tro·pic
he·mo·tym·pa·num
he·mo·zo·ic

he·mo·zo·on
HEMPAS
  cells
hem·u·re·sis
hen·bane
hen-cluck
  ster·tor
Henderson-Hasselbalch
  equa·tion
Hen·der·so·nu·la to·ru·loi·dea
Henke's
  space
Henle's
  am·pul·la
  an·sa
  fis·sures
  glands
  lay·er
  loop
  mem·brane
  re·ac·tion
  sheath
  spine
  tu·bules
  warts
Henle's fen·es·trat·ed elas·tic
  mem·brane
Henle's fi·ber
  lay·er
Henle's ner·vous
  lay·er
hen·na
Henoch's
  cho·rea
  pur·pu·ra
Henoch-Schönlein
  pur·pu·ra
  syn·drome
hen·pu·ye
hen·ry
Henry-Gauer
  re·sponse
Henry's
  law
Hensen's
  ca·nal
  cell
  disk
  duct
  knot
  line
  node
  stripe
Hensing's
  lig·a·ment
HEP
  vac·cine

he·par
  h. lo·ba·tum
hep·a·ran sul·fate
hep·a·rin
  h. elim·i·nase
  h. ly·ase
  h. so·di·um
hep·a·rin
  unit
hep·a·rin·ase
hep·a·ri·ne·mia
hep·a·rin·ic ac·id
hep·a·rin·ize
hep·a·rit·in sul·fate
hep·a·tal·gia
hep·a·ta·tro·phia
hep·a·tat·ro·phy
hep·a·tec·to·my
he·pa·tic
  am·e·bi·a·sis
  cap·su·li·tis
  col·ic
  co·ma
  cords
  cysts
  duct
  en·ceph·a·lop·a·thy
  fis·tu·la
  flex·ure
  in·fan·ti·lism
  in·suf·fi·cien·cy
  lam·i·nae
  lob·ule
  plex·us
  por·phyr·ia
  prom·i·nence
  seg·ments
  ste·a·to·sis
  tri·ad
  veins
he·pa·tic in·ter·mit·tent
  fe·ver
he·pa·tic lymph
  nodes
he·pat·i·co·do·chot·o·my
he·pat·i·co·du·o·de·nos·to·my
he·pat·i·co·en·ter·os·to·my
he·pat·i·co·gas·tros·to·my
he·pat·i·co·li·thot·o·my
he·pat·i·co·lith·o·trip·sy
he·pat·i·co·pul·mo·nary
he·pat·i·cos·to·my
he·pat·i·cot·o·my
he·pa·tic por·tal
  vein
he·pa·tic ve·nous
  seg·ments
hep·a·tin

hep·a·tis
hep·a·tit·ic
hep·a·ti·tis
  h. A
  ac·tive chron·ic h.
  acute par·en·chym·a·tous h.
  an·ic·ter·ic vi·rus h.
  h. B
  chol·an·gi·o·lit·ic h.
  cho·le·stat·ic h.
  chron·ic h.
  chron·ic in·ter·sti·tial h.
  h. con·ta·gi·o·sa ca·nis
  del·ta h.
  drug-in·duced h.
  ep·i·dem·ic h.
  equine se·rum h.
  h. ex·ter·na
  gi·ant cell h.
  hal·o·thane h.
  in·fec·tious h.
  in·fec·tious ca·nine h.
  in·fec·tious ne·crot·ic h. of
    sheep
  long in·cu·ba·tion h.
  lu·poid h.
  mouse h.
  mu·rine h.
  NANB h.
  ne·o·na·tal h.
  non-A h.'s
  non-B h.
  pe·li·o·sis h.
  per·sis·tent chron·ic h.
  plas·ma cell h.
  se·rum h.
  short in·cu·ba·tion h.
  sub·a·cute h.
  sup·pu·ra·tive h.
  trans·fu·sion h.
  vi·ral h.
  vi·ral h. type A
  vi·ral h. type B
  vi·ral h. type D
  vi·rus h.
  vi·rus A h.
  vi·rus B h.
  vi·rus h. of ducks
hep·a·ti·tis A
  vi·rus
hep·a·ti·tis-as·so·ci·at·ed
  an·ti·gen
hep·a·ti·tis B
  vac·cine
  vi·rus
hep·a·ti·tis B core
  an·ti·gen

hep·a·ti·tis B e
   an·ti·gen
hep·a·ti·tis B sur·face
   an·ti·gen
hep·a·ti·tis del·ta
   vi·rus
hep·a·ti·za·tion
   gray h.
   red h.
   yel·low h.
he·pa·to·blas·to·ma
he·pa·to·car·ci·no·ma
he·pa·to·cele
he·pa·to·cel·lu·lar
   car·ci·no·ma
   jaun·dice
he·pa·to·chol·an·gi·o·en·ter·os·
   to·my
he·pa·to·chol·an·gi·o·je·ju·nos·
   to·my
he·pa·to·chol·an·gi·os·to·my
he·pa·to·chol·an·gi·tis
he·pa·to·co·lic
   lig·a·ment
he·pa·to·cu·pre·in
he·pa·to·cys·tic
   duct
He·pa·to·cys·tis
he·pa·to·cyte
he·pa·to·du·o·de·nal
   lig·a·ment
he·pa·to·du·o·de·nos·to·my
he·pa·to·dyn·ia
he·pa·to·dys·en·tery
he·pa·to·en·ter·ic
   re·cess
he·pa·to·e·soph·a·ge·al
   lig·a·ment
hep·a·to·fu·gal
he·pa·to·gas·tric
   lig·a·ment
he·pa·to·gen·ic
he·pa·tog·e·nous
   jaun·dice
   pig·ment
he·pa·tog·raphy
he·pa·to·he·mia
he·pa·toid
he·pa·to·jug·u·lar
   re·flex
   re·flux
he·pa·to·jug·u·la·rom·e·ter
he·pa·to·len·tic·u·lar
   de·gen·er·a·tion
   dis·ease
he·pa·to·li·en·og·ra·phy
he·pa·to·li·en·o·meg·a·ly
he·pa·to·lith

he·pa·to·li·thec·to·my
he·pa·to·li·thi·a·sis
he·pa·tol·o·gist
he·pa·tol·o·gy
he·pa·tol·y·sin
he·pa·to·ma
   ma·lig·nant h.
he·pa·to·ma·la·cia
he·pa·to·me·ga·lia
he·pa·to·meg·a·ly
he·pa·to·mel·a·no·sis
he·pa·tom·pha·lo·cele
he·pa·tom·pha·los
he·pa·to·ne·cro·sis
hep·a·to·ne·pho·ric
   syn·drome
he·pa·to·neph·ric
he·pa·to·neph·ro·meg·a·ly
he·pa·to·path·ic
he·pa·top·a·thy
he·pa·to·per·i·to·ni·tis
hep·a·to·pet·al
he·pa·to·pex·y
he·pa·to·phos·phor·y·lase de·fi·
   cien·cy
   gly·co·ge·no·sis
he·pa·to·phy·ma
he·pa·to·pleu·ral
   fis·tu·la
he·pa·to·pneu·mon·ic
he·pa·to·por·tal
he·pa·to·pto·sis
he·pa·to·pul·mo·nary
he·pa·to·re·nal
   lig·a·ment
   pouch
   re·cess
   syn·drome
he·pa·tor·rha·gia
he·pa·tor·rha·phy
he·pa·tor·rhea
he·pa·tor·rhex·is
he·pa·tos·co·py
he·pa·to·sple·ni·tis
he·pa·to·sple·nog·ra·phy
he·pa·to·splen·o·meg·a·ly
he·pa·to·sple·nop·a·thy
he·pa·tos·to·my
he·pa·to·ther·a·py
he·pa·tot·o·my
he·pa·to·tox·e·mia
he·pa·to·tox·ic
he·pa·to·tox·in
He·pa·to·zo·on
hep·ta·bar·bi·tal
hep·tad
hep·tam·i·nol
hep·ta·nal

hep·ta·zone hy·dro·chlo·ride
hep·tose
hep·tu·lose
D-*manno*-hep·tu·lose
her·ald
   patch
Herbert's
   op·er·a·tion
her·biv·o·rous
Herbst's
   cor·pus·cles
he·red·i·tary
   cho·rea
   he·mo·chro·ma·to·sis
   lymph·e·de·ma
   met·he·mo·glo·bi·ne·mia
   my·o·ky·mia
   ne·phri·tis
   pho·to·my·oc·lo·nus
   sphe·ro·cy·to·sis
   syph·i·lis
he·red·i·tary an·gi·o·neu·rot·ic
   ede·ma
he·red·i·tary cer·e·bel·lar
   atax·ia
he·red·i·tary de·form·ing
   chon·dro·dys·pla·sia
   chon·dro·dys·tro·phy
he·red·i·tary fruc·tose
   in·tol·er·ance
he·red·i·tary hem·or·rhag·ic
   tel·an·gi·ec·ta·sia
   throm·bas·the·nia
he·red·i·tary hy·per·tro·phic
   neu·rop·a·thy
he·red·i·tary met·he·mo·glo·bi·
  ne·mic
   cy·a·no·sis
he·red·i·tary mul·ti·ple
   ex·os·to·ses
   trich·o·ep·i·the·li·o·ma
he·red·i·tary opal·es·cent
   den·tin
he·red·i·tary pro·gress·ive
   ar·thro-oph·thal·mop·a·thy
he·red·i·tary re·nal-ret·i·nal
   dys·pla·sia
he·red·i·tary sen·so·ry ra·dic·
  u·lar
   neu·rop·a·thy
he·red·i·tary spi·nal
   atax·ia
he·red·i·ty
her·e·do·a·tax·ia
her·e·do·fa·mil·i·al
   trem·or
her·e·do·mac·u·lar
   de·gen·er·a·tion

her·e·do·path·ia atac·ti·ca pol·
  y·neu·ri·ti·for·mis
He·rel·lea
Hering-Breuer
   re·flex
Hering's
   test
   the·o·ry of col·or vi·sion
Hering's si·nus
   nerve
her·i·ta·bil·i·ty
her·i·tage
Her·litz
   syn·drome
Hermann's
   fix·a·tive
her·maph·ro·dism
her·maph·ro·dite
her·maph·ro·dit·ism
   ad·re·nal h.
   bi·lat·er·al h.
   di·mid·i·ate h.
   false h.
   fe·male h.
   lat·er·al h.
   male h.
   trans·verse h.
   true h.
   uni·lat·e·ral h.
her·met·ic
her·nia
   ab·dom·i·nal h.
   an·te·ves·i·cal h.
   Barth's h.
   Béclard's h.
   bi·loc·u·lar fem·o·ral h.
   Bochdalek's h.
   h. of the broad lig·a·ment
    of the uter·us
   ce·cal h.
   ce·re·bral h.
   Clo·quet's h.
   com·plete h.
   con·cealed h.
   con·gen·i·tal di·a·phrag·
    mat·ic h.
   Cooper's h.
   cru·ral h.
   di·a·phrag·mat·ic h.
   di·rect in·gui·nal h.
   dou·ble loop h.
   dry h.
   du·o·de·no·je·ju·nal h.
   h. en bis·sac
   ep·i·gas·tric h.
   ex·tra·sac·cu·lar h.
   fas·cial h.
   fat·ty h.

her·nia *(continued)*
  fem·o·ral h.
  gas·tro·e·soph·a·ge·al h.
  glu·te·al h.
  Hesselbach's h.
  Hey's h.
  hi·a·tal h.
  hi·a·tus h.
  Holthouse's h.
  il·i·a·co·sub·fas·cial h.
  in·car·cer·at·ed h.
  in·ci·sion·al h.
  in·di·rect in·gui·nal h.
  in·fan·tile h.
  in·gui·nal h.
  in·gui·no·cru·ral h.
  in·gui·no·fem·o·ral h.
  in·gui·no·la·bi·al h.
  in·gui·no·scro·tal h.
  in·gui·no·su·per·fi·cial h.
  in·ter·sig·moid h.
  in·ter·sti·tial h.
  in·tra·ep·i·plo·ic h.
  in·tra·il·i·ac h.
  in·tra·pel·vic h.
  ir·re·duc·i·ble h.
  is·chi·at·ic h.
  Krönlein's h.
  la·bi·al h.
  lat·er·al ven·tral h.
  Laugier's h.
  le·va·tor h.
  Littre's h.
  lum·bar h.
  Malgaigne's h.
  me·nin·ge·al h.
  mes·en·ter·ic h.
  ob·tu·ra·tor h.
  or·bi·tal h.
  pan·nic·u·lar h.
  par·a·e·soph·a·ge·al h.
  par·a·per·i·to·ne·al h.
  par·a·sac·cu·lar h.
  par·a·ster·nal h.
  pa·ri·e·tal h.
  per·i·ne·al h.
  Petit's h.
  pos·te·ri·or vag·i·nal h.
  pro·per·i·to·ne·al in·gui·nal h.
  pu·den·dal h.
  re·duc·i·ble h.
  ret·ro·grade h.
  ret·ro·per·i·to·ne·al h.
  ret·ro·pu·bic h.
  ret·ro·ster·nal h.
  Richter's h.
  Rokitansky's h.

  sci·at·ic h.
  scro·tal h.
  slid·ing h.
  slid·ing esoph·a·ge·al hi·a·tal h.
  slid·ing hi·a·tal h.
  slipped h.
  spi·ge·li·an h.
  stran·gu·lat·ed h.
  syn·o·vi·al h.
  Treitz' h.
  um·bil·i·cal h.
  Velpeau's h.
  ven·tral h.
  ves·i·cle h.
  vit·re·ous h.
  "w" h.
her·nia
  knife
her·nial
  an·eu·rysm
  sac
her·ni·at·ed
  disk
her·ni·a·tion
  cau·dal trans·ten·to·ri·al h.
  cin·gu·late h.
  fo·ram·i·nal h.
  ros·tral trans·ten·to·ri·al h.
  sphe·noi·dal h.
  sub·fal·cial h.
  ton·sil·lar h.
  trans·ten·to·ri·al h.
  un·cal h.
her·ni·o·en·ter·ot·o·my
her·ni·og·ra·phy
her·ni·oid
her·ni·o·lap·a·rot·o·my
her·ni·o·plas·ty
her·ni·o·punc·ture
her·ni·or·rha·phy
her·ni·o·tome
  Cooper's h.
her·ni·ot·o·my
  Petit's h.
he·ro·ic
her·o·in
her·pan·gi·na
her·pes
  en·ceph·a·li·tis
  vi·rus
her·pes
  h. ca·tar·rha·lis
  h. cir·ci·na·tus bul·lo·sus
  h. cor·ne·ae
  h. des·qua·mans
  h. dig·i·tal·is
  h. fa·ci·a·lis

h. fe·bri·lis
h. ge·ne·ra·li·sa·tus
gen·i·tal h.
h. gen·i·tal·is
h. ges·ta·tio·nis
h. iris
h. la·bi·a·lis
ne·o·na·tal h.
h. sim·plex
trau·mat·ic h.
h. zos·ter
h. zos·ter oph·thal·mi·cus
h. zos·ter va·ri·cel·lo·sus
her·pes sim·plex
vi·rus
Her·pes·vi·rus
H. su·is
H. var·i·cel·lae
her·pes·vi·rus
her·pes·vi·rus type 1
her·pes·vi·rus type 2
her·pes zos·ter
vi·rus
her·pet·ic
fe·ver
ker·a·ti·tis
ker·a·to·con·junc·ti·vi·tis
me·nin·go·en·ceph·a·li·tis
ul·cer
whit·low
her·pet·i·form
aph·thae
Her·pe·to·mo·nas
Her·pe·to·vir·i·dae
her·pe·to·vi·rus
ca·nine h.
cap·rine h.
Herring
bod·ies
her·ring-worm
dis·ease
Herrmann's
syn·drome
Hers'
dis·ease
her·sage
Hertwig's
sheath
hertz
hertz·i·an
ex·per·i·ments
Herxheimer's
re·ac·tion
herz
hor·mone
herz·stoss
Heschl's
gy·ri

hes·i·tan·cy
hes·per·e·tin
hes·per·i·din
Hess
screen
Hess'
test
Hesselbach's
fas·cia
her·nia
lig·a·ment
tri·an·gle
het·a·cil·lin
het·er·a·del·phus
het·er·a·kid
Het·er·a·kis
het·er·a·li·us
het·er·ax·i·al
het·er·e·cious
het·er·e·cism
het·er·es·the·sia
het·er·o·ag·glu·ti·nin
het·er·o·al·leles
het·er·o·an·ti·body
het·er·o·an·ti·se·rum
het·er·o·at·om
het·er·o·blas·tic
het·er·o·cel·lu·lar
het·er·o·cen·tric
het·er·o·ceph·a·lus
het·er·o·chei·ral
het·er·o·chi·ral
het·er·o·chro·mat·ic
het·er·o·chro·ma·tin
con·sti·tu·tive h.
fac·ul·ta·tive h.
sat·el·lite-rich h.
het·er·o·chro·mia
atroph·ic h.
bin·oc·u·lar h.
h. ir·i·dis
h. of iris
mo·noc·u·lar h.
sim·ple h.
sym·pa·thet·ic h.
het·er·o·chro·mic
cy·cli·tis
uve·i·tis
het·er·o·chro·mo·some
het·er·o·chro·mous
het·er·o·chron
het·er·o·chro·nia
het·er·o·chron·ic
het·er·och·ro·nous
het·er·o·clad·ic
anas·to·mo·sis
het·er·o·crine
het·er·o·cri·sis

het·er·o·cy·clic
  com·pound
het·er·o·cy·to·tro·pic
  an·ti·body
het·er·o·der·mic
het·er·o·dis·perse
het·er·o·dont
Het·er·o·dox·us spi·ni·ger
het·er·od·ro·mous
het·er·o·du·plex
het·er·od·y·mus
het·er·o·e·rot·ic
het·er·o·er·o·tism
het·er·o·ga·met·ic
  em·bryo
het·er·og·a·mous
het·er·og·a·my
het·er·o·ge·ne·ic
het·er·o·ge·ne·i·ty
  ge·net·ic h.
het·er·o·ge·neous
  nu·cle·a·tion
  ra·di·a·tion
  RNA
  sys·tem
het·er·o·ge·net·ic
  an·ti·body
  an·ti·gen
  par·a·site
het·er·o·gen·ic
het·er·o·gen·ic en·ter·o·bac·te·ri·al
  an·ti·gen
het·er·o·ge·note
het·er·og·e·nous
  ker·a·to·plas·ty
  vac·cine
het·er·o·graft
het·er·o·hyp·no·sis
het·er·o·kar·y·on
het·er·o·kar·y·ot·ic
het·er·o·ker·a·to·plas·ty
het·er·o·ki·ne·sia
het·er·o·ki·ne·sis
het·er·o·la·lia
het·er·o·lat·er·al
het·er·o·lip·ids
het·er·o·lit·er·al
het·er·ol·o·gous
  an·ti·se·rum
  de·sen·si·tiz·a·tion
  graft
  in·sem·i·na·tion
  pro·tein
  stim·u·lus
  tu·mor
  twins
het·er·ol·o·gy

het·er·o·ly·sin
het·er·ol·y·sis
het·er·o·lyt·ic
het·er·o·mas·ti·gote
het·er·om·er·al
het·er·o·mer·ic
  cell
  pep·tide
het·er·om·er·ous
het·er·o·me·tab·o·lous
  met·a·mor·pho·sis
het·er·o·met·a·pla·sia
het·er·o·met·ric
  au·to·reg·u·la·tion
het·er·o·me·tro·pia
het·er·o·mor·phism
het·er·o·mor·pho·sis
het·er·o·mor·phous
het·er·on·o·mous
  psy·cho·ther·a·py
het·er·on·o·my
het·er·o·nu·cle·ar
het·er·on·y·mous
  di·plo·pia
  hem·i·a·nop·sia
  im·age
  par·al·lax
het·er·o-os·te·o·plas·ty
het·er·op·a·gus
het·er·op·a·thy
het·er·oph·a·gy
het·er·o·pha·sia
het·er·o·phe·mia
het·er·o·phe·my
het·er·o·phil
  an·ti·body
  an·ti·gen
  he·mo·ly·sin
het·er·o·phile
  an·ti·body
het·er·o·pho·nia
het·er·o·pho·ria
het·er·oph·thal·mus
het·er·oph·thon·gia
Het·er·o·phy·es
  H. brev·i·cae·ca
  H. het·er·o·phy·es
  H. kat·sur·a·dai
het·er·o·phy·i·a·sis
het·er·o·phy·id
Het·er·o·phy·i·dae
het·er·o·phy·id·i·a·sis
het·er·o·pla·sia
het·er·o·plas·tic
  graft
het·er·o·plas·tid
het·er·o·plas·ty
het·er·o·ploid

het·er·o·ploi·dy
het·er·o·pol·y·sac·cha·ride
het·er·o·pro·te·ose
het·er·o·psy·cho·log·ic
het·er·o·pyk·no·sis
het·er·o·pyk·not·ic
   chro·ma·tin
het·er·o·sac·cha·ride
het·er·o·sex·u·al
het·er·o·sex·u·al·i·ty
het·er·o·sis
het·er·o·some
het·er·o·spe·cif·ic
   graft
het·er·o·sug·ges·tion
het·er·o·tax·ia
   car·di·ac h.
het·er·o·tax·ic
het·er·o·tax·is
het·er·o·taxy
het·er·o·thal·lic
het·er·o·therm
het·er·o·ther·mic
het·er·ot·ic
het·er·o·to·nia
het·er·o·to·pia
het·er·o·top·ic
   bones
   graft
   pain
   preg·nan·cy
het·er·ot·o·pous
het·er·o·trans·plan·ta·tion
het·er·o·tri·cho·sis
het·er·o·troph
het·er·o·tro·phic
het·er·o·tro·pia
   h. mac·u·lae
het·er·o·tro·pic
   chro·mo·some
het·er·ot·ro·py
het·er·o·type
   mi·to·sis
het·er·o·typ·ic
   cor·tex
het·er·o·typ·i·cal
   chro·mo·some
het·er·o·vac·cine
   ther·a·py
het·er·o·xan·thine
het·er·ox·e·nous
   par·a·site
het·er·o·zo·ic
het·er·o·zy·go·sis
het·er·o·zy·gos·i·ty
het·er·o·zy·gote
   com·pound h.
   man·i·fest·ing h.

het·er·o·zy·gous
   dou·bly h.
Heuser's
   mem·brane
hex·a·bi·one
hex·a·canth
   em·bryo
hex·a·car·ba·cho·line bro·mide
hex·a·chlo·ro·cy·clo·hex·ane
hex·a·chlo·ro·phane
hex·a·chlo·ro·phene
hex·a·co·sa·nol
hex·a·co·syl
hex·ad
hex·a·dac·tyl·ism
hex·a·dac·ty·ly
hex·a·dec·a·no·ic ac·id
hex·a·di·phane
hex·a·flu·o·ren·i·um bro·mide
hex·a·mer
hex·a·meth·one bro·mide
hex·a·me·tho·ni·um chlo·ride
hex·am·i·dine is·e·thi·o·nate
hex·a·mine
Hex·am·i·ta
hex·am·i·ti·a·sis
hex·ane
hex·a·no·ate
hex·a·no·ic ac·id
hex·a·no·yl
hex·a·ploi·dy
Hex·a·po·da
hex·ax·i·al ref·er·ence
   sys·tem
hex·a·zo·ni·um
   salts
hex·es·trol
hex·et·i·dine
hex·i·tol
hex·o·bar·bi·tal so·di·um
hex·o·ben·dine
hex·o·cyc·li·um meth·yl·sul·fate
hex·o·ki·nase
   meth·od
hex·on
   an·ti·gen
hex·one
   ba·ses
hex·on·ic ac·id
hex·os·a·mine
hex·os·a·min·i·dase
hex·o·sans
hex·ose
hex·ose bis·phos·pha·tase
hex·ose di·phos·pha·tase
hex·ose mon·o·phos·phate
   shunt
hex·ose phos·pha·tase

hex·ose·phos·phate isom·er·ase
hex·u·lose
hex·u·ron·ic ac·id
hex·yl
hex·yl·caine hy·dro·chlo·ride
hex·yl·res·or·cin·ol
Heyer-Pudenz
  valve
Heyns' ab·dom·i·nal de·com·
  pres·sion
  ap·pa·ra·tus
Hey's
  am·pu·ta·tion
  her·nia
  lig·a·ment
Hey's in·ter·nal
  de·range·ment
HFR
  strain
Hfr
  strain
HG
  fac·tor
hi·a·tal
  her·nia
hi·a·tus
  her·nia
hi·a·tus
  Breschet's h.
  h. of ca·nal for great·er
    pe·tro·sal nerve
  h. ca·na·lis fa·ci·a·lis
  h. of ca·nal of less·er pe·
    tro·sal nerve
  h. eth·moi·da·lis
  fal·lo·pi·an h.
  max·il·lary h.
  pleu·ro·per·i·car·di·al h.
  pleu·ro·per·i·to·ne·al h.
  sa·cral h.
  Scarpa's h.
  sem·i·lu·nar h.
  h. sub·ar·cu·a·tus
  h. to·ta·lis sa·cra·lis
hi·a·tus
hi·ber·nat·ing
  gland
hi·ber·na·tion
  ar·ti·fi·cial h.
hi·ber·no·ma
  in·ter·scap·u·lar h.
hic·cough
hic·cup
  ep·i·dem·ic h.
hid·den
  part
hide·bound
  dis·ease

hi·drad·e·ni·tis
  h. ax·il·la·ris of Verneuil
  h. sup·pu·ra·ti·va
hi·drad·e·no·ma
  clear cell h.
  nod·u·lar h.
  pap·il·lary h.
hi·droa
hi·dro·cys·to·ma
hi·dro·mei·o·sis
hi·dro·poi·e·sis
hi·dro·poi·et·ic
hi·dro·sad·e·ni·tis
hi·dros·che·sis
hi·dro·sis
hi·drot·ic
hi·drot·ic ec·to·der·mal
  dys·pla·sia
hi·er·ar·chy
  dom·i·nance h.
  Maslow's h.
  re·sponse h.
hi·er·o·ma·nia
hi·er·o·pho·bia
hi·er·o·ther·a·py
high
  con·vex
  en·e·ma
  li·thot·o·my
  wine
high al·ti·tude
  cham·ber
high cal·o·rie
  di·et
high-egg-pas·sage
  vac·cine
high en·do·the·li·al post·cap·
  il·lary
  ven·ules
high en·er·gy
  com·pounds
  phos·phates
high en·er·gy phos·phate
  bond
high·er or·der
  con·di·tion·ing
high·est
  con·cha
high·est in·ter·cos·tal
  ar·tery
  vein
high·est nu·chal
  line
high·est tho·rac·ic
  ar·tery
high·est tur·bi·nat·ed
  bone

high fat
di·et
high for·ceps
de·liv·ery
high fre·quen·cy
cur·rent
deaf·ness
trans·duc·tion
high lip
line
Highmore's
body
high out·put
fail·ure
high pres·sure
ox·y·gen
high-res·o·lu·tion
band·ing
high spi·nal
an·es·the·sia
high step·page
gait
Higoumenakia
sign
hi·la
hi·lar
dance
hi·lar cell
tu·mor of ova·ry
hi·li·tis
Hill
op·er·a·tion
re·ac·tion
Hillis-Müller
ma·neu·ver
hil·lock
ax·on h.
fa·cial h.
sem·i·nal h.
Hill's
equa·tion
phe·nom·e·non
sign
Hill-Sachs
le·sion
Hilton's
law
meth·od
sac
Hilton's white
line
hi·lum
h. of den·tate nu·cle·us
h. of kid·ney
h. of lung
h. of lymph node
h. lym·pho·no·di
h. of ol·i·vary nu·cle·us

h. of ova·ry
h. of spleen
hi·lus
cells
hi·man·to·sis
hind
kid·ney
hind·brain
ves·i·cle
hind·gut
hind·quar·ter
am·pu·ta·tion
hind·wa·ter
hinge
ax·is
joint
move·ment
po·si·tion
re·gion
hinge-bow
hinged
flap
Hinman
syn·drome
Hinton
test
hip
bone
joint
phe·nom·e·non
hip
snap·ping h.
hip-flex·ion
phe·nom·e·non
Hippelates
Hippel-Lindau
dis·ease
Hippel's
dis·ease
Hip·po·bos·ca
Hip·po·bos·ci·dae
hip·po·cam·pal
com·mis·sure
con·vo·lu·tion
fis·sure
gy·rus
scle·ro·sis
hip·po·cam·pus
h. ma·jor
h. mi·nor
hip·po·crat·ic
face
fa·ci·es
fin·gers
nails
suc·cus·sion
hip·po·crat·ic suc·cus·sion
sound

hip·pu·rate
hip·pu·ria
hip·pu·ric ac·id
hip·pu·ri·case
hip·pus
  res·pi·ra·to·ry h.
hir·ci
hir·cis·mus
hir·cus
Hirschberg's
  meth·od
Hirschfeld's
  ca·nals
Hirschowitz
  syn·drome
Hirsch-Peiffer
  stain
Hirschsprung's
  dis·ease
hir·sute
hir·su·ti·es
hir·sut·ism
  Apert's h.
  con·sti·tu·tion·al h.
  id·i·o·path·ic h.
hir·tel·lous
hir·u·di·cide
hir·u·din
Hir·u·din·ea
hir·u·di·ni·a·sis
Hir·u·do
His'
  band
  bun·dle
  cop·u·la
  line
  rule
  spin·dle
His bun·dle
  elec·tro·gram
His' per·i·vas·cu·lar
  space
Hiss'
  stain
His·ta·log
  test
his·ta·mi·nase
his·ta·mine
  h. phos·phate
his·ta·mine
  lib·er·a·tors
  shock
  test
his·ta·mine-fast
his·ta·mi·ne·mia
his·ta·min·ic
  ceph·a·lal·gia
  head·ache

his·ta·mi·nu·ria
his·tan·gic
His-Tawara
  sys·tem
his·ti·dase
his·ti·din·al
his·ti·di·nase
his·ti·dine
  h. am·mo·nia-ly·ase
  h. de·am·i·nase
  h. de·car·box·yl·ase
his·ti·di·ne·mia
his·ti·dino
his·ti·di·nol
his·ti·di·nu·ria
his·ti·dyl
his·ti·o·blast
his·ti·o·cyte
  car·di·ac h.
  sea-blue h.
his·ti·o·cyt·ic
  lym·pho·ma
his·ti·o·cyt·ic med·ul·lary
  re·tic·u·lo·sis
his·ti·o·cy·to·ma
  fi·brous h.
  gen·er·al·ized erup·tive h.
  ma·lig·nant fi·brous h.
his·ti·o·cy·to·sis
  ker·a·sin h.
  lip·id h.
  ma·lig·nant h.
  nod·u·lar non-X h.
  non·lip·id h.
  re·gress·ing atyp·i·cal h.
  si·nus h. with mas·sive
    lym·phad·e·nop·a·thy
  h. X
  h. Y
his·ti·o·gen·ic
his·ti·oid
his·ti·o·ma
his·ti·on·ic
his·to·an·gic
his·to·blast
his·to·chem·is·try
his·to·com·pat·i·bil·i·ty
  gene
his·to·com·pat·i·bil·i·ty test·ing
his·to·cyte
his·to·cy·to·sis
his·to·dif·fer·en·ti·a·tion
his·to·flu·o·res·cence
his·to·gen·e·sis
his·to·ge·net·ic
his·tog·e·nous
his·tog·e·ny
his·to·gram

his·toid
  lep·ro·sy
  ne·o·plasm
  tu·mor
his·to·in·com·pat·i·bil·i·ty
his·to·log·ic
  ac·com·mo·da·tion
his·to·log·i·cal
his·tol·o·gist
his·tol·o·gy
  path·o·log·ic h.
his·tol·y·sis
his·to·ma
his·to·met·a·plas·tic
His·to·mo·nas me·le·ag·ri·dis
his·tom·o·ni·a·sis
his·to·mor·phom·e·try
his·tone
  ba·ses
his·to·nec·to·my
his·to·neu·rol·o·gy
his·ton·o·my
his·to·nu·ria
his·to·path·o·gen·e·sis
his·to·pa·thol·o·gy
his·to·phys·i·ol·o·gy
His·to·plas·ma cap·su·la·tum
his·to·plas·min
his·to·plas·min-la·tex
  test
his·to·plas·mo·ma
his·to·plas·mo·sis
  Af·ri·can h.
  pre·sumed oc·u·lar h.
his·to·ra·di·og·ra·phy
his·tor·rhex·is
his·to·tome
his·tot·o·my
his·to·tox·ic
  an·ox·ia
his·to·troph
his·to·tro·phic
his·to·tro·pic
his·to·zo·ic
his·to·zyme
his·tri·on·ic
  per·son·al·i·ty
  spasm
hitch·hik·er
  thumbs
Hitzig's
  gir·dle
hives
  gi·ant h.
Hjärre's
  dis·ease
HL-A
  an·ti·gens

HLA
  com·plex
Ho
  an·ti·gen
hoarse
hoarse·ness
hob·nail
  cells
  liv·er
  tongue
Hoboken's
  gem·mules
  nod·ules
  valves
Hoche's
  bun·dle
  tract
hock
  capped h.
  curby h.
Hodgen
  splint
Hodge's
  pes·sa·ry
Hodgkin-Key
  mur·mur
Hodgkin's
  dis·ease
Hodgson's
  dis·ease
ho·do·neu·ro·mere
ho·do·pho·bia
hoe
  ex·ca·va·tor
  scal·er
Hofbauer
  cell
Hoffa's
  op·er·a·tion
Hoffmann's
  duct
  phe·nom·e·non
  re·flex
  sign
Hoffmann's mus·cu·lar
  at·ro·phy
Hofmann's
  ba·cil·lus
Hofmeister
  se·ries
Hofmeister-Pólya
  anas·to·mo·sis
Hofmeister's
  op·er·a·tion
hog
  chol·era

hog chol·era
  vac·cines
  vi·rus
Hoglund's
  sign
Hogness
  box
hol·an·dric
  gene
  in·her·i·tance
hol·ar·thrit·ic
hol·ar·thri·tis
Holden's
  line
hole of ret·i·na
hol·i·day
  syn·drome
hol·i·day heart
  syn·drome
ho·lism
ho·lis·tic
  med·i·cine
  psy·chol·o·gy
Hollander
  test
Hollenhorst
  plaques
hol·low
  back
  bone
hol·low
  Sebileau's h.
Holl's
  lig·a·ment
Holmes'
  stain
Holmes-Adie
  pu·pil
  syn·drome
Holmes-Rahe
  ques·tion·naire
Holmgren
  meth·od
Holmgrén-Golgi
  ca·nals
Holmgren's
  test
hol·mi·um
hol·o·a·car·di·us
  h. aceph·a·lus
  h. amor·phus
ho·lo-ACP syn·thase
hol·o·a·cra·nia
hol·o·an·en·ceph·a·ly
hol·o·blas·tic
  cleav·age
hol·o·ce·phal·ic
hol·o·cord

hol·o·crine
  gland
hol·o·di·a·stol·ic
hol·o·en·dem·ic
hol·o·en·zyme
hol·o·gas·tros·chi·sis
hol·o·gram
hol·o·gyn·ic
  in·her·i·tance
hol·o·mas·ti·gote
hol·o·me·tab·o·lous
  met·a·mor·pho·sis
hol·o·mor·pho·sis
hol·o·phyt·ic
hol·o·pros·en·ceph·a·ly
hol·o·ra·chis·chi·sis
hol·o·sys·tol·ic
  mur·mur
hol·o·tel·en·ceph·a·ly
ho·lot·ri·chous
hol·o·zo·ic
Holter
  mon·i·tor
Holthouse's
  her·nia
Holth's
  op·er·a·tion
Holt-Oram
  syn·drome
Holzknecht
  unit
hom·a·lo·ceph·a·lous
Ho·ma·lo·my·ia
hom·a·lu·ria
Homans'
  sign
ho·mat·ro·pine
hom·ax·i·al
ho·me·o·cyte
ho·me·o·met·ric
  au·to·reg·u·la·tion
ho·me·o·mor·phous
ho·me·o·path
ho·me·o·path·ic
ho·me·op·a·thist
ho·me·op·a·thy
ho·me·o·pla·sia
ho·me·o·plas·tic
ho·me·or·rhe·sis
ho·me·o·sis
ho·me·o·sta·sis
  Bernard-Cannon h.
  ge·net·ic h.
  Lerner h.
  on·to·gen·ic h.
  phys·i·o·log·i·cal h.
  wad·ding·to·ni·an h.

ho·me·o·stat·ic
 equi·lib·ri·um
ho·me·o·ther·a·peu·tic
ho·me·o·ther·a·peu·tics
ho·me·o·ther·a·py
ho·me·o·therm
ho·me·o·ther·mal
ho·me·o·ther·mic
ho·me·ot·ic
ho·me·o·typ·i·cal
hom·er·gy
Home's
 lobe
hom·i·cid·al
hom·i·cide
ho·mid·i·um bro·mide
ho·mi·grade
 scale
hom·i·nal
 phys·i·ol·o·gy
hom·ing
 val·ue
Ho·min·i·dae
Ho·mi·noi·dea
ho·mo·bi·o·tin
ho·mo·blas·tic
ho·mo·car·no·sine
ho·mo·cen·tric
ho·mo·chlor·cy·cli·zine
ho·moch·ro·nous
 in·her·i·tance
ho·mo·clad·ic
 anas·to·mo·ses
ho·mo·cy·clic
 com·pound
ho·mo·cys·te·ine
ho·mo·cys·tine
ho·mo·cys·ti·ne·mia
ho·mo·cys·ti·nu·ria
ho·mo·cy·to·tro·pic
 an·ti·body
ho·mo·dont
ho·mod·ro·mous
ho·mo·e·rot·i·cism
ho·mo·er·ot·ism
ho·mo·ga·met·ic
 em·bryo
ho·mog·a·my
ho·mog·e·nate
ho·mo·ge·neous
 im·mer·sion
 nu·cle·a·tion
 ra·di·a·tion
 sys·tem
ho·mo·gen·e·sis
ho·mog·e·ni·za·tion
ho·mog·e·nize

ho·mog·e·nous
 ker·a·to·plas·ty
ho·mo·gen·tis·ic ac·id
 h. a. ox·i·dase
ho·mo·gen·tis·i·case
ho·mo·gen·ti·su·ria
ho·mog·e·ny
ho·mo·graft
ho·moi·o·pla·sia
ho·moi·o·ther·mal
ho·mo·kar·y·on
ho·mo·kar·y·ot·ic
ho·mo·ker·a·to·plas·ty
ho·mo·lat·er·al
ho·mo·lec·i·thal
 egg
ho·mo·lip·ids
ho·mol·o·gous
 an·ti·se·rum
 chro·mo·somes
 de·sen·si·tiz·a·tion
 graft
 in·sem·i·na·tion
 se·ries
 stim·u·lus
 tu·mor
ho·mol·o·gous se·rum
 jaun·dice
ho·mo·logue
ho·mol·o·gy
 h. of chains
 DNA h.
 h. of strands
ho·mol·y·sin
ho·mol·y·sis
ho·mo·mor·phic
ho·mon·o·mous
ho·mon·o·my
ho·mo·nu·cle·ar
ho·mon·y·mous
 di·plo·pia
 hem·i·a·nop·sia
 im·ag·es
 par·al·lax
ho·mo·phenes
ho·mo·phil
ho·mo·plas·tic
 graft
ho·mo·plas·ty
ho·mo·pol·y·mer
ho·mo·pro·line
ho·mo·pro·to·cat·e·chu·ic ac·id
hom·or·gan·ic
ho·mo·sal·ate
Ho·mo sa·pi·ens
ho·mo·ser·ine
 h. de·am·i·nase
 h. de·hy·dra·tase

475

ho·mo·sex·u·al
  pan·ic
ho·mo·sex·u·al·i·ty
  ego-dys·ton·ic h.
  la·tent h.
  overt h.
  un·con·scious h.
ho·mo·thal·lic
ho·mo·ther·mal
ho·mo·ton·ic
ho·mo·top·ic
  pain
ho·mo·trans·plan·ta·tion
ho·mo·type
ho·mo·typ·ic
  cor·tex
ho·mo·typ·i·cal
ho·mo·va·nil·lic ac·id
  test
ho·mo·zo·ic
ho·mo·zy·go·sis
ho·mo·zy·gos·i·ty
ho·mo·zy·gote
ho·mo·zy·gous
  achon·dro·pla·sia
ho·mo·zy·gous by de·scent
Hon·du·ras bark
hon·ey
  urine
hon·ey·comb
  lung
  mac·u·la
  ring·worm
  scall
  tet·ter
Hong Kong
  foot
  in·flu·en·za
  toe
honk
  sys·tol·ic h.
hood
hoof-and-mouth
  dis·ease
hook
  cal·var·i·al h.
  h. of ha·mate bone
  pal·ate h.
  slid·ing h.
  h. of spi·ral lam·i·na
  squint h.
  tra·che·ot·o·my h.
hook·e·an
  be·hav·ior
hooked
  bone
  bun·dle of Russell
  fas·cic·u·lus

Hooker-Forbes
  test
Hooke's
  law
hook·lets
hook-shaped
  cat·a·ract
hook·worm
  ane·mia
  dis·ease
hoose
Hoover's
  signs
Hop·lop·syl·lus anom·a·lus
Hopmann's
  pap·il·lo·ma
  pol·yp
Hoppe-Goldflam
  dis·ease
hops
hor·de·o·lum
  h. ex·ter·num
  h. in·ter·num
  h. mei·bo·mi·a·num
hor·i·zon·tal
  at·ro·phy
  cell of Cajal
  cells of ret·i·na
  fis·sure of cer·e·bel·lum
  fis·sure of right lung
  frac·ture
  heart
  os·te·ot·o·my
  over·lap
  part
  plane
  plate of pal·a·tine bone
  re·sorp·tion
  trans·mis·sion
  ver·ti·go
hor·i·zon·ta·lis
hor·mi·on
Hor·mo·den·drum
hor·mo·nal
  gin·gi·vi·tis
hor·mone
  ad·i·po·ki·net·ic h.
  adre·no·cor·ti·cal h.'s
  adre·no·cor·ti·co·tro·pic h.
  adre·no·tro·pic h.
  an·dro·gen·ic h.
  an·te·ri·or pi·tu·i·tary-
    like h.
  an·ti·di·u·ret·ic h.
  car·di·ac h.
  cho·ri·on·ic go·nad·o·tro·
    phic h.

cho·ri·on·ic go·nad·o·tro·pic h.

cho·ri·on·ic "growth h.-pro·lac·tin"

chro·mat·o·pho·ro·tro·pic h.

cor·pus lu·te·um h.

cor·ti·cal h.'s

cor·ti·co·tro·pic h.

cor·ti·co·tro·pin-re·leas·ing h.

ec·top·ic h.

eryth·ro·poi·et·ic h.

es·tro·gen·ic h.

fol·li·cle-stim·u·lat·ing h.

fol·li·cle-stim·u·lat·ing h.-re·leas·ing h.

fol·lic·u·lar h.

ga·lac·to·poi·et·ic h.

ga·me·to·ki·net·ic h.

gas·tro·in·tes·ti·nal h.

go·nad·o·tro·pic h.

go·nad·o·tro·pin-re·leas·ing h.

growth h.

growth h.-re·leas·ing h.

heart h.

herz h.

hu·man cho·ri·on·ic so·ma·to·mam·mo·tro·pic h.

hy·po·phys·i·o·tro·pic h.

in·ap·pro·pri·ate h.

in·ter·sti·tial cell-stim·u·lat·ing h.

lac·to·gen·ic h.

lip·id-mo·bi·liz·ing h.

lip·o·tro·pic h.

lip·o·tro·pic pi·tu·i·tary h.

lu·te·i·niz·ing h.

lu·te·i·niz·ing hor·mone-re·leas·ing h.

lu·te·o·tro·pic h.

mam·mo·tro·pic h.

mel·a·no·cyte-stim·u·lat·ing h.

pan·cre·at·ic hy·per·gly·ce·mic h.

par·a·thy·roid h.

pi·tu·i·tary go·nad·o·tro·pic h.

pi·tu·i·tary growth h.

pla·cen·tal growth h.

pro·ges·ta·tion·al h.

pro·lac·tin in·hib·it·ing h.

pro·lac·tin re·leas·ing h.

re·leas·ing h.

sal·i·vary gland h.

sex h.'s

so·ma·to·tro·pic h.

ste·roid h.'s

sym·pa·thet·ic h.

thy·roid-stim·u·lat·ing h.

thy·ro·tro·pic h.

thy·rot·ro·pin-re·leas·ing h.

tro·phic h.'s

tro·pic h.'s

hor·mo·no·gen·e·sis

hor·mo·no·gen·ic

hor·mo·no·poi·e·sis

hor·mo·no·poi·et·ic

hor·mo·no·priv·ia

hor·mo·no·ther·a·py

horn

Ammon's h.

an·te·ri·or h.

cic·a·tri·cial h.

coc·cyg·eal h.

cu·ta·ne·ous h.

dor·sal h.

fron·tal h.

great·er h.

h.'s of hy·oid bone

il·i·ac h.

in·fe·ri·or h.

in·fe·ri·or h. of lat·er·al ven·tri·cle

in·fe·ri·or h. of sa·phe·nous open·ing

in·fe·ri·or h. of thy·roid car·ti·lage

lat·er·al h.

less·er h.

nail h.

oc·cip·i·tal h.

pos·te·ri·or h.

pulp h.

sa·cral h.

se·ba·ceous h.

su·pe·ri·or h.

su·pe·ri·or h. of sa·phe·nous open·ing

su·pe·ri·or h. of thy·roid car·ti·lage

tem·po·ral h.

uter·ine h.

h. of uter·us

ven·tral h.

warty h.

Horner's

mus·cle

pu·pil

syn·drome

teeth

Hor·ner-Tran·tas

dots

hor·ni·fi·ca·tion

horny
    lay·er of ep·i·der·mis
    lay·er of nail
ho·rop·ter
hor·rip·i·la·tion
hor·ror
    h. au·to·tox·i·cus
    h. fu·sio·nis
horse·fly
horse·pow·er
horse·pox
    vi·rus
horse·rad·ish
    per·ox·i·das·es
horse·shoe
    fis·tu·la
    kid·ney
    pla·cen·ta
Horsley's bone
    wax
Hortega
    cells
Hortega's neu·rog·lia
    stain
Horton's
    ar·te·ri·tis
    ceph·a·lal·gia
    head·ache
hos·pice
hos·pi·tal
    closed h.
    day h.
    gen·er·al h.
    gov·ern·ment h.
    group h.
    ma·ter·ni·ty h.
    men·tal h.
    mu·nic·i·pal h.
    night h.
    open h.
    phil·an·throp·ic h.
    pri·vate h.
    pro·pri·e·tary h.
    pub·lic h.
    spe·cial h.
    state h.
    teach·ing h.
    vol·un·tary h.
    week·end h.
hos·pi·tal
    fe·ver
    for·mu·lary
    gan·grene
    rec·ord
hos·pi·tal·ism
hos·pi·tal·i·za·tion
host
    am·pli·fi·er h.

    dead-end h.
    de·fin·i·tive h.
    fi·nal h.
    in·ter·me·di·ary h.
    in·ter·me·di·ate h.
    par·a·ten·ic h.
    res·er·voir h.
    sec·on·dary h.
    trans·port h.
hot
    ab·scess
    eye
    flash
    flush
    gan·grene
    nod·ule
    pack
    snare
    spot
hot·foot
hot salt
    ster·il·iz·er
Hot·ten·tot
    tea
Hot·ten·tot apron
hot·ten·tot·ism
Hotz-Anagnostakis
    op·er·a·tion
hound-dog
    fa·ci·es
Hounsfield
    unit
hour·glass
    con·trac·tion
    head
    mur·mur
    pat·tern
    stom·ach
    ver·te·brae
house·fly
house·maid's
    knee
Houssay
    an·i·mal
    phe·nom·e·non
    syn·drome
Houston's
    folds
    mus·cle
    valves
Howard
    test
Howell
    unit
Howell-Jolly
    bod·ies
Howship's
    la·cu·nae

Hoyer's
anas·to·mo·ses
ca·nals
H-R con·duc·tion
time
H-tet·a·nase
HTLV
Hu
an·ti·gens
Hubrecht's pro·to·chor·dal
knot
Hucker-Conn
stain
Hudson's
line
Hudson-Stähli
line
Hueck's
lig·a·ment
Hueter's
ma·neu·ver
sign
Hufner's
equa·tion
Huggins'
op·er·a·tion
Huguier's
ca·nal
cir·cle
si·nus
Huhner
test
Hull's
tri·ad
hum
ve·nous h.
hu·man
ba·be·si·o·sis
bot·fly
e·col·o·gy
fi·brin·o·gen
ge·net·ics
in·su·lin
se·rum
throm·bin
hu·man an·ti·he·mo·phil·ic
fac·tor
frac·tion
hu·man bot·fly
my·i·a·sis
hu·man cho·ri·on·ic
go·nad·o·tro·pin
so·ma·to·mam·mo·tro·pin
hu·man cho·ri·on·ic so·ma·to·mam·mo·tro·pic
hor·mone
hu·man dip·loid cell ra·bies
vac·cine

hu·man fi·brin
foam
hu·man gam·ma
glob·u·lin
hu·man im·mu·no·de·fi·cien·cy
vi·rus
hu·man leu·ke·mia-as·so·ci·at·ed
an·ti·gens
hu·man lym·pho·cyte
an·ti·gens
hu·man mea·sles im·mune
se·rum
hu·man men·o·pau·sal
go·nad·o·tro·pin
hu·man nor·mal
im·mu·no·glob·u·lin
hu·man pap·il·lo·ma
vi·rus
hu·man per·tus·sis im·mune
se·rum
hu·man pla·cen·tal
lac·to·gen
hu·man plas·ma pro·tein
frac·tion
hu·man scar·let fe·ver im·mune
se·rum
hu·man T-cell lym·pho·ma/leu·ke·mia
vi·rus
hu·man T-cell lym·pho·trop·ic
vi·rus
hu·mec·tant
hu·mec·ta·tion
hu·mer·al
ar·tery
ar·tic·u·la·tion
head
hu·meri
hu·mer·o·ra·di·al
ar·tic·u·la·tion
joint
hu·mer·o·scap·u·lar
hu·mer·o·ul·nar
head
joint
hu·mer·us
hu·mid
tet·ter
hu·mid·i·ty
ab·so·lute h.
rel·a·tive h.
hu·min
Hummelsheim's
op·er·a·tion
hu·mor
aque·ous h.
Morgagni's h.

hu·mor *(continued)*
   oc·u·lar h.
   pec·cant hu·mors
   thun·der h.
   vit·re·ous h.
hu·mor·al
   doc·trine
   im·mu·ni·ty
   pa·thol·o·gy
hu·mor·is
hump
   Hampton h.
hump·back
Humphry's
   lig·a·ment
hu·mu·lin
hu·mu·lus
hunch·back
hun·ger
   af·fect h.
   nar·cot·ic h.
hun·ger
   con·trac·tions
   pain
   swell·ing
Hung's
   meth·od
Hunner's
   stric·ture
   ul·cer
Hunter's
   ca·nal
   glos·si·tis
   gu·ber·nac·u·lum
   lig·a·ment
   line
   mem·brane
   op·er·a·tion
   syn·drome
Hunter-Schreger
   bands
   lines
hunt·ing
   phe·nom·e·non
   re·ac·tion
Huntington's
   cho·rea
   dis·ease
Hunt's
   at·ro·phy
   neu·ral·gia
   syn·drome
Hunt's par·a·dox·i·cal
   phe·nom·e·non
Hurler's
   dis·ease
   syn·drome

hur·loid
   fa·ci·es
Hurst
   bou·gies
Hürthle
   cell
Hürthle cell
   ad·e·no·ma
   car·ci·no·ma
   tu·mor
Huschke's
   car·ti·lag·es
   fo·ra·men
   valve
Huschke's au·di·to·ry
   teeth
Hutchinson-Gilford
   dis·ease
   syn·drome
Hutchinson's
   fa·ci·es
   freck·le
   mask
   patch
   pu·pil
   teeth
   tri·ad
Hutchinson's cres·cen·tic
   notch
Hutchison
   syn·drome
Huxley's
   lay·er
   mem·brane
   sheath
Huygens'
   oc·u·lar
H-V
   in·ter·val
HVA
   test
H-V con·duc·tion
   time
H-Y
   an·ti·gen
hy·a·lin
   al·co·hol·ic h.
hy·a·line
   bod·ies
   bod·ies of pi·tu·i·tary
   car·ti·lage
   cast
   de·gen·er·a·tion
   leu·ko·cyte
   mem·brane
   throm·bus
   tu·ber·cle

hy·a·line mem·brane
  dis·ease of the new·born
hy·a·lin·i·za·tion
hy·a·li·no·sis
  sys·tem·ic h.
hy·a·li·nu·ria
hy·a·li·tis
  sup·pu·ra·tive h.
hy·a·lo·bi·u·ron·ic ac·id
hy·a·lo·cap·su·lar
  lig·a·ment
hy·a·lo·cyte
hy·al·o·gens
hy·a·lo·hy·pho·my·co·sis
hy·a·loid
  ar·tery
  body
  ca·nal
  fos·sa
  mem·brane
hy·a·loi·de·o·ret·i·nal
  de·gen·er·a·tion
hy·al·o·mere
Hy·a·lom·ma
  H. an·a·to·li·cum
  H. mar·gi·na·tum
  H. va·ri·e·ga·tum
hy·a·lo·pha·gia
hy·a·loph·a·gy
hy·a·lo·pho·bia
hy·al·o·plasm
  nu·cle·ar h.
hy·a·lo·plas·ma
hy·a·lo·se·ro·si·tis
hy·a·lo·sis
  as·ter·oid h.
  punc·tate h.
hy·al·o·some
hy·a·lu·rate
hy·al·u·ro·nate
  h. ly·ase
hy·al·u·ron·ic ac·id
hy·al·u·ron·ic ly·ase
hy·al·u·ron·i·dase
hy·al·u·ron·o·glu·cos·a·min·i·dase
hy·al·u·ron·o·glu·cu·ron·i·dase
hy·bar·ox·ia
hy·ben·zate
hy·brid
  pros·the·sis
hy·brid·ism
hy·brid·i·za·tion
  cell h.
  cross h.
  DNA h.
  so·mat·ic cell h.
hy·brid·o·ma

hy·can·thone
hy·clate
hy·dan·to·in
hy·dan·to·in·ate
hy·da·tid
  Morgagni's h.
  non·pe·dun·cu·lat·ed h.
  pe·dun·cu·lat·ed h.
  ses·sile h.
  stalked h.
hy·da·tid
  cyst
  dis·ease
  frem·i·tus
  mole
  pol·yp
  preg·nan·cy
  rash
  res·o·nance
  sand
  thrill
hy·da·tid·i·form
  mole
hy·da·tid·o·cele
hy·da·ti·do·ma
hy·da·tid·o·sis
hy·da·ti·dos·to·my
Hy·da·tig·e·ra tae·ni·ae·for·mis
hy·da·toid
Hyde's
  dis·ease
hyd·no·car·pus oil
hy·drac·e·tin
hy·drad·e·ni·tis
hy·drad·e·no·ma
hy·dra·gogue
hy·dral·a·zine
  syn·drome
hy·dral·a·zine hy·dro·chlo·ride
hy·dral·lo·stane
hy·dra·mine
hy·dra·mi·tra·zine tar·trate
hy·dram·ni·on
hy·dram·ni·os
hy·dran·en·ceph·a·ly
hy·drar·gyr·ia
hy·drar·gy·rism
hy·drar·gy·rum
hy·drar·thro·di·al
hy·drar·thron
hy·drar·thro·sis
  in·ter·mit·tent h.
hy·drar·thrus
hy·drase
hy·dras·tine
hy·dras·ti·nine
hy·dras·tis
hy·dra·tase

hy·drate
  crys·tal
hy·drat·ed
  alu·mi·na
hy·drate mi·cro·crys·tal
  the·o·ry of an·es·the·sia
hy·dra·tion
  ab·so·lute h.
hy·drau·lic
  con·duc·tiv·i·ty
hy·dra·zide
hy·dra·zine
hy·dra·zine yel·low
hy·dra·zi·nol·y·sis
hy·dra·zone
hy·dre·mia
hy·dre·mic
  ede·ma
hy·dren·ceph·a·lo·cele
hy·dren·ceph·a·lo·me·nin·go·cele
hy·dren·ceph·a·lus
hy·dri·a·tic
hy·dri·at·ric
hy·dric
hy·dride
  ion
hy·drin·dan·tin
hy·droa
  h. aes·ti·va·le
  h. feb·rile
  h. ges·ta·tio·nis
  h. her·pet·i·for·me
  h. pu·er·or·um
  h. vac·ci·ni·for·me
  h. ve·si·cu·lo·sum
hy·dro·a·dip·sia
hy·dro·al·co·hol·ic
  ex·tract
  tinc·ture
hy·dro·ap·pen·dix
hy·dro·bil·i·ru·bin
hy·dro·bleph·a·ron
hy·dro·bro·mate
hy·dro·bro·mic ac·id
hy·dro·cal·y·co·sis
hy·dro·car·bon
  Diels h.
  sat·u·rat·ed h.
hy·dro·cele
  cer·vi·cal h.
  h. col·li
  con·gen·i·tal h.
  Dupuytren's h.
  h. fe·mi·nae
  fi·lar·i·al h.
  fu·nic·u·lar h.
  h. mu·li·e·bris

Nuck's h.
  h. spi·na·lis
hy·dro·ce·lec·to·my
hy·dro·ce·phal·ic
hy·dro·ceph·a·lo·cele
hy·dro·ceph·a·loid
hy·dro·ceph·a·lus
  com·mu·ni·cat·ing h.
  con·gen·i·tal h.
  dou·ble com·part·ment h.
  ex·ter·nal h.
  h. ex vac·uo
  in·ter·nal h.
  non·com·mu·ni·cat·ing h.
  nor·mal pres·sure h.
  ob·struc·tive h.
  oc·cult h.
  otit·ic h.
  post·men·in·git·ic h.
  post·trau·mat·ic h.
  pri·mary h.
  sec·on·dary h.
  throm·bot·ic h.
  tox·ic h.
hy·dro·ceph·a·ly
hy·dro·chlo·ric ac·id
  di·lut·ed h. a.
hy·dro·chlo·ride
hy·dro·chlo·ro·thi·a·zide
hy·dro·cho·le·cys·tis
hy·dro·cho·le·re·sis
hy·dro·cho·le·ret·ic
hy·dro·cir·so·cele
hy·dro·co·done
hy·dro·col·loid
  ir·re·vers·i·ble h.
  re·vers·i·ble h.
hy·dro·col·po·cele
hy·dro·col·pos
hy·dro·cor·ta·mate hy·dro·chlo·ride
hy·dro·cor·ti·sone
  h. ac·e·tate
  h. cy·clo·pen·tyl·pro·pi·on·ate
  h. cyp·i·o·nate
  h. hy·dro·gen suc·ci·nate
  h. so·di·um phos·phate
  h. so·di·um suc·ci·nate
hy·dro·co·tar·nine
hy·dro·cu·pre·ine
hy·dro·cy·an·ic ac·id
hy·dro·cy·an·ism
hy·dro·cyst
hy·dro·cys·to·ma
hy·dro·dip·sia
hy·dro·dip·so·ma·nia
hy·dro·di·u·re·sis

hy·dro·dy·nam·ics
hy·dro·e·lec·tric
 bath
hy·dro·en·ceph·a·lo·cele
hy·dro·flu·me·thi·a·zide
hy·dro·flu·o·ric ac·id
hy·dro·gel
hy·dro·gen
 ac·ti·vat·ed h.
 ar·sen·iu·ret·ed h.
 h. bro·mide
 h. chlo·ride
 h. cy·a·nide
 h. de·hy·dro·gen·ase
 h. di·ox·ide
 heavy h.
 h. per·ox·ide
 h. phos·phide
 phos·phu·ret·ed h.
 h. sul·fide
 sul·fu·ret·ed h.
hy·dro·gen
 ac·cep·tor
 bond
 car·ri·er
 do·nor
 elec·trode
 ion
 num·ber
 trans·port
hy·dro·gen·ase
hy·dro·gen·a·tion
hy·dro·gen ex·po·nent
hy·dro·gen·ly·ase
hy·dro·ki·net·ic
hy·dro·ki·net·ics
hy·dro·la·bile
hy·dro·la·bil·i·ty
hy·dro·lab·y·rinth
hy·dro·las·es
hy·dro-ly·as·es
hy·dro·lymph
hy·drol·y·sate
hy·drol·y·sis
hy·dro·lyt·ic
 cleav·age
hy·dro·lyze
hy·dro·lyz·ing
 en·zymes
hy·dro·ma
hy·dro·mas·sage
hy·dro·me·nin·go·cele
hy·drom·e·ter
hy·dro·me·tra
hy·dro·met·ric
hy·dro·me·tro·col·pos
hy·drom·e·try
hy·dro·mi·cro·ceph·a·ly

hy·dro·mor·phone hy·dro·chlo·
 ride
hy·drom·pha·lus
hy·dro·my·e·lia
hy·dro·my·e·lo·cele
hy·dro·my·o·ma
hy·dro·ne·phro·sis
hy·dro·ne·phrot·ic
hy·dro·ni·um
 ion
hy·dro·par·a·sal·pinx
hy·dro·path·ic
hy·drop·a·thy
hy·dro·pe·nia
hy·dro·pe·nic
hy·dro·per·i·car·di·tis
hy·dro·per·i·car·di·um
hy·dro·per·i·to·ne·um
hy·dro·per·i·to·nia
hy·dro·per·ox·i·das·es
hy·dro·per·ox·ide
hy·dro·phil
 col·loid
hy·dro·phile
hy·dro·phil·ia
hy·dro·phil·ic
 col·loid
 pe·tro·la·tum
hy·droph·i·lous
hy·dro·pho·bia
hy·dro·pho·bic
 col·loid
 tet·a·nus
hy·dro·pho·ro·graph
hy·droph·thal·mia
hy·droph·thal·mos
hy·droph·thal·mus
Hy·dro·phy·i·dae
hy·drop·ic
 de·gen·er·a·tion
hy·dro·pneu·ma·to·sis
hy·dro·pneu·mo·go·ny
hy·dro·pneu·mo·per·i·car·di·um
hy·dro·pneu·mo·per·i·to·ne·um
hy·dro·pneu·mo·tho·rax
hy·dro·po·sia
hy·drops
 h. ar·tic·u·li
 en·do·lym·phat·ic h.
 fe·tal h.
 h. fe·ta·lis
 h. fol·lic·u·li
 im·mune fe·tal h.
 h. lab·y·rin·thi
 non·im·mune fe·tal h.
 h. ova·rii
 h. tu·bae
 h. tu·bae pro·flu·ens

hy·dro·py·o·ne·phro·sis
hy·dro·quin·ol
hy·dro·qui·none
hy·dror·chis
hy·dro·rhe·o·stat
hy·dror·rhea
   h. grav·i·dae
   h. grav·i·dar·um
   na·sal h.
hy·dro·sal·pinx
   in·ter·mit·tent h.
hy·dro·sar·ca
hy·dro·sar·co·cele
hy·dro·sol
hy·dro·sphyg·mo·graph
hy·dro·stat
hy·dro·stat·ic
   di·la·tor
   pres·sure
hy·dro·su·dop·a·thy
hy·dro·su·do·ther·a·py
hy·dro·sy·rin·go·my·e·lia
hy·dro·tax·is
hy·dro·ther·a·peu·tic
hy·dro·ther·a·peu·tics
hy·dro·ther·a·py
hy·dro·ther·mal
hy·dro·thi·o·ne·mia
hy·dro·thi·o·nu·ria
hy·dro·tho·rax
   chy·lous h.
hy·drot·o·my
hy·drot·ro·pism
hy·dro·tu·ba·tion
hy·dro·u·re·ter
hy·drous
   wool fat
hy·dro·va·ri·um
hy·drox·am·ic ac·ids
hy·drox·ide
hy·drox·o·co·bal·a·min
hy·drox·o·co·be·mine
hy·drox·y ac·id
hy·drox·y·a·cyl·glu·ta·thi·one
   hy·dro·lase
hy·drox·y·am·phet·a·mine hy·
   dro·bro·mide
hy·drox·y·ap·a·tite
hy·drox·y·car·bam·ide
hy·drox·y·chlo·ro·quine sul·fate
hy·drox·y·chro·man
hy·drox·y·chro·mene
hy·drox·y·eph·ed·rine
hy·drox·y·he·min
hy·drox·y·ky·nu·re·ni·nu·ria
hy·drox·yl
hy·drox·yl·a·mine
   h. re·duc·tase

hy·drox·yl·a·mi·no
hy·drox·yl·ap·a·tite
hy·drox·y·las·es
hy·drox·yl·a·tion
p-hy·drox·y·mer·cur·i·ben·zo·
   ate
hy·drox·y·ner·vone
hy·drox·y·phen·a·mate
hy·drox·y·phen·yl·u·ria
hy·drox·y·pro·ges·ter·one hex·
   a·no·ate
hy·drox·y·pro·line
hy·drox·y·pro·li·ne·mia
hy·drox·y·stil·bam·i·dine is·e·
   thi·o·nate
hy·drox·y·to·lu·ic ac·id
hy·drox·y·tryp·to·phan de·car·
   box·yl·ase
hy·drox·y·u·rea
hy·drox·y·zine
Hy·dro·zoa
hy·dru·ria
hy·dru·ric
hy·giei·ol·a·try
hy·giei·ol·o·gy
hy·gie·ist
hy·giene
   crim·i·nal h.
   men·tal h.
   oral h.
hy·gien·ic
hy·gien·ic lab·o·ra·tory
   co·ef·fi·cient
hy·gien·ist
   den·tal h.
hy·gric
hy·gric ac·id
hy·gro·ma
   h. ax·il·la·re
   cer·vi·cal h.
   h. col·li cys·ti·cum
   sub·du·ral h.
hy·grom·e·ter
hy·grom·e·try
hy·gro·pho·bia
hy·gro·scop·ic
   ex·pan·sion
hy·gro·sto·mia
hy·la
hy·le·pho·bia
hy·lic
   tu·mor
hy·lo·ma
   me·sen·chy·mal h.
   mes·o·the·li·al h.
hy·men
   h. bi·fe·nes·tra·tus
   h. bi·fo·ris

crib·ri·form h.
den·tic·u·late h.
im·per·fo·rate h.
in·fun·dib·u·li·form h.
h. sculp·ta·tus
sep·tate h.
h. sub·sep·tus
ver·ti·cal h.
hy·men·al
hy·me·nec·to·my
hy·me·ni·tis
hy·men·oid
hy·me·no·le·pi·a·sis
hy·me·no·lep·i·did
Hy·men·o·lep·i·di·dae
Hy·me·nol·e·pis
    H. di·mi·nu·ta
    H. lan·ce·o·la·ta
    H. na·na
    H. na·na, var. fra·ter·na
hy·me·nol·o·gy
Hy·me·nop·tera
hy·me·nor·rha·phy
hy·men·ot·o·my
hy·o·bran·chi·al
    cleft
hy·o·ep·i·glot·tic
    lig·a·ment
hy·o·ep·i·glot·tid·e·an
hy·o·glos·sal
    mem·brane
    mus·cle
hy·o·glos·sus
hy·oid
    ap·pa·ra·tus
    arch
    bone
hy·o·man·dib·u·lar
    cleft
hy·o·pha·ryn·ge·us
hy·o·scine
    h. hy·dro·bro·mide
hy·o·scy·a·mine
    h. sul·fate
dl-hy·o·scy·a·mine
hy·o·scy·a·mus
Hy·o·stron·gy·lus ru·bi·dus
hy·o·thy·roid
hyp·a·cu·sia
hyp·a·cu·sis
hyp·al·bu·mi·ne·mia
hyp·al·ge·sia
hyp·al·ge·sic
hyp·al·get·ic
hyp·al·gia
hyp·am·ni·on
hyp·am·ni·os
hyp·an·a·ki·ne·sia

hyp·an·a·ki·ne·sis
hyp·ar·te·ri·al
    bron·chi
hyp·ax·i·al
hyp·az·o·tu·ria
hyp·en·ceph·a·lon
hyp·en·gy·o·pho·bia
hy·per·ab·duc·tion
    syn·drome
hy·per·ac·an·tho·sis
hy·per·ac·id
hy·per·a·cid·i·ty
hy·per·ac·tiv·i·ty
hy·per·a·cu·sia
hy·per·a·cu·sis
hy·per·a·cute
    re·jec·tion
hy·per·ad·e·no·sis
hy·per·ad·i·po·sis
hy·per·ad·i·pos·i·ty
hy·per·ad·re·nal·cor·ti·cal·ism
hy·per·a·dre·no·cor·ti·cal·ism
hy·per·al·do·ste·ron·ism
hy·per·al·ge·sia
    au·di·to·ry h.
hy·per·al·ge·sic
hy·per·al·get·ic
hy·per·al·gia
hy·per·al·i·men·ta·tion
    par·en·ter·al h.
hy·per·al·lan·to·in·u·ria
hy·per·a·mi·no·ac·i·du·ria
hy·per·am·mo·ne·mia
    cer·e·bro·a·troph·ic h.
hy·per·am·y·la·se·mia
hy·per·an·a·ci·ne·sia
hy·per·an·a·ci·ne·sis
hy·per·an·a·ki·ne·sia
hy·per·an·a·ki·ne·sis
hy·per·a·phia
hy·per·aph·ic
hy·per·bar·ic
    an·es·the·sia
    cham·ber
    ox·y·gen
    ox·y·gen·a·tion
hy·per·bar·ic ox·y·gen
    ther·a·py
hy·per·bar·ic spi·nal
    an·es·the·sia
hy·per·bar·ism
hy·per·be·ta·lip·o·pro·tein·e·
mia
    fa·mil·i·al h.
    fa·mil·i·al h. and hy·per·
    pre·be·ta·lip·o·pro·tein·e·
    mia
hy·per·bil·i·ru·bi·ne·mia

hy·per·brach·y·ceph·a·ly
hy·per·cal·ce·mia
  id·i·o·path·ic h. of in·fants
hy·per·cal·ce·mic
  sar·coid·o·sis
  ure·mia
hy·per·cal·ci·nu·ria
hy·per·cal·ci·u·ria
hy·per·cal·cu·ria
hy·per·cap·nia
hy·per·car·bia
hy·per·car·dia
hy·per·ca·thar·sis
hy·per·ca·thar·tic
hy·per·ca·thex·is
hy·per·ce·men·to·sis
hy·per·chlor·e·mia
hy·per·chlor·hy·dria
hy·per·chlo·ride
hy·per·chlor·u·ria
hy·per·cho·les·ter·e·mia
hy·per·cho·les·ter·in·e·mia
hy·per·cho·les·ter·ol·e·mia
  fa·mil·i·al h.
  fa·mil·i·al h. with hy·per·
    li·pe·mia
hy·per·cho·les·ter·o·lia
hy·per·cho·lia
hy·per·chro·ma·sia
hy·per·chro·mat·ic
  ane·mia
  mac·ro·cy·the·mia
hy·per·chro·ma·tism
hy·per·chro·mia
  mac·ro·cyt·ic h.
hy·per·chro·mic
  ane·mia
hy·per·chy·lia
hy·per·chy·lo·mi·cro·ne·mia
  fa·mil·i·al h.
  fa·mil·i·al h. with hy·per·
    pre·be·ta·lip·o·pro·tein·e·
    mia
hy·per·ci·ne·sia
hy·per·ci·ne·sis
hy·per·cor·ti·coid·ism
hy·per·cor·ti·sol·ism
hy·per·cry·al·ge·sia
hy·per·cry·es·the·sia
hy·per·cu·pre·mia
hy·per·cy·a·not·ic
  an·gi·na
hy·per·cy·e·sia
hy·per·cy·e·sis
hy·per·cy·the·mia
hy·per·cy·to·chro·mia
hy·per·cy·to·sis
hy·per·dac·tyl·ia

hy·per·dac·tyl·ism
hy·per·dac·ty·ly
hy·per·di·as·to·le
hy·per·di·crot·ic
hy·per·di·cro·tism
hy·per·dip·sia
hy·per·dis·ten·tion
hy·per·dy·nam·ia
  h. uter·i
hy·per·dy·nam·ic
hy·per·e·che·ma
hy·per·em·e·sis
  h. grav·i·dar·um
  h. lac·ten·ti·um
hy·per·e·met·ic
hy·per·e·mia
  ac·tive h.
  ar·te·ri·al h.
  Bier's h.
  col·lat·er·al h.
  con·stric·tion h.
  flux·ion·ary h.
  pas·sive h.
  per·i·stat·ic h.
  re·ac·tive h.
  ve·nous h.
hy·per·e·mia
  test
hy·per·e·mic
hy·per·en·ceph·a·ly
hy·per·e·o·sin·o·phil·ia
hy·per·e·o·sin·o·phil·ic
  syn·drome
hy·per·eph·i·dro·sis
hy·per·ep·i·thy·mia
hy·per·er·ga·sia
hy·per·er·gia
hy·per·er·gic
  en·ceph·a·li·tis
hy·per·e·ryth·ro·cy·the·mia
hy·per·es·o·pho·ria
hy·per·es·the·sia
  au·di·to·ry h.
  ce·re·bral h.
  cer·vi·cal h.
  gus·ta·to·ry h.
  mus·cu·lar h.
  h. ol·fac·to·ria
  ol·fac·to·ry h.
  h. op·ti·ca
  tac·tile h.
hy·per·es·thet·ic
hy·per·eu·ry·pro·so·pic
hy·per·ex·o·pho·ria
hy·per·ex·ten·sion
hy·per·ex·ten·sion-hy·per·flex·
  ion
  in·ju·ry

hy·per·fer·re·mia
hy·per·fi·brin·o·ge·ne·mia
hy·per·fi·bri·nol·y·sis
hy·per·flex·ion
hy·per·fol·lic·u·loid·ism
hy·per·func·tion·al
  oc·clu·sion
hy·per·gal·ac·to·sis
hy·per·gam·ma·glob·u·lin·e·mia
hy·per·ga·sia
hy·per·gen·e·sis
hy·per·ge·net·ic
hy·per·gen·ic
  ter·a·to·sis
hy·per·gen·i·tal·ism
hy·per·geu·sia
hy·per·gia
hy·per·gic
hy·per·glan·du·lar
hy·per·glob·u·lia
hy·per·glob·u·lin·e·mia
hy·per·glob·u·lin·e·mic
  pur·pu·ra
hy·per·glob·u·lism
hy·per·gly·ce·mia
  non·ke·tot·ic h.
  post·hy·po·gly·ce·mic h.
hy·per·gly·ce·mic-gly·co·gen·o·
  lyt·ic
  fac·tor
hy·per·glyc·er·i·de·mia
  en·dog·e·nous h.
  ex·og·e·nous h.
hy·per·gly·ci·ne·mia
hy·per·gly·ci·nu·ria
  h. with hy·per·gly·ci·ne·mia
hy·per·gly·co·gen·ol·y·sis
hy·per·gly·cor·rha·chia
hy·per·gly·co·se·mia
hy·per·gly·co·su·ria
hy·per·gly·ox·yl·e·mia
hy·per·gno·sis
hy·per·go·nad·ism
hy·per·go·nad·o·tro·pic
  eu·nuch·oid·ism
hy·per·gran·u·lo·sis
hy·per·guan·i·di·ne·mia
hy·per·gy·ne·cos·mia
hy·per·he·do·nia
hy·per·he·do·nism
hy·per·he·mo·glo·bi·ne·mia
hy·per·hep·a·ri·ne·mia
hy·per·hi·dro·sis
  gus·ta·to·ry h.
  h. ole·o·sa
hy·per·hy·dra·tion
hy·per·hy·dro·chlo·ria
hy·per·hy·dro·pex·is

hy·per·hy·dro·pexy
hy·per·i·cin
hy·per·i·dro·sis
hy·per·im·mu·no·glob·u·lin E
  syn·drome
hy·per·in·di·can·e·mia
hy·per·in·fec·tion
hy·per·i·no·se·mia
hy·per·i·no·sis
hy·per·in·su·li·ne·mia
hy·per·in·su·lin·ism
  al·i·men·ta·ry h.
hy·per·in·vo·lu·tion
hy·per·i·so·ton·ic
hy·per·ka·le·mia
hy·per·ka·le·mic pe·ri·od·ic
  pa·ral·y·sis
hy·per·kal·i·e·mia
hy·per·kal·u·re·sis
hy·per·ker·a·tin·i·za·tion
hy·per·ker·a·to·my·co·sis
hy·per·ker·a·to·sis
  bo·vine h.
  h. con·gen·i·ta
  h. ec·cen·tri·ca
  ep·i·der·mo·lyt·ic h.
  h. fig·ur·a·ta cen·tri·fu·ga
  atro·phi·ca
  h. fol·lic·u·la·ris et pa·ra·
  fol·li·cu·la·ris
  h. len·tic·u·lar·is per·stans
  h. pen·e·trans
  h. sub·un·gua·lis
hy·per·ke·to·ne·mia
hy·per·ke·ton·u·ria
hy·per·ki·ne·mia
hy·per·ki·ne·sia
hy·per·ki·ne·sis
hy·per·ki·net·ic
  syn·drome
hy·per·lac·ta·tion
hy·per·leu·ko·cy·to·sis
hy·per·lex·ia
hy·per·li·pe·mia
  car·bo·hy·drate-in·duced h.
  com·bined fat- and car·bo·
  hy·drate-in·duced h.
  fa·mil·i·al fat-in·duced h.
  id·i·o·path·ic h.
  mixed h.
hy·per·lip·id·e·mia
hy·per·lip·oi·de·mia
hy·per·lip·o·pro·tein·e·mia
  ac·quired h.
  fa·mil·i·al h.
  type I fa·mil·i·al h.
  type II fa·mil·i·al h.
  type III fa·mil·i·al h.

hy·per·lip·o·pro·tein·e·mia
(continued)
    type IV fa·mil·i·al h.
    type V fa·mil·i·al h.
hy·per·li·po·sis
hy·per·li·thu·ria
hy·per·lo·gia
hy·per·lor·do·sis
hy·per·lu·cent
    lung
hy·per·ly·si·ne·mia
hy·per·ly·si·nu·ria
hy·per·mag·ne·se·mia
hy·per·mas·tia
hy·per·ma·ture
    cat·a·ract
hy·per·men·or·rhea
hy·per·me·tab·o·lism
hy·per·met·a·mor·pho·sis
hy·per·me·tria
hy·per·met·rope
hy·per·me·tro·pia
    in·dex h.
hy·per·mim·ia
hy·perm·ne·sia
hy·per·mo·bil·i·ty
hy·per·morph
hy·per·my·es·the·sia
hy·per·my·o·to·nia
hy·per·my·ot·ro·phy
hy·per·na·tre·mia
hy·per·na·tre·mic
    en·ceph·a·lop·a·thy
hy·per·ne·o·cy·to·sis
hy·per·neph·roid
hy·per·ne·phro·ma
hy·per·noia
hy·per·nom·ic
hy·per·nu·tri·tion
hy·per·on·cot·ic
hy·per·o·nych·ia
hy·per·ope
hy·per·o·pia
    ab·so·lute h.
    ax·i·al h.
    cur·va·ture h.
    fac·ul·ta·tive h.
    la·tent h.
    man·i·fest h.
    to·tal h.
hy·per·o·pic
    astig·ma·tism
hy·per·o·ral·i·ty
hy·per·or·chi·dism
hy·per·o·rex·ia
hy·per·or·tho·cy·to·sis
hy·per·os·mia
hy·per·os·mo·lal·i·ty

hy·per·os·mo·lar hy·per·gly·ce·mic non·ke·ton·ic
    co·ma
hy·per·os·mo·lar·i·ty
hy·per·os·mot·ic
hy·per·os·phre·sia
hy·per·os·phre·sis
hy·per·os·te·oi·do·sis
hy·per·os·to·sis
    an·ky·los·ing h.
    h. cor·ti·ca·lis de·for·mans
    dif·fuse id·i·o·path·ic skel·e·tal h.
    flow·ing h.
    h. fron·ta·lis in·ter·na
    gen·er·al·ized cor·ti·cal h.
    in·fan·tile cor·ti·cal h.
    streak h.
hy·per·os·tot·ic
    spon·dy·lo·sis
hy·per·o·var·i·an·ism
hy·per·ox·al·u·ria
    pri·mary h. and ox·a·lo·sis
hy·per·ox·ia
hy·per·ox·i·da·tion
hy·per·ox·ide
hy·per·pan·cre·a·tism
hy·per·par·a·site
hy·per·par·a·sit·ism
hy·per·par·a·thy·roid·ism
    pri·mary h.
    sec·on·dary h.
hy·per·pa·rot·i·dism
hy·per·path·ia
hy·per·pep·sia
hy·per·pep·sin·ia
hy·per·per·i·stal·sis
hy·per·pha·gia
hy·per·pha·lan·gism
hy·per·phen·yl·al·a·ni·ne·mia
hy·per·pho·ne·sis
hy·per·pho·nia
hy·per·pho·ria
hy·per·phos·pha·ta·se·mia
hy·per·phos·pha·ta·sia
hy·per·phos·pha·te·mia
hy·per·phos·pha·tu·ria
hy·per·phre·nia
hy·per·pi·e·sia
hy·per·pi·e·sis
hy·per·pi·et·ic
hy·per·pig·men·ta·tion
hy·per·pip·e·co·la·te·mia
hy·per·pi·tu·i·ta·rism
hy·per·pla·sia
    an·gi·o·fol·lic·u·lar me·di·as·ti·nal lymph node h.

an·gi·o·lym·phoid h. with
eo·sin·o·phil·ia
atyp·i·cal me·la·no·cyt·ic h.
ba·sal cell h.
be·nign me·di·as·ti·nal
lymph node h.
ce·men·tum h.
con·gen·i·tal ad·re·nal h.
con·gen·i·tal se·ba·ceous h.
cys·tic h.
cys·tic h. of the breast
den·ture h.
duc·tal h.
fi·bro·mus·cu·lar h.
fo·cal ep·i·the·li·al h.
gin·gi·val h.
in·flam·ma·to·ry fi·brous h.
in·flam·ma·to·ry pap·il·lary
h.
in·tra·vas·cu·lar pap·il·lary
en·do·the·li·al h.
nod·u·lar h. of pros·tate
nod·u·lar re·gen·er·a·tive h.
pseu·do·car·ci·nom·a·tous h.
pseu·do·ep·i·the·li·om·a·
tous h.
se·nile se·ba·ceous h.
ver·ru·cous h.
hy·per·plas·tic
ar·te·ri·o·scle·ro·sis
gin·gi·vi·tis
graft
in·flam·ma·tion
os·te·o·ar·thri·tis
pol·yp
pulp·i·tis
hy·per·ploid
hy·per·ploi·dy
hy·per·pnea
hy·per·po·lar·i·za·tion
hy·per·po·ne·sis
hy·per·po·tas·se·mia
hy·per·pra·gia
hy·per·prax·ia
hy·per·pre·be·ta·lip·o·pro·tein·
e·mia
fa·mil·i·al h.
hy·per·pro·chor·e·sis
hy·per·pro·in·su·li·ne·mia
hy·per·pro·lac·ti·ne·mia
hy·per·pro·lac·ti·ne·mic
amen·or·rhea
hy·per·pro·li·ne·mia
hy·per·pro·sex·ia
hy·per·pro·tein·e·mia
hy·per·pro·te·o·sis
hy·per·py·ret·ic

hy·per·py·rex·ia
ful·mi·nant h.
heat h.
ma·lig·nant h.
hy·per·py·rex·i·al
hy·per·quan·ti·va·lent
idea
hy·per·re·ac·tive ma·lar·i·ous
sple·no·meg·a·ly
hy·per·re·flex·ia
hy·per·res·o·nance
hy·per·sal·e·mia
hy·per·sa·line
hy·per·sal·i·va·tion
hy·per·sar·co·si·ne·mia
hy·per·se·cre·tion
glau·co·ma
hy·per·seg·ment·ed
neu·tro·phil
hy·per·sen·si·tive
den·tin
hy·per·sen·si·tive·ness
hy·per·sen·si·tive xi·phoid
syn·drome
hy·per·sen·si·tiv·i·ty
an·gi·i·tis
pneu·mo·ni·tis
re·ac·tion
hy·per·sen·si·tiv·i·ty
de·layed h.
hy·per·sen·si·ti·za·tion
hy·per·se·ro·to·ne·mia
hy·per·ske·o·cy·to·sis
hy·per·so·ma·to·tro·pism
hy·per·so·mia
hy·per·som·nia
hy·per·son·ic
hy·per·sphyx·ia
hy·per·splen·ism
hy·per·ste·a·to·sis
hy·per·ste·re·o·roent·gen·og·ra·
phy
hy·per·sthe·nia
hy·per·sthen·ic
hy·per·sthen·u·ria
hy·per·sus·cep·ti·bil·i·ty
hy·per·sys·to·le
hy·per·sys·tol·ic
hy·per·ta·rach·ia
hy·per·tel·or·ism
can·thal h.
oc·u·lar h.
hy·per·ten·sin
hy·per·ten·sin·ase
hy·per·ten·sin·o·gen
hy·per·ten·sion
ad·re·nal h.
be·nign h.

hy·per·ten·sion *(continued)*
  es·sen·tial h.
  Goldblatt's h.
  id·i·o·path·ic h.
  ma·lig·nant h.
  pale h.
  por·tal h.
  post·par·tum h.
  pri·mary h.
  pul·mo·nary h.
  re·nal h.
  re·no·vas·cu·lar h.
hy·per·ten·sive
  ar·te·ri·op·a·thy
  ar·te·ri·o·scle·ro·sis
  en·ceph·a·lop·a·thy
  ir·i·do·cy·cli·tis
  ret·i·nop·a·thy
hy·per·ten·sor
hy·per·tes·toid·ism
hy·per·the·co·sis
  stro·mal h.
  tes·toid h.
hy·per·the·lia
hy·per·ther·mal·ge·sia
hy·per·ther·mia
  ma·lig·nant h.
hy·per·ther·mo·es·the·sia
hy·per·throm·bi·ne·mia
hy·per·thy·mia
hy·per·thy·mic
hy·per·thy·mism
hy·per·thy·mi·za·tion
hy·per·thy·roid·ism
  io·dine-in·duced h.
  oph·thal·mic h.
  pri·mary h.
  sec·on·dary h.
hy·per·thy·rox·i·ne·mia
hy·per·to·nia
  h. po·ly·cy·the·mi·ca
  sym·pa·thet·ic h.
hy·per·ton·ic
  ab·sence
hy·per·to·nic·i·ty
hy·per·tri·chi·a·sis
hy·per·trich·o·phry·dia
hy·per·tri·cho·sis
  h. la·nu·gi·no·sa
  h. la·nu·gi·no·sa ac·qui·si·ta
  ne·void h.
  h. par·ti·a·lis
  h. uni·ver·sa·lis
hy·per·tri·glyc·er·i·de·mia
  fa·mil·i·al h.
hy·per·troph
hy·per·tro·phia

hy·per·tro·phic
  ar·thri·tis
  car·di·o·my·op·a·thy
  gas·tri·tis
  pulp·i·tis
  rhi·ni·tis
  ring·worm
  ro·sa·cea
  scar
hy·per·tro·phic cer·vi·cal
  pach·y·men·in·gi·tis
hy·per·tro·phic hy·per·se·cre·to·ry
  gas·trop·a·thy
hy·per·tro·phic in·ter·sti·tial
  neu·rop·a·thy
hy·per·tro·phic pul·mo·nary
  os·te·o·ar·throp·a·thy
hy·per·tro·phic py·lor·ic
  ste·no·sis
hy·per·tro·phied fren·u·la
  syn·drome
hy·per·tro·phy
  adap·tive h.
  be·nign pros·tat·ic h.
  com·pen·sa·to·ry h.
  com·pen·sa·to·ry h. of the heart
  com·ple·men·ta·ry h.
  con·cen·tric h.
  ec·cen·tric h.
  en·dem·ic h.
  false h.
  func·tion·al h.
  gi·ant h. of gas·tric mu·co·sa
  he·man·gi·ec·tat·ic h.
  li·po·ma·tous h.
  nu·mer·i·cal h.
  phys·i·o·log·ic h.
  pseu·do·mus·cu·lar h.
  quan·ti·ta·tive h.
  sim·ple h.
  sim·u·lat·ed h.
  true h.
  vi·car·i·ous h.
hy·per·tro·pia
hy·per·ty·ro·si·ne·mia
hy·per·u·re·sis
hy·per·u·ri·ce·mia
hy·per·u·ri·ce·mic
hy·per·u·ri·cu·ria
hy·per·vac·ci·na·tion
hy·per·val·i·ne·mia
hy·per·vas·cu·lar
hy·per·ven·ti·la·tion
  syn·drome

test
tet·a·ny
hy·per·vis·cos·i·ty
   syn·drome
hy·per·vi·ta·min·o·sis
hy·per·vo·le·mia
hy·per·vo·le·mic
hy·per·vo·lia
hyp·es·the·sia
   ol·fac·to·ry h.
hy·pha
   rac·quet h.
   spi·ral hy·phae
hy·phae
hyp·he·do·nia
hy·phe·ma
hy·phe·mia
   in·ter·trop·i·cal h.
   trop·i·cal h.
hyp·hi·dro·sis
Hy·pho·my·ces des·tru·ens
Hy·pho·my·ce·tes
hy·pho·my·co·sis
hyp·na·gog·ic
   hal·lu·ci·na·tion
   im·age
hyp·na·gogue
hyp·nal·gia
hyp·nap·a·gog·ic
hyp·nes·the·sia
hyp·nic
hyp·no·a·nal·y·sis
hyp·no·an·a·lyt·ic
hyp·no·ca·thar·sis
hyp·no·cin·e·mat·o·graph
hyp·no·cyst
hyp·no·don·tics
hyp·no·gen·e·sis
hyp·no·gen·ic
   spot
hyp·nog·e·nous
hyp·noi·dal
hyp·no·lep·sy
hyp·nol·o·gist
hyp·nol·o·gy
hyp·no·pho·bia
hyp·no·pom·pic
   im·age
hyp·no·sis
   le·thar·gic h.
   ma·jor h.
   mi·nor h.
hyp·no·ther·a·py
hyp·not·ic
   psy·cho·ther·a·py
   re·la·tion·ship
   sleep
   state

hyp·no·tism
hyp·no·tist
hyp·no·tize
hyp·no·toid
hyp·no·zo·ite
hy·po·a·cid·i·ty
hy·po·a·cu·sis
hy·po·a·de·nia
hy·po·a·dre·nal·ism
hy·po·al·bu·mi·ne·mia
hy·po·al·dos·ter·on·ism
   hy·po·ren·i·nem·ic h.
   iso·lat·ed h.
   se·lec·tive h.
hy·po·al·do·ster·on·u·ria
hy·po·al·ge·sia
hy·po·al·i·men·ta·tion
hy·po·az·o·tu·ria
hy·po·bar·ia
hy·po·bar·ic
hy·po·bar·ic spi·nal
   an·es·the·sia
hy·po·bar·ism
hy·po·ba·rop·a·thy
hy·po·be·ta·lip·o·pro·tein·e·mia
hy·po·blast
hy·po·blas·tic
hy·po·bran·chi·al
   em·i·nence
hy·po·bro·mite
hy·po·bro·mous ac·id
hy·po·cal·ce·mia
hy·po·cal·ce·mic
   cat·a·ract
hy·po·cal·ci·fi·ca·tion
   enam·el h.
hy·po·cap·nia
hy·po·car·bia
hy·po·ce·lom
hy·po·chlor·e·mia
hy·po·chlor·e·mic
hy·po·chlor·hy·dria
hy·po·chlo·rite
hy·po·chlo·rous ac·id
hy·po·chlor·u·ria
hy·po·cho·les·ter·e·mia
hy·po·cho·les·ter·in·e·mia
hy·po·cho·les·ter·ol·e·mia
hy·po·cho·lia
hy·po·chon·dria
hy·po·chon·dri·ac
   re·gion
hy·po·chon·dri·a·cal
   mel·an·cho·lia
hy·po·chon·dri·al
   re·flex
hy·po·chon·dri·a·sis
hy·po·chon·dri·um

hy·po·chon·dro·pla·sia
hy·po·chord·al
hy·po·chro·ma·sia
hy·po·chro·mat·ic
hy·po·chro·ma·tism
hy·po·chro·mia
hy·po·chro·mic
  ane·mia
hy·po·chro·mic mi·cro·cyt·ic
  ane·mia
hy·po·chro·sis
hy·po·chy·lia
hy·po·ci·ne·sia
hy·po·ci·ne·sis
hy·po·cit·ra·tur·ia
hy·po·com·ple·men·te·mia
hy·po·com·ple·men·te·mic
  glo·mer·u·lo·ne·phri·tis
hy·po·cone
hy·po·con·id
hy·po·con·ule
hy·po·con·u·lid
hy·po·cor·ti·coid·ism
hy·po·cu·pre·mia
hy·po·cy·cloi·dal
  to·mog·ra·phy
hy·po·cys·tot·o·my
hy·po·cy·the·mia
  pro·gress·ive h.
hy·po·cy·to·sis
hy·po·dac·tyl·ia
hy·po·dac·tyl·ism
hy·po·dac·ty·ly
hy·po·derm
Hy·po·der·ma
hy·po·der·mat·ic
hy·po·der·mat·oc·ly·sis
hy·po·der·mat·o·my
hy·po·der·ma·to·sis
hy·po·der·mic
  in·jec·tion
  nee·dle
  sy·ringe
  tab·let
hy·po·der·mis
hy·po·der·moc·ly·sis
hy·po·der·mo·li·thi·a·sis
hy·po·dip·sia
hy·po·don·tia
hy·po·dy·nam·ia
  h. cor·dis
hy·po·dy·nam·ic
hy·po·ec·cri·sis
hy·po·ec·crit·ic
hy·po·e·o·sin·o·phil·ia
hy·po·er·gia
hy·po·er·gy
hy·po·es·o·pho·ria

hy·po·es·the·sia
hy·po·ex·o·pho·ria
hy·po·fer·re·mia
hy·po·fer·ric
  ane·mia
hy·po·fi·brin·o·ge·ne·mia
hy·po·func·tion
hy·po·ga·lac·tia
hy·po·ga·lac·tous
hy·po·gam·ma·glo·bi·ne·mia
hy·po·gam·ma·glob·u·lin·e·mia
  ac·quired h.
  pri·mary h.
  sec·on·dary h.
  tran·sient h. of in·fan·cy
  X-linked h.
  X-linked in·fan·tile h.
hy·po·gan·gli·o·no·sis
hy·po·gas·tric
  ar·tery
  gan·glia
  nerve
  re·flex
  vein
hy·po·gas·tri·um
hy·po·gas·tro·cele
hy·po·gas·trop·a·gus
hy·po·gas·tros·chi·sis
hy·po·gen·e·sis
  po·lar h.
hy·po·ge·net·ic
hy·po·gen·i·tal·ism
hy·po·geu·sia
hy·po·glob·u·lia
hy·po·glos·sal
  ca·nal
  em·i·nence
  nerve
  nu·cle·us
hy·po·glos·sis
hy·po·glos·sus
hy·po·glot·tis
hy·po·gly·ce·mia
  leu·cine h.
  ne·o·na·tal h.
hy·po·gly·ce·mic
hy·po·gly·co·gen·ol·y·sis
hy·po·gly·cor·rha·chia
hy·pog·na·thous
hy·pog·na·thus
hy·po·go·nad·ism
  fa·mil·i·al hy·po·go·nad·o·
    tro·pic h.
  hy·po·go·nad·o·tro·pic h.
  male h.
  pri·mary h.
  sec·on·dary h.
  h. with an·os·mia

hy·po·go·nad·o·tro·pic
 eu·nuch·oid·ism
 hy·po·go·nad·ism
hy·po·gran·u·lo·cy·to·sis
hy·po·he·pat·ia
hy·po·hi·dro·sis
hy·po·hi·drot·ic
hy·po·hi·drot·ic ec·to·der·mal
 dys·pla·sia
hy·po·hy·dre·mia
hy·po·hy·dro·chlo·ria
hy·po·hy·lo·ma
hy·po·hyp·not·ic
hy·po·i·dro·sis
hy·po·i·so·ton·ic
hy·po·ka·le·mia
hy·po·ka·le·mic
 ne·phrop·a·thy
hy·po·ka·le·mic pe·ri·od·ic
 pa·ral·y·sis
hy·po·ki·ne·mia
hy·po·ki·ne·sia
hy·po·ki·ne·sis
hy·po·ki·net·ic
hy·po·lep·i·do·ma
hy·po·leu·ke·mia
hy·po·ley·dig·ism
hy·po·li·po·sis
hy·po·lo·gia
hy·po·lym·phe·mia
hy·po·mag·ne·se·mia
hy·po·ma·nia
hy·po·mas·tia
hy·po·ma·zia
hy·po·mel·an·cho·lia
hy·po·mel·a·no·sis
 h. of Ito
hy·po·me·lia
hy·po·men·or·rhea
hy·po·mere
hy·po·met·a·bol·ic
 state
 syn·drome
hy·po·me·tab·o·lism
 eu·thy·roid h.
hy·po·met·ria
hy·pom·ne·sia
hy·po·morph
hy·po·mo·til·i·ty
hy·po·my·e·li·na·tion
hy·po·my·e·lin·o·gen·e·sis
hy·po·my·o·to·nia
hy·po·myx·ia
hy·po·na·tre·mia
hy·po·ne·o·cy·to·sis
hy·po·noia
hy·po·nych·i·al
hy·po·nych·i·um

hy·pon·y·chon
hy·po·on·cot·ic
hy·po·or·tho·cy·to·sis
hy·po·o·var·i·an·ism
hy·po·pan·cre·a·tism
hy·po·pan·cre·or·rhea
hy·po·par·a·thy·roid
 tet·a·ny
hy·po·par·a·thy·roid·ism
 syn·drome
hy·po·par·a·thy·roid·ism
 fa·mil·i·al h.
hy·po·pep·sia
hy·po·per·i·stal·sis
hy·po·pha·lan·gism
hy·po·pha·ryn·ge·al
 di·ver·tic·u·lum
hy·po·pha·ryn·go·scope
hy·po·phar·ynx
hy·po·pho·ne·sis
hy·po·pho·nia
hy·po·pho·ria
hy·po·phos·pha·ta·se·mia
hy·po·phos·pha·ta·sia
 con·gen·i·tal h.
hy·po·phos·pha·te·mia
hy·po·phos·pha·tu·ria
hy·po·phos·pho·rous ac·id
hy·po·phra·sia
hy·po·phy·se·al
 pouch
hy·po·phy·sec·to·mize
hy·poph·y·sec·to·my
hy·po·phys·e·o·priv·ic
hy·po·phys·e·o·tro·pic
hy·po·phy·si·al
 amen·or·rhea
 ca·chex·ia
 duct
 fos·sa
 syn·drome
hy·poph·y·sin
hy·po·phys·i·o·priv·ic
hy·po·phys·i·o-sphe·noi·dal
 syn·drome
hy·po·phys·i·o·tro·pic
 hor·mone
hy·poph·y·sis
 h. ce·re·bri
 pha·ryn·ge·al h.
 h. sic·ca
hy·poph·y·si·tis
 lym·phoid h.
hy·po·pi·e·sis
 or·tho·stat·ic h.
hy·po·pi·tu·i·ta·rism
hy·po·pla·sia
 car·ti·lage-hair h.

hy·po·pla·sia *(continued)*
  enam·el h.
  fo·cal der·mal h.
  op·tic nerve h.
  re·nal h.
  right ven·tric·u·lar h.
  thy·mic h.
hy·po·plas·tic
  ane·mia
  heart
hy·po·plas·tic left heart
  syn·drome
hy·po·pnea
hy·po·po·sia
hy·po·po·tas·se·mia
hy·po·prax·ia
hy·po·pro·ac·cel·er·i·ne·mia
hy·po·pro·con·ver·ti·ne·mia
hy·po·pro·tein·e·mia
hy·po·pro·tein·o·sis
hy·po·pro·throm·bin·e·mia
hy·pop·ty·a·lism
hy·po·py·on
  re·cur·rent h.
hy·po·py·on
  ker·a·ti·tis
  ul·cer
hy·po·re·flex·ia
hy·po·ren·i·ne·mia
hy·po·ren·i·nem·ic
  hy·po·al·dos·ter·on·ism
hy·po·ri·bo·fla·vin·o·sis
hy·po·sal·e·mi·a
hy·po·sal·i·va·tion
hy·po·sar·ca
hy·pos·che·ot·o·my
hy·po·scle·ral
hy·po·sen·si·tiv·i·ty
hy·po·si·al·ad·e·ni·tis
hy·po·ske·o·cy·to·sis
hy·pos·mia
hy·pos·mo·sis
hy·pos·mot·ic
hy·po·so·ma·to·tro·pism
hy·po·so·mia
hy·po·som·ni·ac
hy·po·spa·di·ac
hy·po·spa·di·as
  ba·lan·ic h.
  pe·no·scro·tal h.
  per·i·ne·al h.
hy·pos·phre·sia
hy·po·sphyx·ia
hy·pos·ta·sis
  post·mor·tem h.
  pul·mo·nary h.
hy·po·stat·ic
  ab·scess

con·ges·tion
ec·ta·sia
pneu·mo·nia
hy·po·sthe·nia
hy·pos·the·ni·ant
hy·po·sthen·ic
hy·pos·the·nu·ria
hy·po·stome
hy·po·sto·mia
hyp·os·to·sis
hy·po·styp·sis
hy·po·styp·tic
hy·po·sys·to·le
hy·po·tax·ia
hy·po·tel·or·ism
hy·po·ten·sion
  ar·te·ri·al h.
  con·trolled h.
  in·duced h.
  in·tra·cra·ni·al h.
  or·tho·stat·ic h.
  pos·tur·al h.
hy·po·ten·sive
  an·es·the·sia
  ret·i·nop·a·thy
hy·po·ten·sor
hy·po·tha·lam·ic
  amen·or·rhea
  in·fun·dib·u·lum
  obe·si·ty
  sul·cus
hy·po·thal·a·mo·hy·po·phy·si·al
  tract
hy·po·thal·a·mo·hy·po·phy·si·al
  por·tal
  sys·tem
hy·po·thal·a·mus
hy·po·the·nar
  em·i·nence
  prom·i·nence
hy·po·ther·mal
hy·po·ther·mia
  ac·ci·den·tal h.
  mod·er·ate h.
  pro·found h.
  re·gion·al h.
  to·tal body h.
hy·po·ther·mic
  an·es·the·sia
hy·poth·e·sis
  au·to·crine h.
  Avogadro's h.
  frus·tra·tion-ag·gres·sion h.
  gate-con·trol h.
  Gompertz' h.
  in·su·lar h.
  Lyon h.
  Makeham's h.

Michaelis-Menten h.
mne·mic h.
null h.
se·quence h.
slid·ing fil·a·ment h.
Starling's h.
zwit·ter h.
hy·po·thet·i·cal mean
or·ga·nism
strain
hy·po·throm·bi·ne·mia
hy·po·throm·bo·plas·ti·ne·mia
hy·po·thy·mia
hy·po·thy·mic
hy·po·thy·mism
hy·po·thy·roid
dwarf·ism
in·fan·ti·lism
hy·po·thy·roid·ism
in·fan·tile h.
sec·on·dary h.
hy·po·thy·rox·i·ne·mia
hy·po·to·nia
hy·po·ton·ic
hy·po·to·nic·i·ty
hy·po·to·nus
hy·pot·o·ny
hy·po·tox·ic·i·ty
hy·po·tri·chi·a·sis
hy·po·tri·cho·sis
h. con·gen·i·ta
hy·po·tro·pia
hy·po·tym·pa·not·o·my
hy·po·tym·pa·num
hy·po·u·re·sis
hy·po·u·ri·ce·mia
hy·po·u·ri·cu·ria
hy·po·var·i·an·ism
hy·po·ven·ti·la·tion
hy·po·vi·ta·min·o·sis
hy·po·vo·le·mia
hy·po·vo·le·mic
shock
hy·po·vo·lia
hy·po·xan·thine
h. gua·nine phos·pho·ri·bo·
syl·trans·fer·ase
h. ox·i·dase
h. phos·pho·ri·bo·syl·trans·
fer·ase
hy·pox·e·mia
test
hy·pox·ia
ane·mic h.
dif·fu·sion h.
hy·pox·ic h.
is·che·mic h.

ox·y·gen af·fin·i·ty h.
stag·nant h.
hy·pox·ia warn·ing
sys·tem
hy·pox·ic
hy·pox·ia
ne·phro·sis
hyp·sa·rhyth·mia
hyp·sar·rhyth·mia
hyp·si·brach·y·ce·phal·ic
hyp·si·ce·phal·ic
hyp·si·ceph·a·ly
hyp·si·con·chous
hyp·si·loid
an·gle
car·ti·lage
lig·a·ment
hyp·si·sta·phyl·ia
hyp·si·sten·o·ce·phal·ic
hyp·so·ceph·a·ly
hyp·so·chro·mic
hyp·so·dont
hy·pur·gia
Hyrtl's
anas·to·mo·sis
fo·ra·men
loop
sphinc·ter
Hyrtl's ep·i·tym·pan·ic
re·cess
hys·ter·al·gia
hys·ter·a·tre·sia
hys·ter·ec·to·my
ab·dom·i·nal h.
ab·dom·i·no·vag·i·nal h.
ce·sar·e·an h.
mod·i·fied rad·i·cal h.
par·a·vag·i·nal h.
Porro h.
rad·i·cal h.
sub·to·tal h.
su·pra·cer·vi·cal h.
vag·i·nal h.
hys·ter·e·sis
stat·ic h.
hys·ter·eu·ry·sis
hys·te·ria
anx·i·e·ty h.
ca·nine h.
con·ver·sion h.
ep·i·dem·ic h.
ma·jor h.
mass h.
mi·nor h.
hys·ter·ic
hys·ter·i·cal
am·bly·o·pia
an·es·the·sia

hys·ter·i·cal *(continued)*
  apho·nia
  cho·rea
  con·vul·sion
  deaf·ness
  joint
  nys·tag·mus
  per·son·al·i·ty
  pol·y·dip·sia
  psy·cho·sis
  syn·co·pe
hys·ter·i·co·neu·ral·gic
hys·ter·ics
hys·ter·o·cat·a·lep·sy
hys·ter·o·cele
hys·ter·o·clei·sis
hys·ter·o·col·po·scope
hys·ter·o·cys·to·pexy
hys·ter·o·dyn·ia
hys·ter·o·ep·i·lep·sy
hys·ter·o·gen·ic
hys·ter·og·en·ous
hys·ter·o·gram
hys·ter·o·graph
hys·ter·og·ra·phy
hys·ter·oid
  con·vul·sion
hys·ter·o·lith
hys·ter·ol·y·sis
hys·ter·om·e·ter
hys·ter·o·my·o·ma
hys·ter·o·my·o·mec·to·my

hys·ter·o·my·ot·o·my
hys·ter·o·nar·co·lep·sy
hys·tero-oo·pho·rec·to·my
hys·ter·op·a·thy
hys·ter·o·pex·y
  ab·dom·i·nal h.
hys·ter·o·phore
hys·ter·o·pia
hys·ter·o·plas·ty
hys·ter·or·rha·phy
hys·ter·or·rhex·is
hys·ter·o·sal·pin·gec·to·my
hys·ter·o·sal·pin·gog·ra·phy
hys·ter·o·sal·pin·go-oo·pho·rec·to·my
hys·ter·o·sal·pin·gos·to·my
hys·ter·o·scope
hys·ter·os·co·py
hys·ter·o·spasm
hys·ter·o·sys·to·le
hys·ter·o·ther·mom·e·try
hys·ter·ot·o·my
  ab·dom·i·nal h.
  vag·i·nal h.
hys·ter·o·to·nin
hys·ter·o·trach·e·lec·to·my
hys·ter·o·trach·e·lo·plas·ty
hys·ter·o·tra·che·lor·rha·phy
hys·ter·o·trach·e·lot·o·my
hys·ter·o·tris·mus
hys·ter·o·tu·bog·ra·phy

I

I
band
cell
disk
pi·li

i
an·ti·gens
ia·tra·lip·tic
ia·tra·lip·tics
iat·ric
iat·ro·gen·ic
trans·mis·sion
ia·trol·o·gy
iat·ro·phys·ics
iat·ro·tech·nique
Iba·ra·ki
vi·rus
IBR
vi·rus
ibu·fe·nac
ibu·pro·fen
ICAO stan·dard
at·mo·sphere
Ice·land
dis·ease
moss
I-cell
dis·ease
ich·no·gram
ichor
icho·re·mia
icho·roid
ichor·ous
pus
ichor·rhea
ichor·rhe·mia
ich·tham·mol
ich·thy·ism
ich·thy·is·mus
i. ex·an·the·ma·ti·cus
ich·thy·o·a·can·tho·tox·ism
ich·thy·o·col·la
ich·thy·o·he·mo·tox·in
ich·thy·o·he·mo·tox·ism
ich·thy·oid
ich·thy·o·o·tox·in
ich·thy·oph·a·gous
ich·thy·o·pho·bia
ich·thy·o·sar·co·tox·in

ich·thy·o·sar·co·tox·ism
ich·thy·o·si·form
eryth·ro·der·ma
ich·thy·o·sis
ac·quired i.
i. con·gen·i·ta ne·o·na·to·rum
i. cor·nea
i. fe·ta·lis
i. fol·lic·u·la·ris
i. hys·trix
i. in·tra·u·te·ri·na
lam·el·lar i.
i. li·ne·a·ris cir·cum·scrip·ta
na·cre·ous i.
i. pal·mar·is et plan·tar·is
i. sau·ro·der·ma
i. scu·tu·la·ta
i. se·ba·cea
i. se·ba·cea cor·nea
i. sim·plex
i. spi·no·sa
i. uter·i
i. vul·ga·ris
X-linked i.
ich·thy·ot·ic
ich·thy·o·tox·i·col·o·gy
ich·thy·o·tox·i·con
ich·thy·o·tox·in
ich·thy·o·tox·ism
ic·ing
heart
liv·er
icon·ic
signs
icon·o·ma·nia
ico·sa·he·dral
n-ico·sa·no·ic ac·id
ic·tal
ic·ter·ic
in·dex
ic·ter·o·a·ne·mia
swine i.
ic·ter·o·gen·ic
ic·ter·o·he·ma·tu·ric
ic·ter·o·he·mo·glo·bi·nu·ria
ic·ter·o·he·mo·lyt·ic
ane·mia

ic·ter·o·hep·a·ti·tis
ic·ter·oid
ic·ter·us
   ac·quired he·mo·lyt·ic i.
   be·nign fa·mil·i·al i.
   chron·ic fa·mil·i·al i.
   con·gen·i·tal he·mo·lyt·ic i.
   cy·the·mo·lyt·ic i.
   i. gra·vis
   in·fec·tious i.
   i. me·las
   i. ne·o·na·to·rum
   phys·i·o·log·ic i.
   i. pre·cox
ic·ter·us
   in·dex
ic·tom·e·ter
ic·tus
   i. cor·dis
   i. ep·i·lep·ti·cus
   i. pa·ra·ly·ti·cus
   i. so·lis
ICU
   psy·cho·sis
id
   re·ac·tion
idea
   au·toch·thon·ous i.'s
   com·pul·sive i.
   dom·i·nant i.
   fixed i.
   hy·per·quan·ti·va·lent i.
   per·ma·nent dom·i·nant i.
   i. of ref·er·ence
ide·al
   ego i.
ide·al al·ve·o·lar
   gas
ide·a·tion
ide·a·tion·al
   ag·no·sia
   aprax·ia
ide·a·tory
   aprax·ia
idée fixe
iden·ti·cal
   twins
iden·ti·fi·ca·tion
iden·ti·ty
   ego i.
   gen·der i.
   sense of i.
iden·ti·ty
   cri·sis
   dis·or·der
ide·o·ki·net·ic
   aprax·ia
ide·ol·o·gy

ide·o·mo·tion
ide·o·mo·tor
   aprax·ia
ide·o·pho·bia
ide·o·plas·tia
id·i·o·ag·glu·ti·nin
id·i·o·chro·mo·some
id·i·o·cy
   am·au·rot·ic fa·mil·i·al i.
id·i·o·dy·nam·ic
   con·trol
id·i·og·a·mist
id·i·o·gen·e·sis
id·i·o·glos·sia
id·i·o·glot·tic
id·i·o·gram
id·i·o·graph·ic
   ap·proach
id·i·o·het·er·o·ag·glu·ti·nin
id·i·o·het·er·o·ly·sin
id·i·o·hyp·no·tism
id·i·o·i·so·ag·glu·ti·nin
id·i·o·i·sol·y·sin
id·i·o·la·lia
id·i·ol·y·sin
id·i·o·mus·cu·lar
   con·trac·tion
id·i·o·nod·al
   rhythm
id·i·o·pa·thet·ic
id·i·o·path·ic
   al·do·ste·ron·ism
   bra·dy·car·dia
   car·di·o·my·op·a·thy
   dwarf·ism
   ep·i·lep·sy
   he·mo·chro·ma·to·sis
   hir·sut·ism
   hy·per·cal·ce·mia of in·fants
   hy·per·li·pe·mia
   hy·per·ten·sion
   in·fan·ti·lism
   meg·a·co·lon
   neu·ral·gia
   proc·ti·tis
   ro·se·o·la
id·i·o·path·ic **Bamberger-Marie**
   dis·ease
id·i·o·path·ic fi·brous
   me·di·as·ti·ni·tis
   ret·ro·per·i·to·ni·tis
id·i·o·path·ic hy·per·cal·ce·mic
   scle·ro·sis of in·fants
id·i·o·path·ic hy·per·tro·phic
   os·te·o·ar·throp·a·thy
id·i·o·path·ic hy·per·tro·phic
   sub·a·or·tic
   ste·no·sis

id·i·o·path·ic mus·cu·lar
  at·ro·phy
id·i·o·path·ic par·ox·ys·mal
  rhab·do·my·ol·y·sis
id·i·o·path·ic pul·mo·nary
  he·mo·sid·er·o·sis
id·i·o·path·ic ret·ro·per·i·to·
  ne·al
  fi·bro·sis
id·i·o·path·ic throm·bo·cy·to·
  pe·nic
  pur·pu·ra
id·i·op·a·thy
id·i·o·phren·ic
id·i·o·psy·cho·log·ic
id·i·o·re·flex
id·i·o·some
id·i·o·spasm
id·i·o·syn·cra·sy
id·i·o·syn·crat·ic
  sen·si·tiv·i·ty
id·i·ot-prod·i·gy
id·i·o·tro·phic
id·i·o·tro·pic
id·i·ot-sa·vant
id·i·o·type
  an·ti·body
  au·to·an·ti·body
id·i·o·typ·ic an·ti·gen·ic
  de·ter·mi·nant
id·i·o·var·i·a·tion
id·i·o·ven·tric·u·lar
  kick
  rhythm
id·i·tol
id·ose
idox·ur·i·dine
idro·sis
idur·on·ic ac·id
IgA
  ne·phrop·a·thy
IgM
  ne·phrop·a·thy
ig·na·tia
ig·ni·pe·di·tes
ig·ni·punc·ture
ig·no·tine
IKI
  cat·gut
iko·ta
il·e·ac
il·e·a·del·phus
il·e·al
  ar·ter·ies
  blad·der
  con·duit
  in·tus·sus·cep·tion

sphinc·ter
  veins
il·e·ec·to·my
il·e·i·tis
  back·wash i.
  dis·tal i.
  re·gion·al i.
  ter·mi·nal i.
il·e·o·ce·cal
  em·i·nence
  fold
  in·tus·sus·cep·tion
  open·ing
  valve
il·e·o·ce·co·co·lic
  sphinc·ter
il·e·o·ce·cos·to·my
il·e·o·ce·cum
il·e·o·co·lic
  ar·tery
  in·tus·sus·cep·tion
  valve
  vein
il·e·o·co·lic lymph
  nodes
il·e·o·co·li·tis
il·e·o·co·lon·ic
il·e·o·co·los·to·my
il·e·o·cys·to·plas·ty
il·e·o·en·tec·tro·py
il·e·o·il·e·os·to·my
il·e·o·je·ju·ni·tis
il·e·o·pexy
il·e·o·proc·tos·to·my
il·e·o·rec·tos·to·my
il·e·or·rha·phy
il·e·o·sig·moid·os·to·my
il·e·os·to·my
  Brooke i.
  Kock i.
il·e·ot·o·my
il·e·o·trans·ver·sos·to·my
il·e·um
  i. du·plex
il·e·us
  ady·nam·ic i.
  dy·nam·ic i.
  gall·stone i.
  me·chan·i·cal i.
  me·co·ni·um i.
  oc·clu·sive i.
  par·a·lyt·ic i.
  spas·tic i.
  i. sub·par·ta
  ter·mi·nal i.
  ver·min·ous i.
Ilhé·us
  en·ceph·a·li·tis

Ilhé·us *(continued)*
  fe·ver
  vi·rus
il·ia
il·i·ac
  bone
  bur·sa
  co·lon
  crest
  fas·cia
  fos·sa
  horn
  mus·cle
  plex·us
  re·gion
  roll
  spine
  steal
  tu·ber·cle
  tu·ber·os·i·ty
  veins
il·i·a·co·sub·fas·cial
  fos·sa
  her·nia
il·i·a·cus
il·i·a·del·phus
il·i·o·coc·cyg·e·al
  mus·cle
il·i·o·co·lot·o·my
il·i·o·cos·tal
  mus·cle
il·i·o·cos·ta·lis
il·i·o·fem·o·ral
  lig·a·ment
  tri·an·gle
il·i·o·fem·o·ro·plas·ty
il·i·o·hy·po·gas·tric
  nerve
il·i·o·in·gui·nal
  nerve
il·i·o·lum·bar
  ar·tery
  lig·a·ment
  vein
il·i·om·e·ter
il·i·op·a·gus
il·i·o·pec·tin·e·al
  arch
  bur·sa
  em·i·nence
  fas·cia
  fos·sa
  lig·a·ment
  line
il·i·o·pel·vic
  sphinc·ter
il·i·o·pso·as
  mus·cle

il·i·o·pu·bic
  em·i·nence
il·i·o·sa·cral
il·i·o·sci·at·ic
  notch
il·i·o·spi·nal
il·i·o·tho·ra·cop·a·gus
il·i·o·tib·i·al
  band
il·i·o·tro·chan·ter·ic
  lig·a·ment
il·i·o·xi·phop·a·gus
il·i·um
ill
  joint i.
  loup·ing i.
  na·vel i.
il·lic·i·um
il·lin·i·tion
ill·ness
  func·tion·al i.
  men·tal i.
il·lu·mi·na·tion
  ax·i·al i.
  cen·tral i.
  con·tact i.
  crit·i·cal i.
  dark-field i.
  dark-ground i.
  di·rect i.
  erect i.
  fo·cal i.
  Köhler i.
  lat·er·al i.
  ob·lique i.
  ver·ti·cal i.
il·lu·mi·nism
il·lu·sion
  i. of dou·bles
  i. of move·ment
  oc·u·lo·grav·ic i.
  oc·u·lo·gy·ral i.
  op·ti·cal i.
il·lu·sion·al
Ilosvay
  re·a·gent
im·age
  ac·ci·den·tal i.
  body i.
  cat·a·tro·pic i.
  di·rect i.
  ei·det·ic i.
  false i.
  het·er·on·y·mous i.
  ho·mon·y·mous i.'s
  hyp·na·gog·ic i.
  hyp·no·pom·pic i.
  in·ci·den·tal i.

in·vert·ed i.
men·tal i.
mir·ror i.
mo·tor i.
op·ti·cal i.
Purkinje i.'s
Purkinje-Sanson i.'s
real i.
ret·i·nal i.
Sanson's i.'s
sen·so·ry i.
spec·u·lar i.
tac·tile i.
un·e·qual ret·i·nal i.
vir·tu·al i.
vi·su·al i.
im·ag·e·ry
imag·i·nal
imag·ines
imag·ing
mag·net·ic res·o·nance i.
NMR i.
nu·cle·ar mag·net·ic res·o·
nance i.
ima·go
im·bal·ance
au·to·nom·ic i.
oc·clu·sal i.
sex chro·mo·some i.
sym·pa·thet·ic i.
va·so·mo·tor i.
im·be·cile
im·bed
im·bi·bi·tion
im·bri·cate
im·bri·cat·ed
im·bri·ca·tion
lines of von Ebner
im·id·a·zole
im·id·az·o·lyl
im·ide
im·i·do·di·pep·ti·dase
im·i·dole
im·in·az·ole
im·in·az·o·lyl
im·i·no ac·ids
im·i·no·car·bon·yl
im·i·no·di·pep·ti·dase
im·i·no·gly·ci·nu·ria
im·i·no·hy·dro·las·es
im·i·pen·em
imip·ra·mine hy·dro·chlo·ride
im·i·ta·tive
tet·a·nus
Imlach's
fat-pad
ring

im·ma·ture
cat·a·ract
gran·u·lo·cyte
neu·tro·phil
im·me·di·ate
al·ler·gy
am·pu·ta·tion
aus·cul·ta·tion
con·ta·gion
den·ture
flap
per·cus·sion
re·ac·tion
trans·fu·sion
im·me·di·ate in·ser·tion
den·ture
im·me·di·ate post·trau·mat·ic
au·tom·a·tism
con·vul·sion
im·me·di·ca·ble
im·mer·sion
ho·mo·ge·neous i.
oil i.
wa·ter i.
im·mer·sion
foot
lens
mi·cros·co·py
ob·jec·tive
im·mi·nent
abor·tion
im·mis·ci·ble
im·mit·tance
im·mo·bi·li·za·tion
im·mo·bi·lize
im·mo·bi·liz·ing
an·ti·body
im·mor·tal·i·za·tion
im·mo·tile cil·ia
syn·drome
im·mov·a·ble
ban·dage
joint
im·mune
ad·sorp·tion
ag·glu·ti·na·tion
ag·glu·ti·nin
body
com·plex
de·fi·cien·cy
de·vi·a·tion
he·mo·ly·sin
he·mol·y·sis
in·flam·ma·tion
in·ter·fer·on
op·so·nin
pre·cip·i·ta·tion
pro·tein

im·mune *(continued)*
  re·ac·tion
  re·sponse
  se·rum
  sur·veil·lance
  sys·tem
  throm·bo·cy·to·pe·nia
im·mune ad·her·ence
  phe·nom·e·non
im·mune ad·he·sion
  test
im·mune com·plex
  dis·ease
  dis·or·der
  ne·phri·tis
im·mune elec·tron
  mi·cros·co·py
im·mune fe·tal
  hy·drops
im·mune re·sponse
  genes
im·mune se·rum
  glob·u·lin
im·mune throm·bo·cy·to·pe·nic
  pur·pu·ra
im·mu·ni·fa·cient
im·mu·ni·ty
  ac·quired i.
  ac·tive i.
  adop·tive i.
  an·ti·vi·ral i.
  ar·ti·fi·cial ac·tive i.
  ar·ti·fi·cial pas·sive i.
  bac·te·ri·o·phage i.
  cell-me·di·at·ed i.
  cel·lu·lar i.
  con·com·i·tant i.
  gen·er·al i.
  ge·net·ic i.
  group i.
  hu·mor·al i.
  in·fec·tion i.
  in·her·ent i.
  in·nate i.
  lo·cal i.
  nat·u·ral i.
  non·spe·cif·ic i.
  pas·sive i.
  rel·a·tive i.
  spe·cif·ic i.
  spe·cif·ic ac·tive i.
  spe·cif·ic pas·sive i.
  stress i.
im·mu·ni·ty
  de·fi·cien·cy
im·mu·ni·za·tion
  ac·tive i.
  pas·sive i.

im·mu·nize
im·mu·no·ad·ju·vant
im·mu·no·ag·glu·ti·na·tion
im·mu·no·as·say
  dou·ble an·ti·body i.
  en·zyme-mul·ti·plied i.
  sol·id phase i.
  thin-lay·er i.
im·mu·no·blast
im·mu·no·blas·tic
  lym·phad·e·nop·a·thy
  lym·pho·ma
  sar·co·ma
im·mu·no·chem·i·cal
  as·say
im·mu·no·chem·is·try
im·mu·no·com·pe·tence
im·mu·no·com·pe·tent
im·mu·no·com·pro·mised
im·mu·no·con·glu·ti·nin
im·mu·no·cyte
im·mu·no·cy·to·chem·is·try
im·mu·no·de·fi·cien·cy
  cel·lu·lar i. with ab·nor·mal
    im·mu·no·glob·u·lin syn·
    the·sis
  com·bined i.
  com·mon var·i·a·ble i.
  sec·on·dary i.
  se·vere com·bined i.
  i. with hy·po·par·a·thy·
    roid·ism
im·mu·no·de·fi·cien·cy
  syn·drome
im·mu·no·de·fi·cient
im·mu·no·de·pres·sant
im·mu·no·de·pres·sor
im·mu·no·di·ag·no·sis
im·mu·no·dif·fu·sion
  dou·ble i.
  ra·di·al i.
  sin·gle i.
im·mu·no·e·lec·tro·pho·re·sis
  crossed i.
  rock·et i.
  two-di·men·sion·al i.
im·mu·no·en·hance·ment
im·mu·no·en·hanc·er
im·mu·no·fer·ri·tin
im·mu·no·flu·o·res·cence
  meth·od
  mi·cros·co·py
im·mu·no·flu·o·res·cent
  stain
im·mu·no·gen
  be·hav·ior·al i.
im·mu·no·ge·net·ics
im·mu·no·gen·ic

im·mu·no·ge·nic·i·ty
im·mu·no·glob·u·lin
   an·ti-D i.
   chick·en·pox i.
   hu·man nor·mal i.
   mea·sles i.
   mon·o·clo·nal i.
   per·tus·sis i.
   po·li·o·my·e·li·tis i.
   ra·bies i.
   $Rh_o(D)$ i.
   tet·a·nus i.
im·mu·no·he·ma·tol·o·gy
im·mu·no·his·to·chem·is·try
im·mu·no·log·i·cal
   com·pe·tence
   de·fi·cien·cy
   en·hance·ment
   mech·a·nism
   pa·ral·y·sis
   sur·veil·lance
   tol·er·ance
im·mu·no·log·i·cal de·fi·cien·cy
   syn·drome
im·mu·no·log·i·cal·ly ac·ti·vat·
  ed
   cell
im·mu·no·log·i·cal·ly com·pe·
  tent
   cell
im·mu·no·log·ic preg·nan·cy
   test
im·mu·nol·o·gist
im·mu·nol·o·gy
im·mu·no·pa·thol·o·gy
im·mu·no·per·ox·i·dase
   tech·nique
im·mu·no·po·ten·ti·a·tion
im·mu·no·po·ten·ti·a·tor
im·mu·no·pre·cip·i·ta·tion
im·mu·no·pro·lif·er·a·tive
   dis·or·ders
im·mu·no·pro·lif·er·a·tive small
  in·tes·ti·nal
   dis·ease
im·mu·no·ra·di·o·met·ric
   as·say
im·mu·no·re·ac·tion
im·mu·no·re·ac·tive
   in·su·lin
im·mu·no·se·lec·tion
im·mu·no·sor·bent
im·mu·no·sup·pres·sant
im·mu·no·sup·pres·sion
im·mu·no·sup·pres·sive
im·mu·no·sym·pa·thec·to·my
im·mu·no·ther·a·py
   adop·tive i.

im·mu·no·tol·er·ance
im·mu·no·trans·fu·sion
imol·a·mine
im·pact
   re·sis·tance
im·pact·ed
   fe·tus
   frac·ture
   tooth
im·pac·tion
   den·tal i.
   fe·cal i.
   food i.
   mu·cus i.
im·pair·ment
   func·tion·al aer·o·bic i.
   men·tal i.
im·par·i·dig·i·tate
IMP-as·par·tate li·gase
im·pat·ent
im·ped·ance
   an·gle
   meth·od
   pleth·ys·mog·ra·phy
im·per·a·tive
   con·cep·tion
im·per·cep·tion
im·per·fect
   fun·gus
   stage
   state
im·per·fo·rate
   anus
   hy·men
im·per·fo·ra·tion
im·per·me·a·ble
im·per·me·ant
im·per·sis·tence
   mo·tor i.
im·per·vi·ous
im·pe·tig·i·ni·za·tion
im·pe·tig·i·nous
   chei·li·tis
   syph·i·lid
im·pe·ti·go
   Bockhart's i.
   i. bul·lo·sa
   bul·lous i. of new·born
   i. cir·ci·na·ta
   i. con·ta·gi·o·sa
   i. ec·ze·ma·todes
   fol·lic·u·lar i.
   i. her·pet·i·for·mis
   i. ne·o·na·to·rum
   i. vul·ga·ris
im·pe·tus
im·plant
   bag-gel i.

im·plant *(continued)*
  car·ci·nom·a·tous i.'s
  co·chle·ar i.
  en·do·me·tri·al i.'s
  en·do·os·se·ous i.
  en·dos·te·al i.
  in·flat·a·ble i.
  in·tra·oc·u·lar i.
  mag·net·ic i.
  or·bi·tal i.
  pe·nile i.
  pin i.
  post i.
  sub·mu·co·sal i.
  sub·per·i·os·te·al i.
  su·pra·per·i·os·te·al i.
  tri·plant i.
im·plant
  den·ture
im·plan·ta·tion
  cone
  cyst
  der·moid
  graft
  the·o·ry of the pro·duc·tion
    of en·do·me·tri·o·sis
im·plan·ta·tion
  cen·tral i.
  cir·cum·fer·en·tial i.
  cor·ti·cal i.
  de·layed i.
  ec·cen·tric i.
  in·ter·sti·tial i.
  nerve i.
  pel·let i.
  per·i·os·te·al i.
  sub·cu·ta·ne·ous i.
  su·per·fi·cial i.
im·plant den·ture
  sub·struc·ture
  su·per·struc·ture
im·plant·ed
  su·ture
im·ple·tion
im·plo·sion
im·plo·sive
  ther·a·py
im·po·tence
  aton·ic i.
  pa·ret·ic i.
  psy·chic i.
  symp·to·mat·ic i.
im·po·ten·cy
im·preg·nate
im·preg·na·tion
im·pres·sio
  i. pe·tro·sa pal·lii

im·pres·sion
  bas·i·lar i.
  car·di·ac i. of liv·er
  car·di·ac i. of lung
  col·ic i.
  com·plete den·ture i.
  i. for cos·to·cla·vic·u·lar
    lig·a·ment
  del·toid i.
  dig·i·tate i.'s
  di·rect bone i.
  du·o·de·nal i.
  esoph·a·ge·al i.
  fi·nal i.
  gas·tric i.
  men·tal i.
  par·tial den·ture i.
  pe·tro·sal i. of the pal·li·
    um
  pre·lim·i·nary i.
  pri·mary i.
  re·nal i.
  rhom·boid i.
  sec·tion·al i.
  su·pra·re·nal i.
  tri·gem·i·nal i.
im·pres·sion
  ar·ea
  com·pound
  ma·te·ri·al
  tray
im·pres·si·o·nes
im·pres·sive
  apha·sia
im·print
im·print·ing
im·pulse
  car·di·ac i.
  ec·top·ic i.
  es·cape i.
  ir·re·sist·i·ble i.
  mor·bid i.
im·pulse con·trol
  dis·or·der
im·pul·sion
im·pul·sive
  ob·ses·sion
im·pure
  flut·ter
imus
in·ac·tion
in·ac·ti·vate
in·ac·ti·vat·ed po·li·o·vi·rus
  vac·cine
in·ac·ti·va·tion
in·ac·tive
  mu·tant

re·pres·sor
tu·ber·cu·lo·sis
in·ad·e·quate
per·son·al·i·ty
stim·u·lus
in·an·i·mate
in·a·ni·tion
fe·ver
in·ap·par·ent
in·ap·pe·tence
in·ap·pro·pri·ate
af·fect
hor·mone
in·ar·tic·u·late
in·as·sim·i·la·ble
in·at·ten·tion
se·lec·tive i.
sen·so·ry i.
vi·su·al i.
in·born
er·rors of me·tab·o·lism
in·bred
in·breed·ing
in·car·cer·at·ed
her·nia
pla·cen·ta
in·car·cer·a·tion
symp·tom
in·ca·ri·al
bone
in·car·nant
in·car·na·tive
in·case·ment
the·o·ry
in·cen·di·a·rism
in·cen·tive
in·cer·tae se·dis
in·cest
bar·ri·er
in·ces·tu·ous
in·ci·dence
in·ci·dent
an·gle
point
ray
in·ci·den·tal
col·or
im·age
learn·ing
par·a·site
in·cip·i·ent
abor·tion
car·ies
in·ci·sal
edge
em·bra·sure
guid·ance
guide

mar·gin
path
point
rest
sur·face
in·ci·sal guide
an·gle
in·cise
in·cised
wound
in·ci·sion
bi·op·sy
in·ci·sion
Agnew-Verhoeff i.
buck·et-han·dle i.
ce·li·ot·o·my i.
chev·ron i.
Deaver's i.
Dührssen's i.'s
end·au·ral i.
Fergusson's i.
flank i.
Kocher's i.
McBurney's i.
par·a·me·di·an i.
Pfannenstiel's i.
in·ci·sion·al
her·nia
in·ci·sive
bone
ca·nal
duct
fo·ra·men
fos·sa
pa·pil·la
su·ture
in·ci·sor
ca·nal
crest
fo·ra·men
tooth
in·ci·sor
cen·tral i.
lat·er·al i.
scal·pri·form i.'s
sec·ond i.
in·ci·su·ra
i. ce·re·bel·li an·te·ri·or
i. ce·re·bel·li pos·te·ri·or
i. ri·vini
in·ci·su·rae san·to·ri·ni
i. sem·i·lu·na·ris ul·nae
i. tra·gi·ca
i. um·bi·li·ca·lis
in·ci·su·rae
in·ci·sure
Lanterman's i.'s
Rivinus' i.

in·ci·sure *(continued)*
  Santorini's i.'s
  Schmidt-Lanterman i.'s
  tym·pan·ic i.
in·cli·na·tio
in·cli·na·tion
  con·dy·lar guid·ance i.
  enam·el rod i.
  lat·er·al con·dy·lar i.
  i. of pel·vis
in·cli·na·ti·o·nes
in·cli·nom·e·ter
in·clu·sion
  cell i.'s
  Döhle i.'s
  fe·tal i.
  leu·ko·cyte i.'s
in·clu·sion
  blen·nor·rhea
  bod·ies
  cell
  com·pound
  con·junc·ti·vi·tis
  cyst
  der·moid
in·clu·sion body
  dis·ease
  en·ceph·a·li·tis
in·clu·sion cell
  dis·ease
in·clu·sion con·junc·ti·vi·tis
  vi·rus·es
in·co·er·ci·ble
in·co·her·ent
in·com·i·tant
  stra·bis·mus
in·com·pat·i·bil·i·ty
  phys·i·o·log·ic i.
  ther·a·peu·tic i.
in·com·pat·i·ble
in·com·pat·i·ble blood trans·fu·sion
  re·ac·tion
in·com·pe·tence
  aor·tic i.
  car·di·ac i.
  mi·tral i.
  mus·cu·lar i.
  pul·mo·nary i.
  pul·mon·ic i.
  py·lor·ic i.
  rel·a·tive i.
  tri·cus·pid i.
  val·vu·lar i.
in·com·pe·ten·cy
in·com·pe·tent cer·vi·cal
  os

in·com·plete
  abor·tion
  achro·ma·top·sia
  alex·ia
  an·ti·body
  an·ti·gen
  as·cer·tain·ment
  cleav·age
  dis·in·fec·tant
  fis·tu·la
  frac·ture
  hem·i·a·nop·sia
  met·a·mor·pho·sis
  neu·ro·fi·bro·ma·to·sis
  tet·a·nus
in·com·plete atri·o·ven·tric·u·lar
  dis·so·ci·a·tion
in·com·plete A-V
  dis·so·ci·a·tion
in·com·plete con·joined
  twins
in·com·plete foot
  pre·sen·ta·tion
in·com·plete knee
  pre·sen·ta·tion
in·con·gru·ent
  nys·tag·mus
in·con·gru·ous
  hem·i·a·nop·sia
in·con·stant
in·con·ti·nence
  i. of milk
  over·flow i.
  par·a·dox·i·cal i.
  pas·sive i.
  i. of pig·ment
  re·flex i.
  urge i.
  ur·gen·cy i.
  uri·nary ex·er·tion·al i.
  uri·nary stress i.
in·con·ti·nent
in·con·ti·nen·tia
  i. pig·men·ti
  i. pig·men·ti achro·mi·ens
in·co·or·di·na·tion
in·cor·po·ra·tion
in·crease
  ab·so·lute cell i.
in·cre·ment
in·cre·men·tal
  lines
  lines of von Ebner
in·cre·tion
in·crus·ta·tion
in·cu·ba·tion
  pe·ri·od

in·cu·ba·tive
   stage
in·cu·ba·tor
in·cu·ba·to·ry
   car·ri·er
in·cu·bus
in·cu·dal
   fold
   fos·sa
in·cu·dec·to·my
in·cu·des
in·cu·di·form
   uter·us
in·cu·dis
in·cu·do·mal·le·al
in·cu·do·mal·le·o·lar
   joint
in·cu·do·sta·pe·di·al
   ar·tic·u·la·tion
   joint
in·cur·a·ble
in·cur·va·tion
in·cus
in·cy·clo·duc·tion
in·cy·clo·pho·ria
in·dan·e·di·ones
in·dap·a·mide
in·de·cid·u·ate
in·den·i·za·tion
in·den·ta·tion
   hard·ness
in·de·pen·dent
   as·sort·ment
   var·i·a·ble
in·de·ter·mi·nate
   cleav·age
   lep·ro·sy
in·dex
   am·bly·o·pia
   am·e·tro·pia
   case
   fin·ger
   hy·per·me·tro·pia
   my·o·pia
in·dex
   ab·sorb·an·cy i.
   al·ve·o·lar i.
   an·es·thet·ic i.
   an·ti·tryp·tic i.
   Arneth i.
   au·ric·u·lar i.
   Ayala's i.
   bas·i·lar i.
   Bödecker i.
   body mass i.
   buff·er i.
   car·di·ac i.
   car·di·o·tho·rac·ic i.

cen·tro·mer·ic i.
ce·phal·ic i.
ceph·a·lo-or·bit·al i.
ceph·a·lor·rha·chid·i·an i.
ce·re·bral i.
cer·e·bro·spi·nal i.
che·mo·ther·a·peu·tic i.
chest i.
col·or i.
cra·ni·al i.
Dean's flu·o·ro·sis i.
DEF car·ies i.
def car·ies i.
de·gen·er·a·tive i.
den·tal i.
DF car·ies i.
df car·ies i.
DMF car·ies i.
dmf car·ies i.
DMFS car·ies i.
dmfs car·ies i.
ef·fec·tive tem·per·a·ture i.
em·path·ic i.
en·dem·ic i.
eryth·ro·cyte in·di·ces
fa·cial i.
Flower's den·tal i.
free thy·rox·ine i.
gnath·ic i.
height-length i.
ic·ter·ic i.
ic·ter·us i.
iron i.
kar·y·o·pyk·not·ic i.
length-breadth i.
length-height i.
leu·ko·pe·nic i.
mat·u·ra·tion i.
met·a·car·pal i.
mi·tot·ic i.
mo·lar ab·sorb·an·cy i.
na·sal i.
nu·cle·o·plas·mic i.
obe·si·ty i.
op·son·ic i.
or·bi·tal i.
or·bi·to·na·sal i.
pal·a·tal i.
pal·a·tine i.
pal·a·to·max·il·lary i.
pel·vic i.
phag·o·cyt·ic i.
PMA i.
pon·der·al i.
pres·sure-vol·ume i.
re·frac·tive i.
Robinson i.
Röhrer's i.

in·di·rect nu·cle·ar
di·vi·sion
in·di·rect o·vu·lar
trans·mi·gra·tion
in·di·rect pulp
cap·ping
in·di·rect pu·pil·lary
re·ac·tion
in·di·rect re·act·ing
bil·i·ru·bin
in·dis·po·si·tion
in·di·um
in·di·um-111
in·di·vid·u·al
dif·fer·enc·es
psy·chol·o·gy
ther·a·py
tol·er·ance
in·di·vid·u·a·tion
field
in·do·cy·a·nine green
in·do·cy·bin
in·dol·ac·e·tu·ria
in·dol·a·mine
in·dole
in·do·lent
bu·bo
ul·cer
in·dol·ic ac·ids
in·do·log·e·nous
in·do·lu·ria
in·do·lyl
in·do·meth·a·cin
in·do·phe·nol
meth·od
in·do·phe·nol·ase
in·do·phe·nol ox·i·dase
in·do·pro·fen
in·dox·yl
in·dox·yl·u·ria
in·duce
in·duced
abor·tion
ap·nea
en·zyme
hy·po·ten·sion
ma·lar·ia
mu·ta·tion
phag·o·cy·to·sis
ra·di·o·ac·tiv·i·ty
sen·si·tiv·i·ty
symp·tom
trance
in·duc·er
cell
in·duc·i·ble
en·zyme
in·duc·tance

in·duc·tion
elec·tro·mag·net·ic i.
ly·so·gen·ic i.
spi·nal i.
in·duc·tion
che·mo·ther·a·py
pe·ri·od
in·duc·tive
re·sis·tance
in·duc·tor
in·duc·to·ri·um
in·duc·to·therm
in·duc·to·ther·my
in·du·lin
in·du·lin·o·phil
in·du·lin·o·phile
in·du·rat·ed
in·du·ra·tion
brown i. of the lung
cy·a·not·ic i.
Froriep's i.
gray i.
pig·ment i. of the lung
plas·tic i.
red i.
in·du·ra·tive
my·o·car·di·tis
in·du·sia
in·du·si·um
in·dus·tri·al
deaf·ness
dis·ease
psy·chol·o·gy
in·dus·tri·al meth·yl·at·ed
spir·it
in·dwell·ing
cath·e·ter
in·e·bri·ant
in·e·bri·a·tion
in·e·bri·e·ty
in·ert
gas·es
in·er·tia
time
in·er·tia
mag·net·ic i.
pri·mary uter·ine i.
psy·chic i.
sec·on·dary uter·ine i.
true uter·ine i.
uter·ine i.
in·ev·i·ta·ble
abor·tion
in·fan·cy
in·fant
death
in·fant
i. Hercules

in·fant *(continued)*
    live·born i.
    post-term i.
    pre·term i.
    still·born i.
    term i.
in·fan·ti·cide
in·fan·tile
    ac·ro·pus·tu·lo·sis
    au·tism
    cat·a·ract
    con·vul·sion
    di·ple·gia
    dwarf·ism
    ec·ze·ma
    fi·bro·sar·co·ma
    gas·tro·en·ter·i·tis
    hem·i·ple·gia
    her·nia
    hy·po·thy·roid·ism
    leish·man·i·a·sis
    myx·e·de·ma
    os·te·o·ma·la·cia
    pel·lag·ra
    scur·vy
    sex·u·al·i·ty
    spasm
    tet·a·ny
in·fan·tile cor·ti·cal
    hy·per·os·to·sis
in·fan·tile dig·i·tal
    fi·bro·ma·to·sis
in·fan·tile gas·tro·en·ter·i·tis
    vi·rus
in·fan·tile mus·cu·lar
    at·ro·phy
in·fan·tile neu·ro·ax·o·nal
    dys·tro·phy
in·fan·tile neu·ro·nal
    de·gen·er·a·tion
in·fan·tile pro·gress·ive spi·nal
mus·cu·lar
    at·ro·phy
in·fan·tile pu·ru·lent
    con·junc·ti·vi·tis
in·fan·tile spas·tic
    par·a·ple·gia
in·fan·ti·lism
    Brissaud's i.
    dys·thy·roi·dal i.
    he·pa·tic i.
    hy·po·thy·roid i.
    id·i·o·path·ic i.
    Lorain-Lévi i.
    myx·e·dem·a·tous i.
    pan·cre·at·ic i.
    pi·tu·i·tary i.
    pro·por·tion·ate i.

    re·nal i.
    sex·u·al i.
    stat·ic i.
    tub·al i.
    uni·ver·sal i.
in·fant mor·tal·i·ty
    rate
in·farct
    ane·mic i.
    bland i.
    bone i.
    Brewer's i.'s
    em·bol·ic i.
    hem·or·rhag·ic i.
    pale i.
    red i.
    sep·tic i.
    throm·bot·ic i.
    uric ac·id i.
    white i.
    Zahn's i.
in·farc·tion
    an·te·ri·or my·o·car·di·al i.
    an·ter·o·in·fe·ri·or my·o·car·di·al i.
    an·ter·o·lat·er·al my·o·car·di·al i.
    an·ter·o·sep·tal my·o·car·di·al i.
    car·di·ac i.
    di·a·phrag·mat·ic my·o·car·di·al i.
    in·fe·ri·or my·o·car·di·al i.
    in·fe·ro·lat·er·al my·o·car·di·al i.
    lat·er·al my·o·car·di·al i.
    my·o·car·di·al i.
    my·o·car·di·al i. in H-form
    non·trans·mu·ral my·o·car·di·al i.
    pos·te·ri·or my·o·car·di·al i.
    si·lent my·o·car·di·al i.
    sub·en·do·car·di·al my·o·car·di·al i.
    through-and-through my·o·car·di·al i.
    trans·mu·ral my·o·car·di·al i.
    wa·ter·shed i.
in·fect
in·fect·ed
    abor·tion
in·fec·tion
    im·mu·ni·ty
in·fec·tion
    ag·o·nal i.
    ap·i·cal i.

cross i.
cryp·to·gen·ic i.
drop·let i.
en·dog·e·nous i.
fo·cal i.
la·tent i.
mass i.
mixed i.
py·o·gen·ic i.
scalp i.
sec·on·dary i.
ter·mi·nal i.
Vincent's i.
zo·o·not·ic i.
in·fec·tion-ex·haus·tion
psy·cho·sis
in·fec·tion-im·mu·ni·ty
in·fec·ti·os·i·ty
in·fec·tious
ane·mia
dis·ease
en·do·car·di·tis
en·ter·o·hep·a·ti·tis
gran·u·lo·ma
hep·a·ti·tis
ic·ter·us
jaun·dice
mon·o·nu·cle·o·sis
my·o·si·tis
nu·cle·ic ac·id
oph·thal·mo·ple·gia
pap·il·lo·ma of cat·tle
plas·mid
pol·y·neu·ri·tis
si·nus·i·tis of tur·keys
warts
in·fec·tious ar·te·ri·tis
vi·rus of hors·es
in·fec·tious avi·an
bron·chi·tis
in·fec·tious bo·vine
ker·a·ti·tis
rhi·no·tra·che·i·tis
in·fec·tious bo·vine rhi·no·tra·che·i·tis
vi·rus
in·fec·tious bron·chi·tis
vi·rus
in·fec·tious bul·bar
pa·ral·y·sis
in·fec·tious bur·sal
dis·ease
in·fec·tious ca·nine
hep·a·ti·tis
in·fec·tious ca·nine hep·a·ti·tis
vi·rus
in·fec·tious ec·tro·me·lia
vi·rus

in·fec·tious ec·ze·ma·toid
der·ma·ti·tis
in·fec·tious hep·a·ti·tis
vi·rus
in·fec·tious ne·crot·ic
hep·a·ti·tis of sheep
in·fec·tious·ness
in·fec·tious pap·il·lo·ma
vi·rus
in·fec·tious por·cine
en·ceph·a·lo·my·e·li·tis
in·fec·tious por·cine en·ceph·a·lo·my·e·li·tis
vi·rus
in·fec·tive
dis·ease
em·bo·lism
en·do·car·di·tis
throm·bus
in·fec·tiv·i·ty
in·fe·cun·di·ty
in·fer·en·tial
sta·tis·tics
in·fe·ri·or
an·gle of scap·u·la
bor·der
bur·sa of bi·ceps fe·mo·ris
col·lic·u·lus
con·cha
ex·trem·i·ty
fas·cia of pel·vic di·a·phragm
fas·cia of uro·gen·i·tal di·a·phragm
flex·ure of du·o·de·num
gan·gli·on of glos·so·pha·ryn·ge·al nerve
gan·gli·on of va·gus
horn
horn of lat·er·al ven·tri·cle
horn of sa·phe·nous open·ing
horn of thy·roid car·ti·lage
lar·yn·got·o·my
lig·a·ment of ep·i·did·y·mis
limb
lobe of lung
mar·gin
ol·ive
part
part of ves·tib·u·lo·co·chle·ar nerve
pole
po·li·o·en·ceph·a·li·tis
ret·i·nac·u·lum of ex·ten·sor mus·cles
root
root of cer·vi·cal loop

in·fe·ri·or *(continued)*
    root of ves·tib·u·lo·co·chle·
      ar nerve
    seg·ment
    sur·face of cer·e·bel·lar
      hem·i·sphere
    sur·face of pan·cre·as
    sur·face of pet·rous part of
      tem·po·ral bone
    sur·face of tongue
    trunk
    veins of cer·e·bel·lar hem·
      i·sphere
    vein of ver·mis
    ve·na ca·va
    wall of or·bit
    wall of tym·pan·ic cav·i·ty
in·fe·ri·or al·ve·o·lar
    ar·tery
    nerve
in·fe·ri·or anas·to·mot·ic
    vein
in·fe·ri·or ar·tic·u·lar
    pit of at·las
    sur·face of tib·ia
in·fe·ri·or ba·sal
    vein
in·fe·ri·or cal·ca·ne·o·na·vic·u·
  lar
    lig·a·ment
in·fe·ri·or car·di·ac
    vein
in·fe·ri·or ca·rot·id
    tri·an·gle
in·fe·ri·or cer·e·bel·lar
    pe·dun·cle
in·fe·ri·or ce·re·bral
    veins
in·fe·ri·or cer·vi·cal
    gan·gli·on
in·fe·ri·or cer·vi·cal car·di·ac
    nerve
in·fe·ri·or cho·roid
    vein
in·fe·ri·or clu·ne·al
    nerves
in·fe·ri·or con·stric·tor
    mus·cle of phar·ynx
in·fe·ri·or cos·tal
    pit
in·fe·ri·or den·tal
    arch
    ar·tery
    ca·nal
    fo·ra·men
    nerve
    plex·us

in·fe·ri·or du·o·de·nal
    fold
    fos·sa
    re·cess
in·fe·ri·or ep·i·gas·tric
    ar·tery
    vein
in·fe·ri·or ep·i·gas·tric lymph
    nodes
in·fe·ri·or fron·tal
    con·vo·lu·tion
    gy·rus
    sul·cus
in·fe·ri·or ge·mel·lus
    mus·cle
in·fe·ri·or glu·te·al
    ar·tery
    nerve
    veins
in·fe·ri·or hem·or·rhoi·dal
    ar·tery
    nerves
    plex·us·es
    veins
in·fe·ri·or hy·po·gas·tric
    plex·us
in·fe·ri·or hy·po·phy·si·al
    ar·tery
in·fe·ri·or il·e·o·ce·cal
    re·cess
in·fe·ri·or in·ter·nal pa·ri·e·tal
    ar·tery
in·fe·ri·or·i·ty
    com·plex
in·fe·ri·or la·bi·al
    ar·tery
    vein
in·fe·ri·or la·ryn·ge·al
    ar·tery
    nerve
    vein
in·fe·ri·or lin·gual
    mus·cle
in·fe·ri·or lin·gu·lar
    seg·ment
in·fe·ri·or lon·gi·tu·di·nal
    fas·cic·u·lus
    si·nus
in·fe·ri·or mac·u·lar
    ar·te·ri·ole
    ven·ule
in·fe·ri·or max·il·lary
    nerve
in·fe·ri·or med·ul·lary
    ve·lum
in·fe·ri·or mes·en·ter·ic
    ar·tery
    gan·gli·on

plex·us
vein
in·fe·ri·or mes·en·ter·ic lymph
nodes
in·fe·ri·or my·o·car·di·al
in·farc·tion
in·fe·ri·or na·sal
ar·te·ri·ole of ret·i·na
ven·ule of ret·i·na
in·fe·ri·or nu·chal
line
in·fe·ri·or ob·lique
mus·cle
mus·cle of head
in·fe·ri·or oc·cip·i·tal
gy·rus
tri·an·gle
in·fe·ri·or ol·i·vary
nu·cle·us
in·fe·ri·or omen·tal
re·cess
in·fe·ri·or oph·thal·mic
vein
in·fe·ri·or or·bi·tal
fis·sure
in·fe·ri·or pan·cre·at·ic
ar·tery
in·fe·ri·or pan·cre·at·i·co·du·o·
de·nal
ar·tery
in·fe·ri·or pa·ri·e·tal
gy·rus
lob·ule
in·fe·ri·or pe·tro·sal
groove
si·nus
sul·cus
in·fe·ri·or phren·ic
ar·tery
vein
in·fe·ri·or phren·ic lymph
nodes
in·fe·ri·or pos·te·ri·or ser·ra·
tus
mus·cle
in·fe·ri·or pu·bic
lig·a·ment
in·fe·ri·or quad·ri·gem·i·nal
bra·chi·um
in·fe·ri·or ra·di·o·ul·nar
joint
in·fe·ri·or rec·tal
ar·tery
nerves
plex·us·es
veins
in·fe·ri·or rec·tus
mus·cle

in·fe·ri·or sag·it·tal
si·nus
in·fe·ri·or sal·i·vary
nu·cle·us
in·fe·ri·or sem·i·lu·nar
lob·ule
In·fe·ri·or strait
in·fe·ri·or su·pra·re·nal
ar·tery
in·fe·ri·or tar·sal
mus·cle
in·fe·ri·or tem·po·ral
ar·te·ri·ole of ret·i·na
con·vo·lu·tion
gy·rus
line
sul·cus
ven·ule of ret·i·na
in·fe·ri·or tha·lam·ic
pe·dun·cle
in·fe·ri·or thal·a·mo·stri·ate
veins
in·fe·ri·or tho·rac·ic
ap·er·ture
in·fe·ri·or thy·roid
ar·tery
notch
plex·us
tu·ber·cle
vein
in·fe·ri·or tib·i·o·fib·u·lar
joint
in·fe·ri·or tra·che·o·bron·chi·al
lymph
nodes
in·fe·ri·or trans·verse scap·u·
lar
lig·a·ment
in·fe·ri·or tur·bi·nat·ed
bone
in·fe·ri·or tym·pan·ic
ar·tery
in·fe·ri·or ul·nar col·lat·er·al
ar·tery
in·fe·ri·or ven·tric·u·lar
vein
in·fe·ri·or ves·i·cal
ar·tery
nerves
plex·us
in·fe·ri·or ves·tib·u·lar
ar·ea
nu·cle·us
in·fe·ro·lat·er·al
mar·gin
sur·face of pros·tate
in·fe·ro·lat·er·al my·o·car·di·al
in·farc·tion

in·fer·o·me·di·al
  mar·gin
in·fer·til·i·ty
in·fest
in·fes·ta·tion
in·fil·trate
  Assmann's tu·ber·cu·lous i.
  in·fra·cla·vic·u·lar i.
in·fil·trat·ing
  li·po·ma
in·fil·tra·tion
  an·es·the·sia
in·fil·tra·tion
  ad·i·pose i.
  cal·car·e·ous i.
  cel·lu·lar i.
  ep·i·tu·ber·cu·lous i.
  fat·ty i.
  ge·lat·i·nous i.
  gray i.
  li·po·ma·tous i.
  par·a·neu·ral i.
  per·i·neu·ral i.
in·fi·nite
  dis·tance
in·fin·i·ty
in·firm
in·fir·ma·ry
in·fir·mi·ty
in·flamed
  ul·cer
in·flam·ma·ble
in·flam·ma·tion
  acute i.
  ad·he·sive i.
  al·ler·gic i.
  al·ter·a·tive i.
  atroph·ic i.
  ca·tarrh·al i.
  chron·ic i.
  croup·ous i.
  de·gen·er·a·tive i.
  ex·ud·a·tive i.
  fi·bri·no·pu·ru·lent i.
  fi·brin·ous i.
  fi·broid i.
  gran·u·lom·a·tous i.
  hy·per·plas·tic i.
  im·mune i.
  in·ter·sti·tial i.
  ne·crot·ic i.
  nec·ro·tiz·ing i.
  pro·duc·tive i.
  pro·lif·er·a·tive i.
  pseu·do·mem·bra·nous i.
  pu·ru·lent i.
  scle·ros·ing i.
  se·ro·fi·brin·ous i.

  se·rous i.
  sub·a·cute i.
  sup·pu·ra·tive i.
in·flam·ma·to·ry
  car·ci·no·ma
  cor·pus·cle
  ede·ma
  lymph
  pol·yp
  pseu·do·tu·mor
  rheu·ma·tism
in·flam·ma·to·ry fi·brous
  hy·per·pla·sia
in·flam·ma·to·ry pap·il·lary
  hy·per·pla·sia
in·flat·a·ble
  im·plant
  splint
in·fla·tion
in·fla·tor
in·flec·tion
in·flex·ion
in·flu·en·za
  i. A
  Asian i.
  avi·an i.
  i. B
  i. C
  en·dem·ic i.
  equine i.
  Hong Kong i.
  i. nos·tras
  Span·ish i.
  swine i.
in·flu·en·za
  ba·cil·lus
  vi·rus·es
in·flu·en·zal
  pneu·mo·nia
In·flu·en·za·vi·rus
in·flu·en·za vi·rus
  vac·cines
in·fold
in·for·ma·tion
  the·o·ry
in·for·ma·tion·al
  RNA
in·formed con·sent
in·for·mo·somes
in·fra·au·ric·u·lar sub·fas·cial
  pa·rot·id lymph
  nodes
in·fra-ax·il·lary
in·fra·bony
  pock·et
in·fra·bulge
in·fra·car·di·ac
  bur·sa

in·fra·ce·re·bral
in·fra·cla·vic·u·lar
  fos·sa
  in·fil·trate
  part of brach·i·al plex·us
  tri·an·gle
in·fra·cli·noid
  an·eu·rysm
in·fra·clu·sion
in·fra·cor·ti·cal
in·fra·cos·tal
  line
in·fra·cot·y·loid
in·fra·cris·tal
in·frac·tion
in·frac·ture
in·fra·den·ta·le
in·fra·di·an
in·fra·di·a·phrag·mat·ic
in·fra·duc·tion
in·fra·du·o·de·nal
  fos·sa
in·fra·gle·noid
  tu·ber·cle
  tu·ber·os·i·ty
in·fra·glot·tic
  space
in·fra·gran·u·lar
  lay·er
in·fra·he·pa·tic
in·fra·hy·oid
  bur·sa
  mus·cles
in·fra·lo·bar
  part
in·fra·mam·il·lary
in·fra·mam·ma·ry
  re·gion
in·fra·man·dib·u·lar
in·fra·mar·gin·al
in·fra·max·il·lary
in·fra·na·tant
  flu·id
in·fra·nod·al
  ex·tra·sys·to·le
in·fra·oc·clu·sion
in·fra·or·bit·al
  ar·tery
  ca·nal
  fo·ra·men
  groove
  mar·gin
  nerve
  re·gion
  su·ture
in·fra·or·bi·to·me·a·tal
  plane
in·fra·pa·tel·lar

in·fra·pa·tel·lar fat
  body
in·fra·pa·tel·lar syn·o·vi·al
  fold
in·fra·psy·chic
in·fra·red
  cat·a·ract
  light
  mi·cro·scope
  ray
  spec·tros·co·py
  spec·trum
  ther·mog·ra·phy
in·fra·scap·u·lar
  ar·tery
  re·gion
in·fra·seg·men·tal
  part
  veins
in·fra·son·ic
in·fra·spi·na·tus
  bur·sa
  fas·cia
  mus·cle
in·fra·spi·nous
  fos·sa
in·fra·splen·ic
in·fra·ster·nal
  an·gle
in·fra·sub·spe·cif·ic
in·fra·tem·po·ral
  crest
  fos·sa
  sur·face of max·il·la
in·fra·tho·rac·ic
in·fra·ton·sil·lar
in·fra·troch·le·ar
  nerve
in·fra·um·bil·i·cal
in·fra·ver·sion
in·fric·tion
in·fun·dib·u·la
in·fun·dib·u·lar
  part of an·te·ri·or lobe of
    hy·poph·y·sis
  re·cess
  stalk
  stem
  ste·no·sis
in·fun·dib·u·lec·to·my
in·fun·dib·u·li·form
  fas·cia
  hy·men
  sheath
in·fun·dib·u·lin
in·fun·dib·u·lo·fol·lic·u·li·tis
  dis·sem·i·nat·ed re·cur·rent
  i.

in·fun·dib·u·lo·ma
in·fun·dib·u·lo-ovar·i·an
   lig·a·ment
in·fun·dib·u·lo·pel·vic
   lig·a·ment
in·fun·dib·u·lum
   eth·moid i.
   hy·po·tha·lam·ic i.
   i. of lungs
   i. of teeth
   i. of uter·ine tube
in·fu·si·ble
in·fu·sion
   graft
in·fu·sion-as·pi·ra·tion
   drain·age
in·fu·so·de·coc·tion
In·fu·so·ria
in·fu·so·ri·an
in·ges·ta
in·ges·tion
in·ges·tive
Ingrassia's
   apoph·y·sis
   wing
in·gra·ves·cent
   ap·o·plexy
in·grow·ing
   toe·nail
in·grown
   hairs
   nail
in·guen
in·gui·nal
   ca·nal
   crest
   fold
   fos·sa
   glands
   her·nia
   lig·a·ment
   lig·a·ment of the kid·ney
   plex·us
   re·gion
   tri·an·gle
   tri·gone
in·gui·nal ap·o·neu·rot·ic
   fold
in·gui·no·cru·ral
   her·nia
in·gui·no·dyn·ia
in·gui·no·fem·o·ral
   her·nia
in·gui·no·la·bi·al
   her·nia
in·gui·no·per·i·to·ne·al
in·gui·no·scro·tal
   her·nia

in·gui·no·su·per·fi·cial
   her·nia
in·hal·ant
in·ha·la·tion
   sol·vent i.
in·ha·la·tion
   an·al·ge·sia
   an·es·the·sia
   an·es·thet·ic
   ther·a·py
in·hale
in·hal·er
in·her·ent
   im·mu·ni·ty
in·her·i·tance
   al·ter·na·tive i.
   blend·ing i.
   co·dom·i·nant i.
   col·lat·er·al i.
   cy·to·plas·mic i.
   dom·i·nant i.
   ex·tra·chro·mo·som·al i.
   ex·tra·nu·cle·ar i.
   gal·to·ni·an i.
   hol·an·dric i.
   hol·o·gyn·ic i.
   ho·moch·ro·nous i.
   ma·ter·nal i.
   men·de·li·an i.
   mo·sa·ic i.
   mul·ti·fac·to·ri·al i.
   pol·y·gen·ic i.
   re·ces·sive i.
   sex-in·flu·enced i.
   sex-lim·it·ed i.
   sex-linked i.
   X-linked i.
   Y-linked i.
in·her·it·ed
   char·ac·ter
in·her·it·ed al·bu·min
   var·i·ants
in·hib·in
in·hib·it
in·hib·i·tine
in·hib·it·ing
   an·ti·body
in·hi·bi·tion
   fac·tor
in·hi·bi·tion
   al·lo·ge·ne·ic i.
   cen·tral i.
   com·pet·i·tive i.
   con·tact i.
   feed·back i.
   hap·ten i. of pre·cip·i·ta·tion
   he·mag·glu·ti·na·tion i.

non·com·pet·i·tive i.
po·tas·si·um i.
pro·ac·tive i.
re·cip·ro·cal i.
re·flex i.
re·sid·u·al i.
ret·ro·ac·tive i.
se·lec·tive i.
Wedensky i.
in·hib·i·tor
an·gi·o·ten·sin con·vert·ing
  en·zyme i.
car·bon·ate de·hy·dra·tase i.
car·bon·ic an·hy·drase i.
cho·lin·es·ter·ase i.
mon·o·am·ine ox·i·dase i.
re·sid·u·al i.
tryp·sin i.
in·hib·i·to·ry
fi·bers
nerve
ob·ses·sion
in·hib·i·to·ry post·syn·ap·tic
po·ten·tial
in·i·ac
in·i·ad
in·i·al
in·i·en·ceph·a·ly
in·i·on
in·i·op·a·gus
in·i·ops
in·i·tial
con·tact
dose
heat
he·ma·tu·ria
in·i·ti·a·ting
agent
co·don
in·i·ti·a·tion
fac·tor
in·i·tis
in·ject
in·ject·a·ble
in·ject·ed
in·jec·tion
de·pot i.
hy·po·der·mic i.
in·su·lin i.
in·tra·the·cal i.
in·tra·ven·tric·u·lar i.
jet i.
lac·tat·ed Ringer's i.
reg·u·lar in·su·lin i.
Ringer's i.
sen·si·tiz·ing i.
Z-tract i.

in·jec·tion
flask
mass
mold·ing
in·jec·tor
jet i.
in·jure
in·ju·ry
blast i.
closed head i.
con·tre·coup i. of brain
coup i. of brain
cur·rent of i.
de·glov·ing i.
egg-white i.
hy·per·ex·ten·sion-hy·per·
  flex·ion i.
i. of in·ter·ver·te·bral disk
open head i.
pneu·mat·ic tire i.
whip·lash i.
in·ju·ry
po·ten·tial
in·lay
graft
wax
in·lay
ep·i·the·li·al i.
gold i.
por·ce·lain i.
in·let
pel·vic i.
in·nate
im·mu·ni·ty
re·flex
in·ner
mal·le·o·lus
ta·ble of skull
in·ner cell
mass
in·ner cone
fi·ber
in·ner den·tal
ep·i·the·li·um
in·ner ear
in·ner enam·el
ep·i·the·li·um
in·ner·most in·ter·cos·tal
mus·cle
in·ner·va·tion
aprax·ia
in·ner·va·tion
re·cip·ro·cal i.
in·nid·i·a·tion
in·no·cent
mur·mur
tu·mor
in·noc·u·ous

in·nom·i·na·tal
in·nom·i·nate
  ar·tery
  bone
  car·ti·lage
  fos·sa
  sub·stance
  veins
in·nom·i·nate car·di·ac
  veins
in·nox·ious
in·oc·u·la·bil·i·ty
in·oc·u·la·ble
in·oc·u·late
in·oc·u·la·tion
  stress i.
in·oc·u·lum
In·o·cy·be
in·o·pec·tic
in·op·er·a·ble
in·or·gan·ic
  ac·id
  cat·a·lyst
  chem·is·try
  com·pound
  mur·mur
  or·tho·phos·phate
  py·ro·phos·pha·tase
in·or·gan·ic den·tal
  ce·ment
in·os·a·mine
in·os·co·py
in·os·cu·late
in·os·cu·la·tion
in·ose
in·o·se·mia
in·o·si·nate
in·o·sine
in·o·sine pran·o·bex
in·o·sin·ic ac·id
in·o·sin·yl
in·o·site
in·o·si·tide
in·o·si·tol
  i. ni·a·cin·ate
meso-in·o·si·tol
myo-in·o·si·tol
in·o·si·tu·ria
in·os·ose
in·o·su·ria
in·o·tro·pic
  neg·a·tive·ly i.
  pos·i·tive·ly i.
Ino·vir·i·dae
in·quest
in·qui·line
  par·a·site
in·sal·i·vate

in·sal·i·va·tion
in·sa·lu·bri·ous
in·sane
in·san·i·tary
in·san·i·ty
  ba·se·dow·i·an i.
  crim·i·nal i.
in·scrip·tio
  i. ten·din·ea
in·scrip·tion
  ten·di·nous i.
in·sect
  vi·rus·es
In·sec·ta
in·sec·tar·i·um
in·sec·ti·cide
in·sec·ti·fuge
In·sec·tiv·o·ra
in·sec·tiv·o·rous
in·se·cu·ri·ty
in·sem·i·na·tion
  ar·ti·fi·cial i.
  het·er·ol·o·gous i.
  ho·mol·o·gous i.
in·se·nes·cence
in·sen·si·ble
  pers·pi·ra·tion
  thirst
in·ser·tion
  se·quence
in·ser·tion
  par·a·sol i.
  vel·a·men·tous i.
in·ser·tion·al
  mu·ta·gen·e·sis
in·sheathed
in·sid·i·ous
in·sight
in·so·la·tion
in·sol·u·ble
  soap
in·som·nia
in·som·ni·ac
in·sorp·tion
in·spec·tion·ism
in·sper·sion
in·spi·ra·tion
  crow·ing i.
in·spi·ra·to·ry
  ca·pac·i·ty
  cen·ter
  stri·dor
in·spi·ra·to·ry re·serve
  vol·ume
in·spire
in·spired
  gas
in·spi·rom·e·ter

in·spis·sate
in·spis·sat·ed
 ce·ru·men
in·spis·sa·tion
in·spis·sa·tor
in·sta·bil·i·ty
 ver·te·bral cer·vi·cal i.
in·stan·ta·ne·ous
 vec·tor
in·stan·ta·ne·ous elec·tri·cal
 ax·is
in·star
in·step
in·stil·la·tion
in·stil·la·tor
in·stinct
 ag·gres·sive i.
 death i.
 ego i.'s
 life i.
 sex·u·al i.
 so·cial i.
in·stinc·tive
in·stinc·tu·al
in·stru·ment
 di·a·mond cut·ting i.'s
 Krueger i. stop
 plug·ging i.
 purse-string i.
 Sabouraud-Noiré i.
 ster·e·o·tac·tic i.
 ster·e·o·tax·ic i.
 test han·dle i.
in·stru·men·tal
 con·di·tion·ing
in·stru·men·tar·i·um
in·stru·men·ta·tion
in·suc·ca·tion
in·su·date
in·suf·fi·cien·cy
 acute adre·no·cor·ti·cal i.
 adre·no·cor·ti·cal i.
 aor·tic i.
 car·di·ac i.
 chron·ic adre·no·cor·ti·cal i.
 con·ver·gence i.
 cor·o·nary i.
 di·ver·gence i.
 i. of eye·lids
 he·pa·tic i.
 la·tent adre·no·cor·ti·cal i.
 mi·tral i.
 mus·cu·lar i.
 my·o·car·di·al i.
 par·a·thy·roid i.
 par·tial adre·no·cor·ti·cal i.
 pri·mary adre·no·cor·ti·cal
  i.

pul·mo·nary i.
py·lor·ic i.
re·nal i.
res·pi·ra·to·ry i.
sec·on·dary adre·no·cor·ti·
 cal i.
tri·cus·pid i.
uter·ine i.
val·vu·lar i.
vel·o·pha·ryn·ge·al i.
ve·nous i.
in·suf·flate
in·suf·fla·tion
 per·i·re·nal i.
 tub·al i.
in·suf·fla·tion
 an·es·the·sia
in·suf·fla·tor
in·su·la
 Haller's i.
in·su·lae
in·su·lar
 ar·ea
 ar·ter·ies
 cor·tex
 hy·poth·e·sis
 part
 scle·ro·sis
 sco·to·ma
 veins
in·su·late
in·su·la·tion
in·su·la·tor
in·su·lin
 atyp·i·cal i.
 bi·pha·sic i.
 glo·bin zinc i.
 hu·man i.
 im·mu·no·re·ac·tive i.
 iso·phane i.
 len·te i.
 NPH i.
 prot·a·mine zinc i.
 sem·i·len·te i.
 ul·tra·len·te i.
in·su·lin
 an·tag·o·nist
 in·jec·tion
 lip·o·at·ro·phy
 lip·o·dys·tro·phy
 re·sis·tance
 shock
 unit
in·su·lin-an·tag·o·niz·ing
 fac·tor
in·su·lin co·ma
 ther·a·py
 treat·ment

in·su·lin-de·pen·dent
di·a·be·tes mel·li·tus
in·su·li·ne·mia
in·su·lin hy·po·gly·ce·mia
test
in·su·lin-like
ac·tiv·i·ty
in·su·lin-like growth
fac·tor
in·su·lin·o·gen·e·sis
in·su·lin·o·gen·ic
in·su·li·no·ma
in·su·lin·o·pe·nic
di·a·be·tes
in·su·lin zinc
sus·pen·sion
in·su·li·tis
in·su·lo·gen·ic
in·su·lo·ma
in·sult
in·sus·cep·ti·bil·i·ty
in·te·gra·tion
per·son·al·i·ty i.
in·teg·ri·ty
mar·gi·nal i. of amal·gam
in·teg·u·ment
in·teg·u·men·ta·ry
sys·tem
in·teg·u·men·tum com·mune
in·tel·lec·tu·al
au·ra
in·tel·lec·tu·al·i·za·tion
in·tel·li·gence
ab·stract i.
mea·sured i.
me·chan·i·cal i.
so·cial i.
in·tel·li·gence
quo·tient
test
in·tem·per·ance
in·ten·si·fi·ca·tion
che·mo·ther·a·py
in·ten·sim·eter
in·ten·si·ty
lu·mi·nous i.
i. of sound
in·ten·sive
care
psy·cho·ther·a·py
in·ten·sive care
unit
in·ten·tion
spasm
trem·or
in·ten·tion·al
re·plan·ta·tion
in·ter·ac·i·nar

in·ter·ac·i·nous
in·ter·ac·tion pro·cess
anal·y·sis
in·ter·al·ve·o·lar
pores
sep·tum
space
in·ter·an·nu·lar
seg·ment
in·ter·arch
dis·tance
in·ter·ar·tic·u·lar
fi·bro·car·ti·lage
joints
in·ter·ar·y·te·noid
notch
in·ter·as·ter·ic
in·ter·a·tri·al
fo·ra·men pri·mum
fo·ra·men se·cun·dum
sep·tum
in·ter·au·ric·u·lar
in·ter·body
in·ter·ca·dence
in·ter·ca·dent
in·ter·ca·lary
neu·ron
staph·y·lo·ma
in·ter·ca·lat·ed
disk
ducts
nu·cle·us
in·ter·can·a·lic·u·lar
in·ter·cap·il·lary
cell
glo·mer·u·lo·scle·ro·sis
in·ter·cap·i·tal
lig·a·ment
in·ter·ca·pit·u·lar
veins
in·ter·ca·rot·ic
in·ter·ca·rot·id
body
in·ter·car·pal
joints
lig·a·ments
in·ter·car·ti·lag·i·nous
part of glot·tic open·ing
in·ter·cav·ern·ous
si·nus·es
in·ter·cel·lu·lar
bridg·es
can·a·lic·u·lus
ce·ment
di·ges·tion
junc·tions
lymph
in·ter·cen·tra

in·ter·cen·tral
in·ter·cen·trum
in·ter·cep·tive oc·clu·sal
  con·tact
in·ter·ce·re·bral
in·ter·chon·dral
  ar·tic·u·la·tions
  joints
in·ter·cil·i·um
in·ter·cla·vic·u·lar
  lig·a·ment
  notch
in·ter·cli·noid
  lig·a·ment
in·ter·coc·cyg·e·al
in·ter·co·lum·nar
  fas·ci·ae
  fi·bers
in·ter·con·dy·lar
  em·i·nence
  fos·sa
  line
  tu·ber·cle
in·ter·con·dyl·ic
  fos·sa
in·ter·con·dy·loid
  em·i·nence
  fos·sa
  notch
in·ter·cor·nu·al
  lig·a·ment
in·ter·cos·tal
  an·es·the·sia
  lig·a·ments
  mem·branes
  nerves
  neu·ral·gia
  space
  veins
in·ter·cos·tal lymph
  nodes
in·ter·cos·to·brach·i·al
  nerves
in·ter·cos·to·hu·mer·al
  nerves
in·ter·cos·to·hu·me·ra·lis
in·ter·course
  sex·u·al i.
in·ter·cri·co·thy·rot·o·my
in·ter·cris·tal
in·ter·cross
in·ter·cru·ral
  fi·bers
  gan·gli·on
in·ter·cu·ne·i·form
  joints
  lig·a·ments
in·ter·cur·rent

in·ter·cus·pal
  po·si·tion
in·ter·cus·pa·tion
in·ter·cusp·ing
in·ter·cu·ta·ne·o·mu·cous
in·ter·de·fer·en·tial
in·ter·den·tal
  ca·nals
  car·ies
  pa·pil·la
  sep·tum
  splint
in·ter·den·ti·um
in·ter·dig·it
in·ter·dig·i·tal
in·ter·dig·i·ta·tion
in·ter·dis·ci·pli·nary
in·ter·ec·top·ic
  in·ter·val
in·ter·face
  crys·tal·line i.
  der·mo·ep·i·der·mal i.
  met·al i.
  struc·tur·al i.
in·ter·fa·cial
  ca·nals
in·ter·fa·cial sur·face
  ten·sion
in·ter·fas·cial
  space
in·ter·fas·cic·u·lar
  fas·cic·u·lus
in·ter·fem·o·ral
in·ter·fer·ence
  bac·te·ri·al i.
  cus·pal i.
in·ter·fer·ence
  beat
  dis·so·ci·a·tion
  mi·cro·scope
in·ter·fer·om·e·ter
  elec·tron i.
in·ter·fer·o·me·try
  elec·tron i.
in·ter·fer·on
  i. al·pha
  an·ti·gen i.
  i. be·ta
  fi·bro·blast i.
  i. gam·ma
  im·mune i.
  leu·ko·cyte i.
in·ter·fi·bril·lar
in·ter·fi·bril·lary
in·ter·fi·brous
in·ter·fil·a·men·tous
in·ter·fo·ve·o·lar
  lig·a·ment

in·ter·fron·tal
in·ter·gan·gli·on·ic
in·ter·gem·mal
in·ter·gen·ic
   com·ple·men·ta·tion
in·ter·glob·u·lar
   space
   space of Owen
in·ter·glu·te·al
in·ter·go·ni·al
in·ter·gy·ral
in·ter·hem·i·ce·re·bral
in·ter·ic·tal
in·ter·il·i·ac lymph
   nodes
in·ter·il·i·o·ab·dom·i·nal
   am·pu·ta·tion
in·ter·im
   den·ture
in·te·ri·or
in·ter·is·chi·ad·ic
in·ter·judge
   re·li·a·bil·i·ty
in·ter·ki·ne·sis
in·ter·la·mel·lar
in·ter·lam·i·nar
   jel·ly
in·ter·lo·bar
   ar·ter·ies
   duct
   sur·fac·es of lung
   veins of kid·ney
in·ter·lo·bi·tis
in·ter·lob·u·lar
   ar·ter·ies
   duct
   duc·tules
   em·phy·se·ma
   pleu·ri·sy
   veins of kid·ney
   veins of liv·er
in·ter·lo·cal
   ad·di·tiv·i·ty
in·ter·lock·ing
   gy·ri
in·ter·mal·le·o·lar
in·ter·mam·ma·ry
in·ter·mam·mil·lary
in·ter·mar·riage
in·ter·max·il·la
in·ter·max·il·lary
   an·chor·age
   bone
   elas·tic
   fix·a·tion
   re·la·tion
   seg·ment

   su·ture
   trac·tion
in·ter·me·di·ary
   host
   move·ments
   nerve
   sys·tem
in·ter·me·di·ate
   abut·ment
   am·pu·ta·tion
   body of Flemming
   bron·chus
   car·ci·no·ma
   disk
   fil·a·ments
   gan·glia
   heart
   hem·or·rhage
   host
   junc·tion
   la·mel·la
   lay·er
   line of il·i·ac crest
   mes·o·derm
   nerve
   part
   rays
   trait
   vein of fore·arm
in·ter·me·di·ate an·te·brach·i·al
   vein
in·ter·me·di·ate ba·sil·ic
   vein
in·ter·me·di·ate ce·phal·ic
   vein
in·ter·me·di·ate cu·bi·tal
   vein
in·ter·me·di·ate cu·ne·i·form
   bone
in·ter·me·di·ate dor·sal cu·ta·ne·ous
   nerve
in·ter·me·di·ate great
   mus·cle
in·ter·me·di·ate la·cu·nar
   node
in·ter·me·di·ate lum·bar lymph
   nodes
in·ter·me·di·ate sa·cral
   crests
in·ter·me·di·ate su·pra·cla·vic·u·lar
   nerve
in·ter·me·di·ate tem·po·ral
   ar·tery
in·ter·me·di·ate vas·tus
   mus·cle

in·ter·me·din
in·ter·me·di·o·lat·er·al
  nu·cle·us
in·ter·me·di·o·lat·er·al cell
  col·umn of spi·nal cord
in·ter·me·di·o·me·di·al
  nu·cle·us
in·ter·me·di·us
in·ter·mem·bra·nous
  part of glot·tic open·ing
in·ter·me·nin·ge·al
in·ter·men·stru·al
  pain
in·ter·mes·en·ter·ic
  plex·us
in·ter·met·a·car·pal
  joints
  lig·a·ments
in·ter·met·a·mer·ic
in·ter·met·a·tar·sal
  ar·tic·u·la·tions
  joints
  lig·a·ments
in·ter·met·a·tar·se·um
in·ter·mis·sion
in·ter·mit
in·ter·mit·tence
in·ter·mit·ten·cy
in·ter·mit·tent
  al·bu·min·ur·ia
  ar·thral·gia
  clau·di·ca·tion
  cramp
  hy·drar·thro·sis
  hy·dro·sal·pinx
  ma·lar·ia
  pulse
  ster·il·i·za·tion
  tet·a·nus
  tor·ti·col·lis
in·ter·mit·tent acute
  por·phyr·ia
in·ter·mit·tent ex·plo·sive
  dis·or·der
in·ter·mit·tent ma·lar·i·al
  fe·ver
in·ter·mit·tent man·da·to·ry
  ven·ti·la·tion
in·ter·mit·tent pos·i·tive pres·
  sure
  breath·ing
  ven·ti·la·tion
in·ter·mit·tent re·in·force·ment
  sched·ule
in·ter·mus·cu·lar
  sep·tum
in·ter·mus·cu·lar glu·te·al
  bur·sa

in·tern
in·ter·nal
  an·ti·gen
  at·tach·ment
  ax·is of eye
  base of skull
  can·thus
  cap·sule
  con·ju·gate
  de·com·pres·sion
  fis·tu·la
  fix·a·tion
  hem·or·rhage
  hem·or·rhoids
  hy·dro·ceph·a·lus
  lip of il·i·ac crest
  mal·le·o·lus
  med·i·cine
  men·in·gi·tis
  nos·tril
  oph·thal·mop·a·thy
  phase
  py·o·ceph·a·lus
  re·sorp·tion
  res·pi·ra·tion
  squint
  stra·bis·mus
  sur·face
  sur·face of fron·tal bone
  sur·face of pa·ri·e·tal bone
  trac·tion
  ure·throt·o·my
  ver·sion
in·ter·nal acous·tic
  fo·ra·men
  me·a·tus
  pore
in·ter·nal ad·he·sive
  per·i·car·di·tis
in·ter·nal ar·cu·ate
  fi·bers
in·ter·nal au·di·to·ry
  ar·tery
  fo·ra·men
  me·a·tus
  veins
in·ter·nal cap·sule
  syn·drome
in·ter·nal ca·rot·id
  ar·tery
  nerve
  plex·us
in·ter·nal ca·rot·id ve·nous
  plex·us
in·ter·nal ce·re·bral
  veins
in·ter·nal col·lat·er·al
  lig·a·ment of the wrist

in·ter·nal con·ver·sion
  elec·tron
in·ter·nal ear
in·ter·nal il·i·ac
  ar·tery
  vein
in·ter·nal il·i·ac lymph
  nodes
in·ter·nal in·gui·nal
  ring
in·ter·nal in·ter·cos·tal
  mus·cle
in·ter·nal·i·za·tion
in·ter·nal jug·u·lar
  vein
in·ter·nal lac·ri·mal
  fis·tu·la
in·ter·nal lim·it·ing
  mem·brane
in·ter·nal mam·ma·ry
  ar·tery
  plex·us
in·ter·nal max·il·lary
  ar·tery
  plex·us
in·ter·nal ob·lique
  line
in·ter·nal ob·tu·ra·tor
  mus·cle
in·ter·nal oc·cip·i·tal
  crest
  pro·tu·ber·ance
in·ter·nal o·vu·lar
  trans·mi·gra·tion
in·ter·nal pil·lar
  cells
in·ter·nal pter·y·goid
  mus·cle
in·ter·nal pu·den·dal
  ar·tery
  vein
in·ter·nal root
  sheath
in·ter·nal sal·i·vary
  gland
in·ter·nal sa·phe·nous
  nerve
in·ter·nal sem·i·lu·nar
  fi·bro·car·ti·lage of knee
   joint
in·ter·nal sper·mat·ic
  ar·tery
  fas·cia
in·ter·nal sphinc·ter
  mus·cle of anus
in·ter·nal spi·ral
  sul·cus

in·ter·nal tho·rac·ic
  ar·tery
  plex·us
  vein
in·ter·nal ure·thral
  open·ing
in·ter·na·ri·al
in·ter·na·sal
  su·ture
In·ter·na·tion·al
  Sys·tem of Units
in·ter·na·tion·al
  unit
In·ter·na·tion·al Com·mit·tee
  of the Red Cross
In·ter·na·tion·al Sys·tem of
  Units
in·ter·neu·ro·mer·ic
  clefts
in·ter·neu·rons
in·tern·ist
in·ter·nod·al
  seg·ment
in·ter·node
in·ter·nu·cle·ar
in·ter·nun·ci·al
  neu·ron
in·ter·nus
in·ter·oc·clu·sal
  clear·ance
  dis·tance
  gap
  rec·ord
in·ter·oc·clu·sal rest
  space
in·ter·o·cep·tive
in·ter·o·cep·tor
in·ter·o·fec·tive
  sys·tem
in·ter·ol·i·vary
in·ter·or·bit·al
in·ter·os·se·al
in·ter·os·sei
in·ter·os·se·ous
  bur·sa of el·bow
  car·ti·lage
  crest
  fas·cia
  groove
  mar·gin
  mem·brane of fore·arm
  mem·brane of leg
  nerve of leg
in·ter·os·se·ous cu·ne·o·cu·boid
  lig·a·ment
in·ter·os·se·ous cu·ne·o·met·a·
  tar·sal
  lig·a·ments

in·ter·os·se·ous met·a·car·pal
   lig·a·ments
in·ter·os·se·ous met·a·tar·sal
   lig·a·ments
in·ter·os·se·ous sa·cro·il·i·ac
   lig·a·ments
in·ter·os·se·ous ta·lo·cal·ca·ne·
al
   lig·a·ment
in·ter·os·se·us
in·ter·pal·pe·bral
   zone
in·ter·pap·il·lary
   ridg·es
in·ter·pa·ri·e·tal
   bone
   sul·cus
   su·ture
in·ter·par·ox·ys·mal
in·ter·pec·to·ral lymph
   nodes
in·ter·pe·dic·u·late
in·ter·pe·dun·cu·lar
   cis·tern
   fos·sa
   gan·gli·on
   nu·cle·us
in·ter·pel·vi·ab·dom·i·nal
   am·pu·ta·tion
in·ter·per·son·al
in·ter·pha·lan·ge·al
   ar·tic·u·la·tions
   joints
in·ter·phase
in·ter·phy·let·ic
in·ter·plant
in·ter·plant·ing
in·ter·pleu·ral
   space
in·ter·po·lat·ed
   ex·tra·sys·to·le
in·ter·po·si·tion
   ar·thro·plas·ty
in·ter·pre·ta·tion
in·ter·prox·i·mal
   pa·pil·la
   space
in·ter·pu·bic
   disk
in·ter·pul·mo·nary
   sep·tum
in·ter·pu·pil·lary
in·ter·ra·di·al
in·ter·ra·dic·u·lar
   al·ve·o·lo·plas·ty
   sep·ta
   space

in·ter·re·nal
   bod·ies
   glands
in·ter·ridge
   dis·tance
in·ter·rupt·ed
   res·pi·ra·tion
   su·ture
in·ter·scap·u·lar
   gland
   hi·ber·no·ma
   re·flex
in·ter·scap·u·lo·tho·rac·ic
   am·pu·ta·tion
in·ter·scap·u·lum
in·ter·sci·at·ic
in·ter·sec·tio
in·ter·sec·tion
   ten·di·nous i.
in·ter·sec·ti·o·nes
in·ter·seg·men·tal
   fas·cic·u·li
   part
   veins
in·ter·sep·tal
in·ter·sep·to·val·vu·lar
   space
in·ter·sep·tum
in·ter·sex·u·al
in·ter·sex·u·al·i·ty
in·ter·sheath
   spac·es of op·tic nerve
in·ter·sig·moid
   her·nia
   re·cess
in·ter·space
in·ter·spe·cif·ic
   graft
in·ter·spi·nal
   line
   mus·cles
   plane
in·ter·spi·na·lis
in·ter·spi·nous
   lig·a·ment
in·ter·spon·gi·o·plas·tic
   sub·stance
in·ter·ster·ne·bral
   joints
in·ter·stice
in·ter·stic·es
in·ter·sti·tial
   ab·sorp·tion
   cells
   cys·ti·tis
   de·le·tion
   dis·ease
   em·phy·se·ma

in·ter·sti·tial *(continued)*
flu·id
gas·tri·tis
gland
growth
her·nia
im·plan·ta·tion
in·flam·ma·tion
ker·a·ti·tis
la·mel·la
mas·ti·tis
my·o·si·tis
ne·phri·tis
neu·ri·tis
nu·cle·us of Cajal
preg·nan·cy
tis·sue
in·ter·sti·tial cell
tu·mor of tes·tis
in·ter·sti·tial cell-stim·u·lat·ing
hor·mone
in·ter·sti·tial gi·ant cell
pneu·mo·nia
in·ter·sti·tial plas·ma cell
pneu·mo·nia
in·ter·stit·i·um
in·ter·sys·to·le
in·ter·sys·tol·ic
pe·ri·od
in·ter·tar·sal
ar·tic·u·la·tions
joints
in·ter·ten·di·ne·us
con·nec·tions
in·ter·tha·lam·ic
ad·he·sion
in·ter·trag·ic
notch
in·ter·trans·ver·sa·lis
in·ter·trans·verse
lig·a·ment
mus·cles
in·ter·trig·i·nous
in·ter·tri·go
in·ter·tro·chan·ter·ic
crest
line
in·ter·trop·i·cal
ane·mia
hy·phe·mia
in·ter·tu·ber·cu·lar
bur·si·tis
groove
line
plane
sheath
sul·cus

in·ter·tu·bu·lar
zone
in·ter·u·re·ter·al
in·ter·u·re·ter·ic
fold
in·ter·val
gout
op·er·a·tion
scale
in·ter·val
a-c i.
A-H i.
A-N i.
atri·o·ca·rot·id i.
A-V i.
BH i.
c-a i.
car·di·o·ar·te·ri·al i.
cou·pling i.
es·cape i.
fo·cal i.
H-V i.
in·ter·ec·top·ic i.
iso·met·ric i.
lu·cid i.
P-A i.
pas·sive i.
P-J i.
post·sphyg·mic i.
P-P i.
P-Q i.
P-R i.
pre·sphyg·mic i.
Q-R i.
Q-RB i.
QRS i.
Q-T i.
R-R i.
sphyg·mic i.
Sturm's i.
sys·tol·ic time i.'s
in·ter·vas·cu·lar
in·ter·ven·ing
se·quence
var·i·a·ble
in·ter·ve·nous
tu·ber·cle
in·ter·ven·tion
cri·sis i.
in·ter·ven·tric·u·lar
fo·ra·men
grooves
sep·tum
in·ter·ver·te·bral
car·ti·lage
disk
fo·ra·men
gan·gli·on

notch
sym·phy·sis
vein
in·ter·vil·lous
   la·cu·na
   spac·es
in·ter·zon·al
   mes·en·chyme
in·tes·ti·na
in·tes·ti·nal
   anas·to·mo·sis
   an·gi·na
   an·thrax
   ar·ter·ies
   atre·sia
   cal·cu·lus
   ca·pil·la·ri·a·sis
   di·ges·tion
   em·phy·se·ma
   fis·tu·la
   fol·li·cles
   glands
   hem·or·rhage
   in·tox·i·ca·tion
   juice
   lip·o·dys·tro·phy
   lym·phan·gi·ec·ta·sis
   met·a·pla·sia
   my·i·a·sis
   por·tals
   ro·ta·tion
   sand
   schis·to·so·mi·a·sis
   sep·sis
   ste·a·tor·rhea
   sur·face of uter·us
   trunks
   vil·li
in·tes·tine
   large i.
   small i.
in·tes·ti·no·tox·in
in·tes·ti·num
   i. ce·cum
   i. il·e·um
   i. je·ju·num
   i. rec·tum
   i. te·nue mes·en·te·ri·a·le
in·ti·ma
in·ti·mal
in·ti·mi·tis
   pro·lif·er·a·tive i.
in·toe
in·tol·er·ance
   he·red·i·tary fruc·tose i.
   lac·tose i.
in·tor·sion
in·tor·tor

in·tox·a·tion
in·tox·i·cant
in·tox·i·ca·tion
   ac·id i.
   an·a·phy·lac·tic i.
   cit·rate i.
   in·tes·ti·nal i.
   sep·tic i.
   wa·ter i.
in·tra-ab·dom·i·nal
in·tra-ac·i·nous
in·tra-ad·e·noi·dal
in·tra-a·or·tic bal·loon
   de·vice
   pump
in·tra-ar·te·ri·al
in·tra-ar·tic·u·lar
   car·ti·lage
   frac·ture
   lig·a·ment of cos·tal head
in·tra-ar·tic·u·lar ster·no·cos·
tal
   lig·a·ment
in·tra-a·tri·al
   block
   con·duc·tion
in·tra-a·tri·al con·duc·tion
   time
in·tra-au·ral
in·tra-au·ric·u·lar
in·tra·bony
   pock·et
in·tra·bron·chi·al
in·tra·buc·cal
in·tra·bul·bar
   fos·sa
in·tra·can·a·lic·u·lar
   fi·bro·ad·e·no·ma
in·tra·ca·nic·u·lar
   part of op·tic nerve
in·tra·cap·su·lar
   an·ky·lo·sis
   frac·ture
   lig·a·ments
in·tra·cap·su·lar tem·po·ro·
man·dib·u·lar joint
   ar·thro·plas·ty
in·tra·car·di·ac
   cath·e·ter
   lead
in·tra·car·di·ac pres·sure
   curve
in·tra·car·pal
in·tra·car·ti·lag·i·nous
in·tra·cath·e·ter
in·tra·cav·i·tary
in·tra·ce·li·al

in·tra·cel·lu·lar
  can·a·lic·u·lus
  di·ges·tion
  en·zyme
  flu·id
  tox·in
in·tra·cer·e·bel·lar
in·tra·ce·re·bral
  hem·or·rhage
in·tra·cer·vi·cal
in·tra·cis·ter·nal
in·tra·co·lic
in·tra·cor·dal
in·tra·cor·o·nal
  re·tain·er
in·tra·cor·po·re·al
in·tra·cor·pus·cu·lar
in·tra·cos·tal
in·tra·cra·ni·al
  an·eu·rysm
  cav·i·ty
  gan·gli·on
  he·ma·to·ma
  hem·or·rhage
  hy·po·ten·sion
  part
  pneu·ma·to·cele
  pneu·mo·cele
  pres·sure
in·trac·ta·ble
  pain
in·tra·cu·ta·ne·ous
  re·ac·tion
in·tra·cys·tic
  pap·il·lo·ma
in·trad
in·tra·der·mal
  ne·vus
  re·ac·tion
in·tra·der·mic
in·tra·duct
in·tra·duc·tal
  car·ci·no·ma
  pap·il·lo·ma
in·tra·du·ral
in·tra·em·bry·on·ic
  mes·o·derm
in·tra·ep·i·der·mal
  car·ci·no·ma
in·tra·ep·i·der·mic bul·la
in·tra·ep·i·phys·i·al
in·tra·ep·i·plo·ic
  her·nia
in·tra·ep·i·the·li·al
  ac·an·tho·ma
  car·ci·no·ma
  dys·ker·a·to·sis
  glands

in·tra·far·a·di·za·tion
in·tra·fas·cic·u·lar
in·tra·fe·brile
in·tra·fi·lar
in·tra·fu·sal
  fi·bers
in·tra·gal·va·ni·za·tion
in·tra·gas·tric
in·tra·gem·mal
in·tra·gen·ic
  com·ple·men·ta·tion
in·tra·glan·du·lar
in·tra·glan·du·lar pa·rot·id lymph
  nodes
in·tra·glob·u·lar
in·tra·gy·ral
in·tra·he·pat·ic
in·tra·hy·oid
in·tra·il·i·ac
  her·nia
in·tra·jug·u·lar
  pro·cess
in·tra·lam·i·nar
  nu·clei of thal·a·mus
  part of op·tic nerve
in·tra·la·ryn·ge·al
in·tra·le·sion·al
  ther·a·py
in·tra·lig·a·men·ta·ry
  preg·nan·cy
in·tra·lig·a·men·tous
in·tra·lo·bar
  part
in·tra·lob·u·lar
  duct
in·tra·loc·u·lar
in·tra·lu·mi·nal
in·tra·max·il·lary
  an·chor·age
in·tra·med·ul·lary
  an·es·the·sia
  ream·er
  trac·tot·o·my
in·tra·mem·bra·nous
  os·si·fi·ca·tion
in·tra·me·nin·ge·al
in·tra·mo·lec·u·lar
in·tra·mu·ral
  he·ma·to·ma
  prac·tice
  preg·nan·cy
in·tra·mus·cu·lar
in·tra·my·o·car·di·al
in·tra·my·o·me·tri·al
in·tra·na·sal
  an·es·the·sia
in·tra·na·tal

in·tra·neu·ral
in·tra·nu·cle·ar
in·tra·oc·u·lar
   flu·id
   im·plant
   neu·ri·tis
   part of op·tic nerve
   pres·sure
in·tra·o·ral
   an·chor·age
   an·es·the·sia
   an·tros·to·my
in·tra·o·ral frac·ture
   ap·pli·ance
in·tra·or·bit·al
in·tra·os·se·ous
   an·es·the·sia
   fix·a·tion
in·tra·os·te·al
in·tra·o·var·i·an
in·tra·ov·u·lar
in·tra·pa·ri·e·tal
   sul·cus
   sul·cus of Turner
in·tra·par·tum
   hem·or·rhage
   pe·ri·od
in·tra·pel·vic
   her·nia
in·tra·per·i·car·di·ac
in·tra·per·i·car·di·al
in·tra·per·i·os·te·al
   frac·ture
in·tra·per·i·to·ne·al
   preg·nan·cy
in·tra·per·son·al
in·tra·pi·al
in·tra·pleu·ral
in·tra·pon·tine
in·tra·pros·tat·ic
in·tra·pro·to·plas·mic
in·tra·psy·chic
in·tra·pul·mo·nary
in·tra·py·ret·ic
   am·pu·ta·tion
in·tra·ra·chid·i·an
in·tra·rec·tal
in·tra·re·nal
in·tra·ret·i·nal
   space
in·trar·rha·chid·i·an
in·tra·scro·tal
in·tra·seg·men·tal
   part
   veins
in·tra·sep·tal
   al·ve·o·lo·plas·ty

in·tra·spi·nal
   an·es·the·sia
in·tra·splen·ic
in·tra·stro·mal
in·tra·syn·ov·i·al
in·tra·tar·sal
in·tra·ten·di·nous
   bur·sa of el·bow
in·tra·the·cal
   in·jec·tion
in·tra·tho·rac·ic
in·tra·thy·roid
   car·ti·lage
in·tra·ton·sil·lar
in·tra·tra·che·al
   an·es·the·sia
   in·tu·ba·tion
   tube
in·tra·tub·al
in·tra·tu·bu·lar
in·tra·tym·pan·ic
in·tra·u·ter·ine
   am·pu·ta·tion
   con·tra·cep·tive de·vice
   de·vic·es
   frac·ture
   pneu·mo·nia
in·tra·u·ter·ine con·tra·cep·tive
   de·vic·es
in·trav·a·sa·tion
in·tra·vas·cu·lar
   lig·a·ture
   lymph
in·tra·vas·cu·lar pap·il·lary en·do·the·li·al
   hy·per·pla·sia
in·tra·ve·na·tion
in·tra·ve·nous
   an·es·the·sia
   an·es·thet·ic
   bo·lus
   drip
   urog·ra·phy
in·tra·ve·nous re·gion·al
   an·es·the·sia
in·tra·ven·tric·u·lar
   block
   con·duc·tion
   hem·or·rhage
   in·jec·tion
in·tra·ven·tric·u·lar
in·tra·ves·i·cal
in·tra·vi·tal
   stain
   ul·tra·vi·o·let
in·tra vi·tam
in·tra·vi·tel·line
in·tra·vit·re·ous

in·trin·sic
  asth·ma
  col·or
  de·flec·tion
  dys·men·or·rhea
  fac·tor
  fi·bers
  mo·ti·va·tion
  re·flex
  sphinc·ter
in·trin·si·coid
  de·flec·tion
in·tro·duc·er
in·tro·flec·tion
in·tro·flex·ion
in·tro·gas·tric
in·tro·i·tus
in·tro·jec·tion
in·tro·mis·sion
in·tro·mit·tent
  or·gan
in·tron
in·tro·spec·tion
in·tro·spec·tive
  meth·od
in·tro·sus·cep·tion
in·tro·ver·sion
in·tro·vert
in·tu·bate
in·tu·ba·tion
  al·ter·cur·sive i.
  aq·ue·duct·al i.
  blind na·so·tra·che·al i.
  en·do·tra·che·al i.
  in·tra·tra·che·al i.
  na·so·tra·che·al i.
  or·o·tra·che·al i.
in·tu·ba·tor
in·tu·i·tive
  stage
in·tu·mesce
in·tu·mes·cence
  tym·pan·ic i.
in·tu·mes·cent
  cat·a·ract
in·tu·mes·cen·tia
  i. gan·gli·o·for·mis
  i. tym·pa·ni·ca
in·tus·sus·cep·tion
  col·ic i.
  dou·ble i.
  il·e·al i.
  il·e·o·ce·cal i.
  il·e·o·co·lic i.
  je·ju·no·gas·tric i.
  ret·ro·grade i.
in·tus·sus·cep·tive
  growth

in·tus·sus·cep·tum
in·tus·sus·cip·i·ens
in·u·lase
in·u·lin
  clear·ance
in·u·lin·ase
in·u·lol
in·unc·tion
in·un·da·tion
  fe·ver
in·vac·ci·na·tion
in·vag·i·nate
  plan·u·la
in·vag·i·na·tion
  bas·i·lar i.
in·vag·i·na·tor
in·va·lid
in·va·lid·ism
in·va·sin
in·va·sion
in·va·sive
  as·per·gil·lo·sis
  car·ci·no·ma
  mole
in·ven·to·ry
  per·son·al·i·ty i.
in·ver·mi·na·tion
in·verse
  an·a·phy·lax·is
  sym·me·try
  syn·tro·py
in·versed jaw-wink·ing
  syn·drome
in·verse oc·u·lar
  bob·bing
in·ver·sion
  i. of chro·mo·somes
  par·a·cen·tric i.
  per·i·cen·tric i.
  i. of the uter·us
  vis·cer·al i.
in·vert
  sug·ar
in·vert·ase
In·ver·te·bra·ta
in·ver·te·brate
in·vert·ed
  im·age
  pap·il·lo·ma
  pel·vis
  re·flex
  tes·tis
in·vert·ed cone
  bur
in·vert·ed fol·lic·u·lar
  ker·a·to·sis
in·vert·ed ra·di·al
  re·flex

in·ver·tin
in·ver·tor
in·ves·ti·ga·to·ry
  re·flex
in·vest·ing
  car·ti·lage
  tis·sues
in·vest·ing
  vac·u·um i.
in·vest·ment
  cast
in·vest·ment
  re·frac·to·ry i.
in·vet·er·ate
in·vis·ca·tion
in·vis·i·ble
  dif·fer·en·ti·a·tion
  spec·trum
in·vo·lu·cra
in·vo·lu·cre
in·vo·lu·crin
in·vo·lu·crum
in·vol·un·tary
  mus·cles
in·vol·un·tary ner·vous
  sys·tem
in·vo·lu·tion
  cyst
  form
in·vo·lu·tion
  se·nile i.
  i. of the uter·us
in·vo·lu·tion·al
  mel·an·cho·lia
  psy·cho·sis
io·ben·zam·ic ac·id
io·ce·tam·ic ac·id
io·da·mide
Iod·a·moe·ba
  I. bütsch·lii
io·date
  re·ac·tion of ep·i·neph·rine
iod·ic
  pur·pu·ra
iod·ic ac·id
io·dide
  i. per·ox·i·dase
io·dide
  ac·ne
io·dide trans·port
  de·fect
io·dim·e·try
io·di·nase
io·di·nate
io·di·nat·ed
  ca·sein
  glyc·er·ol

io·dine
  cysts
  erup·tion
  num·ber
  re·ac·tion of ep·i·neph·rine
  stain
  val·ue
io·dine
  bu·ta·nol-ex·tract·a·ble i.
  Gram's i.
  pro·tein-bound i.
  ra·di·o·ac·tive i.
  tamed i.
io·dine-fast
io·dine-in·duced
  hy·per·thy·roid·ism
io·din·o·phil
io·din·o·phile
io·din·oph·i·lous
io·dip·a·mide
  i. so·di·um
io·dism
io·dize
iodized
  col·lo·di·on
iodized oil
io·do·a·cet·a·mide
io·do·al·phi·on·ic ac·id
io·do·ca·sein
io·do·chlor·hy·drox·y·quin
io·do·chlo·ro·hy·drox·y·quin·o·line
io·do·chlo·rol
io·do·der·ma
io·do·form
io·do·glob·u·lin
io·do·gor·go·ic ac·id
io·do·hip·pu·rate so·di·um
io·do·meth·a·mate so·di·um
io·do·met·ric
io·dom·e·try
io·do·pa·no·ic ac·id
io·do·phen·dyl·ate
io·do·phil
  gran·ule
io·do·phil·ia
io·do·phor
io·do·phtha·lein
io·do·pro·teins
io·dop·sin
io·do·pyr·a·cet
io·do·ther·a·py
io·do·thy·ro·nines
io·do·ty·ro·sine
  i. de·i·o·dase
io·do·ty·ro·sine de·i·o·di·nase
  de·fect
io·dox·a·mate meg·lu·mine

io·dum
io·du·ria
io·gly·cam·ic ac·id
io·hex·ol
iom·e·ter
ion
    aq·uo-i.
    di·po·lar i.'s
    gram-i.
    hy·dride i.
    hy·dro·gen i.
    hy·dro·ni·um i.
    ox·o·ni·um i.
    sul·fo·ni·um i.
ion
    chan·nel
ion-ex·change
    res·in
ion ex·change
ion ex·chang·er
ion·ic
    med·i·ca·tion
    strength
io·ni·um
ion·i·za·tion
    cham·ber
ion·ize
ion·ized
    at·om
ion·iz·ing
    ra·di·a·tion
ion·o·gram
io·none
ion·o·pher·o·gram
ion·o·phore
ion·o·pho·re·sis
ion·o·pho·ret·ic
ion-se·lec·tive
    elec·trodes
ion·to·pho·re·sis
ion·to·pho·ret·ic
ion·to·quan·tim·e·ter
ion·to·ther·a·py
io·pam·i·dol
io·pa·no·ic ac·id
io·phen·dyl·ate
io·phen·ox·ic ac·id
io·pho·bia
io·ta·cism
io·thal·a·mate so·di·um
io·tha·lam·ic ac·id
io·thi·o·u·ra·cil so·di·um
iox·ag·late
ip·e·cac
    pow·dered i.
ip·e·cac·u·a·nha
    de-e·met·in·ized i.
    pre·pared i.

ipo·date so·di·um
ip·o·mea
    res·in
Ip·o·moea
    I. ru·bro·coe·ru·lea var.
      prae·cox
    I. ver·si·col·or
ipra·tro·pi·um
ipro·ni·a·zid
ipro·ni·da·zole
ipro·ver·a·tril
ip·se·fact
ip·si·lat·er·al
    re·flex
Ir
    genes
ir·i·dal
ir·i·dec·to·my
    but·ton·hole i.
    op·ti·cal i.
    pe·riph·e·ral i.
    sec·tor i.
    sten·o·pe·ic i.
    ther·a·peu·tic i.
ir·i·dec·tro·pi·um
ir·i·den·clei·sis
ir·i·den·tro·pi·um
ir·i·der·e·mia
ir·i·des
ir·i·des·cent
irid·e·sis
irid·i·al
    part of ret·i·na
irid·i·an
irid·ic
ir·i·din
irid·i·um
ir·i·do·a·vul·sion
ir·i·do·cele
ir·i·do·cho·roid·i·tis
ir·i·do·col·o·bo·ma
ir·i·do·cor·ne·al
    an·gle
ir·i·do·cor·ne·al en·do·the·li·al
    syn·drome
ir·i·do·cor·ne·al mes·o·der·mal
    dys·gen·e·sis
ir·i·do·cy·clec·to·my
ir·i·do·cy·cli·tis
    hy·per·ten·sive i.
    i. sep·ti·ca
ir·i·do·cy·clo·cho·roid·i·tis
ir·i·do·cys·tec·to·my
ir·i·dod·e·sis
ir·i·do·di·ag·no·sis
ir·i·do·di·al·y·sis
ir·i·do·di·as·ta·sis
ir·i·do·di·la·tor

ir·i·do·do·ne·sis
ir·i·do·ki·ne·sia
ir·i·do·ki·ne·sis
ir·i·do·ki·net·ic
ir·i·dol·o·gy
ir·i·do·ma·la·cia
ir·i·do·mes·o·di·al·y·sis
ir·i·do·mo·tor
ir·i·don·co·sis
ir·i·don·cus
ir·i·do·pa·ral·y·sis
ir·i·dop·a·thy
ir·i·do·ple·gia
   com·plete i.
   re·flex i.
   sym·pa·thet·ic i.
ir·i·dop·to·sis
ir·i·dor·rhex·is
ir·i·dos·chi·sis
ir·i·do·schis·ma
ir·i·do·scle·rot·o·my
ir·i·do·ste·re·sis
ir·i·dot·a·sis
ir·i·dot·o·my
Ir·i·do·vir·i·dae
Ir·i·do·vi·rus
IRI/G
   ra·tio
iri·gen·in
iris
   i. bom·bé
   pla·teau i.
   trem·u·lous i.
iris
   de·his·cence
   freck·les
   pits
iris frill
Irish moss
   gel·a·tin
iri·sin
iris-ne·vus
   syn·drome
iri·sop·sia
irit·ic
iri·ti·des
iri·tis
   i. blen·or·rha·gique à re·
   chutes
   i. cat·a·me·ni·a·lis
   Doyne's gut·tate i.
   fi·brin·ous i.
   fol·lic·u·lar i.
   i. glau·co·ma·to·sa
   hem·or·rhag·ic i.
   nod·u·lar i.
   i. ob·tur·ans
   plas·tic i.

   qui·et i.
   i. re·ci·di·vans staph·y·lo·
   coc·co-al·ler·gi·ca
   se·rous i.
   spongy i.
   sym·pa·thet·ic i.
irit·o·my
iron
   i. al·bu·mi·nate
   al·bu·mi·nized i.
   i. al·um
   i. dex·trin
   pep·to·nized i.
   i. pro·to·por·phy·rin
   i. py·ri·tes
   i. sor·bi·tex
   i. sor·bi·tol
iron
   al·um
   he·ma·tox·y·lin
   in·dex
   lung
iron-bind·ing
   ca·pac·i·ty
iron de·fi·cien·cy
   ane·mia
iron-dex·tran
   com·plex
iron-stor·age
   dis·ease
irot·o·my
ir·ra·di·ate
ir·ra·di·at·ed vi·ta·min D
   milk
ir·ra·di·a·tion
ir·ra·tion·al
ir·re·duc·i·ble
   her·nia
ir·reg·u·lar
   astig·ma·tism
   bone
   den·tin
   nys·tag·mus
ir·re·sist·i·ble
   im·pulse
ir·re·spir·a·ble
ir·re·spon·si·bil·i·ty
   crim·i·nal i.
ir·re·sus·ci·ta·ble
ir·re·vers·i·ble
   col·loid
   hy·dro·col·loid
   pulp·i·tis
   re·ac·tion
   shock
ir·ri·gate
ir·ri·ga·tion
   drip-suck i.

ir·ri·ga·tor
ir·ri·ta·bil·i·ty
  elec·tric i.
  my·o·tat·ic i.
ir·ri·ta·ble
  breast
  co·lon
  heart
  tes·tis
ir·ri·tant
  pri·mary i.
ir·ri·ta·tion
  cell
  den·tin
  fi·bro·ma
ir·ri·ta·tive
ir·ru·ma·tion
ir·rup·tion
  ca·nal
ir·rup·tive
Irvine-Gass
  syn·drome
Is·a·mine blue
is·aux·e·sis
is·che·mia
  my·o·car·di·al i.
  pos·tur·al i.
  i. ret·i·nae
  si·lent i.
is·che·mic
  con·trac·ture of the left
    ven·tri·cle
  hy·pox·ia
  lum·ba·go
  ne·cro·sis
is·che·mic mus·cu·lar
  at·ro·phy
is·che·mic op·tic
  neu·rop·a·thy
is·che·sis
is·chia
is·chi·ad·ic
  plex·us
  spine
is·chi·a·di·cus
is·chi·al
  bone
  bur·sa
  tu·ber·os·i·ty
is·chi·al·gia
is·chi·at·ic
  her·nia
  notch
is·chi·dro·sis
is·chii
is·chi·o·a·nal
is·chi·o·bul·bar

is·chi·o·cap·su·lar
  lig·a·ment
is·chi·o·cav·er·no·sus
is·chi·o·cav·ern·ous
  mus·cle
is·chi·o·cele
is·chi·o·coc·cyg·e·al
is·chi·o·coc·cyg·e·us
is·chi·o·dyn·ia
is·chi·o·fem·o·ral
  lig·a·ment
is·chi·o·fib·u·lar
is·chi·o·me·lus
is·chi·o·neu·ral·gia
is·chi·o·ni·tis
is·chi·op·a·gus
is·chi·o·per·i·ne·al
is·chi·o·pu·bic
  ra·mus
is·chi·o·rec·tal
  ab·scess
  fos·sa
is·chi·o·sa·cral
is·chi·o·tho·ra·cop·a·gus
is·chi·o·tib·i·al
is·chi·o·vag·i·nal
is·chi·o·ver·te·bral
is·chi·um
is·cho·chy·mia
is·chu·ret·ic
is·chu·ria
is·e·thi·o·nate
is·e·thi·on·ic ac·id
Ishihara
  test
isin·glass
is·land
  blood i.
  bone i.
  i.'s of Calleja
  Langerhans' i.'s
  pan·cre·at·ic i.'s
  i. of Reil
is·land
  dis·ease
  fe·ver
  flap
is·let
  cell
  tis·sue
is·let
  blood i.
  i.'s of Langerhans
  pan·cre·at·ic i.'s
  prin·ci·pal i.'s
is·let cell
  ad·e·no·ma
iso·ag·glu·ti·na·tion

iso·ag·glu·ti·nin
iso·ag·glu·tin·o·gen
iso·al·lele
iso·al·lo·typ·ic
   de·ter·mi·nants
iso·al·lox·a·zine
iso·am·i·done
iso·am·i·nile
iso·am·yl
iso·am·y·lase
iso·am·yl·hy·dro·cu·pre·ine
iso·an·dros·ter·one
iso·an·ti·body
iso·an·ti·gen
iso·bar
iso·bar·ic
iso·bar·ic spi·nal
   an·es·the·sia
iso·bes·tic
iso·bor·nyl thi·o·cy·a·no·ac·e·
   tate
iso·bu·caine hy·dro·chlo·ride
iso·bu·te·ine
iso·bu·tyl al·co·hol
iso·bu·tyl ni·trite
iso·bu·tyr·ic ac·id
iso·bu·zole
iso·cap·nia
iso·car·box·az·id
iso·cel·lu·lar
iso·chor·ic
iso·chro·mat·ic
iso·chro·mat·o·phil
iso·chro·mat·o·phile
iso·chro·mic
   ane·mia
iso·chro·mo·some
iso·chro·nia
isoch·ro·nous
isoch·ro·ous
iso·cit·rase
iso·cit·ra·tase
iso·cit·rate de·hy·dro·gen·ase
iso·cit·rate ly·ase
iso·cit·ric ac·id
   i. a. de·hy·dro·gen·ase
iso·cit·ri·tase
iso·cline
iso·co·ria
iso·cor·tex
iso·cy·a·nate
iso·cy·an·ic ac·id
iso·cy·a·nide
iso·cy·clic
   com·pound
iso·cy·tol·y·sin
iso·dac·tyl·ism
iso·dense

iso·di·pha·sic
   com·plex
iso·dul·cit
iso·dy·nam·ic
   law
iso·dy·na·mo·gen·ic
iso·e·lec·tric
   elec·tro·en·ceph·a·lo·gram
   line
   pe·ri·od
   point
   zone
iso·en·er·get·ic
iso·en·zyme
   elec·tro·pho·re·sis
iso·e·ryth·rol·y·sis
   ne·o·na·tal i.
iso·eth·a·rine
iso·fluor·phate
iso·flu·rane
iso·ga·mete
isog·a·my
iso·ge·ne·ic
   graft
iso·gen·e·sis
iso·gen·ic
   strain
isog·e·nous
   chon·dro·cytes
iso·gen·ti·o·bi·ose
iso·glu·ta·mine
iso·gna·thous
iso·graft
iso·he·mag·glu·ti·na·tion
iso·he·mag·glu·ti·nin
iso·he·mo·ly·sin
iso·he·mol·y·sis
iso·hy·dric
iso·hy·dru·ria
iso·hy·per·cy·to·sis
iso·hy·po·cy·to·sis
iso·i·co·nia
iso·i·con·ic
iso·im·mune
   throm·bo·cy·to·pe·nia
iso·im·mu·ni·za·tion
iso·i·on·ic
   point
iso·late
   ge·net·ic i.
   mat·ing i.
iso·lat·ed
   abut·ment
   dex·tro·car·dia
   dys·ker·a·to·sis fol·lic·u·la·
   ris
   hy·po·al·dos·ter·on·ism
   pro·tein·u·ria

iso·lat·ed ex·plo·sive
  dis·or·der
iso·lat·ed pa·ri·e·tal
  en·do·car·di·tis
iso·la·tion
iso·lec·i·thal
  egg
  ovum
iso·leu·cine
iso·leu·cyl
iso·leu·ko·ag·glu·ti·nin
isol·o·gous
  graft
isol·y·sin
isol·y·sis
iso·lyt·ic
iso·malt·ase
iso·malt·ose
iso·mas·ti·gote
iso·mer
isom·er·ase
iso·mer·ic
  func·tion
  tran·si·tion
isom·er·ism
  ge·o·met·ric i.
  op·ti·cal i.
  ster·e·o·chem·i·cal i.
  struc·tur·al i.
isom·er·i·za·tion
isom·er·ous
iso·meth·a·done
iso·meth·ep·tene
iso·met·ric
  ex·er·cise
  in·ter·val
  pe·ri·od
  pe·ri·od of car·di·ac cy·cle
  re·lax·a·tion
  rul·er
  trac·tion
iso·me·tro·pia
iso·mor·phic
  re·sponse
iso·mor·phism
iso·mor·phous
  gli·o·sis
iso·naph·thol
ison·cot·ic
iso·ni·a·zid
  neu·rop·a·thy
iso·nic·o·tin·ic ac·id
iso·ni·trile
iso·ni·tro·so·ac·e·tone
iso·nor·mo·cy·to·sis
iso-os·mot·ic
isop·a·thy
iso·pen·tyl

iso·pen·tyl·hy·dro·cu·pre·ine
iso·per·i·stal·tic
  anas·to·mo·sis
isoph·a·gy
iso·phane
  in·su·lin
iso·pho·ria
iso·pia
iso·plas·sonts
iso·plas·tic
  graft
iso·pleth
iso·po·ten·tial
iso·pre·cip·i·tin
iso·pren·a·line hy·dro·chlo·ride
iso·pren·a·line sul·phate
iso·prene
  rule
iso·pre·noids
iso·pro·pa·mide io·dide
iso·pro·pa·nol
iso·pro·pa·nol pre·cip·i·ta·tion
  test
iso·pro·phen·a·mine hy·dro·chlo·ride
iso·pro·pyl al·co·hol
iso·pro·pyl·ar·te·re·nol hy·dro·chlo·ride
iso·pro·pyl·car·bi·nol
iso·pro·pyl myr·is·tate
iso·pro·pyl·thi·o·ga·lac·to·side
iso·pro·te·re·nol hy·dro·chlo·ride
iso·pro·te·re·nol sul·fate
isop·ter
iso·py·ro·cal·cif·er·ol
iso·quin·o·line
iso·rhyth·mic
  dis·so·ci·a·tion
iso·ri·bo·fla·vin
isor·rhea
isos·best·ic
  point
iso·sen·si·tize
iso·se·rum
  treat·ment
iso·sex·u·al
is·os·mot·ic
iso·sor·bide di·ni·trate
Isos·po·ra
  I. bel·li
  I. bi·gem·i·na
  I. ca·nis
  I. fe·lis
  I. riv·ol·ta
  I. su·is
iso·spore
isos·po·ri·a·sis

iso·stere
isos·the·nu·ria
iso·suc·cin·ic ac·id
iso·sul·fa·mer·a·zine
iso·sul·fan blue
iso·ther·mal
iso·thi·o·cy·a·nate
iso·thi·pen·dyl
iso·tone
iso·to·nia
iso·ton·ic
   co·ef·fi·cient
   trac·tion
iso·to·nic·i·ty
iso·tope
   ra·di·o·ac·tive i.
   sta·ble i.
iso·tope
   clear·ance
iso·to·pic
iso·trans·plan·ta·tion
iso·tret·i·noin
iso·tro·pic
   disk
   lip·id
isot·ro·pous
iso·type
iso·typ·ic
iso·va·ler·ic ac·id
iso·va·ler·ic·ac·i·de·mia
iso·val·thine
iso·vol·ume
iso·vol·ume pres·sure-flow
   curve
iso·vol·u·met·ric
   re·lax·a·tion
iso·vol·u·mic
   re·lax·a·tion
isox·sup·rine hy·dro·chlo·ride
iso·zyme
is·sue
   na·ture-nur·ture i.
isth·mec·to·my
isth·mi
isth·mi·an
isth·mic
isth·mo·pa·ral·y·sis
isth·mo·ple·gia
isth·mus
   i. of aor·ta
   i. of au·di·to·ry tube
   i. of car·ti·lage of ear
   i. of cin·gu·lar gy·rus
   i. of eu·sta·chi·an tube
   i. of ex·ter·nal acous·tic
    me·a·tus
   i. of fau·ces
   Guyon's i.

   i. of gy·rus for·ni·ca·tus
   i. of His
   Krönig's i.
   i. of lim·bic lobe
   i. me·a·tus acus·ti·ci ex·
    ter·ni
   pha·ryn·ge·al i.
   i. pha·ryn·go·na·sa·lis
   i. of pros·tate
   rhomb·en·ce·phal·ic i.
   i. of thy·roid
   i. of uter·ine tube
   i. of uter·us
   Vieussens' i.
isth·mus·es
it·a·con·ic ac·id
Itai-Itai
   dis·ease
Ital·ian
   meth·od
   op·er·a·tion
   rhi·no·plas·ty
itch
   azo i.
   bak·er's i.
   bar·ber's i.
   bath i.
   coo·lie i.
   co·pra i.
   Cu·ban i.
   dew i.
   dho·bie i.
   frost i.
   grain i.
   gro·cer's i.
   ground i.
   jock i.
   ka·bu·re i.
   lum·ber·man's i.
   mad i.
   Mal·a·bar i.
   Nor·way i.
   poul·try·man's i.
   prai·rie i.
   rice i.
   Saint Ignatius' i.
   straw i.
   straw-bed i.
   sum·mer i.
   swamp i.
   swim·mer's i.
   toe i.
   ware·house·man's i.
   wash·er·wom·an's i.
   wa·ter i.
   win·ter i.
itch·ing

iter
  i. chor·dae an·te·ri·us
  i. chor·dae pos·te·ri·us
  i. den·tis
  i. den·ti·um
  i. a ter·tio ad quar tum
   ven·tri·cu·lum
iter·al
ith·y·cy·pho·sis
ith·y·ky·pho·sis
ith·y·lor·do·sis
Ito
  cells
Ito-Reenstierna
  test
Ito's
  ne·vus
itra·min tos·yl·ate
I-V
  block
Ivemark's
  syn·drome
iver·mec·tin
ivo·ry
  ex·os·to·sis
  mem·brane

Ivy loop
  wir·ing
Iwanoff's
  cysts
Ix·o·des
  I. bi·cor·nis
  I. cookei
  I. dam·mini
  I. hol·o·cy·clus
  I. pa·ci·fi·cus
  I. per·sul·ca·tus
  I. pi·lo·sus
  I. ric·i·nus
  I. sca·pu·la·ris
  I. spi·ni·pal·pis
ix·o·di·a·sis
ix·od·ic
ix·o·did
Ix·od·i·dae
Ix·o·doi·dea
ix·o·my·e·li·tis

J
chain
point
jaag·ziek·te
Jaboulay
py·lo·ro·plas·ty
Jaboulay's
am·pu·ta·tion
meth·od
Jaccoud's
ar·thri·tis
ar·throp·a·thy
jack·et
crown
jack·et
Minerva j.
Sayre's j.
straight j.
jack·screw
jack·so·ni·an
ep·i·lep·sy
Jackson's
law
mem·brane
rule
sign
veil
Jacobaeus
op·er·a·tion
Jacobson's
anas·to·mo·sis
ca·nal
car·ti·lage
nerve
or·gan
plex·us
re·flex
Jacod's
syn·drome
Jacquart's fa·cial
an·gle
Jacquemet's
re·cess
Jacquemin's
test
Jacques'
plex·us
Jacquet's
er·y·the·ma

jac·ti·ta·tion
Jadassohn-Lewandowski
syn·drome
Jadassohn-Pellizzari
an·e·to·der·ma
Jadassohn's
ne·vus
Jadassohn-Tièche
ne·vus
Jaeger's
test types
Jaffe
re·ac·tion
Jaffe-Lichtenstein
dis·ease
Jaffe's
test
Jahnke's
syn·drome
jail
fe·ver
jake
pa·ral·y·sis
Jakob-Creutzfeldt
dis·ease
jal·ap
res·in
jal·ap
Ja·mai·can vom·it·ing
sick·ness
James
fi·bers
tracts
James-Lange
the·o·ry
James·town Can·yon
vi·rus
Janet's
test
Janeway
le·sion
jan·i·ceps
j. asym·me·trus
j. pa·ra·si·ti·cus
Jansen's
op·er·a·tion
Jansky-Bielschowsky
dis·ease

Jansky's
clas·si·fi·ca·tion
Janus green B
Ja·pan
wax
Jap·a·nese
dys·en·tery
schis·to·so·mi·a·sis
Jap·a·nese B
en·ceph·a·li·tis
Jap·a·nese B en·ceph·a·li·tis
vi·rus
Jap·a·nese riv·er
fe·ver
jar
heel j.
jar·gon
apha·sia
Jarisch-Herxheimer
re·ac·tion
Jarjavay's
lig·a·ment
Ja·tro·pha
J. cur·cas
J. glan·du·lif·era
J. urens
jaun·dice
achol·u·ric j.
black j.
ca·tarrh·al j.
cho·le·stat·ic j.
chron·ic achol·u·ric j.
chron·ic fa·mil·i·al j.
chron·ic id·i·o·path·ic j.
con·gen·i·tal he·mo·lyt·ic j.
fa·mil·i·al non·he·mo·lyt·ic j.
he·ma·tog·e·nous j.
he·mo·lyt·ic j.
he·pa·to·cel·lu·lar j.
he·pa·tog·e·nous j.
ho·mol·o·gous se·rum j.
in·fec·tious j.
lep·to·spi·ral j.
ma·lig·nant j.
me·chan·i·cal j.
j. of the new·born
non·ob·struc·tive j.
nu·cle·ar j.
ob·struc·tive j.
pain·less j.
phys·i·o·log·ic j.
re·gur·gi·ta·tion j.
re·ten·tion j.
sphe·ro·cyt·ic j.
tox·e·mic j.
jaun·dice root

jaw
crack·ling j.
Hapsburg j. and lip
lock-j.
low·er j.
lumpy j.
par·rot j.
up·per j.
jaw
bone
jerk
joint
move·ments
re·flex
re·po·si·tion·ing
sep·a·ra·tion
skel·e·ton
Jaworski's
bod·ies
jaw-wink·ing
phe·nom·e·non
syn·drome
jaw-work·ing
re·flex
JC
vi·rus
Jeanselme's
nod·ules
jec·o·ris
jec·ur
Jeghers-Peutz
syn·drome
je·ju·nal
ar·ter·ies
je·ju·nal and il·e·al
veins
je·ju·nec·to·my
je·ju·ni·tis
je·ju·no·co·los·to·my
je·ju·no·gas·tric
in·tus·sus·cep·tion
je·ju·no·il·e·al
by·pass
shunt
je·ju·no·il·e·i·tis
je·ju·no·il·e·os·to·my
je·ju·no·je·ju·nos·to·my
je·ju·no·plas·ty
je·ju·nos·to·my
je·ju·not·o·my
je·ju·num
Jellinek's
sign
jel·ly
car·di·ac j.
in·ter·lam·i·nar j.
Wharton's j.
jel·ly·fish

Jem·bra·na
dis·ease
Jendrassik's
ma·neu·ver
Jenner-Kay
unit
Jenner's
stain
Jensen's
dis·ease
sar·co·ma
Jer·i·cho
boil
jerk
fin·ger
jerk
an·kle j.
chin j.
crossed j.
crossed ad·duc·tor j.
crossed knee j.
el·bow j.
jaw j.
knee j.
su·pi·na·tor j.
jerks
jerky
nys·tag·mus
res·pi·ra·tion
Jervell and Lange-Nielsen
syn·drome
Jes·u·it
tea
Jes·u·its'
bark
jet
in·jec·tion
in·jec·tor
neb·u·liz·er
jet ejec·tor
pump
jet lag
Jeune's
syn·drome
jew·el·ler's
for·ceps
Jewett
sound
Jewett and Strong
stag·ing
j-g
com·plex
JH
vi·rus
jig·ger
jim·son weed
jird

Jk
an·ti·gens
Jk blood group
Job
syn·drome
Jobbins
an·ti·gen
Jobert de Lamballe's
fos·sa
su·ture
Jocasta
com·plex
jock
itch
Jod-Basedow
phe·nom·e·non
Joest
bod·ies
Joffroy's
re·flex
sign
jog·ger's
amen·or·rhea
Johne's
ba·cil·lus
dis·ease
joh·nin
Johnson's
meth·od
joint
cap·sule
evil
ga·mete
ill
oil
sense
joint
acro·mi·o·cla·vic·u·lar j.
an·kle j.
an·te·ri·or in·tra·oc·cip·i·tal
j.
ar·thro·di·al j.
at·lan·to-oc·cip·i·tal j.
ball-and-sock·et j.
bi·ax·i·al j.
bi·con·dy·lar j.
bi·loc·u·lar j.
Budin's ob·stet·ri·cal j.
cal·ca·ne·o·cu·boid j.
ca·pit·u·lar j.
car·pal j.'s
car·po·met·a·car·pal j.'s
car·po·met·a·car·pal j. of
thumb
car·ti·lag·i·nous j.
Charcot's j.
Chopart's j.
Clut·ton's j.'s

joint *(continued)*
coc·cyg·eal j.
co·chle·ar j.
cof·fin j.
com·pound j.
con·dy·lar j.
cos·to·chon·dral j.
cos·to·trans·verse j.
cos·to·ver·te·bral j.'s
cot·y·loid j.
cri·co·ar·y·te·noid j.
cri·co·thy·roid j.
Cruveilhier's j.
cu·bi·tal j.
cu·boi·de·o·na·vic·u·lar j.
cu·ne·o·cu·boid j.
cu·ne·o·met·a·tar·sal j.'s
cu·ne·o·na·vic·u·lar j.
den·to·al·ve·o·lar j.
di·ar·thro·di·al j.
dig·i·tal j.'s
DIP j.'s
dis·tal in·ter·pha·lan·ge·al
  j.'s
j.'s of ear bones
el·bow j.
el·lip·soi·dal j.
en·ar·thro·di·al j.
false j.
fem·o·ro·pa·tel·lar j.
fi·brous j.
flail j.
j.'s of free in·fe·ri·or limb
j.'s of free su·pe·ri·or limb
gin·gly·moid j.
glid·ing j.
gom·phol·ic j.
j. of head of rib
he·mo·phil·ic j.
hinge j.
hip j.
hu·mer·o·ra·di·al j.
hu·mer·o·ul·nar j.
hys·ter·i·cal j.
im·mov·a·ble j.
in·cu·do·mal·le·o·lar j.
in·cu·do·sta·pe·di·al j.
j.'s of in·fe·ri·or limb gir·
  dle
in·fe·ri·or ra·di·o·ul·nar j.
in·fe·ri·or tib·i·o·fib·u·lar
  j.
in·ter·ar·tic·u·lar j.'s
in·ter·car·pal j.'s
in·ter·chon·dral j.'s
in·ter·cu·ne·i·form j.'s
in·ter·met·a·car·pal j.'s
in·ter·met·a·tar·sal j.'s

in·ter·pha·lan·ge·al j.'s
in·ter·ster·ne·bral j.'s
in·ter·tar·sal j.'s
jaw j.
knee j.
lat·er·al at·lan·to·ax·i·al j.
lat·er·al at·lan·to·ep·i·
  stroph·ic j.
Lisfranc's j.'s
lum·bo·sa·cral j.
Luschka's j.'s
man·dib·u·lar j.
ma·nu·bri·o·ster·nal j.
me·di·an at·lan·to·ax·i·al j.
met·a·car·po·pha·lan·ge·al
  j.'s
met·a·tar·so·pha·lan·ge·al
  j.'s
mid·dle at·lan·to·ep·i·
  stroph·ic j.
mid·dle car·pal j.
mid·tar·sal j.
mor·tise j.
mov·a·ble j.
MP j.'s
mul·ti·ax·i·al j.
neu·ro·cen·tral j.
neu·ro·path·ic j.
peg-and-sock·et j.
pet·ro·oc·cip·i·tal j.
pha·lan·ge·al j.'s
PIP j.'s
pi·so·tri·que·tral j.
piv·ot j.
plane j.
pol·y·ax·i·al j.
pos·te·ri·or in·tra·oc·cip·i·
  tal j.
prox·i·mal in·ter·pha·lan·
  ge·al j.'s
ra·di·o·car·pal j.
ro·ta·ry j.
ro·ta·to·ry j.
sa·cro·coc·cyg·e·al j.
sa·cro·il·i·ac j.
sad·dle j.
schin·dy·let·ic j.
screw j.
shoul·der j.
sim·ple j.
sock·et j.
sphe·no·oc·cip·i·tal j.
sphe·roid j.
spi·ral j.
ster·nal j.'s
ster·no·cla·vic·u·lar j.
ster·no·cos·tal j.'s
sti·fle j.

sub·ta·lar j.
j.'s of su·pe·ri·or limb gir·
dle
su·pe·ri·or ra·di·o·ul·nar j.
su·pe·ri·or tib·i·o·
fib·u·lar j.
su·ture j.
syn·ar·thro·di·al j.
syn·chon·dro·di·al j.
syn·des·mo·di·al j.
syn·des·mot·ic j.
syn·o·vi·al j.
ta·lo·cal·ca·ne·al j.
ta·lo·cal·ca·ne·o·na·
vic·u·lar j.
tar·sal j.'s
tar·so·met·a·tar·sal j.'s
tem·po·ro·man·dib·u·lar j.
thigh j.
tib·i·o·fib·u·lar j.,
in·fe·ri·or
tib·i·o·fib·u·lar j.,
su·pe·ri·or
trans·verse tar·sal j.
tro·choid j.
un·co·ver·te·bral j.'s
uni·ax·i·al j.
uni·loc·u·lar j.
wedge-and-groove j.
wrist j.
xiph·i·ster·nal j.
zyg·a·poph·y·si·al j.'s
joint mice
Jolles'
test
Jolly
bod·ies
Jolly's
re·ac·tion
Jonnesco's
fos·sa
Jonston's
al·o·pe·cia
ar·ea
Joseph
rhi·no·plas·ty
Joubert's
syn·drome
joule
Joule's
equiv·a·lent
Js
an·ti·gen
J-sel·la
de·for·mi·ty
juc·cu·ya
Judkins
tech·nique

ju·ga
ju·gal
bone
lig·a·ment
point
ju·ga·le
ju·go·max·il·lary
jug·u·lar
duct
em·bry·o·car·dia
fo·ra·men
fos·sa
gan·gli·on
gland
nerve
notch
plex·us
pro·cess
pulse
si·nus
trunk
tu·ber·cle
veins
wall of mid·dle ear
jug·u·lar fo·ra·men
syn·drome
jug·u·lar ve·nous
arch
jug·u·lo·di·gas·tric
node
jug·u·lo-o·mo·hy·oid
node
jug·u·lum
ju·gum
juice
ap·pe·tite j.
can·cer j.
gas·tric j.
in·tes·ti·nal j.
pan·cre·at·ic j.
jump
flap
jump·er
dis·ease
dis·ease of Maine
jump·ing
gene
throm·bo·sis
jump·ing the
bite
junc·tion
ne·vus
junc·tion
am·e·lo·den·tal j.
am·e·lo·den·tin·al j.
am·ni·o·em·bry·on·ic j.
ano·rec·tal j.
ce·ment·o·den·tin·al j.

junc·tion *(continued)*
ce·men·to·e·nam·el j.
cho·led·o·cho·du·o·de·nal j.
den·tin·o·ce·ment·al j.
den·tin·o·e·nam·el j.
elec·tro·ton·ic j.
esoph·a·go·gas·tric j.
gap j.
in·ter·cel·lu·lar j.'s
in·ter·me·di·ate j.
j. of lips
mu·co·cu·ta·ne·ous j.
mus·cle-ten·don j.
my·o·neu·ral j.
neu·ro·ec·to·der·mal j.
neu·ro·mus·cu·lar j.
neu·ro·so·mat·ic j.
sa·cro·coc·cyg·e·al j.
scle·ro·cor·ne·al j.
squa·mo·co·lum·nar j.
ST j.
tight j.
tym·pa·no·sta·pe·di·al j.
junc·tion·al
com·plex
cyst
ep·i·the·li·um
ex·tra·sys·to·le
junc·tu·ra
j. car·ti·la·gi·nea
junc·tu·rae cin·gu·li mem·
bri su·pe·ri·o·ris
j. fi·bro·sa
j. lum·bo·sa·cra·lis
junc·tu·rae mem·bri in·fe·
ri·o·ris li·be·ri
junc·tu·rae mem·bri su·pe·
ri·o·ris li·be·ri
junc·tu·rae os·si·um
j. sa·cro·coc·cy·gea
j. syn·o·vi·a·lis
junc·tu·rae ten·di·num
junc·tu·rae zy·ga·po·phy·se·
a·les
junc·tu·rae
junc·ture
jung·i·an
psy·cho·a·nal·y·sis
jun·gle
fe·ver
jun·gle yel·low
fe·ver
Jüngling's
dis·ease
Jung's
mus·cle
Ju·nin
vi·rus

ju·ni·per
j. ber·ry oil
j. tar
Junod's
boot
jur·is·pru·dence
den·tal j.
med·i·cal j.
jus·ti·fi·a·ble
abor·tion
jus·to ma·jor
jus·to mi·nor
ju·ve·nile
an·gi·o·fi·bro·ma
ar·rhyth·mia
ar·thri·tis
car·ci·no·ma
cat·a·ract
cell
cho·rea
cir·rho·sis
elas·to·ma
he·man·gi·o·fi·bro·ma
ky·pho·sis
neu·tro·phil
os·te·o·ma·la·cia
os·te·o·po·ro·sis
pap·il·lo·ma·to·sis
pat·tern
pel·vis
per·i·o·don·ti·tis
pol·yp
ret·i·nos·chi·sis
xan·tho·gran·u·lo·ma
ju·ve·nile ep·i·the·li·al
dys·tro·phy
ju·ve·nile hy·a·lin
fi·bro·ma·to·sis
ju·ve·nile mus·cu·lar
at·ro·phy
ju·ve·nile my·o·clon·ic
ep·i·lep·sy
ju·ve·nile-on·set
di·a·be·tes
ju·ve·nile pal·mo-plan·tar
fi·bro·ma·to·sis
ju·ve·nile rheu·ma·toid
ar·thri·tis
jux·ta-ar·tic·u·lar
nod·ules
jux·ta·cor·ti·cal
chon·dro·ma
jux·ta·cor·ti·cal os·te·o·gen·ic
sar·co·ma
jux·ta·ep·i·phys·i·al
jux·ta-e·soph·a·ge·al lymph
nodes

jux·ta-e·soph·a·ge·al pul·mo·
  nary lymph
  nodes
jux·ta·glo·mer·u·lar
  ap·pa·ra·tus
  body
  cells
  com·plex
  gran·ules

jux·ta·in·tes·ti·nal lymph
  nodes
jux·tal·lo·cor·tex
jux·ta·po·si·tion
jux·ta·pu·pil·lary
  cho·roid·i·tis
jux·ta·res·ti·form
  body

K

K
 cells
 com·plex
 re·gion
 vi·rus
K-ra·di·a·tion
k
 an·ti·gens
ka·bu·re
 itch
Kaf·fir
 pox
ka·fin·do
Kaiserling's
 fix·a·tive
kak·ké
ka·la azar
ka·le·mia
ka·li·o·pe·nia
ka·li·o·pe·nic
ka·li·um
ka·li·u·re·sis
ka·li·u·ret·ic
kal·lak
kal·li·din
 k. I
 k. II
kal·li·kre·in
 sys·tem
Kallmann's
 syn·drome
kal·u·re·sis
kal·u·ret·ic
ka·na·my·cin sul·fate
kang
 can·cer
kan·gri
 can·cer
kan·gri burn
 car·ci·no·ma
Kanner's
 syn·drome
kan·yem·ba
ka·o·lin
ka·o·lin·o·sis
Kaposi's
 sar·co·ma
Kaposi's var·i·cel·li·form
 erup·tion

kap·pa
 an·gle
 gran·ule
 par·ti·cles
kap·pa·cism
ka·ra·ya
 gum
Karmen
 can·nu·la
 unit
Karnofsky
 scale
Kartagener's
 syn·drome
 tri·ad
kar·y·o·chrome
 cell
kar·y·oc·la·sis
kar·y·o·cyte
kar·y·o·gam·ic
kar·y·og·a·my
kar·y·o·gen·e·sis
kar·y·o·gen·ic
kar·y·o·go·nad
kar·y·o·gram
kar·y·o·ki·ne·sis
kar·y·o·ki·net·ic
kar·y·o·lymph
kar·y·ol·y·sis
kar·y·o·lyt·ic
kar·y·o·mi·cro·some
kar·y·o·mi·to·sis
kar·y·o·mi·tot·ic
kar·y·o·mor·phism
kar·y·on
kar·y·o·phage
kar·y·o·plasm
kar·y·o·plas·mol·y·sis
kar·y·o·plast
kar·y·o·pyk·no·sis
kar·y·o·pyk·not·ic
 in·dex
kar·y·o·rrhex·is
kar·y·o·some
kar·y·os·ta·sis
kar·y·o·the·ca
kar·y·o·type
kar·y·o·zo·ic

Kasabach-Merritt
syn·drome
Kasai
op·er·a·tion
ka·sai
Kashin-Bek
dis·ease
Kasten's flu·o·res·cent Feulgen
stain
Kasten's flu·o·res·cent PAS
stain
Kasten's flu·o·res·cent Schiff
re·a·gents
kat·al
kat·a·ther·mom·e·ter
Katayama
dis·ease
syn·drome
Katayama's
test
kath·o·dal
kath·ode
kat·i·on
ka·va
Kawasaki
dis·ease
Kayser-Fleischer
ring
Kazanjian's
op·er·a·tion
K blood group
k blood group
Kearns-Sayre
syn·drome
Keating-Hart's
meth·od
ke·da·ni
fe·ver
keel
keeled
chest
Keen's
op·er·a·tion
sign
Kegel's
ex·er·cis·es
Kehr's
sign
kei·ro·spasm
Keith and Flack
node
Keith's
bun·dle
node
ke·lec·tome
Ke·lev strain ra·bies
vi·rus
ke·lis

Kell blood group
Keller
bun·ion·ec·to·my
Kelly
clamp
Kelly's
op·er·a·tion
Kelly's rec·tal
spec·u·lum
ke·loid
ac·ne k.
ke·loi·do·sis
ke·lo·plas·ty
ke·lo·so·mia
Kelvin
scale
kel·vin
Kennedy
clas·si·fi·ca·tion
Kennedy's
syn·drome
ken·nel
cough
Kenny's
treat·ment
Kent-His
bun·dle
Kent's
bun·dle
keph·a·lin
Kerandel's
symp·tom
ker·a·phyl·lo·cele
ker·a·sin
his·ti·o·cy·to·sis
ker·a·tan sul·fate
ker·a·tec·ta·sia
ker·a·tec·to·my
ker·a·te·in
ker·a·ti·a·sis
ke·rat·ic
pre·cip·i·tates
ker·a·tin
fil·a·ments
pearl
ker·a·tin·as·es
ker·a·tin·i·za·tion
ker·a·tin·ized
ke·rat·i·no·cyte
ke·rat·i·no·some
ke·rat·i·nous
cyst
ker·a·ti·tis
ac·tin·ic k.
al·pha·bet·i·cal k.
deep punc·tate k.
den·dri·form k.
den·drit·ic k.

dif·fuse deep k.
Dimmer's k.
k. dis·ci·for·mis
ex·po·sure k.
fas·cic·u·lar k.
k. fil·a·men·to·sa
ge·o·graph·ic k.
her·pet·ic k.
hy·po·py·on k.
in·fec·tious bo·vine k.
in·ter·sti·tial k.
lag·oph·thal·mic k.
let·ter-shaped k.
k. li·ne·a·ris mi·grans
mar·gi·nal k.
met·a·her·pet·ic k.
my·cot·ic k.
nec·ro·gran·u·lo·ma·tous k.
neu·ro·par·a·lyt·ic k.
k. num·mu·la·ris
par·en·chym·a·tous k.
k. pe·ri·o·di·ca fu·gax
phlyc·ten·u·lar k.
pol·y·mor·phic su·per·fi·cial k.
k. pro·fun·da
k. punc·ta·ta
punc·tate k.
scle·ros·ing k.
scrof·u·lous k.
ser·pig·i·nous k.
k. sic·ca
su·per·fi·cial lin·e·ar k.
su·per·fi·cial punc·tate k.
tra·chom·a·tous k.
vas·cu·lar k.
ve·sic·u·lar k.
xe·rot·ic k.
ker·a·to·ac·an·tho·ma
ker·a·to·an·gi·o·ma
ker·a·to·at·ro·pho·der·ma
ker·a·to·cele
ker·a·to·con·junc·ti·vi·tis
atop·ic k.
ep·i·dem·ic k.
flash k.
her·pet·ic k.
k. sic·ca
su·pe·ri·or lim·bic k.
ul·tra·vi·o·let k.
ver·nal k.
vi·rus k.
ker·a·to·co·nus
ker·a·to·cri·coid
ker·a·to·cyst
ker·a·to·cyte
ker·a·to·der·ma
k. blen·nor·rha·gi·ca

k. ec·cen·tri·ca
lymph·e·dem·a·tous k.
mu·ti·lat·ing k.
k. pal·mar·is et plan·tar·is
pal·mo·plan·tar k.
k. plan·ta·re sul·ca·tum
punc·tate k.
se·nile k.
k. sym·me·tri·ca
ker·a·to·der·ma·ti·tis
ker·a·to·ec·ta·sia
ker·a·to·ep·i·the·li·o·plas·ty
ker·a·to·gen·e·sis
ker·a·to·ge·net·ic
ker·a·tog·e·nous
mem·brane
ker·a·to·glo·bus
ker·a·to·glos·sus
ker·a·to·hy·al
ker·a·to·hy·a·lin
gran·ules
ker·a·toid
ex·an·the·ma
ker·a·to·lep·tyn·sis
ker·a·to·leu·ko·ma
ker·a·tol·y·sis
k. ex·fo·li·a·ti·va
pit·ted k.
ker·a·to·lyt·ic
ker·a·to·ma
k. dis·se·mi·na·tum
k. he·re·di·ta·ria mu·ti·lans
k. ma·lig·num
k. plan·ta·re sul·ca·tum
se·nile k.
ker·a·to·ma·la·cia
ker·a·tome
ker·a·tom·e·ter
ker·a·tom·e·try
ker·a·to·mi·leu·sis
ker·a·to·my·co·sis
ker·a·to·no·sis
ker·a·to·pach·y·der·ma
ker·a·top·a·thy
band-shaped k.
bul·lous k.
cli·mat·ic k.
fil·a·men·ta·ry k.
Lab·ra·dor k.
lip·id k.
stri·ate k.
ve·sic·u·lar k.
ker·a·to·pha·kia
ker·a·to·phak·ic
ker·a·to·plas·ty
ker·a·to·plas·ty
al·lo·path·ic k.
au·tog·e·nous k.

ker·a·to·plas·ty *(continued)*
  ep·i·ker·a·to·phak·ic k.
  het·er·og·e·nous k.
  ho·mog·e·nous k.
  ker·a·to·phak·ic k.
  lam·el·lar k.
  lay·ered k.
  non·pen·e·trat·ing k.
  op·ti·cal k.
  pen·e·trat·ing k.
  per·fo·rat·ing k.
  tec·ton·ic k.
  to·tal k.
ker·a·to·pros·the·sis
ker·a·to·rhex·is
ker·a·tor·rhex·is
ker·a·to·rus
ker·a·to·scle·ri·tis
ker·a·to·scope
ker·a·tos·co·py
ker·a·tose
ker·a·to·ses
ker·a·to·sic
  cones
ker·a·to·sis
  ac·tin·ic k.
  ar·sen·i·cal k.
  k. blen·nor·rha·gi·ca
  k. dif·fu·sa fe·ta·lis
  k. fol·lic·u·la·ris
  k. fol·lic·u·la·ris con·ta·gi·
    o·sa
  in·vert·ed fol·lic·u·lar k.
  k. la·bi·a·lis
  li·chen·oid k.
  k. ni·gri·cans
  k. ob·tur·ans
  k. pal·mar·is et plan·tar·is
  k. pi·lo·ris atroph·i·cans fa·
    ci·ei
  k. punc·ta·ta
  k. ru·bra fig·ur·a·ta
  seb·or·rhe·ic k.
  k. seb·or·rhe·i·ca
  se·nile k.
  k. se·ni·lis
  so·lar k.
  tar k.
  k. ve·ge·tans
ker·a·to·sul·fate
ker·a·to·tome
ker·a·tot·o·my
  de·lim·it·ing k.
  ra·di·al k.
  re·frac·tive k.
ke·rau·no·pho·bia
Kerckring's
  cen·ter

  folds
  os·si·cle
  valves
ke·ri·on
  Celsus k.
Kerley B
  lines
ker·nic·ter·us
Kernig's
  sign
Kernohan's
  notch
kern-plas·ma re·la·tion
  the·o·ry
ker·oid
ker·o·sene
ker·o·ther·a·py
Kestenbaum's
  sign
ke·tal
ket·a·mine
ke·tene
ke·to ac·id
ke·to·ac·i·do·sis
ke·to·ac·i·du·ria
  branched chain k.
ke·to·bem·i·done
ke·to·con·a·zole
ke·to·gen·e·sis
ke·to·gen·ic
  di·et
ke·to·gen·ic-an·ti·ke·to·gen·ic
  ra·ti·o
ke·to·gen·ic cor·ti·coids
  test
ke·to·hep·tose
ke·to·hex·ose
ke·to·hy·drox·y·es·trin
ke·tol
ke·tole
ke·tole group
ke·to·lyt·ic
ke·tone
  body
ke·tone al·co·hol
ke·tone-al·de·hyde mu·tase
ke·to·ne·mia
ke·ton·ic
ke·ton·i·mine
  dyes
ke·to·ni·za·tion
ke·ton·u·ria
  branched chain k.
ke·to·pan·to·ic ac·id
ke·to·pen·tose
ke·to·pro·fen
ke·tose
ke·tose re·duc·tase

ke·to·sis
  bo·vine k.
ke·to·suc·ci·nic ac·id
Kew Gar·dens
  fe·ver
key
  at·tach·ment
  ridge
  vein
key·hole
  de·for·mi·ty
  pu·pil
key-in-lock
  ma·neu·ver
Key-Retzius
  cor·pus·cles
key·way
  at·tach·ment
khat
khel·lin
kick
  atri·al k.
  id·i·o·ven·tric·u·lar k.
Kidd blood group
kid·ney
  am·y·loid k.
  Armanni-Ebstein k.
  ar·te·ri·o·lo·scle·rot·ic k.
  ar·te·ri·o·scle·rot·ic k.
  ar·ti·fi·cial k.
  Ask-Up·mark k.
  atroph·ic k.
  cake k.
  con·tract·ed k.
  cow k.
  crush k.
  cys·tic k.
  disk k.
  du·plex k.
  fat·ty k.
  flea-bit·ten k.
  float·ing k.
  Formad's k.
  fused k.
  Goldblatt k.
  gran·u·lar k.
  head k.
  hind k.
  horse·shoe k.
  med·ul·lary sponge k.
  mid·dle k.
  mor·tar k.
  mov·a·ble k.
  pan·cake k.
  pel·vic k.
  pol·y·cys·tic k.
  pri·mor·di·al k.
  put·ty k.

py·e·lo·ne·phrit·ic k.
Rose-Bradford k.
scle·rot·ic k.
su·per·nu·mer·ary k.
wan·der·ing k.
waxy k.
kid·ney
  ba·sin
  car·bun·cle
Kiel
  clas·si·fi·ca·tion
Kienböck's
  at·ro·phy
  dis·ease
  dis·lo·ca·tion
  unit
Kiernan's
  space
Kiesselbach's
  ar·ea
Kilham rat
  vi·rus
Kilian's
  line
kill·er
  cells
Killian's
  bun·dle
  op·er·a·tion
kil·o·base
kil·o·cal·o·rie
kil·o·cy·cle
kil·o·gram
  cal·o·rie
kil·o·gram-me·ter
kil·o·roent·gen
kil·o·volt
kil·o·volt·me·ter
Kimmelstiel-Wilson
  dis·ease
  syn·drome
Kimura's
  dis·ease
kin·an·es·the·sia
ki·nase
ki·nase II
kin·dling
kin·dred
kin·e·mat·ic
  face-bow-b.
  vis·cos·i·ty
kin·e·mat·ics
kin·e·mom·e·ter
kin·e·plas·tic
  am·pu·ta·tion
kin·e·plas·tics
kin·e·sal·gia
kin·e·scope

ki·ne·sia
ki·ne·si·al·gia
ki·ne·si·at·rics
ki·ne·sics
kin·e·sim·e·ter
ki·ne·si·ol·o·gy
ki·ne·si·om·e·ter
ki·ne·si·o·neu·ro·sis
kin·e·sip·a·thist
kin·e·sip·a·thy
ki·ne·sis
ki·ne·si·ther·a·py
ki·ne·so·pho·bia
kin·es·the·sia
kin·es·the·si·om·e·ter
kin·es·thet·ic
   au·ra
   sense
ki·net·ic
   an·a·lyz·er
   atax·ia
   drive
   en·er·gy
   mea·sure·ment
   pe·rim·e·try
   stra·bis·mus
   sys·tem
   trem·or
ki·net·ics
   chem·i·cal k.
ki·ne·to·car·di·o·gram
ki·ne·to·car·di·o·graph
ki·ne·to·chore
ki·ne·to·gen·ic
ki·ne·to·plasm
ki·ne·to·plast
ki·ne·to·scope
ki·net·o·some
King
   unit
King-Armstrong
   unit
king's
   evil
Kingsley
   splint
kin·ic ac·id
ki·nin
ki·nin·o·gen
ki·nin·o·ge·nase
ki·nin·o·gen·in
kink
   Lane's k.
kinked
   aor·ta
Kin·ki·ang
   fe·ver

kinky
   hair
kinky-hair
   dis·ease
kin·o·cen·trum
ki·no·cil·i·um
kin·o·hapt
kin·o·mom·e·ter
kin·o·plasm
kin·o·plas·mic
kin·ship
Kinyoun
   stain
ki·on
Kirkland
   knife
Kirk's
   am·pu·ta·tion
Kirschner's
   ap·pa·ra·tus
   wire
Kisch's
   re·flex
Ki·sen·yi sheep dis·ease
   vi·rus
Kitasato's
   ba·cil·lus
Kittrich's
   stain
Kjeldahl
   ap·pa·ra·tus
   meth·od
Kjelland's
   for·ceps
Klapp's
   meth·od
Kleb·si·el·la
   K. ozae·nae
   K. pneu·mo·ni·ae
   K. rhi·no·scle·ro·ma·tis
Klebs-Loeffler
   ba·cil·lus
klee·blatt·schä·del
Kleihauer's
   stain
Kleine-Levin
   syn·drome
Klein-Gumprecht shad·ow
   nu·clei
Klein's
   mus·cle
klep·to·lag·nia
klep·to·ma·nia
klep·to·ma·ni·ac
klep·to·pho·bia
Klinefelter's
   syn·drome

Klinger-Ludwig ac·id-thi·o·nin
stain for sex chro·ma·tin
Klippel-Feil
syn·drome
Klippel's
dis·ease
Klippel-Trenaunay-Weber
syn·drome
Klumpke-Dejerine
syn·drome
Klumpke's
pa·ral·y·sis
Klüver-Barrera Lux·ol fast blue
stain
Klüver-Bucy
syn·drome
Knapp's
streaks
stri·ae
knee
jerk
joint
phe·nom·e·non
pre·sen·ta·tion
re·flex
knee
Brodie's k.
capped k.
house·maid's k.
locked k.
knee·cap
knee-chest
po·si·tion
knee-el·bow
po·si·tion
knee-jerk
re·flex
Kne·mi·do·kop·tes
Knies'
sign
Kniest
syn·drome
knife
nee·dle
knife
Beer's k.
car·ti·lage k.
cau·tery k.
chem·i·cal k.
elec·trode k.
fis·tu·la k.
free-hand k.
Goldman-Fox knives
Graefe's k.
her·nia k.
Kirkland k.
len·tic·u·lar k.
Liston's knives

Merrifield k.
val·vot·o·my k.
knife-rest
crys·tal
knis·mo·gen·ic
knis·mo·lag·nia
knit·ting
knives
knob
Engelmann's ba·sal k.'s
ma·lar·i·al k.'s
knock
per·i·car·di·al k.
knock-knee
knock-out
drops
Knoll's
glands
Knoop hard·ness
num·ber
test
Knoop's
the·o·ry
knot
false k.'s
false k.'s of um·bil·i·cal
cord
Hensen's k.
Hubrecht's pro·to·chor·dal
k.
net k.
prim·i·tive k.
pro·to·chor·dal k.
syn·cy·tial k.
true k.
true k. of um·bil·i·cal cord
vi·tal k.
knuck·le
cer·vi·cal aor·tic k.
knuck·le
pads
knuck·ling
Kobelt's
tu·bules
Kober
test
Köbner's
phe·nom·e·non
Kocher
clamp
Kocher's
in·ci·sion
sign
Koch's
ba·cil·lus
law
node
phe·nom·e·non

Koch's *(continued)*
  pos·tu·lates
  tri·an·gle
Koch's blue
  bod·ies
Koch's old
  tu·ber·cu·lin
Koch's orig·i·nal
  tu·ber·cu·lin
Koch-Weeks
  ba·cil·lus
  con·junc·ti·vi·tis
Kock
  il·e·os·to·my
  pouch
Koenen's
  tu·mor
Koenig's
  syn·drome
Koerber-Salus-Elschnig
  syn·drome
Koerte-Ballance
  op·er·a·tion
Koettstorfer
  num·ber
Köhler
  il·lu·mi·na·tion
Köhler's
  dis·ease
Köhlmeier-Degos
  dis·ease
Kohlrausch's
  mus·cle
  valves
Kohn's
  pores
Kohnstamm's
  phe·nom·e·non
koi·lo·cyte
koi·lo·cy·to·sis
koi·lo·nych·ia
koil·o·ster·nia
Kojewnikoff's
  ep·i·lep·sy
ko·jic ac·id
ko·koi
  ven·om
ko·la
Kölliker's
  lay·er
  re·tic·u·lum
Kollmann's
  di·la·tor
Kolmer
  test
ko·lyt·ic
Kondoleon
  op·er·a·tion

ko·ni·o·cor·tex
Koongol
  vi·rus·es
Koplik's
  spots
kop·o·pho·bia
Ko·re·an hem·or·rhag·ic
  fe·ver
Korff's
  fi·bers
ko·ro
ko·ro·ni·on
Korotkoff
  sounds
Korotkoff's
  test
Korsakoff's
  psy·cho·sis
  syn·drome
Kossa
  stain
Krabbe's
  dis·ease
  syn·drome
krait
kra-kra
Kraske's
  op·er·a·tion
krau·ro·sis vul·vae
Krause
  graft
Krause's
  bone
  glands
  lig·a·ment
  meth·od
  mus·cle
  syn·drome
  valve
Krause's end
  bulbs
Krause's res·pi·ra·to·ry
  bun·dle
Krebs
  cy·cle
Krebs-Henseleit
  cy·cle
Krebs or·ni·thine
  cy·cle
Krebs-Ringer
  so·lu·tion
Krebs urea
  cy·cle
Kretschmann's
  space
Kreysig's
  sign

Krogh
spi·rom·e·ter
Kromayer's
lamp
Kronecker's
stain
Krönig's
isth·mus
steps
Krönlein
op·er·a·tion
Krönlein's
her·nia
Krueger
in·stru·ment stop
Krukenberg's
am·pu·ta·tion
spin·dle
tu·mor
veins
Kruse's
brush
kryp·ton
ku·bi·sa·ga·ri
ku·bi·sa·ga·ru
Kuersteiner's
ca·nals
Kufs
dis·ease
Kugelberg-Welander
dis·ease
Kugel's
ar·tery
Kühne's
fi·ber
meth·yl·ene blue
phe·nom·e·non
plate
spin·dle
Kuhnt-Junius
de·gen·er·a·tion
dis·ease
Kuhnt's
op·er·a·tion
spac·es
Kulchitsky
cells
Külz's
cyl·in·der
Kümmell's
spon·dy·li·tis
Küntscher
nail
Kupffer
cells
kur·chi bark
Kurloff's
bod·ies

Kürsteiner's
ca·nals
ku·ru
Ku·ru·ne·ga·la
ul·cers
Kurzrok-Ratner
test
Kus·ko·kwim
syn·drome
Kussmaul
res·pi·ra·tion
Kussmaul-Kien
res·pi·ra·tion
Kussmaul-Landry
pa·ral·y·sis
Kussmaul's
apha·sia
co·ma
dis·ease
sign
symp·tom
Kussmaul's par·a·dox·i·cal
pulse
Kveim
an·ti·gen
test
Kveim-Stilz·bach
an·ti·gen
test
kwa·shi·or·kor
Ky·as·a·nur For·est
dis·ease
Ky·as·a·nur For·est dis·ease
vi·rus
kyl·lo·sis
ky·ma·tism
ky·mo·gram
ky·mo·graph
ky·mog·ra·phy
ky·mo·scope
kyn·u·ren·ic ac·id
kyn·u·ren·i·nase
kyn·u·ren·ine
kyn·u·ren·ine for·mam·i·dase
ky·phos
ky·pho·sco·li·o·sis
ky·pho·sco·li·ot·ic
pel·vis
ky·pho·sis
ju·ve·nile k.
ky·phot·ic
pel·vis
ky·pho·tone
Kyrle's
dis·ease

L
  chain
  dos·es
  form
  unit of strep·to·my·cin
L⁺
  dose
L₊
  dose
L_f
  dose
L₀
  dose
L_r
  dose
L-
  mer·o·my·o·sin
  ra·di·a·tion
Laband's
  syn·drome
Labbé's
  tri·an·gle
  vein
Labbé's neu·ro·cir·cu·la·to·ry
  syn·drome
la·beled
  at·om
la belle in·dif·fer·ence
la·bet·a·lol hy·dro·chlo·ride
la·bia
la·bi·al
  arch
  bar
  em·bra·sure
  flange
  gin·gi·va
  glands
  her·nia
  oc·clu·sion
  pa·ral·y·sis
  part
  splint
  sul·cus
  sur·face
  swell·ing
  tu·ber·cle
  veins
  ves·ti·bule
la·bi·al·ism

la·bi·al·ly
la·bii
la·bile
  af·fect
  cur·rent
  el·e·ments
  fac·tor
la·bil·i·ty
la·bi·o·cer·vi·cal
la·bi·o·cho·rea
la·bi·o·cli·na·tion
la·bi·o·den·tal
la·bi·o·gin·gi·val
  lam·i·na
la·bi·o·glos·so·la·ryn·ge·al
la·bi·o·glos·so·pha·ryn·ge·al
la·bi·o·graph
la·bi·o·lin·gual
  ap·pli·ance
  plane
la·bi·o·men·tal
la·bi·o·my·co·sis
la·bi·o·na·sal
la·bi·o·pal·a·tine
la·bi·o·place·ment
la·bi·o·plas·ty
la·bi·o·scro·tal
  folds
  swell·ings
la·bi·o·ver·sion
lab·i·tome
la·bi·um
  l. ure·thrae
  la·bia uter·i
  l. vo·ca·le
  la·bia vo·ca·lia
la·bor
  dry l.
  missed l.
  pre·cip·i·tate l.
  pre·ma·ture l.
la·bor
  pains
lab·o·ra·to·ri·an
lab·o·ra·tory
  per·son·al growth l.
lab·o·ra·tory
  di·ag·no·sis
la·bra

Lab·ra·dor
ker·a·top·a·thy
la·bra·le in·fe·ri·us
la·bra·le su·pe·ri·us
lab·ro·cyte
la·brum
lab·y·rinth
bony l.
co·chle·ar l.
eth·moi·dal l.
Ludwig's l.
mem·bra·nous l.
os·se·ous l.
re·nal l.
Santorini's l.
ves·tib·u·lar l.
lab·y·rin·thec·to·my
lab·y·rin·thine
an·gi·o·spasm
deaf·ness
nys·tag·mus
pla·cen·ta
re·flex·es
tor·ti·col·lis
veins
ver·ti·go
wall of mid·dle ear
lab·y·rin·thine right·ing
re·flex·es
lab·y·rin·thi·tis
lab·y·rin·thot·o·my
lab·y·rin·thus
lac
l. sul·fu·ris
l. vac·ci·num
lac·ca
lac·case
lac·er·a·ble
lac·er·at·ed
fo·ra·men
lac·er·a·tion
brain l.
scalp l.
vag·i·nal l.
la·cer·tus
l. cor·dis
l. fi·bro·sus
l. of lat·er·al rec·tus mus·
cle
l. me·di·us
lach·ry·mal
la·cin·i·ae tu·bae
la·cin·i·ate
lig·a·ment
la·cis
cell
lac·ri·mal
ap·pa·ra·tus

ar·tery
bay
bone
cal·cu·lus
can·a·lic·u·lus
con·junc·ti·vi·tis
duct
fas·cia
fis·tu·la
fold
fos·sa
gland
groove
ham·u·lus
lake
mar·gin
nerve
notch
open·ing
pa·pil·la
pro·cess
punc·tum
re·flex
sac
vein
lac·ri·ma·tion
lac·ri·ma·tor
lac·ri·ma·to·ry
lac·ri·mo·con·chal
su·ture
lac·ri·mo-gus·ta·to·ry
re·flex
lac·ri·mo·max·il·lary
su·ture
lac·ri·mo·tome
lac·ri·mot·o·my
La Crosse
vi·rus
lac·tac·i·de·mia
lac·tac·i·do·sis
lact·ac·id ox·y·gen
debt
lac·tal·bu·min
lac·tam
lac·tase
lac·tate
l. de·hy·dro·gen·ase
ex·cess l.
lac·tate de·hy·dro·gen·ase
vi·rus
lac·tat·ed Ringer's
in·jec·tion
so·lu·tion
lac·tat·ing
ad·e·no·ma
lac·ta·tion
amen·or·rhea

lac·ta·tion·al
  mas·ti·tis
lac·te·al
  cyst
  fis·tu·la
  ves·sel
lac·te·al
  cen·tral l.
lac·te·nin
lac·tes·cent
lac·tic
  ac·i·do·sis
lac·tic ac·id
  ba·cil·lus
  fer·men·ta·tion
lac·tic ac·id de·hy·dro·gen·ase
lac·tic·ac·i·de·mia
lac·tic ac·id ox·i·da·tive de·
  car·box·yl·ase
lac·tif·er·ous
  ducts
  gland
  si·nus
lac·tif·u·gal
lac·ti·fuge
lac·tig·e·nous
lac·tig·er·ous
lac·tim
lac·ti·mor·bus
lac·ti·nat·ed
lac·tis
Lac·to·bac·il·la·ce·ae
lac·to·bac·il·la·ry
  milk
lac·to·ba·cil·li
lac·to·ba·cil·lic ac·id
Lac·to·ba·cil·lus
  L. ac·i·doph·i·lus
  L. bif·i·dus
  L. bif·i·dus subsp. *penn·syl·*
  van·i·cus
  L. bre·vis
  L. buch·neri
  L. bul·gar·i·cus
  L. ca·sei
  L. ca·te·na·for·me
  L. cel·lo·bi·o·sus
  L. cop·roph·i·lus
  L. co·ry·ni·for·mis
  L. cur·va·tus
  L. del·bruec·kii
  L. de·si·di·o·sus
  L. fer·men·ti
  L. fer·men·tum
  L. fruc·ti·vo·rans
  L. hel·ve·ti·cus
  L. het·er·o·hi·o·chi
  L. hil·gar·dii

  L. ho·mo·hi·o·chi
  L. jen·se·nii
  L. lac·tis
  L. leich·man·nii
  L. pas·to·ri·a·nus
  L. plan·tar·um
  L. sa·li·va·ri·us
  L. ther·mo·phi·lus
  L. trich·o·des
  L. vi·ri·des·cens
lac·to·ba·cil·lus
Lac·to·ba·cil·lus bul·gar·i·cus
  fac·tor
Lac·to·ba·cil·lus ca·sei
  fac·tor
lac·to·bu·ty·rom·e·ter
lac·to·cele
lac·to·chrome
lac·to·crit
lac·to·den·sim·e·ter
lac·to·fer·rin
lac·to·fla·vin
lac·to·gen
  hu·man pla·cen·tal l.
lac·to·gen·e·sis
lac·to·gen·ic
  fac·tor
  hor·mone
lac·to·glob·u·lin
lac·tom·e·ter
lac·to·nase
lac·tone
lac·to·per·ox·i·dase
lac·to·pro·tein
lac·tor·rhea
lac·to·scope
lac·tose
  in·tol·er·ance
lac·tose-lit·mus
  agar
lac·tos·u·ria
lac·to·ther·a·py
lac·to·tro·pin
lac·to·veg·e·tar·i·an
lac·to·yl·glu·ta·thi·one ly·ase
lac·tu·lose
la·cu·na
  car·ti·lage l.
  l. ce·re·bri
  Howship's la·cu·nae
  in·ter·vil·lous l.
  l. mag·na
  Morgagni's l.
  mus·cu·lar l.
  os·se·ous l.
  l. pha·ryn·gis
  re·sorp·tion la·cu·nae
  troph·o·blas·tic l.

la·cu·na *(continued)*
  ure·thral l.
  vas·cu·lar l.
la·cu·nae
la·cu·nar
  ab·scess
  am·ne·sia
  lig·a·ment
  ton·sil·li·tis
la·cu·nule
la·cus
  l. se·mi·na·lis
la·cus
lad·der
  splint
Ladd-Franklin
  the·o·ry
Ladd's
  band
  op·er·a·tion
Lae·laps echid·ni·nus
Laënnec's
  cir·rho·sis
  pearls
la·e·trile
Lafora
  body
Lafora body
  dis·ease
Lafora's
  dis·ease
lag
  phase
lag
  an·a·phase l.
la·ge·na
la·ge·nae
lag·ging
lag·o·morph
Lag·o·mor·pha
lag·oph·thal·mia
lag·oph·thal·mic
  ker·a·ti·tis
lag·oph·thal·mos
Lagrange's
  op·er·a·tion
Lahey
  for·ceps
lake
  cap·il·lary l.
  lac·ri·mal l.
  lat·er·al l.'s
  sem·i·nal l.
  sub·cho·ri·al l.
  ve·nous l.'s
Laki-Lorand
  fac·tor

laky
  blood
la·li·a·try
lal·i·o·pho·bia
Lallemand's
  bod·ies
lal·ling
Lallouette's
  pyr·a·mid
lal·o·che·zia
lal·og·no·sis
la·lo·ple·gia
Lamaze
  meth·od
LAMB
  syn·drome
lamb
  dys·en·tery
lamb·da
lamb·da·cism
lamb·doid
  mar·gin
  su·ture
lam·bert
Lambert-Eaton
  syn·drome
lamb·ing
  pa·ral·y·sis
  sick·ness
Lam·blia in·tes·ti·na·lis
lam·bli·a·sis
lam·bo lam·bo
Lam·bri·nu·di
  op·er·a·tion
la·mel·la
  an·nu·late la·mel·lae
  ar·tic·u·lar l.
  l. of bone
  cir·cum·fer·en·tial l.
  con·cen·tric l.
  cor·noid l.
  elas·tic l.
  enam·el l.
  glan·du·lo·pre·pu·tial l.
  ground l.
  ha·ver·si·an l.
  in·ter·me·di·ate l.
  in·ter·sti·tial l.
  tri·an·gu·lar l.
  vit·re·ous l.
la·mel·lae
lam·el·lar
  bone
  cat·a·ract
  gran·ule
  ich·thy·o·sis
  ker·a·to·plas·ty
lam·el·late

lam·el·lat·ed
cor·pus·cles
la·mel·li·po·dia
la·mel·li·po·di·um
lam·i·na
alar l. of neu·ral tube
ba·sal l.
ba·sal l. of cho·roid
ba·sal l. of neu·ral tube
base·ment l.
bas·i·lar l.
l. cho·ri·o·cap·il·la·ris
l. cho·roi·dea
l. cho·roi·dea ep·i·the·li·a·lis
l. ci·ne·rea
l. cri·bro·sa scler·ae
l. of cri·coid car·ti·lage
l. den·sa
den·tal l.
l. den·ta·ta
den·to·gin·gi·val l.
l. dor·sa·lis
l. du·ra
l. elas·ti·ca an·te·ri·or
l. elas·ti·ca pos·te·ri·or
elas·tic lam·i·nae of ar·ter·ies
ep·i·scle·ral l.
ep·i·the·li·al l.
l. fi·bro·car·ti·la·gi·nea in·ter·pu·bi·ca
l. fi·bro·re·ti·cu·la·ris
he·pa·tic lam·i·nae
la·bi·o·gin·gi·val l.
lat·er·al med·ul·lary l. of cor·pus stri·a·tum
l. of lens
l. lu·ci·da
me·di·al med·ul·lary l. of cor·pus stri·a·tum
lam·i·nae me·dul·la·res ce·re·bel·li
or·bi·tal l. of eth·moid bone
os·se·ous spi·ral l.
l. pap·y·ra·cea
per·i·claus·tral l.
pri·mary den·tal l.
pter·y·goid lam·i·nae
l. quad·ri·gem·i·na
l. ra·ra
re·tic·u·lar l.
Rexed l.
ros·tral l.
l. ros·tra·lis
l. of sep·tum pel·lu·ci·dum
l. su·pra·neu·ro·po·ri·ca

l. of thy·roid car·ti·lage
l. of tra·gus
l. ven·tra·lis
l. of ver·te·bral arch
l. vi·trea
lam·i·nae
lam·i·na·gram
lam·i·na·graph
lam·i·nag·ra·phy
lam·i·nar
lam·i·nar cor·ti·cal
ne·cro·sis
scle·ro·sis
lam·i·nar·ia
lam·i·nar·in
l. sul·fate
lam·i·nat·ed
clot
cor·tex
ep·i·the·li·um
throm·bus
lam·i·nat·ed ep·i·the·li·al
plug
lam·i·na·tion
lam·i·nec·to·my
lam·i·nin
lam·i·ni·tis
lam·i·not·o·my
lam·ins
lamp
an·neal·ing l.
Edridge-Green l.
heat l.
Kromayer's l.
mi·gnon l.
spir·it l.
ul·tra·vi·o·let l.
uvi·ol l.
Wood's l.
lamp·brush
chro·mo·some
Lan
an·ti·gen
la·na
la·nae
la·nat·o·side D
la·nat·o·sides A, B and C
lance
Lancefield
clas·si·fi·ca·tion
lan·cet
gum l.
spring l.
thumb l.
lan·ci·nat·ing
Lancisi's
sign

land
scur·vy
Landau-Kleffner
syn·drome
Landolfi's
sign
Landolt's
bod·ies
Landouzy-Dejerine
dys·tro·phy
Landouzy-Grasset
law
Landry
syn·drome
Landry-Guillain-Barré
syn·drome
Landry's
pa·ral·y·sis
Landschutz
tu·mor
Landsteiner-Donath
test
Landström's
mus·cle
Landzert's
fos·sa
Lane's
band
dis·ease
kink
plates
Langenbeck's
tri·an·gle
Langendorff's
meth·od
Langerhans'
cells
gran·ule
is·lands
Langer's
arch
lines
mus·cle
Lange's
so·lu·tion
test
Langhans'
cells
lay·er
stri·a
Langhans'-type gi·ant
cells
Langley's
gran·ules
Langmuir
trough

lan·guage
game
zone
lan·guage
body l.
lan·i·ary
Lannelongue's
fo·ram·i·na
lig·a·ments
lan·o·lin
an·hy·drous l.
Lanterman's
in·ci·sures
seg·ments
lan·tha·nic
lan·tha·nides
lan·tha·num
l. ni·trate
lan·thi·o·nine
la·nu·gi·nous
la·nu·go
hair
Lanz's
line
lap·a·rec·to·my
lap·a·ro·cele
lap·a·ro·gas·tros·co·py
lap·a·ro·hys·ter·ec·to·my
lap·a·ro·hys·tero-o·o·pho·rec·
to·my
lap·a·ro·hys·ter·o·pexy
lap·a·ro·hys·ter·o·sal·pin·go-o·
o·pho·rec·to·my
lap·a·ro·hys·ter·ot·o·my
lap·a·ro·my·o·mec·to·my
lap·a·ro·my·o·si·tis
lap·a·ror·rha·phy
lap·a·ro·sal·pin·gec·to·my
lap·a·ro·sal·pin·go-o·o·pho·rec·
to·my
lap·a·ro·sal·pin·got·o·my
lap·a·ro·scope
lap·a·ros·co·py
lap·a·rot·o·my
pad
lap·a·ro·trach·e·lot·o·my
lap·a·ro·u·ter·ot·o·my
Lapicque's
law
lap·i·ni·za·tion
lap·i·nized
Laplace's
for·ceps
law
Laquer's
stain for al·co·hol·ic hy·a·
lin
lar·bish

larch
  tur·pen·tine
lard
lar·da·ceous
  liv·er
  spleen
large
  cal·o·rie
  in·tes·tine
  mus·cle of he·lix
  pel·vis
  vein
large cell
  car·ci·no·ma
  lym·pho·ma
large in·ter·arch
  dis·tance
large pu·den·dal
  lip
large sa·phe·nous
  vein
lark·spur
Laron type
  dwarf·ism
Laroyenne's
  op·er·a·tion
Larrey's
  am·pu·ta·tion
  cleft
  li·ga·tion
Larrey-Weil
  dis·ease
Larsen's
  syn·drome
lar·va
  fi·lar·i·form l.
  l. mi·grans
lar·va·ceous
lar·va cur·rens
lar·vae
lar·val
  con·junc·ti·vi·tis
  plague
lar·va mi·grans
  cu·ta·ne·ous l. m.
  oc·u·lar l. m.
  spi·ru·roid l. m.
  vis·cer·al l. m.
lar·vate
lar·vi·cid·al
lar·vi·cide
lar·vip·a·rous
lar·vi·phag·ic
la·ryn·ge·al
  atre·sia
  bur·sa
  cho·rea
  cri·sis

ep·i·lep·sy
glands
gran·u·lo·ma
pap·il·lo·ma·to·sis
part of phar·ynx
phar·ynx
pol·yp
pouch
prom·i·nence
re·flex
si·nus
ste·no·sis
stri·dor
syn·co·pe
ton·sils
veins
ven·tri·cle
ver·ti·go
la·ryn·gec·to·my
la·ryn·gem·phrax·is
la·ryn·ges
lar·yn·gis·mus
  l. stri·du·lus
lar·yn·git·ic
lar·yn·gi·tis
  chron·ic sub·glot·tic l.
  croup·ous l.
  mem·bra·nous l.
  spas·mod·ic l.
  l. stri·du·lo·sa
la·ryn·go·cele
la·ryn·go·fis·sure
la·ryn·go·graph
lar·yn·gol·o·gy
la·ryn·go·ma·la·cia
la·ryn·go·pa·ral·y·sis
lar·yn·gop·a·thy
la·ryn·go·phan·tom
la·ryn·go·pha·ryn·ge·al
la·ryn·go·phar·yn·gec·to·my
la·ryn·go·pha·ryn·ge·us
la·ryn·go·phar·yn·gi·tis
la·ryn·go·phar·ynx
lar·yn·goph·o·ny
la·ryn·go·phthi·sis
la·ryn·go·plas·ty
la·ryn·go·ple·gia
la·ryn·go·pto·sis
la·ryn·go·rhi·nol·o·gy
la·ryn·go·scope
la·ryn·go·scop·ic
lar·yn·gos·co·pist
lar·yn·gos·co·py
  sus·pen·sion l.
la·ryn·go·spasm
la·ryn·go·spas·tic
  re·flex
la·ryn·go·ste·no·sis

lar·yn·gos·to·my
la·ryn·go·stro·bo·scope
la·ryn·go·tome
  di·lat·ing l.
lar·yn·got·o·my
  in·fe·ri·or l.
  me·di·an l.
  su·pe·ri·or l.
la·ryn·go·tra·che·al
  groove
la·ryn·go·tra·che·i·tis
  avi·an in·fec·tious l.
la·ryn·go·tra·che·o·bron·chi·tis
la·ryn·go·tra·che·ot·o·my
la·ryn·go·xe·ro·sis
lar·ynx
lase
Lasègue's
  dis·ease
  sign
  syn·drome
la·ser
  mi·cro·scope
  pho·to·co·ag·u·la·tor
  tra·bec·u·lo·plas·ty
lash
Lash's
  op·er·a·tion
las·ing
La·si·o·he·lea
Lassa
  fe·ver
  vi·rus
Lassa hem·or·rhag·ic
  fe·ver
las·si·tude
la·tah
Latarget's
  nerve
  vein
late
  de·cel·er·a·tion
  ep·i·lep·sy
  re·ac·tion
  rick·ets
  sys·to·le
late ap·i·cal sys·tol·ic
  mur·mur
lat·e·bra
late di·a·stol·ic
  mur·mur
la·ten·cy
  pe·ri·od
  phase
late ne·o·na·tal
  death
la·tent
  al·ler·gy

car·ci·no·ma
coc·cid·i·oi·do·my·co·sis
con·tent
di·a·be·tes
em·py·e·ma
en·er·gy
gout
heat
ho·mo·sex·u·al·i·ty
hy·per·o·pia
in·fec·tion
learn·ing
mi·cro·bism
nys·tag·mus
pe·ri·od
re·flex
scar·la·ti·na
schiz·o·phre·nia
stage
tet·a·ny
ty·phoid
zone
la·tent adre·no·cor·ti·cal
  in·suf·fi·cien·cy
la·tent rat
  vi·rus
late-phase
  re·sponse
la·te·ra
lat·er·ad
lat·er·al
  ab·er·ra·tion
  an·gle of eye
  an·gle of scap·u·la
  an·gle of uter·us
  ap·er·ture of the fourth
    ven·tri·cle
  ca·nal
  can·thus
  car·ti·lage
  car·ti·lage of nose
  col·umn of spi·nal cord
  con·dyle
  con·dyle of fe·mur
  con·dyle of tib·ia
  cord of brach·i·al plex·us
  cur·va·ture
  ep·i·con·dyle
  ep·i con·dyle of fe·mur
  ep·i·con·dyle of hu·mer·us
  ex·cur·sion
  fil·let
  folds
  fos·sa of brain
  fu·nic·u·lus of spi·nal cord
  gin·gly·mus
  head
  her·maph·ro·dit·ism

horn
il·lu·mi·na·tion
in·ci·sor
lakes
lay·er
lig·a·ment of an·kle
lig·a·ment of el·bow
lig·a·ment of knee
lig·a·ment of mal·le·us
lig·a·ments of the blad·der
lig·a·ment of tem·po·ro·
  man·dib·u·lar joint
lig·a·ment of wrist
limb
line
lip of lin·ea as·pe·ra
li·thot·o·my
mal·le·o·lus
mar·gin
mass of at·las
mass of eth·moid bone
me·nis·cus
mes·o·derm
move·ment
nu·cle·us of me·dul·la ob·
  lon·ga·ta
nu·cle·us of thal·a·mus
nys·tag·mus
oc·clu·sion
part
plate
plate of pter·y·goid pro·cess
pole
pro·cess of cal·ca·ne·al tu·
  ber·os·i·ty
pro·cess of mal·le·us
pro·cess of ta·lus
re·cess of fourth ven·tri·cle
re·gion
re·gion of neck
ret·i·nac·u·lum of pa·tel·la
root of me·di·an nerve
root of op·tic tract
seg·ment
si·nus
sur·face
sur·face of leg
sur·face of ova·ry
tu·ber·cle of pos·te·ri·or
  pro·cess of ta·lus
vein of lat·er·al ven·tri·cle
ven·tri·cle
ver·ti·go
wall of mid·dle ear
wall of or·bit
lat·er·al ab·er·rant thy·roid
  car·ci·no·ma

lat·er·al al·ve·o·lar
  ab·scess
lat·er·al am·pul·lar
  nerve
lat·er·al an·te·ri·or tho·rac·ic
  nerve
lat·er·al ar·cu·ate
  lig·a·ment
lat·er·al at·lan·to·ax·i·al
  joint
lat·er·al at·lan·to·ep·i·stroph·ic
  joint
lat·er·al atri·al
  vein
lat·er·al ax·il·lary lymph
  nodes
lat·er·al ba·sal
  seg·ment
lat·er·al bi·cip·i·tal
  groove
lat·er·al car·ti·lag·i·nous
  lay·er
lat·er·al ce·re·bral
  fis·sure
  fos·sa
  sul·cus
lat·er·al cir·cum·flex
  ar·tery of thigh
lat·er·al cir·cum·flex fem·o·ral
  veins
lat·er·al con·dy·lar
  in·cli·na·tion
lat·er·al cor·ti·co·spi·nal
  tract
lat·er·al cos·to·trans·verse
  lig·a·ment
lat·er·al cri·co·ar·y·te·noid
  mus·cle
lat·er·al cu·ne·ate
  nu·cle·us
lat·er·al cu·ne·i·form
  bone
lat·er·al cu·ta·ne·ous
  nerve of calf
  nerve of fore·arm
  nerve of thigh
lat·er·al di·rect
  veins
lat·er·al ep·i·con·dy·lar
  crest
  ridge
lat·er·al fem·o·ral
  tu·ber·os·i·ty
lat·er·al fron·to·ba·sal
  ar·tery
lat·er·al ge·nic·u·late
  body

lat·er·al glos·so·ep·i·glot·tic
fold
lat·er·al great
mus·cle
lat·er·al ground
bun·dle
lat·er·al ham·string
lat·er·al hu·mer·al
ep·i·con·dy·li·tis
lat·er·al in·fe·ri·or ge·nic·u·lar
ar·tery
lat·er·al in·gui·nal
fos·sa
lat·er·al in·ter·oc·clu·sal
rec·ord
la·te·ra·lis
lat·er·al·i·ty
crossed l.
lat·er·al jug·u·lar lymph
nodes
lat·er·al la·cu·nar
node
lat·er·al line
sys·tem
lat·er·al line sense
or·gan
lat·er·al lin·gual
swell·ings
lat·er·al lon·gi·tu·di·nal
arch
stri·a
lat·er·al lum·bar in·ter·trans·
verse
mus·cles
lat·er·al lum·bo·cos·tal
arch
lat·er·al mal·le·o·lar
lig·a·ment
net·work
sur·face of ta·lus
lat·er·al mal·le·o·lus
bur·sa
lat·er·al med·ul·lary
lam·i·na of cor·pus stri·a·
tum
syn·drome
lat·er·al my·o·car·di·al
in·farc·tion
lat·er·al na·sal
ar·tery
el·e·va·tion
fold
pro·cess
lat·er·al ob·lique
roent·gen·o·gram
lat·er·al oc·cip·i·tal
ar·tery
sul·cus

lat·er·al oc·cip·i·to·tem·po·ral
gy·rus
lat·er·al pal·pe·bral
com·mis·sure
lig·a·ment
ra·phe
lat·er·al pec·to·ral
nerve
lat·er·al per·i·car·di·ac lymph
nodes
lat·er·al per·i·o·don·tal
ab·scess
cyst
lat·er·al pha·ryn·ge·al
space
lat·er·al plan·tar
ar·tery
nerve
lat·er·al plate
mes·o·derm
lat·er·al pop·lit·e·al
nerve
lat·er·al pre·op·tic
nu·cle·us
lat·er·al pter·y·goid
mus·cle
lat·er·al pu·bo·pros·tat·ic
lig·a·ment
lat·er·al py·ram·i·dal
tract
lat·er·al ra·mus
roent·gen·o·gram
lat·er·al rec·tus
mus·cle
mus·cle of the head
lat·er·al re·cum·bent
po·si·tion
lat·er·al re·tic·u·lar
nu·cle·us
lat·er·al sa·cral
ar·tery
crests
veins
lat·er·al sa·cro·coc·cyg·e·al
lig·a·ment
lat·er·al sem·i·cir·cu·lar
ca·nals
lat·er·al skull
roent·gen·o·gram
lat·er·al spi·nal
scle·ro·sis
lat·er·al spi·no·tha·lam·ic
tract
lat·er·al splanch·nic
ar·ter·ies
lat·er·al stri·ate
ar·ter·ies

lat·er·al su·pe·ri·or ge·nic·u·
lar
ar·tery
lat·er·al su·pra·cla·vic·u·lar
nerve
lat·er·al su·pra·con·dy·lar
crest
ridge
lat·er·al sym·pa·thet·ic
line
lat·er·al ta·lo·cal·ca·ne·al
lig·a·ment
lat·er·al tar·sal
ar·tery
lat·er·al tha·lam·ic
pe·dun·cle
lat·er·al tho·rac·ic
ar·tery
vein
lat·er·al thy·ro·hy·oid
lig·a·ment
lat·er·al tu·be·ral
nu·clei
lat·er·al um·bil·i·cal
fold
lig·a·ment
lat·er·al vag·i·nal wall
smear
lat·er·al vas·tus
mus·cle
lat·er·al ven·tral
her·nia
lat·er·al ves·tib·u·lar
nu·cle·us
late rep·li·cat·ing
chro·mo·some
lat·er·i·flec·tion
lat·er·i·flex·ion
la·te·ris
lat·er·o·ab·dom·i·nal
lat·er·o·de·vi·a·tion
lat·er·o·duc·tion
lat·er·o·flec·tion
lat·er·o·flex·ion
lat·er·o·po·si·tion
lat·er·o·pul·sion
lat·er·o·tor·sion
lat·er·o·tru·sion
lat·er·o·ver·sion
la·tex ag·glu·ti·na·tion
test
la·tex fix·a·tion
test
lathe
lath·y·rism
lath·y·ro·gen
La·tro·dec·tus
L. mac·tans

lat·tice
lat·tice cor·ne·al
dys·tro·phy
lat·ticed
lay·er
la·tus
Latzko's ce·sar·e·an
sec·tion
laud·a·ble
pus
lau·da·nine
lau·da·no·sine
lau·da·num
laugh·ing
dis·ease
gas
sick·ness
laugh·ter
re·flex
Laugier's
her·nia
sign
Laumonier's
gan·gli·on
Launois-Bensaude
syn·drome
Launois-Cléret
syn·drome
lau·rel
fe·ver
Laurence-Biedl
syn·drome
Laurence-Moon
syn·drome
Laurence-Moon-Bardet-Biedl
syn·drome
Laurer's
ca·nal
lau·ric ac·id
Lauth's
ca·nal
lig·a·ment
Lauth's vi·o·let
la·vage
Lavdovsky's
nu·cle·oid
La·ver·an·ia
la·veur
law
all or none l.
Ambard's l.'s
Angström's l.
Arndt's l.
Arrhenius l.
l.'s of as·so·ci·a·tion
l. of av·er·age lo·cal·i·za·
tion
Avogadro's l.

law *(continued)*

Baer's l.
Baruch's l.
Beer's l.
Behring's l.
Bell-Magendie l.
Bell's l.
Bernoulli's l.
Berthollet's l.
l. of bi·o·gen·e·sis
bi·o·ge·net·ic l.
Blagden's l.
Bowditch's l.
Boyle's l.
Broadbent's l.
Bunsen-Roscoe l.
Charles l.
l. of con·stant num·bers in o·vu·la·tion
l. of con·ti·gu·i·ty
l. of con·trary in·ner·va·tion
Coppet's l.
Courvoisier's l.
Dale-Feldberg l.
Dalton-Henry l.
Dalton's l.
l. of def·i·nite pro·por·tions
l. of de·ner·va·tion
Descartes' l.
Donders' l.
Draper's l.
Du Bois-Reymond's l.
Dulong-Petit l.
Einthoven's l.
Elliott's l.
l. of ex·ci·ta·tion
Faraday's l.'s
Farr's l.
Fechner-Weber l.
Ferry-Porter l.
Flatau's l.
Galton's l.
Gay-Lussac's l.
Gerhardt-Semon l.
Godélier's l.
Graham's l.
Grasset's l.
l. of grav·i·ta·tion
Guldberg-Waage l.
Haeckel's l.
Halsted's l.
Hamburger's l.
l. of the heart
Heidenhain's l.
Hellin's l.
Henry's l.

Hilton's l.
Hooke's l.
l. of in·de·pen·dent as·sort·ment
l. of in·i·tial val·ue
l. of in·tes·tine
l. of in·verse square
l. of isoch·ro·nism
iso·dy·nam·ic l.
Jackson's l.
Koch's l.
Landouzy-Grasset l.
Lapicque's l.
Laplace's l.
Le Chatelier's l.
Listing's l.
Louis' l.
Magendie's l.
Marey's l.
Marfan's l.
Mariotte's l.
mass l.
l. of mass ac·tion
Meltzer's l.
Mendeléeff's l.
Mendel's l.'s
l. of the min·i·mum
Müller's l.
l. of mul·ti·ple pro·por·tions
Nasse's l.
Neumann's l.
Newton's l.
Nysten's l.
Ochoa's l.
Ohm's l.
l. of par·tial pres·sures
Pascal's l.
pe·ri·od·ic l.
Pflüger's l.
Plateau-Talbot l.
Poiseuille's l.
l. of po·lar ex·ci·ta·tion
l. of pri·or·i·ty
Profeta's l.
Proust's l.
Raoult's l.
l. of re·ca·pi·tu·la·tion
l. of re·cip·ro·cal pro·por·tions
rec·i·proc·i·ty l.
l. of re·ferred pain
l. of re·frac·tion
l. of re·gres·sion to mean
Riccò's l.
Ritter's l.
Roscoe-Bunsen l.
Rosenbach's l.

Rubner's l.'s of growth
Schütz' l.
sec·ond l. of ther·mo·dy·nam·ics
l. of seg·re·ga·tion
Semon's l.
Sherrington's l.
l. of sim·i·lars
Snell's l.
Spallanzani's l.
Starling's l.
Stokes' l.
Tait's l.
Thoma's l.'s
van der Kolk's l.
van't Hoff's l.
Virchow's l.
Vogel's l.
wal·le·ri·an l.
Weber-Fechner l.
Weber's l.
Weigert's l.
Wilder's l. of in·i·tial val·ue
Williston's l.
Wolff's l.
Lawford's
syn·drome
Lawless'
stain
Lawrence-Seip
syn·drome
law·ren·ci·um
lax·a·tion
lax·a·tive
la·xa·tor tym·pa·ni
lay·er
am·e·lo·blas·tic l.
an·te·ri·or elas·tic l.
an·te·ri·or lim·it·ing l. of cor·nea
an·te·ri·or l. of rec·tus ab·do·mi·nis sheath
bac·il·la·ry l.
ba·sal l.
ba·sal cell l.
ba·sal l. of cho·roid
ba·sal l. of cil·i·ary body
l. of Bechterew
blas·to·der·mic l.'s
brown l.
cam·bi·um l.
l.'s of cer·e·bel·lar cor·tex
l.'s of ce·re·bral cor·tex
ce·re·bral l. of ret·i·na
Chievitz' l.
cho·ri·o·cap·il·la·ry l.

cir·cu·lar l.'s of mus·cu·lar tu·nics
cir·cu·lar l. of tym·pan·ic mem·brane
claus·tral l.
clear l. of ep·i·der·mis
co·lum·nar l.
con·junc·ti·val l. of bulb
con·junc·ti·val l. of eye·lids
cor·ne·al l. of ep·i·der·mis
cor·ni·fied l. of nail
cu·ta·ne·ous l. of tym·pan·ic mem·brane
deep l.
elas·tic l.'s of ar·ter·ies
elas·tic l.'s of cor·nea
enam·el l.
ep·en·dy·mal l.
ep·i·the·li·al l.'s
ep·i·the·li·al cho·roid l.
ep·i·trich·i·al l.
fi·brous l.
fil·let l.
fu·si·form l.
gan·gli·on·ic l. of cer·e·bel·lar cor·tex
gan·gli·on·ic l. of ce·re·bral cor·tex
gan·gli·on·ic l. of op·tic nerve
gan·gli·on·ic l. of ret·i·na
germ l.
ger·mi·na·tive l.
ger·mi·na·tive l. of nail
glo·mer·u·lar l. of ol·fac·to·ry bulb
gran·u·lar l. of cer·e·bel·lar cor·tex
gran·u·lar l.'s of ce·re·bral cor·tex
gran·u·lar l. of ep·i·der·mis
gran·u·lar l.'s of ret·i·na
gran·u·lar l. of a ve·sic·u·lar ovar·i·an fol·li·cle
gray l. of su·pe·ri·or col·lic·u·lus
half-val·ue l.
Henle's l.
Henle's fi·ber l.
Henle's ner·vous l.
horny l. of ep·i·der·mis
horny l. of nail
Huxley's l.
in·fra·gran·u·lar l.
in·ter·me·di·ate l.
Kölliker's l.
Langhans' l.
lat·er·al l.

lay·er *(continued)*
 lat·er·al car·ti·lag·i·nous l.
 lat·ticed l.
 lim·it·ing l.'s of cor·nea
 lon·gi·tu·di·nal l.'s of mus·cu·lar tu·nics
 mal·pi·ghi·an l.
 man·tle l.
 mar·gi·nal l.
 me·di·al l.
 me·di·al car·ti·lag·i·nous l.
 med·ul·lary l.'s of thal·a·mus
 mem·bra·nous l.
 Meynert's l.
 mo·lec·u·lar l.
 mo·lec·u·lar l. of cer·e·bel·lar cor·tex
 mo·lec·u·lar l. of ce·re·bral cor·tex
 mo·lec·u·lar l.'s of ol·fac·to·ry bulb
 mo·lec·u·lar l. of ret·i·na
 mul·ti·form l.
 mus·cu·lar l. of mu·co·sa
 neu·ral l. of ret·i·na
 neu·ro·ep·i·the·li·al l. of ret·i·na
 Nitabuch's l.
 nu·cle·ar l.'s of ret·i·na
 odon·to·blas·tic l.
 op·tic l.
 or·bi·tal l. of eth·moid bone
 os·te·o·ge·net·ic l.
 pal·i·sade l.
 pap·il·lary l.
 pa·ri·e·tal l.
 per·fo·rat·ed l. of scle·ra
 pig·ment·ed l. of cil·i·ary body
 pig·ment·ed l. of iris
 pig·ment·ed l. of ret·i·na
 l. of pir·i·form neu·rons
 plas·ma l.
 plex·i·form l.
 plex·i·form l. of ce·re·bral cor·tex
 plex·i·form l.'s of ret·i·na
 pol·y·mor·phous l.
 pos·te·ri·or elas·tic l.
 pos·te·ri·or lim·it·ing l. of cor·nea
 pos·te·ri·or l. of rec·tus ab·do·mi·nis sheath
 pre·tra·che·al l.
 pre·ver·te·bral l.
 prick·le cell l.

 Purkinje's l.
 py·ram·i·dal cell l.
 ra·di·ate l. of tym·pan·ic mem·brane
 Rauber's l.
 re·tic·u·lar l. of co·ri·um
 l.'s of ret·i·na
 l. of rods and cones
 ros·tral l.
 Sattler's elas·tic l.
 l.'s of skin
 slug·gish l.
 so·mat·ic l.
 spin·dle-celled l.
 spi·nous l.
 splanch·nic l.
 still l.
 sub·en·do·car·di·al l.
 sub·en·do·the·li·al l.
 sub·pap·il·lary l.
 su·per·fi·cial l.
 su·pra·cho·roid l.
 Tomes' gran·u·lar l.
 vas·cu·lar l.
 vas·cu·lar l. of cho·roid coat of eye
 ven·tric·u·lar l.
 vis·cer·al l.
 Waldeyer's zon·al l.
 Weil's ba·sal l.
 zo·nu·lar l.
lay·ered
 ker·a·to·plas·ty
laz·a·ret
laz·a·ret·to
laz·a·rine
 lep·ro·sy
LCAT
 de·fi·cien·cy
L-chain
 dis·ease
 my·e·lo·ma
LCM
 vi·rus
l-cone
L-D
 body
LDH
 agent
LE
 cell
 fac·tors
 phe·nom·e·non
L.E.
 body
Le
 an·ti·gens
leach·ing

lead
    ABC l.'s
    bi·po·lar l.
    CB l.
    CF l.
    chest l.'s
    CL l.
    CR l.
    di·rect l.
    esoph·a·ge·al l.
    in·di·rect l.
    in·tra·car·di·ac l.
    limb l.
    pre·cor·di·al l.'s
    sem·i·di·rect l.'s
    stan·dard l.
    uni·po·lar l.'s
    V l.
lead
    l. ac·e·tate
    black l.
    l. car·bon·ate
    l. chro·mate
    l. mon·ox·ide
    l. ox·ide (yel·low)
    red l.
    red ox·ide of l.
    l. sul·fide
    l. tet·ra·eth·yl
    l. te·trox·ide
    white l.
lead
    ane·mia
    col·ic
    en·ceph·a·li·tis
    en·ceph·a·lop·a·thy
    gout
    line
    neu·rop·a·thy
    pal·sy
    pa·ral·y·sis
    poi·son·ing
    sto·ma·ti·tis
lead hy·drox·ide
    stain
lead·ing
    edge
lead-pipe
    co·lon
    ri·gid·i·ty
leap·frog
    po·si·tion
Lear
    com·plex
learned
    drive
learned help·less·ness

learn·ing
    in·ci·den·tal l.
    la·tent l.
    pas·sive l.
    rote l.
    state-de·pen·dent l.
learn·ing
    dis·a·bil·i·ty
    set
    the·o·ry
least dif·fu·sion
    cir·cle
leath·er-bot·tle
    stom·ach
Le Bel-van't Hoff
    rule
Leber's
    plex·us
Leber's he·red·i·tary op·tic
    at·ro·phy
Leber's id·i·o·path·ic stel·late
    ret·i·nop·a·thy
Le Blood Group
LE cell
    test
Le Chatelier's
    law
    prin·ci·ple
lech·e·guil·la
    poi·son·ing
lec·i·thal
lec·i·thin
    l. ac·yl·trans·fer·ase
lec·i·thi·nase
    l. A
    l. B
    l. C
    l. D
**lec·i·thin-cho·les·ter·ol ac·yl·
    trans·fer·ase**
lec·i·thin/sphin·go·my·e·lin
    ra·ti·o
lec·i·tho·blast
lec·i·tho·pro·tein
lec·tin
Lederer's
    ane·mia
ledge
    den·tal l.
    enam·el l.
leech
Lee's
    gan·gli·on
Leeuwenhoek's
    ca·nals
lee·way
    space

Lee-White
meth·od
Le Fort
sound
Le Fort I
frac·ture
Le Fort II
frac·ture
Le Fort III
frac·ture
Le Fort's
am·pu·ta·tion
left
atri·um
au·ri·cle
crus of atri·o·ven·tric·u·lar
trunk
crus of di·a·phragm
duct of cau·date lobe
heart
lobe
lobe of liv·er
plate of thy·roid car·ti·lage
ven·tri·cle
left atri·o·ven·tric·u·lar
valve
left au·ric·u·lar
ap·pend·age
left ax·is
de·vi·a·tion
left col·ic
ar·tery
flex·ure
vein
left col·ic lymph
nodes
left cor·o·nary
ar·tery
vein
left-eyed
left fi·brous
tri·gone
left-foot·ed
left gas·tric
ar·tery
vein
left gas·tric lymph
nodes
left gas·tro·ep·i·plo·ic
ar·tery
vein
left gas·tro·ep·i·plo·ic lymph
nodes
left gas·tro·o·men·tal
vein
left gas·tro-o·men·tal
ar·tery
nodes

left-hand·ed
left he·pa·tic
duct
veins
left in·fe·ri·or pul·mo·nary
vein
left lum·bar lymph
nodes
left main
bron·chus
left ovar·i·an
vein
left pul·mo·nary
ar·tery
left sag·it·tal
fis·sure
left-sid·ed·ness
bi·lat·er·al l.
left su·pe·ri·or in·ter·cos·tal
vein
left su·pe·ri·or pul·mo·nary
vein
left su·pra·re·nal
vein
left tes·tic·u·lar
vein
left-to-right
shunt
left tri·an·gu·lar
lig·a·ment
left um·bil·i·cal
vein
left ven·tric·u·lar
fail·ure
left ven·tric·u·lar ejec·tion
time
leg
phe·nom·e·non
leg
l. of an·ti·he·lix
Bar·ba·dos l.
bow-l.
el·e·phant l.
milk l.
rest·less l.'s
rid·er's l.
scaly l.
ten·nis l.
white l.
le·gal
blind·ness
den·tis·try
med·i·cine
psy·chi·a·try
Legal's
test
Legendre's
sign

Legg-Calvé-Perthes
dis·ease
Legg-Perthes
dis·ease
Legg's
dis·ease
Le·gion·el·la
  L. boze·man·ii
  L. mic·da·dei
  L. pneu·mo·phi·la
le·gi·o·nel·lo·sis
Le·gion·naires'
dis·ease
le·gu·min
le·gu·mi·niv·o·rous
Leichtenstern's
phe·nom·e·non
sign
Leigh's
dis·ease
Leiner's
dis·ease
lei·o·der·mia
lei·o·my·o·fi·bro·ma
lei·o·my·o·ma
  l. cu·tis
  par·a·sit·ic l.
  vas·cu·lar l.
lei·o·my·o·ma·to·sis
lei·o·my·o·sar·co·ma
lei·ot·ri·chous
Leipzig yel·low
Leishman-Donovan
body
Leish·man·ia
  L. ae·thi·o·pi·ca
  L. bra·zil·i·en·sis
  L. bra·zil·i·en·sis bra·zil·i·en·sis
  L. bra·zil·i·en·sis guy·an·en·sis
  L. bra·zil·i·en·sis pan·a·men·sis
  L. don·o·vani
  L. don·o·vani ar·chi·baldi
  L. don·o·vani cha·gasi
  L. don·o·vani don·o·vani
  L. don·o·vani in·fan·tum
  L. fu·run·cu·lo·sa
  L. ma·jor
  L. mex·i·cana
  L. mex·i·cana am·a·zo·nen·sis
  L. mex·i·cana garn·hami
  L. mex·i·cana mex·i·cana
  L. mex·i·cana pi·fa·noi
  L. mex·i·cana ve·ne·zu·e·len·sis

  L. pe·ru·vi·ana
  L. pi·fa·noi
  L. tro·pi·ca
  L. tro·pi·ca ma·jor
  L. tro·pi·ca mex·i·cana
leish·man·i·a·sis
  acute cu·ta·ne·ous l.
  Amer·i·can l.
  l. amer·i·cana
  an·er·gic l.
  an·thro·po·not·ic cu·ta·ne·ous l.
  ca·nine l.
  chron·ic cu·ta·ne·ous l.
  cu·ta·ne·ous l.
  dif·fuse l.
  dif·fuse cu·ta·ne·ous l.
  dis·sem·i·nat·ed cu·ta·ne·ous l.
  dry cu·ta·ne·ous l.
  in·fan·tile l.
  lu·poid l.
  mu·co·cu·ta·ne·ous l.
  na·so·pha·ryn·ge·al l.
  New World l.
  Old World l.
  pseu·do·lep·ro·ma·tous l.
  l. re·ci·di·vans
  ru·ral cu·ta·ne·ous l.
  l. teg·u·men·ta·ria dif·fu·sa
  ur·ban cu·ta·ne·ous l.
  vis·cer·al l.
  wet cu·ta·ne·ous l.
  zo·o·not·ic cu·ta·ne·ous l.
leish·man·i·o·sis
leish·man·oid
  der·mal l.
  post-ka·la azar der·mal l.
Leishman's
stain
Leishman's chrome
cells
Lei·ter In·ter·na·tion·al Per·form·ance
Scale
Lejeune
syn·drome
le·ma
Lembert
su·ture
le·mic
lem·mo·blast
lem·mo·cyte
lem·nis·ci
lem·nis·cus
  acous·tic l.
  au·di·to·ry l.
  gus·ta·to·ry l.

lem·nis·cus *(continued)*
  me·di·al l.
  tri·gem·i·nal l.
lem·on
lem·on yel·low
Lendrum's phlox·ine-tar·tra·zine
  stain
Le·nègre's
  dis·ease
  syn·drome
length
  arch l.
  avail·a·ble arch l.
  crown-heel l.
  crown-rump l.
  re·quired arch l.
length-breadth
  in·dex
length·en·ing
  re·ac·tion
length-height
  in·dex
Lenhossék's
  pro·cess·es
len·i·tive
Lennert
  clas·si·fi·ca·tion
Lennert's
  le·sion
  lym·pho·ma
Lennox
  syn·drome
Lennox-Gastaut
  syn·drome
Lenoir's
  fac·et
lens
  pits
  plac·odes
  stars
  su·tures
  ves·i·cle
lens
  ach·ro·mat·ic l.
  ap·la·nat·ic l.
  ap·o·chro·mat·ic l.
  aspher·ic l.
  as·tig·mat·ic l.
  bi·con·cave l.
  bi·con·vex l.
  bi·fo·cal l.
  cat·a·ract l.
  com·pound l.
  con·cave l.
  con·ca·vo·con·cave l.
  con·ca·vo·con·vex l.
  con·tact l.
  con·vex l.

  con·vex·o·con·cave l.
  con·vex·o·con·vex l.
  cor·ne·al l.
  crys·tal·line l.
  cy·lin·dri·cal l.
  de·cen·tered l.
  dou·ble con·cave l.
  dou·ble con·vex l.
  eye l.
  field l.
  Fresnel l.
  im·mer·sion l.
  me·nis·cus l.
  mi·nus l.
  mul·ti·fo·cal l.
  oc·u·lar l.
  om·ni·fo·cal l.
  or·tho·scop·ic l.
  per·i·scop·ic l.
  pho·to·chro·mic l.
  pla·no·con·cave l.
  pla·no·con·vex l.
  plus l.
  safe·ty l.
  slab-off l.
  spher·i·cal l.
  sphe·ro·cy·lin·dri·cal l.
  to·ric l.
  tri·al l.'s
  tri·fo·cal l.
lens·ec·to·my
lens-in·duced
  uve·i·tis
lens·om·e·ter
lens·op·a·thy
len·te
  in·su·lin
len·ti·co·nus
len·tic·u·la
len·tic·u·lar
  an·sa
  apoph·y·sis
  astig·ma·tism
  bone
  cap·sule
  col·o·ny
  fos·sa
  gan·gli·on
  knife
  loop
  nu·cle·us
  pa·pil·lae
  pro·cess of in·cus
  syph·i·lid
  ves·i·cle
len·tic·u·lar pro·gress·ive
  de·gen·er·a·tion
len·tic·u·li

len·tic·u·lo-op·tic
len·tic·u·lo·pap·u·lar
len·tic·u·lo·stri·ate
  ar·ter·ies
len·tic·u·lo·tha·lam·ic
len·tic·u·lus
len·ti·form
  bone
  nu·cle·us
len·tig·i·nes
len·tig·i·no·sis
  cen·tro·fa·cial l.
  gen·er·al·ized l.
  per·i·or·i·fi·cial l.
len·ti·glo·bus
len·ti·go
  ma·lig·nant l.
  se·nile l.
len·ti·go·mel·a·no·sis
Len·ti·vir·i·nae
len·ti·vi·rus
len·to·gen·ic
len·tu·la
len·tu·lo
le·o·nine
  fa·ci·es
le·on·ti·a·sis
  l. os·sea
leop·ard
  fun·dus
  ret·i·na
leop·ard's bane
Leopold's
  ma·neu·vers
LEP
  vac·cine
Lepehne-Pickworth
  stain
lep·er
le·pid·ic
Lep·i·dop·tera
lep·i·do·sis
Le·pore
  thal·as·se·mia
Lep·or·i·pox·vi·rus
lep·o·thrix
lep·ra
  cells
lep·re·chaun·ism
lep·rid
le·prol·o·gist
le·prol·o·gy
le·pro·ma
lep·rom·a·tous
  lep·ro·sy
lep·ro·min
  re·ac·tion
  test

lep·ro·sar·i·um
lep·rose
lep·ro·sery
lep·ro·stat·ic
lep·ro·sy
  an·es·thet·ic l.
  ar·tic·u·lar l.
  bor·der·line l.
  cu·ta·ne·ous l.
  di·mor·phous l.
  dry l.
  his·toid l.
  in·de·ter·mi·nate l.
  laz·a·rine l.
  lep·rom·a·tous l.
  Lucio's l.
  mac·u·lar l.
  Mal·a·bar l.
  mouse l.
  mu·rine l.
  mu·ti·lat·ing l.
  nod·u·lar l.
  rat l.
  smooth l.
  troph·o·neu·rot·ic l.
  tu·ber·cu·loid l.
lep·ro·sy
  ba·cil·lus
lep·rot·ic
lep·rous
  neu·rop·a·thy
lep·to·ceph·a·lous
lep·to·ceph·a·ly
lep·to·chroa
lep·to·chro·mat·ic
lep·to·cyte
lep·to·cy·to·sis
lep·to·dac·ty·lous
lep·to·der·mic
lep·to·me·nin·ge·al
  car·ci·no·ma
  car·ci·no·ma·to·sis
  fi·bro·sis
lep·to·me·nin·ges
lep·to·men·in·gi·tis
  bas·i·lar l.
lep·to·me·ninx
lep·to·mere
lep·to·mo·nad
Lep·tom·o·nas
lep·to·ne·ma
lep·to·pho·nia
lep·to·phon·ic
lep·to·po·dia
lep·to·pro·so·pia
lep·to·pro·so·pic
lep·tor·rhine
lep·to·scope

lep·to·so·mat·ic
lep·to·som·ic
Lep·to·spi·ra
 L. in·ter·ro·gans
lep·to·spi·ral
 jaun·dice
lep·to·spire
lep·to·spi·ro·sis
lep·to·spi·ru·ria
lep·to·tene
lep·to·thri·co·sis
Lep·to·thrix
Lep·to·trich·ia
 L. buc·ca·lis
Lep·to·trom·bid·i·um
 L. ak·a·mu·shi
Leriche's
 op·er·a·tion
 syn·drome
Leris
 ple·on·os·te·o·sis
Leri's
 sign
Leri-Weill
 dis·ease
 syn·drome
Lermoyez'
 syn·drome
Lerner
 ho·me·o·sta·sis
les·bi·an
les·bi·an·ism
Lesch-Nyhan
 syn·drome
Leser-Trélat
 sign
le·sion
 Baehr-Lohlein l.
 be·nign lym·pho·ep·i·the·li·al l.
 Bracht-Wachter l.
 cav·i·ar l.
 coin l.'s of lungs
 Councilman's l.
 Duret's l.
 Ghon's pri·mary l.
 gross l.
 Hill-Sachs l.
 Janeway l.
 Lennert's l.
 Lohlein-Baehr l.
 Mallory-Weiss l.
 pre·can·cer·ous l.
 ra·di·al scle·ros·ing l.
 ring-wall l.
 su·pra·nu·cle·ar l.
 up·per mo·tor neu·ron l.
 wire-loop l.

less·er
 cir·cu·la·tion
 cul-de-sac
 cur·va·ture of stom·ach
 horn
 omen·tum
 pan·cre·as
 tro·chan·ter
 tu·ber·cle of hu·mer·us
 tu·ber·os·i·ty of hu·mer·us
 wing of sphe·noid bone
less·er alar
 car·ti·lag·es
less·er ar·te·ri·al
 cir·cle of iris
less·er in·ter·nal cu·ta·ne·ous
 nerve
less·er mult·ang·u·lar
 bone
less·er oc·cip·i·tal
 nerve
less·er pal·a·tine
 ar·tery
 fo·ram·i·na
 nerves
less·er per·i·to·ne·al
 cav·i·ty
 sac
less·er pe·tro·sal
 nerve
less·er rhom·boid
 mus·cle
Lesser's
 tri·an·gle
less·er sci·at·ic
 notch
less·er splanch·nic
 nerve
less·er su·per·fi·cial pe·tro·sal
 nerve
less·er su·pra·cla·vic·u·lar
 fos·sa
less·er tym·pan·ic
 spine
less·er ves·tib·u·lar
 glands
less·er zy·go·mat·ic
 mus·cle
Lesshaft's
 tri·an·gle
le·thal
 co·ef·fi·cient
 dose
 dwarf·ism
 equiv·a·lent
 fac·tor
 gene
 mu·ta·tion

le·thal
   clin·i·cal l.
   ge·net·ic l.
le·thal·i·ty
   rate
le·thal mid·line
   gran·u·lo·ma
le·thar·gic
   hyp·no·sis
leth·ar·gy
let·ter
   blind·ness
Letterer-Siwe
   dis·ease
let·ter-shaped
   ker·a·ti·tis
leu·cin
leu·cine
   hy·po·gly·ce·mia
leu·cine ami·no·pep·ti·dase
leu·ci·no·sis
leu·cin·u·ria
leu·ci·tis
Leu·co·cy·to·zo·on
   L. mar·choux·i
   L. sa·bra·zesi
   L. si·mon·di
   L. smithi
leu·co·cy·to·zo·o·no·sis
leu·co·har·mine
leu·co·line
leu·co·meth·yl·ene blue
Leu·co·nos·toc
   L. ci·trov·o·rum
   L. mes·en·te·roi·des
leu·co pa·tent blue
leu·co·vo·rin
   l. cal·ci·um
Leudet's
   tin·ni·tus
leu·en·keph·a·lin
leuk·a·ne·mia
leuk·a·phe·re·sis
leu·kas·mus
leu·ke·mia
   acute pro·my·e·lo·cyt·ic l.
   adult T-cell l.
   aleu·ke·mic l.
   ba·so·phil·ic l.
   ba·so·phil·o·cyt·ic l.
   l. cu·tis
   em·bry·o·nal l.
   eo·sin·o·phil·ic l.
   eo·sin·o·phil·o·cyt·ic l.
   fe·line l.
   l. of fowls
   gran·u·lo·cyt·ic l.
   hairy cell l.

   leu·ke·mic l.
   leu·ko·pe·nic l.
   lym·phat·ic l.
   lym·pho·blas·tic l.
   lym·pho·cyt·ic l.
   lym·phoid l.
   mast cell l.
   ma·ture cell l.
   meg·a·kar·y·o·cyt·ic l.
   me·nin·ge·al l.
   mi·cro·my·el·o·blas·tic l.
   mixed l.
   mixed cell l.
   mon·o·cyt·ic l.
   my·e·lo·blas·tic l.
   my·e·lo·cyt·ic l.
   my·e·lo·gen·ic l.
   my·e·log·e·nous l.
   my·e·loid l.
   my·e·lo·mon·o·cyt·ic l.
   Naegeli type of mon·o·cyt·ic l.
   neu·tro·phil·ic l.
   plas·ma cell l.
   pol·y·mor·pho·cyt·ic l.
   Rieder cell l.
   Schilling type of mon·o·cyt·ic l.
   splen·ic l.
   stem cell l.
   sub·leu·ke·mic l.
leu·ke·mic
   leu·ke·mia
   my·e·lo·sis
   re·tic·u·lo·en·do·the·li·o·sis
   re·tic·u·lo·sis
   ret·i·ni·tis
   ret·i·nop·a·thy
leu·ke·mic hy·per·plas·tic
   gin·gi·vi·tis
leu·ke·mid
leu·ke·mo·gen
leu·ke·mo·gen·e·sis
leu·ke·mo·gen·ic
leu·ke·moid
   re·ac·tion
leu·ke·moid re·ac·tion
   lym·pho·cyt·ic l. r.
   mon·o·cyt·ic l. r.
   my·e·lo·cyt·ic l. r.
   plas·mo·cyt·ic l. r.
leu·kin
leu·ko·ag·glu·ti·nin
leu·ko·bil·in
leu·ko·blast
   gran·u·lar l.
leu·ko·blas·to·sis
leu·ko·chlo·ro·ma

leu·ko·ci·din
leu·ko·co·ria
leu·ko·cy·tac·tic
leu·ko·cy·tal
leu·ko·cy·tax·ia
leu·ko·cy·tax·is
leu·ko·cyte
  ac·i·do·phil·ic l.
  agran·u·lar l.
  ba·so·phil·ic l.
  cys·ti·not·ic l.
  en·do·the·li·al l.
  eo·sin·o·phil·ic l.
  fil·a·ment pol·y·mor·pho·nu·cle·ar l.
  glob·u·lar l.
  gran·u·lar l.
  hy·a·line l.
  mast l.
  mo·tile l.
  mul·ti·nu·cle·ar l.
  neu·tro·phil·ic l.
  non·fil·a·ment pol·y·mor·pho·nu·cle·ar l.
  non·gran·u·lar l.
  non·mo·tile l.
  ox·y·phil·ic l.
  pol·y·mor·pho·nu·cle·ar l.
  pol·y·nu·cle·ar l.
  seg·ment·ed l.
  tran·si·tion·al l.
  Türk's l.
leu·ko·cyte
  cream
  in·clu·sions
  in·ter·fer·on
leu·ko·cyte ad·her·ence as·say
  test
leu·ko·cyte bac·te·ri·cid·al as·say
  test
leu·ko·cy·the·mia
leu·ko·cyt·ic
  sar·co·ma
leu·ko·cy·to·blast
leu·ko·cy·toc·la·sis
leu·ko·cy·to·clas·tic
  an·gi·i·tis
  vas·cu·li·tis
leu·ko·cy·to·gen·e·sis
leu·ko·cy·toid
leu·ko·cy·tol·y·sin
leu·ko·cy·tol·y·sis
leu·ko·cy·to·lyt·ic
leu·ko·cy·to·ma
leu·ko·cy·tom·e·ter
leu·ko·cy·to·pe·nia
leu·ko·cy·to·pla·nia

leu·ko·cy·to·poi·e·sis
leu·ko·cy·to·sis
  ab·so·lute l.
  ag·o·nal l.
  ba·so·phil·ic l.
  di·ges·tive l.
  dis·tri·bu·tion l.
  emo·tion·al l.
  eo·sin·o·phil·ic l.
  lym·pho·cyt·ic l.
  mon·o·cyt·ic l.
  neu·tro·phil·ic l.
  l. of the new·born
  phys·i·o·log·ic l.
  rel·a·tive l.
  ter·mi·nal l.
leu·ko·cy·to·sis-pro·mot·ing fac·tor
leu·ko·cy·to·tac·tic
leu·ko·cy·to·tax·ia
leu·ko·cy·to·tox·in
Leu·ko·cy·to·zo·on
leu·ko·cy·to·zo·o·no·sis
leu·ko·cy·tu·ria
leu·ko·der·ma
  ac·quired l.
  l. ac·quis·i·tum cen·tri·fu·gum
  l. col·li
  con·gen·i·tal l.
  syph·i·lit·ic l.
leu·ko·der·ma·tous
leu·ko·don·tia
leu·ko·dys·tro·phia
  l. ce·re·bri pro·gres·si·va
leu·ko·dys·tro·phy
  glo·boid cell l.
  met·a·chro·mat·ic l.
leu·ko·e·de·ma
leu·ko·en·ceph·a·li·tis
  acute ep·i·dem·ic l.
  sub·a·cute scle·ros·ing l.
leu·ko·en·ceph·a·lop·a·thy
  pro·gress·ive mul·ti·fo·cal l.
leu·ko·e·ryth·ro·blas·tic ane·mia
leu·ko·e·ryth·ro·blas·to·sis
leu·ko·ker·a·to·sis
leu·ko·ko·ria
leu·ko·krau·ro·sis
leu·ko·lymph·o·sar·co·ma
leu·kol·y·sin
leu·kol·y·sis
leu·ko·lyt·ic
leu·ko·ma
  ad·her·ent l.
leu·ko·ma·tous
leu·ko·my·e·lop·a·thy

leu·kon
leu·ko·ne·cro·sis
leu·ko·nych·ia
leu·ko·path·ia
   ac·quired l.
   con·gen·i·tal l.
   l. un·guis
leu·kop·a·thy
leu·ko·pe·de·sis
leu·ko·pe·nia
   ba·so·phil·ic l.
   eo·sin·o·phil·ic l.
   lym·pho·cyt·ic l.
   mon·o·cyt·ic l.
   neu·tro·phil·ic l.
leu·ko·pe·nic
   fac·tor
   in·dex
   leu·ke·mia
   my·e·lo·sis
leu·ko·phleg·ma·sia
   l. do·lens
leu·ko·pla·kia
   hairy l.
   l. vul·vae
leu·ko·plak·ic
   vul·vi·tis
leu·ko·poi·e·sis
leu·ko·poi·et·ic
leu·ko·pro·te·ase
leu·ko·ri·bo·fla·vin
leu·kor·rha·gia
leu·kor·rhea
   men·stru·al l.
leu·kor·rhe·al
leu·ko·sar·co·ma
leu·ko·sar·co·ma·to·sis
leu·ko·sis
   avi·an l.
   en·zo·ot·ic bo·vine l.
   fowl l.
   spo·rad·ic bo·vine l.
leu·ko·tac·tic
leu·ko·tax·ia
leu·ko·tax·ine
leu·ko·tax·is
leu·kot·ic
leu·ko·tome
leu·kot·o·my
   pre·fron·tal l.
   trans·or·bit·al l.
leu·ko·tox·in
leu·ko·trich·ia
   l. an·nu·la·ris
leu·kot·ri·chous
leu·ko·tri·enes
Leu·ko·vi·rus
leu·pro·lide ac·e·tate

Levaditi
   stain
lev·al·lor·phan tar·trate
lev·an
lev·an·su·crase
lev·ar·te·re·nol
   l. bi·tar·trate
le·va·tor
   cush·ion
   her·nia
   swell·ing
Levay
   an·ti·gen
LeVeen
   shunt
lev·el
   acous·tic ref·er·ence l.
   l. of as·pi·ra·tion
   Clark's l.
   hear·ing l.
   sound pres·sure l.
   win·dow l.
le·ver
   den·tal l.
le·ver·age
Levin
   tube
Levinea
   L. ama·lo·na·ti·ca
   L. mal·o·na·ti·ca
lev·i·ta·tion
Le·vi·vir·i·dae
le·vo·a·trio-car·di·nal
   vein
le·vo·bu·no·lol hy·dro·chlo·ride
le·vo·car·dia
le·vo·car·di·o·gram
le·vo·cli·na·tion
le·vo·cy·clo·duc·tion
le·vo·do·pa
le·vo·duc·tion
le·vo·form
le·vo·glu·cose
le·vo·gram
le·vo·gy·rate
le·vo·gy·rous
le·vo·nor·def·rin
le·vo·pha·ce·top·er·ane
le·vo·pho·bia
le·vo·pro·pox·y·phene nap·syl·ate
le·vo·ro·ta·tion
le·vo·ro·ta·to·ry
lev·or·pha·nol tar·trate
le·vo·tor·sion
le·vo·ver·sion
Levret's
   for·ceps

Lev's
  dis·ease
  syn·drome
lev·u·lan
lev·u·lic ac·id
lev·u·lin
lev·u·li·nate
lev·u·lin·ic ac·id
lev·u·lo·san
lev·u·lose
lev·u·lo·se·mia
lev·u·lo·su·ria
Lewandowski-Lutz
  dis·ease
Lewis Blood Group
lew·is·ite
Lewy
  bod·ies
Leyden-Möbius mus·cu·lar
  dys·tro·phy
Leyden's
  atax·ia
  crys·tals
  neu·ri·tis
ley·dig·ar·che
Leydig cell
  ad·e·no·ma
Leydig's
  cells
Lf
  dose
Lhermitte-Duclos
  dis·ease
Lhermitte's
  sign
lib·er·a·tor
  his·ta·mine l.'s
lib·er·o·mo·tor
li·bid·i·ni·za·tion
li·bid·i·nous
li·bi·do
  ob·ject l.
li·bi·do
  the·o·ry
Libman-Sacks
  en·do·car·di·tis
  syn·drome
Liborius'
  meth·od
lice
li·chen
  l. acu·mi·na·tus
  l. ag·ri·us
  l. al·bus
  l. an·nu·la·ris
  l. hem·or·rha·gi·cus
  l. in·fan·tum
  l. iris

  l. myx·e·de·ma·to·sus
  l. ni·ti·dus
  l. nu·chae
  l. ob·tu·sus
  oral (ero·sive) l. pla·nus
  oral (non·e·ro·sive) l. pla·
    nus
  l. pla·no·pi·la·ris
  l. pla·nus
  l. pla·nus an·nu·la·ris
  l. pla·nus et acu·mi·na·tus
    atroph·i·cans
  l. pla·nus fol·lic·u·la·ris
  l. pla·nus hy·per·tro·phi·cus
  l. pla·nus ver·ru·co·sus
  l. ru·ber
  l. ru·ber mo·nil·i·for·mis
  l. ru·ber pla·nus
  l. ru·ber ver·ru·co·sus
  l. scle·ro·sus et atro·phi·cus
  l. scrof·u·lo·so·rum
  l. sim·plex
  l. spi·nu·lo·sus
  l. stri·a·tus
  l. stroph·u·lo·sus
  l. syph·i·li·ti·cus
  trop·i·cal l.
  l. tro·pi·cus
  l. ur·ti·ca·tus
  l. va·ri·e·ga·tus
  Wilson's l.
li·chen
  am·y·loi·do·sis
li·chen·i·fi·ca·tion
li·chen·in
li·chen·i·za·tion
li·chen·oid
  der·ma·to·sis
  ec·ze·ma
  ker·a·to·sis
Lichtheim's
  sign
lic·o·rice
lid
  gran·u·lar l.'s
lid
  re·flex
lid clo·sure
  re·ac·tion
Liddell-Sherrington
  re·flex
li·do·caine hy·dro·chlo·ride
li·do·fla·zine
lie
  lon·gi·tu·di·nal l.
  ob·lique l.
  trans·verse l.
lie·ber·kühn

Lieberkühn's
 crypts
 fol·li·cles
 glands
Liebermann-Burchard
 test
Liebermeister's
 rule
Liebig's
 the·o·ry
lie de·tec·tor
li·en
 l. ac·ces·so·ri·us
 l. mo·bi·lis
 l. suc·cen·tu·ri·a·tus
li·e·nal
 ar·tery
li·en·cu·lus
li·e·nec·to·my
li·e·no·med·ul·lary
li·e·no·my·e·log·e·nous
li·e·no·pan·cre·at·ic
li·e·no·phren·ic
 lig·a·ment
li·e·no·re·nal
 lig·a·ment
li·en·ter·ic
 di·ar·rhea
li·en·tery
li·en·un·cu·lus
Liesegang
 rings
Lieutaud's
 body
 tri·an·gle
 tri·gone
 uvu·la
life
 cy·cle
 in·stinct
 stress
 ta·ble
life
 half-l.
 post·na·tal l.
 pre·na·tal l.
 sex·u·al l.
 veg·e·ta·tive l.
life-belt
 cat·a·ract
life e·vents
life-span
 de·vel·op·ment
life-style
Li-Fraumeni can·cer
 syn·drome
lig·a·ment
 ac·ces·so·ry l.'s

ac·ces·so·ry plan·tar l.'s
ac·ces·so·ry vo·lar l.'s
acro·mi·o·cla·vic·u·lar l.
alar l.'s
al·ve·o·lo·den·tal l.
an·nu·lar l.
an·nu·lar l. of the ra·di·us
an·nu·lar l. of the sta·pes
an·nu·lar l.'s of the tra·
 chea
ano·coc·cyg·e·al l.
an·te·ri·or cos·to·trans·verse
 l.
an·te·ri·or cru·ci·ate l.
an·te·ri·or l. of head of
 fib·u·la
an·te·ri·or lon·gi·tu·di·nal
 l.
an·te·ri·or l. of mal·le·us
an·te·ri·or me·nis·co·fem·o·
 ral l.
an·te·ri·or sa·cro·coc·cyg·e·
 al l.
an·te·ri·or sa·cro·il·i·ac l.'s
an·te·ri·or sa·cro·sci·at·ic l.
an·te·ri·or ster·no·cla·vic·u·
 lar l.
an·te·ri·or ta·lo·fib·u·lar l.
an·te·ri·or ta·lo·tib·i·al l.
an·te·ri·or tib·i·o·fib·u·lar
 l.
ap·i·cal l. of dens
Arantius' l.
ar·cu·ate pop·lit·e·al l.
ar·cu·ate pu·bic l.
ar·te·ri·al l.
l.'s of au·di·to·ry os·si·cles
au·ric·u·lar l.'s
ax·is l. of mal·le·us
Bardinet's l.
Barkow's l.
Bellini's l.
Berry's l.
Bertin's l.
Bichat's l.
bi·fur·cat·ed l.
Bigelow's l.
Botallo's l.
Bourgery's l.
broad l. of the uter·us
Brodie's l.
Burns' l.
cal·ca·ne·o·cu·boid l.
cal·ca·ne·o·fib·u·lar l.
cal·ca·ne·o·na·vic·u·lar l.
cal·ca·ne·o·tib·i·al l.
Caldani's l.
Campbell's l.

lig·a·ment *(continued)*

Camper's l.
cap·su·lar l.
car·di·nal l.
ca·rot·i·co·cli·noid l.
car·po·met·a·car·pal l.'s
cau·dal l.
cer·a·to·cri·coid l.
cer·vi·cal l. of uter·us
check l.'s of eye·ball, me·di·al and lat·er·al
check l.'s of odon·toid
chon·dro·xi·phoid l.
cil·i·ary l.
Civinini's l.
Clado's l.
col·lat·er·al l.
Colles' l.
con·ju·gate l.
co·noid l.
Cooper's l.'s
cor·a·co·a·cro·mi·al l.
cor·a·co·cla·vic·u·lar l.
cor·a·co·hu·mer·al l.
cor·nic·u·lo·pha·ryn·ge·al l.
cor·o·nary l. of knee
cor·o·nary l. of liv·er
cos·to·cla·vic·u·lar l.
cos·to·col·ic l.
cos·to·trans·verse l.
cos·to·xi·phoid l.
cot·y·loid l.
Cowper's l.
cri·co·pha·ryn·ge·al l.
cri·co·san·to·ri·ni·an l.
cri·co·thy·roid l.
cri·co·tra·che·al l.
cru·cial l.
cru·ci·ate l. of the at·las
cru·ci·ate l.'s of knee
cru·ci·ate l. of leg
cru·ci·form l. of at·las
Cruveilhier's l.'s
cu·boi·de·o·na·vic·u·lar l.
cu·ne·o·cu·boid l.
cu·ne·o·na·vic·u·lar l.'s
cys·to·du·o·de·nal l.
deep dor·sal sa·cro·coc·cyg·e·al l.
deep pos·te·ri·or sa·cro·coc·cyg·e·al l.
deep trans·verse met·a·car·pal l.
deep trans·verse met·a·tar·sal l.
del·toid l.
Denonvilliers' l.
den·tic·u·late l.

Denucé's l.
di·a·phrag·mat·ic l. of the mes·o·neph·ros
dor·sal car·pal l.
dor·sal car·po·met·a·car·pal l.'s
dor·sal cu·boi·de·o·na·vic·u·lar l.
dor·sal cu·ne·o·cu·boid l.
dor·sal cu·ne·o·na·vic·u·lar l.'s
dor·sal met·a·car·pal l.'s
dor·sal met·a·tar·sal l.'s
dor·sal ra·di·o·car·pal l.
dor·sal sa·cro·il·i·ac l.'s
du·o··de·no·re·nal l.
l. of ep·i·did·y·mis
ep·i·hy·al l.
ex·ter·nal col·lat·er·al l. of wrist
ex·tra·cap·su·lar l.'s
fal·ci·form l.
fal·ci·form l. of liv·er
fal·lo·pi·an l.
Ferrein's l.
fib·u·lar col·lat·er·al l.
Flood's l.
fun·di·form l. of foot
fun·di·form l. of pe·nis
gas·tro·co·lic l.
gas·tro·di·a·phrag·mat·ic l.
gas·tro·li·e·nal l.
gas·tro·phren·ic l.
gas·tro·splen·ic l.
gen·i·tal l.
gen·i·to·in·gui·nal l.
Gerdy's l.
Gillette's sus·pen·so·ry l.
Gimbernat's l.
gin·gi·vo·den·tal l.
gle·no·hu·mer·al l.'s
gle·noid l.
glos·so·ep·i·glot·tic l.
Günz' l.
ham·mock l.
l. of head of fe·mur
l.'s of head of fib·u·la
Helmholtz' ax·is l.
Hensing's l.
he·pa·to·co·lic l.
he·pa·to·du·o·de·nal l.
he·pa·to·e·soph·a·ge·al l.
he·pa·to·gas·tric l.
he·pa·to·re·nal l.
Hesselbach's l.
Hey's l.
Holl's l.
Hueck's l.

Humphry's l.
Hunter's l.
hy·a·lo·cap·su·lar l.
hy·o·ep·i·glot·tic l.
hyp·si·loid l.
il·i·o·fem·o·ral l.
il·i·o·lum·bar l.
il·i·o·pec·tin·e·al l.
il·i·o·tro·chan·ter·ic l.
l. of in·cus
in·fe·ri·or cal·ca·ne·o·na·vic·u·lar l.
in·fe·ri·or l. of ep·i·did·y·mis
in·fe·ri·or pu·bic l.
in·fe·ri·or trans·verse scap·u·lar l.
in·fun·dib·u·lo-ovar·i·an l.
in·fun·dib·u·lo·pel·vic l.
in·gui·nal l.
in·gui·nal l. of the kid·ney
in·ter·cap·i·tal l.
in·ter·car·pal l.'s
in·ter·cla·vic·u·lar l.
in·ter·cli·noid l.
in·ter·cor·nu·al l.
in·ter·cos·tal l.'s
in·ter·cu·ne·i·form l.'s
in·ter·fo·ve·o·lar l.
in·ter·met·a·car·pal l.'s
in·ter·met·a·tar·sal l.'s
in·ter·nal col·lat·er·al l. of the wrist
in·ter·os·se·ous cu·ne·o·cu·boid l.
in·ter·os·se·ous cu·ne·o·met·a·tar·sal l.'s
in·ter·os·se·ous met·a·car·pal l.'s
in·ter·os·se·ous met·a·tar·sal l.'s
in·ter·os·se·ous sa·cro·il·i·ac l.'s
in·ter·os·se·ous ta·lo·cal·ca·ne·al l.
in·ter·spi·nous l.
in·ter·trans·verse l.
in·tra-ar·tic·u·lar l. of cos·tal head
in·tra-ar·tic·u·lar ster·no·cos·tal l.
in·tra·cap·su·lar l.'s
is·chi·o·cap·su·lar l.
is·chi·o·fem·o·ral l.
Jarjavay's l.
ju·gal l.
Krause's l.
la·cin·i·ate l.

la·cu·nar l.
Lannelongue's l.'s
lat·er·al l. of an·kle
lat·er·al ar·cu·ate l.
lat·er·al l.'s of the blad·der
lat·er·al cos·to·trans·verse l.
lat·er·al l. of el·bow
lat·er·al l. of knee
lat·er·al mal·le·o·lar l.
lat·er·al l. of mal·le·us
lat·er·al pal·pe·bral l.
lat·er·al pu·bo·pros·tat·ic l.
lat·er·al sa·cro·coc·cyg·e·al l.
lat·er·al ta·lo·cal·ca·ne·al l.
lat·er·al l. of tem·po·ro·man·dib·u·lar joint
lat·er·al thy·ro·hy·oid l.
lat·er·al um·bil·i·cal l.
lat·er·al l. of wrist
Lauth's l.
l. of left su·pe·ri·or ve·na ca·va
left tri·an·gu·lar l.
li·e·no·phren·ic l.
li·e·no·re·nal l.
Lisfranc's l.'s
Lockwood's l.
lon·gi·tu·di·nal l.
long plan·tar l.
lum·bo·cos·tal l.
Luschka's l.'s
Mackenrodt's l.
l.'s of mal·le·us
Mauchart's l.'s
Meckel's l.
me·di·al l.
me·di·al ar·cu·ate l.
me·di·al cal·ca·ne·o·cu·boid l.
me·di·al l. of el·bow
me·di·al l. of knee
me·di·al pal·pe·bral l.
me·di·al pu·bo·pros·tat·ic l.
me·di·al ta·lo·cal·ca·ne·al l.
me·di·al um·bil·i·cal l.
me·di·al l. of wrist
me·di·an ar·cu·ate l.
me·di·an thy·ro·hy·oid l.
me·nis·co·fem·o·ral l.'s
met·a·car·pal l.'s
met·a·tar·sal l.'s
mid·dle cos·to·trans·verse l.
mid·dle um·bil·i·cal l.
nu·chal l.
ob·lique l. of el·bow joint
ob·lique pop·lit·e·al l.
oc·cip·i·to·ax·i·al l.'s

lig·a·ment *(continued)*

odon·toid l.

or·bic·u·lar l.

or·bic·u·lar l. of ra·di·us

ovar·i·an l.

pal·mar l.'s

pal·mar car·po·met·a·car·pal l.'s

pal·mar met·a·car·pal l.'s

pal·mar ra·di·o·car·pal l.

pal·mar ul·no·car·pal l.

pa·tel·lar l.

pec·ti·nate l. of ir·i·do·cor·ne·al an·gle

pec·ti·nate l. of iris

pec·tin·e·al l.

per·i·den·tal l.

per·i·o·don·tal l.

Petit's l.

phren·i·co·col·ic l.

phren·i·co·li·e·nal l.

phren·i·co·splen·ic l.

phren·o·gas·tric l.

phren·o·splen·ic l.

pi·so·ha·mate l.

pi·so·met·a·car·pal l.

pis·oun·ci·form l.

pis·oun·ci·nate l.

plan·tar l.'s

plan·tar cal·ca·ne·o·cu·boid l.

plan·tar cal·ca·ne·o·na·vic·u·lar l.

plan·tar cu·boi·de·o·na·vic·u·lar l.

plan·tar cu·ne·o·cu·boid l.

plan·tar cu·ne·o·na·vic·u·lar l.'s

plan·tar met·a·tar·sal l.'s

pos·te·ri·or cos·to·trans·verse l.

pos·te·ri·or cri·co·ar·y·te·noid l.

pos·te·ri·or cru·ci·ate l.

pos·te·ri·or l. of head of fib·u·la

pos·te·ri·or l. of in·cus

pos·te·ri·or l. of knee

pos·te·ri·or lon·gi·tu·di·nal l.

pos·te·ri·or me·nis·co·fem·o·ral l.

pos·te·ri·or oc·cip·i·to·ax·i·al l.

pos·te·ri·or sa·cro·il·i·ac l.'s

pos·te·ri·or sa·cro·sci·at·ic l.

pos·te·ri·or ster·no·cla·vic·u·lar l.

pos·te·ri·or ta·lo·fib·u·lar l.

pos·te·ri·or ta·lo·tib·i·al l.

pos·te·ri·or tib·i·o·fib·u·lar l.

Poupart's l.

prop·er l. of ova·ry

pter·y·go·man·dib·u·lar l.

pter·y·go·spi·nal l.

pter·y·go·spi·nous l.

pu·bo·cap·su·lar l.

pu·bo·fem·o·ral l.

pu·bo·pros·tat·ic l.

pu·bo·ves·i·cal l.

pul·mo·nary l.

quad·rate l.

ra·di·al col·lat·er·al l.

ra·di·al col·lat·er·al l. of wrist

ra·di·ate l. of rib

ra·di·ate ster·no·cos·tal l.'s

ra·di·ate l. of wrist

re·flex l.

Retzius' l.

rhom·boid l.

right tri·an·gu·lar l.

ring l.

round l. of el·bow joint

round l. of fe·mur

round l. of liv·er

round l. of uter·us

sa·cro·du·ral l.

sa·cro·spi·nous l.

sa·cro·tu·ber·ous l.

se·rous l.

sheath l.'s

Simonart's l.'s

Soemmering's l.

sphe·no·man·dib·u·lar l.

spi·no·gle·noid l.

spi·ral l. of co·chlea

sple·no·re·nal l.

spring l.

Stanley's cer·vi·cal l.'s

stel·late l.

ster·no·cla·vic·u·lar l.

ster·no·per·i·car·di·al l.

sty·lo·hy·oid l.

sty·lo·man·dib·u·lar l.

sty·lo·max·il·lary l.

su·per·fi·cial dor·sal sa·cro·coc·cyg·e·al l.

su·per·fi·cial pos·te·ri·or sa·cro·coc·cyg·e·al l.

su·per·fi·cial trans·verse met·a·car·pal l.

su·per·fi·cial trans·verse met·a·tar·sal l.

su·pe·ri·or cos·to·trans·verse l.

su·pe·ri·or l. of ep·i·did·y·mis

su·pe·ri·or l. of in·cus

su·pe·ri·or l. of mal·le·us

su·pe·ri·or pu·bic l.

su·pe·ri·or trans·verse scap·u·lar l.

su·pra·scap·u·lar l.

su·pra·spi·nous l.

sus·pen·so·ry l. of ax·il·la

sus·pen·so·ry l.'s of breast

sus·pen·so·ry l. of clit·o·ris

sus·pen·so·ry l.'s of Cooper

sus·pen·so·ry l. of esoph·a·gus

sus·pen·so·ry l. of eye·ball

sus·pen·so·ry l. of go·nad

sus·pen·so·ry l. of lens

sus·pen·so·ry l. of ova·ry

sus·pen·so·ry l. of pe·nis

sus·pen·so·ry l. of tes·tis

sus·pen·so·ry l. of thy·roid gland

su·tur·al l.

syn·o·vi·al l.

ta·lo·cal·ca·ne·al l.

ta·lo·na·vic·u·lar l.

tar·sal l.'s

tar·so·met·a·tar·sal l.'s

tem·po·ro·man·dib·u·lar l.

Teutleben's l.

thy·ro·ep·i·glot·tic l.

thy·ro·e·pi·glot·tid·e·an l.

tib·i·al col·lat·er·al l.

tib·i·o·fib·u·lar l.

tib·i·o·na·vic·u·lar l.

trans·verse l. of ac·e·tab·u·lum

trans·verse l. of at·las

trans·verse car·pal l.

trans·verse cru·ral l.

trans·verse l. of el·bow

trans·verse hu·mer·al l.

trans·verse l. of knee

trans·verse l. of leg

trans·verse met·a·car·pal l.

trans·verse met·a·tar·sal l.

trans·verse l. of pel·vis

trans·verse l. of per·i·ne·um

trans·verse tib·i·o·fib·u·lar l.

trap·e·zoid l.

Treitz' l.

tri·an·gu·lar l.

tri·an·gu·lar l.'s of liv·er

ul·nar col·lat·er·al l.

ul·nar col·lat·er·al l. of wrist

ura·chal l.

uter·o·sa·cral l.

Valsalva's l.'s

ve·nous l.

ven·tral sa·cro·coc·cyg·e·al l.

ven·tral sa·cro·il·i·ac l.'s

ven·tric·u·lar l.

ver·te·bro·pel·vic l.'s

ves·i·co·um·bi·li·cal l.

ves·i·co·u·ter·ine l.

ves·tib·u·lar l.

vo·cal l.

vo·lar car·pal l.

Weitbrecht's l.

Winslow's l.

Wrisberg's l.

yel·low l.

Y-shaped l.

Zaglas' l.

Zinn's l.

lig·a·men·ta

lig·a·men·to·pex·is

lig·a·men·to·pexy

lig·a·men·tous

lig·a·men·tum

l. an·nu·la·re

l. an·nu·la·re bul·bi

l. an·nu·la·re di·gi·to·rum

lig·a·men·ta ba·si·um

l. cal·ca·ne·o·ti·bi·a·le

lig·a·men·ta ca·pi·tu·lo·rum trans·ver·sa

l. cap·su·la·re

l. car·pi dor·sa·le

l. car·pi trans·ver·sum

l. car·pi vo·la·re

l. cau·da·le

l. cer·a·to·cri·coi·de·um

l. col·li cos·tae

l. con·ju·ga·le

l. cor·nic·u·lo·pha·ryn·ge·um

l. cos·to·trans·ver·sa·ri·um an·te·ri·us

l. cos·to·trans·ver·sa·ri·um pos·te·ri·us

l. co·ty·loi·de·um

lig·a·men·ta cru·ci·a·ta di·gi·to·rum

l. cru·ci·a·tum at·lan·tis

l. cru·ci·a·tum cru·ris

lig·a·men·tum *(continued)*
l. cru·ci·a·tum ter·ti·um ge·nus
l. duc·tus ve·no·si
l. du·o·de·no·re·na·le
l. fal·ci·for·me
l. gle·noi·da·le
l. he·pa·to·e·soph·a·ge·um
l. hy·a·loi·deo-cap·su·la·rio
l. hy·o·thy·roi·de·um la·te·ra·le
l. hy·o·thy·roi·de·um me·di·um
l. il·i·o·pec·ti·ne·a·le
l. in·ter·ca·pi·ta·le
lig·a·men·ta in·ter·cos·ta·lia
l. is·chi·o·cap·su·la·re
l. ju·ga·le
l. la·ci·ni·a·tum
l. la·tum pul·mo·nis
l. mal·le·o·li la·te·ra·lis
l. me·nis·ci la·te·ra·lis
l. na·ta·to·ri·um
lig·a·men·ta na·vi·cu·la·ri·cu·nei·for·mia
l. or·bic·u·la·re ra·dii
l. pal·pe·bra·le ex·ter·num
l. pec·ti·na·tum an·gu·li ir·i·do·cor·ne·a·lis
l. pec·ti·na·tum ir·i·dis
l. phren·i·co·sple·ni·cum
l. pu·bo·cap·su·la·re
l. pu·bo·pros·ta·ti·cum la·te·ra·le
l. pu·bo·pros·ta·ti·cum me·di·a·le
l. ra·di·a·tum
l. sa·cro·du·ra·le
l. sa·cro·il·i·a·cum pos·te·ri·us
l. sa·cro·spi·no·sum
l. sa·cro·tu·be·ro·sum
l. se·ro·sum
l. ta·lo·ti·bi·a·le an·te·ri·us
l. ta·lo·ti·bi·a·le pos·te·ri·us
l. tar·sa·le ex·ter·num
l. tar·sa·le in·ter·num
l. tem·po·ro·man·di·bu·la·re
l. te·res fe·mo·ris
l. tes·tis
l. tib·i·o·fib·u·la·re me·di·um
l. tib·i·o·na·vic·u·la·re
l. trans·ver·sa·lis col·li
l. trans·ver·sum cru·ris
l. trans·ver·sum pel·vis
l. tri·an·gu·la·re
l. tu·ber·cu·li cos·tae
l. um·bi·li·ca·le la·te·ra·le
l. ve·nae ca·vae si·nis·trae
l. ven·tri·cu·la·re

lig·and
lig·and-gat·ed
chan·nel
li·gase
li·gate
li·ga·tion
Larrey's l.
pole l.
sur·gi·cal l.
tooth l.
tub·al l.
li·ga·tor
lig·a·ture
Desault's l.
elas·tic l.
in·tra·vas·cu·lar l.
non·ab·sorb·a·ble l.
oc·clud·ing l.
pro·vi·sion·al l.
sol·u·ble l.
Stannius l.
sub·oc·clud·ing l.
su·ture l.
lig·a·ture
wire
light
ad·ap·ta·tion
bath
cells of thy·roid
chain
dif·fer·ence
met·al
re·flex
sense
sleep
treat·ment
light
cold l.
Finsen l.
in·fra·red l.
min·i·mum l.
po·lar·ized l.
re·flect·ed l.
re·fract·ed l.
Simpson l.
trans·mit·ted l.
Wood's l.
light-adapt·ed
eye
light dif·fer·en·tial
thresh·old
light·en·ing
light green SF yel·low·ish

light liq·uid
pe·tro·la·tum
light·ning
strip
light·ning eye
move·ments
light-touch
pal·pa·tion
light wire
ap·pli·ance
Lignac-Fanconi
syn·drome
lig·ne·ous
con·junc·ti·vi·tis
stru·ma
thy·roid·i·tis
lig·nin
lig·no·cer·ic ac·id
Lillie's al·lo·chrome con·nec·tive tis·sue
stain
Lillie's az·ure-e·o·sin
stain
Lillie's fer·rous iron
stain
Lillie's sul·fu·ric ac·id Nile blue
stain
lil·li·pu·tian
hal·lu·ci·na·tion
limb
bud
lead
limb
am·pul·la·ry l.'s of sem·i·cir·cu·lar ducts
an·a·crot·ic l.
an·te·ri·or l. of in·ter·nal cap·sule
an·te·ri·or l. of sta·pes
l.'s of bony sem·i·cir·cu·lar ca·nals
com·mon l. of mem·bra·nous sem·i·cir·cu·lar ducts
l. of he·lix
in·fe·ri·or l.
lat·er·al l.
me·di·al l.
pel·vic l.
phan·tom l.
pos·te·ri·or l. of in·ter·nal cap·sule
pos·te·ri·or l. of sta·pes
ret·ro·len·tic·u·lar l. of in·ter·nal cap·sule
sim·ple mem·bra·nous l. of sem·i·cir·cu·lar duct

sub·len·tic·u·lar l. of in·ter·nal cap·sule
su·pe·ri·or l.
tho·rac·ic l.
limb-gir·dle mus·cu·lar
dys·tro·phy
lim·bi
lim·bic
lobe
sys·tem
limb-ki·net·ic
aprax·ia
lim·bus
l. al·ve·o·la·ris
l. mem·bra·nae tym·pa·ni
l. pe·ni·cil·la·tus
l. stri·a·tus
Vieussens' l.
lime
air-slaked l.
chlo·ri·nat·ed l.
slaked l.
sul·fu·rat·ed l.
li·men
limes
li·mi·na
lim·i·nal
stim·u·lus
trait
lim·i·nom·e·ter
lim·it
dex·trin
dex·tri·nase
dex·tri·no·sis
lim·it
elas·tic l.
Hayflick's l.
pro·por·tion·al l.
quan·tum l.
short-term ex·po·sure l.
lim·it·ed range
au·di·om·e·ter
lim·it·ing
an·gle
lay·ers of cor·nea
mem·brane of neu·ral tube
mem·brane of ret·i·na
sul·cus of Reil
sul·cus of rhom·boid fos·sa
Lim·na·tis ni·lot·i·ca
lim·ne·mia
lim·ne·mic
lim·nol·o·gy
li·mon
li·mo·nis
li·mo·phoi·tas
li·moph·thi·sis
li·mo·sis

587

limp
li·mu·lus ly·sate
  test
lin·co·my·cin
linc·ture
linc·tus
lin·dane
Lindau's
  dis·ease
  tu·mor
Lindemann's
  can·nu·la
Lindner's
  bod·ies
  op·er·a·tion
line
  an·gle
  test
line
  ab·sorp·tion l.'s
  ac·cre·tion l.'s
  al·ve·o·lo·na·sal l.
  Amberg's lat·er·al si·nus l.
  ano·cu·ta·ne·ous l.
  an·te·ri·or ax·il·lary l.
  an·te·ri·or me·di·an l.
  ar·cu·ate l.
  ar·te·ri·al l.
  ax·il·lary l.
  az·y·gos ve·nous l.
  Baillarger's l.'s
  base l.
  ba·si·na·sal l.
  Beau's l.'s
  l. of Bechterew
  bis·muth l.
  black l.
  blue l.
  Bolton-na·si·on l.
  Brödel's blood·less l.
  Burton's l.
  cal·ci·fi·ca·tion l.'s of
    Retzius
  Camper's l.
  cell l.
  ce·ment l.
  cer·vi·cal l.
  Chamberlain's l.
  Chaussier's l.
  Clapton's l.
  cleav·age l.'s
  Conradi's l.
  con·tour l.'s of Owen
  Correra's l.
  cos·to·cla·vic·u·lar l.
  cos·to·phren·ic sep·tal l.'s
  Crampton's l.
  Daubenton's l.

  l. of de·mar·ca·tion
  de·mar·ca·tion l. of ret·i·na
  Dennie's l.
  den·tate l.
  de·vel·op·men·tal l.'s
  Douglas' l.
  Eberth's l.'s
  Egger's l.
  Ehrlich-Türk l.
  ep·i·phys·i·al l.
  es·tab·lished cell l.
  Farre's l.
  Feiss l.
  l. of fix·a·tion
  Fleischner l.'s
  Fraunhofer's l.'s
  ful·crum l.
  Futcher's l.
  l. of Gennari
  germ l.
  glu·te·al l.
  Granger's l.
  growth l.'s
  Gubler's l.
  gum l.
  Haller's l.
  Hampton l.
  Harris' l.'s
  Head's l.'s
  Hensen's l.
  high·est nu·chal l.
  high lip l.
  Hilton's white l.
  His' l.
  Holden's l.
  Hudson's l.
  Hudson-Stähli l.
  Hunter's l.
  Hunter-Schreger l.'s
  il·i·o·pec·tin·e·al l.
  im·bri·ca·tion l.'s of von
    Ebner
  in·cre·men·tal l.'s
  in·cre·men·tal l.'s of von
    Ebner
  in·fe·ri·or nu·chal l.
  in·fe·ri·or tem·po·ral l.
  in·fra·cos·tal l.
  in·ter·con·dy·lar l.
  in·ter·me·di·ate l. of il·i·ac
    crest
  in·ter·nal ob·lique l.
  in·ter·spi·nal l.
  in·ter·tro·chan·ter·ic l.
  in·ter·tu·ber·cu·lar l.
  iso·e·lec·tric l.
  l. of Kaes
  Kerley B l.'s

Kilian's l.
Langer's l.'s
Lanz's l.
lat·er·al l.
lat·er·al sym·pa·thet·ic l.
lead l.
low lip l.
M l.
mam·il·lary l.
mam·ma·ry l.
McKee's l.
me·di·al sym·pa·thet·ic l.
me·di·an l.
Mees' l.'s
mer·cu·ri·al l.
Meyer's l.
mid·ax·il·lary l.
mid·cla·vic·u·lar l.
mid·dle ax·il·lary l.
milk l.
Monro-Richter l.
Monro's l.
Muehrcke's l.'s
my·lo·hy·oid l.
na·so·bas·i·lar l.
Nélaton's l.
ne·o·na·tal l.
nip·ple l.
Obersteiner-Redlich l.
ob·lique l.
l. of oc·clu·sion
Ogston's l.
Ohngren's l.
Owen's l.'s
par·a·ster·nal l.
par·a·ver·te·bral l.
Par·is l.
pec·ti·nate l.
pec·tin·e·al l.
pec·tin·e·al l. of pu·bis
pleu·ro·e·soph·a·ge·al l.
Poirier's l.
pop·lit·e·al l.
post·ax·il·lary l.
pos·te·ri·or ax·il·lary l.
pos·te·ri·or me·di·an l.
Poupart's l.
pre·ax·il·lary l.
pure l.
Reid's base l.
re·ten·tive ful·crum l.
l.'s of Retzius
Richter-Monro l.
Roser-Nélaton l.
sag·it·tal l.
Salter's in·cre·men·tal l.'s
S-BP l.
scap·u·lar l.

Schreger's l.'s
sem·i·cir·cu·lar l.
sem·i·lu·nar l.
Sergent's white l.
Shenton's l.
S-N l.
so·le·al l.
l. for so·le·us mus·cle
Spigelius' l.
spi·ral l.
sta·bi·liz·ing ful·crum l.
Stahl's l.
ster·nal l.
Stocker's l.
sub·cos·tal l.
su·pe·ri·or nu·chal l.
su·pe·ri·or tem·po·ral l.
su·pra·crest·al l.
sur·vey l.
Sydney l.
syl·vi·an l.
tem·po·ral l.
ten·der l.'s
ter·mi·nal l.
tho·ra·co·lum·bar ve·nous l.
Topinard's l.
trans·verse l.
trap·e·zoid l.
Ullmann's l.
Vesling's l.
vi·brat·ing l.
l. of vi·sion
Voigt's l.'s
Wegner's l.
white l.
white l. of anal ca·nal
Z l.
l.'s of Zahn
Zöllner's l.'s

lin·ea
l. ad·mi·nic·u·lum
lin·e·ae al·bi·can·tes
lin·e·ae atro·phi·cae
l. cor·ne·ae se·ni·lis
l. nig·ra
l. nu·chae me·di·a·na
l. pop·li·tea
l. sem·i·cir·cu·la·ris
l. spi·ra·lis
l. splen·dens

lin·e·ae
lin·e·ar
ac·cel·er·a·tion
ac·cel·er·a·tor
am·pu·ta·tion
at·ro·phy
cra·ni·ec·to·my

lin·e·ar *(continued)*
  frac·ture
  pho·no·car·di·o·graph
lin·e·ar ab·sorp·tion
  co·ef·fi·cient
lin·e·ar IgA bul·lous
  dis·ease in chil·dren
lin·e·ar skull
  frac·ture
line·breed·ing
lined
  flap
li·ner
  as·bes·tos l.
  cav·i·ty l.
Lineweaver-Burk
  equa·tion
Lin·gel·sheim·ia
  L. an·i·tra·ta
ling·ism
Ling's
  meth·od
lin·gua
  l. ce·re·bel·li
  l. dis·sec·ta
  l. fis·su·ra·ta
  l. fre·na·ta
  l. ge·o·gra·phi·ca
  l. nig·ra
  l. pli·ca·ta
lin·guae
lin·gual
  ap·o·neu·ro·sis
  arch
  ar·tery
  bar
  bone
  crypt
  em·bra·sure
  flange
  flap
  fol·li·cles
  gin·gi·va
  goi·ter
  gy·rus
  lobe
  nerve
  oc·clu·sion
  pa·pil·la
  plate
  plex·us
  quin·sy
  rest
  splint
  sur·face
  ton·sil
  troph·o·neu·ro·sis
  vein

lin·gual sal·i·vary gland
  de·pres·sion
Lin·guat·u·la
  L. rhi·nar·ia
  L. ser·ra·ta
lin·guat·u·li·a·sis
Lin·gua·tu·li·dae
lin·gui·form
lin·gu·la
  l. of left lung
  l. of man·di·ble
lin·gu·lae
lin·gu·lar
lin·gu·lec·to·my
lin·guo·cer·vi·cal
  ridge
lin·guo·cli·na·tion
lin·guo·clu·sion
lin·guo·dis·tal
lin·guo·gin·gi·val
  fis·sure
  groove
  ridge
lin·guo-oc·clu·sal
lin·guo·pap·il·li·tis
lin·guo·plate
lin·guo·ver·sion
lin·i·ment
li·nin
  net·work
lin·ing
  cell
li·ni·tis
  l. plas·ti·ca
link·age
  ge·net·ic l.
  med·i·cal rec·ord l.
  sex l.
link·age
  anal·y·sis
  dis·e·qui·lib·ri·um
  group
  mark·er
link·age map
linked
link·er
lin·nae·an
  sys·tem of no·men·cla·ture
Li·nog·na·thus
li·no·le·ate
lin·o·le·ic ac·id
lin·o·len·ic ac·id
lin·o·lic ac·id
lin·seed
  l. oil
lint
li·on-jaw bone-hold·ing
  for·ceps

li·o·thy·ro·nine
  l. so·di·um
li·o·trix
lip
  ac·e·tab·u·lar l.
  an·te·ri·or l.
  ar·tic·u·lar l.
  cleft l.
  ex·ter·nal l. of il·i·ac crest
  gle·noi·dal l.
  Hapsburg l.
  in·ter·nal l. of il·i·ac crest
  large pu·den·dal l.
  lat·er·al l. of lin·ea as·pe·ra
  low·er l.
  me·di·al l. of lin·ea as·pe·ra
  l.'s of mouth
  pos·te·ri·or l.
  rhom·bic l.
  small pu·den·dal l.
  tym·pan·ic l.
  up·per l.
  ves·tib·u·lar l.
lip
  re·flex
  sul·cus
li·pan·cre·a·tin
lip·a·ro·cele
li·pase
lip·ec·to·my
lip·e·de·ma
li·pe·de·ma·tous
  al·o·pe·cia
li·pe·mia
  al·i·men·ta·ry l.
  di·a·bet·ic l.
  post·pran·di·al l.
  l. re·ti·na·lis
li·pe·mic
  ret·i·nop·a·thy
lip·id
  gran·u·lo·ma·to·sis
  his·ti·o·cy·to·sis
  ker·a·top·a·thy
  pneu·mo·nia
  pro·tein·o·sis
lip·id
  an·i·so·tro·pic l.
  brain l.
  com·pound l.'s
  iso·tro·pic l.
  sim·ple l.'s
lip·i·de·mia
lip·id-mo·bi·liz·ing
  hor·mone
lip·i·do·ses

lip·i·do·sis
  ce·re·bral l.
  cer·e·bro·side l.
  gan·gli·o·side l.
  gly·co·lip·id l.
  sphin·go·my·e·lin l.
  sul·fa·tide l.
lip·in
lip and leg
  ul·cer·a·tion
lip·o·am·ide
lip·o·am·ide de·hy·dro·gen·ase
lip·o·am·ide di·sul·fide
lip·o·am·ide re·duc·tase
lip·o·ar·thri·tis
lip·o·ate
lip·o·ate ace·tyl·trans·fer·ase
lip·o·a·tro·phia
  l. an·nu·la·ris
  l. cir·cum·scrip·ta
lip·o·a·tro·phic
  di·a·be·tes
lip·o·at·ro·phy
  in·su·lin l.
  par·tial l.
lip·o·blast
lip·o·blas·tic
  li·po·ma
lip·o·blas·to·ma
lip·o·blas·to·ma·to·sis
lip·o·car·di·ac
lip·o·cat·a·bol·ic
lip·o·cele
lip·o·cer·a·tous
lip·o·cere
lip·o·chon·dro·dys·tro·phy
lip·o·chrome
li·poc·la·sis
lip·o·clas·tic
lip·o·crit
lip·o·cyte
lip·o·der·moid
lip·o·di·er·e·sis
lip·o·dys·tro·phia
  l. in·tes·ti·na·lis
  l. pro·ges·si·va su·pe·ri·or
lip·o·dys·tro·phy
  con·gen·i·tal to·tal l.
  in·su·lin l.
  in·tes·ti·nal l.
  mem·bra·nous l.
  pro·gress·ive l.
lip·o·e·de·ma
li·pof·er·ous
lip·o·fi·bro·ma
lip·o·fus·cin
lip·o·fus·ci·no·sis
  ce·roid l.

lip·o·gen·e·sis
lip·o·gen·ic
li·pog·e·nous
    di·a·be·tes
lip·o·gran·u·lo·ma
lip·o·gran·u·lo·ma·to·sis
    dis·sem·i·nat·ed l.
lip·o·he·mia
li·po·ic ac·id
lip·oid
    der·mat·o·ar·thri·tis
    gran·u·lo·ma
    gran·u·lo·ma·to·sis
    ne·phro·sis
    pneu·mo·nia
    the·o·ry of nar·co·sis
lip·oi·de·mia
lip·oi·do·sis
    l. cor·ne·ae
    l. cu·tis et mu·co·sae
lip·o·lip·oi·do·sis
li·pol·y·sis
lip·o·lyt·ic
li·po·ma
    l. an·nu·la·re col·li
    l. ar·bo·res·cens
    atyp·i·cal l.
    l. cap·su·la·re
    l. ca·ver·no·sum
    l. fi·bro·sum
    in·fil·trat·ing l.
    lip·o·blas·tic l.
    l. myx·o·ma·to des
    l. os·sif·i·cans
    l. pet·ri·fi·cans
    ple·o·mor·phic l.
    l. sar·co·ma·to·des
    l. sar·co·ma·to·sum
    spin·dle cell l.
    tel·an·gi·ec·tat·ic l.
li·po·ma·toid
lip·o·ma·to·sis
    en·ceph·a·lo·cra·ni·o·cu·ta·
    ne·ous l.
    mul·ti·ple sym·met·ric l.
    l. neu·ro·ti·ca
li·po·ma·tous
    hy·per·tro·phy
    in·fil·tra·tion
    pol·yp
lip·o·me·lan·ic
    re·tic·u·lo·sis
lip·o·me·nin·go·cele
lip·o·mu·co·pol·y·sac·cha·ri·do·
  sis
lip·o·nu·cle·o·pro·teins
Lip·o·nys·sus
lip·o·pe·nia

lip·o·pe·nic
lip·o·pep·tid
lip·o·phage
lip·o·pha·gia
    l. gran·u·lo·ma·to·sis
lip·o·phag·ic
    gran·u·lo·ma
lip·o·phag·ic in·tes·ti·nal
    gran·u·lo·ma·to·sis
lip·oph·a·gy
lip·o·phan·er·o·sis
lip·o·phil
lip·o·phil·ic
lip·o·phos·pho·di·es·ter·ase I
lip·o·phos·pho·di·es·ter·ase II
lip·o·pol·y·sac·cha·ride
lip·o·pro·tein
    elec·tro·pho·re·sis
    pol·y·mor·phism
lip·o·pro·tein li·pase
lip·o·pro·tein-X
lip·o·sar·co·ma
li·po·sis
li·pos·i·tol
lip·o·sol·u·ble
lip·o·some
lip·o·suc·tion·ing
lip·o·thi·am·ide py·ro·phos·
  phate
lip·o·tro·phic
li·pot·ro·phy
lip·o·tro·pic
    fac·tor
    hor·mone
lip·o·tro·pic pi·tu·i·tary
    hor·mone
lip·o·tro·pin
li·pot·ro·py
lip·o·vac·cine
lip·o·vi·tel·lin
li·pox·e·nous
li·pox·e·ny
li·pox·i·dase
li·pox·y·ge·nase
lip·o·yl
lip·o·yl de·hy·dro·gen·ase
lip·ping
lip·pi·tude
lip·pi·tu·do
Lipschütz
    cell
Lipschütz'
    ul·cer
li·pu·ria
li·pur·ic
liq·ue·fa·cient
liq·ue·fac·tion
    de·gen·er·a·tion

liq·ue·fac·tive
    ne·cro·sis
liq·ue·fied
    phe·nol
li·ques·cent
li·queur
liq·uid
    Cotunnius' l.
liq·uid
    air
    ex·tract
    glu·cose
    par·af·fin
    pe·tro·le·um
    pitch
liq·uid crys·tal
    ther·mog·ra·phy
liq·uid hu·man
    se·rum
liq·uid-liq·uid
    chro·ma·tog·ra·phy
li·quor
    l. am·nii
    l. co·tun·nii
    l. en·ter·i·cus
    l. fol·lic·u·li
    malt l.
    Morgagni's l.
    moth·er l.
    Scarpa's l.
    spir·i·tu·ous l.
    vi·nous l.
li·quo·res
li·quo·rice
li·quor·is
li·quor·rhea
Lisch
    nod·ule
Lisfranc's
    am·pu·ta·tion
    joints
    lig·a·ments
    op·er·a·tion
    tu·ber·cle
lis·in·o·pril
Lison-Dunn
    stain
lisp·ing
Lissauer's
    bun·dle
    fas·cic·u·lus
    tract
Lissauer's mar·gi·nal
    zone
lis·sen·ce·pha·lia
lis·sen·ce·phal·ic
lis·sen·ceph·a·ly
lis·sive

lis·so·sphinc·ter
lis·so·trich·ic
lis·sot·ri·chous
Lis·ter·el·la
Lis·te·ria
    L. de·ni·tri·fi·cans
    L. grayi
    L. mon·o·cy·to·genes
lis·te·ria
    men·in·gi·tis
lis·te·ri·o·sis
lis·ter·ism
Lister's
    dress·ing
    meth·od
    tu·ber·cle
Listing's
    law
Listing's re·duced
    eye
Liston's
    knives
    shears
    splint
li·sur·ide
li·ter
lit·er·al
    agraph·ia
lith·a·gogue
lith·arge
li·thec·to·my
li·thi·a·sis
    l. con·junc·ti·vae
    pan·cre·at·ic l.
li·thi·a·sis
    con·junc·ti·vi·tis
lith·ic ac·id
lith·i·um
    l. bro·mide
    l. car·bon·ate
    l. cit·rate
    ef·fer·ves·cent l. cit·rate
    l. tung·state
Lith·o·bi·us
lith·o·cho·lic ac·id
lith·o·clast
lith·o·cys·tot·o·my
lith·o·di·al·y·sis
lith·o·gen·e·sis
lith·o·gen·ic
lith·og·e·nous
li·thog·e·ny
lith·oid
lith·o·kel·y·pho·pe·di·on
lith·o·kel·y·pho·pe·di·um
lith·o·kel·y·phos
lith·o·labe
li·thol·a·paxy

li·thol·y·sis
lith·o·lyte
lith·o·lyt·ic
li·thom·e·ter
lith·o·myl
lith·o·ne·phri·tis
lith·o·pe·di·on
lith·o·pe·di·um
lith·o·phone
lith·o·scope
lith·o·tome
li·thot·o·mist
li·thot·o·my
   bi·lat·er·al l.
   high l.
   lat·er·al l.
   mar·i·an l.
   me·di·an l.
   per·i·ne·al l.
   pre·rec·tal l.
   su·pra·pu·bic l.
   vag·i·nal l.
   ves·i·cal l.
li·thot·o·my
   po·si·tion
lith·o·tre·sis
   ul·tra·son·ic l.
lith·o·trip·sy
lith·o·trip·tic
lith·o·trip·tor
lith·o·trip·to·scope
lith·o·trip·tos·co·py
lith·o·trite
li·thot·ri·ty
lith·o·troph
lith·u·re·sis
lith·u·re·te·ria
li·thu·ria
li·ti·gious
   par·a·noia
lit·mus
Litten's
   phe·nom·e·non
lit·ter
lit·tle
   fin·ger
   fos·sa of the co·chle·ar
     win·dow
   fos·sa of the ves·tib·u·lar
     round win·dow
   fos·sa of the ves·tib·u·lar
     win·dow
   head of hu·mer·us
Little Leagu·er's
   el·bow
Little's
   ar·ea
   dis·ease

lit·to·ral
   cell
Littre's
   glands
   her·nia
lit·tri·tis
Litzmann
   ob·liq·ui·ty
live
   vac·cine
live·birth
live birth
live·born
   in·fant
li·ve·do
   vas·cu·li·tis
li·ve·do
   post·mor·tem l.
   l. ra·ce·mo·sa
   l. re·tic·u·la·ris
   l. re·tic·u·la·ris id·i·o·path·
     i·ca
   l. re·tic·u·la·ris symp·to·
     ma·ti·ca
   l. tel·an·gi·ec·ta·ti·ca
liv·e·doid
   der·ma·ti·tis
live oral po·li·o·vi·rus
   vac·cine
liv·er
   ac·i·nus
   bud
   flap
   palm
   spot
   starch
liv·er of
   sul·fur
liv·er
   car·di·ac l.
   des·ic·cat·ed l.
   fat·ty l.
   frost·ed l.
   hob·nail l.
   ic·ing l.
   lar·da·ceous l.
   nut·meg l.
   pol·y·cys·tic l.
   sug·ar·ic·ing l.
   wan·der·ing l.
   waxy l.
liv·er cell
   car·ci·no·ma
liv·er fil·trate
   fac·tor
liv·er Lac·to·ba·cil·lus ca·sei
   fac·tor
liv·e·tin

α-liv·e·tin
β-liv·e·tin
γ-liv·e·tin
liv·id
li·vid·i·ty
  post·mor·tem l.
liv·ing
  anat·o·my
li·vor
lix·iv·i·a·tion
lix·iv·i·um
L-L
  fac·tor
Lloyd's
  re·a·gent
Lo
  dose
load
  elec·tron·ic pace·mak·er l.
  ge·net·ic l.
load·ing
  salt l.
load·ing
  dose
Loa loa
lo·bar
  bron·chi
  pneu·mo·nia
  scle·ro·sis
lo·bate
lobe
  an·te·ri·or l. of hy·poph·y·
    sis
  cau·date l.
  l.'s of cer·e·brum
  cu·ne·i·form l.
  ear l.
  fal·ci·form l.
  floc·cu·lo·nod·u·lar l.
  fron·tal l.
  Home's l.
  in·fe·ri·or l. of lung
  left l.
  left l. of liv·er
  lim·bic l.
  lin·gual l.
  low·er l. of lung
  l.'s of mam·ma·ry gland
  mid·dle l. of pros·tate
  mid·dle l. of right lung
  ner·vous l.
  oc·cip·i·tal l.
  pa·ri·e·tal l.
  pla·cen·tal l.
  pos·te·ri·or l. of hy·poph·
    y·sis
  l. of pros·tate

py·ram·i·dal l. of thy·roid
  gland
quad·rate l.
re·nal l.
Riedel's l.
right l.
right l. of liv·er
Spigelius' l.
su·pe·ri·or l. of lung
sup·ple·men·tal l.
tem·po·ral l.
l.'s of thy·roid gland
up·per l. of lung
lo·bec·to·my
lo·be·lia
lo·be·line
  l. sul·fate
lo·bi
lo·bi·tis
Lo·boa lo·boi
lo·bo·my·co·sis
lo·bo·po·dia
lo·bo·po·di·um
Lobo's
  dis·ease
lo·bose
lo·bot·o·my
  pre·fron·tal l.
  trans·or·bit·al l.
lo·bous
Lobry de Bruyn-van Ekenstein
  trans·for·ma·tion
Lobstein's
  gan·gli·on
  syn·drome
lob·ster-claw
  de·for·mi·ty
lob·u·lar
  car·ci·no·ma
  car·ci·no·ma in si·tu
  glo·mer·u·lo·ne·phri·tis
lob·u·late
lob·u·lat·ed
lob·ule
  an·si·form l.
  an·te·ri·or lu·nate l.
  l. of au·ri·cle
  bi·ven·tral l.
  cen·tral l.
  cres·cen·tic l.'s of the cer·
    e·bel·lum
  l.'s of ep·i·did·y·mis
  he·pa·tic l.
  in·fe·ri·or pa·ri·e·tal l.
  in·fe·ri·or sem·i·lu·nar l.
  l.'s of mam·ma·ry gland
  par·a·cen·tral l.
  por·tal l. of liv·er

lob·ule *(continued)*
  pos·te·ri·or lu·nate l.
  pri·mary pul·mo·nary l.
  qua·dran·gu·lar l.
  quad·rate l.
  re·nal cor·ti·cal l.
  res·pi·ra·to·ry l.
  sec·on·dary pul·mo·nary l.
  sim·ple l.
  slen·der l.
  su·pe·ri·or pa·ri·e·tal l.
  su·pe·ri·or sem·i·lu·nar l.
  l.'s of tes·tis
  l.'s of thy·mus
  l.'s of thy·roid gland
lob·u·let
lob·u·lette
lob·u·li
lob·u·lus
  l. bi·ven·tra·lis
  l. cli·vi
  l. cul·mi·nis
  l. cu·ne·i·for·mis
  l. fo·lii
  l. fu·si·for·mis
  l. grac·i·lis
  l. quad·ra·tus
lo·bus
  l. ap·pen·di·cu·la·ris
  l. az·y·gos
  l. cli·vi
  l. fal·ci·for·mis
  l. glan·du·la·ris hy·po·phys·
   e·os
  l. lin·gui·for·mis
  l. ner·vo·sus
lo·cal
  an·a·phy·lax·is
  ane·mia
  an·es·the·sia
  an·es·thet·ic
  as·phyx·ia
  blood·let·ting
  death
  ep·i·lep·sy
  flap
  glo·mer·u·lo·ne·phri·tis
  im·mu·ni·ty
  re·ac·tion
  sign
  stim·u·lant
  symp·tom
  syn·co·pe
  tet·a·nus
  tic
lo·cal an·es·thet·ic
  re·ac·tion

lo·cal ex·cit·a·to·ry
  state
lo·cal·i·za·tion
  ag·no·sia
lo·cal·i·za·tion
  au·di·to·ry l.
  ce·re·bral l.
  ger·mi·nal l.
  pneu·mo·tax·ic l.
  spa·tial l.
  ster·e·o·tax·ic l.
lo·cal·ized
  am·ne·sia
  os·te·i·tis fi·bro·sa
  per·i·to·ni·tis
  scle·ro·der·ma
lo·cal·ized mu·ci·no·sis
lo·cal·ized nod·u·lar
  ten·o·syn·o·vi·tis
lo·cal·iz·ing
  elec·trode
  symp·tom
lo·cant
lo·ca·tor
lo·chia
  l. al·ba
  l. cru·en·ta
  l. pu·ru·len·ta
  l. ru·bra
  l. san·gui·no·len·ta
  l. se·ro·sa
lo·chi·al
lo·chi·o·me·tra
lo·chi·o·me·tri·tis
lo·chi·o·per·i·to·ni·tis
lo·chi·or·rha·gia
lo·chi·or·rhea
lo·ci
lock
  fin·ger
lock-jaw
locked
  bite
  fac·ets
  knee
locked-in
  syn·drome
Locke-Ringer
  so·lu·tion
Locke's
  so·lu·tions
lock·jaw
Lockwood's
  lig·a·ment
lo·co
lo·co·mo·tive
lo·co·mo·tor
  atax·ia

lo·co·mo·to·ri·al
lo·co·mo·to·ri·um
lo·co·mo·to·ry
lo·co·weed
  dis·ease
loc·u·lar
loc·u·late
loc·u·lat·ed
  em·py·e·ma
loc·u·la·tion
  syn·drome
loc·u·li
loc·u·lus
lo·cus
  l. ci·ne·re·us
  com·plex l.
  l. of con·trol
  l. fer·ru·gi·ne·us
  ge·net·ic l.
  l. ni·ger
  l. per·fo·ra·tus an·ti·cus
  l. per·fo·ra·tus pos·ti·cus
  sex-linked l.
  X-linked l.
  Y-linked l.
lo·cust
  gum
lod
  meth·od
Loeb's
  de·cid·u·o·ma
Loeffler's
  ba·cil·lus
  meth·yl·ene blue
  stain
Loeffler's blood cul·ture
  me·di·um
Loeffler's caus·tic
  stain
Loevit's
  cells
Loewenthal's
  bun·dle
  re·ac·tion
  tract
Loewi's
  sign
lo·fen·ta·nil
Löffler's
  dis·ease
  en·do·car·di·tis
  syn·drome
Löffler's fi·bro·plas·tic
  en·do·car·di·tis
log·ag·no·sia
log·a·graph·ia
log·am·ne·sia

Logan's
  bow
log·a·pha·sia
log·a·rith·mic
  phase
  pho·no·car·di·o·graph
log·as·the·nia
lo·get·ro·nog·ra·phy
lo·gis·tic
  curve
lo·git
  trans·for·ma·tion
log·op·a·thy
log·o·pe·dia
log·o·pe·dics
log·o·ple·gia
log·or·rhea
log·o·spasm
log·o·ther·a·py
Lohlein-Baehr
  le·sion
lo·i·a·sis
loin
lo·li·ism
Lombard voice-re·flex
  test
lo·mus·tine
London
  forc·es
long
  ax·is
  ax·is of body
  bone
  chain
  crus of in·cus
  gy·rus of in·su·la
  head
  mus·cle of head
  mus·cle of neck
  pro·cess of mal·le·us
  pulse
  root of cil·i·ary gan·gli·on
  sight
  vin·cu·lum
long ab·duc·tor
  mus·cle of thumb
long-act·ing thy·roid
  stim·u·la·tor
long ad·duc·tor
  mus·cle
long buc·cal
  nerve
long cen·tral
  ar·tery
long-chain fat·ty ac·id–CoA li·gase
long cil·i·ary
  nerve

long cone
  tech·nique
lon·gev·i·ty
long ex·ten·sor
  mus·cle of great toe
  mus·cle of thumb
  mus·cle of toes
long fib·u·lar
  mus·cle
long flex·or
  mus·cle of great toe
  mus·cle of thumb
  mus·cle of toes
long in·cu·ba·tion
  hep·a·ti·tis
lon·gis·si·mus ca·pi·tis
  mus·cle
lon·gi·tu·di·nal
  ab·er·ra·tion
  arch of foot
  arc of skull
  ca·nals of mo·di·o·lus
  dis·so·ci·a·tion
  duct of ep·o·oph·o·ron
  fis·sure of cer·e·brum
  fold of du·o·de·num
  frac·ture
  lay·ers of mus·cu·lar tu·nics
  lie
  lig·a·ment
  meth·od
  si·nus
  study
  sul·cus of heart
lon·gi·tu·di·na·lis
lon·gi·tu·di·nal oval
  pel·vis
lon·gi·tu·di·nal pon·tine
  bun·dles
lon·gi·type
long-leg
  ar·throp·a·thy
Longmire's
  op·er·a·tion
long pal·mar
  mus·cle
long per·o·ne·al
  mus·cle
long plan·tar
  lig·a·ment
long pos·te·ri·or cil·i·ary
  ar·tery
long ra·di·al ex·ten·sor
  mus·cle of wrist
Long's
  co·ef·fi·cient
  for·mu·la

long sa·phe·nous
  nerve
  vein
long sub·scap·u·lar
  nerve
long-term
  mem·o·ry
long tho·rac·ic
  ar·tery
  nerve
  vein
loop
  di·u·ret·ic
  sto·ma
loop
  Biebl l.
  bul·bo·ven·tric·u·lar l.
  cap·il·lary l.'s
  cer·vi·cal l.
  gam·ma l.
  Gerdy's in·ter·a·tri·al l.
  Granit's l.
  Henle's l.
  Hyrtl's l.
  len·tic·u·lar l.
  mem·o·ry l.
  Meyer-Archambault l.
  neph·ron·ic l.
  pe·dun·cu·lar l.
  l.'s of spi·nal nerves
  sub·cla·vi·an l.
  vec·tor l.
  ven·tric·u·lar l.
  Vieussens' l.
loose
  body
  car·ti·lage
  skin
loos·en·ing of as·so·ci·a·tion
Looser's
  zones
lop-ear
lo·per·am·ide hy·dro·chlo·ride
loph·o·dont
Lo·phoph·o·ra wil·liam·sii
lo·phot·ri·chate
lo·phot·ri·chous
lo·pre·mone
Lorain-Lévi
  dwarf·ism
  in·fan·ti·lism
  syn·drome
Lorain's
  dis·ease
lor·a·ze·pam
lor·do·sco·li·o·sis
lor·do·sis
  re·flex

lor·dot·ic
  al·bu·min·ur·ia
  pel·vis
Lorenz'
  sign
Loschmidt's
  num·ber
lo·tion
Louis'
  an·gle
  law
Louis-Bar
  syn·drome
loupe
  bin·oc·u·lar l.
loup·ing
  ill
loup·ing-ill
  vi·rus
louse
  flies
louse
  bit·ing l.
  chew·ing l.
  feath·er l.
  suck·ing l.
louse-borne
  ty·phus
lous·i·ness
lousy
lo·va·stat·in
Lovén
  re·flex
Lovibond's
  an·gle
Lovibond's pro·file
  sign
low
  con·vex
  de·lir·i·um
  fe·ver
  wine
low cal·o·rie
  di·et
low cer·vi·cal ce·sar·e·an
  sec·tion
low-com·pli·ance
  blad·der
low-egg-pas·sage
  vac·cine
Löwenberg's
  ca·nal
  for·ceps
  sca·la
low·er
  air·way
  ex·trem·i·ty
  eye·lid

jaw
lip
lobe of lung
low·er ab·dom·i·nal per·i·os·te·al
  re·flex
low·er al·ve·o·lar
  point
low·er lat·er·al cu·ta·ne·ous
  nerve of arm
low·er mo·tor
  neu·ron
low·er neph·ron
  ne·phro·sis
low·er no·dal
  ex·tra·sys·to·le
  rhythm
low·er res·pi·ra·to·ry tract
  smear
low·er ridge
  slope
Lower's
  ring
  tu·ber·cle
low·er uter·ine
  seg·ment
Lowe's
  syn·drome
Löwe's
  ring
low·est lum·bar
  ar·tery
low·est splanch·nic
  nerve
low·est thy·roid
  ar·tery
Lowe-Terrey-MacLachlan
  syn·drome
low fat
  di·et
low flow
  prin·ci·ple
low for·ceps
  de·liv·ery
low fre·quen·cy
  trans·duc·tion
low lip
  line
Lown-Ganong-Levine
  syn·drome
low out·put
  fail·ure
low salt
  syn·drome
Lowsley
  trac·tor
low so·di·um
  syn·drome

low spi·nal
 an·es·the·sia
low ten·sion
 glau·co·ma
low tone
 deaf·ness
lox·a·pine
lox·ia
lox·oph·thal·mus
Lox·os·ce·les
lox·os·ce·lism
Lox·o·tre·ma ova·tum
loz·enge
L-phase
 var·i·ants
Lr
 dose
Lu
 an·ti·gens
Lubarsch's
 crys·tals
Lu Blood Group
lu·bri·cat·ing
 cream
lu·can·thone hy·dro·chlo·ride
Lucas'
 groove
lu·cen·so·my·cin
lu·cent
Lu·ci·bac·te·ri·um
 L. har·veyi
lu·cid
 in·ter·val
lu·cid·i·fi·ca·tion
lu·cid·i·ty
lu·cif·er·as·es
lu·cif·er·ins
lu·cif·u·gal
Lu·cil·ia
 L. cae·sar
 L. cu·pri·na
 L. il·lus·tris
 L. ser·i·ca·ta
lu·ci·my·cin
Lucio's
 lep·ro·sy
Lucio's lep·ro·sy
 phe·nom·e·non
lu·cip·e·tal
Lucké
 car·ci·no·ma
Lüc·ken·schä·del
Lucké's
 ad·e·no·car·ci·no·ma
 vi·rus
Lücke's
 test
lu·co·ther·a·py

Luc's
 op·er·a·tion
lud·ic
Ludloff's
 sign
Ludwig's
 an·gi·na
 an·gle
 gan·gli·on
 lab·y·rinth
 nerve
 stro·muhr
Luer
 sy·ringe
Luer-Lok
 sy·ringe
lu·es
 l. ve·ne·rea
lu·et·ic
 mask
Luft's
 dis·ease
Luft's po·tas·si·um per·man·ga·nate
 fix·a·tive
Lu·gol's io·dine
 so·lu·tion
Lukes-Collins
 clas·si·fi·ca·tion
lu·lib·er·in
lum·ba·go
 is·che·mic l.
lum·bar
 ap·pen·di·ci·tis
 ar·tery
 en·large·ment of spi·nal cord
 flex·ure
 gan·glia
 her·nia
 ne·phrec·to·my
 nerves
 part
 part of di·a·phragm
 part of spi·nal cord
 plex·us
 punc·ture
 re·gion
 rheu·ma·tism
 rib
 tri·an·gle
 trunks
 veins
 ver·te·brae
lum·bar il·i·o·cos·tal
 mus·cle
lum·bar in·ter·spi·nal
 mus·cle

lum·bar·i·za·tion
lum·bar lymph
  nodes
lum·bar punc·ture
  nee·dle
lum·bar quad·rate
  mus·cle
lum·bar ro·ta·tor
  mus·cles
lum·bar splanch·nic
  nerves
lum·ber·man's
  itch
lum·bi
lum·bo·ab·dom·i·nal
lum·bo·co·los·to·my
lum·bo·co·lot·o·my
lum·bo·cos·tal
  lig·a·ment
lum·bo·cos·to·ab·dom·i·nal
  tri·an·gle
lum·bo·dor·sal
  fas·cia
lum·bo·il·i·ac
lum·bo·in·gui·nal
  nerve
lum·bo-ova·ri·an
lum·bo·sa·cral
  an·gle
  joint
  plex·us
  trunk
lum·bri·cal
  mus·cle of foot
  mus·cle of hand
lum·bri·ca·lis
lum·bri·ci·dal
lum·bri·cide
lum·bri·coid
lum·bri·co·sis
lum·bri·cus
lum·bus
lu·men
  re·sid·u·al l.
lu·mens
lu·mi·chrome
lu·mi·fla·vin
lu·mi·na
lu·mi·nal
lu·mi·nes·cence
lu·mi·nif·er·ous
lu·mi·no·phore
lu·mi·nous
  flux
  in·ten·si·ty
  ret·i·no·scope
lu·mi·rho·dop·sin
lump·ec·to·my

lumpy
  jaw
lumpy skin
  dis·ease
lumpy skin dis·ease
  vi·rus·es
lu·na·cy
Luna-Ishak
  stain
lu·nar
  per·i·o·dic·i·ty
lu·na·re
lu·nate
  bone
  fis·sure
  sul·cus
  sur·face of ac·e·tab·u·lum
lu·na·tic
lu·na·to·ma·la·cia
lung
  air-con·di·tion·er l.
  bird-breed·er's l.
  bird-fan·ci·er's l.
  black l.
  but·ter·fly l.
  car·di·ac l.
  cheese work·er's l.
  col·lier's l.
  farm·er's l.
  fi·broid l.
  hon·ey·comb l.
  hy·per·lu·cent l.
  iron l.
  malt-work·er's l.
  ma·son's l.
  min·er's l.
  mush·room-work·er's l.
  post·per·fu·sion l.
  pump l.
  qui·et l.
  shock l.
  thresh·er's l.
  trench l.
  ure·mic l.
  van·ish·ing l.
  weld·er's l.
  wet l.
  white l.
lung
  bud
  unit
lung·worms
lu·nu·la
  az·ure l. of nails
lu·nu·lae
Lun·yo
  vi·rus
lu·pi·form

601

lu·pin·i·dine
lu·pi·no·sis
lu·poid
  hep·a·ti·tis
  leish·man·i·a·sis
  sy·co·sis
  ul·cer
lu·pous
lu·pu·lin
lu·pus
  chron·ic dis·coid l. er·y·
    the·ma·to·sus
  dis·coid l. er·y·the·ma·to·
    sus
  dis·sem·i·nat·ed l. er·y·the·
    ma·to·sus
  l. er·y·the·ma·todes
  l. er·y·the·ma·to·sus
  l. er·y·the·ma·to·sus pro·
    fun·dus
  l. hy·per·tro·phi·cus
  l. li·vi·do
  l. lym·pha·ti·cus
  l. mil·i·a·ris dis·se·mi·na·
    tus fa·ci·ei
  l. mu·ti·lans
  l. pa·pil·lo·ma·to·sus
  l. per·nio
  l. pso·ri·a·sis
  l. scle·ro·sus
  l. se·ba·ceus
  l. ser·pi·gi·no·sus
  l. su·per·fi·ci·a·lis
  sys·tem·ic l. er·y·the·ma·
    to·sus
  l. tu·ber·cu·lo·sus
  l. tu·mi·dus
  l. ver·ru·co·sus
  l. vul·ga·ris
  l. vul·ga·ris er·y·the·ma·
    toi·des
lu·pus
  ne·phri·tis
lu·pus band
  test
lu·pus er·y·the·ma·to·sus
  cell
lu·pus er·y·the·ma·to·sus cell
  test
lu·ra
lu·ral
Luschka's
  bur·sa
  car·ti·lage
  ducts
  gland
  joints
  lig·a·ments

  si·nus
  ton·sil
Luschka's cys·tic
  glands
Luse
  bod·ies
lu·sus na·tu·rae
lute
lu·te·al
  cell
  phase
lu·te·al phase
  de·fect
  de·fi·cien·cy
lu·te·ci·um
lu·te·in
  cell
lu·te·in·i·za·tion
lu·te·i·nize
lu·te·i·niz·ing
  hor·mone
  prin·ci·ple
lu·te·i·niz·ing hor·mone/fol·li·
  cle-stim·u·lat·ing hor·mone-
  re·leas·ing
  fac·tor
lu·te·i·niz·ing hor·mone-re·leas·
  ing
  fac·tor
  hor·mone
lu·te·i·no·ma
Lutembacher's
  syn·drome
lu·te·o·gen·ic
lu·te·o·hor·mone
lu·te·ol
lu·te·ole
lu·te·o·lin
lu·te·ol·y·sin
lu·te·ol·y·sis
lu·te·o·lyt·ic
lu·te·o·ma
  preg·nan·cy l.
lu·te·o·pla·cen·tal
  shift
lu·te·o·tro·phic
lu·te·o·tro·pic
  hor·mone
lu·te·o·tro·pin
lu·te·ti·um
lu·te·us
Lu·ther·an Blood Group
lut·ing
  agent
lu·tro·pin
lu·tu·trin
Lutz·o·my·ia
  L. fla·vis·cu·tel·la·ta

L. in·ter·me·di·us
L. lon·gi·pal·pis
L. pe·ru·en·sis
Lutz-Splendore-Almeida
dis·ease
lux·a·tio
l. erec·ta
l. pe·ri·ne·al·is
lux·a·tion
Malgaigne's l.
Lux·ol fast blue
lux·us
heart
Luys'
body
ly·ase
ly·can·thro·py
ly·coc·to·nine
ly·co·pene
ly·co·pe·ne·mia
Ly·co·per·don
ly·co·per·do·no·sis
ly·coph·o·ra
ly·co·po·di·um
Lyell's
dis·ease
syn·drome
ly·go·phil·ia
Lyme
ar·thri·tis
dis·ease
ly·me·cy·cline
Lym·naea
lymph
aplas·tic l.
blood l.
cor·pus·cu·lar l.
croup·ous l.
den·tal l.
eu·plas·tic l.
fi·brin·ous l.
in·flam·ma·to·ry l.
in·ter·cel·lu·lar l.
in·tra·vas·cu·lar l.
plas·tic l.
tis·sue l.
vac·cine l.
vac·cin·ia l.
lymph
cap·il·lary
cell
cir·cu·la·tion
cor·pus·cle
em·bo·lism
fol·li·cle
gland
node
nodes of el·bow

nod·ule
sacs
scro·tum
si·nus
space
var·ix
ves·sels
lym·pha
lym·pha·den
lym·phad·e·nec·to·my
lym·phad·e·ni·tis
ca·se·ous l.
der·mat·o·path·ic l.
par·a·tu·ber·cu·lous l.
re·gion·al gran·u·lom·a·tous l.
tu·ber·cu·lous l.
lym·phad·e·nog·ra·phy
lym·phad·e·noid
goi·ter
lym·phad·e·no·ma
lym·phad·e·no·ma·to·sis
lym·phad·e·nop·a·thy
an·gi·o·im·mu·no·blas·tic l.
der·mat·o·path·ic l.
im·mu·no·blas·tic l.
lymph·ad·e·nop·a·thy-as·so·ci·at·ed
vi·rus
lym·phad·e·no·sis
be·nign l.
ma·lig·nant l.
lym·phad·e·no·va·rix
lym·pha·gogue
lym·phan·ge·i·tis
lym·phan·gi·al
lym·phan·gi·ec·ta·sia
lym·phan·gi·ec·ta·sis
cav·ern·ous l.
cys·tic l.
in·tes·ti·nal l.
sim·ple l.
lym·phan·gi·ec·tat·ic
lym·phan·gi·ec·to·des
lym·phan·gi·ec·to·my
lym·phan·gi·i·tis
lym·phan·gi·o·en·do·the·li·o·ma
lym·phan·gi·og·ra·phy
lym·phan·gi·ol·o·gy
lym·phan·gi·o·ma
l. ca·pil·la·re va·ri·co·sum
l. ca·ver·no·sum
l. cir·cum·scrip·tum
l. cys·ti·cum
l. sim·plex
l. su·per·fi·ci·um sim·plex
l. tu·be·ro·sum mul·ti·plex
l. xan·the·las·moi·de·um

lym·phan·gi·o·ma·tous
lym·phan·gi·on
lym·phan·gi·o·phle·bi·tis
lym·phan·gi·o·plas·ty
lym·phan·gi·o·sar·co·ma
lym·phan·gi·ot·o·my
lym·phan·gi·tis
 l. car·ci·no·ma·to·sa
 ep·i·zo·ot·ic l.
 l. ep·i·zo·o·ti·ca
lym·pha·phe·re·sis
lym·phat·ic
 af·fer·ent l.
 ef·fer·ent l.
lym·phat·ic
 an·gi·na
 cor·pus·cle
 duct
 ede·ma
 fis·tu·la
 fol·li·cle
 fol·li·cles of lar·ynx
 fol·li·cles of rec·tum
 leu·ke·mia
 plex·us
 ring of car·dia
 sar·co·ma
 si·nus
 stro·ma
 sys·tem
 tis·sue
 val·vule
 ves·sels
lym·phat·ic dis·sem·i·na·tion
 the·o·ry of en·do·me·tri·o·
  sis
lym·phat·i·cos·to·my
lym·pha·ti·tis
lym·pha·tol·o·gy
lym·pha·tol·y·sis
lym·pha·to·lyt·ic
lym·phec·ta·sia
lymph·e·de·ma
 con·gen·i·tal l.
 he·red·i·tary l.
 l. pre·cox
 pri·mary l.
lymph·e·dem·a·tous
 ker·a·to·der·ma
lym·phe·mia
lym·phi·za·tion
lymph node per·me·a·bil·i·ty
 fac·tor
lym·pho·ad·e·no·ma
lym·pho·blast
lym·pho·blas·tic
 leu·ke·mia
 lym·pho·ma

lym·pho·blas·to·ma
 gi·ant fol·lic·u·lar l.
lym·pho·blas·to·sis
lym·pho·cele
lym·pho·cer·as·tism
lym·pho·ci·ne·sia
lym·pho·ci·ne·sis
lym·pho·cyst
lym·pho·cy·ta·phe·re·sis
lym·pho·cyte
 B l.
 Rieder's l.
 T l.
 trans·formed l.
lym·pho·cyte
 trans·for·ma·tion
lym·pho·cyte-me·di·at·ed
 cy·to·tox·ic·i·ty
lym·pho·cy·the·mia
lym·pho·cyt·ic
 ad·e·no·hy·poph·y·si·tis
 cho·ri·o·men·in·gi·tis
 leu·ke·mia
 leu·ke·moid re·ac·tion
 leu·ko·cy·to·sis
 leu·ko·pe·nia
 se·ries
lym·pho·cyt·ic cho·ri·o·men·in·
 gi·tis
 vi·rus
lym·pho·cy·to·blast
lym·pho·cy·to·ma
 be·nign l. cu·tis
lym·pho·cy·to·pe·nia
lym·pho·cy·to·poi·e·sis
lym·pho·cy·to·sis
lym·pho·cy·to·tox·ic
 an·ti·bod·ies
lym·pho·der·ma
 l. per·ni·ci·o·sa
lym·pho·duct
lym·pho·ep·i·the·li·o·ma
lym·pho·gen·e·sis
lym·pho·gen·ic
lym·phog·e·nous
 em·bo·lism
lym·phog·e·nous me·tas·ta·sis
lym·pho·glan·du·la
lym·pho·gran·u·lo·ma
 l. be·nig·num
 l. in·gui·na·le
 l. ma·lig·num
 Schaumann's l.
 ve·ne·re·al l.
 l. ve·ne·re·um
lym·pho·gran·u·lo·ma·to·sis

lym·pho·gran·u·lo·ma ve·ne·re·um
  an·ti·gen
  vi·rus
lym·phog·ra·phy
lym·pho·his·ti·o·cy·to·sis
lym·phoid
  cell
  cor·pus·cle
  he·mo·blast of Pappenheim
  hy·poph·y·si·tis
  leu·ke·mia
  pol·yp
  ring
  se·ries
  tis·sue
lym·phoi·dec·to·my
lym·phoi·do·cyte
lym·pho·kines
lym·pho·ki·ne·sis
lym·pho·leu·ko·cyte
lym·phol·o·gy
lym·pho·ma
  adult T cell l.
  be·nign l. of the rec·tum
  Burkitt's l.
  dif·fuse small cleaved cell l.
  fol·lic·u·lar l.
  fol·lic·u·lar pre·dom·i·nant·ly large cell l.
  fol·lic·u·lar pre·dom·i·nant·ly small cleaved cell l.
  his·ti·o·cyt·ic l.
  im·mu·no·blas·tic l.
  large cell l.
  Lennert's l.
  lym·pho·blas·tic l.
  ma·lig·nant l.
  Med·i·ter·ra·ne·an l.
  nod·u·lar l.
  nod·u·lar his·ti·o·cyt·ic l.
  non-Hodgkin's l.
  poor·ly dif·fer·en·ti·at·ed lym·pho·cyt·ic l.
  small lym·pho·cyt·ic l.
  well dif·fer·en·ti·at·ed lym·pho·cyt·ic l.
lym·pho·ma·toid
  gran·u·lo·ma·to·sis
  pa·pu·lo·sis
lym·pho·ma·to·sis
  avi·an l.
  fowl l.
  oc·u·lar l.
  vis·cer·al l.
lym·pho·ma·tous
lym·pho·my·e·lo·ma
lym·pho·myx·o·ma

lym·pho·no·di
lym·pho·no·dus
  lym·pho·no·di bron·cho·pul·mo·na·les
  lym·pho·no·di co·mi·tan·tes ner·vi ac·ces·so·rii
  lym·pho·no·di pan·cre·a·ti·co·li·e·na·les
  lym·pho·no·di pul·mo·na·les
lym·pho·path·ia
  l. ve·ne·re·um
lym·phop·a·thy
lym·pho·pe·nia
lym·pho·pe·nic thy·mic
  dys·pla·sia
lym·pho·plas·ma·phe·re·sis
lym·pho·plas·ty
lym·pho·poi·e·sis
lym·pho·poi·et·ic
lym·pho·re·tic·u·lo·sis
  be·nign in·oc·u·la·tion l.
lym·phor·rha·gia
lym·phor·rhea
lym·phor·rhoid
lym·pho·sar·co·ma
  bo·vine l.
lym·pho·sar·co·ma·to·sis
lym·pho·sis
lym·phos·ta·sis
lym·pho·stat·ic
  ver·ru·co·sis
lym·pho·tax·is
lym·pho·tox·ic·i·ty
lym·pho·tox·in
lym·phot·ro·phy
lym·phu·ria
lyn·es·tre·nol
ly·o·en·zyme
ly·ol·y·sis
Lyon
  hy·poth·e·sis
ly·on·i·za·tion
ly·o·phil
ly·o·phile
ly·o·phil·ic
  col·loid
ly·oph·i·li·za·tion
ly·o·phobe
ly·o·pho·bic
  col·loid
ly·o·sorp·tion
ly·o·tro·pic
  se·ries
ly·pres·sin
ly·ra
  l. da·vi·dis
  lyre of David
  l. ute·ri·na

ly·sate
lyse
ly·se·mia
ly·serg·am·ide
ly·ser·gic ac·id
    l. a. am·ide
    l. a. di·eth·yl·am·ide
    l. a. mon·o·eth·yl·am·ide
ly·ser·gide
ly·sin
ly·sine
    l. de·car·box·yl·ase
ly·si·ne·mia
ly·sin·o·gen
ly·si·no·gen·ic
ly·sin·u·ria
ly·sis
ly·so·ceph·a·lin
ly·so·gen
ly·so·gen·e·sis
ly·so·gen·ic
    bac·te·ri·um
    in·duc·tion
    strain
ly·so·ge·nic·i·ty
ly·so·ge·ni·za·tion
ly·sog·e·ny

ly·so·ki·nase
ly·so·lec·i·thin
ly·so·lec·i·thin·ase
ly·so·phos·pha·tid·ic ac·id
ly·so·phos·pha·ti·dyl·cho·line
ly·so·phos·pha·ti·dyl·ser·ine
ly·so·phos·pho·li·pase
ly·so·so·mal
    dis·ease
ly·so·some
    de·fin·i·tive l.'s
    pri·mary l.'s
    sec·on·dary l.'s
ly·so·zyme
lys·sa
Lys·sa·vi·rus
ly·syl
ly·syl-brad·y·ki·nin
lyt·ic
    cock·tail
lyt·ta
lyx·i·tol
lyx·o·fla·vin
lyx·ose
lyx·u·lose
lyze

M

an·ti·gen
band
con·cen·tra·tion
line
pro·tein
Ma·ca·ca
ma·caque
Macchiavello's
stain
MacConkey
agar
mac·er·ate
mac·er·a·tion
Macewen's
sign
symp·tom
tri·an·gle
Mach
num·ber
Machado-Guerreiro
test
Machado-Joseph
dis·ease
Mache
unit
ma·chine
an·es·the·sia m.
heart-lung m.
pan·o·ram·ic ro·tat·ing m.
ma·chin·ery
mur·mur
Mach's
band
Ma·chu·po
vi·rus
Macintosh
block·ers
Mackay-Marg
to·nom·e·ter
Mackenrodt's
lig·a·ment
Mackenzie's
am·pu·ta·tion
pol·y·graph
Macleod's
rheu·ma·tism
syn·drome
ma·clur·in

MacNeal's tet·ra·chrome blood
stain
Mac·ra·can·tho·rhyn·chus
M. hir·u·di·na·ce·us
mac·ren·ce·pha·lia
mac·ren·ceph·a·ly
mac·ro·ad·e·no·ma
mac·ro·ag·gre·ga·ted
al·bu·min
mac·ro·am·y·lase
mac·ro·am·y·la·se·mia
mac·ro·bac·te·ri·um
mac·ro·bi·o·sis
mac·ro·bi·ote
mac·ro·bi·ot·ic
di·et
mac·ro·bi·ot·ics
mac·ro·blast
mac·ro·ble·pha·ria
mac·ro·bra·chia
mac·ro·car·dia
mac·ro·ce·pha·lia
mac·ro·ce·phal·ic
mac·ro·ceph·a·lous
mac·ro·ceph·a·ly
mac·ro·chei·lia
mac·ro·chei·ria
mac·ro·chem·is·try
mac·ro·chi·lia
mac·ro·chi·ria
mac·ro·chy·lo·mi·cron
mac·ro·cne·mia
mac·ro·coc·cus
mac·ro·co·lon
mac·ro·co·nid·ia
mac·ro·co·nid·i·um
mac·ro·cor·nea
mac·ro·cra·ni·um
mac·ro·cry·o·glob·u·lin
mac·ro·cry·o·glob·u·li·ne·mia
mac·ro·cyst
mac·ro·cy·tase
mac·ro·cyte
mac·ro·cy·the·mia
hy·per·chro·mat·ic m.
mac·ro·cyt·ic
ane·mia
ane·mia of preg·nan·cy
hy·per·chro·mia

mac·ro·cyt·ic achy·lic
  ane·mia
mac·ro·cy·to·sis
mac·ro·dac·tyl·ia
mac·ro·dac·tyl·ism
mac·ro·dac·ty·ly
mac·ro·dont
mac·ro·don·tia
mac·ro·don·tism
mac·ro·dys·tro·phia li·po·ma·
  to·sa
mac·ro·en·ceph·a·lon
mac·ro·e·ryth·ro·blast
mac·ro·e·ryth·ro·cyte
mac·ro·es·the·sia
mac·ro·fol·lic·u·lar
  ad·e·no·ma
mac·ro·ga·mete
mac·ro·ga·me·to·cyte
mac·ro·gam·ont
ma·crog·a·my
mac·ro·gas·tria
mac·ro·gen·i·to·so·mia
  m. pre·cox
  m. pre·cox su·pra·re·na·lis
ma·crog·lia
  cell
mac·ro·glob·u·lin
mac·ro·glob·u·lin·e·mia
  Waldenström's m.
mac·ro·glos·sia
mac·ro·gna·thia
ma·crog·ra·phy
mac·ro·gy·ria
mac·ro-Kjel·dahl
  meth·od
mac·ro·la·bia
mac·ro·leu·ko·blast
mac·ro·lides
mac·ro·ma·nia
mac·ro·mas·tia
mac·ro·ma·zia
mac·ro·mel·a·no·some
mac·ro·me·lia
mac·ro·mere
mac·ro·mer·o·zo·ite
mac·ro·mo·lec·u·lar
  chem·is·try
mac·ro·mol·e·cule
mac·ro·mon·o·cyte
mac·ro·my·e·lo·blast
mac·ro·nor·mo·blast
mac·ro·nor·mo·chro·mo·blast
mac·ro·nu·cle·us
mac·ro·nu·tri·ents
mac·ro·nych·ia
mac·ro·par·a·site
mac·ro·pa·thol·o·gy

mac·ro·pe·nis
mac·ro·phage
  al·ve·o·lar m.
  fixed m.
  free m.
  Hansemann m.
mac·ro·phage mi·gra·tion in·
  hi·bi·tion
  test
mac·ro·phag·o·cyte
mac·ro·phal·lus
mac·roph·thal·mia
mac·ro·po·dia
mac·ro·pol·y·cyte
mac·ro·pro·my·e·lo·cyte
mac·ro·pro·so·pia
mac·ro·pro·so·pous
ma·crop·sia
mac·ro·rhin·ia
mac·ro·sce·lia
mac·ro·scop·ic
  anat·o·my
  sphinc·ter
ma·cros·co·py
mac·ro·sig·moid
ma·cro·sis
mac·ros·mat·ic
mac·ro·so·mia
mac·ro·splanch·nic
mac·ro·spore
mac·ro·ster·e·og·no·sis
mac·ro·sto·mia
mac·ro·tia
mac·ro·tome
mac·u·la
  mac·u·lae acus·ti·cae
  m. ad·he·rens
  m. al·bi·da
  mac·u·lae al·bi·dae
  m. atro·phi·ca
  m. ce·ru·lea
  m. com·mu·ni·cans
  m. com·mu·nis
  m. cor·ne·ae
  m. den·sa
  false m.
  m. fla·va
  m. ger·mi·na·ti·va
  m. gon·or·rho·i·ca
  hon·ey·comb m.
  m. lac·tea
  m. lu·tea
  mon·go·li·an m.
  m. pel·lu·ci·da
  Saenger's m.
  m. ten·din·ea
mac·u·lae

mac·u·lar
 am·y·loi·do·sis
 ar·ea
 ar·ter·ies
 at·ro·phy
 col·o·bo·ma
 de·gen·er·a·tion
 er·y·the·ma
 eva·sion
 lep·ro·sy
 ret·i·nop·a·thy
 syph·i·lid
mac·u·late
mac·u·la·tion
mac·ule
mac·u·lo·ce·re·bral
mac·u·lo·er·y·the·ma·tous
mac·u·lo·pap·u·lar
 eryth·ro·der·ma
mac·u·lo·pap·ule
mac·u·lop·a·thy
 bull's-eye m.
 cys·toid m.
 fa·mil·i·al pseu·do·in·flam·
  ma·to·ry m.
 nic·o·tin·ic ac·id m.
mad
 itch
mad·a·ro·sis
mad·der
Maddox's
 rod
Madelung's
 de·for·mi·ty
 dis·ease
 neck
ma·des·cent
Mad Hat·ter
 syn·drome
ma·di·dans
Madlener
 op·er·a·tion
mad·ness
Madura
 boil
 foot
Mad·u·rel·la
ma·du·ro·my·co·sis
mae·di
 vi·rus
ma·fe·nide
Maffucci's
 syn·drome
mag·al·drate
Magendie-Hertwig
 sign
 syn·drome

Magendie's
 fo·ra·men
 law
 spac·es
ma·gen·stras·se
ma·gen·ta
 tongue
mag·got
 cheese m.
 sur·gi·cal m.
 wool m.
mag·i·cal
 think·ing
mag·is·tral
mag·ma
 m. re·ti·cu·la·re
Magnan's
 sign
Magnan's trom·bone
 move·ment
mag·ne·sia
 cal·cined m.
 m. mag·ma
mag·ne·sia and alu·mi·na oral
 sus·pen·sion
mag·ne·si·um
 m. alu·mi·num sil·i·cate
 m. bac·ter·i·o·phe·o·phy·
  tin·ate
 m. ben·zo·ate
 m. car·bon·ate
 m. chlo·ride
 m. cit·rate
 dried m. sul·fate
 ef·fer·ves·cent m. cit·rate
 ef·fer·ves·cent m. sul·fate
 m. hy·drox·ide
 m. lac·tate
 m. ox·ide
 m. per·ox·ide
 m. phy·tin·ates
 m. sa·lic·y·late
 m. ste·a·rate
 m. sul·fate
 tri·ba·sic m. phos·phate
 m. tri·sil·i·cate
mag·net
 re·ac·tion
 re·flex
mag·net
 Haab's m.
mag·net·ic
 at·trac·tion
 field
 im·plant
 in·er·tia
mag·net·ic res·o·nance
 imag·ing

mag·ne·tism
mag·ne·to·car·di·og·ra·phy
mag·ne·to·en·ceph·a·lo·gram
mag·ne·to·en·ceph·a·log·ra·phy
mag·ne·tom·e·ter
mag·ne·ton
    Bohr m.
    elec·tron m.
    nu·cle·ar m.
mag·ne·to·ther·a·py
mag·ni·fi·ca·tion
    ra·di·og·ra·phy
mag·ni·tude
    av·er·age pulse m.
    peak m.
mag·no·cel·lu·lar
mag·num
Magnus'
    sign
mag·nus
Mahaim
    fi·bers
Ma-huang
maid·en·head
mai·dism
Maier's
    si·nus
maim
main
    m. d'ac·cou·cheur
    m. en cro·chet
    m. en griffe
    m. en lor·gnette
    m. four·ché
main sen·so·ry
    nu·cle·us of the tri·gem·i·nus
main·stream·ing
main·tain·er
    space m.
main·te·nance
    dose
main·te·nance drug
    ther·a·py
maise oil
Maissiat's
    band
Majocchi
    gran·u·lo·mas
Majocchi's
    dis·ease
ma·jor
    ag·glu·ti·nin
    am·bly·o·scope
    am·pu·ta·tion
    ca·li·ces
    con·nec·tor
    ep·i·lep·sy

hyp·no·sis
hys·te·ria
op·er·a·tion
sur·gery
tran·quil·iz·er
ma·jor du·o·de·nal
    pa·pil·la
ma·jor his·to·com·pat·i·bil·i·ty
    com·plex
ma·jor sal·i·vary
    glands
ma·jor sub·lin·gual
    duct
Makeham's
    hy·poth·e·sis
mal
    m. de ca·de·ras
    m. de Cay·enne
    m. de la ro·sa
    m. de los pin·tos
    m. de Me·le·da
    m. de mer
    m. de San La·za·ro
    grand m.
    m. mor·a·do
    m. per·fo·rant
    pe·tit m.
    m. ros·so
ma·la
Mal·a·bar
    itch
    lep·ro·sy
mal·ab·sorp·tion
    syn·drome
Malacarne's
    pyr·a·mid
    space
mal·a·chite green
ma·la·cia
ma·la·cic
mal·a·co·pla·kia
mal·a·co·sis
mal·a·cot·ic
mal·a·cot·o·my
ma·lac·tic
ma·la·die
    m. de Roger
mal·ad·just·ment
    so·cial m.
mal·a·dy
ma·lag·ma
mal·aise
mal·a·lign·ment
ma·lar
    arch
    bone
    flush
    fold

fo·ra·men
node
point
pro·cess
ma·lar·ia
  acute m.
  al·gid m.
  au·toch·thon·ous m.
  avi·an m.
  be·nign ter·tian m.
  bil·ious re·mit·tent m.
  ce·re·bral m.
  chron·ic m.
  m. co·ma·to·sa
  dou·ble ter·tian m.
  dys·en·ter·ic al·gid m.
  fal·cip·a·rum m.
  gas·tric al·gid m.
  in·duced m.
  in·ter·mit·tent m.
  ma·lar·i·ae m.
  ma·lig·nant ter·tian m.
  mon·key m.
  no·nan m.
  ova·le m.
  ova·le ter·tian m.
  per·ni·cious m.
  quar·tan m.
  quo·tid·i·an m.
  re·laps·ing m.
  re·mit·tent m.
  sim·i·an m.
  ter·tian m.
  ther·a·peu·tic m.
  vi·vax m.
ma·lar·i·ae
  ma·lar·ia
ma·lar·i·al
  ca·chex·ia
  cres·cent
  fe·ver
  he·mo·glo·bi·nu·ria
  knobs
  per·i·o·dic·i·ty
  pig·ment
ma·lar·i·al pig·ment
  stain
ma·lar·i·ol·o·gy
ma·lar·i·ous
Malassez' ep·i·the·li·al
  rests
Ma·las·sez·ia
  M. fur·fur
  M. ova·lis
mal·as·sim·i·la·tion
ma·late
ma·late-con·dens·ing
  en·zyme

ma·late de·hy·dro·gen·ase
ma·late syn·thase
mal·a·thi·on
mal·ax·a·tion
mal·di·ges·tion
Maldonado-San Jose
  stain
male
  breast
  go·nad
  her·maph·ro·dit·ism
  hy·po·go·nad·ism
  pseu·do·her·maph·ro·dit·ism
  ste·ril·i·ty
  ure·thra
male
  ge·net·ic m.
  XX m.
  XXY m.
  XYY m.
Malecot
  cath·e·ter
ma·le·ic ac·id
mal·e·mis·sion
male pat·tern
  al·o·pe·cia
  bald·ness
male pro·nu·cle·us
mal·e·rup·tion
male Turner's
  syn·drome
mal·for·ma·tion
  Arnold-Chiari m.
mal·func·tion
Malgaigne's
  am·pu·ta·tion
  fos·sa
  her·nia
  lux·a·tion
  tri·an·gle
Malherbe's
  dis·ease
Malherbe's cal·ci·fy·ing
  ep·i·the·li·o·ma
mal·ic
  en·zyme
mal·ic ac·id
mal·ic ac·id de·hy·dro·gen·ase
mal·ic de·hy·dro·gen·ase
ma·lig·nan·cy
ma·lig·nant
  ane·mia
  bu·bo
  ca·tarrh of cat·tle
  down
  dys·en·tery
  dys·ker·a·to·sis
  ede·ma

ma·lig·nant *(continued)*
  en·do·car·di·tis
  ex·oph·thal·mos
  glau·co·ma
  gran·u·lo·ma
  he·pa·to·ma
  his·ti·o·cy·to·sis
  hy·per·py·rex·ia
  hy·per·ten·sion
  hy·per·ther·mia
  jaun·dice
  len·ti·go
  lym·phad·e·no·sis
  lym·pho·ma
  mal·nu·tri·tion
  mel·a·no·ma
  mel·a·no·ma in si·tu
  my·o·pia
  neph·ro·scle·ro·sis
  pus·tule
  scle·ri·tis
  small·pox
  stu·por
  syn·o·vi·o·ma
  tu·mor
ma·lig·nant atroph·ic
  pa·pu·lo·sis
ma·lig·nant car·ci·noid
  syn·drome
ma·lig·nant ca·tarrh·al
  fe·ver
ma·lig·nant ca·tarrh·al fe·ver
  vi·rus
ma·lig·nant cil·i·ary
  ep·i·the·li·o·ma
ma·lig·nant fi·brous
  his·ti·o·cy·to·ma
ma·lig·nant len·ti·go
  mel·a·no·ma
ma·lig·nant mes·en·chy·mo·ma
ma·lig·nant ovine and cap·rine
  thei·le·ri·o·sis
ma·lig·nant ter·tian
  fe·ver
  ma·lar·ia
ma·lig·nant ter·tian ma·lar·i·al
  par·a·site
ma·lin·ger
ma·lin·ger·er
ma·lin·ger·ing
mal·in·ter·dig·i·ta·tion
mal·le·a·ble
mal·le·ar
  fold
  prom·i·nence
  stripe
mal·le·a·tion
mal·le·brin

mal·lei
mal·le·in
mal·le·in·i·za·tion
mal·le·o·in·cu·dal
mal·le·o·lar
  sul·cus
mal·le·o·lar ar·tic·u·lar
  sur·face of fib·u·la
  sur·face of tib·ia
mal·le·o·li
mal·le·o·lus
  ex·ter·nal m.
  in·ner m.
  in·ter·nal m.
  lat·er·al m.
  me·di·al m.
  out·er m.
mal·le·ot·o·my
mal·let
  fin·ger
mal·le·us
Mal·loph·a·ga
Mallory
  bod·ies
Mallory's
  stain for ac·ti·no·my·ces
  stain for he·mo·fuch·sin
Mallory's an·i·line blue
  stain
Mallory's col·la·gen
  stain
Mallory's io·dine
  stain
Mallory's phlox·ine
  stain
Mallory's phos·pho·tung·stic
  ac·id he·ma·tox·y·lin
  stain
Mallory's tri·chrome
  stain
Mallory's tri·ple
  stain
Mallory-Weiss
  le·sion
  syn·drome
  tear
Mall's
  for·mu·la
  ridg·es
mal·nu·tri·tion
  ma·lig·nant m.
mal·oc·clu·sion
Maloney
  bou·gies
ma·lo·nic ac·id
mal·o·nyl
  m. trans·ac·yl·ase
mal·o·nyl-CoA

mal·o·nyl·co·en·zyme A
mal·o·nyl·u·rea
mal·pi·ghi·an
  bod·ies
  cap·sule
  cell
  cor·pus·cles
  glands
  glo·mer·u·lus
  lay·er
  nod·ules
  pyr·a·mid
  re·te
  stig·mas
  stra·tum
  tu·bules
  tuft
  ves·i·cles
mal·po·si·tion
mal·prac·tice
mal·pre·sen·ta·tion
mal·ro·ta·tion
malt
  li·quor
  sug·ar
Mal·ta
  fe·ver
malt·ase
  ac·id m.
mal·to·bi·ose
mal·tose
mal·to·tet·rose
malt-work·er's
  lung
ma·lum
  m. ar·ti·cu·lo·rum se·ni·lis
  m. cor·dis
  m. cox·ae
  m. cox·ae se·nile
  m. per·fo·rans pe·dis
  m. ve·ne·re·um
  m. ver·te·bra·le sub·oc·ci·
    pi·ta·le
mal·un·ion
ma·man·pi·an
mam·e·lon
mam·e·lon·at·ed
mam·e·lo·na·tion
ma·mil·la
ma·mil·lae
ma·mil·la·re
mam·il·lar·ia
mam·il·lary
  body
  ducts
  line
  pro·cess
  tu·ber·cle

tu·ber·cle of hy·po·thal·a·
  mus
mam·il·late
mam·il·lat·ed
mam·il·la·tion
ma·mil·li·form
ma·mil·lo·teg·men·tal
  fas·cic·u·lus
mam·il·lo·tha·lam·ic
  fas·cic·u·lus
  tract
mam·ma
  m. er·ra·ti·ca
  su·per·nu·mer·ary m.
  m. vi·ri·lis
mam·mae
mam·mal
mam·mal·gia
Mam·ma·lia
mam·ma·plas·ty
  aug·men·ta·tion m.
  re·con·struc·tive m.
  re·duc·tion m.
mam·ma·ry
  cal·cu·lus
  ducts
  dys·pla·sia
  fis·tu·la
  fold
  gland
  line
  neu·ral·gia
  plex·us
  re·gion
  ridge
  souf·fle
mam·ma·ry can·cer
  vi·rus of mice
mam·ma·ry duct
  ec·ta·sia
mam·ma·ry tu·mor
  vi·rus of mice
mam·mec·to·my
mam·mi·form
mam·mil·la·plas·ty
mam·mil·li·tis
  bo·vine her·pes m.
  bo·vine ul·cer·a·tive m.
  bo·vine vac·cin·ia m.
mam·mi·tis
mam·mo·gram
mam·mog·ra·phy
mam·mo·plas·ty
mam·mose
mam·mo·so·ma·to·troph
mam·mot·o·my
mam·mo·troph
mam·mo·tro·phic

mam·mo·tro·phin
mam·mo·tro·pic
  fac·tor
  hor·mone
mam·mo·tro·pin
Man·ches·ter
  op·er·a·tion
  ovoid
man·chette
Man·chu·ri·an
  fe·ver
Man·chu·ri·an hem·or·rhag·ic
  fe·ver
man·del·ate
man·del·ic ac·id
Mandelin's
  re·a·gent
man·de·lyt·ro·pine
man·di·ble
man·dib·u·la
man·dib·u·lae
man·dib·u·lar
  arch
  ax·is
  ca·nal
  car·ti·lage
  con·dyle
  den·ti·tion
  disk
  fo·ra·men
  fos·sa
  glide
  joint
  move·ment
  nerve
  nodes
  notch
  pro·cess
  pro·trac·tion
  re·flex
  re·trac·tion
  tongue
  to·rus
man·dib·u·lar guide
  pros·the·sis
man·dib·u·lar hinge
  po·si·tion
man·dib·u·lec·to·my
man·dib·u·lo·ac·ral
  dys·os·to·sis
man·dib·u·lo·fa·cial
  dys·os·to·sis
  dys·pla·sia
man·dib·u·lo·fa·cial dys·o·to·sis
  syn·drome
man·dib·u·lo·max·il·lary
  fix·a·tion

man·dib·u·lo-oc·u·lo·fa·cial
  dys·mor·phia
  syn·drome
man·dib·u·lo·pha·ryn·ge·al
man·dib·u·lum
man·drag·o·ra
man·drake
man·drel
man·dril
man·drill
man·drin
ma·neu·ver
  Adson m.
  Bill's m.
  Bracht m.
  Brandt-Andrews m.
  Buzzard's m.
  Credé's m.'s
  DeLee's m.
  Ejrup m.
  Hampton m.
  Heimlich m.
  Hillis-Müller m.
  Hueter's m.
  Jendrassik's m.
  key-in-lock m.
  Leopold's m.'s
  Mauriceau-Levret m.
  Mauriceau's m.
  McDonald's m.
  Müller's m.
  Pajot's m.
  Pinard's m.
  Prague m.
  Ritgen's m.
  Scanzoni's m.
  Sellick's m.
  Valsalva m.
  Wigand m.
man·ga·nese
man·gan·ic
man·ga·nous
man·ga·num
mange
  cho·ri·op·tic m.
  dem·o·dec·tic m.
  ear m.
  fol·lic·u·lar m.
  no·to·ed·ric m.
  oto·dec·tic m.
  pso·rop·tic m.
  red m.
  sar·cop·tic m.
man·go
  der·ma·ti·tis
man·grove
  fly
ma·nia

ma·ni·ac
ma·ni·a·cal
man·ic
  ex·cite·ment
man·ic-de·pres·sive
  psy·cho·sis
man·i·cy
man·i·fest
  con·tent
  hy·per·o·pia
  stra·bis·mus
  tet·a·ny
  vec·tor
man·i·fes·ta·tion
  be·hav·ior·al m.
  neu·rot·ic m.
  psy·cho·phys·i·o·log·ic m.
  psy·chot·ic m.
man·i·fest·ing
  car·ri·er
  het·er·o·zy·gote
man·i·kin
man·i·pha·lanx
man·na
  sug·ar
man·na can·nel·la·ta
man·na com·mu·nis
man·na in lac·ri·mis
man·nans
man·na in sor·tis
Mann-Bollman
  fis·tu·la
man·ner·ism
man·nite
man·ni·tol
  m. hex·a·ni·trate
Mannkopf's
  sign
man·no·hep·tu·lose
man·no·mus·tine
man·no·sans
man·nose
man·no·side
man·no·si·do·sis
Mann's meth·yl blue-e·o·sin
  stain
man·nu·ron·ic ac·id
Mann-Williamson
  op·er·a·tion
  ul·cer
ma·nom·e·ter
  an·er·oid m.
  di·al m.
  dif·fer·en·tial m.
  mer·cu·ri·al m.
man·o·met·ric
ma·nom·e·try
  esoph·a·ge·al m.

ma·nos·co·py
Man·son·el·la
  M. dem·ar·quayi
  M. oz·zar·di
  M. per·stans
  M. strep·to·cer·ca
  M. tu·cu·ma·na
man·so·nel·li·a·sis
Man·so·nia
Man·so·noi·des
Manson's
  dis·ease
  py·o·sis
  schis·to·so·mi·a·sis
Manson's eye
  worm
man·tle
  lay·er
  ra·di·o·ther·a·py
  scle·ro·sis
  zone
man·tle
  brain m.
  my·o·ep·i·car·di·al m.
Mantoux
  pit
  test
man·u·al
  pel·vim·e·try
  ven·ti·la·tion
ma·nu·bria
ma·nu·bri·o·ster·nal
  joint
  sym·phy·sis
ma·nu·bri·um
man·u·dy·na·mom·e·ter
ma·nus
  m. ca·va
  m. ex·ten·sa
  m. flexa
  m. pla·na
  m. su·per·ex·ten·sa
  m. val·ga
  m. va·ra
ma·nus
many-tailed
  ban·dage
map dis·tance
map-dot-fin·ger·print
  dys·tro·phy
ma·ple
  sug·ar
ma·ple bark
  dis·ease
ma·ple syr·up
  urine
ma·ple syr·up urine
  dis·ease

map·like
skull
map·pine
map·ping func·tion
ma·pro·ti·line
Ma·ra·ñón's
sign
syn·drome
ma·ran·tic
at·ro·phy
ede·ma
en·do·car·di·tis
throm·bo·sis
throm·bus
ma·ras·mic
throm·bo·sis
throm·bus
ma·ras·moid
ma·ras·mus
mar·a·thon group
psy·cho·ther·a·py
mar·ble
bones
mar·ble bone
dis·ease
mar·ble cut·ters'
phthi·sis
Marburg
vi·rus
Marburg vi·rus
dis·ease
marc
Marcacci's
mus·cle
march
frac·ture
he·mo·glo·bi·nu·ria
Marchand's
ad·re·nals
rest
Marchand's wan·der·ing
cell
Marchant's
zone
Marchesani
syn·drome
Marchiafava-Bignami
dis·ease
Marchiafava-Micheli
ane·mia
syn·drome
Marchi's
fix·a·tive
re·ac·tion
stain
tract
mar·cid

Marcille's
tri·an·gle
mar·cor
Marcus Gunn
phe·nom·e·non
pu·pil
syn·drome
Marcus Gunn's
sign
Marek's
dis·ease
Marek's dis·ease
vi·rus
Marey's
law
mar·fan·oid
Marfan's
dis·ease
law
syn·drome
mar·ga·rine
dis·ease
Mar·gar·o·pus
M. win·themi
mar·gin
m. of ac·e·tab·u·lum
an·te·ri·or m.
ar·tic·u·lar m.
cav·i·ty m.
cer·vi·cal m.
cil·i·ary m.
cor·ne·al m.
m. of eye·lid
fal·ci·form m.
fib·u·lar m. of foot
m. of fos·sa ova·lis
free m.
fron·tal m.
gin·gi·val m.
in·ci·sal m.
in·fe·ri·or m.
in·fe·ro·lat·er·al m.
in·fer·o·me·di·al m.
in·fra·or·bit·al m.
in·ter·os·se·ous m.
lac·ri·mal m.
lamb·doid m.
lat·er·al m.
mas·toid m.
me·di·al m.
mes·o·va·ri·an m.
na·sal m.
oc·cip·i·tal m.
pa·ri·e·tal m.
pos·te·ri·or m.
pu·pil·lary m.
right m. of heart
m. of safe·ty

squa·mous m.
su·pe·ri·or m.
su·per·o·me·di·al m.
su·pra·or·bit·al m.
m. of the tongue
ul·nar m.
zy·go·mat·ic m.

mar·gi·nal
ar·tery of co·lon
bleph·a·ri·tis
crest
gin·gi·vi·tis
gy·rus
in·teg·ri·ty of amal·gam
ker·a·ti·tis
lay·er
part
rays
ridge
si·nus of pla·cen·ta
sphinc·ter
tu·ber·cle
zone

mar·gi·nal cor·ne·al
de·gen·er·a·tion

**Mar·gi·nal Line Cal·cu·lus In·
dex**

mar·gi·nal ring
ul·cer of cor·nea

mar·gin·a·tion
m. of pla·cen·ta

mar·gi·nes

mar·gi·nis

mar·gi·no·plas·ty

mar·go
m. pal·pe·brae

mar·i·an
li·thot·o·my

Marie-Robinson
syn·drome

Marie's
atax·ia

Marie-Strümpell
dis·ease

mar·i·hua·na

ma·rine
phar·ma·col·o·gy
soap

Marinesco-Garland
syn·drome

Marinesco-Sjögren
syn·drome

Marinesco's suc·cu·lent
hand

mar·i·no·bu·fo·tox·in

Marion's
dis·ease

Mariotte
bot·tle

Mariotte's
ex·per·i·ment
law

Mariotte's blind
spot

mar·i·po·sia

mar·i·tal
coun·sel·ing

Marjolin's
ul·cer

mar·jo·ram

mark
align·ment m.
dho·bie m.
port-wine m.
straw·ber·ry m.
Unna's m.
wash·er·man's m.

mark·er
trait

mark·er
al·lo·typ·ic m.
Amsler's m.
cell m.
ge·net·ic m.
link·age m.
on·co·fe·tal m.
time m.
tu·mor m.

mark·er X
chro·mo·some

Marme's
re·a·gent

mar·mo·rat·ed

mar·mo·set
vi·rus

mar·mot

Maroteaux-Lamy
syn·drome

Marquis'
re·a·gent

mar·riage
ther·a·py

mar·row
ca·nal
cell

mar·row
bone m.
red bone m.
spi·nal m.
yel·low bone m.

mar·row-lymph
gland

Mar·seilles
fe·ver

marsh
fe·ver
gas
Marshall
syn·drome
Mar·shal·la·gia mar·shalli
Marshall-Marchetti-Krantz
op·er·a·tion
Marshall's
meth·od
Marshall's ob·lique
vein
Marshall's ves·tig·i·al
fold
marsh·mal·low root
mar·su·pi·al
notch
mar·su·pi·al·i·za·tion
mar·su·pi·um
Martegiani's
ar·ea
fun·nel
Martinotti's
cell
Martin's
ban·dage
dis·ease
tube
mar·ti·us yel·low
Martorell's
syn·drome
Mar·y·land co·ma scale
mas·chal·ad·e·ni·tis
mas·cha·le
mas·chal·eph·i·dro·sis
mas·chal·on·cus
mas·chal·y·per·i·dro·sis
mas·cu·line
pel·vis
uter·us
mas·cu·line pro·test
mas·cu·lin·i·ty
mas·cu·lin·i·ty-fem·i·nin·i·ty
scale
mas·cu·lin·i·za·tion
mas·cu·li·nize
mas·cu·lin·o·vo·blas·to·ma
mas·cu·li·nus
Masini's
sign
mask
ec·chy·mot·ic m.
Hutchinson's m.
lu·et·ic m.
non·re·breath·ing m.
m. of preg·nan·cy
trop·i·cal m.

masked
ep·i·lep·sy
gout
vi·rus
mask·ing
mask·like
face
Maslow's
hi·er·ar·chy
mas·och·ism
mas·och·ist
mas·och·is·tic
per·son·al·i·ty
Mason
op·er·a·tion
ma·son's
lung
masque bil·ia·ire
mass
ap·per·cep·tive m.
fi·lar m.
in·jec·tion m.
in·ner cell m.
lat·er·al m. of at·las
lat·er·al m. of eth·moid
bone
pil·u·lar m.
scle·rot·ic ce·ment·al m.
tu·bu·lar ex·cre·to·ry m.
mass
hys·te·ria
in·fec·tion
law
move·ment
num·ber
per·i·stal·sis
re·flex
spec·tro·graph
mas·sa
m. in·ter·me·dia
mass ac·tion
the·o·ry
mas·sae
mas·sage
car·di·ac m.
closed chest m.
ex·ter·nal car·di·ac m.
gin·gi·val m.
nerve-point m.
open chest m.
pros·tat·ic m.
vi·bra·to·ry m.
Masselon's
spec·ta·cles
mas·se·ter
re·flex
mas·se·ter·ic
ar·tery

fas·cia
nerve
tu·ber·os·i·ty
veins
mas·seur
mas·seuse
mas·si·cot
mas·sive
col·lapse
mas·sive bow·el re·sec·tion
syn·drome
Masson-Fontana am·mo·ni·a·cal
sil·ver
stain
Masson's
pseu·do·an·gi·o·sar·co·ma
Masson's ar·gen·taf·fin
stain
Masson's tri·chrome
stain
mas·so·ther·a·py
mast
cell
leu·ko·cyte
mast·ad·e·ni·tis
mast·ad·e·no·ma
Mast·ad·e·no·vi·rus
mas·tal·gia
mas·ta·tro·phia
mas·tat·ro·phy
mas·tauxe
mast cell
leu·ke·mia
mas·tec·to·my
ex·tend·ed rad·i·cal m.
mod·i·fied rad·i·cal m.
rad·i·cal m.
sim·ple m.
sub·cu·ta·ne·ous m.
to·tal m.
mas·ter
cast
eye
gland
mas·ter-dom·i·nant
eye
Master's
test
Master's two-step ex·er·cise
test
mas·tery
mo·tive
mas·tic
mas·ti·cate
mas·ti·cat·ing
cy·cles
sur·face
mas·ti·ca·tion

mas·ti·ca·tor
nerve
mas·ti·ca·to·ry
ap·pa·ra·tus
di·ple·gia
force
nu·cle·us
spasm
sur·face
sys·tem
mas·ti·ca·to·ry si·lent
pe·ri·od
mas·tich
mas·ti·che
Mas·ti·goph·o·ra
mas·ti·gote
mas·ti·tis
bo·vine m.
chron·ic cys·tic m.
gar·gan·tuan m.
glan·du·lar m.
gran·u·lom·a·tous m.
in·ter·sti·tial m.
lac·ta·tion·al m.
m. ne·o·na·to·rum
ovine m.
par·en·chym·a·tous m.
phleg·mon·ous m.
plas·ma cell m.
pu·er·per·al m.
ret·ro·mam·ma·ry m.
stag·na·tion m.
sub·mam·ma·ry m.
sup·pu·ra·tive m.
mas·toc·cip·i·tal
mas·to·cyte
mas·to·cy·to·gen·e·sis
mas·to·cy·to·ma
mas·to·cy·to·sis
mas·to·dyn·ia
mas·toid
ab·scess
an·gle of pa·ri·e·tal
an·trum
ar·tery
bone
can·a·lic·u·lus
cells
em·py·e·ma
fon·ta·nel
fo·ra·men
fos·sa
groove
mar·gin
notch
part
pro·cess

mas·toid *(continued)*
si·nus·es
wall of mid·dle ear
mas·toi·dal
mas·toi·da·le
mas·toid·ec·to·my
rad·i·cal m.
mas·toid em·is·sary
vein
mas·toi·de·o·cen·te·sis
mas·toid·i·tis
Bezold's m.
scle·ros·ing m.
mas·toid lymph
nodes
mas·toi·dot·o·my
mas·ton·cus
mas·to-oc·cip·i·tal
mas·to·pa·ri·e·tal
mas·top·a·thy
mas·to·pexy
mas·to·pla·sia
mas·to·plas·ty
mas·top·to·sis
mas·tor·rha·gia
mas·to·scir·rhus
mas·to·squa·mous
mas·to·syr·inx
mas·tot·o·my
mas·tur·bate
mas·tur·ba·tion
false m.
Masugi's
ne·phri·tis
mat
burn
gold
Matas'
op·er·a·tion
matched
groups
match·ing
maté
ma·te·ria
m. al·ba
m. med·i·ca
ma·te·ri·al
base m.
cross-re·act·ing m.
den·tal m.
im·pres·sion m.
plas·tic res·to·ra·tion m.
re·stor·a·tive den·tal m.'s
ma·te·ri·es mor·bi
ma·ter·nal
cot·y·le·don
death
dys·to·cia

in·her·i·tance
pla·cen·ta
ma·ter·nal death
rate
ma·ter·ni·ty
hos·pi·tal
math·e·mat·i·cal
ge·net·ics
mat·ing
iso·late
sea·son
mat·ing
as·sort·a·tive m.
cross m.
ran·dom m.
mat·rass
mat·ri·cal
mat·ri·ca·ria
ma·tri·ces
ma·tri·cial
mat·ri·cide
mat·ri·lin·e·al
ma·trix
amal·gam m.
bone m.
car·ti·lage m.
cell m.
cy·to·plas·mic m.
mi·to·chon·dri·al m.
m. mi·to·chon·dri·a·lis
nail m.
ter·ri·to·ri·al m.
ma·trix
band
cal·cu·lus
re·tain·er
mat·ter
gray m.
pon·tine gray m.
white m.
mat·tress
su·ture
mat·u·rate
mat·u·ra·tion
ar·rest
fac·tor
in·dex
val·ue
ma·ture
bac·te·ri·o·phage
cat·a·ract
neu·tro·phil
ma·ture cell
leu·ke·mia
ma·ture ovar·i·an
fol·li·cle
ma·tu·ri·ty

ma·tu·ri·ty-on·set
  di·a·be·tes
ma·tu·ti·nal
  ep·i·lep·sy
Mauchart's
  lig·a·ments
Maurer's
  clefts
  dots
Mauriac's
  syn·drome
Mauriceau-Levret
  ma·neu·ver
Mauriceau's
  ma·neu·ver
Mauthner's
  cell
  sheath
  test
max·il·la
max·il·lae
max·il·lary
  an·gle
  an·trum
  ar·tery
  den·ti·tion
  em·i·nence
  gland
  hi·a·tus
  nerve
  plex·us
  pro·cess
  pro·cess of em·bryo
  pro·trac·tion
  si·nus
  sur·face
  tu·ber·os·i·ty
  vein
max·il·lary si·nus
  roent·gen·o·gram
max·il·lec·to·my
max·il·li·tis
max·il·lo·den·tal
max·il·lo·fa·cial
  pros·thet·ics
max·il·lo·ju·gal
max·il·lo·man·dib·u·lar
  fix·a·tion
  rec·ord
  reg·is·tra·tion
  re·la·tion
  trac·tion
max·il·lo·pal·a·tine
max·il·lot·o·my
max·il·lo·tur·bi·nal
max·i·mal
  dose
  stim·u·lus

max·i·mal His·ta·log
  test
max·i·mal per·mis·si·ble
  dose
Maximow's
  stain for bone mar·row
max·i·mum
  tem·per·a·ture
  ve·loc·i·ty
max·i·mum
  glu·cose trans·port m.
  trans·port m.
  tu·bu·lar m.
max·i·mum breath·ing
  ca·pac·i·ty
max·i·mum oc·cip·i·tal
  point
max·i·mum urea
  clear·ance
max·i·mum vol·un·tary
  ven·ti·la·tion
Maxwell's
  ring
  spot
May ap·ple
Mayaro
  vi·rus
Mayer-Rokitansky-Küster-Hauser
  syn·drome
Mayer's
  pes·sa·ry
  re·flex
Mayer's he·mal·um
  stain
Mayer's mu·ci·car·mine
  stain
Mayer's mu·ci·he·ma·te·in
  stain
May-Grünwald
  stain
May-Hegglin
  anom·a·ly
may·id·ism
Mayo
  bun·ion·ec·to·my
Mayo-Robson's
  point
  po·si·tion
Mayo's
  op·er·a·tion
  vein
May-White
  syn·drome
ma·za·mor·ra
maze
ma·zin·dol
ma·zo·dyn·ia
ma·zol·y·sis

ma·zo·path·ia
ma·zop·a·thy
ma·zo·pexy
ma·zo·pla·sia
Mazzoni's
   cor·pus·cle
Mazzotti
   re·ac·tion
   test
McArdle's
   dis·ease
McArdle-Schmid-Pearson
   dis·ease
McBurney's
   in·ci·sion
   point
McCarthy's
   re·flex·es
McCrea
   sound
Mc·Cune-Al·bright
   syn·drome
McDonald's
   ma·neu·ver
McGoon's
   tech·nique
McKee's
   line
McMurray
   test
m-cone
McPhail
   test
McReynolds'
   op·er·a·tion
McVay's
   op·er·a·tion
M:E
   ra·ti·o
mead·ow
   der·ma·ti·tis
   saf·fron
mead·ow grass
   der·ma·ti·tis
Mead·ows'
   syn·drome
meal
   worm
meal
   Boyden m.
   test m.
mean
   arith·me·tic m.
   ge·o·met·ric m.
   har·mon·ic m.
   stan·dard er·ror of the m.
mean
   cal·o·rie

tem·per·a·ture
vec·tor
mean cell
   he·mo·glo·bin
   vol·ume
mean cell he·mo·glo·bin
   con·cen·tra·tion
mean elec·tri·cal
   ax·is
mean foun·da·tion
   plane
Means'
   sign
mea·sle
mea·sles
   atyp·i·cal m.
   black m.
   Ger·man m.
   hem·or·rhag·ic m.
   three-day m.
   trop·i·cal m.
mea·sles
   im·mu·no·glob·u·lin
   vi·rus
mea·sles con·va·les·cent
   se·rum
mea·sles im·mune
   glob·u·lin (hu·man)
mea·sles, mumps, and ru·bel·la
   vac·cine
mea·sles vi·rus
   vac·cine
mea·sly
mea·sured
   in·tel·li·gence
mea·sure·ment
   end-point m.
   ki·net·ic m.
   na·si·on-po·go·ni·on m.
me·a·tal
   car·ti·lage
   spine
me·a·to·mas·toid·ec·to·my
me·a·tom·e·ter
me·a·to·plas·ty
me·a·tor·rha·phy
me·at·o·scope
me·a·tos·co·py
me·at·o·tome
me·a·tot·o·my
me·a·tus
   ex·ter·nal acous·tic m.
   ex·ter·nal au·di·to·ry m.
   fish-mouth m.
   in·ter·nal acous·tic m.
   in·ter·nal au·di·to·ry m.
   ure·ter·al m.
   m. uri·na·ri·us

me·a·tus
me·ban·a·zine
me·ben·da·zole
me·bev·er·ine hy·dro·chlo·ride
meb·hy·dro·line
me·bro·phen·hy·dra·mine
me·but·a·mate
mec·a·myl·a·mine hy·dro·chlo·
  ride
Mec·ca
  bal·sam
me·chan·i·cal
  abra·sion
  al·ter·na·tion
  an·ti·dote
  dys·men·or·rhea
  il·e·us
  in·tel·li·gence
  jaun·dice
  stra·bis·mus
  vec·tor
  ven·ti·la·tion
  ver·ti·go
me·chan·i·cal·ly bal·anced
  oc·clu·sion
me·chan·i·cal mix·ture
me·chan·i·co·re·cep·tor
me·chan·ics
  body m.
mech·a·nism
  as·so·ci·a·tion m.
  count·er·cur·rent m.
  de·fense m.
  Douglas m.
  Duncan's m.
  gat·ing m.
  im·mu·no·log·i·cal m.
  ping-pong m.
  pres·so·re·cep·tive m.
  pro·pri·o·cep·tive m.
  Schultze's m.
mech·a·no·car·di·og·ra·phy
mech·a·no·cyte
mech·a·no·pho·bia
mech·a·no·re·cep·tor
mech·a·no·re·flex
mech·a·no·ther·a·py
mèche
mech·lor·eth·a·mine hy·dro·
  chlo·ride
me·cil·li·nam
me·cism
Me·cis·to·cir·rus
Meckel
  scan
  syn·drome
Meckel-Gruber
  syn·drome

Meckel's
  band
  car·ti·lage
  cav·i·ty
  di·ver·tic·u·lum
  gan·gli·on
  lig·a·ment
  plane
  space
Mecke's
  re·a·gent
me·clas·tine
mec·li·zine hy·dro·chlo·ride
mec·lo·fen·a·mate so·di·um
mec·lo·fen·ox·ate
mec·lo·qua·lone
mec·lo·zine hy·dro·chlo·ride
me·com·e·ter
mec·o·nate
me·co·ni·al
  col·ic
me·con·ic ac·id
mec·o·nin
me·co·ni·or·rhea
me·co·nism
me·co·ni·um
  as·pi·ra·tion
  il·e·us
  per·i·to·ni·tis
me·co·ni·um block·age
  syn·drome
me·daz·e·pam hy·dro·chlo·ride
med·fal·an
me·di
  vi·rus
me·dia
me·di·ad
me·di·al
  an·gle of eye
  ar·te·ri·ole of ret·i·na
  ar·te·ri·o·scle·ro·sis
  can·thus
  con·dyle
  con·dyle of fe·mur
  con·dyle of tib·ia
  cord of brach·i·al plex·us
  crest
  em·i·nence
  ep·i·con·dyle
  ep·i·con·dyle of fe·mur
  ep·i·con·dyle of hu·mer·us
  fil·let
  lay·er
  lem·nis·cus
  lig·a·ment
  lig·a·ment of el·bow
  lig·a·ment of knee
  lig·a·ment of wrist

me·di·al *(continued)*
  limb
  lip of lin·ea as·pe·ra
  mal·le·o·lus
  mar·gin
  me·nis·cus
  nu·cle·us of thal·a·mus
  part
  plate of pter·y·goid pro·cess
  pole
  pro·cess of cal·ca·ne·al tu·
   ber·os·i·ty
  ret·i·nac·u·lum of pa·tel·la
  root of me·di·an nerve
  root of op·tic tract
  ro·ta·tor
  seg·ment
  sur·face
  sur·face of ar·y·te·noid car·
   ti·lage
  sur·face of ce·re·bral hem·
   i·sphere
  sur·face of fib·u·la
  sur·face of lung
  sur·face of ova·ry
  sur·face of tes·tis
  sur·face of tib·ia
  sur·face of ul·na
  tu·ber·cle of pos·te·ri·or
   pro·cess of ta·lus
  vein of lat·er·al ven·tri·cle
  ven·ule of ret·i·na
  wall of mid·dle ear
  wall of or·bit
me·di·al ac·ces·so·ry ol·i·vary
  nu·cle·us
me·di·al an·te·ri·or tho·rac·ic
  nerve
me·di·al ar·cu·ate
  lig·a·ment
me·di·al atri·al
  vein
me·di·al ba·sal
  seg·ment
me·di·al bi·cip·i·tal
  groove
me·di·al cal·ca·ne·o·cu·boid
  lig·a·ment
me·di·al car·ti·lag·i·nous
  lay·er
me·di·al cen·tral
  nu·cle·us of thal·a·mus
me·di·al cir·cum·flex
  ar·tery of thigh
me·di·al cir·cum·flex fem·o·ral
  veins
me·di·al cu·ne·i·form
  bone

me·di·al cu·ta·ne·ous
  nerve of arm
  nerve of fore·arm
  nerve of leg
me·di·a·lec·i·thal
me·di·al ep·i·con·dy·lar
  crest
  ridge
me·di·al fem·o·ral
  tu·ber·os·i·ty
me·di·al fore·brain
  bun·dle
me·di·al fron·to·ba·sal
  ar·tery
me·di·al ge·nic·u·late
  body
me·di·al great
  mus·cle
me·di·al ham·string
me·di·al in·fe·ri·or ge·nic·u·lar
  ar·tery
me·di·al in·gui·nal
  fos·sa
me·di·a·lis
me·di·al la·cu·nar
  node
me·di·al lon·gi·tu·di·nal
  arch
  bun·dle
  fas·cic·u·lus
  stri·a
me·di·al lum·bar in·ter·trans·
  verse
  mus·cles
me·di·al lum·bo·cos·tal
  arch
me·di·al mal·le·o·lar
  bur·sa
  net·work
  sur·face of ta·lus
me·di·al med·ul·lary
  lam·i·na of cor·pus stri·a·
   tum
me·di·al na·sal
  el·e·va·tion
  fold
  pro·cess
me·di·al oc·cip·i·tal
  ar·tery
me·di·al oc·cip·i·to·tem·po·ral
  gy·rus
me·di·al pal·pe·bral
  com·mis·sure
  lig·a·ment
me·di·al pec·to·ral
  nerve

me·di·al plan·tar
  ar·tery
  nerve
me·di·al pop·lit·e·al
  nerve
me·di·al pre·op·tic
  nu·cle·us
me·di·al pter·y·goid
  mus·cle
me·di·al pu·bo·pros·tat·ic
  lig·a·ment
me·di·al rec·tus
  mus·cle
me·di·al stri·ate
  ar·ter·ies
me·di·al su·pe·ri·or ge·nic·u·
  lar
  ar·tery
me·di·al su·pra·cla·vic·u·lar
  nerve
me·di·al su·pra·con·dy·lar
  crest
  ridge
me·di·al sym·pa·thet·ic
  line
me·di·al ta·lo·cal·ca·ne·al
  lig·a·ment
me·di·al tar·sal
  ar·tery
me·di·al um·bil·i·cal
  fold
  lig·a·ment
me·di·al vas·tus
  mus·cle
me·di·al ves·tib·u·lar
  nu·cle·us
me·di·an
  ap·er·ture of the fourth
    ven·tri·cle
  ar·tery
  bar of Mercier
  em·i·nence
  groove of tongue
  lar·yn·got·o·my
  line
  li·thot·o·my
  nerve
  plane
  re·la·tion
  rhi·nos·co·py
  stru·mec·to·my
  sul·cus of fourth ven·tri·cle
  vein of fore·arm
  vein of neck
me·di·an an·te·brach·i·al
  vein
me·di·an ar·cu·ate
  lig·a·ment

me·di·an at·lan·to·ax·i·al
  joint
me·di·an ba·sil·ic
  vein
me·di·an ce·phal·ic
  vein
me·di·an cu·bi·tal
  vein
me·di·an fron·tal
  sul·cus
me·di·an lon·gi·tu·di·nal
  ra·phe of tongue
me·di·an man·dib·u·lar
  point
me·di·an pal·a·tine
  su·ture
me·di·an re·trud·ed
  re·la·tion
me·di·an rhom·boid
  glos·si·tis
me·di·an sa·cral
  ar·tery
  crest
  vein
me·di·an thy·ro·hy·oid
  lig·a·ment
me·di·an tongue
  bud
me·di·a·nus
me·di·as·ti·nal
  em·phy·se·ma
  fi·bro·sis
  part
  space
  veins
me·di·as·ti·ni·tis
  id·i·o·path·ic fi·brous m.
me·di·as·ti·nog·ra·phy
  gas·e·ous m.
me·di·as·tin·o·per·i·car·di·tis
me·di·as·tin·o·scope
me·di·as·ti·nos·co·py
me·di·as·ti·not·o·my
me·di·as·ti·num
me·di·as·ti·num an·te·ri·us
me·di·as·ti·num in·fe·ri·us
me·di·as·ti·num me·di·um
me·di·as·ti·num pos·te·ri·us
me·di·as·ti·num su·pe·ri·us
me·di·ate
  aus·cul·ta·tion
  con·ta·gion
  per·cus·sion
  trans·fu·sion
me·di·a·tion
me·di·a·tor
  phar·ma·co·log·ic m.'s of
    an·a·phy·lax·is

med·i·ca·ble
med·i·cal
  anat·o·my
  care
  chem·is·try
  di·a·ther·my
  eth·ics
  ex·am·in·er
  ge·net·ics
  jur·is·pru·dence
  mod·el
  my·col·o·gy
  pa·thol·o·gy
  psy·chol·o·gy
  rec·ord
  se·lec·tion
  treat·ment
med·i·cal rec·ord
  link·age
med·i·cal tran·scrip·tion·ist
me·dic·a·ment
med·i·ca·men·to·sus
med·i·cate
med·i·cat·ed
med·i·ca·tion
  ar·rhen·ic m.
  ion·ic m.
  pre·an·es·thet·ic m.
med·i·ca·tor
me·di·ce·phal·ic
me·dic·i·nal
  char·coal
  chem·is·try
  erup·tion
  zinc per·ox·ide
me·dic·i·nal scar·let red
me·dic·i·nal soft
  soap
med·i·cine
  ad·o·les·cent m.
  aer·o·space m.
  avi·a·tion m.
  be·hav·ior·al m.
  clin·i·cal m.
  de·fen·sive m.
  ex·per·i·men·tal m.
  fam·i·ly m.
  fe·tal m.
  folk m.
  fo·ren·sic m.
  ho·lis·tic m.
  in·ter·nal m.
  le·gal m.
  mil·i·tary m.
  ne·o·na·tal m.
  nu·cle·ar m.
  os·te·o·path·ic m.
  pa·tent m.

per·i·na·tal m.
phys·i·cal m.
po·di·a·tric m.
pre·ven·tive m.
pro·pri·e·tary m.
psy·cho·so·mat·ic m.
quack m.
so·cial·ized m.
space m.
sports m.
trop·i·cal m.
vet·er·i·nary m.
med·i·co·bi·o·log·ic
med·i·co·bi·o·log·i·cal
med·i·co·chi·rur·gi·cal
med·i·co·le·gal
med·i·co·me·chan·i·cal
med·i·co·phys·i·cal
med·i·co·psy·chol·o·gy
me·di·o·car·pal
me·di·oc·cip·i·tal
me·di·o·col·ic
  sphinc·ter
me·di·o·dens
me·di·o·dor·sal
  nu·cle·us
me·di·o·lat·er·al
me·di·o·ne·cro·sis
  m. of the aor·ta
  m. aor·tae id·i·o·path·i·ca
    cys·ti·ca
me·di·o·pu·bic
  re·flex
me·di·o·tar·sal
  am·pu·ta·tion
me·di·o·tru·sion
me·di·o·type
me·di·sect
Med·i·ter·ra·ne·an
  ane·mia
  fe·ver
  lym·pho·ma
  thei·le·ri·o·sis
Med·i·ter·ra·ne·an ex·an·them·
  a·tous
  fe·ver
Med·i·ter·ra·ne·an-he·mo·glo·
  bin E
  dis·ease
me·di·um
  ar·tery
  vein
me·di·um
  clear·ing m.
  com·plete m.
  con·trast m.
  cul·ture m.
  Czapek-Dox m.

dis·per·sion m.
Dorset's cul·ture egg m.
Eagle's ba·sal m.
Eagle's min·i·mum es·sen·tial m.
Endo's m.
ex·ter·nal m.
Loeffler's blood cul·ture m.
mo·til·i·ty test m.
mount·ing m.
pas·sive m.
se·lec·tive m.
sep·a·rat·ing m.
Simmons' cit·rate m.
sup·port m.
Thayer-Martin m.
trans·port m.
me·di·us
me·dor·rhea
med·pha·lan
med·ro·ges·tone
me·drox·y·pro·ges·ter·one ac·e·tate
med·ryl·a·mine
med·ry·sone
me·dul·la
    m. of ad·re·nal gland
    m. glan·du·lae su·pra·re·na·lis
    m. of hair shaft
    m. of kid·ney
    m. of lymph node
    m. no·di lym·pha·ti·ci
me·dul·lae
me·dul·lar
med·ul·lary
    ar·ter·ies of brain
    bone
    cal·lus
    car·ci·no·ma
    cav·i·ty
    cen·ter
    che·mo·re·cep·tor
    cone
    cords
    groove
    lay·ers of thal·a·mus
    mem·brane
    plate
    pyr·a·mid
    py·ram·i·dot·o·my
    ray
    sar·co·ma
    sheath
    space
    stri·ae of the fourth ven·tri·cle
    stri·a of the thal·a·mus

    sub·stance
    te·ni·ae
    tube
med·ul·lary sponge
    kid·ney
med·ul·lat·ed
med·ul·lat·ed nerve
    fi·ber
med·ul·la·tion
med·ul·lec·to·my
med·ul·li·za·tion
me·dul·lo·ar·thri·tis
me·dul·lo·blas·to·ma
me·dul·lo·cell
me·dul·lo·ep·i·the·li·o·ma
    adult m.
    em·bry·o·nal m.
me·dul·lo·my·o·blas·to·ma
Me·du·sa
    head
Meeh
    for·mu·la
Meeh-Dubois
    for·mu·la
Mees'
    lines
    stripes
Meesman
    dys·tro·phy
mef·e·nam·ic ac·id
me·fen·o·rex hy·dro·chlo·ride
me·fex·a·mide
meg·a·bac·te·ri·um
meg·a·blad·der
meg·a·car·dia
meg·a·car·y·o·blast
meg·a·car·y·o·cyte
meg·a·ce·pha·lia
meg·a·ce·phal·ic
meg·a·ceph·a·lous
meg·a·ceph·a·ly
meg·a·cins
meg·a·coc·ci
meg·a·coc·cus
meg·a·co·lon
    con·gen·i·tal m.
    m. con·ge·ni·tum
    id·i·o·path·ic m.
    tox·ic m.
meg·a·cy·cle
meg·a·cys·tic
    syn·drome
meg·a·cys·tis
meg·a·dac·tyl·ia
meg·a·dac·tyl·ism
meg·a·dac·ty·ly
meg·a·dol·i·cho·co·lon
meg·a·dont

meg·a·don·tism
meg·a·dyne
meg·a·e·soph·a·gus
meg·a·ga·mete
meg·a·gna·thia
meg·a·hertz
meg·a·kar·y·o·blast
meg·a·kar·y·o·cyte
meg·a·kar·y·o·cyt·ic
  leu·ke·mia
meg·a·lec·i·thal
meg·al·gia
meg·a·lo·blast
meg·a·lo·blas·tic
  ane·mia
meg·a·lo·car·dia
meg·a·lo·ce·pha·lia
meg·a·lo·ceph·a·ly
meg·a·lo·chei·ria
meg·a·lo·chi·ria
meg·a·lo·cor·nea
meg·a·lo·cys·tis
meg·a·lo·cyte
meg·a·lo·cy·the·mia
meg·a·lo·cyt·ic
  ane·mia
meg·a·lo·cy·to·sis
meg·a·lo·dac·tyl·ia
meg·a·lo·dac·tyl·ism
meg·a·lo·dac·ty·ly
meg·a·lo·dont
meg·a·lo·don·tia
meg·a·lo·en·ce·phal·ic
meg·a·lo·en·ceph·a·lon
meg·a·lo·en·ceph·a·ly
meg·a·lo·en·ter·on
meg·a·lo·gas·tria
meg·a·lo·glos·sia
meg·a·lo·graph·ia
meg·a·lo·he·pat·ia
meg·a·lo·kar·y·o·cyte
meg·a·lo·ma·nia
meg·a·lo·ma·ni·ac
meg·a·lo·me·lia
meg·a·lon·y·cho·sis
meg·a·lo·pe·nis
meg·a·lo·phal·lus
meg·a·loph·thal·mus
  an·te·ri·or m.
meg·a·lo·pia
meg·a·lo·po·dia
meg·a·lop·sia
meg·a·lo·splanch·nic
meg·a·lo·sple·nia
meg·a·lo·spore
meg·a·lo·syn·dac·tyl·ia
meg·a·lo·syn·dac·ty·ly
meg·a·lo·u·re·ter

meg·a·lo·u·re·thra
meg·a·mer·o·zo·ite
meg·a·nu·cle·us
meg·a·pro·so·pia
meg·a·pros·o·pous
meg·a·rec·tum
meg·a·seme
meg·a·sig·moid
meg·a·so·mia
meg·a·spore
meg·a·throm·bo·cyte
meg·a·u·re·ter
meg·a·u·re·thra
meg·a·volt
meg·a·volt·age
me·ges·trol ac·e·tate
meg·lu·mine
  m. ac·e·tri·zo·ate
  m. di·a·tri·zo·ate
  m. io·thal·a·mate
meg·ohm
meg·oph·thal·mus
meg·ox·y·cyte
meg·ox·y·phil
meg·ox·y·phile
me·grim
mei·bo·mi·an
  bleph·a·ri·tis
  con·junc·ti·vi·tis
  cyst
  glands
  sty
mei·bo·mi·a·ni·tis
mei·bo·mi·tis
Meige's
  dis·ease
Meigs'
  syn·drome
Meinicke
  test
mei·o·sis
mei·ot·ic
  di·vi·sion
  drive
  phase
Meissel
Meissner's
  cor·pus·cle
  plex·us
me·lag·ra
me·lal·gia
mel·a·mine
  res·in
mel·a·mine form·al·de·hyde
mel·an·cho·lia
  hy·po·chon·dri·a·cal m.
  in·vo·lu·tion·al m.
mel·an·chol·ic

mel·an·choly
mel·an·e·de·ma
mel·a·ne·mia
mel·an·i·dro·sis
mel·a·nif·er·ous
mel·a·nin
    ar·ti·fi·cial m.
    fac·ti·tious m.
mel·a·nism
mel·a·no·am·e·lo·blas·to·ma
mel·a·no·blast
mel·a·no·blas·to·ma
mel·a·no·car·ci·no·ma
mel·a·noc·o·mous
mel·a·no·cyte
mel·a·no·cyte-stim·u·lat·ing
    hor·mone
mel·a·no·cy·to·ma
mel·a·no·den·dro·cyte
mel·a·no·der·ma
    m. ca·chec·ti·co·rum
    m. chlo·as·ma
    par·a·sit·ic m.
    ra·cial m.
    se·nile m.
mel·a·no·der·ma·ti·tis
mel·a·no·der·mic
me·la·no·gen
mel·a·no·ge·ne·mia
mel·a·no·gen·e·sis
mel·a·no·glos·sia
mel·a·noid
mel·a·no·ker·a·to·sis
mel·a·no·leu·ko·der·ma
    m. col·li
mel·a·no·ma
    ac·ral len·tig·i·nous m.
    amel·a·not·ic m.
    be·nign ju·ve·nile m.
    Cloudman m.
    ha·lo m.
    Harding-Passey m.
    ma·lig·nant m.
    ma·lig·nant len·ti·go m.
    ma·lig·nant m. in si·tu
    min·i·mal de·vi·a·tion m.
    nod·u·lar m.
    sub·un·gual m.
    su·per·fi·cial spread·ing m.
mel·a·no·ma·to·sis
mel·a·no·nych·ia
mel·a·nop·a·thy
mel·a·no·phage
mel·a·no·phore
mel·a·no·phore-ex·pand·ing
    prin·ci·ple
mel·a·no·pla·kia
mel·a·no·pro·tein

mel·a·nor·rha·gia
mel·a·nor·rhea
mel·a·no·sis
    m. cir·cum·scrip·ta pre·can·
      ce·ro·sa
    m. co·li
    m. co·rii de·ge·ne·ra·ti·va
    neu·ro·cu·ta·ne·ous m.
    oc·u·lo·der·mal m.
    pre·can·cer·ous m. of
      Dubreuilh
    Riehl's m.
mel·a·nos·i·ty
mel·a·no·some
    gi·ant m.
mel·a·not·ic
    car·ci·no·ma
    freck·le
    pig·ment
    pro·gon·o·ma
    whit·low
mel·a·not·ic neu·ro·ec·to·der·
    mal
    tu·mor
mel·a·not·ri·chous
mel·a·no·troph
me·la·no·tro·pin
mel·a·nu·ria
mel·a·nu·ric
mel·ar·so·prol
me·las·ma
    m. grav·i·dar·um
    m. uni·ver·sa·le
mel·a·ton·in
Melchior
me·le·na
    m. ne·o·na·to·rum
    m. spu·ria
    m. ve·ra
mel·e·nem·e·sis
Meleney's
    gan·grene
    ul·cer
mel·en·ges·trol ac·e·tate
mel·e·tin
mel·i·bi·ase
mel·i·bi·ose
mel·i·ce·ra
mel·i·ce·ris
mel·i·oi·do·sis
me·lis·sa
me·lis·so·pho·bia
me·li·tis
mel·i·tose
mel·i·tra·cen hy·dro·chlo·ride
mel·i·tri·ose
mel·i·tu·ria

Melkersson-Rosenthal
  syn·drome
mel·li·ta
mel·li·ti
mel·li·tum
Melnick-Needles
  syn·drome
mel·o·cer·vi·co·plas·ty
mel·o·ma·nia
mel·o·me·lia
me·lon·o·plas·ty
mel·on-seed
  body
Me·loph·a·gus
  M. ovi·nus
mel·o·plas·ty
mel·o·rhe·os·to·sis
mel·o·sal·gia
me·los·chi·sis
me·lo·tia
mel·pha·lan
melt·ing
  point
  tem·per·a·ture
  tem·per·a·ture of DNA
Meltzer-Lyon
  test
Meltzer's
  law
mem·ber
  vir·ile m.
mem·bra
mem·bra·na
  m. ab·do·mi·nis
  m. ad·a·man·ti·na
  m. ad·ven·ti·tia
  m. bas·i·la·ris
  m. cap·su·lar·is
  m. cap·su·lo·pu·pil·la·ris
  m. car·no·sa
  m. ce·re·bri
  m. cho·ri·o·cap·il·la·ris
  m. cor·dis
  m. cri·co·thy·roi·dea
  m. e·bor·is
  m. flac·ci·da
  m. fus·ca
  m. ger·mi·na·ti·va
  m. gran·u·lo·sa
  m. hy·a·loi·dea
  m. hy·o·thy·roi·dea
  m. lim·i·tans
  m. lim·i·tans gli·ae
  m. mu·co·sa
  m. nic·ti·tans
  m. pi·tu·i·to·sa
  m. pre·for·ma·ti·va
  m. se·ro·sa

  m. ser·o·ti·na
  m. stri·a·ta
  m. suc·cin·gens
  m. ten·sa
  m. ver·si·col·or
  m. vi·brans
  m. vit·el·li·na
mem·bra·na·ceous
mem·bra·nae
mem·bra·nate
mem·brane
  ad·a·man·tine m.
  al·lan·toid m.
  al·ve·o·lo·den·tal m.
  anal m.
  an·te·ri·or at·lan·to-oc·cip·
   i·tal m.
  arach·noid m.
  at·lan·to-oc·cip·i·tal m.
  base·ment m.
  bas·i·lar m.
  Bichat's m.
  Bogros' se·rous m.
  Bowman's m.
  Bruch's m.
  Brunn's m.
  buc·co·na·sal m.
  buc·co·pha·ryn·ge·al m.
  cell m.
  cho·ri·o·al·lan·to·ic m.
  clo·a·cal m.
  clos·ing m.'s
  Corti's m.
  cri·co·thy·roid m.
  cri·co·tra·che·al m.
  cri·co·vo·cal m.
  croup·ous m.
  de·cid·u·ous m.
  Descemet's m.
  diph·the·rit·ic m.
  drum m.
  Duddell's m.
  dys·men·or·rhe·al m.
  egg m.
  elas·tic m.
  em·bry·on·ic m.
  enam·el m.
  ep·i·pap·il·lary m.
  ep·i·ret·i·nal m.
  ex·o·ce·lom·ic m.
  false m.
  fen·es·trat·ed m.
  fer·til·i·za·tion m.
  fe·tal m.
  fi·brous m.
  Fielding's m.
  flac·cid m.
  germ m.

ger·mi·nal m.
glas·sy m.
Henle's m.
Henle's fen·es·trat·ed elas·
 tic m.
Heuser's m.
Hunter's m.
Huxley's m.
hy·a·line m.
hy·a·loid m.
hy·o·glos·sal m.
in·ter·cos·tal m.'s
in·ter·nal lim·it·ing m.
in·ter·os·se·ous m. of fore·
 arm
in·ter·os·se·ous m. of leg
ivo·ry m.
Jackson's m.
ker·a·tog·e·nous m.
lim·it·ing m. of neu·ral
 tube
lim·it·ing m. of ret·i·na
med·ul·lary m.
mu·cous m.'s
Nasmyth's m.
nic·ti·tat·ing m.
Nitabuch's m.
nu·cle·ar m.
ob·tu·ra·tor m.
ol·fac·to·ry m.
oral m.
or·o·na·sal m.
or·o·pha·ryn·ge·al m.
oto·lith·ic m.
out·er lim·it·ing m.
o·vu·lar m.
Payr's m.
per·i·car·di·o·pleur·al m.
per·i·den·tal m.
per·i·ne·al m.
per·i·o·don·tal m.
per·i·or·bi·tal m.
pha·ryn·ge·al m.'s
pi·al-gli·al m.
pi·tu·i·tary m.
pla·cen·tal m.
plas·ma m.
pleu·ro·per·i·car·di·al m.
pleu·ro·per·i·to·ne·al m.
pos·te·ri·or at·lan·to-oc·cip·
 i·tal m.
post·syn·ap·tic m.
pre·syn·ap·tic m.
pri·mary egg m.
pro·lig·er·ous m.
pro·phy·lac·tic m.
pu·pil·lary m.
py·o·gen·ic m.

qua·dran·gu·lar m.
Reissner's m.
re·tic·u·lar m.
Rivinus' m.
Ruysch's m.
Scarpa's m.
schnei·de·ri·an m.
Schultze's m.
sec·on·dary egg m.
sec·on·dary tym·pan·ic m.
sem·i·per·me·a·ble m.
se·rous m.
Shrapnell's m.
spi·ral m.
sta·pe·di·al m.
stat·o·co·ni·al m.
ster·nal m.
stri·at·ed m.
su·pra·pleu·ral m.
syn·o·vi·al m.
tec·to·ri·al m.
tec·to·ri·al m. of co·chle·ar
 duct
ter·ti·ary egg m.
thy·ro·hy·oid m.
Toldt's m.
Tourtual's m.
tym·pan·ic m.
m. of tym·pa·num
un·du·lat·ing m.
un·du·la·to·ry m.
unit m.
uro·gen·i·tal m.
uro·rec·tal m.
uter·o·ep·i·cho·ri·al m.
vag·i·nal syn·o·vi·al m.
ves·tib·u·lar m.
vir·gin·al m.
vi·tel·line m.
vit·re·ous m.
Wachendorf's m.
yolk m.
Zinn's m.
mem·brane
 bone
 po·ten·tial
mem·brane at·tack
 com·plex
mem·brane-coat·ing
 gran·ule
mem·bra·nec·to·my
mem·brane ex·pan·sion
 the·o·ry
mem·bra·nelle
mem·bra·ni·form
mem·bra·no·car·ti·lag·i·nous
mem·bra·noid

631

mem·bra·no·pro·lif·er·a·tive
  glo·mer·u·lo·ne·phri·tis
mem·bra·nous
  am·pul·la
  cat·a·ract
  co·chlea
  con·junc·ti·vi·tis
  dys·men·or·rhea
  glo·mer·u·lo·ne·phri·tis
  lab·y·rinth
  lar·yn·gi·tis
  lay·er
  lip·o·dys·tro·phy
  neu·ro·cra·ni·um
  os·si·fi·ca·tion
  part
  part of male ure·thra
  part of na·sal sep·tum
  phar·yn·gi·tis
  rhi·ni·tis
  sep·tum
  ure·thra
  vis·cer·o·cra·ni·um
  wall of mid·dle ear
  wall of tra·chea
mem·brum
  m. mu·li·e·bre
  m. vir·ile
mem·o·ry
  af·fect m.
  an·ter·o·grade m.
  long-term m.
  re·mote m.
  ret·ro·grade m.
  screen m.
  se·lec·tive m.
  se·nile m.
  short-term m.
  sub·con·scious m.
mem·o·ry
  loop
  span
  trace
mem·o·tine hy·dro·chlo·ride
men·ac·me
men·a·di·ol di·ac·e·tate
men·a·di·ol so·di·um di·phos·phate
men·a·di·one
  m. re·duc·tase
  m. so·di·um bi·sul·fite
men·aph·thone
men·a·quin·one
men·ar·che
men·ar·che·al
men·ar·chi·al
Mendel-Bechterew
  re·flex

Mendeléeff's
  law
men·de·le·vi·um
men·de·li·an
  char·ac·ter
  ge·net·ics
  in·her·i·tance
  ra·ti·o
men·del·ism
men·del·iz·ing
Mendel's
  laws
Mendel's in·step
  re·flex
Mendelson's
  syn·drome
Ménétrièr's
  dis·ease
  syn·drome
Menge's
  pes·sa·ry
Men·go
  en·ceph·a·li·tis
  vi·rus
Ménière's
  dis·ease
  syn·drome
me·nin·ge·al
  car·ci·no·ma
  car·ci·no·ma·to·sis
  her·nia
  leu·ke·mia
  plex·us
  veins
me·nin·ge·o·cor·ti·cal
me·nin·ge·or·rha·phy
me·nin·ges
me·nin·gi·o·ma
  cu·ta·ne·ous m.
  psam·mo·ma·tous m.
me·nin·gi·o·ma·to·sis
me·nin·gis
me·nin·gism
men·in·git·ic
  streak
men·in·git·i·des
men·in·gi·tis
  bas·i·lar m.
  cer·e·bro·spi·nal m.
  eo·sin·o·phil·ic m.
  ep·i·dem·ic cer·e·bro·spi·nal m.
  ep·i·du·ral m.
  ex·ter·nal m.
  in·ter·nal m.
  lis·te·ria m.
  me·nin·go·coc·cal m.
  ne·o·plas·tic m.

oc·clu·sive m.
otit·ic m.
se·rous m.
tu·ber·cu·lous m.
me·nin·go·cele
spu·ri·ous m.
trau·mat·ic m.
me·nin·go·ce·re·bral
cic·a·trix
me·nin·go·coc·cal
men·in·gi·tis
me·nin·go·coc·ce·mia
me·nin·go·coc·ci
me·nin·go·coc·cus
me·nin·go·cor·ti·cal
me·nin·go·cyte
me·nin·go·en·ceph·a·li·tis
acute pri·mary hem·or·rhag·
ic m.
bi·un·du·lant m.
eo·sin·o·phil·ic m.
her·pet·ic m.
mumps m.
pri·mary ame·bic m.
syph·i·lit·ic m.
me·nin·go·en·ceph·a·lo·cele
**me·nin·go·en·ceph·a·lo·my·e·li·
tis**
me·nin·go·en·ceph·a·lop·a·thy
me·nin·go·my·e·li·tis
me·nin·go·my·e·lo·cele
me·nin·go-os·te·o·phle·bi·tis
me·nin·go·ra·dic·u·lar
me·nin·go·ra·dic·u·li·tis
me·nin·gor·rha·chid·i·an
me·nin·gor·rha·gia
men·in·go·sis
me·nin·go·ty·phoid
fe·ver
me·nin·go·vas·cu·lar
syph·i·lis
men·in·gu·ria
me·ninx
m. fi·bro·sa
m. pri·mi·ti·va
m. se·ro·sa
m. ten·u·is
m. vas·cu·lo·sa
men·is·cec·to·my
me·nis·ci
men·is·ci·tis
me·nis·co·cyte
me·nis·co·cy·to·sis
me·nis·co·fem·o·ral
lig·a·ments
me·nis·co·pexy
men·is·cor·rha·phy
me·nis·co·tome

me·nis·cus
ar·tic·u·lar m.
con·verg·ing m.
di·verg·ing m.
lat·er·al m.
me·di·al m.
neg·a·tive m.
per·i·scop·ic m.
pos·i·tive m.
tac·tile m.
me·nis·cus
lens
Menkes'
syn·drome
men·o·ce·lis
men·o·me·tror·rha·gia
men·o·pau·sal
syn·drome
men·o·pause
men·o·pha·nia
Men·o·pon
men·or·rha·gia
men·or·rhal·gia
me·nos·che·sis
men·o·sta·sia
me·nos·ta·sis
men·o·stax·is
men·o·tro·pins
men·o·u·ria
men·o·xe·nia
men·ses
men·strua
men·stru·al
col·ic
cy·cle
ede·ma
leu·kor·rhea
mo·lim·i·na
pe·ri·od
scle·ro·sis
men·stru·al ex·trac·tion
abor·tion
men·stru·ant
men·stru·ate
men·stru·a·tion
an·ov·u·lar m.
an·ov·u·la·tion·al m.
non·ov·u·la·tion·al m.
re·tained m.
ret·ro·grade m.
sup·ple·men·tary m.
sup·pressed m.
vi·car·i·ous m.
men·stru·um
men·su·al
men·su·ra·tion
men·tag·ra

men·tal
  ab·er·ra·tion
  age
  agraph·ia
  ap·pa·ra·tus
  ar·tery
  ca·nal
  chro·nom·e·try
  de·fi·cien·cy
  dis·ease
  dis·or·der
  dis·tur·bance
  fo·ra·men
  health
  hos·pi·tal
  hy·giene
  ill·ness
  im·age
  im·pair·ment
  im·pres·sion
  nerve
  point
  pro·cess
  pro·tu·ber·ance
  re·gion
  re·tar·da·tion
  sco·to·ma
  spine
  struc·ture
  sym·phy·sis
  tu·ber·cle
men·tal
men·ta·lis
men·tal·i·ty
men·ta·tion
Men·tha
men·thane
men·thol
  cam·phor·at·ed m.
men·ti
men·to·an·te·ri·or
  po·si·tion
men·to·la·bi·al
  fur·row
men·to·la·bi·a·lis
men·ton
men·to·plas·ty
men·to·pos·te·ri·or
  po·si·tion
men·to·trans·verse
  po·si·tion
men·tum
men·yan·thes
mep·a·crine hy·dro·chlo·ride
me·par·fy·nol
mep·a·zine ac·e·tate
me·pen·zo·late bro·mide
me·per·i·dine hy·dro·chlo·ride

me·phen·e·sin
me·phen·ox·a·lone
me·phen·ter·mine
  m. sul·fate
me·phen·y·to·in
me·phit·ic
meph·o·bar·bi·tal
me·piv·a·caine hy·dro·chlo·ride
me·pred·ni·sone
me·pro·ba·mate
me·pyr·a·mine ma·le·ate
me·pyr·a·pone
me·ral·gia
  m. par·a·es·thet·i·ca
mer·al·lu·ride
mer·bro·min
mer·cap·tal
mer·cap·tan
  meth·yl m.
mer·cap·to·a·ce·tic ac·id
mer·cap·tol
mer·cap·tom·er·in so·di·um
mer·cap·to·pu·rine
mer·cap·tu·ric ac·id
Mercier's
  bar
  sound
  valve
mer·co·cre·sols
mer·cu·ma·til·in
mer·cu·ra·mide
mer·cu·ri·al
  line
  ma·nom·e·ter
  sto·ma·ti·tis
  trem·or
mer·cu·ri·a·len·tis
mer·cu·ri·a·lism
p-mer·cur·i·ben·zo·ate
mer·cu·ric
mer·cu·ric chlo·ride
  am·mo·ni·at·ed m. c.
mer·cu·ric io·dide
mer·cu·ric ole·ate
mer·cu·ric ox·ide
mer·cu·ric sa·lic·y·late
mer·cu·ro·phen
mer·cu·ro·phyl·line so·di·um
mer·cu·rous
mer·cu·rous chlo·ride
mer·cu·rous io·dide
mer·cu·ry
  am·mo·ni·at·ed m.
  m. bi·chlo·ride
  m. bin·i·o·dide
  cor·ro·sive m. chlo·ride
  m. deu·to·i·o·dide
  m. per·chlo·ride

m. pro·to·i·o·dide
m. sub·sa·lic·y·late
yel·low m. io·dide
mer·cu·ry
arc
poi·son·ing
Merendino's
tech·nique
mer·e·prine
mer·e·thox·yl·line pro·caine
me·rid·i·an
m. of cor·nea
m.'s of eye
me·rid·i·ani
me·rid·i·a·nus
me·rid·i·o·nal
ab·er·ra·tion
cleav·age
fi·bers
mer·i·spore
mer·i·ste·mat·ic
me·ris·tic
var·i·a·tion
Merkel cell
tu·mor
Merkel's
cor·pus·cle
fil·trum ven·tric·u·li
fos·sa
mus·cle
Merkel's tac·tile
cell
disk
mer·maid
de·for·mi·ty
mer·o·a·cra·nia
mer·o·an·en·ceph·a·ly
mer·o·blas·tic
cleav·age
mer·o·cele
mer·o·crine
gland
mer·o·di·a·stol·ic
mer·o·gen·e·sis
mer·o·ge·net·ic
mer·o·gen·ic
me·rog·o·ny
mer·o·me·lia
mer·o·mi·cro·so·mia
mer·o·my·o·sin
H-m.
L-m.
mer·ont
mer·o·ra·chis·chi·sis
mer·or·rha·chis·chi·sis
me·ros·mia
mer·o·sys·tol·ic
me·rot·o·my

mer·o·zo·ite
me·ro·zy·gote
mer·pha·lan
Merrifield
knife
mer·sa·lyl
m. ac·id
m. the·o·phyl·line
Méry's
gland
Merzbacher-Pelizaeus
dis·ease
me·sad
me·sal
me·sal·a·mine
mes·a·me·boid
mes·an·gi·al
cell
ne·phri·tis
mes·an·gi·al pro·lif·er·a·tive
glo·mer·u·lo·ne·phri·tis
mes·an·gi·o·cap·il·lary
glo·mer·u·lo·ne·phri·tis
mes·an·gi·um
ex·tra·glo·mer·u·lar m.
mes·a·or·ti·tis
mes·a·ra·ic
mes·a·re·ic
mes·ar·ter·i·tis
me·sat·i·ce·phal·ic
me·sat·i·pel·lic
pel·vis
me·sat·i·pel·vic
mes·ax·on
mes·cal but·tons
mes·ca·line
me·sec·tic
mes·ec·to·derm
mes·en·ce·phal·ic
flex·ure
nu·cle·us of the tri·gem·i·nus
teg·men·tum
tract of tri·gem·i·nal nerve
veins
mes·en·ceph·a·li·tis
mes·en·ceph·a·lon
mes·en·ceph·a·lot·o·my
me·sen·chy·ma
me·sen·chy·mal
cells
ep·i·the·li·um
hy·lo·ma
tis·sue
mes·en·chyme
in·ter·zon·al m.
syn·o·vi·al m.
mes·en·chy·mo·ma

mes·en·ter·ic
  glands
  her·nia
  veins
mes·en·ter·ic ar·tery
  oc·clu·sion
mes·en·ter·ic lymph
  nodes
mes·en·ter·i·co·pa·ri·e·tal
  fos·sa
  re·cess
mes·en·ter·i·o·lum
  m. pro·ces·sus ver·mi·for·
    mis
mes·en·ter·i·o·pexy
mes·en·ter·i·or·rha·phy
mes·en·ter·i·pli·ca·tion
mes·en·ter·i·tis
mes·en·te·ri·um
  m. dor·sa·le com·mune
mes·en·ter·on
mes·en·tery
  m. of ap·pen·dix
  uro·gen·i·tal m.
mes·eth·moid
  bone
mesh
  graft
mesh·work
  tra·bec·u·lar m.
me·si·ad
me·si·al
  an·gle
  car·ies
  dis·place·ment
  oc·clu·sion
  sur·face of tooth
me·si·o·buc·cal
me·si·o·buc·co-oc·clu·sal
me·si·o·buc·co·pul·pal
me·si·o·cer·vi·cal
me·si·o·clu·sion
me·si·o·dens
me·si·o·dis·tal
me·si·o·dis·toc·clu·sal
me·si·o·gin·gi·val
me·si·o·gnath·ic
me·si·o·in·ci·sal
me·si·o·la·bi·al
me·si·o·lin·gual
me·si·o·lin·guo-oc·clu·sal
me·si·o·lin·guo·pul·pal
me·si·on
me·sio-oc·clu·sal
me·sio-oc·clu·sion
me·si·o·place·ment
me·si·o·pul·pal
me·si·o·ver·sion

mes·mer·ism
mes·mer·ize
meso
  com·pounds
mes·o·ap·pen·dix
mes·o·ar·i·um
mes·o·bi·lane
mes·o·bi·lene
mes·o·bil·i·ru·bin
mes·o·bil·i·ru·bin·o·gen
mes·o·bil·i·vi·o·lin
mes·o·blast
mes·o·blas·te·ma
mes·o·blas·tem·ic
mes·o·blas·tic
  ne·phro·ma
  seg·ment
  sen·si·bil·i·ty
mes·o·car·dia
mes·o·car·di·um
  dor·sal m.
  ven·tral m.
mes·o·car·pal
mes·o·ca·val
  shunt
mes·o·ce·cal
mes·o·ce·cum
mes·o·ce·phal·ic
mes·o·ceph·a·lous
mes·o·col·ic
mes·o·col·ic lymph
  nodes
mes·o·co·lon
mes·o·co·lon as·cen·dens
mes·o·co·lon de·scen·dens
mes·o·co·lon sig·moi·de·um
mes·o·co·lon trans·ver·sum
mes·o·co·lo·pexy
mes·o·co·lo·pli·ca·tion
mes·o·cord
mes·o·cu·ne·i·form
mes·o·derm
  bran·chi·al m.
  ex·tra·em·bry·on·ic m.
  gas·tral m.
  in·ter·me·di·ate m.
  in·tra·em·bry·on·ic m.
  lat·er·al m.
  lat·er·al plate m.
  par·ax·i·al m.
  pri·mary m.
  pro·sto·mi·al m.
  sec·on·dary m.
  so·mat·ic m.
  so·mit·ic m.
  splanch·nic m.
  vis·cer·al m.
mes·o·der·mic

mes·o·di·a·stol·ic
mes·o·dont
mes·o·du·o·de·nal
mes·o·du·o·de·num
mes·o·en·te·ri·o·lum
mes·o·ep·i·did·y·mis
mes·o·gas·ter
mes·o·gas·tric
mes·o·gas·tri·um
mes·o·gen·ic
mes·o·ge·ni·ta·le
me·sog·lia
me·sog·li·al
   cells
mes·o·glu·te·al
mes·o·glu·te·us
mes·o·gnath·ic
mes·o·gna·thi·on
me·sog·na·thous
mes·o·il·e·um
mes·o·je·ju·num
mes·o·lep·i·do·ma
me·sol·o·bus
mes·o·lym·pho·cyte
mes·o·me·lia
mes·o·mel·ic
   dwarf·ism
mes·o·mere
mes·o·mer·ic
me·som·er·ism
mes·o·met·a·neph·ric
   car·ci·no·ma
mes·o·met·ric
   preg·nan·cy
mes·o·me·tri·tis
mes·o·me·tri·um
mes·o·morph
mes·o·mor·phic
me·son
mes·o·neph·ric
   ad·e·no·car·ci·no·ma
   duct
   fold
   rest
   ridge
   tis·sue
   tu·bule
mes·o·neph·roi
mes·o·neph·roid
   tu·mor
mes·o·ne·phro·ma
mes·o·neph·ros
mes·o·neu·ri·tis
   nod·u·lar m.
meso-on·to·morph
mes·o·pexy
mes·o·phil
mes·o·phile

mes·o·phil·ic
mes·o·phle·bi·tis
mes·o·phrag·ma
me·soph·ry·on
me·sop·ic
   pe·rim·e·try
mes·o·por·phy·rins
mes·o·pro·sop·ic
mes·o·pul·mon·um
me·sor·chi·al
me·sor·chi·um
mes·o·rec·tum
mes·o·rid·a·zine be·syl·ate
mes·or·rha·chis·chi·sis
mes·or·rha·phy
mes·or·rhine
mes·o·sal·pinx
mes·o·scope
mes·o·seme
mes·o·sig·moid
mes·o·sig·moid·i·tis
mes·o·sig·moid·o·pexy
mes·o·so·ma·tous
mes·o·so·mia
mes·o·ste·ni·um
mes·o·ster·num
mes·o·syph·i·lis
mes·o·sys·tol·ic
mes·o·tar·sal
mes·o·ten·di·ne·um
mes·o·ten·don
mes·o·the·lia
mes·o·the·li·al
   cell
   hy·lo·ma
mes·o·the·li·o·ma
   be·nign m. of gen·i·tal tract
mes·o·the·li·um
mes·o·tho·ri·um
mes·o·tro·pic
mes·o·u·ran·ic
mes·o·va·ria
mes·o·va·ri·an
   mar·gin
mes·o·va·ri·um
Mes·o·zoa
mes·sen·ger
   first m.
   sec·ond m.
mes·sen·ger
   RNA
mes·tan·o·lone
mes·tene·di·ol
mes·tra·nol
me·sul·phen
me·su·ran·ic
me·tab·a·sis
met·a·bi·o·sis

met·a·bi·sul·fite
  test
met·a·bol·ic
  ac·i·do·sis
  al·ka·lo·sis
  co·ma
  cra·ni·op·a·thy
  en·ceph·a·lop·a·thy
  equiv·a·lent
  in·di·can
  pool
met·a·bol·ic mu·ci·no·sis
met·a·bo·lim·e·ter
me·tab·o·lin
me·tab·o·lism
  ba·sal m.
  car·bo·hy·drate m.
  elec·tro·lyte m.
  fat m.
  pro·tein m.
  res·pi·ra·to·ry m.
me·tab·o·lite
me·tab·o·lize
me·tab·o·lized vi·ta·min D
  milk
met·a·bu·teth·am·ine hy·dro·
  chlo·ride
met·a·bu·tox·y·caine hy·dro·
  chlo·ride
met·a·car·pal
  in·dex
  lig·a·ments
  veins
met·a·car·pec·to·my
met·a·car·pi
met·a·car·po·hy·po·the·nar
  re·flex
met·a·car·po·pha·lan·ge·al
  ar·tic·u·la·tions
  joints
met·a·car·po·the·nar
  re·flex
met·a·car·pus
met·a·cen·tric
  chro·mo·some
met·a·cer·ca·ria
met·a·cer·ca·ri·ae
met·a·ces·tode
met·a·chlo·ral
met·a·chro·ma·sia
met·a·chro·mat·ic
  bod·ies
  gran·ules
  leu·ko·dys·tro·phy
  stain
met·a·chro·ma·tism
met·a·chrom·ing
met·a·chro·mo·phil

met·a·chro·mo·phile
me·tach·ro·nous
met·a·chro·sis
met·a·cone
met·a·co·nid
met·a·con·trast
met·a·con·ule
met·a·cre·sol
met·a·cryp·to·zo·ite
met·a·cy·e·sis
met·a·dys·en·tery
met·a·fa·cial
  an·gle
met·a·gen·e·sis
Met·a·gon·i·mus
met·a·her·pet·ic
  ker·a·ti·tis
met·a·hy·po·phy·si·al
  di·a·be·tes
met·a·ic·ter·ic
met·a·in·fec·tive
met·a·ki·ne·sia
met·a·ki·ne·sis
met·al
  al·ka·li m.
  al·ka·li earth m.
  Babbitt m.
  base m.
  ba·sic m.
  col·loi·dal m.
  d'Arcet's m.
  fu·si·ble m.
  light m.
  no·ble m.
  rare earth m.
  res·pi·ra·to·ry m.
met·al
  base
  in·ter·face
met·al·de·hyde
met·al fume
  fe·ver
met·al in·sert
  teeth
me·tal·lic
  rale
  trem·or
me·tal·lo·cy·a·nide
me·tal·lo·en·zyme
me·tal·lo·fla·vo·de·hy·drog·e·
  nase
met·al·loid
me·tal·lo·phil·ia
me·tal·lo·pho·bia
me·tal·lo·por·phy·rin
me·tal·lo·pro·tein
met·al·los·co·py
me·tal·lo·thi·o·nein

met·a·lu·et·ic
met·a·mer
met·a·mere
met·a·mer·ic
met·a·mer·ic ner·vous
   sys·tem
me·tam·er·ism
met·a·mor·phop·sia
met·a·mor·pho·sis
   com·plete m.
   fat·ty m.
   het·er·o·me·tab·o·lous m.
   hol·o·me·tab·o·lous m.
   in·com·plete m.
   ret·ro·grade m.
met·a·mor·phot·ic
met·a·my·el·o·cyte
met·a·neph·ric
   bud
   cap
   di·ver·tic·u·lum
   duct
   tu·bule
met·a·neph·rine
met·a·neph·ro·gen·ic
   tis·sue
met·a·ne·phrog·e·nous
met·a·neph·roi
met·a·neph·ros
met·a·neu·tro·phil
met·a·neu·tro·phile
met·a·nil yel·low
met·a·phase
met·a·phos·phor·ic ac·id
met·a·phy·se·al
me·taph·y·ses
met·a·phy·si·al
   dys·os·to·sis
   dys·pla·sia
met·a·phy·si·al fi·brous cor·ti·
cal
   de·fect
me·taph·y·sis
me·taph·y·si·tis
met·a·pla·sia
   ag·no·gen·ic my·e·loid m.
   ap·o·crine m.
   au·to·par·en·chym·a·tous m.
   in·tes·ti·nal m.
   my·e·loid m.
   pri·mary my·e·loid m.
   sec·on·dary my·e·loid m.
   squa·mous m.
   squa·mous m. of am·ni·on
   symp·to·mat·ic my·e·loid
   m.
me·tap·la·sis
met·a·plasm

met·a·plas·tic
   ane·mia
   car·ci·no·ma
   os·si·fi·ca·tion
   pol·yp
met·a·plex·us
met·a·poph·y·sis
met·a·pore
met·a·pro·tein
met·a·pro·ter·e·nol sul·fate
met·a·psy·chol·o·gy
met·a·py·ret·ic
met·a·py·ro·cat·e·chase
met·a·ram·i·nol bi·tar·trate
met·ar·te·ri·ole
met·a·ru·bri·cyte
   per·ni·cious ane·mia type
   m.
met·a·sta·ble
me·tas·ta·ses
me·tas·ta·sis
   bi·o·chem·i·cal m.
   cal·car·e·ous m.
   pul·sat·ing me·tas·ta·ses
   sat·el·lite m.
me·tas·ta·size
met·a·stat·ic
   ab·scess
   cal·ci·fi·ca·tion
   car·ci·no·ma
   cho·roid·i·tis
   mumps
   oph·thal·mia
   pneu·mo·nia
   ret·i·ni·tis
met·a·stat·ic car·ci·noid
   syn·drome
met·a·ster·num
met·a·stron·gyle
Met·a·stron·gy·lus
   M. ap·ri
   M. elon·ga·tus
   M. pu·den·do·tec·tus
   M. sal·mi
met·a·syph·i·lis
met·a·syph·i·lit·ic
met·a·tar·sal
   ar·tery
   lig·a·ments
   re·flex
met·a·tar·sal·gia
met·a·tar·sec·to·my
me·ta·tar·si
met·a·tar·so·pha·lan·ge·al
   ar·tic·u·la·tions
   joints
met·a·tar·sus
   m. ad·duc·to·var·us

met·a·tar·sus *(continued)*
   m. ad·duc·tus
   m. at·a·vi·cus
   m. la·tus
   m. var·us
met·a·thal·a·mus
me·tath·e·sis
met·a·troph
met·a·tro·phic
met·a·tro·pic
   dwarf·ism
met·a·typ·i·cal
   car·ci·no·ma
me·tax·a·lone
Met·a·zoa
met·a·zo·o·no·sis
Metchnikoff's
   the·o·ry
met·en·ce·phal·ic
met·en·ceph·a·lon
Metenier's
   sign
met·en·keph·a·lin
me·te·or·ism
me·te·or·op·a·thy
me·te·or·o·tro·pic
me·ter
   at·om m.
   rate m.
   ven·ti·la·tion m.
   Venturi m.
me·ter
   an·gle
me·ter-can·dle
met·er·ga·sia
me·ter-kil·o·gram-sec·ond
   sys·tem
   unit
met·es·trum
met·es·trus
met·for·min
meth·a·cho·line chlo·ride
meth·ac·ry·late
   res·in
meth·a·cryl·ic ac·id
meth·a·cy·cline hy·dro·chlo·ride
meth·a·done hy·dro·chlo·ride
meth·al·len·es·tril
meth·am·phet·a·mine hy·dro·
   chlo·ride
meth·am·py·rone
meth·an·di·e·none
meth·an·dri·ol
meth·an·dro·sten·o·lone
meth·ane
Meth·a·no·bac·te·ri·a·ce·ae
meth·an·o·gen

meth·a·nol
   fix·a·tive
meth·an·the·line bro·mide
meth·a·pyr·i·lene
meth·a·qua·lone
meth·ar·bi·tal
meth·ar·gen
meth·a·zo·la·mide
meth·dil·a·zine hy·dro·chlo·ride
met·hem·al·bu·min
met·hem·al·bu·mi·ne·mia
met·he·mo·glo·bin
   m. re·duc·tase
met·he·mo·glo·bi·ne·mia
   ac·quired m.
   con·gen·i·tal m.
   en·ter·og·e·nous m.
   he·red·i·tary m.
   pri·mary m.
   sec·on·dary m.
met·he·mo·glo·bi·nu·ria
meth·en·a·mine
   m. hip·pu·rate
   m. man·del·ate
   m. sa·lic·y·late
meth·en·a·mine-sil·ver
meth·ene
meth·i·cil·lin so·di·um
meth·im·a·zole
me·thi·o·dal so·di·um
me·thi·o·nine
   ac·tive m.
   m. aden·o·syl·trans·fer·ase
   m. sulf·ox·ime
me·thi·o·nine-ac·ti·vat·ing
   en·zyme
me·thi·o·nyl
   di·pep·ti·dase
me·this·a·zone
me·thix·ene hy·dro·chlo·ride
meth·o·car·ba·mol
meth·od
   Abbott's m.
   Abell-Kendall m.
   ac·ti·vat·ed sludge m.
   Altmann-Gersh m.
   Anel's m.
   Antyllus' m.
   ar·is·to·te·lian m.
   Ashby m.
   aux·an·o·graph·ic m.
   Barraquer's m.
   Beck's m.
   Bier's m.
   Born m. of wax plate re·
   con·struc·tion
   Brasdor's m.

broad mar·gi·nal con·fron·ta·tion m.
Callahan's m.
Carpue's m.
Charters' m.
Chayes' m.
chlo·ro·per·cha m.
closed cir·cuit m.
con·fron·ta·tion m.
cooled-knife m.
cop·per sul·fate m.
cor·re·la·tion·al m.
Credé's m.'s
cross-sec·tion·al m.
de·fin·i·tive m.
Dick m.
Dieffenbach's m.
dif·fu·sion m.
di·rect m. for mak·ing in·lays
disk sen·si·tiv·i·ty m.
dou·ble an·ti·body m.
Edman m.
Eggleston m.
Eicken's m.
ex·per·i·men·tal m.
flash m.
flo·ta·tion m.
Gärtner's m.
Gerota's m.
glu·cose ox·i·dase m.
Gräupner's m.
Gruber's m.
Hammerschlag's m.
hex·o·ki·nase m.
Hilton's m.
Hirschberg's m.
Holmgren m.
Hung's m.
im·mu·no·flu·o·res·cence m.
im·ped·ance m.
In·di·an m.
in·di·rect m. for mak·ing in·lays
in·do·phe·nol m.
in·tro·spec·tive m.
Ital·ian m.
Jaboulay's m.
Johnson's m.
Keating-Hart's m.
Kjeldahl m.
Klapp's m.
Krause's m.
Lamaze m.
Langendorff's m.
Lee-White m.
Liborius' m.
Ling's m.

Lister's m.
lod m.
lon·gi·tu·di·nal m.
mac·ro-Kjeldahl m.
Marshall's m.
mi·cro-Astrup m.
mi·cro-Kjeldahl m.
Moore's m.
Müller's m.
Needles' split cast m.
Nikiforoff's m.
Ochsner's m.
Ollier's m.
open cir·cuit m.
Orsi-Grocco m.
Pachon's m.
par·a·cel·si·an m.
par·al·lax m.
Pavlov m.
Politzer m.
Porges m.
Purmann's m.
Quick's m.
ref·er·ence m.
Rehfuss m.
Reverdin's m.
rhythm m.
Rideal-Walker m.
Roux's m.
Scarpa's m.
Schäfer's m.
Schede's m.
Schick m.
Schmidt-Thannhauser m.
Shaffer-Hartman m.
Somogyi m.
split cast m.
Stas-Otto m.
Stroganoff's m.
Thane's m.
Theden's m.
Thiersch's m.
thi·o·chrome m.
ul·tro·paque m.
Wardrop's m.
Westergren m.
Wheeler m.
Wilson's m.
Wolfe's m.
zinc sul·fate flo·ta·tion cen·trif·u·ga·tion m.
me·thod·i·cal
cho·rea
meth·o·hex·i·tal so·di·um
meth·o·in
me·tho·ni·um
com·pounds
meth·o·phen·a·zine

meth·o·pho·line
meth·op·ter·in
meth·or·phi·nan
meth·o·ser·pi·dine
meth·o·trex·ate
meth·o·tri·mep·ra·zine
me·thox·a·mine hy·dro·chlo·ride
me·thox·sa·len
me·thox·y·flu·rane
me·thox·yl
me·thox·y·phen·a·mine hy·dro·chlo·ride
meth·sco·pol·a·mine bro·mide
meth·sux·i·mide
meth·y·clo·thi·a·zide
meth·yl
  ac·tive m.
  m. al·co·hol
  m. al·de·hyde
  an·gu·lar m.
  m. chlo·ride
  m. cys·te·ine hy·dro·chlo·ride
  m. hy·drox·y·ben·zo·ate
  m. iso·bu·tyl ke·tone
  m. meth·ac·ry·late
  m. nic·o·tin·ate
  m. sa·lic·y·late
meth·yl
  mer·cap·tan
meth·yl·a·cryl·ic ac·id
meth·yl·am·phet·a·mine hy·dro·chlo·ride
meth·yl·ate
meth·yl·at·ed
  spir·it
meth·yl·a·tion
meth·yl·at·ro·pine bro·mide
meth·yl·ben·zene
meth·yl·ben·ze·tho·ni·um chlo·ride
meth·yl blue
meth·yl·car·no·sine
meth·yl·cel·lu·lose
meth·yl·chlo·ro·form
meth·yl·cys·te·ine syn·thase
meth·yl·di·hy·dro·mor·phi·none hy·dro·chlo·ride
meth·yl·do·pa
meth·yl·ene
meth·yl·ene az·ure
meth·yl·ene blue
  Kühne's m. b.
  Loeffler's m. b.
  new m. b.
  pol·y·chrome m. b.

meth·yl·ene·suc·cin·ic ac·id
meth·yl·ene white
meth·yl·en·o·phil
meth·yl·en·o·phile
meth·yl·en·o·phil·ic
meth·yl·e·noph·i·lous
meth·yl·er·go·met·rine ma·le·ate
meth·yl·er·go·no·vine ma·le·ate
meth·yl·glu·ca·mine
  m. di·a·tri·zo·ate
  m. io·dip·a·mide
meth·yl·gly·ox·al
  m. bis(gua·nl·hy·dra·zone)
meth·yl·gly·ox·a·lase
meth·yl green
meth·yl green-py·ro·nin
  stain
meth·yl·hex·ane·a·mine
meth·yl·ki·nase
meth·yl·ma·lon·ic ac·id
meth·yl·ma·lon·ic ac·i·de·mia
meth·yl·ma·lon·ic ac·i·du·ria
meth·yl·mal·o·nyl-CoA mu·tase
meth·yl·mor·phine
meth·yl·nor·tes·tos·ter·one
meth·yl·ol
  ri·bo·fla·vin
meth·yl or·ange
meth·y·lose
meth·yl·par·a·ben
meth·yl·pen·tose
meth·yl·phen·i·date hy·dro·chlo·ride
meth·yl·pred·nis·o·lone
  m. ac·e·tate
  so·di·um m. suc·ci·nate
meth·yl red
meth·yl·ros·an·i·line chlo·ride
meth·yl·tes·tos·ter·one
meth·yl·thi·o·a·den·o·sine
meth·yl·thi·o·u·ra·cil
meth·yl·to·col
meth·yl·trans·fer·ase
meth·yl vi·o·let
meth·yl yel·low
meth·y·pry·lon
meth·y·pry·lone
meth·y·ser·gide ma·le·ate
me·thys·ti·cum
met·my·o·glo·bin
met·o·clo·pra·mide hy·dro·chlo·ride
met·o·cur·ine io·dide
me·tol·a·zone
me·ton·y·my
me·top·a·gus

me·top·ic
  point
  su·ture
me·to·pi·on
met·o·pism
met·o·pon hy·dro·chlo·ride
met·o·po·plas·ty
met·o·pos·co·py
me·to·pro·lol tar·trate
Met·or·chis
me·tox·e·nous
me·tox·e·ny
me·tra
me·tra·to·nia
me·tra·tro·phia
me·trat·ro·phy
me·tria
me·tri·al
  gland
met·ric
  sys·tem
me·tri·fo·nate
met·ri·o·ce·phal·ic
me·tri·tis
  con·ta·gious equine m.
me·triz·a·mide
met·ri·zo·ate so·di·um
me·tro·cyte
me·tro·dy·na·mom·e·ter
me·tro·dyn·ia
me·tro·fi·bro·ma
me·trog·ra·phy
me·tro·lym·phan·gi·tis
me·tro·ma·la·cia
me·tro·ma·la·co·ma
me·tro·mal·a·co·sis
met·ro·ma·nia
met·ro·ni·da·zole
me·tron·o·scope
me·tro·pa·ral·y·sis
me·tro·path·ia
  m. hem·or·rha·gi·ca
me·tro·path·ic
me·trop·a·thy
me·tro·per·i·to·ne·al
  fis·tu·la
me·tro·per·i·to·ni·tis
me·tro·phle·bi·tis
met·ro·plas·ty
me·tror·rha·gia
  m. my·o·path·i·ca
me·tror·rhea
me·tror·rhex·is
me·tro·sal·pin·gi·tis
me·tro·sal·pin·gog·ra·phy
me·tro·scope
me·tro·stax·is
me·tro·ste·no·sis

me·trot·o·my
me·tro·tro·phic
  test
me·tyr·a·pone
me·ty·ro·sine
mev·a·lon·ic ac·id
me·vin·o·lin
mex·e·none
Mex·i·can
  tea
Mex·i·can hat
  cell
  cor·pus·cle
Mex·i·can spot·ted
  fe·ver
mex·il·e·tin hy·dro·chlo·ride
Meyenburg-Altherr-Uehlinger
  syn·drome
Meyenburg's
  com·plex
  dis·ease
Meyer-Archambault
  loop
Meyer-Betz
  syn·drome
Meyer-Overton
  the·o·ry of nar·co·sis
Meyer's
  car·ti·lag·es
  dis·ease
  line
  re·a·gent
  si·nus
Meyer-Schwickerath
  op·er·a·tion
Meyer-Schwickerath and Weyers
  syn·drome
Meynert's
  cells
  com·mis·sures
  de·cus·sa·tion
  fas·cic·u·lus
  lay·er
Meynert's ret·ro·flex
  bun·dle
mez·lo·cil·lin so·di·um
MHA-TP
  test
mi·an·eh
  dis·ease
  fe·ver
mi·an·ser·in hy·dro·chlo·ride
Mibelli's
  an·gi·o·ker·a·to·mas
  dis·ease
mi·cel·lar
mi·celle

Michaelis
  con·stant
Michaelis-Gutmann
  body
Michaelis-Menten
  con·stant
  equa·tion
  hy·poth·e·sis
Michel's
  spur
mi·con·a·zole ni·trate
mi·cra·cou·stic
mi·cren·ce·pha·lia
mi·cren·ceph·a·lous
mi·cren·ceph·a·ly
mi·cro·ab·scess
  Munro's m.
  Pautrier's m.
mi·cro·ad·e·no·ma
mi·cro·ae·ro·bi·on
mi·cro·aer·o·phil
mi·cro·aer·o·phile
mi·cro·aer·o·phil·ic
mi·cro·aer·oph·i·lous
mi·cro·aer·o·sol
mi·cro·a·nal·y·sis
mi·cro·a·nas·to·mo·sis
mi·cro·a·nat·o·mist
mi·cro·a·nat·o·my
mi·cro·an·eu·rysm
mi·cro·an·gi·og·ra·phy
mi·cro·an·gi·o·path·ic he·mo·
  lyt·ic
  ane·mia
mi·cro·an·gi·op·a·thy
  throm·bot·ic m.
mi·cro·an·gi·os·co·py
mi·cro·ar·te·ri·og·ra·phy
mi·cro-As·trup
  meth·od
mi·cro·bal·ance
mi·crobe
mi·cro·bi·al
  ge·net·ics
  per·sis·tence
  RNase II
  vi·ta·min
Mi·cro·bi·al as·so·ci·ates
mi·cro·bic
mi·cro·bi·ci·dal
mi·cro·bi·cide
mi·cro·bid
mi·cro·bi·o·log·ic
mi·cro·bi·ol·o·gist
mi·cro·bi·ol·o·gy
mi·cro·bi·ot·ic
mi·cro·bism
  la·tent m.

mi·cro·blast
mi·cro·ble·pha·ria
mi·cro·bleph·a·rism
mi·cro·bleph·a·ron
mi·cro·body
mi·cro·bra·chia
mi·cro·bren·ner
mi·cro·car·dia
mi·cro·cen·trum
mi·cro·ce·pha·lia
mi·cro·ce·phal·ic
mi·cro·ceph·a·lism
mi·cro·ceph·a·lous
mi·cro·ceph·a·ly
  en·ceph·a·lo·clas·tic m.
  schiz·en·ce·phal·ic m.
mi·cro·chei·lia
mi·cro·chei·ria
mi·cro·chem·is·try
mi·cro·chi·lia
mi·cro·chi·ria
mi·cro·cide
mi·cro·cin·e·ma·tog·ra·phy
mi·cro·cir·cu·la·tion
Mi·cro·coc·ca·ce·ae
mi·cro·coc·cal
  en·do·nu·cle·ase
  nu·cle·ase
mi·cro·coc·ci
Mi·cro·coc·cus
  M. can·di·dus
  M. con·glo·me·ra·tus
  M. cry·o·phi·lus
  M. fla·vus
  M. lu·te·us
  M. mor·rhua
  M. ure·ae
  M. va·ri·ans
mi·cro·coc·cus
mi·cro·co·li·tis
mi·cro·co·lon
mi·cro·co·nid·ia
mi·cro·co·nid·i·um
mi·cro·co·ria
mi·cro·cor·nea
mi·cro·cou·lomb
mi·cro·cou·stic
mi·cro·crys·tal·line
  cel·lu·lose
mi·cro·cu·rie
mi·cro·cyst
mi·cro·cys·tic
  dis·ease of re·nal me·dul·la
mi·cro·cys·tic ep·i·the·li·al
  dys·tro·phy
mi·cro·cyte
mi·cro·cy·the·mia

mi·cro·cyt·ic
   ane·mia
mi·cro·cy·to·sis
mi·cro·dac·tyl·ia
mi·cro·dac·ty·lous
mi·cro·dac·ty·ly
mi·cro·dis·sec·tion
mi·cro·dont
mi·cro·don·tia
mi·cro·don·tism
mi·cro·dose
mi·cro·drep·a·no·cyt·ic
   ane·mia
mi·cro·drep·a·no·cy·to·sis
mi·cro·dys·ge·ne·sia
mi·cro·e·lec·tric
   waves
mi·cro·e·lec·trode
mi·cro·en·ceph·a·ly
mi·cro·e·ryth·ro·cyte
mi·cro·ev·o·lu·tion
mi·cro·fi·bril
mi·cro·fil·a·ment
mi·cro·fil·a·re·mia
mi·cro·fi·lar·ia
mi·cro·fi·lar·i·ae
mi·cro·fi·lar·i·al
   sheath
mi·cro·fol·lic·u·lar
   ad·e·no·ma
   goi·ter
mi·cro·ga·mete
mi·cro·ga·me·to·cyte
mi·cro·gam·ont
mi·crog·a·my
mi·cro·gas·tria
mi·cro·gen·ia
mi·cro·gen·i·tal·ism
mi·cro·glan·du·lar
   ad·e·no·sis
mi·crog·lia
   cells
mi·crog·li·a·cyte
mi·crog·li·al
   cells
mi·crog·li·o·ma
mi·cro·gli·o·ma·to·sis
mi·crog·li·o·sis
mi·cro·glos·sia
mi·cro·gna·thia
   m. with pe·ro·me·lia
mi·cro·gram
mi·cro·graph
   elec·tron m.
mi·crog·ra·phy
mi·cro·gy·ria

mi·cro·he·mag·glu·ti·na·tion-
   Trep·o·ne·ma pal·li·dum
   test
mi·cro·he·pat·ia
mi·crohm
mi·cro·in·cin·er·a·tion
mi·cro·in·cis·ion
mi·cro·in·va·sion
mi·cro·in·va·sive
   car·ci·no·ma
mi·cro-Kjeldahl
   meth·od
mi·cro·ky·mat·o·ther·a·py
mi·cro·lec·i·thal
   egg
mi·cro·leu·ko·blast
mi·cro·li·ter
mi·cro·lith
mi·cro·li·thi·a·sis
   pul·mo·nary al·ve·o·lar m.
mi·crol·o·gy
mi·cro·ma·nia
mi·cro·ma·nip·u·la·tion
mi·cro·ma·nip·u·la·tor
mi·cro·ma·zia
mi·cro·me·lia
mi·cro·mel·ic
   dwarf·ism
mi·cro·mere
mi·cro·mer·o·zo·ite
mi·cro·me·tas·ta·sis
mi·cro·met·a·stat·ic
   dis·ease
mi·crom·e·ter
   cal·i·per m.
   fi·lar m.
   oc·u·lar m.
   slide m.
mi·crom·e·try
mi·cro·mi·cro·gram
mi·cro·mi·cron
mi·cro·mo·lar
mi·cro·mole
mi·cro·mo·to·scope
mi·cro·my·e·lia
mi·cro·my·el·o·blast
mi·cro·my·el·o·blas·tic
   leu·ke·mia
mi·cron
mi·cro·nee·dle
mi·cro·neme
mi·cro·neu·ro·vas·cu·lar
   anas·to·mo·sis
mi·cron·ic
mi·cro·nod·u·lar
mi·cro·nu·cle·us
mi·cro·nu·tri·ents
mi·cro·nych·ia

mi·cro·nys·tag·mus
mi·cro-ohm
mi·cro·or·gan·ism
mi·cro·par·a·site
mi·cro·pa·thol·o·gy
mi·cro·pe·nis
mi·cro·phage
mi·cro·phag·o·cyte
mi·cro·phal·lus
mi·cro·pho·bia
mi·cro·phone
mi·cro·pho·nia
mi·cro·pho·no·scope
mi·croph·o·ny
mi·cro·pho·to·graph
mi·croph·thal·mia
mi·croph·thal·mos
mi·cro·pi·pet
mi·cro·pi·pette
mi·cro·pla·nia
mi·cro·pla·sia
mi·cro·pleth·ys·mog·ra·phy
mi·cro·po·dia
mi·cro·pore
mi·cro·pre·cip·i·ta·tion
   test
mi·cro·pro·my·el·o·cyte
mi·cro·pro·so·pia
mi·crop·sia
mi·cro·punc·ture
mi·cro·pyle
mi·cro·ra·di·og·ra·phy
mi·cro·re·frac·tom·e·ter
mi·cro·res·pi·rom·e·ter
mi·cro·sac·cades
mi·cro·scin·tig·ra·phy
mi·cro·scope
  bin·oc·u·lar m.
  col·or-con·trast m.
  com·par·a·tor m.
  com·pound m.
  dark-field m.
  elec·tron m.
  flu·o·res·cence m.
  fly·ing spot m.
  Greenough m.
  in·fra·red m.
  in·ter·fer·ence m.
  la·ser m.
  opaque m.
  op·er·at·ing m.
  phase m.
  phase-con·trast m.
  po·lar·iz·ing m.
  Rheinberg m.
  scan·ning elec·tron m.
  sim·ple m.
  sin·gle m.

  ster·e·o·scop·ic m.
  stro·bo·scop·ic m.
  sur·gi·cal m.
  tel·e·vi·sion m.
  ultra-m.
  ul·tra·son·ic m.
  ul·tra·vi·o·let m.
  x-ray m.
mi·cro·scop·ic
  anat·o·my
  field
  he·ma·tu·ria
  sec·tion
  sphinc·ter
mi·cro·scop·i·cal
mi·cros·co·py
  elec·tron m.
  flu·o·res·cence m.
  im·mer·sion m.
  im·mune elec·tron m.
  im·mu·no·flu·o·res·cence m.
mi·cro·seme
mi·cro·sides
mi·cros·mat·ic
mi·cro·some
mi·cro·so·mia
mi·cro·spec·tro·pho·tom·e·try
mi·cro·spec·tro·scope
mi·cro·sphe·ro·cy·to·sis
mi·cro·sphyg·my
mi·cro·sphyx·ia
mi·cro·splanch·nic
mi·cro·sple·nia
Mi·cro·spo·ra
Mi·cro·spo·ra·si·da
Mi·cro·spo·rida
Mi·cros·po·rum
  M. au·dou·i·nii
  M. ca·nis
  M. dis·tor·tum
  M. fer·ru·gi·ne·um
  M. ful·vum
  M. gal·li·nae
  M. gyp·se·um
  M. na·num
  M. per·si·col·or
  M. van·breu·se·ghe·mi
mi·cro·steth·o·phone
mi·cro·steth·o·scope
mi·cro·sto·mia
mi·cro·sur·gery
mi·cro·su·ture
mi·cro·sy·ringe
mi·cro·the·lia
mi·cro·tia
mi·cro·tome
mi·crot·o·my
mi·cro·to·nom·e·ter

Mi·cro·trom·bid·i·um
mi·cro·tro·pia
mi·cro·tu·bule
 sub·pel·lic·u·lar m.
mi·cro·vas·cu·lar
 anas·to·mo·sis
mi·cro·ves·i·cle
mi·cro·vil·li
mi·cro·vil·lus
Mi·cro·vir·i·dae
mi·cro·volt
mi·cro·wave
 ther·a·py
mi·cro·waves
mi·cro·weld·ing
mi·crox·y·phil
mi·cro·zo·on
mi·crur·gi·cal
mic·tion
mic·tu·rate
mic·tu·ri·tion
 re·flex
 syn·co·pe
mid·ax·il·lary
 line
mi·daz·o·lam
mi·daz·o·lam hy·dro·chlo·ride
mid·body
mid·brain
 deaf·ness
 teg·men·tum
 ves·i·cle
mid·car·pal
mid·cla·vic·u·lar
 line
mid·di·a·stol·ic
 mur·mur
mid·dle
 cells
 con·cha
 fin·ger
 kid·ney
 lobe of pros·tate
 lobe of right lung
 pain
 piece
 si·nus·es
 trunk
mid·dle at·lan·to·ep·i·stroph·ic
 joint
mid·dle ax·il·lary
 line
mid·dle cal·ca·ne·al ar·tic·u·lar
 sur·face
mid·dle car·di·ac
 vein
mid·dle car·pal
 joint

mid·dle cer·e·bel·lar
 pe·dun·cle
mid·dle ce·re·bral
 ar·tery
mid·dle cer·vi·cal
 fas·cia
 gan·gli·on
mid·dle cer·vi·cal car·di·ac
 nerve
mid·dle clu·ne·al
 nerves
mid·dle col·ic
 ar·tery
 vein
mid·dle col·ic lymph
 nodes
mid·dle col·lat·er·al
 ar·tery
mid·dle con·stric·tor
 mus·cle of phar·ynx
mid·dle cos·to·trans·verse
 lig·a·ment
mid·dle cra·ni·al
 fos·sa
mid·dle cu·ne·i·form
 bone
mid·dle ear
mid·dle fron·tal
 con·vo·lu·tion
 gy·rus
 sul·cus
mid·dle ge·nic·u·lar
 ar·tery
mid·dle glos·so·ep·i·glot·tic
 fold
mid·dle hem·or·rhoi·dal
 ar·tery
 plex·us·es
 veins
mid·dle he·pa·tic
 veins
mid·dle lobe
 syn·drome
mid·dle me·nin·ge·al
 ar·tery
 nerve
 veins
mid·dle rec·tal
 ar·tery
 node
 plex·us·es
 veins
mid·dle sa·cral
 ar·tery
 plex·us
mid·dle sca·lene
 mus·cle

mid·dle su·pra·cla·vic·u·lar
  nerve
mid·dle su·pra·re·nal
  ar·tery
mid·dle tem·po·ral
  ar·tery
  con·vo·lu·tion
  gy·rus
  sul·cus
  vein
mid·dle thy·roid
  vein
mid·dle tur·bi·nat·ed
  bone
mid·dle um·bil·i·cal
  fold
  lig·a·ment
mid·for·ceps
  de·liv·ery
mid·gas·tric trans·verse
  sphinc·ter
midg·et bi·po·lar
  cells
mid·grac·ile
mid·gut
mid·life
  cri·sis
mid·line
  my·e·lot·o·my
mid·men·stru·al
mid·no·dal
  ex·tra·sys·to·le
  rhythm
mid·oc·cip·i·tal
mid·pain
mid·plane
mid·riff
mid·sag·it·tal
  plane
mid·sec·tion
mid·sig·moid
  sphinc·ter
mid·ster·num
mid·tar·sal
  joint
mid·wife
mid·wife·ry
Miescher's
  elas·to·ma
  gran·u·lo·ma·to·sis
  tubes
mi·gnon
  lamp
mi·graine
  head·ache
mi·graine
  ab·dom·i·nal m.
  clas·sic m.

com·mon m.
ful·gu·rat·ing m.
Harris' m.
hem·i·ple·gic m.
oph·thal·mic m.
oph·thal·mo·ple·gic m.
mi·grat·ing
  ab·scess
  teeth
mi·gra·tion
  the·o·ry
mi·gra·tion
  ep·i·the·li·al m.
  m. of ovum
mi·gra·tion in·hi·bi·tion
  test
mi·gra·tion-in·hib·i·tory
  fac·tor
mi·gra·to·ry
  oph·thal·mia
  pneu·mo·nia
mi·ka
  op·er·a·tion
Mikulicz
  clamp
Mikulicz'
  aph·thae
  cells
  dis·ease
  drain
  op·er·a·tion
  syn·drome
Mikulicz-Vladimiroff
  am·pu·ta·tion
mild
  sil·ver pro·tein
Miles
  re·sec·tion
Miles'
  op·er·a·tion
mil·ia
Milian's
  dis·ease
  er·y·the·ma
mil·i·a·ria
  m. al·ba
  ap·o·crine m.
  m. cry·stal·li·na
  m. pro·fun·da
  pus·tu·lar m.
  m. ru·bra
mil·i·a·ry
  ab·scess
  an·eu·rysm
  em·bo·lism
  fe·ver
  tu·ber·cu·lo·sis

mil·i·a·ry pap·u·lar
  syph·i·lid
mil·ieu
  ther·a·py
mil·ieu
  m. in·té·ri·eur
  m. in·terne
mil·i·tar·y
  med·i·cine
  neu·ro·sis
mil·i·um
  col·loid m.
milk
  ac·i·doph·i·lus m.
  m. of bis·muth
  bud·de·ized m.
  cer·ti·fied m.
  cer·ti·fied pas·teur·ized m.
  con·densed m.
  crop m.
  for·ti·fied vi·ta·min D m.
  ir·ra·di·at·ed vi·ta·min D
   m.
  lac·to·bac·il·la·ry m.
  m. of mag·ne·sia
  me·tab·o·lized vi·ta·min D
   m.
  mod·i·fied m.
  per·hy·drase m.
  pi·geon's m.
  skim m.
  skimmed m.
  m. of sul·fur
  uter·ine m.
  vi·ta·min D m.
  witch's m.
milk
  ane·mia
  col·ic
  cor·pus·cle
  crust
  cyst
  ducts
  fac·tor
  fe·ver
  gland
  leg
  line
  ridge
  scall
  sick·ness
  spots
  sug·ar
  tet·ter
  tooth
milk-al·ka·li
  syn·drome

milk-e·jec·tion
  re·flex
milk·ers'
  nodes
  nod·ules
Milkman's
  syn·drome
milk·pox
milk-ring
  test
milky
  as·ci·tes
  urine
mill
  fe·ver
Millard-Gubler
  syn·drome
milled-in
  curves
  paths
Miller-Abbott
  tube
mill·er's
  asth·ma
Miller's chem·i·co·par·a·sit·ic
  the·o·ry
Milles'
  syn·drome
mil·let seed
mil·li·am·pere
mil·li·bar
mil·li·cu·rie
mil·li·e·quiv·a·lent
mil·li·gram
mil·li·gram·age
mil·li·gram hour
mil·li·lam·bert
mil·li·li·ter
mil·li·me·ter
mil·li·mi·cron
mil·li·mole
mil·ling-in
mil·li·os·mole
mil·li·pede
mil·li·sec·ond
mil·li·volt
Millon
  re·ac·tion
Millon-Nasse
  test
Millon's
  re·a·gent
mill wheel
  mur·mur
mil·pho·sis
Milroy's
  dis·ease

Milton's
dis·ease
mi·me·sis
mi·met·ic
cho·rea
mus·cles
pa·ral·y·sis
mim·ic
con·vul·sion
genes
spasm
tic
mim·ma·tion
Minamata
dis·ease
mind
blind·ness
pain
mind
pre·log·i·cal m.
sub·con·scious m.
mind-read·ing
min·er·al
wa·ter
wax
min·er·al·o·coid
min·er·al·o·cor·ti·coid
min·er·al oil
min·er's
asth·ma
cramps
dis·ease
el·bow
lung
nys·tag·mus
Minerva
jack·et
min·i·a·ture
stom·ach
min·i·a·ture scar·let
fe·ver
min·i·lap·a·rot·o·my
min·im
min·i·mal
air
dose
min·i·mal al·ve·o·lar
con·cen·tra·tion
min·i·mal al·ve·o·lar an·es·
thet·ic
con·cen·tra·tion
min·i·mal am·pli·tude
nys·tag·mus
min·i·mal brain
dys·func·tion
min·i·mal-change
dis·ease

min·i·mal-change neph·rot·ic
syn·drome
min·i·mal de·vi·a·tion
mel·a·no·ma
min·i·mal in·fect·ing
dose
min·i·mal in·hib·i·to·ry
con·cen·tra·tion
min·i·mal le·thal
dose
min·i·mal re·act·ing
dose
min·i·mum
light
tem·per·a·ture
min·i·mum light
thresh·old
mink en·ter·i·tis
vi·rus
Min·ne·so·ta mul·ti·pha·sic
per·son·al·i·ty in·ven·to·ry
test
min·o·cy·cline
mi·nor
ag·glu·ti·nin
am·pu·ta·tion
ca·li·ces
con·nec·tor
hyp·no·sis
hys·te·ria
op·er·a·tion
sur·gery
tran·quil·iz·er
mi·nor du·o·de·nal
pa·pil·la
mi·nor sal·i·vary
glands
mi·nor sub·lin·gual
ducts
mi·nox·i·dil
mint
mi·nus
lens
strand
min·ute
out·put
vol·ume
mi·o·car·dia
mi·o·did·y·mus
mi·od·y·mus
mi·o·lec·i·thal
mi·o·nec·tic
mi·o·pra·gia
mi·o·pus
mi·o·sis
par·a·lyt·ic m.
spas·tic m.
mi·o·sphyg·mia

mi·o·stag·min
  re·ac·tion
mi·ot·ic
mi·ra·cid·ia
mi·ra·cid·i·um
Mirchamp's
  sign
mire
Mirrizzi's
  syn·drome
mir·ror
  hap·lo·scope
  im·age
  speech
mir·ror
  con·cave m.
  con·vex m.
  head m.
  mouth m.
  van Helmont's m.
mir·ror-im·age
  cell
mir·ror-writ·ing
mir·yach·it
mis·an·dry
mis·an·thro·py
mis·car·riage
mis·car·ry
mis·ce·ge·na·tion
mis·ci·ble
mis·di·ag·no·sis
mis·di·rec·tion
  phe·nom·e·non
mis·e·ro·tia
mi·sog·a·my
mi·sog·y·ny
mis·o·lo·gia
mis·o·ne·ism
mis·o·pe·dia
mis·op·e·dy
missed
  abor·tion
  la·bor
  pe·ri·od
mis·sense
  mu·ta·tion
mist
  ba·cil·lus
mis·tle·toe
Mitchell's
  dis·ease
  treat·ment
mite
  ty·phus
mi·tel·la
mith·ra·my·cin
mith·ri·da·tism
mi·ti·ci·dal

mi·ti·cide
mit·i·gate
mi·tis
mi·to·chon·dria
mi·to·chon·dri·al
  gene
  ma·trix
  my·op·a·thy
  sheath
mi·to·chon·dri·on
  m. of he·mo·flag·el·lates
mi·to·gen
  poke·weed m.
mi·to·gen·e·sis
mi·to·ge·net·ic
mi·to·gen·ic
mi·to·my·cin
mi·to·ses
mi·to·sis
  het·er·o·type m.
  mul·ti·po·lar m.
  so·mat·ic m.
mi·to·tane
mi·tot·ic
  di·vi·sion
  fig·ure
  in·dex
  pe·ri·od
  rate
  spin·dle
mi·to·xan·trone hy·dro·chlo·ride
mi·tral
  ar·ea
  cells
  click
  com·mis·sur·ot·o·my
  fa·ci·es
  gra·di·ent
  in·com·pe·tence
  in·suf·fi·cien·cy
  mur·mur
  or·i·fice
  re·gur·gi·ta·tion
  ste·no·sis
  tap
  valve
mi·tral·i·za·tion
mi·tral valve
  pro·lapse
mit·ra·my·cin
Mitsuda
  an·ti·gen
  re·ac·tion
mit·tel·schmerz
Mitzuo's
  phe·nom·e·non

mixed
ag·glu·ti·na·tion
apha·sia
astig·ma·tism
beat
chan·cre
es·o·tro·pia
gland
gli·o·ma
glyc·er·ides
hy·per·li·pe·mia
in·fec·tion
leu·ke·mia
nerve
pa·ral·y·sis
throm·bus
to·coph·er·ols con·cen·trate
tu·mor
tu·mor of sal·i·vary gland
tu·mor of skin
mixed ag·glu·ti·na·tion
re·ac·tion
test
mixed cell
leu·ke·mia
mixed con·nec·tive-tis·sue
dis·ease
mixed ex·pired
gas
mixed lym·pho·cyte
cul·ture
mixed lym·pho·cyte cul·ture
re·ac·tion
test
mixed mes·o·der·mal
tu·mor
mix·ing
phe·no·typ·ic m.
mix·ture
Bordeaux m.
ex·tem·po·ra·ne·ous m.
Miyagawa
bod·ies
Mi·ya·ga·wa·nel·la
MKS
unit
mks
unit
MLC
test
MM
vi·rus
M-mode
M'Naghten
rule
mne·me
mne·men·ic

mne·mic
hy·poth·e·sis
the·o·ry
mne·mism
mne·mon·ic
mne·mon·ics
MNSs
an·ti·gens
MNSs blood group
mo·bile
spasm
mo·bi·li·za·tion
sta·pes m.
mo·bi·lize
Mobitz types of atri·o·ven·tric·u·lar
block
Möbius
dis·ease
Möbius'
sign
syn·drome
mo·dal
al·ter·a·tion
mo·dal·i·ty
mode
mod·el
an·i·mal m.
Bingham m.
com·put·er m.
med·i·cal m.
mod·el
game
mod·el·ing
com·po·si·tion
com·pound
plas·tic
mod·er·ate
hy·po·ther·mia
mod·er·a·tor
band
mod·i·fi·ca·tion
be·hav·ior m.
mod·i·fied
milk
small·pox
mod·i·fied rad·i·cal
hys·ter·ec·to·my
mas·tec·to·my
mod·i·fied zinc ox·ide-eu·ge·nol
ce·ment
mod·i·fi·er
gene
mo·di·o·li
mo·di·o·lus
m. la·bii
mod·u·la·tion

mod·u·la·tion trans·fer
  func·tion
mo·du·lus
  bulk m.
  m. of elas·tic·i·ty
  m. of vol·ume elas·tic·i·ty
  Young's m.
Moeller's
  glos·si·tis
Moeller's grass
  ba·cil·lus
mo·fe·bu·ta·zone
mo·gen
  clamp
mog·i·ar·thria
mog·i·graph·ia
mog·i·la·lia
mog·i·pho·nia
Mohrenheim's
  fos·sa
  space
Mohs
  scale
Mohs' fresh tis·sue che·mo·
  sur·gery
  tech·nique
moi·e·ty
moist
  gan·grene
  pap·ule
  rale
  tet·ter
  wart
Mo·ko·la
  vi·rus
mo·lal
mo·lal·i·ty
mo·lar
  first m.
  first per·ma·nent m.
  Moon's m.'s
  mul·ber·ry m.
  sec·ond m.
  sixth-year m.
  third m.
  twelfth-year m.
mo·lar
  ab·sorp·tiv·i·ty
  be·hav·ior
  con·cen·tra·tion
  glands
  preg·nan·cy
  tooth
mo·lar ab·sorb·an·cy
  in·dex
mo·lar ab·sorp·tion
  co·ef·fi·cient

mo·lar ex·tinc·tion
  co·ef·fi·cient
mo·lar·i·form
mo·lar·i·ty
mold
  guide
mold·ing
  bor·der m.
  com·pres·sion m.
  in·jec·tion m.
  tis·sue m.
mole
  blood m.
  Breus m.
  car·ne·ous m.
  cys·tic m.
  false m.
  fleshy m.
  grape m.
  hairy m.
  hy·da·tid m.
  hy·da·tid·i·form m.
  in·va·sive m.
  spi·der m.
  ve·sic·u·lar m.
mole
  frac·tion
mo·lec·u·lar
  ane·mia
  be·hav·ior
  bi·ol·o·gy
  dis·ease
  dis·per·sion
  dis·til·la·tion
  for·mu·la
  ge·net·ics
  heat
  lay·er
  lay·er of cer·e·bel·lar cor·
    tex
  lay·er of ce·re·bral cor·tex
  lay·er of ret·i·na
  lay·ers of ol·fac·to·ry bulb
  move·ment
  pa·thol·o·gy
  ro·ta·tion
  sieve
  weight
mo·lec·u·lar dis·persed
  so·lu·tion
mo·lec·u·lar dis·so·ci·a·tion
  the·o·ry
mo·lec·u·lar weight
  ra·ti·o
mol·e·cule
mol·i·la·lia

mo·li·men
  m. cli·mac·te·re·i·um vir·ile
  men·stru·al mo·lim·i·na
mo·lim·i·na
mo·lin·done hy·dro·chlo·ride
Molisch's
  test
mol·li·ti·es
Moll's
  glands
mol·lusc
Mol·lus·ca
mol·lus·cous
mol·lus·cum
  m. con·ta·gi·o·sum
  m. fi·bro·sum
  m. fi·bro·sum grav·i·dar·um
  m. ver·ru·co·sum
mol·lus·cum
  body
  con·junc·ti·vi·tis
  cor·pus·cle
mol·lus·cum con·ta·gi·o·sum
  vi·rus
mol·lusk
Moloney
  test
Moloney's
  vi·rus
molt
mo·lyb·date
mo·lyb·den·ic
mo·lyb·de·nous
mo·lyb·de·num
mo·lyb·dic
mo·lyb·dic ac·id
mo·lyb·dous
mo·lys·mo·pho·bia
mom·ism
mo·nad
Monakow's
  bun·dle
  nu·cle·us
  syn·drome
  tract
mon·am·ide
mon·am·ine
mon·am·i·nu·ria
mon·an·gle
mon·ar·da
mon·ar·thric
mon·ar·thri·tis
mon·ar·tic·u·lar
mon·as·ter
mon·ath·e·to·sis
mon·a·tom·ic
mon·au·ral
mon·ax·on·ic

Mönckeberg's
  ar·te·ri·o·scle·ro·sis
  cal·ci·fi·ca·tion
  de·gen·er·a·tion
  scle·ro·sis
Mon·day morn·ing
  sick·ness
Mondini
  deaf·ness
  dys·pla·sia
Mondonesi's
  re·flex
Mondor's
  dis·ease
mo·ner
Mo·ne·ra
mo·ne·ran
mon·es·thet·ic
mon·es·trous
Monge's
  dis·ease
mon·gol
mon·go·li·an
  fold
  mac·u·la
  spot
mon·go·lism
  trans·lo·ca·tion m.
mon·go·loid
Mo·ni·e·zia ex·pan·sa
mon·i·lat·ed
mo·nil·e·thrix
Mo·nil·i·a
Mo·nil·i·a·ce·ae
mo·nil·i·al
mon·i·li·a·sis
  pneu·mo·nia
mo·nil·i·form
  hair
Mo·nil·i·for·mis
mo·nil·i·id
mon·ism
mo·nis·tic
mon·i·tor
  car·di·ac m.
  elec·tron·ic fe·tal m.
  Holter m.
mon·key
  ma·lar·ia
mon·key B
  vi·rus
mon·key-paw
mon·key pox
  vi·rus
monks·hood
mon·o-a·me·lia
mon·o·am·ide
mon·o·am·ine

mon·o·am·ine ox·i·dase
  in·hib·i·tor
mon·o·am·i·ner·gic
mon·o·am·i·nu·ria
mon·o·am·ni·ot·ic
  twins
mon·o·as·so·ci·at·ed
mon·o·bac·tam
mon·o·ba·sic
  ac·id
  am·mo·ni·um phos·phate
  po·tas·si·um phos·phate
mon·o·ben·zone
mon·o·blast
mon·o·bra·chi·us
mon·o·bro·mat·ed
  cam·phor
mon·o·bro·mi·nat·ed
mon·o·car·di·an
mon·o·ceph·a·lus
mon·o·chlor·phen·am·ide
mon·o·chord
mon·o·cho·rea
mon·o·cho·ri·al
  twins
mon·o·cho·ri·on·ic
mon·o·cho·ri·on·ic di·am·
  ni·ot·ic
  pla·cen·ta
mon·o·cho·ri·on·ic mon·o·am·
  ni·ot·ic
  pla·cen·ta
mon·o·chro·ic
mon·o·chro·ma·sia
mon·o·chro·ma·sy
  blue cone m.
  pi cone m.
  rod m.
mon·o·chro·mat·ic
  ab·er·ra·tion
  rays
mon·o·chro·ma·tism
mon·o·chro·mat·o·phil
mon·o·chro·mat·o·phile
mon·o·chro·ma·tor
mon·o·chro·mic
mon·o·chro·mo·phil
mon·o·chro·mo·phile
mon·o·cle
mon·o·clin·ic
mon·o·clo·nal
  an·ti·body
  gam·mop·a·thy
  im·mu·no·glob·u·lin
  pro·tein
mon·o·clo·nal peak
mon·o·cra·ni·us
mon·o·cro·ta·line

mon·o·crot·ic
  pulse
mon·oc·ro·tism
mo·noc·u·lar
  di·plo·pia
  het·er·o·chro·mia
  stra·bis·mus
mo·no·cu·lus
mon·o·cyte
mon·o·cyt·ic
  an·gi·na
  leu·ke·mia
  leu·ke·moid re·ac·tion
  leu·ko·cy·to·sis
  leu·ko·pe·nia
mon·o·cy·toid
  cell
mon·o·cy·to·pe·nia
mon·o·cy·to·sis
  avi·an m.
mon·o·dac·tyl·ism
mon·o·dac·ty·ly
mon·o·der·mo·ma
mon·o·di·plo·pia
mon·o·dis·perse
mon·o·eth·a·nol·a·mine
mon·o·ga·met·ic
mo·nog·a·my
mon·o·gen·e·sis
mon·o·ge·net·ic
mon·o·gen·ic
mo·nog·e·nous
mon·o·ger·mi·nal
mon·o·graph
mon·o·hy·drat·ed
mon·o·hy·dric
  al·co·hol
mon·o·i·de·ism
mon·o·in·fec·tion
mon·o·i·so·ni·tro·so·ac·e·tone
mon·o·lay·ers
mon·o·lep·tic
  fe·ver
mon·o·loc·u·lar
mon·o·ma·nia
mon·o·ma·ni·ac
mon·o·mas·ti·gote
mon·o·mel·ic
mon·o·mer
mon·o·mer·ic
mon·o·me·tal·lic
mon·o·mi·cro·bic
mon·o·mo·lec·u·lar
  re·ac·tion
mon·o·mor·phic
  ad·e·no·ma
mon·om·pha·lus
mon·o·my·o·ple·gia

mon·o·my·o·si·tis
mon·o·neme
mon·o·neu·ral
mon·o·neu·ral·gia
mon·o·neu·ric
mon·o·neu·ri·tis
   m. mul·ti·plex
mon·o·neu·rop·a·thy
   m. mul·ti·plex
mon·o·noea
mon·o·nu·cle·ar
mon·o·nu·cle·ar phag·o·cyte
   sys·tem
mon·o·nu·cle·o·sis
   in·fec·tious m.
mon·o·nu·cle·o·tide
mon·o·oc·tan·o·in
mon·o·ox·y·ge·na·ses
mon·o·pa·re·sis
mon·o·par·es·the·sia
mon·o·path·ic
mo·nop·a·thy
mo·noph·a·gism
mon·o·pha·sia
mon·o·pha·sic
   com·plex
mon·o·phe·nol mon·o·ox·y·gen·ase
mon·o·phe·nol ox·i·dase
mon·o·pho·bia
mon·oph·thal·mos
mon·oph·thal·mus
mon·o·phy·let·ic
   the·o·ry
mon·o·phy·le·tism
mon·o·phy·o·dont
mon·o·plas·mat·ic
mon·o·plast
mon·o·plas·tic
mon·o·ple·gia
   m. mas·ti·ca·to·ria
mon·o·ploid
mon·o·po·dia
mon·o·po·lar
   cau·tery
mon·o·po·tas·si·um
   phos·phate
mon·ops
mon·o·pty·chi·al
mon·or·chia
mon·or·chid
mon·or·chid·ic
mon·or·chid·ism
mon·or·chism
mon·o·rec·i·dive
   chan·cre
mon·o·rhin·ic

mon·o·sac·cha·ride
mon·o·scel·ous
mon·o·sce·nism
mon·ose
mon·o·so·di·um
   phos·phate
mon·o·so·di·um glu·ta·mate
mon·o·some
mon·o·so·mia
mon·o·so·mic
mon·o·so·mous
mon·o·so·my
mon·o·spasm
mon·o·sper·my
Mon·o·spo·ri·um ap·i·o·sper·mum
Mo·nos·to·ma
mon·o·stome
mon·o·stot·ic
mon·o·stot·ic fi·brous
   dys·pla·sia
mon·o·stra·tal
mon·o·sub·sti·tut·ed
mon·o·symp·to·mat·ic
mon·o·sy·nap·tic
mon·o·syph·i·lide
mon·o·ter·penes
mon·o·ther·mia
mon·o·thi·o·glyc·er·ol
mo·not·o·cous
Mon·o·tre·ma·ta
mon·o·treme
mo·not·ri·chate
mo·not·ri·chous
mon·o·va·lence
mon·o·va·len·cy
mon·o·va·lent
   an·ti·se·rum
mon·o·vu·lar
   twins
mon·ox·e·nous
mon·ox·ide
mon·o·zo·ic
mon·o·zy·got·ic
   twins
mon·o·zy·gous
Monro-Kellie
   doc·trine
Monro-Richter
   line
Monro's
   doc·trine
   fo·ra·men
   line
   sul·cus
mons
   m. ure·te·ris
   m. ve·ne·ris

Monson
  curve
mon·ster
Monteggia's
  frac·ture
mon·tes
Montgomery's
  fol·li·cles
  glands
  tu·ber·cles
mon·tic·u·li
mon·tic·u·lus
mon·tis
mood
mood swing
moon
  blind·ness
  face
Moon's
  mo·lars
Mooren's
  ul·cer
Moore's
  meth·od
Moore's light·ning
  streaks
Mooser
  bod·ies
mor·al
  atax·ia
  treat·ment
Morand's
  foot
  spur
Morax-Axenfeld
  con·junc·ti·vi·tis
  dip·lo·ba·cil·lus
Mor·ax·el·la
  M. bo·vis
  M. la·cu·na·ta
  M. non·li·que·fa·ciens
  M. os·lo·en·sis
  M. phe·nyl·py·ru·vi·ca
mor·bid
  im·pulse
  obe·si·ty
  thirst
mor·bid·i·ty
  rate
mor·bid·i·ty
  pu·er·per·al m.
mor·bif·ic
mor·big·e·nous
mor·bil·i·ty
mor·bil·li
mor·bil·li·form
Mor·bil·li·vi·rus
mor·bi·lous

mor·bus
mor·cel
mor·cel·la·tion
  op·er·a·tion
mor·celle·ment
mor·dant
Morel's
  ear
Mo·re·ra·stron·gy·lus cos·tar·i·cen·sis
Morgagni-Adams-Stokes
  syn·drome
mor·ga·gni·an
  cyst
Morgagni's
  ap·pen·dix
  car·ti·lage
  ca·run·cle
  cat·a·ract
  col·umns
  con·cha
  crypts
  dis·ease
  fo·ra·men
  fos·sa
  fo·vea
  fre·num
  glob·ules
  hu·mor
  hy·da·tid
  la·cu·na
  li·quor
  nod·ule
  pro·lapse
  ret·i·nac·u·lum
  si·nus
  spheres
  syn·drome
  tu·ber·cle
  valves
  ven·tri·cle
mor·gan
Morgan's
  ba·cil·lus
  fold
morgue
mo·ria
mor·i·bund
mo·rin
Morison's
  pouch
Morner's
  test
morn·ing
  di·ar·rhea
  sick·ness
  vom·it·ing

morn·ing glo·ry
anom·a·ly
syn·drome
Moro
re·flex
mo·ron
mo·rox·y·dine
mor·pha·zin·a·mide hy·dro·
chlo·ride
mor·phea
m. ac·ro·ter·i·ca
m. al·ba
m. gut·ta·ta
m. her·pet·i·for·mis
m. li·ne·a·ris
m. pig·men·to·sa
mor·pheme
mor·phine
m. hy·dro·chlo·ride
m. sul·fate
mor·pho·gen·e·sis
mor·pho·ge·net·ic
move·ment
mor·pho·log·ic
el·e·ment
mor·phol·o·gy
mor·pho·met·ric
mor·phom·e·try
mor·phon
mor·pho·sis
mor·pho·syn·the·sis
mor·pho·type
Morquio's
dis·ease
syn·drome
Morquio-Ullrich
dis·ease
mor·rhu·ate so·di·um
Morris
syn·drome
mors
m. thy·mi·ca
mor·su·lus
mor·tal
mor·tal·i·ty
rate
mor·tar
kid·ney
Mor·ti·er·el·la
mor·ti·fi·ca·tion
mor·ti·fied
mor·tis
mor·tise
joint
Mor·ton's
neu·ral·gia
plane
syn·drome

mor·tu·ary
mor·u·la
mor·u·la·tion
Mor·u·la·vi·rus
mor·u·loid
Morvan's
cho·rea
dis·ease
mo·sa·ic
fun·gus
in·her·i·tance
wart
mo·sa·i·cism
cel·lu·lar m.
chro·mo·some m.
gene m.
ger·mi·nal m.
go·nad·al m.
Moschcowitz'
dis·ease
mos·chus
Mosler's
di·a·be·tes
mos·qui·to
clamp
for·ceps
Moss
tube
moss
starch
Mossman
fe·ver
Mosso's
er·go·graph
sphyg·mo·ma·nom·e·ter
mossy
cell
fi·bers
foot
Moszkowicz'
test
Motais'
op·er·a·tion
mote
blood m.'s
moth
patch
moth-eat·en
al·o·pe·cia
moth·er
cell
col·o·ny
cyst
li·quor
star
sur·ro·gate
yaw

moth·er
   sur·ro·gate m.
moth·er su·pe·ri·or
   com·plex
moth·er of vin·e·gar
mo·tile
   leu·ko·cyte
mo·til·in
mo·til·i·ty
mo·til·i·ty test
   me·di·um
mo·tion
   sick·ness
mo·tion
   brown·i·an m.
   con·tin·u·ous pas·sive m.
mo·ti·va·tion
   ex·trin·sic m.
   in·trin·sic m.
   per·son·al m.
mo·tive
   achieve·ment m.
   mas·tery m.
mo·to·fa·cient
mo·to·neu·ron
mo·tor
   m. oc·u·li
   plas·tic m.
mo·tor
   ab·re·ac·tion
   agraph·ia
   apha·sia
   aprax·ia
   ar·ea
   atax·ia
   cell
   cor·tex
   de·cus·sa·tion
   end·plate
   fi·bers
   im·age
   im·per·sis·tence
   nerve
   nerve of face
   neu·ron
   nu·clei
   nu·cle·us of fa·cial nerve
   nu·cle·us of tri·gem·i·nus
   pa·ral·y·sis
   plate
   point
   root of cil·i·ary gan·gli·on
   root of tri·gem·i·nal nerve
   unit
   ur·gen·cy
   zone
  mo·tor alex·ia

mo·tor dap·sone
   neu·rop·a·thy
mo·tor·i·al
mo·tor·me·ter
mo·tor neu·ron
   dis·ease
mo·tor speech
   cen·ter
mot·tled
   enam·el
   tooth
mot·tling
Motulsky dye re·duc·tion
   test
mou·lage
mould
moult
mound·ing
Mounier-Kuhn
   syn·drome
moun·tain
   balm
   sick·ness
mount·ing
   me·di·um
mount·ing
   split cast m.
mourn
mouse
   mul·ti·mam·mate m.
   New Zea·land m.'s
   nude m.
mouse
   can·cer
   en·ceph·a·lo·my·e·li·tis
   hep·a·ti·tis
   lep·ro·sy
   po·li·o·my·e·li·tis
   unit
mouse an·ti·al·o·pe·cia
   fac·tor
mouse en·ceph·a·lo·my·e·li·tis
   vi·rus
mouse hep·a·ti·tis
   vi·rus
mouse leu·ke·mia
   vi·rus·es
mouse mam·ma·ry tu·mor
   vi·rus
mouse pa·rot·id tu·mor
   vi·rus
mouse po·li·o·my·e·li·tis
   vi·rus
mouse·pox
   vi·rus
mouse·tail
   pulse

mouse thy·mic
vi·rus
mouse-tooth
for·ceps
mouth
breath·ing
mir·ror
re·ha·bil·i·ta·tion
mouth
carp m.
den·ture sore m.
par·rot m.
sore m.
ta·pir m.
trench m.
m. of the womb
mouth guard
mouth stick
mouth-to-mouth
res·pi·ra·tion
re·sus·ci·ta·tion
mouth·wash
mov·a·ble
heart
joint
kid·ney
pulse
spleen
tes·tis
move·ment
ac·tive m.
ad·ver·sive m.
af·ter-m.
ame·boid m.
as·sist·ive m.
as·so·ci·at·ed m.
Bennett m.
bor·der m.'s
bor·der tis·sue m.'s
brown·i·an m.
brown·i·an-Zsigmondy m.
car·di·nal oc·u·lar m.'s
cho·re·ic m.
cil·i·ary m.
cir·cus m.
cog·wheel oc·u·lar m.'s
con·ju·gate m. of eyes
de·com·po·si·tion of m.
dis·ju·gate m. of eyes
drift m.'s
fe·tal m.
fix·a·tion·al oc·u·lar m.
flick m.'s
free man·dib·u·lar m.'s
func·tion·al man·dib·u·lar
m.'s
fu·sion·al m.
hinge m.

in·ter·me·di·ary m.'s
jaw m.'s
lat·er·al m.
light·ning eye m.'s
Magnan's trom·bone m.
man·dib·u·lar m.
mass m.
mo·lec·u·lar m.
mor·pho·ge·net·ic m.
mus·cu·lar m.
neu·ro·bi·o·tac·tic m.
non-rap·id eye m.
open·ing m.
par·a·dox·i·cal m. of eye·
lids
pas·sive m.
pen·du·lar m.
per·vert·ed oc·u·lar m.
pro·to·plas·mic m.
rap·id eye m.'s
re·flex m.
re·sis·tive m.
sac·cad·ic m.
stream·ing m.
Swed·ish m.'s
trans·la·to·ry m.
ver·mic·u·lar m.
Mowry's col·loi·dal iron
stain
moxa
mox·a·lac·tam di·so·di·um
mox·i·bus·tion
mox·i·sy·lyte
moy·a·moya
dis·ease
Mozart
ear
MP
joints
MSB tri·chrome
stain
Mu
an·ti·gen
mu·case
Mucha-Habermann
dis·ease
syn·drome
Much's
ba·cil·lus
mu·ci·car·mine
mu·cid
mu·cif·er·ous
mu·ci·fi·ca·tion
mu·ci·form
mu·cig·e·nous
mu·ci·he·ma·te·in
mu·ci·lage

mu·ci·lag·i·nous
  gland
mu·cin
  gas·tric m.
mu·cin·ase
mu·cin clot
  test
mu·ci·ne·mia
mu·cin·o·gen
  gran·ules
mu·ci·noid
  de·gen·er·a·tion
mu·ci·no·lyt·ic
mu·ci·no·sis
  fol·lic·u·lar m.
  pap·u·lar m.
  re·tic·u·lar er·y·them·a·
    tous m.
mu·ci·nous
  car·ci·no·ma
  plaque
mu·ci·nu·ria
mu·cip·a·rous
  gland
mu·ci·tis
Muckle-Wells
  syn·drome
mu·co·al·bu·mi·nous
  cells
mu·co·buc·cal
  fold
mu·co·cele
mu·coc·la·sis
mu·co·co·li·tis
mu·co·col·pos
mu·co·cu·ta·ne·ous
  junc·tion
  leish·man·i·a·sis
  mus·cle
mu·co·cu·ta·ne·ous lymph node
  syn·drome
mu·co·en·ter·i·tis
mu·co·ep·i·der·moid
  car·ci·no·ma
  tu·mor
mu·co·ep·i·the·li·al
  dys·pla·sia
mu·co·glob·u·lin
mu·coid
  ad·e·no·car·ci·no·ma
  col·o·ny
  de·gen·er·a·tion
mu·coid me·di·al
  de·gen·er·a·tion
mu·co·lip·i·do·ses
mu·co·lip·i·do·sis
  m. I
  m. II

  m. III
  m. IV
mu·col·y·sis
mu·co·lyt·ic
mu·co·mem·bra·nous
  en·ter·i·tis
mu·co·pep·tide
  m. gly·co·hy·dro·lase
mu·co·per·i·chon·dri·al
  flap
mu·co·per·i·os·te·al
  flap
mu·co·per·i·os·te·um
mu·co·pol·y·sac·cha·ri·dase
mu·co·pol·y·sac·cha·ride
mu·co·pol·y·sac·cha·ri·do·ses
mu·co·pol·y·sac·cha·ri·do·sis
  type I m.
  type II m.
  type III m.
  type IS m.
  type IV m.
  type V m.
  type VI m.
  type VII m.
mu·co·pol·y·sac·cha·ri·du·ria
mu·co·pro·tein
  Tamm-Horsfall m.
mu·co·pu·ru·lent
  con·junc·ti·vi·tis
mu·co·pus
Mu·cor
Mu·co·ra·ce·ae
mu·cor·my·co·sis
mu·co·sa
  al·ve·o·lar m.
  gin·gi·val m.
  ol·fac·to·ry m.
  res·pi·ra·to·ry m.
mu·co·sal
  dis·ease
  folds of gall·blad·der
  graft
  tu·nics
mu·co·sal dis·ease
  vi·rus
mu·co·sal re·lief
  roent·gen·og·ra·phy
mu·co·san·guin·e·ous
mu·co·san·guin·o·lent
mu·co·sec·to·my
mu·co·se·rous
  cells
mu·co·stat·ic
mu·co·sul·fa·ti·do·sis
mu·cous
  cast
  cell

mu·cous *(continued)*
  co·li·tis
  cyst
  di·ar·rhea
  gland
  glands of au·di·to·ry tube
  mem·branes
  oph·thal·mia
  pap·ule
  patch
  plaque
  plug
  pol·yp
  rale
  sheath of ten·don
  tu·nics
mu·cous con·nec·tive
  tis·sue
mu·cous neck
  cell
mu·co·vis·ci·do·sis
mu·cro
  m. cor·dis
  m. ster·ni
mu·cron
mu·cro·nate
mu·cron·es
mu·cus
  glairy m.
mu·cus
  im·pac·tion
mud
  bed
  fe·ver
Muehrcke's
  lines
Mueller elec·tron·ic
  to·nom·e·ter
Muel·le·ri·us cap·il·la·ris
muf·fle
  fur·nace
Muir-Torre
  syn·drome
mul·ber·ry
  cal·cu·lus
  mo·lar
  ova·ry
  spots
Mules'
  op·er·a·tion
mule-spin·ner's
  can·cer
mu·li·e·bria
mül·le·ri·an
  ad·e·no·sar·co·ma
  duct
mül·le·ri·an duct in·hib·i·to·ry
  fac·tor

mül·le·ri·an re·gres·sion
  fac·tor
Müller's
  cap·sule
  duct
  fi·bers
  fix·a·tive
  law
  ma·neu·ver
  meth·od
  mus·cle
  sign
  tri·gone
  tu·ber·cle
Müller's ra·di·al
  cells
mul·ling
mult·ang·u·lar
  bone
mul·ti·ar·tic·u·lar
mul·ti·ax·i·al
  clas·si·fi·ca·tion
  joint
mul·ti·bac·il·lary
mul·ti·cap·su·lar
mul·ti·cel·lu·lar
mul·ti·cen·tric
  re·tic·u·lo·his·ti·o·cy·to·sis
Mul·ti·ceps
  M. mul·ti·ceps
  M. se·ri·a·lis
mul·ti·core
  dis·ease
mul·ti·cus·pid
  tooth
mul·ti·cus·pi·date
mul·ti·fac·to·ri·al
  in·her·i·tance
mul·ti·fe·ta·tion
mul·ti·fid
mul·tif·i·dus
mul·ti·fo·cal
  cho·roid·i·tis
  lens
  os·te·i·tis fi·bro·sa
mul·ti·form
  lay·er
mul·ti·glan·du·lar
mul·ti·grav·i·da
mul·ti·in·farct
  de·men·tia
mul·ti·in·fec·tion
mul·ti·lam·el·lar
  body
mul·ti·lo·bar
mul·ti·lo·bate
mul·ti·lobed
mul·ti·lob·u·lar

mul·ti·lo·cal
mul·ti·loc·u·lar
  cyst
  fat
mul·ti·loc·u·lar ad·i·pose
  tis·sue
mul·ti·loc·u·lar hy·da·tid
  cyst
mul·ti·loc·u·late hy·da·tid
  cyst
mul·ti·mam·mae
mul·ti·mam·mate
  mouse
mul·ti·no·dal
mul·ti·nod·u·lar
  goi·ter
mul·ti·nod·u·late
mul·ti·nu·cle·ar
  leu·ko·cyte
mul·ti·nu·cle·ate
mul·ti·nu·cle·o·sis
mul·tip·a·ra
  grand m.
mul·ti·par·i·ty
mul·tip·a·rous
mul·ti·par·tial
mul·ti·pen·nate
  mus·cle
mul·ti·pha·sic
  screen·ing
mul·ti·ple
  am·pu·ta·tion
  an·chor·age
  em·bo·lism
  en·do·cri·no·ma
  en·do·cri·nop·a·thy
  ex·os·to·sis
  fis·sion
  frac·ture
  my·e·lo·ma
  my·e·lo·ma·to·sis
  my·o·si·tis
  neu·ri·tis
  par·a·sit·ism
  per·son·al·i·ty
  preg·nan·cy
  scle·ro·sis
  se·ro·si·tis
  stain
  vi·sion
mul·ti·ple ego
  states
mul·ti·ple ep·i·phys·i·al
  dys·pla·sia
mul·ti·ple ham·ar·to·ma
  syn·drome

mul·ti·ple id·i·o·path·ic hem·
  or·rhag·ic
  sar·co·ma
mul·ti·ple in·tes·ti·nal
  pol·yp·o·sis
mul·ti·ple len·tig·i·nes
  syn·drome
mul·ti·ple mu·co·sal neu·ro·ma
  syn·drome
mul·ti·ple punc·ture tu·ber·cu·
  lin
  test
mul·ti·ple self-heal·ing squa·
  mous
  ep·i·the·li·o·ma
mul·ti·ple sym·met·ric
  lip·o·ma·to·sis
mul·ti·pli·ca·tive
  di·vi·sion
  growth
mul·ti·po·lar
  cell
  mi·to·sis
  neu·ron
mul·ti·root·ed
mul·ti·ro·ta·tion
mul·ti·sy·nap·tic
mul·ti·va·lence
mul·ti·va·len·cy
mul·ti·va·lent
  vac·cine
mul·ti·var·i·ate
  stud·ies
mul·ti·ve·sic·u·lar
  bod·ies
mum·mi·fi·ca·tion
  ne·cro·sis
mum·mi·fied
  pulp
mumps
  me·nin·go·en·ceph·a·li·tis
  vi·rus
mumps
  met·a·stat·ic m.
mumps sen·si·tiv·i·ty
  test
mumps skin test
  an·ti·gen
mumps vi·rus
  vac·cine
mu·mu
  fe·ver
Munchausen
  syn·drome
mung bean
  nu·cle·ase
mu·nic·i·pal
  hos·pi·tal

Munro's
ab·scess
mi·cro·ab·scess
point
Munson's
sign
mu·ral
an·eu·rysm
cell
en·do·car·di·tis
preg·nan·cy
throm·bo·sis
throm·bus
mu·ram·ic ac·id
mu·ram·i·dase
mu·reins
mu·rex·ide
mu·ri·ate
mu·ri·at·ic
mu·ri·at·ic ac·id
Mu·ri·dae
mu·ri·form
mu·rine
hep·a·ti·tis
lep·ro·sy
ty·phus
mu·rine sar·co·ma
vi·rus
mur·mur
ac·ci·den·tal m.
ane·mic m.
aor·tic m.
ar·te·ri·al m.
atri·o·sys·tol·ic m.
Austin Flint m.
bel·lows m.
brain m.
Cabot-Locke m.
car·di·ac m.
car·di·o·pul·mo·nary m.
car·di·o·res·pi·ra·to·ry m.
Carey Coombs m.
Cole-Cecil m.
con·tin·u·ous m.
Coombs m.
cre·scen·do m.
Cruveilhier-Baumgarten m.
di·a·mond-shaped m.
di·a·stol·ic m.
Duroziez' m.
dy·nam·ic m.
ear·ly di·a·stol·ic m.
ejec·tion m.
en·do·car·di·al m.
ex·o·car·di·al m.
ex·tra·car·di·ac m.
Flint's m.
Fräntzel's m.

func·tion·al m.
Gibson m.
Graham Steell's m.
he·mic m.
Hodgkin-Key m.
hol·o·sys·tol·ic m.
hour·glass m.
in·no·cent m.
in·or·gan·ic m.
late ap·i·cal sys·tol·ic m.
late di·a·stol·ic m.
ma·chin·ery m.
mid·di·a·stol·ic m.
mill wheel m.
mi·tral m.
mus·cu·lar m.
mu·si·cal m.
nun's m.
ob·struc·tive m.
or·gan·ic m.
pan·sys·tol·ic m.
per·i·car·di·al m.
pleu·ro·per·i·car·di·al m.
pre·sys·tol·ic m.
pul·mo·nary m.
pul·mon·ic m.
re·gur·gi·tant m.
res·pi·ra·to·ry m.
Roger's m.
sea gull m.
see·saw m.
Steell's m.
ste·no·sal m.
Still's m.
sys·tol·ic m.
to-and-fro m.
tri·cus·pid m.
vas·cu·lar m.
ve·nous m.
ve·sic·u·lar m.
wa·ter wheel m.
Murphy
drip
Murphy's
but·ton
Murray Val·ley
en·ceph·a·li·tis
rash
Murray Val·ley en·ceph·a·li·tis
vi·rus
mur·ri·na
Mu·ru·tu·cu
vi·rus
Mus·ca
mus·cae vol·i·tan·tes
mus·ca·rine
mus·ca·rin·ic
mus·ca·rin·ism

Mus·ci
mus·ci·cide
Mus·ci·dae
mus·cle
m.'s of ab·do·men
ab·dom·i·nal ex·ter·nal ob·lique m.
ab·dom·i·nal in·ter·nal ob·lique m.
ab·duc·tor m. of great toe
ab·duc·tor m. of lit·tle fin·ger
ab·duc·tor m. of lit·tle toe
ad·duc·tor m. of great toe
ad·duc·tor m. of thumb
Aeby's m.
Albinus' m.
an·co·ne·us m.
an·tag·o·nis·tic m.'s
an·te·ri·or au·ric·u·lar m.
an·te·ri·or cer·vi·cal in·ter·trans·verse m.'s
an·te·ri·or rec·tus m. of head
an·te·ri·or sca·lene m.
an·te·ri·or ser·ra·tus m.
an·te·ri·or tib·i·al m.
an·ti·grav·i·ty m.'s
m. of an·ti·tra·gus
ap·pen·dic·u·lar m.
ar·tic·u·lar m.
ar·tic·u·lar m. of el·bow
ar·tic·u·lar m. of knee
ar·y·ep·i·glot·tic m.
m.'s of au·di·to·ry os·si·cles
ax·i·al m.
Bell's m.
bi·ceps m. of arm
bi·ceps m. of thigh
bi·pen·nate m.
Bochdalek's m.
Bovero's m.
Bowman's m.
brach·i·al m.
bra·chi·o·ce·phal·ic m.
bra·chi·o·ra·di·al m.
bran·chi·o·mer·ic m.'s
Braune's m.
broad·est m. of back
bron·cho·e·soph·a·ge·al m.
Brücke's m.
car·di·ac m.
Casser's per·fo·rat·ed m.
cer·vi·cal il·i·o·cos·tal m.
cer·vi·cal in·ter·spi·nal m.
cer·vi·cal lon·gis·si·mus m.
cer·vi·cal ro·ta·tor m.'s

cheek m.
chin m.
cil·i·ary m.
coc·cyg·eal m.
m.'s of coc·cyx
Coiter's m.
com·pres·sor m. of lips
cor·a·co·brach·i·al m.
cor·ru·ga·tor m.
cowl m.
Crampton's m.
cre·mas·ter m.
cri·co·thy·roid m.
cru·ci·ate m.
cu·ta·ne·o·mu·cous m.
cu·ta·ne·ous m.
dar·tos m.
deep flex·or m. of fin·gers
deep trans·verse m. of per·i·ne·um
del·toid m.
de·pres·sor m. of ep·i·glot·tis
de·pres·sor m. of eye·brow
de·pres·sor m. of low·er lip
de·pres·sor m. of sep·tum
di·gas·tric m.
di·la·tor m.
dor·sal m.'s
dor·sal in·ter·os·se·ous m. of foot
dor·sal in·ter·os·se·ous m. of hand
dor·sal sa·cro·coc·cyg·e·al m.
Dupré's m.
Duverney's m.
el·e·va·tor m. of anus
el·e·va·tor m. of pros·tate
el·e·va·tor m. of rib
el·e·va·tor m. of scap·u·la
el·e·va·tor m. of soft pal·ate
el·e·va·tor m. of thy·roid gland
el·e·va·tor m. of up·per eye·lid
el·e·va·tor m. of up·per lip
el·e·va·tor m. of up·per lip and wing of nose
ep·i·cra·ni·al m.
erec·tor m.'s of the hairs
erec·tor m. of spine
ex·ten·sor m. of fin·gers
ex·ten·sor m. of lit·tle fin·ger
ex·ter·nal in·ter·cos·tal m.
ex·ter·nal ob·tu·ra·tor m.

mus·cle *(continued)*

ex·ter·nal pter·y·goid m.
ex·ter·nal sphinc·ter m. of
  anus
m.'s of eye·ball
fa·cial m.'s
m.'s of fa·cial ex·pres·sion
fem·o·ral m.
fix·a·tor m.
fu·si·form m.
Gantzer's m.
gas·troc·ne·mi·us m.
Gavard's m.
ge·ni·o·glos·sal m.
ge·ni·o·hy·oid m.
glu·te·us max·i·mus m.
glu·te·us me·di·us m.
glu·te·us mi·ni·mus m.
grac·i·lis m.
great ad·duc·tor m.
great·er pec·to·ral m.
great·er pos·te·ri·or rec·tus
  m. of head
great·er pso·as m.
great·er rhom·boid m.
great·er zy·go·mat·ic m.
Guthrie's m.
ham·string m.'s
m.'s of head
m. of heart
Horner's m.
Houston's m.
hy·o·glos·sal m.
il·i·ac m.
il·i·o·coc·cyg·e·al m.
il·i·o·cos·tal m.
il·i·o·pso·as m.
in·dex ex·ten·sor m.
in·fe·ri·or con·stric·tor m.
  of phar·ynx
in·fe·ri·or ge·mel·lus m.
in·fe·ri·or lin·gual m.
in·fe·ri·or ob·lique m.
in·fe·ri·or ob·lique m. of
  head
in·fe·ri·or pos·te·ri·or ser·
  ra·tus m.
in·fe·ri·or rec·tus m.
in·fe·ri·or tar·sal m.
in·fra·hy·oid m.'s
in·fra·spi·na·tus m.
in·ner·most in·ter·cos·tal m.
in·ter·me·di·ate great m.
in·ter·me·di·ate vas·tus m.
in·ter·nal in·ter·cos·tal m.
in·ter·nal ob·tu·ra·tor m.
in·ter·nal pter·y·goid m.

in·ter·nal sphinc·ter m. of
  anus
in·ter·spi·nal m.'s
in·ter·trans·verse m.'s
in·vol·un·tary m.'s
is·chi·o·cav·ern·ous m.
Jung's m.
Klein's m.
Kohlrausch's m.
Krause's m.
Landström's m.
Langer's m.
large m. of he·lix
m.'s of lar·ynx
lat·er·al cri·co·ar·y·te·noid
  m.
lat·er·al great m.
lat·er·al lum·bar in·ter·
  trans·verse m.'s
lat·er·al pter·y·goid m.
lat·er·al rec·tus m.
lat·er·al rec·tus m. of the
  head
lat·er·al vas·tus m.
less·er rhom·boid m.
less·er zy·go·mat·ic m.
long ab·duc·tor m. of
  thumb
long ad·duc·tor m.
long ex·ten·sor m. of great
  toe
long ex·ten·sor m. of
  thumb
long ex·ten·sor m. of toes
long fib·u·lar m.
long flex·or m. of great toe
long flex·or m. of thumb
long flex·or m. of toes
long m. of head
lon·gis·si·mus ca·pi·tis m.
long m. of neck
long pal·mar m.
long per·o·ne·al m.
long ra·di·al ex·ten·sor m.
  of wrist
lum·bar il·i·o·cos·tal m.
lum·bar in·ter·spi·nal m.
lum·bar quad·rate m.
lum·bar ro·ta·tor m.'s
lum·bri·cal m. of foot
lum·bri·cal m. of hand
Marcacci's m.
m.'s of mas·ti·ca·tion
me·di·al great m.
me·di·al lum·bar in·ter·
  trans·verse m.'s
me·di·al pter·y·goid m.
me·di·al rec·tus m.

me·di·al vas·tus m.
Merkel's m.
mid·dle con·stric·tor m. of phar·ynx
mid·dle sca·lene m.
mi·met·ic m.'s
mu·co·cu·ta·ne·ous m.
Müller's m.
mul·ti·pen·nate m.
my·lo·hy·oid m.
na·sal m.
m.'s of neck
m. of notch of he·lix
ob·lique ar·y·te·noid m.
ob·lique m. of au·ri·cle
oc·cip·i·to·fron·tal m.
oc·u·lar m.'s
Oehl's m.'s
omo·hy·oid m.
op·pos·er m. of lit·tle fin·ger
op·pos·er m. of thumb
or·bic·u·lar m.
or·bic·u·lar m. of eye
or·bic·u·lar m. of mouth
or·bi·tal m.
pal·a·to·glos·sus m.
pal·a·to·pha·ryn·ge·al m.
pa·la·to·u·vu·la·ris m.
pal·mar in·ter·os·se·ous m.
pan·nic·u·lus car·no·sus m.
pap·il·lary m.
pec·ti·nate m.'s
pec·tin·e·al m.
pen·nate m.
per·i·ne·al m.'s
pir·i·form m.
plan·tar m.
plan·tar in·ter·os·se·ous m.
plan·tar quad·rate m.
pleu·ro·e·soph·a·ge·al m.
pop·lit·e·al m.
pos·te·ri·or au·ric·u·lar m.
pos·te·ri·or cer·vi·cal in·ter·trans·verse m.'s
pos·te·ri·or cri·co·ar·y·te·noid m.
pos·te·ri·or sca·lene m.
pos·te·ri·or tib·i·al m.
Pozzi's m.
pro·ce·rus m.
pu·bo·coc·cy·ge·al m.
pu·bo·pros·tat·ic m.
pu·bo·rec·tal m.
pu·bo·vag·i·nal m.
pu·bo·ves·i·cal m.
py·ram·i·dal m.
py·ram·i·dal m. of au·ri·cle

quad·rate m.
quad·rate m. of loins
quad·rate pro·na·tor m.
quad·rate m. of sole
quad·rate m. of thigh
quad·rate m. of up·per lip
quad·ri·ceps m. of thigh
ra·di·al flex·or m. of wrist
rec·to·coc·cyg·e·al m.
rec·to·u·re·thral m.
rec·to·ves·i·cal m.
rec·tus m. of ab·do·men
rec·tus m. of thigh
red m.
Reisseisen's m.'s
rid·er's m.'s
Riolan's m.
ri·so·ri·us m.
ro·ta·tor m.'s
Rouget's m.
round pro·na·tor m.
Ruysch's m.
sal·pin·go·pha·ryn·ge·al m.
Santorini's m.
scalp m.
Sebileau's m.
sec·ond tib·i·al m.
sem·i·mem·bra·no·sus m.
sem·i·spi·nal m.
sem·i·spi·nal m. of head
sem·i·spi·nal m. of neck
sem·i·spi·nal m. of tho·rax
sem·i·ten·di·no·sus m.
sem·i·ten·di·nous m.
shawl m.
short ab·duc·tor m. of thumb
short ad·duc·tor m.
short ex·ten·sor m. of great toe
short ex·ten·sor m. of thumb
short ex·ten·sor m. of toes
short fib·u·lar m.
short flex·or m. of great toe
short flex·or m. of lit·tle fin·ger
short flex·or m. of lit·tle toe
short flex·or m. of thumb
short flex·or m. of toes
short pal·mar m.
short per·o·ne·al m.
short ra·di·al ex·ten·sor m. of wrist
Sibson's m.
skel·e·tal m.

mus·cle *(continued)*
small·er m. of he·lix
small·er pec·to·ral m.
small·er pos·te·ri·or rec·tus m. of head
small·er pso·as m.
small·est sca·lene m.
smooth m.
Soemmering's m.
so·le·us m.
sphinc·ter m.
sphinc·ter m. of com·mon bile duct
sphinc·ter m. of pan·cre·at·ic duct
sphinc·ter m. of pu·pil
sphinc·ter m. of py·lo·rus
sphinc·ter m. of ure·thra
sphinc·ter m. of uri·nary blad·der
spi·nal m.
spi·nal m. of head
spi·nal m. of neck
spi·nal m. of tho·rax
spin·dle-shaped m.
sple·ni·us m. of head
sple·ni·us m. of neck
sta·pe·di·us m.
ster·nal m.
ster·no·chon·dro·scap·u·lar m.
ster·no·cla·vic·u·lar m.
ster·no·clei·do·mas·toid m.
ster·no·hy·oid m.
ster·no·mas·toid m.
ster·no·thy·roid m.
strap m.'s
stri·at·ed m.
sty·lo·au·ric·u·lar m.
sty·lo·glos·sus m.
sty·lo·hy·oid m.
sty·lo·pha·ryn·ge·al m.
sub·an·co·ne·us m.
sub·cla·vi·an m.
sub·cos·tal m.
sub·cru·ral m.
sub·oc·cip·i·tal m.'s
sub·quad·ri·cip·i·tal m.
sub·scap·u·lar m.
su·per·fi·cial flex·or m. of fin·gers
su·per·fi·cial lin·gual m.
su·per·fi·cial trans·verse m. of per·i·ne·um
su·pe·ri·or au·ric·u·lar m.
su·pe·ri·or con·stric·tor m. of phar·ynx
su·pe·ri·or ge·mel·lus m.

su·pe·ri·or ob·lique m.
su·pe·ri·or ob·lique m. of head
su·pe·ri·or pos·te·ri·or ser·ra·tus m.
su·pe·ri·or rec·tus m.
su·pe·ri·or tar·sal m.
su·pi·na·tor m.
su·pra·cla·vic·u·lar m.
su·pra·hy·oid m.'s
su·pra·spi·nous m.
sus·pen·so·ry m. of du·o·de·num
syn·er·gis·tic m.'s
tai·lor's m.
tem·po·ral m.
tem·po·ro·pa·ri·e·tal m.
ten·sor m. of fas·cia la·ta
ten·sor m. of soft pal·ate
ten·sor tar·si m.
ten·sor m. of tym·pan·ic mem·brane
te·res ma·jor m.
te·res mi·nor m.
Theile's m.
third per·o·ne·al m.
tho·rac·ic in·ter·spi·nal m.
tho·rac·ic in·ter·trans·verse m.'s
tho·rac·ic lon·gis·si·mus m.
tho·rac·ic ro·ta·tor m.'s
m.'s of tho·rax
thy·ro·ar·y·te·noid m.
thy·ro·ep·i·glot·tic m.
thy·ro·e·pi·glot·tid·e·an m.
thy·ro·hy·oid m.
Tod's m.
m.'s of tongue
Toynbee's m.
trach·e·lo·cla·vic·u·lar m.
m. of tra·gus
trans·verse m. of ab·do·men
trans·verse ar·y·te·noid m.
trans·verse m. of au·ri·cle
trans·verse m. of chin
trans·verse m. of nape
trans·verse m. of tho·rax
trans·verse m. of tongue
trans·ver·so·spi·nal m.
tra·pe·zi·us m.
Treitz' m.
tri·an·gu·lar m.
tri·ceps m. of arm
tri·ceps m. of calf
two-bel·lied m.
ul·nar ex·ten·sor m. of wrist
ul·nar flex·or m. of wrist

uni·pen·nate m.
un·stri·at·ed m.
un·striped m.
m. of uvu·la
Valsalva's m.
ven·tral sa·cro·coc·cyg·e·al
  m.
ver·ti·cal m. of tongue
ves·tig·i·al m.
vo·cal m.
vol·un·tary m.
white m.
Wilson's m.
wrin·kler m. of eye·brow
mus·cle
  bun·dle
  curve
  ep·i·the·li·um
  fas·ci·cle
  he·mo·glo·bin
  plas·ma
  plate
  re·po·si·tion·ing
  re·sec·tion
  se·rum
  sound
  spasm
  spin·dle
mus·cle-bound
mus·cle-ten·don
  at·tach·ment
  junc·tion
mus·cle-trim·ming
mus·cone
mus·cu·la·mine
mus·cu·lar
  an·es·the·sia
  ar·tery
  as·the·no·pia
  at·ro·phy
  dys·tro·phy
  fas·cia of ex·tra·oc·u·lar
   mus·cle
  fi·bril
  hy·per·es·the·sia
  in·com·pe·tence
  in·suf·fi·cien·cy
  la·cu·na
  lay·er of mu·co·sa
  move·ment
  mur·mur
  pro·cess of ar·y·te·noid
   car·ti·lage
  pul·ley
  re·flex
  re·lax·ant
  rheu·ma·tism
  sense

sub·stance of pros·tate
sys·tem
tis·sue
tri·an·gle
troph·o·neu·ro·sis
tu·nics
mus·cu·la·ris
  m. mu·co·sae
mus·cu·lar·i·ty
mus·cu·lar sub·a·or·tic
  ste·no·sis
mus·cu·la·ture
mus·cu·li
mus·cu·lo·ap·o·neu·rot·ic
mus·cu·lo·cu·ta·ne·ous
  am·pu·ta·tion
  flap
  nerve
  nerve of leg
mus·cu·lo·mem·bra·nous
mus·cu·lo·phren·ic
  ar·tery
  veins
mus·cu·lo·skel·e·tal
mus·cu·lo·spi·ral
  groove
  nerve
  pa·ral·y·sis
mus·cu·lo·ten·di·nous
  cuff
mus·cu·lo·tro·pic
mus·cu·lo·tu·bal
  ca·nal
mus·cu·lus
  m. ab·duc·tor di·gi·ti quin·
   ti
  m. ac·ces·so·ri·us glu·te·us
   mi·ni·mus
  m. ad·duc·tor mi·ni·mus
  m. ar·y·vo·ca·lis
  m. at·tol·lens au·rem
  m. at·tol·lens au·ric·u·lam
  m. at·tra·hens au·rem
  m. at·tra·hens au·ric·u·lam
  m. az·y·gos uvu·lae
  m. bi·ceps flex·or cru·ris
  m. bi·ven·ter man·dib·u·lae
  m. bra·chi·o·ce·pha·li·cus
  m. buc·co·pha·ryn·ge·us
  m. bul·bo·cav·er·no·sus
  m. ca·ni·nus
  m. ceph·a·lo·pha·ryn·ge·us
  m. cer·a·to·pha·ryn·ge·us
  m. cer·vi·ca·lis as·cen·dens
  m. chon·dro·pha·ryn·ge·us
  m. clei·do·e·pi·tro·chle·a·ris
  m. clei·do·mas·toi·de·us
  m. clei·do-oc·cip·i·ta·lis

mus·cu·lus *(continued)*

m. com·plex·us

m. com·plex·us mi·nor

m. com·pres·sor na·ris

m. com·pres·sor ure·thrae

m. con·stric·tor ure·thrae

m. cor·ru·ga·tor cu·tis ani

m. cri·co·pha·ryn·ge·us

m. cu·ta·ne·o·mu·co·sus

m. de·tru·sor uri·nae

m. di·a·phrag·ma

m. dil·a·ta·tor

m. di·la·tor

m. di·la·tor ir·i·dis

m. di·la·tor na·ris

m. di·la·tor py·lo·ri gas·tro·du·o·de·na·lis

m. di·la·tor py·lo·ri il·e·a·lis

m. di·la·tor tu·bae

m. ejac·u·la·tor se·mi·nis

m. ep·i·troch·le·o·an·co·ne·us

m. erec·tor cli·to·ri·dis

m. erec·tor pe·nis

m. ex·ten·sor bre·vis di·gi·to·rum

m. ex·ten·sor bre·vis pol·li·cis

m. ex·ten·sor coc·cy·gis

m. ex·ten·sor di·gi·ti quin·ti pro·pri·us

m. ex·ten·sor di·gi·to·rum bre·vis ma·nus

m. ex·ten·sor di·gi·to·rum com·mu·nis

m. ex·ten·sor in·di·cis pro·pri·us

m. ex·ten·sor lon·gus di·gi·to·rum

m. ex·ten·sor lon·gus pol·li·cis

m. ex·ten·sor mi·ni·mi di·gi·ti

m. ex·ten·sor os·sis met·a·car·pi pol·li·cis

m. flex·or bre·vis di·gi·to·rum

m. flex·or bre·vis hal·lu·cis

m. flex·or di·gi·to·rum sub·li·mis

m. flex·or lon·gus di·gi·to·rum

m. flex·or lon·gus hal·lu·cis

m. flex·or lon·gus pol·li·cis

m. flex·or pro·fun·dus

m. flex·or sub·li·mis

m. fron·ta·lis

m. ge·ni·o·hy·o·glos·sus

m. glos·so·pal·a·ti·nus

m. glos·so·pha·ryn·ge·us

m. glu·te·us quar·tus

m. hy·po·pha·ryn·ge·us

m. il·i·a·cus mi·nor

m. il·i·o·cap·su·la·ris

m. il·i·o·cos·ta·lis dor·si

m. in·ci·si·vus la·bii in·fe·ri·o·ris

m. in·ci·si·vus la·bii su·pe·ri·o·ris

mus·cu·li in·fra·cos·ta·les

m. in·fra·cos·ta·lis

m. in·ter·os·se·us vo·la·ris

m. in·ter·tra·gi·cus

m. is·chi·o·coc·cyg·e·us

m. ke·ra·to·pha·ryn·ge·us

m. la·ryn·go·pha·ryn·ge·us

m. le·va·tor alae na·si

m. le·va·tor an·gu·li scap·u·lae

m. le·va·tor la·bii in·fe·ri·o·ris

m. le·va·tor pa·la·ti

m. lon·gis·si·mus dor·si

m. mul·tif·i·dus spi·nae

m. my·lo·pha·ryn·ge·us

m. oc·ci·pi·ta·lis

m. op·po·nens di·gi·ti quin·ti

m. op·po·nens mi·ni·mi di·gi·ti

m. or·bi·cu·la·ris pal·pe·bra·rum

m. or·bi·to·pal·pe·bra·lis

m. pa·la·to·sal·pin·ge·us

m. pa·la·to·sta·phy·li·nus

m. pe·ro·ne·o·cal·ca·ne·us

m. pet·ro·pha·ryn·ge·us

m. pe·tro·sta·phy·li·nus

m. pha·ryn·go·pa·la·ti·nus

m. pla·tys·ma

m. pla·tys·ma my·oi·des

m. pro·na·tor pe·dis

m. pro·na·tor ra·dii te·res

m. pros·ta·ti·cus

m. pte·ry·goi·de·us ex·ter·nus

m. pte·ry·goi·de·us in·ter·nus

m. pte·ry·go·pha·ryn·ge·us

m. pte·ry·go·spi·no·sus

m. py·ra·mi·da·lis na·si

m. pyr·i·for·mis

m. quad·ra·tus la·bii in·fe·ri·o·ris

m. quad·ra·tus la·bii su·pe·ri·o·ris

m. quad·ra·tus men·ti

m. quad·ri·ceps ex·ten·sor fe·mo·ris

m. rec·tus ca·pi·tis an·ti·cus ma·jor

m. rec·tus ca·pi·tis an·ti·cus mi·nor

m. rec·tus ca·pi·tis pos·ti·cus ma·jor

m. rec·tus ca·pi·tis pos·ti·cus mi·nor

m. rec·tus ex·ter·nus

m. rec·tus in·ter·nus

m. rec·tus tho·ra·cis

m. re·tra·hens au·rem

m. re·tra·hens au·ric·u·lam

m. rhom·bo·at·loi·de·us

m. sa·cro·coc·cyg·e·us an·te·ri·or

m. sa·cro·coc·cyg·e·us pos·te·ri·or

m. sa·cro·lum·ba·lis

m. sa·cro·spi·na·lis

m. sca·le·nus an·ti·cus

m. sca·le·nus pos·ti·cus

m. scan·so·ri·us

m. sem·i·spi·na·lis col·li

m. sem·i·spi·na·lis dor·si

m. ser·ra·tus mag·nus

m. ske·le·ti

m. sphe·no·sal·pin·go·staph·y·li·nus

m. sphinc·ter duc·tus pan·cre·a·ti·ci

m. sphinc·ter oris

m. sphinc·ter ure·thrae mem·bra·na·ceae

m. sphinc·ter va·gi·nae

m. sphinc·ter ve·si·cae

m. spi·na·lis col·li

m. spi·na·lis dor·si

m. sple·ni·us col·li

m. ster·no·chon·dro·sca·pu·la·ris

m. ster·no·cla·vi·cu·la·ris

m. ster·no·fas·ci·a·lis

m. sty·lo·au·ri·cu·la·ris

m. sty·lo·la·ryn·ge·us

m. sub·cu·ta·ne·us col·li

m. su·pi·na·tor lon·gus

m. su·pi·na·tor ra·dii bre·vis

m. su·pra·cla·vic·u·lar·is

m. su·pra·spi·na·lis

m. ten·sor fas·ci·ae fe·mo·ris

m. ten·sor pa·la·ti

m. ten·sor tar·si

m. tet·ra·go·nus

m. thy·ro·ar·y·te·noi·de·us ex·ter·nus

m. thy·ro·ar·y·te·noi·de·us in·ter·nus

m. thy·ro·pha·ryn·ge·us

m. tib·i·a·lis an·ti·cus

m. tib·i·a·lis grac·i·lis

m. tib·i·a·lis pos·ti·cus

m. tib·i·a·lis se·cun·dus

m. tib·i·o·fas·ci·a·lis an·te·ri·or

m. tib·i·o·fas·ci·a·lis an·ti·cus

m. trach·e·lo·cla·vi·cu·la·ris

m. trach·e·lo·mas·toi·de·us

m. trans·ver·sa·lis ab·do·mi·nis

m. trans·ver·sa·lis ca·pi·tis

m. trans·ver·sa·lis cer·vis·cis

m. trans·ver·sa·lis col·li

m. trans·ver·sa·lis na·si

m. tri·an·gu·la·ris

m. tri·an·gu·la·ris la·bii in·fe·ri·o·ris

m. tri·an·gu·la·ris la·bii su·pe·ri·o·ris

m. tri·an·gu·la·ris ster·ni

m. tri·ti·ce·o·glos·sus

m. vas·tus ex·ter·nus

m. vas·tus in·ter·nus

m. ven·tric·u·lar·is

m. zy·go·ma·ti·cus

mush·bite

mush·room
poi·son·ing

mush·room-work·er's
lung

mu·sic
blind·ness

mu·si·cal
agraph·ia
alex·ia
mur·mur

mu·si·cian's
cramp

mu·si·co·ther·a·py

mus·keag
moss

Musset's
sign

mus·si·ta·tion

Mustard
op·er·a·tion
pro·ce·dure

mus·tard
  gas
mus·tard oil
  ex·pressed m. o.
  vol·a·tile m. o.
mus·tine hy·dro·chlo·ride
mu·ta·cism
mu·ta·gen
  frame-shift m.
mu·ta·gen·e·sis
  in·ser·tion·al m.
mu·ta·gen·ic
mu·tant
  ac·tive m.
  con·di·tion·al-le·thal m.
  con·di·tion·al·ly le·thal m.
  in·ac·tive m.
  si·lent m.
  sup·pres·sor-sen·si·tive m.
  tem·per·a·ture-sen·si·tive m.
mu·tant
  gene
mu·ta·ro·tase
mu·ta·ro·ta·tion
mu·tase
mu·ta·tion
  ad·di·tion-de·le·tion m.
  am·ber m.
  back m.
  frame-shift m.
  in·duced m.
  le·thal m.
  mis·sense m.
  nat·u·ral m.
  neu·tral m.
  new m.
  non·sense m.
  ochre m.
  point m.
  read·ing-frame-shift m.
  re·verse m.
  si·lent m.
  so·mat·ic m.
  spon·ta·ne·ous m.
  sup·pres·sor m.
  tran·si·tion m.
  trans·ver·sion m.
mu·ta·tion
  rate
mute
mu·tein
mu·ti·lat·ing
  ker·a·to·der·ma
  lep·ro·sy
mu·ti·la·tion
mut·ism
  aki·net·ic m.

elec·tive m.
vol·un·tary m.
mu·ton
mut·ter·ing
  de·lir·i·um
mut·ton-fat ke·rat·ic
  pre·cip·i·tates
mu·tu·al
  re·sis·tance
mu·tu·al·ism
mu·tu·al·ist
muz·zle
MVE
  vi·rus
my·al·gia
  ep·i·dem·ic m.
  m. ther·mi·ca
my·as·the·nia
  m. an·gi·o·scle·ro·ti·ca
  m. cor·dis
  m. gra·vis
my·as·then·ic
  fa·ci·es
  re·ac·tion
my·a·to·nia
  m. con·gen·i·ta
my·at·o·ny
my·at·ro·phy
my·ce·lia
my·ce·li·an
my·ce·li·oid
my·ce·li·um
  aer·i·al m.
  non·sep·tate m.
  sep·tate m.
my·cete
my·ce·tism
  m. ce·re·bra·lis
  m. cho·li·for·mis
  m. gas·tro·in·tes·ti·na·lis
  m. ner·vo·sa
  m. san·gui·na·re·us
my·ce·tis·mus
my·ce·to·ge·net·ic
my·ce·to·gen·ic
my·ce·tog·e·nous
my·ce·to·ma
  Bouffardi's black m.
  Bouffardi's white m.
  Brumpt's white m.
  Carter's black m.
  Nicolle's white m.
  Vincent's white m.
my·cid
my·co·bac·te·ria
  group I m.
  group II m.

group III m.
group IV m.
My·co·bac·te·ri·a·ce·ae
my·co·bac·te·ri·o·sis
My·co·bac·te·ri·um
M. ab·sces·sus
M. avi·um
M. bal·nei
M. bo·vis
M. for·tu·i·tum
M. in·tra·cel·lu·la·re
M. kan·sa·sii
M. lep·rae
M. lep·rae·mu·ri·um
M. mar·i·an·um
M. ma·ri·num
M. mi·cro·ti
M. par·a·tu·ber·cu·lo·sis
M. phlei
M. pla·ty·poe·ci·lus
M. scro·fu·la·ce·um
M. smeg·ma·tis
M. tham·no·phe·os
M. tu·ber·cu·lo·sis
M. tu·ber·cu·lo·sis subsp.
  bo·vis
M. ul·ce·rans
M. xen·o·pei
M. xen·o·pi
my·co·bac·tin
my·co·cide
My·co·der·ma
my·co·der·ma·ti·tis
my·co·gas·tri·tis
my·col·ic ac·ids
my·col·o·gist
my·col·o·gy
  med·i·cal m.
my·co·myr·in·gi·tis
my·co·phage
My·co·plas·ma
M. ag·a·lac·ti·ae
M. buc·ca·le
M. con·junc·ti·vae subsp.
  ovis
M. fau·ci·um
M. fer·men·tans
M. gal·li·sep·ti·cum
M. gran·u·la·rum
M. hom·i·nis
M. hy·o·rhi·nis
M. hy·o·sy·no·vi·ae
M. hy·po·pneu·mo·ni·ae
M. laid·la·wii
M. me·le·ag·ri·dis
M. my·coi·des
M. neu·ro·ly·ti·cum
M. pha·ryn·gis

M. pneu·mo·ni·ae
M. sal·i·var·i·um
M. syn·o·vi·ae
my·co·plas·ma
  pneu·mo·nia of pigs
my·co·plas·mal
  pneu·mo·nia
my·co·plas·ma·ta
My·co·plas·ma·ta·les
my·co·pus
my·cose
my·co·ses
my·co·sis
  m. cu·tis chron·i·ca
  m. fram·boe·si·oi·des
  m. fun·goi·des
  Gilchrist's m.
  m. in·tes·ti·na·lis
my·co·stat·ic
my·cos·ter·ols
my·cot·ic
  ab·scess
  an·eu·rysm
  ker·a·ti·tis
my·co·tox·i·co·sis
my·co·tox·ins
my·co·vi·rus
my·da·le·ine
my·da·tox·in
my·dri·a·sis
  al·ter·nat·ing m.
  am·au·rot·ic m.
  par·a·lyt·ic m.
  spas·mod·ic m.
  spas·tic m.
  spring·ing m.
myd·ri·at·ic
  ri·gid·i·ty
my·ec·to·my
my·ec·to·pia
my·ec·to·py
my·el·ap·o·plexy
my·el·a·te·lia
my·el·auxe
my·e·le·mia
my·el·en·ceph·a·lon
my·el·ic
my·e·lin
  body
  fig·ure
  sheath
my·e·li·nat·ed
my·e·li·nat·ed nerve
  fi·ber
my·e·li·na·tion
my·e·lin·ic
  de·gen·er·a·tion
my·e·lin·i·za·tion

my·e·li·noc·la·sis
my·e·lin·o·gen·e·sis
my·e·li·nol·y·sis
   cen·tral pon·tine m.
my·e·lit·ic
my·e·li·tis
   acute trans·verse m.
   as·cend·ing m.
   bul·bar m.
   con·cus·sion m.
   Foix-Alajouanine m.
   fu·nic·u·lar m.
   sub·a·cute nec·ro·tiz·ing m.
   sys·tem·ic m.
   trans·verse m.
my·e·lo·ar·chi·tec·ton·ics
my·e·lo·blast
my·e·lo·blas·te·mia
my·e·lo·blas·tic
   leu·ke·mia
   pro·tein
my·e·lo·blas·to·ma
my·e·lo·blas·to·sis
   avi·an m.
   fowl m.
my·e·lo·cele
my·e·lo·cyst
my·e·lo·cyst·ic
my·e·lo·cys·to·cele
my·e·lo·cys·to·me·ning·o·cele
my·e·lo·cyte
   m. A
   m. B
   m. C
my·e·lo·cy·the·mia
my·e·lo·cyt·ic
   cri·sis
   leu·ke·mia
   leu·ke·moid re·ac·tion
my·e·lo·cy·to·ma
my·e·lo·cy·to·ma·to·sis
my·e·lo·cy·to·sis
my·e·lo·di·as·ta·sis
my·e·lo·dys·pla·sia
my·e·lo·fi·bro·sis
my·e·lo·gen·e·sis
my·e·lo·ge·net·ic
my·e·lo·gen·ic
   leu·ke·mia
   sar·co·ma
my·e·log·e·nous
   leu·ke·mia
my·e·lo·gone
my·e·lo·go·ni·um
my·e·lo·gram
my·e·log·ra·phy
my·e·lo·ic

my·e·loid
   cell
   leu·ke·mia
   met·a·pla·sia
   re·tic·u·lo·sis
   sar·co·ma
   se·ries
   tis·sue
my·e·loi·do·sis
my·e·lo·leu·ke·mia
my·e·lo·li·po·ma
my·e·lo·lym·pho·cyte
my·e·lol·y·sis
my·e·lo·ma
   Bence Jones m.
   en·do·the·li·al m.
   gi·ant cell m.
   L-chain m.
   mul·ti·ple m.
   m. mul·ti·plex
   non·se·cre·to·ry m.
   plas·ma cell m.
my·e·lo·ma·la·cia
   an·gi·o·dys·ge·net·ic m.
my·e·lo·ma·to·sis
   mul·ti·ple m.
   m. mul·ti·plex
my·e·lo·me·ning·o·cele
my·e·lo·mere
my·e·lo·mon·o·cyte
my·e·lo·mon·o·cyt·ic
   leu·ke·mia
my·e·lo·neu·ri·tis
my·e·lon·ic
my·e·lo·pa·ral·y·sis
my·e·lo·path·ic
   ane·mia
my·e·lop·a·thy
   car·ci·nom·a·tous m.
   com·pres·sive m.
   di·a·bet·ic m.
   par·a·car·ci·nom·a·tous m.
   ra·di·a·tion m.
my·e·lo·per·ox·i·dase
my·e·lop·e·tal
my·e·lo·phthis·ic
   ane·mia
my·e·loph·thi·sis
my·e·lo·plast
my·e·lo·ple·gia
my·e·lo·poi·e·sis
my·e·lo·poi·et·ic
my·e·lo·pro·lif·er·a·tive
   syn·dromes
my·e·lo·ra·dic·u·li·tis
my·e·lo·ra·dic·u·lo·dys·pla·sia
my·e·lo·ra·dic·u·lop·a·thy

my·e·lo·ra·dic·u·lo·pol·y·neu·
  ron·i·tis
my·e·lor·rha·gia
my·e·lor·rha·phy
my·e·lo·sar·co·ma
my·e·lo·sar·co·ma·to·sis
my·e·los·chi·sis
my·e·lo·scle·ro·sis
my·e·lo·sis
  aleu·ke·mic m.
  chron·ic non·leu·ke·mic m.
  er·y·threm·ic m.
  fu·nic·u·lar m.
  leu·ke·mic m.
  leu·ko·pe·nic m.
  sub·leu·ke·mic m.
my·e·lo·spon·gi·um
my·e·lo·syph·i·lis
my·e·lo·sy·rin·go·sis
my·e·lo·tome
my·e·lo·to·mog·ra·phy
my·e·lot·o·my
  Bischof's m.
  com·mis·sur·al m.
  mid·line m.
  T m.
my·e·lo·tox·ic
my·en·ter·ic
  plex·us
  re·flex
my·en·ter·on
my·es·the·sia
my·i·a·sis
  Af·ri·can fu·run·cu·lar m.
  au·ral m.
  creep·ing m.
  hu·man bot·fly m.
  in·tes·ti·nal m.
  m. li·ne·a·ris
  na·sal m.
  oc·u·lar m.
  m. oes·tru·o·sa
  sub·cu·ta·ne·ous m.
  trau·mat·ic m.
  tum·bu der·mal m.
  wound m.
my·i·tis
my·kol
myl·a·bris
my·lo·hy·oid
  fos·sa
  groove
  line
  mus·cle
  nerve
  ridge
my·lo·hy·oi·de·us

my·lo·pha·ryn·ge·al
  part
my·o·al·bu·min
my·o·ar·chi·tec·ton·ic
my·o·at·ro·phy
my·o·blast
my·o·blas·tic
my·o·blas·to·ma
  gran·u·lar cell m.
my·o·bra·dia
my·o·car·dia
my·o·car·di·al
  bridge
  in·farc·tion
  in·farc·tion in H-form
  in·suf·fi·cien·cy
  is·che·mia
  rig·or mor·tis
my·o·car·di·al de·pres·sant
  fac·tor
my·o·car·di·o·graph
my·o·car·di·op·a·thy
my·o·car·di·or·ra·phy
my·o·car·di·tis
  acute iso·lat·ed m.
  Fiedler's m.
  frag·men·ta·tion m.
  gi·ant cell m.
  in·du·ra·tive m.
my·o·car·di·um
my·o·car·do·sis
my·o·cele
my·o·ce·li·al·gia
my·o·ce·li·tis
my·o·cel·lu·li·tis
my·o·ce·ro·sis
my·o·chrome
my·o·chron·o·scope
my·o·cin·e·sim·e·ter
my·o·clo·nia
  fi·bril·lary m.
my·o·clon·ic
  ab·sence
my·o·clon·ic astat·ic
  ep·i·lep·sy
my·oc·lo·nus
  ep·i·lep·sy
my·oc·lo·nus
  m. mul·ti·plex
  noc·tur·nal m.
  oc·u·lar m.
  pal·a·tal m.
  stim·u·lus sen·si·tive m.
my·o·col·pi·tis
my·o·com·ma
my·o·com·ma·ta
my·o·cris·mus

my·o·cu·ta·ne·ous
  flap
my·o·cyte
  Anitschkow m.
my·o·cy·tol·y·sis
  m. of heart
my·o·cy·to·ma
my·o·de·gen·er·a·tion
my·o·de·mia
my·o·der·mal
  flap
my·o·di·as·ta·sis
my·o·dy·na·mia
my·o·dy·nam·ics
my·o·dy·na·mom·e·ter
my·o·dyn·ia
my·o·dys·to·ny
my·o·dys·tro·phia
my·o·dys·tro·phy
my·o·e·de·ma
my·o·e·las·tic
  the·o·ry
my·o·e·lec·tric
my·o·en·do·car·di·tis
my·o·ep·i·car·di·al
  man·tle
my·o·ep·i·the·li·al
  cell
my·o·ep·i·the·li·o·ma
my·o·ep·i·the·li·um
my·o·es·the·sia
my·o·es·the·sis
my·o·fa·cial pain-dys·func·tion
  syn·drome
my·o·fas·ci·al
  syn·drome
my·o·fas·ci·tis
my·o·fi·bril
my·o·fi·bril·la
my·o·fi·bril·lae
my·o·fi·bro·blast
my·o·fi·bro·ma
my·o·fi·bro·sis
  m. cor·dis
my·o·fi·bro·si·tis
my·o·fil·a·ments
my·o·func·tion·al
  ther·a·py
my·o·gen
my·o·gen·e·sis
my·o·ge·net·ic
my·o·gen·ic
  pa·ral·y·sis
  po·ten·tial
  the·o·ry
my·og·e·nous
my·o·glo·bin

my·o·glo·bi·nu·ria
  par·a·lyt·ic m.
my·o·glob·u·lin
my·o·glob·u·li·nu·ria
my·og·na·thus
my·o·gram
my·o·graph
  pal·ate m.
my·o·graph·ic
my·og·ra·phy
my·o·he·mo·glo·bin
my·oid
  cells
my·oi·de·ma
my·o·is·che·mia
my·o·ke·ro·sis
my·o·ki·nase
my·o·kin·e·sim·e·ter
my·o·ky·mia
  he·red·i·tary m.
my·o·lem·ma
my·o·li·po·ma
my·o·lo·gia
my·ol·o·gist
my·ol·o·gy
  de·scrip·tive m.
my·ol·y·sis
  car·di·o·tox·ic m.
my·o·ma
my·o·ma·la·cia
my·o·ma·tous
  pol·yp
my·o·mec·to·my
  ab·dom·i·nal m.
  vag·i·nal m.
my·o·mel·a·no·sis
my·o·mere
my·om·e·ter
my·o·me·tri·al
my·o·me·tri·al ar·cu·ate
  ar·ter·ies
my·o·me·tri·al ra·di·al
  ar·ter·ies
my·o·me·tri·tis
my·o·me·tri·um
my·o·mi·to·chon·dria
my·o·mi·to·chon·dri·on
my·o·mot·o·my
my·on
my·o·ne·cro·sis
  clos·trid·i·al m.
my·o·neme
my·o·neu·ral
  block·ade
  junc·tion
my·o·neu·ral·gia
  pos·tur·al m.
my·o·neu·ras·the·nia

my·o·neu·ro·ma
my·on·o·sus
my·on·y·my
my·o·pa·chyn·sis
my·o·pal·mus
my·o·pa·ral·y·sis
my·o·pa·re·sis
my·o·path·ic
   at·ro·phy
   fa·ci·es
   sco·li·o·sis
my·op·a·thy
   car·ci·nom·a·tous m.
   cen·tro·nu·cle·ar m.
   dis·tal m.
   mi·to·chon·dri·al m.
   my·o·tu·bu·lar m.
   nem·a·line m.
   oc·u·lar m.
   rod m.
   thy·ro·tox·ic m.
my·o·per·i·car·di·tis
my·o·per·i·to·ni·tis
my·o·phone
my·o·phos·phor·y·lase de·fi·cien·cy
   gly·co·ge·no·sis
my·o·pia
   ax·i·al m.
   cur·va·ture m.
   de·gen·er·a·tive m.
   in·dex m.
   ma·lig·nant m.
   night m.
   path·o·log·ic m.
   pre·ma·tu·ri·ty m.
   se·nile len·tic·u·lar m.
   sim·ple m.
   space m.
   tran·sient m.
my·o·pic
   astig·ma·tism
   cho·roi·dop·a·thy
   co·nus
   cres·cent
   de·gen·er·a·tion
my·o·plasm
my·o·plas·tic
my·o·plas·ty
my·o·po·lar
my·o·pro·tein
my·o·rhyth·mia
my·or·rha·phy
my·or·rhex·is
my·o·sal·gia
my·o·sal·pin·gi·tis
my·o·sal·pinx
my·o·sar·co·ma

my·o·scle·ro·sis
my·o·seism
my·o·sep·tum
my·o·sin
   fil·a·ment
my·o·sin·o·gen
my·o·si·nose
my·o·sis
my·o·sit·ic
my·o·si·tis
   acute dis·sem·i·nat·ed m.
   cer·vi·cal m.
   ep·i·dem·ic m.
   m. ep·i·dem·i·ca acu·ta
   m. fi·bro·sa
   in·fec·tious m.
   in·ter·sti·tial m.
   mul·ti·ple m.
   m. os·sif·i·cans
   m. os·sif·i·cans cir·cum·scrip·ta
   m. os·sif·i·cans pro·gres·si·va
   pro·lif·er·a·tive m.
   m. pu·ru·len·ta tro·pi·ca
   trop·i·cal m.
my·o·spasm
   cer·vi·cal m.
my·o·spas·mus
my·o·spher·u·lo·sis
my·o·sthe·nom·e·ter
my·o·stro·ma
my·o·stro·min
my·o·tac·tic
my·ot·a·sis
my·o·tat·ic
   con·trac·tion
   ir·ri·ta·bil·i·ty
   re·flex
my·o·ten·o·si·tis
my·o·te·not·o·my
my·o·ther·mic
my·o·tome
my·ot·o·my
my·o·tone
my·o·to·nia
   m. ac·qui·si·ta
   m. atro·phi·ca
   m. con·gen·i·ta
   m. dys·tro·phi·ca
   m. ne·o·na·to·rum
my·o·ton·ic
   cat·a·ract
   dys·tro·phy
my·ot·o·noid
my·ot·o·nus
my·ot·o·ny
my·ot·ro·phy

my·o·tube
my·o·tu·bu·lar
   my·op·a·thy
my·o·tu·bule
my·o·vas·cu·lar
   sphinc·ter
my·o·ve·nous
   sphinc·ter
My·o·vir·i·dae
myr·ia·chit
myr·i·ca
myr·i·cin
my·rin·ga
myr·in·gec·to·my
myr·in·gi·tis
   m. bul·bo·sa
   bul·lous m.
my·rin·go·dec·to·my
my·rin·go·der·ma·ti·tis
my·rin·go·my·co·sis
my·rin·go·plas·ty
my·rin·go·sta·pe·di·o·pexy
my·rin·go·tome
myr·in·got·o·my
my·rinx
my·ris·ti·ca
   m. oil
my·ris·tic ac·id
my·ris·ti·cin
my·ris·to·le·ic ac·id
myr·me·cia
my·ro·si·nase
myrrh
my·so·phil·ia
my·so·pho·bia
my·ta·cism
my·ur·ous
myx·ad·e·no·ma
myx·as·the·nia
myx·e·de·ma
   cir·cum·scribed m.
   con·gen·i·tal m.
   in·fan·tile m.
   op·er·a·tive m.
   pi·tu·i·tary m.
   pre·tib·i·al m.
myx·e·de·ma
   heart
   voice

myx·e·de·ma·toid
myx·e·dem·a·tous
   in·fan·ti·lism
myx·e·mia
myx·o·chon·dro·fi·bro·sar·co·ma
myx·o·chon·dro·ma
Myx·o·coc·cid·i·um steg·o·my·i·ae
myx·o·cyte
myx·o·fi·bro·ma
myx·o·fi·bro·sar·co·ma
myx·oid
   cyst
   de·gen·er·a·tion
myx·o·li·po·ma
myx·o·ma
   atri·al m.
   m. en·chon·dro·ma·to·sum
   m. fi·bro·sum
   m. li·po·ma·to·sum
   odon·to·gen·ic m.
   m. sar·co·ma·to·sum
myx·o·ma·to·sis
   vi·rus
myx·o·ma·tous
   de·gen·er·a·tion
myx·o·mem·bra·nous
   co·li·tis
myx·o·my·cete
Myx·o·my·ce·tes
myx·o·neu·ro·ma
myx·o·pap·il·lary
   ep·en·dy·mo·ma
myx·o·pap·il·lo·ma
myx·o·poi·e·sis
myx·or·rhea
   m. gas·tri·ca
myx·o·sar·co·ma
Myx·o·spo·ra
myx·o·spore
Myx·o·spo·rea
myx·o·vi·rus
Myx·o·zoa

nab·i·lone
na·both·i·an
    cyst
    fol·li·cle
na·cre·ous
    ich·thy·o·sis
NADH de·hy·dro·gen·ase
NADH-hy·drox·yl·a·mine re·duc·tase
Nadi
    re·ac·tion
na·dide
NAD⁺ nu·cle·o·si·dase
na·do·lol
NADPH de·hy·dro·gen·ase
NAD(P)H de·hy·dro·gen·ase (qui·none)
NADPH de·hy·dro·gen·ase (qui·none)
NADPH di·aph·o·rase
NADPH-fer·ri·he·mo·pro·tein re·duc·tase
NAD(P)⁺ nu·cle·o·si·dase
Naegeli
    syn·drome
Naegeli type of mon·o·cyt·ic leu·ke·mia
Nae·gle·ria
naf·cil·lin
    n. so·di·um
Naffziger
    op·er·a·tion
    syn·drome
naf·ro·nyl ox·a·late
naf·ti·fine hy·dro·chlo·ride
na·ga·na
Nägele
    ob·liq·ui·ty
Nägele's
    pel·vis
    rule
Nagel's
    test
Nageotte
    cells
nail
    bed
    ex·ten·sion
    fold

    horn
    ma·trix
    pits
    plate
    pulse
    skin
nail
    egg shell n.
    half and half n.
    hip·po·crat·ic n.'s
    in·grown n.
    Küntscher n.
    par·rot-beak n.
    pin·cer n.
    rack·et n.
    reedy n.
    shell n.
    Smith-Petersen n.
    spoon n.
    Terry's n.'s
    yel·low n.
nail·ing
nail-pa·tel·la
    syn·drome
Nai·ro·bi sheep
    dis·ease
Nai·ro·bi sheep dis·ease
    vi·rus
Nakanishi's
    stain
na·ked
    vi·rus
nal·bu·phine hy·dro·chlo·ride
na·li·dix·ic ac·id
nal·or·phine
nal·ox·one hy·dro·chlo·ride
nal·trex·one
NAME
    syn·drome
NANB
    hep·a·ti·tis
nan·dro·lone
    n. dec·a·no·ate
    n. phen·pro·pi·o·nate
    n. phen·yl·pro·pi·o·nate
nan·ism
Nan·niz·zia
nan·o·ce·pha·lia
nan·o·ce·phal·ic

nan·o·ceph·a·lous
nan·o·ceph·a·ly
nan·o·cor·mia
nan·o·gram
nan·oid
  enam·el
nan·o·me·lia
nan·o·me·ter
nan·oph·thal·mia
nan·oph·thal·mos
Na·no·phy·e·tus sal·min·co·la
na·nous
Nanta
na·nu·ka·ya·mi
  fe·ver
na·nus
nape
  ne·vus
na·pex
naph·az·o·line hy·dro·chlo·ride
naph·tha
  coal tar n.
  wood n.
naph·tha·lene
naph·thal·e·nol
naph·tha·lin
naph·thaz·o·line hy·dro·chlo·ride
naph·thol
α-naph·thol
β-naph·thol
naph·tho·late
naph·thol yel·low S
naph·tho·qui·none
naph·thyl
na·pi·er
nap·kin
  rash
na·prap·a·thy
na·prox·en
nap·syl·ate
nar·ce·ine
nar·cis·sism
  pri·mary n.
  sec·on·dary n.
nar·co·a·nal·y·sis
nar·co·hyp·nia
nar·co·hyp·no·sis
nar·co·lep·sy
nar·co·lep·tic
  tet·rad
nar·co·sis
  ni·tro·gen n.
nar·co·syn·the·sis
nar·co·ther·a·py
nar·cot·ic
  block·ade

hun·ger
  re·ver·sal
dl-nar·co·tine
nar·co·tism
na·res
na·ris
  an·te·ri·or n.
  pos·te·ri·or n.
nar·row-an·gle
  glau·co·ma
na·sal
  bone
  cal·cu·lus
  cap·sule
  ca·tarrh
  cav·i·ty
  con·cha
  crest
  duct
  feed·ing
  fo·ra·men
  gan·gli·on
  glands
  gli·o·ma
  height
  hem·or·rhage
  hy·dror·rhea
  in·dex
  mar·gin
  mus·cle
  my·i·a·sis
  nerve
  notch
  part
  part of phar·ynx
  phar·ynx
  pits
  plac·odes
  point
  pol·yp
  pro·cess
  re·flex
  re·gion
  ridge
  sacs
  sep·tum
  spine of fron·tal bone
  sur·face of max·il·la
  sur·face of pal·a·tine bone
  valve
  ven·ules of ret·i·na
na·sal ve·nous
  arch
nas·cent
Na·sik
  vib·rio
na·si·o·in·i·ac
na·si·on

na·si·on-po·go·ni·on
  mea·sure·ment
na·si·on-post·con·dy·lar
  plane
na·si·on soft
  tis·sue
Nasmyth's
  cu·ti·cle
  mem·brane
na·so·an·tral
na·so·bas·i·lar
  line
na·so·breg·mat·ic
  arc
na·so·cil·i·ary
  nerve
  root
na·so·fron·tal
  vein
na·so·gas·tric
  tube
na·so·ju·gal
  fold
na·so·la·bi·al
  groove
  node
na·so·lac·ri·mal
  ca·nal
  duct
na·so·man·dib·u·lar
  fix·a·tion
na·so·max·il·lary
  su·ture
na·so·men·tal
  re·flex
na·so-oc·cip·i·tal
  arc
na·so-oral
na·so·pal·a·tine
  groove
  nerve
na·so·pha·ryn·ge·al
  groove
  leish·man·i·a·sis
  pas·sage
na·so·phar·yn·gi·tis
na·so·pha·ryn·go·la·ryn·go·
  scope
na·so·pha·ryn·go·scope
na·so·pha·ryn·gos·co·py
na·so·pha·rynx
na·so·ros·tral
na·so·scope
na·so·si·nu·si·tis
na·so·tra·che·al
  in·tu·ba·tion
  tube

Nasse's
  law
na·sus
na·tal
  cleft
  tooth
na·tal·i·ty
na·ta·my·cin
na·tes
na·ti·mor·tal·i·ty
na·tive
  al·bu·min
  pro·tein
na·tre·mia
na·trex·one hy·dro·chlo·ride
na·tri·e·mia
na·trif·er·ic
na·tri·um
na·tri·u·re·sis
na·tri·u·ret·ic
nat·u·ral
  an·ti·body
  den·ti·tion
  dyes
  fo·cus of in·fec·tion
  he·mo·ly·sin
  im·mu·ni·ty
  mu·ta·tion
  se·lec·tion
nat·u·ral kill·er
  cells
na·ture-nur·ture
  is·sue
na·tur·o·path
na·tur·o·path·ic
na·tur·op·a·thy
Nauheim
  bath
  treat·ment
nau·path·ia
nau·sea
  ep·i·dem·ic n.
  n. grav·i·dar·um
nau·se·ant
nau·se·ate
nau·se·at·ed
nau·seous
Nauta's
  stain
na·vel
  ill
na·vic·u·la
na·vic·u·lar
  ab·do·men
  bone
  bone of hand
  dis·ease
  fos·sa of ure·thra

na·vic·u·lar ar·tic·u·lar
  sur·face of ta·lus
na·vic·u·lar·thri·tis
ND
  vi·rus
ne·al·bar·bi·tal
near
  point
  re·ac·tion
  re·flex
  sight
near point of
  con·ver·gence
near·sight·ed·ness
ne·ar·thro·sis
neb·ra·my·cin
Ne·bras·ka calf scours
  vi·rus
neb·u·la
neb·u·lae
neb·u·la·rine
neb·u·li·za·tion
neb·u·lize
neb·u·liz·er
  jet n.
  spin·ning disk n.
  ul·tra·son·ic n.
neb·u·lous
  urine
Ne·ca·tor
ne·ca·to·ri·a·sis
neck
  re·flex·es
  sign
neck
  an·a·tom·i·cal n. of hu·
    mer·us
  buf·fa·lo n.
  bull n.
  den·tal n.
  n. of fe·mur
  n. of fib·u·la
  n. of gall·blad·der
  n. of glans pe·nis
  n. of hair fol·li·cle
  n. of hu·mer·us
  Madelung's n.
  n. of mal·le·us
  n. of man·di·ble
  n. of ra·di·us
  n. of rib
  n. of scap·u·la
  stiff n.
  sur·gi·cal n. of hu·mer·us
  n. of ta·lus
  n. of thigh bone
  n. of tooth
  n. of uri·nary blad·der

n. of uter·us
webbed n.
n. of womb
wry n.
neck·lace
  Casal's n.
  n. of Venus
nec·rec·to·my
nec·ro·bi·o·sis
  n. li·poi·di·ca
  n. li·poi·di·ca di·a·be·ti·co·
    rum
nec·ro·bi·ot·ic
  xan·tho·gran·u·lo·ma
nec·ro·cy·to·sis
nec·ro·gen·ic
  wart
ne·crog·e·nous
nec·ro·gran·u·lo·ma·tous
  ker·a·ti·tis
ne·crol·o·gist
ne·crol·o·gy
ne·crol·y·sis
  tox·ic ep·i·der·mal n.
nec·ro·lyt·ic mi·gra·to·ry
  er·y·the·ma
nec·ro·ma·nia
ne·crom·e·ter
nec·ro·par·a·site
ne·crop·a·thy
ne·croph·a·gous
nec·ro·phil·ia
ne·croph·i·lism
ne·croph·i·lous
nec·ro·pho·bia
ne·crop·sy
nec·ro·sa·dism
ne·cros·co·py
ne·crose
ne·cro·sis
  asep·tic n.
  avas·cu·lar n.
  bridg·ing he·pa·tic n.
  ca·se·a·tion n.
  ca·se·ous n.
  cen·tral n.
  co·ag·u·la·tion n.
  col·liq·ua·tive n.
  cys·tic me·di·al n.
  ep·i·phys·i·al asep·tic n.
  fat n.
  fi·brin·oid n.
  fo·cal n.
  is·che·mic n.
  lam·i·nar cor·ti·cal n.
  liq·ue·fac·tive n.
  mum·mi·fi·ca·tion n.

pro·gress·ive em·phy·sem·a·
  tous n.
re·nal pap·il·lary n.
sim·ple n.
sub·cu·ta·ne·ous fat n. of
  new·born
sup·pu·ra·tive n.
to·tal n.
Zenker's n.
zon·al n.
ne·cro·sis
  ba·cil·lus
nec·ro·sper·mia
ne·cros·te·on
ne·cros·te·o·sis
ne·crot·ic
  an·gi·na
  cir·rho·sis
  cyst
  in·flam·ma·tion
  pulp
  rhi·ni·tis of pigs
ne·crot·ic in·fec·tious
  con·junc·ti·vi·tis
nec·ro·tiz·ing
  an·gi·i·tis
  ar·ter·i·o·li·tis
  en·ceph·a·li·tis
  en·ceph·a·lo·my·e·lop·a·thy
  en·ter·o·co·li·tis
  fas·ci·i·tis
  in·flam·ma·tion
  pap·il·li·tis
  scle·ri·tis
  si·al·o·met·a·pla·sia
nec·ro·tiz·ing ul·cer·a·tive
  gin·gi·vi·tis
ne·crot·o·my
  os·te·o·plas·tic n.
nee·dle
  an·eu·rysm n.
  ar·tery n.
  as·pi·rat·ing n.
  atrau·mat·ic n.
  bi·op·sy n.
  cat·a·ract n.
  couch·ing n.
  Deschamps n.
  Emmet's n.
  ex·plor·ing n.
  Francke's n.
  Frazier's n.
  Gillmore n.
  Hagedorn n.
  hy·po·der·mic n.
  knife n.
  lum·bar punc·ture n.
  Salah's ster·nal punc·ture n.

spat·u·la n.
stop-n.
Tuohy n.
Vicat n.
nee·dle
  bath
  bi·op·sy
  cul·ture
  for·ceps
nee·dle-car·ri·er
nee·dle-driv·er
nee·dle-hold·er
nee·dle point
  trac·ing
Needles' split cast
  meth·od
nee·dling
ne·en·ceph·a·lon
Neethling
  vi·rus
nef·o·pam hy·dro·chlo·ride
Neftel's
  dis·ease
ne·ga·tion
neg·a·tive
  false n.
neg·a·tive
  ac·com·mo·da·tion
  af·ter·im·age
  an·er·gy
  cat·a·lyst
  chro·not·ro·pism
  con·ver·gence
  elec·trode
  elec·tro·tax·is
  feed·back
  me·nis·cus
  phase
  pol·itz·er·i·za·tion
  pres·sure
  sco·to·ma
  stain
  tax·is
  ther·mo·tax·is
  trans·fer·ence
  va·lence
neg·a·tive base
  ex·cess
neg·a·tive che·mo·tax·is
neg·a·tive cy·to·tax·is
neg·a·tive end-ex·pi·ra·to·ry
  pres·sure
neg·a·tive G
neg·a·tive hy·drot·ro·pism
neg·a·tive leu·ko·cy·to·tax·ia
neg·a·tive·ly
  bath·mo·tro·pic

neg·a·tive·ly *(continued)*
  dro·mo·tro·pic
  in·o·tro·pic
neg·a·tive neu·tro·tax·is
neg·a·tive p
neg·a·tive pho·tod·ro·my
neg·a·tive pho·to·tax·is
neg·a·tive pho·tot·ro·pism
neg·a·tive re·in·forc·er
neg·a·tive S
neg·a·tive ster·e·ot·ro·pism
neg·a·tive strand
  vi·rus
neg·a·tive sup·port·ing
  re·ac·tion's
neg·a·tive tro·pism
neg·a·tiv·ism
neg·a·tron
Ne·gi·shi
  vi·rus
Negri
  bod·ies
  cor·pus·cles
Negro's
  phe·nom·e·non
Neis·se·ria
  N. ca·vi·ae
  N. fla·va
  N. fla·ves·cens
  N. gon·or·rhoe·ae
  N. hae·mo·ly·sans
  N. me·nin·gi·ti·dis
  N. sic·ca
  N. sub·fla·va
neis·se·ria
neis·se·ri·ae
Neisser's
  coc·cus
  stain
  sy·ringe
Nélaton's
  cath·e·ter
  dis·lo·ca·tion
  fi·bers
  line
  sphinc·ter
Nelson
  syn·drome
  tu·mor
nem·a·line
  my·op·a·thy
nem·a·thel·minth
Nem·a·thel·min·thes
nem·a·to·ci·dal
nem·a·to·cide
nem·a·to·cyst
Nem·a·to·da
nem·a·tode

nem·a·to·di·a·sis
  cer·e·bro·spi·nal n.
Nem·a·to·di·rel·la lon·gi·spi·cu·la·ta
Nem·a·to·di·rus
nem·a·toid
nem·a·tol·o·gist
nem·a·tol·o·gy
nem·a·to·sper·mia
ne·o·an·ti·gens
ne·o·ars·phen·a·mine
ne·o·ar·thro·sis
Ne·o·as·ca·ris vi·tu·lo·rum
ne·o·bi·o·gen·e·sis
ne·o·blas·tic
ne·o·cer·e·bel·lum
ne·o·chy·mo·tryp·sin·o·gen
ne·o·cin·cho·phen
ne·o·cor·tex
ne·o·cys·tos·to·my
ne·o·dym·i·um
ne·o·en·ceph·a·lon
ne·o·fe·tal
ne·o·fe·tus
ne·o·for·ma·tion
ne·og·a·la
ne·o·gen·e·sis
ne·o·ge·net·ic
ne·o·ki·net·ic
ne·o·lal·lism
ne·ol·o·gism
ne·o·mem·brane
ne·o·morph
ne·o·mor·phism
ne·o·my·cin sul·fate
ne·on
ne·o·na·tal
  ane·mia
  ap·o·plexy
  ar·thri·tis of foals
  death
  di·ag·no·sis
  hep·a·ti·tis
  her·pes
  hy·po·gly·ce·mia
  iso·e·ryth·rol·y·sis
  line
  med·i·cine
  ring
  screen·ing
  tet·a·ny
  tooth
ne·o·na·tal calf di·ar·rhea
  vi·rus
ne·o·na·tal mor·tal·i·ty
  rate
ne·o·nate
ne·o·na·tol·o·gist

ne·o·na·tol·o·gy
ne·o·pal·li·um
ne·op·a·thy
ne·o·pho·bia
ne·o·phre·nia
ne·o·pla·sia
   cer·vi·cal in·tra·ep·i·the·li·al n.
ne·o·plasm
   his·toid n.
ne·o·plas·tic
   arach·noid·i·tis
   men·in·gi·tis
ne·op·trin
ne·o·pyr·i·thi·a·min
ne·o·ret·i·nene B
Ne·o·rick·ett·sia hel·min·the·ca
ne·o·stig·mine
ne·os·to·my
ne·o·stri·a·tum
ne·o·stro·phin·gic
ne·ot·e·ny
Ne·o·tes·tu·di·na ro·sa·ti
ne·o·thal·a·mus
ne·o·type
   cul·ture
   strain
ne·o·ty·ro·sine
ne·o·vas·cu·lar
   glau·co·ma
ne·o·vas·cu·lar·i·za·tion
ne·per
neph·e·lom·e·ter
neph·e·lom·e·try
neph·rad·e·no·ma
ne·phral·gia
ne·phral·gic
neph·ras·the·nia
neph·ra·to·nia
ne·phrat·o·ny
ne·phrec·ta·sia
ne·phrec·ta·sis
ne·phrec·to·my
   ab·dom·i·nal n.
   an·te·ri·or n.
   lum·bar n.
   par·a·per·i·to·ne·al n.
   pos·te·ri·or n.
neph·re·de·ma
neph·rel·co·sis
neph·ric
   blas·te·ma
   duct
ne·phrid·ia
ne·phrid·i·um
ne·phrit·ic
   cal·cu·lus

fac·tor
syn·drome
ne·phrit·i·des
ne·phri·tis
   acute n.
   acute in·ter·sti·tial n.
   an·al·ge·sic n.
   an·ti-base·ment mem·brane n.
   an·ti-kid·ney se·rum n.
   chron·ic n.
   fo·cal n.
   glo·mer·u·lar n.
   n. grav·i·dar·um
   hem·or·rhag·ic n.
   he·red·i·tary n.
   im·mune com·plex n.
   in·ter·sti·tial n.
   lu·pus n.
   Masugi's n.
   mes·an·gi·al n.
   salt-los·ing n.
   scar·la·ti·nal n.
   se·rum n.
   sub·a·cute n.
   sup·pu·ra·tive n.
   syph·i·lit·ic n.
   trans·fu·sion n.
   trench n.
   tu·ber·cu·lous n.
   tu·bu·lo·in·ter·sti·tial n.
   ura·ni·um n.
ne·phrit·o·gen·ic
neph·ro·blas·te·ma
neph·ro·blas·to·ma
neph·ro·cal·ci·no·sis
neph·ro·cap·sec·to·my
neph·ro·car·di·ac
neph·ro·cele
neph·ro·ce·lom
neph·ro·cys·to·sis
neph·ro·ge·net·ic
neph·ro·gen·ic
   ad·e·no·ma
   cord
   di·a·be·tes in·sip·i·dus
   tis·sue
ne·phrog·e·nous
neph·ro·gram
ne·phrog·ra·phy
neph·ro·hy·dro·sis
neph·roid
neph·ro·lith
neph·ro·li·thi·a·sis
neph·ro·li·thot·o·my
ne·phrol·o·gy
ne·phrol·y·sin
ne·phrol·y·sis

neph·ro·lyt·ic
ne·phro·ma
  mes·o·blas·tic n.
neph·ro·ma·la·cia
neph·ro·meg·a·ly
neph·ro·mere
neph·ron
neph·ron·ic
  loop
neph·ro·path·ia ep·i·dem·i·ca
ne·phrop·a·thy
  an·al·ge·sic n.
  Bal·kan n.
  Da·nu·bi·an en·dem·ic fa·
    mil·i·al n.
  hy·po·ka·le·mic n.
  IgA n.
  IgM n.
neph·ro·pexy
neph·roph·thi·sis
  fa·mil·i·al ju·ve·nile n.
neph·rop·to·sia
neph·rop·to·sis
neph·ro·py·e·li·tis
neph·ro·py·e·lo·plas·ty
neph·ro·py·o·sis
neph·ror·rha·phy
neph·ro·scle·ro·sis
  ar·te·ri·al n.
  ar·te·ri·o·lar n.
  be·nign n.
  ma·lig·nant n.
  se·nile n.
neph·ro·scle·rot·ic
ne·phro·sis
  acute n.
  am·y·loid n.
  cho·lem·ic n.
  fa·mil·i·al n.
  he·mo·glo·bi·nu·ric n.
  hy·pox·ic n.
  lip·oid n.
  low·er neph·ron n.
  os·mot·ic n.
  tox·ic n.
  vac·u·o·lar n.
neph·ro·spa·sia
neph·ros·pa·sis
ne·phros·to·gram
ne·phros·to·ma
neph·ro·stome
ne·phros·to·my
neph·rot·ic
  syn·drome
neph·ro·tome
neph·ro·tom·ic
  cav·i·ty
neph·ro·to·mo·gram

neph·ro·to·mog·ra·phy
ne·phrot·o·my
  an·a·tro·phic n.
neph·ro·tox·ic
neph·ro·tox·ic·i·ty
neph·ro·tox·in
neph·ro·tro·phic
neph·ro·tro·pic
neph·ro·tu·ber·cu·lo·sis
neph·ro·u·re·ter·ec·to·my
neph·ro·u·re·ter·o·cys·tec·to·my
nep·i·ol·o·gy
Neptune's
  gir·dle
nep·tu·ni·um
ne·ri·ine
Néri's
  sign
Nernst's
  equa·tion
  the·o·ry
nerve
  avul·sion
  block
  cell
  con·duc·tion
  deaf·ness
  de·com·pres·sion
  end·ing
  fas·ci·cle
  fi·ber
  field
  force
  gan·gli·on
  graft
  im·plan·ta·tion
  pain
  pa·pil·la
  plex·us
  root
  su·ture
  tract
  trunk
nerve
  ab·du·cent n.
  ac·cel·er·a·tor n.'s
  ac·ces·so·ry n.
  ac·ces·so·ry phren·ic n.'s
  acous·tic n.
  af·fer·ent n.
  Andersch's n.
  ano·coc·cyg·e·al n.'s
  an·te·ri·or am·pul·lar n.
  an·te·ri·or an·te·brach·i·
    al n.
  an·te·ri·or au·ric·u·lar n.'s
  an·te·ri·or cru·ral n.
  an·te·ri·or eth·moi·dal n.

an·te·ri·or in·ter·os·se·ous n.
an·te·ri·or la·bi·al n.'s
an·te·ri·or scro·tal n.'s
an·te·ri·or su·pra·cla·vic·u·lar n.
an·te·ri·or tib·i·al n.
aor·tic n.
Arnold's n.
ar·tic·u·lar n.
au·di·to·ry n.
aug·men·tor n.'s
au·ric·u·lo·tem·po·ral n.
au·to·nom·ic n.
ax·il·lary n.
bar·o·re·cep·tor n.
Bell's res·pi·ra·to·ry n.
Bock's n.
buc·cal n.
buc·ci·na·tor n.
ca·rot·i·co·tym·pan·ic n.
ca·rot·id si·nus n.
cav·ern·ous n.'s of clit·o·ris
cav·ern·ous n.'s of pe·nis
cen·trif·u·gal n.
cen·trip·e·tal n.
cer·vi·cal n.'s
cir·cum·flex n.
coc·cyg·eal n.
co·chle·ar n.
com·mon fib·u·lar n.
com·mon pal·mar dig·i·tal n.'s
com·mon per·o·ne·al n.
com·mon plan·tar dig·i·tal n.'s
cra·ni·al n.'s
cu·bi·tal n.
cu·ta·ne·ous n.
cu·ta·ne·ous cer·vi·cal n.
Cy·on's n.
dead n.
deep fib·u·lar n.
deep per·o·ne·al n.
deep pe·tro·sal n.
deep tem·po·ral n.'s
den·tal n.
de·pres·sor n. of Ludwig
dor·sal n. of clit·o·ris
dor·sal dig·i·tal n.'s
dor·sal dig·i·tal n.'s of foot
dor·sal in·ter·os·se·ous n.
dor·sal lat·er·al cu·ta·ne·ous n.
dor·sal me·di·al cu·ta·ne·ous n.
dor·sal n. of pe·nis
dor·sal n. of scap·u·la

dor·sal n.'s of toes
ef·fer·ent n.
eighth cra·ni·al n.
elev·enth cra·ni·al n.
es·od·ic n.
ex·ci·tor n.
ex·ci·to·re·flex n.
ex·od·ic n.
n. of ex·ter·nal acous·tic me·a·tus
ex·ter·nal ca·rot·id n.'s
ex·ter·nal res·pi·ra·to·ry n. of Bell
ex·ter·nal sa·phe·nous n.
fa·cial n.
fem·o·ral n.
fifth cra·ni·al n.
first cra·ni·al n.
fourth cra·ni·al n.
fourth lum·bar n.
fron·tal n.
fur·cal n.
Galen's n.
gan·gli·at·ed n.
Gaskell's n.'s
gen·i·to·cru·ral n.
gen·i·to·fem·o·ral n.
glos·so·pha·ryn·ge·al n.
great au·ric·u·lar n.
great·er oc·cip·i·tal n.
great·er pal·a·tine n.
great·er pe·tro·sal n.
great·er splanch·nic n.
great·er su·per·fi·cial pe·tro·sal n.
great sci·at·ic n.
hem·or·rhoi·dal n.'s
Hering's si·nus n.
hy·po·gas·tric n.
hy·po·glos·sal n.
il·i·o·hy·po·gas·tric n.
il·i·o·in·gui·nal n.
in·fe·ri·or al·ve·o·lar n.
in·fe·ri·or cer·vi·cal car·di·ac n.
in·fe·ri·or clu·ne·al n.'s
in·fe·ri·or den·tal n.
in·fe·ri·or glu·te·al n.
in·fe·ri·or hem·or·rhoi·dal n.'s
in·fe·ri·or la·ryn·ge·al n.
in·fe·ri·or max·il·lary n.
in·fe·ri·or rec·tal n.'s
in·fe·ri·or ves·i·cal n.'s
in·fra·or·bit·al n.
in·fra·troch·le·ar n.
in·hib·i·to·ry n.
in·ter·cos·tal n.'s

nerve *(continued)*

in·ter·cos·to·brach·i·al n.'s
in·ter·cos·to·hu·mer·al n.'s
in·ter·me·di·ary n.
in·ter·me·di·ate n.
in·ter·me·di·ate dor·sal cu·ta·ne·ous n.
in·ter·me·di·ate su·pra·cla·vic·u·lar n.
in·ter·nal ca·rot·id n.
in·ter·nal sa·phe·nous n.
in·ter·os·se·ous n. of leg
Jacobson's n.
jug·u·lar n.
lac·ri·mal n.
Latarget's n.
lat·er·al am·pul·lar n.
lat·er·al an·te·ri·or tho·rac·ic n.
lat·er·al cu·ta·ne·ous n. of calf
lat·er·al cu·ta·ne·ous n. of fore·arm
lat·er·al cu·ta·ne·ous n. of thigh
lat·er·al pec·to·ral n.
lat·er·al plan·tar n.
lat·er·al pop·lit·e·al n.
lat·er·al su·pra·cla·vic·u·lar n.
less·er in·ter·nal cu·ta·ne·ous n.
less·er oc·cip·i·tal n.
less·er pal·a·tine n.'s
less·er pe·tro·sal n.
less·er splanch·nic n.
less·er su·per·fi·cial pe·tro·sal n.
lin·gual n.
long buc·cal n.
long cil·i·ary n.
long sa·phe·nous n.
long sub·scap·u·lar n.
long tho·rac·ic n.
low·er lat·er·al cu·ta·ne·ous n. of arm
low·est splanch·nic n.
Ludwig's n.
lum·bar n.'s
lum·bar splanch·nic n.'s
lum·bo·in·gui·nal n.
man·dib·u·lar n.
mas·se·ter·ic n.
mas·ti·ca·tor n.
max·il·lary n.
me·di·al an·te·ri·or tho·rac·ic n.

me·di·al cu·ta·ne·ous n. of arm
me·di·al cu·ta·ne·ous n. of fore·arm
me·di·al cu·ta·ne·ous n. of leg
me·di·al pec·to·ral n.
me·di·al plan·tar n.
me·di·al pop·lit·e·al n.
me·di·al su·pra·cla·vic·u·lar n.
me·di·an n.
men·tal n.
mid·dle cer·vi·cal car·di·ac n.
mid·dle clu·ne·al n.'s
mid·dle me·nin·ge·al n.
mid·dle su·pra·cla·vic·u·lar n.
mixed n.
mo·tor n.
mo·tor n. of face
mus·cu·lo·cu·ta·ne·ous n.
mus·cu·lo·cu·ta·ne·ous n. of leg
mus·cu·lo·spi·ral n.
my·lo·hy·oid n.
na·sal n.
na·so·cil·i·ary n.
na·so·pal·a·tine n.
ninth cra·ni·al n.
ob·tu·ra·tor n.
oc·u·lo·mo·tor n.
ol·fac·to·ry n.
oph·thal·mic n.
op·tic n.
or·bi·tal n.
par·a·sym·pa·thet·ic n.
pa·thet·ic n.
pel·vic splanch·nic n.'s
per·i·ne·al n.'s
per·o·ne·al com·mu·ni·cat·ing n.
phren·ic n.
pneu·mo·gas·tric n.
pop·lit·e·al com·mu·ni·cat·ing n.
pos·te·ri·or am·pul·lar n.
pos·te·ri·or an·te·brach·i·al n.
pos·te·ri·or au·ric·u·lar n.
pos·te·ri·or cu·ta·ne·ous n. of arm
pos·te·ri·or cu·ta·ne·ous n. of fore·arm
pos·te·ri·or cu·ta·ne·ous n. of thigh
pos·te·ri·or eth·moi·dal n.

pos·te·ri·or in·ter·os·se·ous n.
pos·te·ri·or la·bi·al n.'s
pos·te·ri·or scap·u·lar n.
pos·te·ri·or scro·tal n.'s
pos·te·ri·or su·pra·cla·vic·u·lar n.
pos·te·ri·or tho·rac·ic n.
pre·sa·cral n.
pres·sor n.
pres·so·re·cep·tor n.
prop·er pal·mar dig·i·tal n.'s
prop·er plan·tar dig·i·tal n.'s
pter·y·goid n.
n. of pter·y·goid ca·nal
pter·y·go·pal·a·tine n.'s
pu·den·dal n.
pu·dic n.
ra·di·al n.
re·cur·rent n.
re·cur·rent la·ryn·ge·al n.
re·cur·rent me·nin·ge·al n.
n. to rhom·boid
sac·cu·lar n.
sa·cral n.'s
sa·cral splanch·nic n.'s
sa·phe·nous n.
sci·at·ic n.
sec·ond cra·ni·al n.
se·cre·to·ry n.
sen·so·ry n.
sev·enth cra·ni·al n.
short cil·i·ary n.
short sa·phe·nous n.
si·nus n. of Hering
si·nu·ver·te·bral n.
sixth cra·ni·al n.
small deep pe·tro·sal n.
small·est splanch·nic n.
small sci·at·ic n.
n. of smell
so·mat·ic n.
space n.
spi·nal n.'s
spi·nal ac·ces·so·ry n.
splanch·nic n.
n. to sta·pe·di·us mus·cle
sub·cla·vi·an n.
sub·cos·tal n.
sub·lin·gual n.
sub·oc·cip·i·tal n.
sub·scap·u·lar n.
su·per·fi·cial cer·vi·cal n.
su·per·fi·cial fib·u·lar n.
su·per·fi·cial per·o·ne·al n.
su·pe·ri·or al·ve·o·lar n.'s

su·pe·ri·or cer·vi·cal car·di·ac n.
su·pe·ri·or clu·ne·al n.'s
su·pe·ri·or den·tal n.'s
su·pe·ri·or glu·te·al n.
su·pe·ri·or la·ryn·ge·al n.
su·pe·ri·or max·il·lary n.
su·pra·or·bit·al n.
su·pra·scap·u·lar n.
su·pra·troch·le·ar n.
su·ral n.
sym·pa·thet·ic n.
tem·po·ro·man·dib·u·lar n.
n. of ten·sor tym·pa·ni mus·cle
n. of ten·sor ve·li pa·la·ti·ni mus·cle
tenth cra·ni·al n.
ten·to·ri·al n.
ter·mi·nal n.'s
third cra·ni·al n.
third oc·cip·i·tal n.
tho·rac·ic n.'s
tho·rac·ic car·di·ac n.'s
tho·ra·co·dor·sal n.
tib·i·al n.
tib·i·al com·mu·ni·cat·ing n.
Tiedemann's n.
trans·verse n. of neck
tri·fa·cial n.
tri·gem·i·nal n.
troch·le·ar n.
twelfth cra·ni·al n.
tym·pan·ic n.
n. of tym·pan·ic mem·brane
ul·nar n.
up·per lat·er·al cu·ta·ne·ous n. of arm
utric·u·lar n.
utric·u·lo·am·pul·lar n.
vag·i·nal n.'s
va·gus n.
Valentin's n.
vas·cu·lar n.
va·so·mo·tor n.
ver·te·bral n.
ves·tib·u·lar n.
ves·tib·u·lo·co·chle·ar n.
vid·i·an n.
vo·lar in·ter·os·se·ous n.
Wrisberg's n.
zy·go·mat·ic n.

nerve block
  an·es·the·sia
nerve cell
  body

nerve con·duc·tion
  ve·loc·i·ty
nerve growth
  fac·tor
nerve growth fac·tor
  an·ti·se·rum
nerve-point
  mas·sage
ner·vi
ner·vi·mo·til·i·ty
ner·vi·mo·tion
ner·vi·mo·tor
ner·vine
ner·vone
ner·von·ic ac·id
ner·vo·sism
ner·vous
  as·the·no·pia
  asth·ma
  blad·der
  dys·pep·sia
  dys·pha·gia
  force
  in·di·ges·tion
  lobe
  sys·tem
  tis·sue
  tu·nic of eye·ball
ner·vous break·down
ner·vous·ness
ner·vus
  n. acus·ti·cus
  n. cer·vi·ca·lis su·per·fi·ci·
    a·lis
  n. com·mu·ni·cans fib·u·la·
    ris
  n. com·mu·ni·cans per·o·
    ne·us
  n. fur·ca·lis
  n. hem·or·rhoi·dal·is
  n. im·par
  n. in·ter·os·se·us dor·sa·lis
  ner·vi ner·vo·rum
  n. oc·ta·vus
  n. pha·ryn·ge·us
  ner·vi pte·ry·go·pa·la·ti·ni
  n. sper·ma·ti·cus ex·ter·nus
  ner·vi sphe·no·pa·la·ti·ni
  n. stat·o·a·cus·ti·cus
  n. ten·to·rii
ne·sid·i·ec·to·my
ne·sid·i·o·blast
ne·sid·i·o·blas·to·ma
ne·sid·i·o·blas·to·sis
ness·ler·ize
Nessler's
  re·a·gent

nest
  Brunn's n.'s
  cell n.'s
  ep·i·the·li·al n.
net
  Chiari's n.
  chro·mid·i·al n.
net
  flux
  knot
Netherton's
  syn·drome
net·il·mi·cin sul·fate
net·tle
  rash
nett·ling
  hairs
net·work
  acro·mi·al n.
  ar·te·ri·al n.
  ar·tic·u·lar n. of el·bow
  ar·tic·u·lar n. of knee
  ar·tic·u·lar vas·cu·lar n.
  chro·ma·tin n.
  dor·sal car·pal n.
  dor·sal ve·nous n. of foot
  dor·sal ve·nous n. of hand
  n. of heel
  lat·er·al mal·le·o·lar n.
  li·nin n.
  me·di·al mal·le·o·lar n.
  pa·tel·lar n.
  per·i·tar·sal n.
  plan·tar ve·nous n.
  Purkinje's n.
  sub·pap·il·lary n.
  tra·bec·u·lar n.
Neubauer's
  ar·tery
Neufeld
  re·ac·tion
Neufeld cap·su·lar
  swell·ing
Neumann's
  cells
  dis·ease
  law
  sheath
neu·rag·mia
neu·ral
  arch
  ax·is
  ca·nal
  crest
  cyst
  deaf·ness
  folds
  gan·gli·on

groove
lay·er of ret·i·na
plate
seg·ment
spine
tube
neu·ral crest
syn·drome
neu·ral·gia
atyp·i·cal fa·cial n.
atyp·i·cal tri·gem·i·nal n.
ep·i·lep·ti·form n.
fa·cial n.
n. fa·ci·a·lis ve·ra
Fothergill's n.
ge·nic·u·late n.
glos·so·pha·ryn·ge·al n.
hal·lu·ci·na·to·ry n.
Hunt's n.
id·i·o·path·ic n.
in·ter·cos·tal n.
mam·ma·ry n.
Morton's n.
oc·cip·i·tal n.
pe·ri·od·ic mi·grain·ous n.
red n.
rem·i·nis·cent n.
sci·at·ic n.
Sluder's n.
sphe·no·pal·a·tine n.
stump n.
sub·oc·cip·i·tal n.
su·pra·or·bit·al n.
symp·to·mat·ic n.
tri·fa·cial n.
tri·gem·i·nal n.
neu·ral·gic
amy·ot·ro·phy
neu·ral·gi·form
neur·am·e·bim·e·ter
neur·a·min·ic ac·id
neur·a·min·i·dase
neur·an·a·gen·e·sis
neur·a·poph·y·sis
neur·a·prax·ia
neur·ar·chy
neur·as·the·nia
an·gi·o·par·a·lyt·ic n.
an·gi·o·path·ic n.
gas·tric n.
n. gra·vis
n. prae·cox
pri·mary n.
pul·sat·ing n.
sex·u·al n.
trau·mat·ic n.
neur·as·then·ic
as·the·no·pia

neur·as·then·ic hel·met
neur·ax·is
neur·ax·on
neur·ax·one
neur·ec·ta·sia
neur·ec·ta·sis
neur·ec·ta·sy
neu·rec·to·my
pre·sa·cral n.
ret·ro·gas·se·ri·an n.
neur·ec·to·pia
neur·ec·to·py
neur·en·ter·ic
ca·nal
neur·ep·i·the·li·um
neu·rer·gic
neur·ex·er·e·sis
neu·ri·at·ria
neu·ri·a·try
neu·ri·dine
neu·ri·lem·ma
cells
neu·ri·le·mo·ma
acous·tic n.
Antoni type A n.
Antoni type B n.
neu·ril·i·ty
neu·ri·mo·til·i·ty
neu·ri·mo·tor
neu·rine
neu·ri·no·ma
acous·tic n.
neu·rit
neu·rite
neu·rit·ic
at·ro·phy
plaque
neu·ri·ti·des
neu·ri·tis
ad·ven·ti·tial n.
as·cend·ing n.
ax·i·al n.
brach·i·al n.
cen·tral n.
de·scend·ing n.
Eichhorst's n.
en·dem·ic n.
fal·lo·pi·an n.
in·ter·sti·tial n.
in·tra·oc·u·lar n.
Leyden's n.
mul·ti·ple n.
oc·cip·i·tal n.
op·tic n.
par·en·chym·a·tous n.
ret·ro·bul·bar n.
sci·at·ic n.
seg·men·tal n.

neu·ri·tis *(continued)*
  sub·oc·cip·i·tal n.
  tox·ic n.
  trau·mat·ic n.
neu·ro·al·ler·gy
neu·ro·an·as·to·mo·sis
neu·ro·a·nat·o·my
neu·ro·ar·throp·a·thy
neu·ro·aug·men·ta·tion
neu·ro·aug·men·tive
neu·ro·bi·o·tac·tic
  move·ment
neu·ro·bi·o·tax·is
neu·ro·blast
neu·ro·blas·to·ma
  ol·fac·to·ry n.
neu·ro·car·di·ac
neu·ro·cele
neu·ro·cen·tral
  joint
  su·ture
  syn·chon·dro·sis
neu·ro·chem·is·try
neu·ro·chi·tin
neu·ro·cho·ri·o·ret·i·ni·tis
neu·ro·cho·roi·di·tis
neu·ro·chro·nax·ic
  the·o·ry
neu·ro·cir·cu·la·to·ry
  as·the·nia
neu·roc·la·dism
neu·ro·cra·ni·um
  car·ti·lag·i·nous n.
  mem·bra·nous n.
neu·ro·cris·top·a·thy
neu·ro·cu·ta·ne·ous
  mel·a·no·sis
  syn·drome
neu·ro·cyte
neu·ro·cy·tol·y·sis
neu·ro·cy·to·ma
neu·ro·den·drite
neu·ro·den·dron
neu·ro·der·ma·ti·tis
neu·ro·der·ma·to·sis
neu·ro·dy·nam·ic
neu·ro·dyn·ia
neu·ro·ec·to·derm
neu·ro·ec·to·der·mal
  junc·tion
neu·ro·ec·to·my
neu·ro·en·ceph·a·lo·my·e·lop·a·thy
neu·ro·en·do·crine
  cell
neu·ro·en·do·crine trans·duc·er
  cell
neu·ro·en·do·crin·ol·o·gy

neu·ro·ep·i·the·li·al
  body
  cells
  lay·er of ret·i·na
neu·ro·ep·i·the·li·um
  n. of am·pul·la·ry crest
  n. of mac·u·la
neu·ro·fi·bril
neu·ro·fi·bril·lar
neu·ro·fi·bril·la·ry
  de·gen·er·a·tion
neu·ro·fi·bro·ma
  plex·i·form n.
  sto·ri·form n.
neu·ro·fi·bro·ma·to·sis
  abor·tive n.
  in·com·plete n.
neu·ro·fil·a·ment
neu·ro·gang·li·on
neu·ro·gas·tric
neu·ro·gen·e·sis
neu·ro·ge·net·ic
neu·ro·gen·ic
  at·ro·phy
  blad·der
  frac·ture
  the·o·ry
neu·rog·e·nous
neu·rog·lia
  cells
neu·rog·li·a·cyte
neu·rog·li·al
neu·rog·li·ar
neu·rog·li·o·ma·to·sis
neu·ro·gram
neu·rog·ra·phy
neu·ro·he·mal
neu·ro·his·tol·o·gy
neu·ro·hor·mone
neu·ro·hu·mor
neu·ro·hu·mor·al
  se·cre·tion
  trans·mis·sion
neu·ro·hy·po·phys·i·al
neu·ro·hy·poph·y·sis
neu·roid
neu·ro·ker·a·tin
neu·ro·lem·ma
  cells
neu·ro·lept·an·al·ge·sia
neu·ro·lept·an·es·the·sia
neu·ro·lep·tic
  agent
neu·ro·lep·tic ma·lig·nant
  syn·drome
neu·ro·lin·guis·tics
neu·rol·o·gist
neu·rol·o·gy

neu·ro·lymph
neu·ro·lym·pho·ma·to·sis
   n. gal·li·na·rum
neu·rol·y·sin
neu·rol·y·sis
neu·ro·lyt·ic
neu·ro·ma
   acous·tic n.
   am·pu·ta·tion n.
   n. cu·tis
   false n.
   fi·bril·lary n.
   plex·i·form n.
   n. tel·an·gi·ec·to·des
   trau·mat·ic n.
   Verneuil's n.
neu·ro·ma·la·cia
neu·ro·mast
   or·gan
neu·ro·ma·to·sis
neu·ro·mel·a·nin
neu·ro·mere
neu·ro·mi·me·sis
neu·ro·mi·met·ic
neu·ro·mus·cu·lar
   cell
   junc·tion
   re·lax·ant
   spin·dle
   sys·tem
neu·ro·mus·cu·lar block·ing
   agent
neu·ro·my·as·the·nia
   ep·i·dem·ic n.
neu·ro·my·e·li·tis
   n. op·ti·ca
neu·ro·my·op·a·thy
   car·ci·nom·a·tous n.
neu·ro·my·o·si·tis
neu·ron
   au·to·nom·ic mo·tor n.
   bi·po·lar n.
   gam·ma mo·tor n.'s
   gan·gli·on·ic mo·tor n.
   Golgi type I n.
   Golgi type II n.
   in·ter·ca·lary n.
   in·ter·nun·ci·al n.
   low·er mo·tor n.
   mo·tor n.
   mul·ti·po·lar n.
   post·gan·gli·on·ic mo·tor n.
   pre·gan·gli·on·ic mo·tor n.
   pseu·do·u·ni·po·lar n.
   so·mat·ic mo·tor n.
   uni·po·lar n.
   up·per mo·tor n.
   vis·cer·al mo·tor n.

neu·ro·nal
neu·rone
neu·ro·neph·ric
neu·ro·ne·vus
neu·ron·i·tis
neu·ro·nop·a·thy
   sen·so·ry n.
neu·ron·o·phage
neu·ron·o·pha·gia
neu·ro·noph·a·gy
neu·ro·nyx·is
neu·ro-on·col·o·gy
neu·ro-oph·thal·mol·o·gy
neu·ro-o·tol·o·gy
neu·ro·pap·il·li·tis
neu·ro·pa·ral·y·sis
neu·ro·par·a·lyt·ic
   ker·a·ti·tis
   oph·thal·mia
neu·ro·path
neu·ro·path·ic
   al·bu·min·ur·ia
   ar·thri·tis
   ar·throp·a·thy
   joint
neu·ro·path·o·gen·e·sis
neu·ro·pa·thol·o·gy
neu·rop·a·thy
   asym·met·ric mo·tor n.
   brach·i·al plex·us n.
   di·a·bet·ic n.
   diph·the·rit·ic n.
   en·trap·ment n.
   fa·mil·i·al am·y·loid n.
   gi·ant ax·o·nal n.
   he·red·i·tary hy·per·tro·phic n.
   he·red·i·tary sen·so·ry ra·dic·u·lar n.
   hy·per·tro·phic in·ter·sti·tial n.
   is·che·mic op·tic n.
   iso·ni·a·zid n.
   lead n.
   lep·rous n.
   mo·tor dap·sone n.
   on·ion bulb n.
   seg·men·tal n.
   sym·met·ric dis·tal n.
neu·ro·pep·tide
neu·ro·phar·ma·col·o·gy
neu·ro·phil·ic
neu·ro·pho·nia
neu·roph·thal·mol·o·gy
neu·ro·phy·sins
neu·ro·phys·i·ol·o·gy
neu·ro·pil
neu·ro·pile

neu·ro·plasm
neu·ro·plas·ty
neu·ro·ple·gic
neu·ro·po·dia
neu·ro·pore
   cau·dal n.
   ros·tral n.
neu·ro·psy·chi·a·try
neu·ro·psy·cho·log·ic
   dis·or·der
neu·ro·psy·cho·log·i·cal
neu·ro·psy·chol·o·gy
neu·ro·psy·cho·path·ic
neu·ro·psy·chop·a·thy
neu·ro·psy·cho·phar·ma·col·o·gy
neu·ro·ra·di·ol·o·gy
neu·ro·rec·i·dive
neu·ro·re·cur·rence
neu·ro·re·lapse
neu·ro·ret·i·ni·tis
neu·ror·rha·phy
neu·ro·sar·co·clei·sis
neu·ro·sar·coid·o·sis
neu·ro·schwan·no·ma
neu·ro·sci·enc·es
neu·ro·se·cre·tion
neu·ro·se·cre·to·ry
   cells
   sub·stance
neu·ro·ses
neu·ro·sis
   ac·ci·dent n.
   anx·i·e·ty n.
   as·so·ci·a·tion n.
   bat·tle n.
   car·di·ac n.
   char·ac·ter n.
   com·pen·sa·tion n.
   com·pul·sive n.
   con·ver·sion hys·te·ria n.
   ex·pec·ta·tion n.
   ex·per·i·men·tal n.
   mil·i·tar·y n.
   no·o·gen·ic n.
   ob·ses·sive-com·pul·sive n.
   oc·cu·pa·tion·al n.
   oe·di·pal n.
   pen·sion n.
   post·con·cus·sion n.
   post·trau·mat·ic n.
   pro·fes·sion·al n.
   n. tar·da
   tor·sion n.
   trans·fer·ence n.
   trau·mat·ic n.
   war n.

neu·ro·so·mat·ic
   junc·tion
neu·ro·spasm
neu·ro·splanch·nic
neu·ro·spon·gi·um
Neu·ros·po·ra
neu·ro·sthe·nia
neu·ro·stim·u·la·tor
neu·ro·sur·geon
neu·ro·sur·gery
   func·tion·al n.
neu·ro·su·ture
neu·ro·syph·i·lis
neu·ro·ta·bes
   Dejerine's pe·riph·e·ral n.
neu·ro·ten·di·nous
   or·gan
   spin·dle
neu·ro·ten·sin
neu·ro·ten·sion
neu·ro·the·ke·o·ma
neu·ro·the·le
neu·ro·ther·a·peu·tics
neu·ro·ther·a·py
neu·ro·thlip·sia
neu·ro·thlip·sis
neu·rot·ic
   ex·co·ri·a·tion
   man·i·fes·ta·tion
neu·rot·i·cism
neu·rot·i·za·tion
neu·ro·tize
neu·rot·me·sis
neu·ro·tol·o·gy
neu·ro·tome
neu·rot·o·my
   ret·ro·gas·se·ri·an n.
neu·ro·ton·ic
   pu·pil
   re·ac·tion
neu·rot·o·ny
neu·ro·tox·ic
neu·ro·tox·in
neu·ro·trans·mis·sion
neu·ro·trans·mit·ter
neu·ro·trau·ma
neu·ro·trip·sy
neu·ro·tro·phic
   at·ro·phy
neu·rot·ro·phy
neu·ro·tro·pic
   at·trac·tion
   vi·rus
neu·rot·ro·pism
neu·rot·ro·py
neu·ro·tro·sis
neu·ro·tu·bule
neu·ro·vac·cine

neu·ro·var·i·co·sis
neu·ro·var·i·cos·i·ty
neu·ro·vas·cu·lar
  flap
neu·ro·veg·e·ta·tive
neu·ro·vi·rus
neu·ro·vis·cer·al
neu·ru·la
neu·ru·lae
neu·ru·la·tion
Neusser's
  gran·ules
neu·tral
  ax·is of straight beam
  el·e·ment
  fat
  mu·ta·tion
  oc·clu·sion
  ox·ide
  point
  re·ac·tion
  stain
  zone
neu·tral buff·ered for·ma·lin
  fix·a·tive
neu·tral·i·za·tion
  plate
  test
neu·tra·lize
neu·tra·liz·ing
  an·ti·body
neu·tral lip·id stor·age
  dis·ease
neu·tral red
neu·tri·no
neu·tro·clu·sion
neu·tron
  ep·i·ther·mal n.
neu·tro·pe·nia
  cy·clic n.
  pe·ri·od·ic n.
neu·tro·pe·nic
  an·gi·na
neu·tro·phil
  gran·ule
neu·tro·phil
  band n.
  hy·per·seg·ment·ed n.
  im·ma·ture n.
  ju·ve·nile n.
  ma·ture n.
  seg·ment·ed n.
  stab n.
neu·tro·phile
neu·tro·phil·ia
neu·tro·phil·ic
  leu·ke·mia
  leu·ko·cyte

leu·ko·cy·to·sis
leu·ko·pe·nia
neu·tro·phil·o·pe·nia
neu·troph·i·lous
neu·tro·tax·is
ne·vi
ne·vo·cyte
ne·void
  amen·tia
  el·e·phan·ti·a·sis
  hy·per·tri·cho·sis
ne·vo·li·po·ma
ne·vose
ne·vous
ne·vo·xan·tho·en·do·the·li·o·ma
ne·vus
  ac·quired n.
  n. ane·mi·cus
  n. an·gi·ec·to·des
  n. an·gi·o·ma·to·des
  n. ar·ach·noi·de·us
  n. ara·ne·us
  bal·loon cell n.
  ba·sal cell n.
  bath·ing trunk n.
  Becker's n.
  blue n.
  blue rub·ber-bleb nevi
  cap·il·lary n.
  n. ca·ver·no·sus
  cel·lu·lar blue n.
  com·e·do n.
  n. co·me·do·ni·cus
  com·pound n.
  con·gen·i·tal n.
  dys·plas·tic n.
  n. elas·ti·cus of
    Lewandowski
  ep·i·der·mic-der·mic n.
  ep·i·the·li·oid cell n.
  faun tail n.
  flame n.
  n. flam·me·us
  n. fol·lic·u·la·ris ker·a·to·
    sis
  gi·ant pig·ment·ed n.
  ha·lo n.
  in·tra·der·mal n.
  Ito's n.
  Jadassohn's n.
  Jadassohn-Tièche n.
  junc·tion n.
  n. li·po·ma·to·des
  n. li·po·ma·to·sus
  n. lu·pus
  n. lym·pha·ti·cus
  nape n.
  oral ep·i·the·li·al n.

ne·vus *(continued)*
  or·gan·oid n.
  Ota's n.
  n. pa·pil·lo·ma·to·sus
  pig·ment·ed hair ep·i·der·
   mal n.
  n. pig·men·to·sus
  n. pi·lo·sus
  n. san·gui·ne·us
  n. se·ba·ceus
  spi·der n.
  n. spi·lus
  spin·dle cell n.
  Spitz n.
  straw·ber·ry n.
  Sutton's n.
  n. sy·rin·go·cyst·ad·e·no·
   ma·to·sus pa·pil·li·fe·rus
  sys·tem·a·tized n.
  n. uni·us la·te·ris
  n. vas·cu·la·ris
  n. vas·cu·lo·sus
  n. ve·no·sus
  ver·ru·cous n.
  white sponge n.
  wool·ly-hair n.
ne·vus
  cell
new
  com·bi·na·tion
  growth
  meth·yl·ene blue
  mu·ta·tion
new·born
New·cas·tle
  dis·ease
New·cas·tle dis·ease
  vi·rus
Newcomer's
  fix·a·tive
New Hampshire
  rule
new·ton
new·to·ni·an
  ab·er·ra·tion
  con·stant of grav·i·ta·tion
  flu·id
  vis·cos·i·ty
new·ton-me·ter
Newton's
  disk
  law
New World
  leish·man·i·a·sis
new yel·low
  en·zyme
New Zea·land
  mice

nex·us
Nezelof
  syn·drome
Nezelof type of thy·mic
  alym·pho·pla·sia
NGF
  an·ti·se·rum
ni·a·cin
  test
ni·a·cin·a·mide
ni·al·a·mide
niche
  enam·el n.
  Haudek's n.
nick
nick·el
  der·ma·ti·tis
Nickerson-Kveim
  test
nick·ing
  ar·te·ri·o·ve·nous n.
Nicklès'
  test
ni·clo·sa·mide
ni·co·fu·ra·nose
Ni·col
  prism
Nicolas-Favre
  dis·ease
Nicolle's
  stain for cap·sules
Nicolle's white
  my·ce·to·ma
nic·o·tin·a·mide
nic·o·tin·a·mide ad·e·nine di·
  nu·cle·o·tide
nic·o·tin·a·mide ad·e·nine di·
  nu·cle·o·tide phos·phate
nic·o·tin·a·mide mon·o·nu·cle·
  o·tide
nic·o·tin·ate
nic·o·tine
nic·o·tine·hy·drox·am·ic ac·id
  me·thi·o·dide
nic·o·tin·ic
nic·o·tin·ic ac·id
  mac·u·lop·a·thy
nic·o·tin·ic ac·id am·ide
nic·o·tin·ic al·co·hol
nic·o·tin·o·mi·met·ic
nic·o·ti·nyl al·co·hol
nic·o·ti·nyl tar·trate
ni·cou·ma·lone
nic·ta·tion
nic·ti·tate
nic·ti·tat·ing
  mem·brane
  spasm

nic·ti·ta·tion
ni·dal
ni·da·tion
ni·di
ni·dus
   n. avis
   n. hir·un·din·is
Nieden's
   syn·drome
Niemann-Pick
   cell
   dis·ease
Niewenglowski
   rays
ni·fed·i·pine
ni·fen·a·zone
ni·fur·al·de·zone
ni·fu·ra·tel
ni·fu·rox·ime
ni·ge·rose
night
   blind·ness
   hos·pi·tal
   my·o·pia
   pain
   pal·sy
   sight
   sweats
   vi·sion
night·guard
night·mare
night·shade
   dead·ly n.
night-ter·rors
nig·ra
ni·gri·cans
ni·gri·ti·es
   n. lin·guae
ni·gro·sin
ni·gro·sine
Ni·gros·po·ra
ni·gro·stri·a·tal
ni·hil·ism
   ther·a·peu·tic n.
ni·hil·is·tic
   de·lu·sion
ni·keth·a·mide
Nikiforoff's
   meth·od
Nikolsky's
   sign
nil
   dis·ease
Nile blue A
nin·hy·drin
   re·ac·tion
nin·hy·drin-Schiff
   stain for pro·teins

ninth cra·ni·al
   nerve
ninth-day
   er·y·the·ma
ni·o·bi·um
nip·ple
   line
   shield
ni·ri·da·zole
nir·va·na
   prin·ci·ple
Nissen's
   op·er·a·tion
Nissl
   bod·ies
   de·gen·er·a·tion
   gran·ules
   sub·stance
Nissl's
   stain
Nitabuch's
   lay·er
   mem·brane
   stri·a
ni·ter
   cu·bic n.
ni·ton
ni·trate
   res·pi·ra·tion
ni·tra·ze·pam
ni·tric ac·id
   fum·ing n. a.
ni·tric-ox·ide re·duc·tase
ni·trid·a·tion
ni·tride
ni·tri·fi·ca·tion
ni·trile
ni·tri·mu·ri·at·ic ac·id
ni·trite
ni·tri·toid
   re·ac·tion
ni·tri·tu·ria
ni·tro
   dyes
ni·tro·blue
   tet·ra·zo·li·um
ni·tro·blue tet·ra·zo·li·um
   test
ni·tro·cel·lu·lose
ni·tro·chlo·ro·form
ni·tro·fu·rans
ni·tro·fu·ran·to·in
ni·tro·fu·ra·zone
ni·tro·gen
   blood urea n.
   fil·trate n.
   heavy n.
   n. mon·ox·ide

ni·tro·gen *(continued)*
  non·pro·tein n.
  n. pen·tox·ide
  rest n.
  un·de·ter·mined n.
  urea n.
  uri·nary n.
ni·tro·gen
  cy·cle
  equiv·a·lent
  mus·tards
  nar·co·sis
ni·tro·ge·nase
ni·tro·gen dis·tri·bu·tion
ni·tro·gen group
ni·tro·gen lag
ni·trog·e·nous
  equi·lib·ri·um
ni·tro·gen par·ti·tion
ni·tro·glyc·er·in
ni·tro·hy·dro·chlo·ric ac·id
ni·troid
  shock
ni·tro·man·ni·tol
ni·tro·mer·sol
ni·trom·e·ter
ni·tron
ni·tro·phen·yl·sul·fen·yl
ni·tro·prus·side
  test
ni·tros·a·mines
ni·tro·syl
ni·trous
ni·trous ac·id
ni·trous ox·ide
ni·tro·xan·thic ac·id
ni·trox·o·line
ni·troxy
ni·trox·yl
ni·tryl
ni·zat·i·dine
njo·ve·ra
NK
  cells
NMR
  imag·ing
no·bel·i·um
no·ble
  cells
  el·e·ment
  gas·es
  met·al
Noble-Collip
  pro·ce·dure
Noble's
  po·si·tion
  stain

No·car·dia
  N. af·ri·ca·na
  N. as·ter·oi·des
  N. bra·sil·i·en·sis
  N. ca·vi·ae
  N. far·ci·ni·ca
  N. gib·so·nii
  N. leish·ma·nii
  N. lu·ri·da
  N. lu·tea
  N. ma·du·rae
  N. med·i·ter·ra·nei
  N. or·i·en·ta·lis
no·car·dia
No·car·di·a·ce·ae
no·car·di·ae
no·car·di·a·sis
no·car·di·o·form
no·car·di·o·sis
  gran·u·lom·a·tous n.
no·ci·cep·tive
  re·flex
no·ci·cep·tor
no·ci·fen·sor
  re·flex
no·ci-in·flu·ence
no·ci·per·cep·tion
noc·tam·bu·la·tion
noc·tam·bu·lism
noc·tu·ria
noc·tur·nal
  am·bly·o·pia
  di·ar·rhea
  en·u·re·sis
  ep·i·lep·sy
  my·oc·lo·nus
  per·i·o·dic·i·ty
  ver·ti·go
noc·tur·nal emis·sion
no·dal
  bi·gem·i·ny
  bra·dy·car·dia
  es·cape
  ex·tra·sys·to·le
  fe·ver
  plane
  point
  rhythm
  tach·y·car·dia
  tis·sue
nod·ding
  spasm
node
  ac·ces·so·ry nerve lymph n.'s
  ano·rec·tal lymph n.'s
  an·te·ri·or cer·vi·cal lymph n.'s

an·te·ri·or jug·u·lar lymph n.'s
an·te·ri·or me·di·as·ti·nal lymph n.'s
an·te·ri·or tib·i·al n.
ap·i·cal lymph n.'s
ap·pen·dic·u·lar lymph n.'s
n. of Aschoff and Tawara
atri·o·ven·tric·u·lar n.
ax·il·lary lymph n.'s
n. of az·y·gos arch
Babès' n.'s
bi·fur·ca·tion lymph n.'s
brach·i·al lymph n.'s
bron·cho·pul·mo·nary lymph n.'s
buc·cal n.
buc·ci·na·tor n.
ce·li·ac lymph n.'s
cen·tral lymph n.'s
cer·vi·cal par·a·tra·che·al lymph n.'s
n. of Cloquet
com·mon il·i·ac lymph n.'s
com·pan·ion lymph n.'s of ac·ces·so·ry nerve
cor·o·nary n.
cu·bi·tal lymph n.'s
cys·tic n.
deep an·te·ri·or cer·vi·cal lymph n.'s
deep in·gui·nal lymph n.'s
deep lat·er·al cer·vi·cal lymph n.'s
deep pa·rot·id lymph n.'s
del·phi·an n.
di·a·phrag·mat·ic n.'s
Dürck's n.'s
ep·i·troch·le·ar n.'s
ex·ter·nal il·i·ac lymph n.'s
fa·cial lymph n.'s
fib·u·lar n.
Flack's n.
fo·ram·i·nal n.
gas·tro·du·o·de·nal lymph n.'s
glu·te·al lymph n.'s
Haygarth's n.'s
Heberden's n.'s
he·mal n.
he·mo·lymph n.
Hensen's n.
he·pa·tic lymph n.'s
il·e·o·co·lic lymph n.'s
in·fe·ri·or ep·i·gas·tric lymph n.'s
in·fe·ri·or mes·en·ter·ic lymph n.'s

in·fe·ri·or phren·ic lymph n.'s
in·fe·ri·or tra·che·o·bron·chi·al lymph n.'s
in·fra-au·ric·u·lar sub·fas·cial pa·rot·id lymph n.'s
in·ter·cos·tal lymph n.'s
in·ter·il·i·ac lymph n.'s
in·ter·me·di·ate la·cu·nar n.
in·ter·me·di·ate lum·bar lymph n.'s
in·ter·nal il·i·ac lymph n.'s
in·ter·pec·to·ral lymph n.'s
in·tra·glan·du·lar pa·rot·id lymph n.'s
jug·u·lo·di·gas·tric n.
jug·u·lo-o·mo·hy·oid n.
jux·ta-e·soph·a·ge·al lymph n.'s
jux·ta-e·soph·a·ge·al pul·mo·nary lymph n.'s
jux·ta·in·tes·ti·nal lymph n.'s
Keith and Flack n.
Keith's n.
Koch's n.
lat·er·al ax·il·lary lymph n.'s
lat·er·al jug·u·lar lymph n.'s
lat·er·al la·cu·nar n.
lat·er·al per·i·car·di·ac lymph n.'s
left col·ic lymph n.'s
left gas·tric lymph n.'s
left gas·tro·ep·i·plo·ic lymph n.'s
left gas·tro-o·men·tal n.'s
left lum·bar lymph n.'s
n. of lig·a·men·tum ar·te·ri·o·sum
lum·bar lymph n.'s
lymph n.
lymph n.'s of el·bow
ma·lar n.
man·dib·u·lar n.'s
mas·toid lymph n.'s
me·di·al la·cu·nar n.
mes·en·ter·ic lymph n.'s
mes·o·col·ic lymph n.'s
mid·dle col·ic lymph n.'s
mid·dle rec·tal n.
milk·ers' n.'s
na·so·la·bi·al n.
ob·tu·ra·tor lymph n.'s
oc·cip·i·tal lymph n.'s
Osler n.
pan·cre·at·ic lymph n.'s

node *(continued)*
pan·cre·at·i·co·du·o·de·nal lymph n.'s
pan·cre·at·i·co·splen·ic lymph n.'s
par·a·mam·ma·ry lymph n.'s
par·a·rec·tal lymph n.'s
par·a·ster·nal lymph n.'s
par·a·tra·che·al lymph n.
par·a·u·ter·ine lymph n.'s
par·a·vag·i·nal lymph n.'s
par·a·ves·i·cal lymph n.'s
pa·ri·e·tal n.'s
pec·to·ral lymph n.'s
per·o·ne·al n.
pop·lit·e·al lymph n.'s
pos·te·ri·or me·di·as·ti·nal lymph n.'s
pos·te·ri·or tib·i·al n.
pre·au·ric·u·lar sub·fas·cial pa·rot·id lymph n.'s
pre·ce·cal lymph n.'s
pre·la·ryn·ge·al lymph n.'s
pre·per·i·car·di·ac lymph n.'s
pre·tra·che·al lymph n.'s
pre·ver·te·bral lymph n.'s
prim·i·tive n.
prom·on·to·ry lymph n.'s
pul·mo·nary lymph n.'s
py·lor·ic lymph n.'s
Ranvier's n.
ret·ro·au·ric·u·lar lymph n.'s
ret·ro·ce·cal lymph n.'s
ret·ro·pha·ryn·ge·al lymph n.'s
ret·ro·py·lor·ic n.'s
right col·ic lymph n.'s
right gas·tric lymph n.'s
right gas·tro·ep·i·plo·ic lymph n.'s
right gas·tro-o·men·tal lymph n.'s
right lum·bar lymph n.'s
Rosenmüller's n.
n. of Rouviere
sa·cral lymph n.'s
sig·moid lymph n.'s
sig·nal n.
sing·er's n.'s
si·no·a·tri·al n.
si·nus n.
splen·ic lymph n.'s
sub·a·or·tic lymph n.'s
sub·di·gas·tric n.

sub·man·dib·u·lar lymph n.'s
sub·men·tal lymph n.'s
sub·py·lor·ic n.
sub·scap·u·lar lymph n.'s
su·per·fi·cial an·te·ri·or cer·vi·cal lymph n.'s
su·per·fi·cial in·gui·nal lymph n.'s
su·per·fi·cial lat·er·al cer·vi·cal lymph n.'s
su·per·fi·cial pa·rot·id lymph n.'s
su·pe·ri·or gas·tric lymph n.'s
su·pe·ri·or mes·en·ter·ic lymph n.'s
su·pe·ri·or phren·ic lymph n.'s
su·pe·ri·or rec·tal lymph n.'s
su·pe·ri·or tra·che·o·bron·chi·al lymph n.'s
su·pra·cla·vic·u·lar lymph n.'s
su·pra·py·lor·ic n.
Tawara's n.
teach·ers' n.'s
thy·roid lymph n.'s
tra·che·al lymph n.'s
Troisier's n.
Virchow's n.
vis·cer·al n.'s
vi·tal n.
no·di
no·dose
gan·gli·on
rheu·ma·tism
no·do·si·tas
n. cri·ni·um
no·dos·i·ty
Haygarth's n.'s
Heberden's n.'s
no·dous
nod·u·lar
am·y·loi·do·sis
ar·te·ri·o·scle·ro·sis
body
dis·ease
ep·i·scle·ri·tis
fas·ci·i·tis
head·ache
hi·drad·e·no·ma
hy·per·pla·sia of pros·tate
iri·tis
lep·ro·sy
lym·pho·ma
mel·a·no·ma

mes·o·neu·ri·tis
pan·en·ceph·a·li·tis
scle·ri·tis
scle·ro·sis
syph·i·lid
trans·for·ma·tion of the liv·
er
tu·ber·cu·lid
vas·cu·li·tis
nod·u·lar his·ti·o·cyt·ic
lym·pho·ma
nod·u·lar non·sup·pur·a·tive
pan·nic·u·li·tis
nod·u·lar non-X
his·ti·o·cy·to·sis
nod·u·lar re·gen·er·a·tive
hy·per·pla·sia
nod·u·lar sub·ep·i·der·mal
fi·bro·sis
nod·u·late
nod·u·lat·ed
nod·u·la·tion
nod·ule
ag·gre·gat·ed lym·phat·ic
n.'s
Albini's n.'s
ap·ple jel·ly n.'s
Arantius' n.
Aschoff n.'s
Bianchi's n.
Bohn's n.'s
Caplan's n.'s
cold n.
Dalen-Fuchs n.'s
enam·el n.
Gamna-Gandy n.'s
Hoboken's n.'s
hot n.
Jeanselme's n.'s
jux·ta-ar·tic·u·lar n.'s
Lisch n.
lymph n.
mal·pi·ghi·an n.'s
milk·ers' n.'s
Morgagni's n.
pri·mary n.
pulp n.
rheu·ma·toid n.'s
Schmorl's n.
sec·on·dary n.
n. of sem·i·lu·nar valve
sid·er·ot·ic n.'s
sing·er's n.'s
Sister Joseph's n.
sol·i·tary n.'s of in·tes·tine
splen·ic lymph n.'s
vo·cal cord n.'s
no·du·li

nod·u·lous
no·du·lus
n. ca·ro·ti·cus
n. lym·pha·ti·cus
no·dus
no·di lym·pha·ti·ci
no·di lym·pha·ti·ci cen·tra·
les
n. lym·pha·ti·cus
n. rec·ta·lis me·dia
no·dus si·nu·a·tri·a·lis
echo
no·e·mat·ic
no·e·sis
no·et·ic
anx·i·e·ty
no·eud vi·tal
No·gu·chia
N. cu·nic·u·li
N. gran·u·lo·sis
N. sim·i·ae
noise
pol·lu·tion
no·ma
Nomarski
op·tics
no·ma·to·pho·bia
no·men·cla·tur·al
type
no·men·cla·ture
bi·na·ry n.
bi·no·mi·al n.
no·mi·fen·sine ma·le·ate
nom·i·nal
apha·sia
no·mo·gen·e·sis
nom·o·gram
blood vol·ume n.
car·te·sian n.
d'Ocagne n.
Radford n.
Siggaard-Andersen n.
nom·o·graph
nom·o·thet·ic
ap·proach
no·mo·top·ic
non-A
hep·a·ti·tis
non·ab·sorb·a·ble
lig·a·ture
non·ab·sorb·a·ble sur·gi·cal
su·ture
non·ac·com·mo·da·tive
es·o·tro·pia
no·nan
ma·lar·ia
non·an·a·tom·ic
teeth

non·an·e·di·o·ic ac·id
n-non·a·no·ic ac·id
non-ar·con
  ar·tic·u·la·tor
non-B
  hep·a·ti·tis
non·bac·te·ri·al throm·bot·ic
  en·do·car·di·tis
non·bac·te·ri·al ver·ru·cous
  en·do·car·di·tis
non·bur·sate
non·car·i·o·gen·ic
non·cel·lu·lar
non·chro·maf·fin
  par·a·gan·gli·o·ma
non·chro·mo·gens
non·clo·no·gen·ic
  cell
non·co·he·sive
  gold
non·com·mu·ni·cat·ing
  hy·dro·ceph·a·lus
non·com·pet·i·tive
  in·hi·bi·tion
non·com·ple·men·ta·ry
  role
non com·pos men·tis
non·con·ju·ga·tive
  plas·mid
non·de·cid·u·ous
  pla·cen·ta
non·de·po·lar·iz·ing
  block
  re·lax·ant
non·de·po·lar·iz·ing neu·ro·
  mus·cu·lar block·ing
  agent
non·di·rec·tive
  psy·cho·ther·a·py
non·dis·ease
non·dis·junc·tion
  pri·mary n.
  sec·on·dary n.
non·e·lec·tro·lyte
non·es·sen·tial
  ami·no ac·ids
non·fen·es·trat·ed
  for·ceps
non·fil·a·ment pol·y·mor·pho·
  nu·cle·ar
  leu·ko·cyte
non·gon·o·coc·cal
  ure·thri·tis
non·gran·u·lar
  leu·ko·cyte
non-Hodgkin's
  lym·pho·ma

non·ho·mol·o·gous
  chro·mo·somes
non·im·mune
  ag·glu·ti·na·tion
  se·rum
non·im·mune fe·tal
  hy·drops
non·im·mun·i·ty
non·in·fil·trat·ing lob·u·lar
  car·ci·no·ma
non·in·flam·ma·to·ry
  ede·ma
non-in·su·lin de·pen·dent
  di·a·be·tes mel·li·tus
non·in·va·sive
non·iso·lat·ed
  pro·tein·u·ria
non·ke·tot·ic
  hy·per·gly·ce·mia
non·la·mel·lar
  bone
non·lip·id
  his·ti·o·cy·to·sis
non·med·ul·lat·ed
  fi·bers
non·mo·tile
  leu·ko·cyte
non·my·e·li·nat·ed
Nonne-Milroy
  dis·ease
non·ne·o·plas·tic
non-new·to·ni·an
  flu·id
non-nu·cle·at·ed
non·ob·struc·tive
  jaun·dice
non·oc·clud·ed
  vi·rus
non·oc·clu·sion
non·ose
non·os·si·fy·ing
  fi·bro·ma
non·os·te·o·gen·ic
  fi·bro·ma
non·ov·u·la·tion·al
  men·stru·a·tion
non·par·ous
non·par·tic·i·pant
  ob·ser·ver
non·pe·dun·cu·lat·ed
  hy·da·tid
non·pen·e·trance
non·pen·e·trant
  trait
non·pen·e·trat·ing
  ker·a·to·plas·ty
  wound

non·pha·sic si·nus
  ar·rhyth·mia
non·po·lar
  com·pound
  sol·vents
non·pre·cip·i·ta·ble
  an·ti·body
non·pre·cip·i·tat·ing
  an·ti·body
non·pro·pri·e·tary name
non·pro·tein
  ni·tro·gen
non-rap·id eye
  move·ment
non·re·breath·ing
  an·es·the·sia
  mask
  valve
non·re·frac·tive ac·com·mo·da·
  tive
  es·o·tro·pia
non·re·nal
  az·o·te·mia
non·re·set no·dus si·nu·a·tri·a·
  lis
non·ro·ta·tion
  n. of in·tes·tine
  n. of kid·ney
non·se·cre·tor
non·se·cre·to·ry
  my·e·lo·ma
non·sense
  mu·ta·tion
  syn·drome
  trip·let
non·sep·tate
  my·ce·li·um
non·sex·u·al
  gen·er·a·tion
non·spe·cif·ic
  an·er·gy
  cho·lin·es·ter·ase
  en·ceph·a·lo·my·e·lo·neu·
    rop·a·thy
  im·mu·ni·ty
  pro·tein
  sys·tem
  ther·a·py
  ure·thri·tis
non·throm·bo·cy·to·pe·nic
  pur·pu·ra
non·tox·ic
  goi·ter
non·trans·mu·ral my·o·car·di·al
  in·farc·tion
non·trop·i·cal
  sprue
non·un·ion

non·va·lent
non·vas·cu·lar
non·ver·bal
non·vi·a·ble
non·vit·al
  pulp
  tooth
no·o·gen·ic
  neu·ro·sis
Noonan's
  syn·drome
NOR-
  band·ing
nor·a·dren·a·line
  n. ac·id tar·trate
  n. bi·tar·trate
nor·def·rin hy·dro·chlo·ride
Nordhausen
  sul·fu·ric ac·id
no re·flow
  phe·nom·e·non
nor·ep·i·neph·rine
  n. bi·tar·trate
nor·eth·an·dro·lone
nor·eth·in·drone
  n. ac·e·tate
nor·eth·is·ter·one
nor·e·thyn·o·drel
nor·flox·a·cin
nor·ges·trel
nor·leu·cine
nor·ma
  n. an·te·ri·or
  n. fron·ta·lis
  n. in·fe·ri·or
  n. pos·te·ri·or
  n. sa·git·ta·lis
  n. su·pe·ri·or
  n. tem·po·ra·lis
  n. ven·tra·lis
nor·mae
nor·mal
  an·i·mal
  an·ti·body
  an·ti·throm·bin
  an·ti·tox·in
  ax·is
  bite
  con·cen·tra·tion
  dis·tri·bu·tion
  hear·ing
  oc·clu·sion
  op·so·nin
  ovar·i·ot·o·my
  phos·phate
  se·rum
  so·lu·tion
  tar·trate

nor·mal *(continued)*
  tox·in
  val·ues
nor·mal bu·tyr·ic ac·id
nor·mal cho·les·ter·e·mic
  xan·tho·ma·to·sis
nor·mal horse
  se·rum
nor·mal hu·man
  plas·ma
  se·rum
nor·mal hu·man se·rum
  al·bu·min
nor·mal·i·za·tion
nor·mal·ize
nor·mal·ly posed
  tooth
nor·mal pres·sure
  hy·dro·ceph·a·lus
nor·met·a·neph·rine
nor·meth·a·done
nor·meth·an·drone
nor·mo·bar·ic
nor·mo·blast
nor·mo·cap·nia
nor·mo·ce·phal·ic
nor·mo·chro·mia
nor·mo·chro·mic
  ane·mia
nor·mo·cyte
nor·mo·cyt·ic
  ane·mia
nor·mo·cy·to·sis
nor·mo·e·ryth·ro·cyte
nor·mo·gly·ce·mia
nor·mo·gly·ce·mic
  gly·cos·ur·ia
nor·mo·ka·le·mia
nor·mo·ka·le·mic pe·ri·od·ic
  pa·ral·y·sis
nor·mo·ka·li·e·mia
nor·mo·li·pe·mic
  xan·tho·ma pla·num
nor·mo·pla·sia
nor·mo·sper·ma·to·gen·ic
  ste·ril·i·ty
nor·mo·sthe·nu·ria
nor·mo·ten·sive
nor·mo·ther·mia
nor·mo·ton·ic
nor·mo·to·pia
nor·mo·top·ic
nor·mo·vol·e·mia
nor·mox·ia
nor·oph·thal·mic ac·id
nor·pi·pa·none
Norrie's
  dis·ease

Norris'
  cor·pus·cles
nor·ster·oids
nor·sym·pa·tol
nor·sy·neph·rine
North Amer·i·can
  blas·to·my·co·sis
North·ern blot
  anal·y·sis
North Queens·land tick
  fe·ver
  ty·phus
Norton's
  op·er·a·tion
nor·trip·ty·line hy·dro·chlo·ride
nor·val·ine
Nor·walk
  agent
Nor·way
  itch
Nor·we·gian
  sca·bies
nos·ca·pine
nose
  bran·dy n.
  cleft n.
  cop·per n.
  dog n.
  ex·ter·nal n.
  ham·mer n.
  po·ta·to n.
  rum n.
  sad·dle n.
  top·er's n.
nose·bleed
nose-bridge-lid
  re·flex
nose-eye
  re·flex
No·se·ma
No·se·mat·i·dae
nose·piece
nos·e·ti·ol·o·gy
nos·och·tho·nog·ra·phy
nos·o·co·mi·al
  gan·grene
nos·o·gen·e·sis
nos·o·gen·ic
no·sog·e·ny
nos·o·ge·og·ra·phy
nos·o·graph·ic
no·sog·ra·phy
nos·o·log·ic
no·sol·o·gy
  psy·chi·at·ric n.
nos·o·ma·nia
no·som·e·try
nos·o·my·co·sis

no·son·o·my
nos·o·phil·ia
nos·o·pho·bia
nos·o·phyte
nos·o·poi·et·ic
Nos·o·psyl·lus
nos·o·taxy
nos·o·tox·ic
nos·o·tox·i·co·sis
nos·o·tox·in
no·sot·ro·phy
nos·o·tro·pic
nos·tal·gia
nos·to·ma·nia
nos·to·pho·bia
nos·tril
  in·ter·nal n.
nos·trum
no·tal
no·tal·gia
  n. pa·res·the·ti·ca
no·tan·ce·pha·lia
no·tan·en·ce·pha·lia
no·ta·tin
notch
  ac·e·tab·u·lar n.
  an·gu·lar n.
  antegonial n.
  an·te·ri·or n. of cer·e·bel·
   lum
  an·te·ri·or n. of ear
  aor·tic n.
  n. of apex of heart
  au·ric·u·lar n.
  car·di·ac n.
  car·di·ac n. of left lung
  n.'s in car·ti·lage of ex·ter·
   nal acous·tic me·a·tus
  cla·vic·u·lar n.
  cos·tal n.
  cot·y·loid n.
  cra·ni·o·fa·cial n.
  di·crot·ic n.
  di·gas·tric n.
  eth·moi·dal n.
  fib·u·lar n.
  fron·tal n.
  great·er sci·at·ic n.
  ham·u·lar n.
  Hutchinson's cres·cen·tic n.
  il·i·o·sci·at·ic n.
  in·fe·ri·or thy·roid n.
  in·ter·ar·y·te·noid n.
  in·ter·cla·vic·u·lar n.
  in·ter·con·dy·loid n.
  in·ter·trag·ic n.
  in·ter·ver·te·bral n.
  is·chi·at·ic n.

jug·u·lar n.
Kernohan's n.
lac·ri·mal n.
less·er sci·at·ic n.
man·dib·u·lar n.
mar·su·pi·al n.
mas·toid n.
na·sal n.
pan·cre·at·ic n.
pa·ri·e·tal n.
pa·rot·id n.
pop·lit·e·al n.
pos·te·ri·or n. of cer·e·bel·
 lum
pre·oc·cip·i·tal n.
pre·ster·nal n.
pter·y·goid n.
pter·y·go·max·il·lary n.
ra·di·al n.
Rivinus' n.
n. for round lig·a·ment of
 liv·er
sa·cro·sci·at·ic n.
scap·u·lar n.
sem·i·lu·nar n.
sig·moid n.
sphe·no·pal·a·tine n.
ster·nal n.
su·pe·ri·or thy·roid n.
su·pra·or·bit·al n.
su·pra·scap·u·lar n.
su·pra·ster·nal n.
n. of ten·to·ri·um
ter·mi·nal n. of au·ri·cle
troch·le·ar n.
tym·pan·ic n.
ul·nar n.
um·bil·i·cal n.
ver·te·bral n.
notched
  teeth
note
  blind·ness
no·ten·ceph·a·lo·cele
Nothnagel's
  syn·drome
no-thresh·old
  con·cept
no·ti·fi·a·ble
  dis·ease
no·to·chord
no·to·chor·dal
  ca·nal
  plate
  pro·cess
  sheath
  ver·te·brate
No·to·ed·res cati

no·to·ed·ric
 mange
nou·men·al
nour·ish·ment
no·vo·bi·o·cin
Novy and MacNeal's blood
 agar
noxa
nox·ious
nox·y·thi·o·lin
NPH
 in·su·lin
NS
 echo
N-ter·mi·nal
nu·bec·u·la
nu·cha
nu·chal
 fas·cia
 lig·a·ment
 plane
 tu·ber·cle
Nuck's
 di·ver·tic·u·lum
 hy·dro·cele
nu·cle·ar
 at·om
 bag
 cat·a·ract
 chem·is·try
 en·er·gy
 en·ve·lope
 fam·i·ly
 fu·sion
 hy·al·o·plasm
 jaun·dice
 lay·ers of ret·i·na
 mag·ne·ton
 med·i·cine
 mem·brane
 oph·thal·mo·ple·gia
 pace·mak·er
 pore
 re·ac·tion
 RNA
 sap
 scle·ro·sis
 spin·dle
 stain
nu·cle·ar bag
 fi·ber
nu·cle·ar chain
 fi·ber
nu·cle·ar-cy·to·plas·mic
 ra·tio
nu·cle·ar in·clu·sion
 bod·ies

nu·cle·ar mag·net·ic
 res·o·nance
nu·cle·ar mag·net·ic res·o·
 nance
 imag·ing
nu·cle·ase
 Azo·to·bac·ter n.
 mi·cro·coc·cal n.
 mung bean n.
nu·cle·ate
 en·do·nu·cle·ase
nu·cle·at·ed
nu·cle·a·tion
 het·er·o·ge·neous n.
 ho·mo·ge·neous n.
nu·clei
nu·cle·ic ac·id
 in·fec·tious n. a.
nu·cle·ic ac·id
 base
 probe
nu·cle·i·form
nu·cle·in·ase
nu·cle·in·ic
 base
nu·cle·o·cap·sid
nu·cle·o·chy·le·ma
nu·cle·o·chyme
nu·cle·of·u·gal
nu·cle·o·his·tone
nu·cle·oid
 Lavdovsky's n.
nu·cle·o·lar
 chro·mo·some
 or·ga·niz·er
 sat·el·lite
 zone
nu·cle·o·li
nu·cle·o·li·form
nu·cle·o·loid
nu·cle·o·lo·ne·ma
nu·cle·o·lus
 chro·ma·tin n.
 false n.
nu·cle·o·mi·cro·some
nu·cle·on
nu·cle·op·e·tal
Nu·cle·oph·a·ga
nu·cle·o·phil
nu·cle·o·phile
nu·cle·o·phil·ic
nu·cle·o·phos·pha·tas·es
nu·cle·o·plasm
nu·cle·o·plas·mic
 in·dex
nu·cle·o·pro·tein
nu·cle·o·re·tic·u·lum
nu·cle·or·rhex·is

nu·cle·o·si·das·es
nu·cle·o·side
  n. bis·phos·phate
  n. di·phos·phate
  n. phos·phate
  n. tri·phos·phate
nu·cle·o·side
  pair
  phos·pho·ryl·as·es
nu·cle·o·side·di·phos·phate ki·nase
nu·cle·o·side·di·phos·phate sug·ars
nu·cle·o·some
nu·cle·o·spin·dle
nu·cle·o·ti·da·ses
nu·cle·o·tide
  de·le·tion
  pair
nu·cle·o·tid·yl·trans·fer·as·es
nu·cle·o·tox·in
nu·cle·us
  ab·du·cens n.
  n. ab·du·cen·tis
  n. of ab·du·cent nerve
  ac·ces·so·ry cu·ne·ate n.
  ac·ces·so·ry ol·i·vary nu·clei
  n. ac·cum·bens sep·ti
  n. acus·ti·cus
  n. alae ci·ne·re·ae
  al·mond n.
  am·big·u·ous n.
  n. amyg·da·lae
  amyg·da·loid n.
  an·te·ri·or nu·clei of thal·a·mus
  ar·cu·ate n.
  ar·cu·ate nu·clei
  n. ar·cu·a·tus
  n. ar·cu·a·tus thal·a·mi
  au·di·to·ry n.
  n. ba·sa·lis of Ganser
  Bechterew's n.
  ben·zene n.
  Blumenau's n.
  bran·chi·o·mo·tor nu·clei
  Burdach's n.
  cau·date n.
  n. cen·tra·lis la·te·ra·lis thal·a·mi
  n. cen·tra·lis teg·men·ti su·pe·ri·or
  cen·tro·me·di·an n.
  Clarke's n.
  co·chle·ar nu·clei
  con·ver·gence n. of Perlia
  nu·clei of cra·ni·al nerves

cu·ne·ate n.
n. of Darkschewitsch
deep cer·e·bel·lar nu·clei
Deiters' n.
den·tate n. of cer·e·bel·lum
de·scend·ing n. of the tri·gem·i·nus
dip·loid n.
dor·sal n.
dor·sal ac·ces·so·ry ol·i·vary n.
n. dor·sa·lis
dor·sal mo·tor n. of va·gus
dor·sal n. of va·gus
dor·so·me·di·al n.
dor·so·me·di·al hy·po·tha·lam·ic n.
drop·let nu·clei
Edinger-Westphal n.
em·bol·i·form n.
ex·ter·nal cu·ne·ate n.
n. fa·ci·a·lis
fa·cial mo·tor n.
n. fas·cic·u·li grac·i·lis
n. fi·bro·sus lin·guae
n. fi·li·for·mis
n. fu·nic·u·li cu·ne·a·ti
n. fu·nic·u·li grac·i·lis
ga·met·ic n.
n. ge·la·ti·no·sus
germ n.
n. gi·gan·to·cel·lu·la·ris me·dul·lae ob·lon·ga·tae
n. of Goll
go·nad n.
Gudden's teg·men·tal nu·clei
gus·ta·to·ry n.
ha·ben·u·lar n.
hy·po·glos·sal n.
n. of hy·po·glos·sal nerve
in·fe·ri·or ol·i·vary n.
in·fe·ri·or sal·i·vary n.
in·fe·ri·or ves·tib·u·lar n.
in·ter·ca·lat·ed n.
in·ter·me·di·o·lat·er·al n.
n. in·ter·me·di·o·la·te·ra·lis
in·ter·me·di·o·me·di·al n.
n. in·ter·me·di·o·me·di·a·lis
in·ter·pe·dun·cu·lar n.
n. in·ter·po·si·tus
in·ter·sti·tial n. of Cajal
in·tra·lam·i·nar nu·clei of thal·a·mus
Klein-Gumprecht shad·ow nu·clei
lat·er·al cu·ne·ate n.
n. of lat·er·al lem·nis·cus

nu·cle·us *(continued)*
lat·er·al n. of me·dul·la ob·lon·ga·ta
lat·er·al pre·op·tic n.
lat·er·al re·tic·u·lar n.
lat·er·al n. of thal·a·mus
lat·er·al tu·be·ral nu·clei
lat·er·al ves·tib·u·lar n.
n. of lens
len·tic·u·lar n.
len·ti·form n.
n. of Luys
main sen·so·ry n. of the tri·gem·i·nus
n. of the mam·il·lary body
n. mas·ti·ca·tori·us
mas·ti·ca·to·ry n.
me·di·al ac·ces·so·ry ol·i·vary n.
me·di·al cen·tral n. of thal·a·mus
n. of me·di·al ge·nic·u·late body
me·di·al pre·op·tic n.
me·di·al n. of thal·a·mus
me·di·al ves·tib·u·lar n.
me·di·o·dor·sal n.
mes·en·ce·phal·ic n. of the tri·gem·i·nus
Monakow's n.
mo·tor nu·clei
mo·tor n. of fa·cial nerve
mo·tor n. of tri·gem·i·nus
nu·clei ner·vi co·chle·a·ris
n. ni·ger
oc·u·lo·mo·tor n.
n. of oc·u·lo·mo·tor nerve
Onuf's n.
nu·clei of or·i·gin
par·a·bra·chi·al nu·clei
nu·clei pa·ra·bra·chi·al·es
n. pa·ra·cen·tra·lis thal·a·mi
par·a·cen·tral n. of thal·a·mus
par·a·ven·tric·u·lar n.
Perlia's n.
phen·an·threne n.
pon·tine nu·clei
pos·te·ri·or hy·po·tha·lam·ic n.
pos·te·ri·or me·di·al n. of thal·a·mus
pos·te·ri·or per·i·ven·tric·u·lar n.
pre·ru·bral n.
n. py·ra·mi·da·lis
pyr·role n.

ra·phe nu·clei
nu·clei ra·phes
red n.
re·duc·tion n.
re·pro·duc·tive n.
re·tic·u·lar nu·clei of the brain·stem
re·tic·u·lar n. of thal·a·mus
rhomb·en·ce·phal·ic gus·ta·to·ry n.
Roller's n.
roof n.
Schwalbe's n.
sec·on·dary sen·so·ry nu·clei
seg·men·ta·tion n.
sem·i·lu·nar n. of Flechsig
n. sen·so·ri·us su·pe·ri·or ner·vi tri·gem·i·ni
shad·ow n.
sole nu·clei
n. of sol·i·tary tract
so·mat·ic n.
so·mat·ic mo·tor nu·clei
spe·cial vis·cer·al ef·fer·ent nu·clei
spe·cial vis·cer·al mo·tor nu·clei
sperm n.
spher·i·cal n.
spi·nal n. of ac·ces·so·ry nerve
spi·nal n. of the tri·gem·i·nus
Spitzka's n.
Staderini's n.
ste·roid n.
Stilling's n.
sub·tha·lam·ic n.
su·pe·ri·or ol·i·vary n.
su·pe·ri·or sal·i·vary n.
su·pe·ri·or ves·tib·u·lar n.
su·pra·op·tic n.
n. tec·ti
ter·mi·nal nu·clei
nu·clei ter·mi·na·les
tet·ra·cy·clic ste·roid n.
tha·lam·ic gus·ta·to·ry n.
tho·rac·ic n.
troch·le·ar n.
n. of troch·le·ar nerve
tro·phic n.
tu·be·ral nu·clei
ven·tral an·te·ri·or n. of thal·a·mus
ven·tral in·ter·me·di·ate n. of thal·a·mus

n. ven·tra·lis an·te·ri·or thal·a·mi
n. ven·tra·lis la·te·ra·lis
n. ven·tra·lis pos·te·ri·or in·ter·me·di·us thal·a·mi
n. ven·tra·lis pos·te·ri·or thal·a·mi
ven·tral lat·er·al n. of thal·a·mus
ven·tral pos·te·ri·or in·ter·me·di·ate n. of thal·a·mus
ven·tral pos·te·ri·or lat·er·al n. of thal·a·mus
ven·tral pos·te·ri·or n. of thal·a·mus
ven·tral pos·ter·o·lat·er·al n. of thal·a·mus
ven·tral pos·ter·o·me·di·al n. of thal·a·mus
ven·tral n. of thal·a·mus
ven·tral tier tha·lam·ic nu·clei
ven·tral n. of trap·e·zoid body
ven·tro·ba·sal n.
ven·tro·me·di·al n. of hy·po·thal·a·mus
ves·tib·u·lar nu·clei

nu·clide

nude
mouse

Nuel's
space

Nuhn's
gland

null
cells
hy·poth·e·sis

null-cell
ad·e·no·ma

nul·li·grav·i·da

nul·lip·a·ra

nul·li·par·i·ty

nul·lip·a·rous

num·ber
atom·ic n.
Avogadro's n.
Brinell hard·ness n.
charge n.
CT n.
elec·tron·ic n.
gold n.
Hehner n.
hy·dro·gen n.
io·dine n.
Knoop hard·ness n.
Koettstorfer n.
Loschmidt's n.

Mach n.
mass n.
Polenské n.
Reichert-Meissl n.
sa·pon·i·fi·ca·tion n.
thi·o·cy·an·o·gen n.
trans·port n.
vol·a·tile fat·ty ac·id n.
wave n.

numb·ness
wak·ing n.

nu·mer·i·cal
ap·er·ture
hy·per·tro·phy
tax·on·o·my

num·mi·form

num·mu·lar
spu·tum
syph·i·lid

num·mu·la·tion

nun·na·tion

nun's
mur·mur

nurse
cells

nurse
charge n.
clin·i·cal n. spe·cial·ist
com·mu·ni·ty health n.
head n.
pri·vate du·ty n.
pub·lic health n.
reg·is·tered n.
scrub n.
vis·it·ing n.
wet n.

nurse anes·the·tist

nurse·maid's
el·bow

nurse-mid·wife

nurse prac·ti·tion·er

nurs·ing

nurs·ing home

Nussbaum's
brace·let
ex·per·i·ment

nu·ta·tion

nut·gall

nut·meg
liv·er

nut·meg oil

nu·tri·ent
agar
ar·ter·ies of hu·mer·us
ar·tery
ar·tery of fe·mur
ar·tery of fib·u·la
ar·tery of the tib·ia

nu·tri·ent *(continued)*
  ca·nal
  en·e·ma
  fo·ra·men
  ves·sel
nu·tri·lites
nu·trit·ion
  to·tal par·en·ter·al n.
nu·trit·ion·al
  am·bly·o·pia
  ane·mia
  cir·rho·sis
  ede·ma
  en·ceph·a·lo·ma·la·cia of
    chicks
  en·er·gy
  he·mo·sid·er·o·sis
  pol·y·neu·rop·a·thy
nu·trit·ion·al type cer·e·bel·lar
  at·ro·phy
nu·tri·tive
  equi·lib·ri·um
  ra·ti·o
nu·tri·ture
Nut·tal·lia
nux vom·i·ca
nyc·tal·gia
nyc·ta·lo·pia
  n. with con·gen·i·tal my·o·
    pia
nyc·ta·no·pia
nyc·ter·ine
nyc·ter·o·hem·er·al
nyc·to·hem·e·ral
nyc·to·phil·ia
nyc·to·pho·bia
Nyc·to·the·rus
nyc·tu·ria
ny·li·drin hy·dro·chlo·ride
nymph
nym·pha
nym·phae
nym·phal
nym·phec·to·my
nym·phi·tis
nym·pho·ca·run·cu·lar
  sul·cus
nym·pho·hy·men·al
  sul·cus
nym·pho·la·bi·al
nym·pho·lep·sy
nym·pho·ma·nia
nym·pho·ma·ni·ac
nym·pho·ma·ni·a·cal
nym·phon·cus
nym·phot·o·my
nys·tag·mic
nys·tag·mi·form

nys·tag·mo·gram
nys·tag·mo·graph
nys·tag·mog·ra·phy
nys·tag·moid
nys·tag·mus
  af·ter-n.
  am·au·rot·ic n.
  atax·ic n.
  ca·lor·ic n.
  cen·tral n.
  cer·vi·cal n.
  Cheyne's n.
  com·pres·sive n.
  con·gen·i·tal n.
  con·ju·gate n.
  de·vi·a·tion·al n.
  dis·so·ci·at·ed n.
  down·beat n.
  dys·junc·tive n.
  end-po·si·tion n.
  fix·a·tion n.
  gal·van·ic n.
  gaze n.
  hys·ter·i·cal n.
  in·con·gru·ent n.
  ir·reg·u·lar n.
  jerky n.
  lab·y·rin·thine n.
  la·tent n.
  lat·er·al n.
  min·er's n.
  min·i·mal am·pli·tude n.
  oc·u·lar n.
  op·ti·co·ki·net·ic n.
  op·to·ki·net·ic n.
  pal·a·tal n.
  pen·du·lar n.
  per·vert·ed n.
  po·si·tion·al n.
  rail·road n.
  re·trac·tion n.
  ro·ta·tion·al n.
  ro·ta·to·ry n.
  see·saw n.
  stra·bis·mic n.
  up·beat n.
  ver·ti·cal n.
  ves·tib·u·lar n.
  vol·un·tary n.
nys·tag·mus
  test
nys·tag·mus block·age
  syn·drome
nys·tat·in
Nysten's
  law
nyx·is

O
  ag·glu·ti·nin
  an·ti·gen
  col·o·ny
oak ap·ple
oar·i·um
oast·house urine
  dis·ease
oat
  cell
oat cell
  car·ci·no·ma
oath
oat·meal-to·ma·to paste
  agar
OAV
  dys·pla·sia
  syn·drome
ob·dor·mi·tion
O'Beirne's
  sphinc·ter
obe·li·ac
obe·li·ad
obe·li·ar
  ar·ea
obe·li·on
Obermayer's
  test
Obermeier's
  spi·ril·lum
Obersteiner-Redlich
  line
  zone
obese
obe·si·ty
  hy·po·tha·lam·ic o.
  mor·bid o.
  sim·ple o.
obe·si·ty
  in·dex
obex
ob·fus·ca·tion
ob·ject
  good o.
  sex o.
  test o.
ob·ject
  blind·ness
  con·stan·cy

  glass
  li·bi·do
  re·la·tion·ship
ob·ject choice
ob·jec·tive
  ach·ro·mat·ic o.
  ap·o·chro·mat·ic o.
  im·mer·sion o.
ob·jec·tive
  op·tom·e·ter
  pe·rim·e·try
  psy·chol·o·gy
  sen·sa·tion
  sign
  symp·tom
  syn·o·nyms
ob·jec·tive ver·ti·go
ob·li·gate
  aer·obe
  an·aer·obe
  par·a·site
ob·lique
  am·pu·ta·tion
  ban·dage
  bun·dle of pons
  cord
  di·am·e·ter
  fi·bers of stom·ach
  fis·sure
  frac·ture
  head
  il·lu·mi·na·tion
  lie
  lig·a·ment of el·bow joint
  line
  mus·cle of au·ri·cle
  part
  ridge
  ridge of tra·pe·zi·um
  si·nus of per·i·car·di·um
  vein of left atri·um
ob·lique ar·y·te·noid
  mus·cle
ob·lique fa·cial
  cleft
ob·lique lat·er·al jaw
  roent·gen·o·gram
ob·lique pop·lit·e·al
  lig·a·ment

ob·liq·ui·ty
   Litzmann o.
   Nägele o.
ob·li·qu·us
ob·lit·er·at·ing
   ar·te·ri·tis
   end·ar·te·ri·tis
ob·lit·er·a·tion
oblit·er·a·tive
   arach·noid·i·tis
   bron·chi·tis
ob·long
   pit of ar·y·te·noid car·ti·
    lage
ob·lon·ga·ta
ob·ser·ver
   non·par·tic·i·pant o.
   par·tic·i·pant o.
ob·ses·sion
   im·pul·sive o.
   in·hib·i·to·ry o.
ob·ses·sive
   be·hav·ior
ob·ses·sive-com·pul·sive
   neu·ro·sis
ob·so·les·cence
ob·sta·cle
   sense
ob·stet·ric
   con·ju·gate
   con·ju·gate of out·let
   po·si·tion
ob·stet·ri·cal
   bind·er
   for·ceps
   hand
   pa·ral·y·sis
ob·ste·tri·cian
ob·stet·rics
ob·sti·nate
ob·sti·pa·tion
ob·struct·ed
   tes·tis
ob·struc·tion
   closed-loop o.
   ure·ter·o·pel·vic o.
   ure·ter·o·ves·i·cal o.
ob·struc·tive
   ap·nea
   ap·pen·di·ci·tis
   dys·men·or·rhea
   hy·dro·ceph·a·lus
   jaun·dice
   mur·mur
   throm·bus
ob·stru·ent
ob·tund

ob·tu·rat·ing
   em·bo·lism
ob·tu·ra·tion
ob·tu·ra·tor
   ap·pli·ance
   ar·tery
   ca·nal
   crest
   fas·cia
   fo·ra·men
   groove
   her·nia
   mem·brane
   nerve
   tu·ber·cle
   vein
ob·tu·ra·tor lymph
   nodes
ob·tuse
ob·tu·sion
oc·cip·i·tal
   an·chor·age
   an·gle of pa·ri·e·tal
   ar·tery
   bel·ly
   bone
   con·dyle
   fon·ta·nel
   groove
   gy·ri
   horn
   lobe
   mar·gin
   neu·ral·gia
   neu·ri·tis
   oper·cu·lum
   plane
   plex·us
   point
   pole
   re·gion of head
   si·nus
   so·mite
   tri·an·gle
   vein
   veins
oc·cip·i·tal em·is·sary
   vein
oc·ci·pi·ta·lis
oc·cip·i·tal·i·za·tion
oc·cip·i·tal lymph
   nodes
oc·cip·i·tis
oc·cip·i·to·an·te·ri·or
   po·si·tion
oc·cip·i·to·at·loid
oc·cip·i·to·ax·i·al
   lig·a·ments

oc·cip·i·to·ax·oid
oc·cip·i·to·breg·mat·ic
oc·cip·i·to·col·lic·u·lar
  tract
oc·cip·i·to·fa·cial
oc·cip·i·to·fron·tal
  di·am·e·ter
  fas·cic·u·lus
  mus·cle
oc·cip·i·to·fron·ta·lis
oc·cip·i·to·mas·toid
  su·ture
oc·cip·i·to·men·tal
  di·am·e·ter
oc·cip·i·to·pa·ri·e·tal
oc·cip·i·to·pon·tine
  tract
oc·cip·i·to·pos·te·ri·or
  po·si·tion
oc·cip·i·to·tec·tal
  tract
oc·cip·i·to·tem·po·ral
  sul·cus
oc·cip·i·to·tha·lam·ic
  ra·di·a·tion
oc·cip·i·to·trans·verse
  po·si·tion
oc·ci·put
oc·clude
oc·clud·ed
  vi·rus
oc·clud·er
oc·clud·ing
  frame
  lig·a·ture
  pa·per
  re·la·tion
oc·clud·ing cen·tric re·la·tion
  rec·ord
oc·clu·sal
  ad·just·ment
  anal·y·sis
  bal·ance
  car·ies
  clear·ance
  cor·rec·tion
  cur·va·ture
  dis·har·mo·ny
  em·bra·sure
  force
  form
  har·mo·ny
  im·bal·ance
  path
  pat·tern
  piv·ot
  plane
  po·si·tion

  pres·sure
  ra·di·o·graph
  rest
  rim
  scheme
  sur·face
  sys·tem
  ta·ble
  trau·ma
  wear
oc·clu·sal rest
  bar
oc·clu·sal ver·ti·cal
  di·men·sion
oc·clu·sion
  rim
oc·clu·sion
  ab·nor·mal o.
  afunc·tion·al o.
  an·te·ri·or o.
  bal·anced o.
  bi·max·il·lary pro·tru·sive
    o.
  buc·cal o.
  cen·tric o.
  cor·o·nary o.
  dis·tal o.
  ec·cen·tric o.
  edge-to-edge o.
  end-to-end o.
  func·tion·al o.
  glid·ing o.
  hy·per·func·tion·al o.
  la·bi·al o.
  lat·er·al o.
  lin·gual o.
  me·chan·i·cal·ly bal·anced
    o.
  mes·en·ter·ic ar·tery o.
  me·si·al o.
  neu·tral o.
  nor·mal o.
  path·o·gen·ic o.
  phys·i·o·log·ic o.
  phys·i·o·log·i·cal·ly bal·
    anced o.
  pos·te·ri·or o.
  post·nor·mal o.
  pro·tru·sive o.
  o. of pu·pil
  re·tru·sive o.
  spher·i·cal form of o.
  tor·sive o.
  trau·mat·ic o.
  trau·ma·to·gen·ic o.
  work·ing o.
oc·clu·sive
  dress·ing

oc·clu·sive *(continued)*
  il·e·us
  men·in·gi·tis
oc·clu·som·e·ter
oc·cult
  bleed·ing
  blood
  bor·der of nail
  car·ci·no·ma
  frac·ture
  hy·dro·ceph·a·lus
oc·cu·pa·tion·al
  deaf·ness
  dis·ease
  neu·ro·sis
  spasm
  ther·a·py
Oce·an·o·spi·ril·lum
ocel·li
ocel·lus
och·lo·pho·bia
Ochoa's
  law
ochre
  mu·ta·tion
ochro·der·mia
ochrom·e·ter
ochro·no·sis
  ex·og·e·nous o.
ochro·not·ic
  ar·thri·tis
Ochsner
  clamp
Ochsner's
  meth·od
oc·ry·late
oc·tad
oc·ta·meth·yl py·ro·phos·phor·
  a·mide
oc·ta·myl·a·mine
oc·tan
oc·ta·no·ate
oc·ta·no·ic ac·id
oc·ta·pep·tide
oc·ta·ploi·dy
oc·ta·pres·sin
oc·ta·va·lent
oc·ta·vus
Oc·to·mit·i·dae
Oc·tom·i·tus hom·i·nis
oc·to·pa·mine
oc·tose
oc·tox·y·nol
oc·tu·lose
oc·tu·lo·son·ic ac·id
oc·tyl gal·late
oc·tyl·phe·noxy pol·y·eth·ox·y·
  eth·a·nol

oc·u·lar
  com·pen·sat·ing o.
  Huygens' o.
  Ramsden's o.
  wide field o.
oc·u·lar
  al·bi·nism
  atax·ia
  bob·bing
  cone
  cri·sis
  cup
  dys·met·ria
  flut·ter
  hu·mor
  hy·per·tel·or·ism
  lar·va mi·grans
  lens
  lym·pho·ma·to·sis
  mi·cro·me·ter
  mus·cles
  my·i·a·sis
  my·oc·lo·nus
  my·op·a·thy
  nys·tag·mus
  on·cho·cer·ci·a·sis
  pa·ral·y·sis
  pem·phi·goid
  pros·the·sis
  ri·gid·i·ty
  sco·li·o·sis
  spar·ga·no·sis
  ten·sion
  tor·ti·col·lis
  ver·ti·go
  ves·i·cle
oc·u·lar·ist
oc·u·lar mo·tor
  aprax·ia
oc·u·lar-mu·cous mem·brane
  syn·drome
o·cu·len·ta
o·cu·len·tum
oc·u·li
oc·u·list
oc·u·lo·au·ric·u·lo·ver·te·bral
  dys·pla·sia
oc·u·lo·buc·co·gen·i·tal
  syn·drome
oc·u·lo·car·di·ac
  re·flex
oc·u·lo·ce·phal·ic
  re·flex
oc·u·lo·ceph·a·lo·gy·ric
  re·flex
oc·u·lo·cer·e·bro·re·nal
  syn·drome

oc·u·lo·cu·ta·ne·ous
  al·bi·nism
  syn·drome
oc·u·lo·den·to·dig·i·tal
  dys·pla·sia
  syn·drome
oc·u·lo·der·mal
  mel·a·no·sis
oc·u·lo·en·ce·phal·ic
  an·gi·o·ma·to·sis
oc·u·lo·fa·cial
oc·u·log·ra·phy
  pho·to·sen·sor o.
oc·u·lo·grav·ic
  il·lu·sion
oc·u·lo·gy·ral
  il·lu·sion
oc·u·lo·gy·ria
oc·u·lo·gy·ric
  cri·ses
oc·u·lo·man·dib·u·lo·dys·ceph·
  a·ly
oc·u·lo·mo·tor
  nerve
  nu·cle·us
  re·sponse
  sys·tem
o·cu·lo·mo·to·ri·us
oc·u·lo·na·sal
oc·u·lop·a·thy
oc·u·lo·pha·ryn·ge·al
  syn·drome
oc·u·lo·pleth·ys·mog·ra·phy
oc·u·lo·pneu·mo·pleth·ys·mog·
  ra·phy
oc·u·lo·pu·pil·lary
oc·u·lo·ver·te·bral
  dys·pla·sia
  syn·drome
oc·u·lo·ves·tib·u·lo-au·di·to·ry
  syn·drome
oc·u·lo·zy·go·mat·ic
oc·u·lus
ocy·toc·in
odax·es·mus
odax·et·ic
ODD
  dys·pla·sia
  syn·drome
odd
  chro·mo·some
Oddi's
  sphinc·ter
od·di·tis
Od·land
  body
odo·gen·e·sis
odon·tag·ra

odon·tal·gia
  o. den·ta·lis
odon·tal·gic
odon·tec·to·my
odon·ter·ism
odon·ti·a·sis
odon·ti·noid
odon·ti·tis
odon·to·am·e·lo·blas·to·ma
odon·to·blast
odon·to·blas·tic
  lay·er
  pro·cess
odon·to·blas·to·ma
odon·to·clast
odon·to·dyn·ia
odon·to·dys·pla·sia
odon·to·gen·e·sis
  o. im·per·fec·ta
odon·to·gen·ic
  cyst
  dys·pla·sia
  fi·bro·ma
  myx·o·ma
odon·tog·e·ny
odon·toid
  lig·a·ment
  pro·cess
  pro·cess of ep·i·stro·phe·us
  ver·te·bra
odon·tol·o·gy
  fo·ren·sic o.
odon·to·lox·ia
odon·to·loxy
odon·tol·y·sis
odon·to·ma
  am·e·lo·blas·tic o.
  com·plex o.
  com·pound o.
odon·to·neu·ral·gia
odon·ton·o·my
odon·to·no·sol·o·gy
odon·to·par·al·lax·is
odon·top·a·thy
odon·to·pho·bia
odon·to·plast
odon·to·plas·ty
odon·top·ri·sis
odon·top·to·sis
odon·tor·rha·gia
odon·to·schism
odon·to·scope
odon·tos·co·py
odon·to·sis
odon·to·ther·a·py
odon·tot·o·my
  pro·phy·lac·tic o.
odor

odor·ant
odor·a·tism
odor·if·er·ous
  gland
odor·im·e·ter
odo·rim·e·try
odor·i·vec·tion
odor·og·ra·phy
odor·ous
O'Dwyer's
  tube
odyn·a·cu·sis
ody·nom·e·ter
odyn·o·pha·gia
odyn·o·pho·nia
oe·di·pal
  neu·ro·sis
  pe·ri·od
  phase
oe·di·pism
Oedipus
  com·plex
Oehler's
  symp·tom
Oehl's
  mus·cles
oe·nan·thal
oer·sted
oe·soph·a·go·sto·mi·a·sis
Oe·soph·a·gos·to·mum
  O. ap·i·o·sto·mum
  O. brev·i·cau·dum
  O. brumpti
  O. co·lum·bi·a·num
  O. den·ta·tum
  O. ge·or·gi·a·num
  O. quad·ri·spi·nu·la·tum
  O. ra·di·a·tum
  O. ste·pha·no·sto·mum
  O. ve·nu·lo·sum
oest·rids
oes·tro·sis
Oes·trus
OFD
  syn·drome
of·fi·cial
  for·mu·la
of·fic·i·nal
Ogino-Knaus
  rule
Ogston-Luc
  op·er·a·tion
Ogston's
  line
Oguchi's
  dis·ease
Ogura
  op·er·a·tion

O'Hara
  for·ceps
ohm·am·me·ter
ohm·me·ter
Ohm's
  law
oh·ne Hauch
Ohngren's
  line
oid·ia
oid·i·o·my·cin
oid·i·um
oil
  es·sen·tial o.'s
  ethe·re·al o.
  fat·ty o.
  fixed o.
  joint o.
  vol·a·tile o.
oil
  bath
  cyst
  em·bo·lism
  glands
  im·mer·sion
  pneu·mo·nia
  sug·ar
  tu·mor
  vac·cine
oil of
  thyme
oil red O
oil re·ten·tion
  en·e·ma
oil of vit·ri·ol
oily
  gran·u·lo·ma
oint·ment
  eye o.
  oph·thal·mic o.
OKT
  cells
ol·a·mine
Old World
  leish·man·i·a·sis
old yel·low
  en·zyme
o·le·ag·i·nous
ole·an·der
ole·an·do·my·cin phos·phate
ole·ate
olec·ra·non
  bur·si·tis
  fos·sa
  pro·cess
  re·flex
ole·fi·ant
  gas

ole·fin
ole·ic ac·id
ole·in
ole·o·go·men·ol
ole·o·gran·u·lo·ma
ole·o·ma
ole·om·e·ter
ole·o·pal·mi·tate
ole·o·res·in
ole·o·sac·cha·ra
ole·o·sac·cha·rum
ole·o·ste·a·rate
ole·o·sus
ole·o·ther·a·py
ole·o·thor·ax
ole·o·vi·ta·min
   o. A and D
ole·yl al·co·hol
ol·fac·tie
ol·fac·tion
ol·fac·tol·o·gy
ol·fac·tom·e·ter
ol·fac·tom·e·try
ol·fac·to·pho·bia
ol·fac·to·ry
   an·es·the·sia
   an·gle
   ar·ea
   bulb
   bun·dle
   cor·tex
   ep·i·the·li·um
   es·the·si·o·neu·ro·blas·to·ma
   fo·ra·men
   glands
   glo·mer·u·lus
   groove
   hy·per·es·the·sia
   hyp·es·the·sia
   mem·brane
   mu·co·sa
   nerve
   neu·ro·blas·to·ma
   or·gan
   pe·dun·cle
   pits
   plac·odes
   pyr·a·mid
   re·gion of tu·ni·ca mu·co·
    sa of nose
   roots
   stri·ae
   sul·cus
   sul·cus of nose
   tract
   tri·gone
   tu·ber·cle

ol·fac·to·ry re·cep·tor
   cells
ol·fac·ty
olib·a·num
ol·i·gam·ni·os
ol·i·ge·mia
ol·i·ge·mic
   shock
ol·ig·he·mia
ol·ig·hid·ria
ol·ig·id·ria
ol·i·go·am·ni·os
ol·i·go·cho·lia
ol·i·go·chy·li·a
ol·i·go·chy·mia
ol·i·go·cys·tic
ol·i·go·dac·tyl·ia
ol·i·go·dac·ty·ly
ol·i·go·den·dria
ol·i·go·den·dro·blast
ol·i·go·den·dro·blas·to·ma
ol·i·go·den·dro·cyte
ol·i·go·den·drog·lia
   cells
ol·i·go·den·dro·gli·o·ma
ol·i·go·dip·sia
ol·i·go·don·tia
ol·i·go·dy·nam·ic
ol·i·go·ga·lac·tia
ol·i·go·glu·can-branch·ing gly·
   co·syl·trans·fer·ase
ol·i·go·hy·dram·ni·os
ol·i·go·hy·dru·ria
ol·i·go·lec·i·thal
ol·i·go·men·or·rhea
ol·i·go·mer
ol·i·go·mor·phic
ol·i·go·neph·ron·ic
ol·i·go·nu·cle·o·tide
ol·i·go·pep·sia
ol·i·go·plas·tic
ol·i·gop·nea
ol·i·go·pty·a·lism
ol·i·gor·ia
ol·i·go·sac·cha·ride
ol·i·go·si·a·lia
ol·i·go·sper·ma·tism
ol·i·go·sper·mia
ol·i·go·symp·to·mat·ic
ol·i·go·sy·nap·tic
ol·i·go·thy·mia
ol·i·go·trich·ia
ol·i·go·tri·cho·sis
ol·i·go·tro·phia
ol·i·got·ro·phy
ol·i·go·zo·o·sper·ma·tism
ol·i·go·zo·o·sper·mia
ol·i·gu·re·sia

ol·i·gu·re·sis
ol·i·gu·ria
oli·va
  o. in·fe·ri·or
  o. su·pe·ri·or
oli·vae
ol·i·vary
  body
  em·i·nence
ol·ive
  in·fe·ri·or o.
  su·pe·ri·or o.
ol·ive oil
ol·ive-tipped
  cath·e·ter
ol·i·vif·u·gal
ol·i·vip·e·tal
ol·i·vo·cer·e·bel·lar
  tract
ol·i·vo·co·chle·ar
  bun·dle
ol·i·vo·pon·to·cer·e·bel·lar
  at·ro·phy
  de·gen·er·a·tion
ol·i·vo·spi·nal
  tract
Ollier
  graft
Ollier's
  dis·ease
  meth·od
  the·o·ry
Ollier-Thiersch
  graft
olo·liu·qui
olo·pho·nia
olym·pi·an
  fore·head
oma·si·tis
oma·sum
Ombrédanne
  op·er·a·tion
om·bro·pho·bia
omega-
  ox·i·da·tion
ome·ga-ox·i·da·tion
  the·o·ry
Omenn's
  syn·drome
omen·ta
omen·tal
  bur·sa
  en·ter·o·clei·sis
  graft
  sac
  tu·ber
omen·tec·to·my
omen·ti·tis

omen·to·fix·a·tion
omen·to·pexy
omen·to·plas·ty
omen·tor·rha·phy
omen·to·vol·vu·lus
omen·tu·lum
omen·tum
  gas·tro·co·lic o.
  gas·tro·he·pat·ic o.
  gas·tro·splen·ic o.
  great·er o.
  less·er o.
omen·tum·ec·to·my
OMM
  dys·pla·sia
  syn·drome
Ommaya
  res·er·voir
om·ni·fo·cal
  lens
om·nip·o·tence of thought
om·niv·o·rous
omo·cla·vic·u·lar
  tri·an·gle
omo·hy·oid
  mus·cle
omo·pha·gia
omo·thy·roid
omo·tra·che·al
  tri·an·gle
om·pha·lec·to·my
om·phal·el·co·sis
om·phal·ic
om·pha·li·tis
om·pha·lo·an·gi·op·a·gous
  twins
om·pha·lo·an·gi·op·a·gus
om·phal·o·cele
om·pha·lo·en·ter·ic
om·pha·lo·mes·en·ter·ic
  ar·tery
  duct
om·pha·lop·a·gus
om·pha·lo·phle·bi·tis
om·pha·lor·rha·gia
om·pha·lor·rhea
om·pha·lor·rhex·is
om·pha·los
om·pha·lo·site
om·pha·lo·spi·nous
om·pha·lot·o·my
om·pha·lo·trip·sy
om·pha·lo·ves·i·cal
om·pha·lus
Omsk hem·or·rhag·ic
  fe·ver
Omsk hem·or·rhag·ic fe·ver
  vi·rus

onan·ism
On·cho·cer·ca
  O. cer·vi·ca·lis
  O. gib·soni
  O. li·e·na·lis
  O. vol·vu·lus
on·cho·cer·ci·a·sis
  oc·u·lar o.
on·cho·cer·cid
On·cho·cer·ci·dae
on·cho·cer·co·sis
On·co·cer·ca
on·co·cer·ci·a·sis
on·co·cyte
on·co·cyt·ic he·pa·to·cel·lu·lar
  tu·mor
on·co·cy·to·ma
on·co·fe·tal
  an·ti·gens
  mark·er
on·co·gene
on·co·gen·e·sis
on·co·gen·ic
  vi·rus
on·cog·en·ous
on·co·graph
on·cog·ra·phy
on·coi·des
on·col·o·gist
on·col·o·gy
on·col·y·sis
on·co·lyt·ic
on·co·ma
On·co·me·la·nia
on·com·e·ter
on·co·met·ric
on·com·e·try
on·co·plas·tic
  car·ci·no·ma
on·cor·na·vi·rus·es
on·co·sis
on·co·sphere
  em·bryo
on·co·ther·a·py
on·cot·ic
  pres·sure
on·cot·o·my
on·co·tro·pic
On·co·vir·i·nae
on·co·vi·rus
Ondine's
  curse
one-car·bon
  frag·ment
one-child
  ste·ril·i·ty
one-horned
  uter·us

onei·ric
onei·rism
onei·ro·crit·i·cal
onei·ro·dyn·ia
  o. ac·ti·va
  o. gra·vis
onei·rog·mus
onei·rol·o·gy
onei·ro·phre·nia
onei·ros·co·py
oni·o·ma·nia
on·ion
  bod·ies
on·ion bulb
  neu·rop·a·thy
oni·ric
on·lay
  graft
on-off
  phe·nom·e·non
on·o·mat·o·ma·nia
on·o·mat·o·pho·bia
on·o·mat·o·poi·e·sis
on·to·gen·e·sis
on·to·ge·net·ic
on·to·gen·ic
  ho·me·o·sta·sis
on·tog·e·ny
Onuf's
  nu·cle·us
on·y·al·ai
on·y·chal·gia
on·y·cha·tro·phia
on·ych·at·ro·phy
on·y·chaux·is
on·y·chec·to·my
onych·ia
  o. la·te·ra·lis
  o. ma·lig·na
  o. pe·ri·un·gua·lis
  o. sic·ca
on·y·chi·tis
on·y·choc·la·sis
on·y·cho·cryp·to·sis
on·y·cho·dys·tro·phy
on·y·cho·graph
on·y·cho·gry·pho·sis
on·y·cho·gry·po·sis
on·y·cho·het·er·o·to·pia
on·y·choid
on·y·chol·o·gy
on·y·chol·y·sis
on·y·cho·ma
on·y·cho·ma·de·sis
on·y·cho·ma·la·cia
on·y·cho·my·co·sis
on·y·chon·o·sus
on·y·cho-os·te·o·dys·pla·sia

on·y·cho·path·ic
on·y·cho·pa·thol·o·gy
on·y·chop·a·thy
on·y·cho·pha·gia
on·y·choph·a·gy
on·y·cho·pho·sis
on·y·cho·phy·ma
on·y·cho·plas·ty
on·y·chop·to·sis
on·y·chor·rhex·is
on·y·cho·schiz·ia
on·y·cho·sis
on·y·cho·stro·ma
on·y·chot·il·lo·ma·nia
on·y·chot·o·my
on·y·chot·ro·phy
O'ny·ong-ny·ong
  fe·ver
  vi·rus
on·yx
on·yx·is
on·yx·i·tis
oo·cy·e·sis
oo·cyst
oo·cyte
  pri·mary o.
  sec·on·dary o.
oo·gen·e·sis
oo·ge·net·ic
oo·gen·ic
oog·e·nous
oo·go·nia
oo·go·ni·um
oo·ki·ne·sia
oo·ki·ne·sis
oo·ki·nete
oo·lem·ma
oo·my·co·sis
oo·pha·gia
ooph·a·gy
ooph·or·al·gia
ooph·o·rec·to·my
ooph·or·it·ic
  cyst
ooph·or·i·tis
ooph·or·o·cys·tec·to·my
ooph·or·o·cys·to·sis
ooph·or·o·hys·ter·ec·to·my
ooph·or·o·ma
ooph·or·on
ooph·or·op·a·thy
ooph·or·o·pel·i·o·pexy
ooph·or·o·pexy
ooph·or·o·plas·ty
ooph·o·ror·rha·phy
ooph·or·o·sal·pin·gec·to·my
ooph·or·o·sal·pin·gi·tis
ooph·or·os·to·my

ooph·or·ot·o·my
ooph·or·rha·gia
oo·plasm
oo·spo·ran·gi·um
oo·spore
oo·the·ca
oo·tid
oo·type
opac·i·fi·ca·tion
opac·i·fy·ing
  gall·stones
opac·i·ty
  snow·ball o.
opal·es·cent
opal·ine
  patch
Opalski
  cell
opaque
  mi·cro·scope
o·pei·do·scope
open
  an·gi·og·ra·phy
  bi·op·sy
  bite
  com·e·do
  cor·dot·o·my
  dis·lo·ca·tion
  drain·age
  flap
  frac·ture
  hos·pi·tal
  pneu·mo·thor·ax
  re·duc·tion of frac·tures
  tu·ber·cu·lo·sis
  wound
open-an·gle
  glau·co·ma
open chain
  com·pound
open chest
  mas·sage
open cir·cuit
  meth·od
open drop
  an·es·the·sia
open head
  in·ju·ry
open heart
  sur·gery
open·ing
  ax·is
  con·trac·tion
  move·ment
  snap
open·ing
  ac·cess o.
  aor·tic o.

car·di·ac o.
esoph·a·ge·al o.
ex·ter·nal ure·thral o.
fem·o·ral o.
il·e·o·ce·cal o.
o. of in·fe·ri·or ve·na ca·
va
in·ter·nal ure·thral o.
lac·ri·mal o.
pha·ryn·ge·al o. of au·di·
to·ry tube
pha·ryn·ge·al o. of eu·sta·
chi·an tube
pir·i·form o.
pul·mo·nary o.
o.'s of pul·mo·nary veins
sa·phe·nous o.
o. of su·pe·ri·or ve·na ca·
va
ten·di·nous o.
tym·pan·ic o. of au·di·to·ry
tube
tym·pan·ic o. of ca·nal for
chor·da tym·pa·ni
tym·pan·ic o. of eu·sta·chi·
an tube
ure·ter·al o.
ure·thral o.'s
o. of uter·us
vag·i·nal o.
ver·ti·cal o.
open skull
frac·ture
op·er·a·ble
op·e·ra-glass
hand
op·er·ant
be·hav·ior
con·di·tion·ing
op·er·ate
op·er·at·ing
mi·cro·scope
ta·ble
op·er·a·tion
Abbe o.
Adams' o. for ec·tro·pi·on
Ammon's o.
Anagnostakis' o.
Arlt's o.
Baldy's o.
Ball's o.
Barkan's o.
Bassini's o.
Baudelocque's o.
Beer's o.
Belsey o.
Billroth's o. I
Billroth's o. II

Blalock-Hanlon o.
Blalock-Taussig o.
Blaskovics' o.
blood·less o.
Bonnet's o.
Bowman's o.
Bozeman's o.
Bricker o.
Brock o.
Brunschwig's o.
Burow's o.
Caldwell-Luc o.
cap·i·tal o.
Carmody-Batson o.
Caslick's o.
ce·sar·e·an o.
com·man·do o.
con·crete o.'s
Cotte's o.
Dana's o.
Dandy o.
Daviel's o.
de·bulk·ing o.
de·com·pres·sion o.'s
de Vincentiis o.
Doyle's o.
Dupuy-Dutemps o.
Elliot's o.
Emmet's o.
Esser o.
Estes o.
Estlander o.
fen·es·tra·tion o.
Filatov's o.
fil·ter·ing o.
Finney's o.
flap o.
Foley o.
Fontan o.
for·mal o.'s
Fothergill's o.
Frazier-Spiller o.
Fredet-Ramstedt o.
Freund's o.
Frost-Lang o.
Gifford's o.
Gigli's o.
Gilliam's o.
Gillies' o.
Gil-Vernet o.
Glenn's o.
Graefe's o.
Gritti's o.
Halsted's o.
Hartmann's o.
Heaney's o.
Heine's o.
Heller o.

op·er·a·tion *(continued)*
Herbert's o.
Hill o.
Hoffa's o.
Hofmeister's o.
Holth's o.
Hotz-Anagnostakis o.
Huggins' o.
Hummelsheim's o.
Hunter's o.
In·di·an o.
in·ter·val o.
Ital·ian o.
Jacobaeus o.
Jansen's o.
Kasai o.
Kazanjian's o.
Keen's o.
Kelly's o.
Killian's o.
Koerte-Ballance o.
Kondoleon o.
Kraske's o.
Krönlein o.
Kuhnt's o.
Ladd's o.
Lagrange's o.
Lambrinudi o.
Laroyenne's o.
Lash's o.
Leriche's o.
Lindner's o.
Lisfranc's o.
Longmire's o.
Luc's o.
Madlener o.
ma·jor o.
Man·ches·ter o.
Mann-Williamson o.
Marshall-Marchetti-Krantz o.
Mason o.
Matas' o.
Mayo's o.
McReynolds' o.
McVay's o.
Meyer-Schwickerath o.
mi·ka o.
Mikulicz' o.
Miles' o.
mi·nor o.
mor·cel·la·tion o.
Motais' o.
Mules' o.
Mustard o.
Naffziger o.
Nissen's o.
Norton's o.
Ogston-Luc o.

Ogura o.
Ombrédanne o.
Payne o.
plas·tic o.
Pólya's o.
Pomeroy's o.
Porro o.
Potts' o.
Putti-Platt o.
rad·i·cal o. for her·nia
Ramstedt o.
Récamier's o.
Ridell's o.
Roux-en-Y o.
Saemisch's o.
Saenger's o.
Schauta vag·i·nal o.
Schroeder's o.
Schuchardt's o.
scle·ral buck·ling o.
Scott o.
sec·ond-look o.
se·ton o.
Shirodkar o.
Sistrunk o.
Smith-Boyce o.
Smith-Indian o.
Smith-Robinson o.
Smith's o.
Soave o.
Spinelli o.
sta·pes mo·bi·li·za·tion o.
Stoffel's o.
Stookey-Scarff o.
Sturmdorf's o.
sub·cu·ta·ne·ous o.
Syme's o.
tag·li·a·co·ti·an o.
talc o.
TeLinde o.
Torek o.
Trendelenburg's o.
Urban's o.
Waters' o.
Webster's o.
Weir's o.
Wertheim's o.
Wheelhouse's o.
Whipple's o.
Whitehead's o.
Ziegler's o.
op·er·a·tive
den·tis·try
myx·e·de·ma
op·er·a·tor
gene
oper·cu·la

oper·cu·lar
    fold
oper·cu·lat·ed
oper·cu·li
oper·cu·li·tis
oper·cu·lum
    o. il·ei
    oc·cip·i·tal o.
    troph·o·blas·tic o.
op·er·on
ophi·a·sis
Ophid·ia
ophi·di·a·sis
ophid·i·o·pho·bia
ophid·ism
oph·ri·tis
oph·ry·i·tis
oph·ry·on
Oph·ry·o·sco·lec·i·dae
oph·ry·o·sis
oph·ry·o·spi·nal
    an·gle
oph·thal·mal·gia
oph·thal·mia
    Bra·zil·ian o.
    ca·tarrh·al o.
    cat·er·pil·lar-hair o.
    o. ec·ze·ma·to·sa
    Egyp·tian o.
    elec·tric o.
    gon·or·rhe·al o.
    gran·u·lar o.
    o. he·pat·i·ca
    o. len·ta
    met·a·stat·ic o.
    mi·gra·to·ry o.
    mu·cous o.
    o. ne·o·na·to·rum
    neu·ro·par·a·lyt·ic o.
    o. ni·va·lis
    o. no·do·sa
    pe·ri·od·ic o.
    phlyc·ten·u·lar o.
    pseu·do·tu·ber·cu·lous o.
    pu·ru·lent o.
    reap·er's o.
    scrof·u·lous o.
    spring o.
    sym·pa·thet·ic o.
    trans·ferred o.
    veg·e·ta·ble o.
oph·thal·mic
    ar·tery
    hy·per·thy·roid·ism
    mi·graine
    nerve
    oint·ment
    plex·us

sco·li·o·sis
so·lu·tions
veins
oph·thal·mic ac·id
oph·thal·mi·tis
oph·thal·mo·di·aph·a·no·scope
oph·thal·mo·dy·na·mom·e·ter
    Bailliart's o.
    suc·tion o.
oph·thal·mo·dy·na·mom·e·try
oph·thal·mo·gram
oph·thal·mo·graph
oph·thal·mog·ra·phy
oph·thal·mo·lith
oph·thal·mol·o·gist
oph·thal·mol·o·gy
oph·thal·mo·ma·la·cia
oph·thal·mo·man·dib·u·lo·mel·
  ic
    dys·pla·sia
oph·thal·mo·mel·a·no·sis
oph·thal·mom·e·ter
oph·thal·mo·my·co·sis
oph·thal·mo·my·i·a·sis
oph·thal·mo·my·i·tis
oph·thal·mop·a·thy
    en·do·crine o.
    ex·ter·nal o.
    in·ter·nal o.
oph·thal·mo·ple·gia
    ex·oph·thal·mic o.
    o. ex·ter·na
    fas·cic·u·lar o.
    in·fec·tious o.
    o. in·ter·na
    o. in·ter·nu·cle·a·ris
    nu·cle·ar o.
    or·bi·tal o.
    Parinaud's o.
    o. par·ti·a·lis
    o. pro·gres·si·va
    o. to·ta·lis
oph·thal·mo·ple·gic
    mi·graine
oph·thal·mo·scope
    bin·oc·u·lar o.
    dem·on·stra·tion o.
    di·rect o.
    in·di·rect o.
oph·thal·mo·scop·ic
oph·thal·mos·co·py
    di·rect o.
    in·di·rect o.
    o. with re·flect·ed light
oph·thal·mo·trope
oph·thal·mo·vas·cu·lar
opi·a·nine
opi·a·nyl

opi·ate
  re·cep·tors
opine
opi·oid
opi·o·mel·a·no·cor·tin
opip·ra·mol hy·dro·chlo·ride
opis·the·nar
opis·thi·o·ba·si·al
opis·thi·on
opis·thi·o·na·si·al
op·is·tho·chei·lia
op·is·tho·chi·lia
opis·tho·mas·ti·gote
opis·tho·po·reia
op·is·thor·chi·a·sis
op·is·thor·chid
Opis·thor·chi·i·dae
Opis·thor·chis
  O. fe·li·ne·us
  O. si·nen·sis
  O. vi·ver·ri·ni
op·is·thotic
op·is·thot·on·ic
op·is·thot·o·noid
op·is·thot·o·nos
op·is·thot·o·nus
opi·um
  Bos·ton o.
  de·nar·co·tized o.
  de·o·dor·ized o.
  gran·u·lat·ed o.
  pow·dered o.
  pud·ding o.
op·o·bal·sa·mum
op·o·did·y·mus
opos·sum
  en·ceph·a·li·tis
Oppenheim's
  dis·ease
  re·flex
  syn·drome
op·pi·la·tion
op·pi·la·tive
op·po·nens
op·po·nent
  col·or
op·por·tun·is·tic
  path·o·gen
op·pos·er
  mus·cle of lit·tle fin·ger
  mus·cle of thumb
op·po·si·tion·al
  dis·or·der
op·sin
op·sin·o·gen
op·si·u·ria
op·so·clo·nus
op·so·gen

op·so·ma·nia
op·son·ic
  in·dex
op·so·nin
  com·mon o.
  im·mune o.
  nor·mal o.
  spe·cif·ic o.
  ther·mo·la·bile o.
  ther·mo·sta·ble o.
op·son·i·za·tion
op·so·no·cy·to·pha·gic
op·so·nom·e·try
op·so·no·phil·ia
op·so·no·phil·ic
op·tes·the·sia
op·tic
  ag·no·sia
  ax·is
  ca·nal
  cap·sule
  chi·asm
  cup
  de·cus·sa·tion
  disk
  fis·sure
  fo·ra·men
  groove
  lay·er
  nerve
  neu·ri·tis
  pa·pil·la
  part of ret·i·na
  plac·odes
  ra·di·a·tion
  re·cess
  stalk
  tract
  ves·i·cle
op·ti·cal
  ab·er·ra·tion
  ac·tiv·i·ty
  al·la·ches·the·sia
  an·ti·pode
  den·si·ty
  il·lu·sion
  im·age
  ir·i·dec·to·my
  isom·er·ism
  ker·a·to·plas·ty
  pa·chym·e·ter
  ro·ta·tion
op·ti·cal alex·ia
op·ti·cal right·ing
  re·flex·es
op·ti·cal ro·ta·to·ry
  dis·per·sion
op·ti·cian

op·ti·cian·ry
op·tic nerve
   dru·sen
   hy·po·pla·sia
op·ti·co·cil·i·a·ry
op·ti·co·fa·cial
   re·flex
op·ti·co·ki·net·ic
   nys·tag·mus
op·ti·co·pu·pil·lary
op·tics
   Nomarski o.
op·ti·mism
   ther·a·peu·tic o.
op·ti·mum
   dose
   pH
   tem·per·a·ture
op·to·ki·net·ic
   nys·tag·mus
op·to·me·ninx
op·tom·e·ter
   ob·jec·tive o.
op·tom·e·trist
op·tom·e·try
op·to·my·om·e·ter
op·to·types
O-R
   sys·tem
ora
or·ad
orae
oral
   bi·ol·o·gy
   cav·i·ty
   cav·i·ty prop·er
   con·tra·cep·tive
   fis·sure
   hy·giene
   mem·brane
   part of phar·ynx
   pa·thol·o·gy
   phar·ynx
   phase
   phys·i·o·ther·a·py
   plate
   pri·ma·cy
   re·gion
   shields
   smear
   ster·e·o·typy
   sur·geon
   sur·gery
   teeth
ora·le
oral ep·i·the·li·al
   ne·vus

oral (ero·sive)
   li·chen pla·nus
Oral Hy·giene In·dex
oral·i·ty
oral lac·tose tol·er·ance
   test
oral (non·e·ro·sive)
   li·chen pla·nus
oral po·li·o·vi·rus
   vac·cine
or·ange
   bit·ter o. peel
   bit·ter o. peel, dried
   bit·ter o. peel, fresh
   bit·ter o. peel oil
or·ange G
or·ange wood
Orbeli
   ef·fect
or·bic·u·lar
   bone
   lig·a·ment
   lig·a·ment of ra·di·us
   mus·cle
   mus·cle of eye
   mus·cle of mouth
   pro·cess
   zone
or·bic·u·la·re
or·bi·cu·la·ris
   phe·nom·e·non
or·bi·cu·la·ris oc·u·li
   re·flex
or·bi·cu·la·ris pu·pil·lary
   re·flex
or·bi·cu·lus cil·i·ar·is
or·bit
or·bi·ta
or·bi·tal
   ab·scess
   apex
   ar·tery
   ax·is
   cav·i·ty
   de·com·pres·sion
   em·i·nence
   ex·en·ter·a·tion
   fas·ci·ae
   gy·ri
   height
   her·nia
   im·plant
   in·dex
   lam·i·na of eth·moid bone
   lay·er of eth·moid bone
   mus·cle
   nerve
   oph·thal·mo·ple·gia

or·bi·tal *(continued)*
  part
  part of op·tic nerve
  per·i·os·ti·tis
  plane
  plate
  pro·cess
  re·gion
  sul·ci
  sur·face
  syn·drome
  tu·ber·cle
  width
or·bi·ta·le
or·bi·to·fron·tal
  ar·tery
  cor·tex
or·bi·tog·ra·phy
or·bi·to·na·sal
  in·dex
or·bi·to·nom·e·ter
or·bi·to·nom·e·try
or·bi·top·a·gus
or·bi·to·sphe·noid
  car·ti·lage
or·bi·tot·o·my
Or·bi·vi·rus
or·ce·in
or·chec·to·my
or·chel·la
or·chi·al·gia
or·chi·at·ro·phy
or·chi·cho·rea
or·chi·dal·gia
or·chi·dec·to·my
or·chid·ic
or·chi·di·tis
or·chi·dom·e·ter
or·chi·dop·to·sis
or·chi·dor·ra·phy
or·chi·ec·to·my
or·chi·ep·i·did·y·mi·tis
or·chil
or·chi·lyt·ic
or·chi·o·cele
or·chi·o·coc·cus
or·chi·o·dyn·ia
or·chi·on·cus
or·chi·o·neu·ral·gia
or·chi·op·a·thy
or·chi·o·pexy
  trans·sep·tal o.
or·chi·o·plas·ty
or·chi·or·rha·phy
or·chi·o·ther·a·py
or·chi·ot·o·my
or·chis
or·chis·es

or·chit·ic
or·chi·tis
  o. pa·ro·ti·dea
  trau·mat·ic o.
  o. va·ri·o·lo·sa
or·chot·o·my
or·cin
or·cin·ol
  test
or·ci·pren·a·line sul·fate
or·deal bean
or·der
  peck·ing o.
or·der·ly
or·di·nate
orec·tic
orex·ia
orex·i·gen·ic
orf
  vi·rus
or·gan
  cul·ture
or·gan
  ac·ces·so·ry o.'s
  ac·ces·so·ry o.'s of eye
  an·nu·lo·spi·ral o.
  Chievitz' o.
  cir·cum·ven·tric·u·lar o.'s
  Corti's o.
  crit·i·cal o.
  enam·el o.
  end o.
  float·ing o.
  flow·er-spray o. of Ruffini
  gen·i·tal o.'s.
  Golgi ten·don o.
  gus·ta·to·ry o.
  o. of hear·ing
  in·tro·mit·tent o.
  Jacobson's o.
  lat·er·al line sense o.
  neu·ro·mast o.
  neu·ro·ten·di·nous o.
  ol·fac·to·ry o.
  pto·tic o.
  o. of Rosenmüller
  sense o.'s
  o. of smell
  spi·ral o.
  sub·com·mis·sur·al o.
  su·per·nu·mer·ary o.'s
  tar·get o.
  o. of taste
  o. of touch
  uri·nary o.'s
  ves·tib·u·lar o.
  ves·tib·u·lo·co·chle·ar o.
  ves·tig·i·al o.

o. of vi·sion
vom·er·o·na·sal o.
wan·der·ing o.
Weber's o.
o.'s of Zuckerkandl
or·ga·na
or·ga·na
or·gan·elle
  cell o.
  paired o.'s
or·gan·ic
  ac·id
  cat·a·lyst
  chem·is·try
  com·pound
  con·trac·ture
  deaf·ness
  dis·ease
  ev·o·lu·tion
  head·ache
  mur·mur
  pain
  phos·phate
  prin·ci·ple
  stric·ture
  ver·ti·go
or·gan·ic brain
  syn·drome
or·gan·ic den·tal
  ce·ment
or·gan·i·cism
or·gan·i·cist
or·gan·ic men·tal
  dis·or·der
  syn·drome
or·gan·i·fi·ca·tion
  de·fect
or·ga·nism
  cal·cu·lat·ed mean o.
  fas·tid·i·ous o.
  hy·po·thet·i·cal mean o.
  pleu·ro·pneu·mo·nia-like o.'s
or·ga·ni·za·tion
  pre·gen·i·tal o.
or·ga·nize
or·ga·nized
  pneu·mo·nia
or·ga·niz·er
  nu·cle·o·lar o.
  pri·mary o.
  pro·cen·tri·ole o.
or·gan·o·fer·ric
or·gan·o·gel
or·ga·no·gen·e·sis
or·ga·no·ge·net·ic
or·ga·no·gen·ic
or·ga·nog·e·ny
or·ga·nog·ra·phy

or·gan·oid
  ne·vus
  tu·mor
or·ga·no·lep·tic
or·ga·nol·o·gy
or·ga·no·ma
or·ga·no·meg·a·ly
or·gan·o·mer·cur·i·al
or·ga·no·me·tal·lic
or·ga·non
or·ga·non·o·my
or·ga·non·y·my
or·ga·nop·a·thy
or·ga·no·pex·ia
or·ga·no·pexy
or·ga·no·phil·ic
or·ga·no·phi·lic·i·ty
or·gan·o·sol
or·ga·no·tax·is
or·ga·no·ther·a·py
or·ga·no·tro·phic
or·ga·no·tro·pic
or·ga·not·ro·pism
or·ga·not·ro·py
or·gan-spe·cif·ic
  an·ti·gen
or·ga·num
  o. au·di·tus
  o. tac·tus
or·gasm
or·gas·mic
or·gas·tic
Ori·bo·ca
  vi·rus
Or·i·en·tal
  boil
  but·ton
  ring·worm
  schis·to·so·mi·a·sis
  sore
  ul·cer
or·i·en·ta·tion
or·i·ent·ing
  re·flex
  re·sponse
or·i·en·to·my·cin
or·i·fice
  anal o.
  esoph·a·go·gas·tric o.
  gas·tro·du·o·de·nal o.
  golf-hole ure·ter·al o.
  mi·tral o.
  py·lor·ic o.
  root ca·nal o.
  tri·cus·pid o.
or·i·fi·cia
or·i·fi·cial

or·i·fi·ci·um
  o. ex·ter·num uter·i
  o. in·ter·num uter·i
  o. ure·te·ris
  o. ure·thrae ex·ter·num
  o. va·gi·nae
orig·a·num oil
or·i·gin
oris
ori·za·ba jal·ap root
Ormond's
  dis·ease
or·nate
or·ni·thine
  o. ace·tyl·trans·fer·ase
  o. car·bam·o·yl·trans·fer·ase
  o. de·car·box·yl·ase
  o. trans·car·bam·o·y·lase
or·ni·thine
  cy·cle
or·ni·thi·ne·mia
or·ni·thi·nu·ria
Or·ni·thod·o·ros
  O. co·ri·a·ce·us
  O. er·ra·ti·cus
  O. herm·si
  O. la·ho·ren·sis
  O. mou·ba·ta com·plex
  O. pap·pi·li·pes
  O. par·keri
  O. ru·dis
  O. sa·vigni
  O. ta·la·jé
  O. tho·lo·za·ni
  O. tu·ri·ca·ta
  O. ve·ne·zu·e·len·sis
  O. ver·ru·co·sus
Or·ni·tho·nys·sus
or·ni·tho·sis
  vi·rus
or·o·an·tral
  fis·tu·la
or·o·dig·i·to·fa·cial
  dys·os·to·sis
or·o·fa·cial
  fis·tu·la
or·o·fa·ci·o·dig·i·tal
  syn·drome
or·o·lin·gual
or·o·na·sal
  fis·tu·la
  mem·brane
or·o·pha·ryn·ge·al
  mem·brane
or·o·pha·ryn·go·lar·yn·gi·tis
or·o·phar·ynx
or·o·so·mu·coid

or·o·tate
  o. phos·pho·ri·bo·syl·trans·
  fer·ase
orot·ic ac·id
orot·ic ac·i·du·ria
orot·i·dine
orot·i·dyl·ate
orot·i·dyl·ic ac·id
  o. a. phos·pho·ryl·ase
or·o·tra·che·al
  in·tu·ba·tion
  tube
Oro·ya
  fe·ver
or·phan
  drugs
  pro·ducts
  vi·rus·es
or·phen·a·drine cit·rate
or·phen·a·drine hy·dro·chlo·ride
or·ris
or·seil·lin BB
Orsi-Grocco
  meth·od
orth·er·ga·sia
or·the·sis
or·thet·ics
or·tho·ac·id
or·tho·ar·te·ri·ot·o·ny
or·tho·bi·o·sis
or·tho·caine
or·tho·ce·phal·ic
or·tho·ceph·a·lous
or·tho·cho·rea
or·tho·chro·mat·ic
or·tho·chro·mo·phil
or·tho·chro·mo·phile
or·tho·cra·sia
or·tho·cy·to·sis
or·tho·den·tin
or·tho·di·gi·ta
or·tho·don·tia
or·tho·don·tic
  ap·pli·ance
  band
  ther·a·py
or·tho·don·tics
  sur·gi·cal o.
or·tho·dont·ist
or·tho·dro·mic
or·tho·gen·e·sis
or·tho·gen·ic
  ev·o·lu·tion
or·tho·gen·ics
or·thog·nath·ia
or·thog·nath·ic
  sur·gery
or·thog·na·thous

or·tho·grade
  de·gen·er·a·tion
or·tho·ker·a·tol·o·gy
or·tho·ker·a·to·sis
or·tho·ki·net·ics
or·tho·me·chan·i·cal
or·tho·me·chan·o·ther·a·py
or·tho·me·lic
or·thom·e·ter
or·tho·mo·lec·u·lar
  ther·a·py
Or·tho·myx·o·vir·i·dae
or·tho·pae·dic
  sur·gery
or·tho·pae·dics
or·tho·pae·dist
or·tho·pe·dic
  sur·gery
or·tho·pe·dics
  den·tal o.
  func·tion·al jaw o.
or·tho·pe·dist
or·tho·per·cus·sion
or·tho·pho·ria
or·tho·phor·ic
or·tho·phos·phate
  in·or·gan·ic o.
or·tho·phos·phor·ic ac·id
or·tho·phre·nia
or·thop·nea
or·thop·ne·ic
Or·tho·pox·vi·rus
or·tho·pros·the·sis
or·tho·psy·chi·a·try
Or·thop·tera
or·thop·tic
or·thop·tics
or·thop·tist
or·tho·scope
or·tho·scop·ic
  lens
  spec·ta·cles
or·thos·co·py
or·tho·ses
or·tho·sis
or·tho·stat·ic
  al·bu·min·ur·ia
  hy·po·pi·e·sis
  hy·po·ten·sion
  pro·tein·u·ria
or·tho·ster·e·o·scope
or·tho·sym·pa·thet·ic
or·tho·tha·na·sia
or·thot·ics
or·tho·tist
or·tho·tol·i·dine
or·thot·o·nos
or·thot·o·nus

or·tho·top·ic
  graft
or·tho·tro·pic
or·tho·vol·tage
Orth's
  fix·a·tive
  stain
os
  o. acro·mi·a·le
  o. bas·i·la·re
  o. cal·cis
  o. cen·tra·le tar·si
  o. clit·o·ris
  os·sa fa·ci·ei
  o. in·cae
  in·com·pe·tent cer·vi·cal o.
  o. in·no·mi·na·tum
  o. in·ter·max·il·la·re
  o. in·ter·me·di·um
  o. in·ter·met·a·tar·se·um
  o. ja·po·ni·cum
  o. mag·num
  o. ma·la·re
  o. mult·ang·u·lum ma·jus
  o. mult·ang·u·lum mi·nus
  o. na·vi·cu·la·re ma·nus
  o. odon·toi·de·um
  o. or·bic·u·la·re
  o. pe·nis
  o. pre·max·il·la·re
  o. pte·ry·goi·de·um
  o. py·ra·mi·da·le
  Scanzoni's sec·ond o.
  o. sub·tib·i·a·le
  o. syl·vii
  o. tib·i·a·le pos·te·ri·us
  o. tib·i·a·le pos·ti·cum
  o. tri·an·gu·la·re
  o. tri·ba·si·la·re
  o. un·guis
  o. uteri ex·ter·num
  o. uteri in·ter·num
  o. ve·sa·li·a·num
osa·zone
os·che·al
os·che·i·tis
osch·el·e·phan·ti·a·sis
os·che·o·hy·dro·cele
os·che·o·plas·ty
os·cil·lat·ing
  vi·sion
os·cil·la·tion
os·cil·la·tor
os·cil·la·to·ry
  po·ten·tial
os·cil·lo·graph
os·cil·log·ra·phy
os·cil·lom·e·ter

os·cil·lo·met·ric
os·cil·lom·e·try
os·cil·lop·sia
os·cil·lo·scope
  cath·ode ray o.
  stor·age o.
os·ci·tate
os·ci·ta·tion
os·cu·la
os·cu·lum
Osgood-Schlatter
  dis·ease
Osler
  node
Osler's
  dis·ease
  sign
Osler-Vaquez
  dis·ease
os·mate
os·mat·ic
os·me·sis
os·mic ac·id
  fix·a·tive
os·mi·cate
os·mi·ca·tion
os·mics
os·mi·dro·sis
os·mi·fi·ca·tion
os·mi·o·phil·ic
os·mi·o·pho·bic
os·mi·um
  o. te·trox·ide
os·mo·cep·tor
os·mo·dys·pho·ria
os·mo·gram
os·mo·lal
  clear·ance
os·mo·lal·i·ty
  cal·cu·lat·ed se·rum
os·mo·lar
os·mo·lar·i·ty
os·mole
os·mol·o·gy
os·mom·e·ter
os·mom·e·try
os·mo·phil
os·mo·phil·ic
os·mo·pho·bia
os·mo·phore
os·mo·re·cep·tor
os·mo·reg·u·la·to·ry
os·mose
os·mo·sis
  re·verse o.
os·mos·i·ty
os·mo·ther·a·py

os·mot·ic
  di·u·re·sis
  ne·phro·sis
  pres·sure
  shock
os·phre·si·o·lag·nia
os·phre·si·o·log·ic
os·phre·si·ol·o·gy
os·phre·si·o·phil·ia
os·phre·si·o·pho·bia
os·phre·sis
os·phret·ic
os·sa
os·se·in
os·se·ine
os·se·let
os·se·o·car·ti·lag·i·nous
os·se·o·mu·cin
os·se·o·mu·coid
os·se·ous
  am·pul·la
  cell
  lab·y·rinth
  la·cu·na
  part of skel·e·tal sys·tem
  pol·yp
  tis·sue
os·se·ous hy·da·tid
  cyst
os·se·ous spi·ral
  lam·i·na
os·si·cle
  Andernach's o.'s
  au·di·to·ry o.'s
  Bertin's o.'s
  epac·tal o.'s
  Kerckring's o.
os·sic·u·la
os·sic·u·lar
  chain
os·sic·u·lec·to·my
os·si·cu·lot·o·my
os·sic·u·lum
  os·sic·u·la men·ta·lia
os·sif·er·ous
os·sif·ic
  cen·ter
os·si·fi·ca·tion
  en·do·chon·dral o.
  in·tra·mem·bra·nous o.
  mem·bra·nous o.
  met·a·plas·tic o.
os·si·form
os·si·fy
os·sis
os·te·al
os·te·al·gia
os·te·al·gic

os·te·an·a·gen·e·sis
os·te·a·naph·y·sis
os·tec·to·my
os·te·in
os·te·ine
os·te·it·ic
os·te·i·tis
  al·ve·o·lar o.
  ca·se·ous o.
  cen·tral o.
  con·dens·ing o.
  cor·ti·cal o.
  o. de·for·mans
  o. fi·bro·sa cir·cum·scrip·ta
  o. fi·bro·sa cys·ti·ca
  o. fi·bro·sa dis·sem·i·na·ta
  he·ma·tog·e·nous o.
  lo·cal·ized o. fi·bro·sa
  mul·ti·fo·cal o. fi·bro·sa
  re·nal o. fi·bro·sa
  scle·ros·ing o.
  o. tu·ber·cu·lo·sa mul·ti·
    plex cys·ti·ca
os·tem·bry·on
os·te·mia
os·tem·py·e·sis
os·te·o·an·a·gen·e·sis
os·te·o·ar·thri·tis
  hy·per·plas·tic o.
os·te·o·ar·throp·a·thy
  hy·per·tro·phic pul·mo·nary
    o.
  id·i·o·path·ic hy·per·tro·
    phic o.
  pneu·mo·gen·ic o.
  pul·mo·nary o.
os·te·o·ar·thro·sis
os·te·o·blast
os·te·o·blas·tic
os·te·o·blas·to·ma
os·te·o·car·ci·no·ma
os·te·o·car·ti·lag·i·nous
os·te·o·chon·dri·tis
  o. de·for·mans ju·ve·ni·lis
  o. de·for·mans ju·ve·ni·lis
    dor·si
  o. dis·se·cans
  syph·i·lit·ic o.
os·te·o·chon·dro·dys·tro·phia
  de·for·mans
os·te·o·chon·dro·dys·tro·phy
os·te·o·chon·dro·gen·ic
  cell
os·te·o·chon·dro·ma
os·te·o·chon·dro·ma·to·sis
  syn·o·vi·al o.
os·te·o·chon·dro·sar·co·ma
os·te·o·chon·dro·sis

os·te·o·chon·drous
os·te·o·cla·sia
os·te·oc·la·sis
os·te·o·clast
os·te·o·clast ac·ti·vat·ing
  fac·tor
os·te·o·clas·tic
os·te·o·clas·to·ma
os·te·o·col·lag·e·nous
  fi·bers
os·te·o·cra·ni·um
os·te·o·cys·to·ma
os·te·o·cyte
os·te·o·den·tin
os·te·o·der·ma·to·poi·ki·lo·sis
os·te·o·der·ma·tous
os·te·o·der·mia
os·te·o·des·mo·sis
os·te·o·di·as·ta·sis
os·te·o·dyn·ia
os·te·o·dys·plas·ty
os·te·o·dys·tro·phia
os·te·o·dys·tro·phy
  Albright's he·red·i·tary o.
  re·nal o.
os·te·o·ec·ta·sia
os·te·o·ec·to·my
os·te·o·e·piph·y·sis
os·te·o·fi·bro·ma
os·te·o·fi·bro·sis
  per·i·ap·i·cal o.
os·te·o·gen
os·te·o·gen·e·sis
  o. im·per·fec·ta
  o. im·per·fec·ta con·gen·i·ta
  o. im·per·fec·ta tar·da
os·te·o·ge·net·ic
  fi·bers
  lay·er
os·te·o·gen·ic
  cell
  sar·co·ma
  tis·sue
os·te·og·e·nous
os·te·og·e·ny
os·te·og·ra·phy
os·te·o·ha·li·ste·re·sis
os·te·o·hy·per·tro·phy
os·te·oid
  os·te·o·ma
  tis·sue
os·te·o·lath·y·rism
os·te·o·lip·o·chon·dro·ma
os·te·o·lo·gia
os·te·ol·o·gist
os·te·ol·o·gy
os·te·ol·y·sis
os·te·o·lyt·ic

os·te·o·ma
  o. cu·tis
  den·tal o.
  gi·ant os·te·oid o.
  o. me·dul·la·re
  os·te·oid o.
  o. spon·gi·o·sum
os·te·o·ma·la·cia
  in·fan·tile o.
  ju·ve·nile o.
  se·nile o.
  X-linked hy·po·phos·pha·
    tem·ic o.
os·te·o·ma·lac·ic
  pel·vis
os·te·o·ma·toid
os·te·o·mere
os·te·om·e·try
os·te·o·my·e·li·tis
os·te·o·my·e·lo·dys·pla·sia
os·te·o·my·e·lo·fi·brot·ic
  syn·drome
os·te·on
os·te·on·cus
os·te·one
os·te·o·ne·cro·sis
os·te·o·path
os·te·o·path·ia
  o. con·den·sans
  o. hem·or·rha·gi·ca in·fan·
    tum
  o. stri·a·ta
os·te·o·path·ic
  med·i·cine
  phy·si·cian
  sco·li·o·sis
os·te·o·pa·thol·o·gy
os·te·op·a·thy
  al·i·men·ta·ry o.
os·te·o·pe·di·on
os·te·o·pe·nia
os·te·o·per·i·os·te·al
  graft
os·te·o·per·i·os·ti·tis
os·te·o·pe·tro·sis
  o. ac·ro-os·te·o·lyt·i·ca
  o. gal·li·na·rum
os·te·o·pe·trot·ic
os·te·o·phage
os·te·o·pha·gia
os·te·o·phle·bi·tis
os·te·oph·o·ny
os·te·o·phy·ma
os·te·o·phyte
os·te·o·plaque
os·te·o·plast
os·te·o·plas·tic
  am·pu·ta·tion

cra·ni·ot·o·my
ne·crot·o·my
os·te·o·plas·ty
os·te·o·poi·ki·lo·sis
os·te·o·po·ro·sis
  o. cir·cum·scrip·ta cra·nii
  ju·ve·nile o.
  post·trau·mat·ic o.
os·te·o·po·rot·ic
os·te·o·pro·gen·i·tor
  cell
os·te·o·ra·di·o·ne·cro·sis
os·te·or·rha·phy
os·te·o·sar·co·ma
os·te·o·scle·ro·sis
  o. con·gen·i·ta
os·te·o·scle·rot·ic
  ane·mia
os·te·o·scope
os·te·o·sis
  o. cu·tis
  o. ebur·ni·sans mo·no·me·
    li·ca
  par·a·thy·roid o.
  re·nal fi·bro·cys·tic o.
os·te·o·spon·gi·o·ma
os·te·o·ste·a·to·ma
os·te·o·su·ture
os·te·o·syn·the·sis
os·te·o·throm·bo·sis
os·te·o·tome
os·te·ot·o·my
  "C" slid·ing o.
  hor·i·zon·tal o.
  sag·it·tal split man·dib·u·lar
    o.
  seg·men·tal al·ve·o·lar o.
  slid·ing ob·lique o.
  ver·ti·cal o.
os·te·o·tribe
os·te·o·trite
os·te·ot·ro·phy
os·te·o·tym·pan·ic
Os·ter·ta·gia
os·tia
os·ti·al
  sphinc·ter
os·ti·tic
os·ti·tis
os·ti·um
  aor·tic o.
  o. ar·te·ri·o·sum
  o. in·ter·num
  o. pri·mum
  o. se·cun·dum
  o. uter·i ex·ter·num
  o. uter·i in·ter·num
  o. ve·no·sum

os·to·mate
os·to·my
os·to·sis
os·tra·ceous
os·tre·o·tox·ism
Ostwald's sol·u·bil·i·ty
  co·ef·fi·cient
Ot
  an·ti·gen
otal·gia
  ge·nic·u·late o.
  re·flex o.
otal·gic
Ota's
  ne·vus
Othello
  syn·drome
o·the·ma·to·ma
o·the·mor·rha·gia
oth·er-di·rect·ed
oti·at·ria
oti·at·rics
otic
  ab·scess
  bar·o·trau·ma
  cap·sule
  gan·gli·on
  plac·odes
  ves·i·cle
otit·ic
  hy·dro·ceph·a·lus
  men·in·gi·tis
oti·tis
  avi·a·tion o.
  o. des·qua·ma·ti·va
  o. diph·the·ri·ti·ca
  o. ex·ter·na
  o. ex·ter·na cir·cum·scrip·ta
  o. ex·ter·na dif·fu·sa
  o. ex·ter·na hem·or·rha·gi·
  ca
  o. fu·run·cu·lo·sa
  o. in·ter·na
  o. in·ti·ma
  o. lab·y·rin·thi·ca
  o. me·dia
  o. me·dia ca·tar·rha·lis
  o. me·dia pu·ru·len·ta
  o. me·dia sup·pu·ra·ti·va
  o. my·co·ti·ca
  par·a·sit·ic o.
  re·flux o. me·dia
  se·cre·to·ry o. me·dia
  se·rous o.
oto·ac·a·ri·a·sis
oto·an·tri·tis
oto·bi·o·sis
Oto·bi·us

oto·ceph·a·ly
oto·cer·e·bri·tis
oto·clei·sis
oto·co·nia
oto·co·ni·um
oto·cra·ni·al
oto·cra·ni·um
oto·cyst
Oto·dec·tes
oto·dec·tic
  mange
oto·dyn·ia
oto·en·ceph·a·li·tis
oto·gang·li·on
oto·gen·ic
otog·e·nous
otog·ra·phy
oto·lar·yn·gol·o·gist
oto·lar·yn·gol·o·gy
oto·lites
oto·lith·ic
  mem·brane
oto·liths
oto·log·ic
otol·o·gist
otol·o·gy
oto·man·dib·u·lar
  dys·os·to·sis
  syn·drome
oto·mas·sage
oto·mu·cor·my·co·sis
oto·my·co·sis
oto·neu·ral·gia
oto·pal·a·to·dig·i·tal
  syn·drome
otop·a·thy
oto·pha·ryn·ge·al
  tube
oto·plas·ty
oto·pol·y·pus
oto·py·or·rhea
oto·rhi·no·lar·yn·gol·o·gy
oto·rhi·nol·o·gy
otor·rha·gia
otor·rhea
  cer·e·bro·spi·nal flu·id o.
oto·sal·pinx
oto·scle·ro·sis
oto·scope
  Siegle's o.
otos·co·py
otos·te·al
otos·te·on
otot·o·my
oto·tox·ic
oto·tox·ic·i·ty
Otto
  pel·vis

Otto's
  dis·ease
Ottoson
  po·ten·tial
oua·ba·in
Ouchterlony
  test
ounce
out·er
  mal·le·o·lus
  ta·ble of skull
out·er cone
  fi·ber
out·er lim·it·ing
  mem·brane
out·let
  pel·vic o.
out·line
  form
out·pa·tient
out of phase
out·put
  car·di·ac o.
  min·ute o.
  pace·mak·er o.
  stroke o.
ova
oval
  am·pu·ta·tion
  ar·ea of Flechsig
  cor·pus·cle
  fas·cic·u·lus
  fo·ra·men
  fos·sa
  win·dow
ov·al·bu·min
ova·le
  ma·lar·ia
ova·le ter·tian
  ma·lar·ia
oval·o·cyte
oval·o·cyt·ic
  ane·mia
oval·o·cy·to·sis
ova·ria
ovar·i·al·gia
ovar·i·an
  amen·or·rhea
  ar·tery
  col·ic
  cy·cle
  cyst
  dys·men·or·rhea
  fim·bria
  fol·li·cle
  fos·sa
  lig·a·ment
  plex·us

  preg·nan·cy
  var·i·co·cele
  veins
ovar·i·an ascor·bic ac·id de·ple·tion
  test
ovar·i·an tu·bu·lar
  ad·e·no·ma
ovar·i·ec·to·my
ovar·i·o·ab·dom·i·nal
  preg·nan·cy
ovar·i·o·cele
ovar·i·o·cen·te·sis
ovar·i·o·cy·e·sis
ovar·i·o·dys·neu·ria
ovar·i·o·gen·ic
ovar·i·o·hys·ter·ec·to·my
ovar·i·o·lyt·ic
ovar·i·on·cus
ovar·i·op·a·thy
ovar·i·or·rhex·is
ovar·i·o·sal·pin·gec·to·my
ovar·i·o·sal·pin·gi·tis
ovar·i·o·ste·re·sis
ovar·i·os·to·my
ovar·i·ot·o·my
  nor·mal o.
ova·ri·tis
ovar·i·um
  o. bi·par·ti·tum
  o. dis·junc·tum
  o. gy·ra·tum
  o. lo·ba·tum
  o. mas·cu·li·num
ova·ry
  mul·ber·ry o.
  pol·y·cys·tic o.
  third o.
over·anx·ious
  dis·or·der
over·bite
over·clo·sure
over·com·pen·sa·tion
over·cor·rec·tion
over·den·ture
over·de·ter·mi·na·tion
over·dom·i·nance
over·dom·i·nant
over·e·rup·tion
over·ex·ten·sion
over·flow
  in·con·ti·nence
  wave
over·hang
over·hang·ing
  res·to·ra·tion
over·hy·dra·tion
over·jet

over·jut
over·lap
   hor·i·zon·tal o.
   ver·ti·cal o.
over·lay
   emo·tion·al o.
over·lay
   den·ture
over·learn·ing
over·pro·duc·tion
   the·o·ry
over·re·sponse
over·rid·ing
   aor·ta
over·ripe
   cat·a·ract
over·shoot
overt
   ho·mo·sex·u·al·i·ty
over·tone
   psy·chic o.
over·ven·ti·la·tion
over·win·ter·ing
ovi
ovi·ci·dal
ovi·du·cal
ovi·duct
ovi·duc·tal
ovif·er·ous
ovi·form
ovi·gen·e·sis
ovi·ge·net·ic
ovi·gen·ic
ovig·e·nous
ovine
   ac·e·ton·e·mia
   mas·ti·tis
ovin·ia
ovi·par·i·ty
ovip·a·rous
ovi·pos·it
ovi·po·si·tion
ovi·pos·i·tor
ovo·cen·ter
ovo·cyte
ovo·fla·vin
ovo·gen·e·sis
ovo·glob·u·lin
ovo·go·ni·um
ovoid
   fe·tal o.
   Man·ches·ter o.
ovo·lar·vip·a·rous
ovo·mu·cin
ovo·mu·coid
ovo·plasm
ovo·pro·to·gen
ovo·tes·tis

ovo·trans·fer·rin
ovo·vi·tel·lin
ovo·vi·vip·ar·ous
ovu·la
o·vu·lar
   mem·brane
   trans·mi·gra·tion
o·vu·la·tion
   an·es·trous o.
   par·a·cy·clic o.
o·vu·la·tion·al
   scle·ro·sis
o·vu·la·to·ry
o·vule
o·vu·lo·cy·clic
   por·phyr·ia
o·vu·lum
ovum
   alec·i·thal o.
   blight·ed o.
   cen·tro·lec·i·thal o.
   fer·til·ized o.
   iso·lec·i·thal o.
   Peters' o.
   tel·o·lec·i·thal o.
Owen's
   lines
own
   con·trols
Owren's
   dis·ease
ox
   bots
ox·a·cil·lin so·di·um
ox·al·al·de·hyde
ox·a·late
   cal·cu·lus
ox·a·le·mia
ox·al·ic ac·id
ox·a·lo
ox·a·lo·ac·e·tate trans·ac·e·tase
ox·a·lo·a·ce·tic ac·id
ox·a·lo·sis
ox·a·lo·suc·cin·ic ac·id
ox·a·lo·suc·cin·ic car·box·yl·
   ase
ox·a·lo·u·rea
ox·a·lu·ria
ox·a·lur·ic ac·id
ox·a·lyl
ox·a·lyl·u·rea
ox·am·ide
ox·am·mon·i·um
ox·am·ni·quine
ox·an·a·mide
ox·an·dro·lone
ox·a·phen·a·mide
ox·a·ze·pam

ox·a·zin
  dyes
ox·a·zole
ox·el·a·din
Ox·ford
  unit
ox·i·dant
ox·i·dase
  di·rect o.
  in·di·rect o.
ox·i·dase
  re·ac·tion
ox·i·da·sis
ox·i·da·tion
  beta-o.
  omega-o.
ox·i·da·tion-re·duc·tion
  elec·trode
  in·di·ca·tor
  re·ac·tion
  sys·tem
ox·i·da·tive
  phos·pho·ryl·a·tion
ox·ide
  ac·id o.
  ba·sic o.
  in·dif·fer·ent o.
  neu·tral o.
ox·i·di·za·tion
ox·i·dize
ox·i·dized
  cel·lu·lose
Ox·i·dized glu·ta·thi·one
ox·i·do·re·duc·tase
ox·ime
  am·ide o.'s
ox·im·e·ter
  cu·vette o.
ox·im·e·try
oxo ac·id
ox·ol·a·mine
ox·o·lin·ic ac·id
ox·o·ni·um
  ion
ox·o·phen·ar·sine hy·dro·chlo·ride
ox·o·suc·cin·ic ac·id
ox·pren·o·lol hy·dro·chlo·ride
ox·tri·phyl·line
ox·y·a·coia
ox·y·a·koia
ox·y·a·phia
ox·y·bar·bi·tu·rates
ox·y·ben·zone
ox·y·bi·o·tin
ox·y·bu·ty·nin chlo·ride
ox·y·cal·o·rim·e·ter
ox·y·cel·lu·lose

ox·y·ce·pha·lia
ox·y·ce·phal·ic
ox·y·ceph·a·lous
ox·y·ceph·a·ly
ox·y·chlo·ride
ox·y·chro·mat·ic
ox·y·chro·ma·tin
ox·y·co·done
ox·y·dase
ox·y·es·the·sia
ox·y·gen
  heavy o.
  high pres·sure o.
  hy·per·bar·ic o.
  sin·glet o.
  trip·let o.
ox·y·gen
  ca·pac·i·ty
  con·sump·tion
  debt
  def·i·cit
  ef·fect
  elec·trode
  poi·son·ing
  tent
  ther·a·py
  tox·ic·i·ty
ox·y·gen af·fin·i·ty
  an·ox·ia
  hy·pox·ia
ox·y·gen·ase
ox·y·gen·ate
ox·y·gen·at·ed
  he·mo·glo·bin
ox·y·gen·a·tion
  ap·ne·ic o.
  hy·per·bar·ic o.
ox·y·gen dep·ri·va·tion
  the·o·ry of nar·co·sis
ox·y·gen·ic
ox·y·gen·ize
ox·y·gen uti·li·za·tion
  co·ef·fi·cient
ox·y·geu·sia
ox·y·heme
ox·y·he·mo·chro·mo·gen
ox·y·he·mo·glo·bin
ox·y·i·o·dide
ox·y·krin·in
ox·y·lon·pro·caine hy·dro·chlo·ride
ox·y·mes·ter·one
ox·y·met·az·o·line hy·dro·chlo·ride
ox·y·meth·o·lone
ox·y·mor·phone hy·dro·chlo·ride
ox·y·my·o·glo·bin

ox·y·ner·vone
ox·y·neu·rine
ox·yn·tic
   cell
   gland
ox·y·os·mia
ox·y·os·phre·sia
ox·y·per·tine
ox·y·phen·bu·ta·zone
ox·y·phen·cy·cli·mine hy·dro·chlo·ride
ox·y·phe·ni·sa·tin ac·e·tate
ox·y·phe·no·ni·um bro·mide
ox·y·phil
   ad·e·no·ma
   cells
   chro·ma·tin
   gran·ule
ox·y·phile
ox·y·phil·ic
   leu·ko·cyte
ox·y·pho·nia
ox·y·pol·y·gel·a·tin
ox·y·pu·rine
ox·y·rhine
ox·y·ryg·mia
Ox·y·spi·ru·ra man·so·ni

ox·y·ta·lan fi·ber
   stain
ox·y·tet·ra·cy·cline
ox·y·thi·a·min
ox·y·to·cia
ox·y·to·cic
ox·y·to·cin
   ar·gi·nine o.
ox·y·u·ri·a·sis
ox·y·u·ri·cide
ox·y·u·rid
Ox·y·u·ri·dae
Ox·y·u·ris
oze·na
oze·nous
ozo·ce·rite
ozo·chro·tia
ozo·ker·ite
   pu·ri·fied o.
ozon·a·tor
ozone
ozo·nide
ozon·ol·y·sis
ozon·om·e·ter
ozo·no·scope
ozo·sto·mia

P
 an·ti·gens
 cell
 en·zyme
 fac·tor
 wave
P-A
 in·ter·val
Paas'
 dis·ease
pab·lum
pab·u·lar
pab·u·lum
pac·chi·o·ni·an
 bod·ies
 cor·pus·cles
 de·pres·sions
 glands
 gran·u·la·tions
pace·fol·low·er
pace·mak·er
 ar·ti·fi·cial p.
 de·mand p.
 ec·top·ic p.
 elec·tric car·di·ac p.
 ex·ter·nal p.
 fixed-rate p.
 nu·cle·ar p.
 per·ve·nous p.
 shift·ing p.
 sub·sid·i·ary atri·al p.
 wan·der·ing p.
pace·mak·er
 fail·ure
 out·put
 sen·si·tiv·i·ty
Pacheco's par·rot dis·ease
 vi·rus
pa·chom·e·ter
Pachon's
 meth·od
 test
pach·y·bleph·a·ron
pach·y·ce·pha·lia
pach·y·ce·phal·ic
pach·y·ceph·a·lous
pach·y·ceph·a·ly
pach·y·chei·lia
pach·y·chi·lia

pach·y·cho·lia
pach·y·chro·mat·ic
pach·y·chy·mia
pach·y·dac·tyl·ia
pach·y·dac·ty·lous
pach·y·dac·ty·ly
pach·y·der·ma
 p. la·ryn·gis
 p. lym·phan·gi·ec·ta·ti·ca
 p. ver·ru·co·sa
 p. ve·si·cae
pach·y·der·mat·o·cele
pach·y·der·ma·to·sis
pach·y·der·ma·tous
pach·y·der·mia
pach·y·der·mic
pach·y·der·mo·per·i·os·to·sis
 syn·drome
pach·y·glos·sia
pa·chyg·na·thous
pach·y·gy·ria
pach·y·hy·me·nia
pach·y·hy·men·ic
pach·y·lep·to·men·in·gi·tis
pach·y·lo·sis
pach·y·me·nia
pach·y·men·ic
pach·y·men·in·gi·tis
 p. ex·ter·na
 hem·or·rhag·ic p.
 hy·per·tro·phic cer·vi·cal p.
 p. in·ter·na
 py·o·gen·ic p.
pach·y·me·nin·gop·a·thy
pach·y·me·ninx
pa·chym·e·ter
 op·ti·cal p.
pach·y·ne·ma
pa·chyn·sis
pa·chyn·tic
pach·y·o·nych·ia
 p. con·gen·i·ta
pach·y·o·tia
pach·y·per·i·os·ti·tis
pach·y·per·i·to·ni·tis
pach·y·pleu·ri·tis
pa·chyp·o·dous
pach·y·sal·pin·gi·tis
pach·y·sal·pin·go-o·va·ri·tis

pach·y·so·mia
pach·y·tene
pach·y·vag·i·nal·i·tis
pach·y·vag·i·ni·tis
   p. cys·ti·ca
pac·ing
   cath·e·ter
pa·ci·ni·an
   cor·pus·cles
pa·cin·i·tis
pack
   cold p.
   dry p.
   hot p.
   wet p.
packed cell
   vol·ume
packed hu·man blood
   cells
pack·er
pack·ing
   den·ture p.
pack·ing
   pro·cess
P-A con·duc·tion
   time
pad
   ab·dom·i·nal p.
   din·ner p.
   fat p.
   knuck·le p.'s
   lap·a·rot·o·my p.
   Passavant's p.
   per·i·ar·te·ri·al p.
   pha·ryn·go·e·soph·a·ge·al
     p.'s
   ret·ro·mo·lar p.
   suck·ing p.
   suc·to·ri·al p.
Padykula-Herman
   stain for my·o·sin ATPase
Pae·ci·lo·my·ces
Pagenstecher's
   cir·cle
Paget-Eccleston
   stain
pa·get·ic
pag·et·oid
   cells
   re·tic·u·lo·sis
Paget's
   cells
   dis·ease
Paget-von Schrötter
   syn·drome
pa·go·pha·gia

Pah·vant Val·ley
   fe·ver
   plague
pai·dol·o·gy
pain
   af·ter-p.'s
   bear·ing-down p.
   dream p.
   ex·pul·sive p.'s
   false p.'s
   gir·dle p.
   grow·ing p.'s
   het·er·o·top·ic p.
   ho·mo·top·ic p.
   hun·ger p.
   in·ter·men·stru·al p.
   in·trac·ta·ble p.
   la·bor p.'s
   mid·dle p.
   mind p.
   nerve p.
   night p.
   or·gan·ic p.
   phan·tom limb p.
   psy·cho·gen·ic p.
   re·ferred p.
   rest p.
   soul p.
   tra·che·al p.
pain
   prin·ci·ple
   re·ac·tion
   thresh·old
   tol·er·ance
pain·ful
   an·es·the·sia
   heel
   he·ma·tu·ria
   par·a·ple·gia
   point
   toe
pain·ful-bruis·ing
   syn·drome
pain·less
   he·ma·tu·ria
   jaun·dice
pain-plea·sure
   prin·ci·ple
paint
   car·bol-fuch·sin p.
   Castellani's p.
paint·er's
   col·ic
pair
   base p.
   buff·er p.
   chro·mo·some p.
   con·ju·gate ac·id-base p.

nu·cle·o·side p.
nu·cle·o·tide p.
paired
al·lo·some
as·so·ci·ates
beats
or·gan·elles
pa·ja·roe·llo
Pajot's
ma·neu·ver
Palade
gran·ule
pal·a·tal
ab·scess
bar
in·dex
my·oc·lo·nus
nys·tag·mus
pap·il·lo·ma·to·sis
plate
pro·cess·es
re·flex
seal
shelf
tri·an·gle
pal·ate
hook
my·o·graph
pal·ate
bony p.
By·zan·tine arch p.
cleft p.
fall·ing p.
Goth·ic p.
hard p.
pen·du·lous p.
pri·mary p.
prim·i·tive p.
sec·on·dary p.
soft p.
pa·la·ti
pa·lat·i·form
pa·lat·i·nase
pal·a·tine
ap·o·neu·ro·sis
bone
crest
glands
groove
in·dex
pa·pil·la
pro·cess
ra·phe
re·flex
ridge
spines
sur·face
ton·sil

to·rus
vein
pa·lat·i·nose
pal·a·ti·tis
pal·a·to·eth·moi·dal
su·ture
pal·a·to·glos·sal
arch
pal·a·to·glos·sus
mus·cle
pal·a·tog·na·thous
pal·a·to·gram
pal·a·to·graph
pal·a·to·max·il·lary
in·dex
su·ture
pal·a·to·my·o·graph
pal·a·to·na·sal
pal·a·to·pha·ryn·ge·al
arch
mus·cle
pal·a·to·pha·ryn·ge·us
pal·a·to·pha·ryn·go·plas·ty
pal·a·to·pha·ryn·gor·rha·phy
pal·a·to·plas·ty
pal·a·to·ple·gia
pal·a·tor·rha·phy
pa·la·to·sal·pin·ge·us
pal·a·tos·chi·sis
pa·la·to·u·vu·la·ris
mus·cle
pal·a·to·vag·i·nal
ca·nal
groove
pa·la·tum
p. fis·sum
pale
globe
hy·per·ten·sion
in·farct
throm·bus
pa·le·en·ceph·a·lon
pa·le·o·cer·e·bel·lum
pa·le·o·cor·tex
pa·le·o·ki·net·ic
pa·le·o·pa·thol·o·gy
pa·le·o·stri·a·tal
syn·drome
pa·le·o·stri·a·tum
pa·le·o·thal·a·mus
Palfyn's
si·nus
pal·i·ci·ne·sia
pal·i·ki·ne·sia
pal·i·la·lia
pal·i·nal
pal·in·drome
pal·in·dro·mia

pal·in·drom·ic
  DNA
  en·ceph·a·lop·a·thy
  se·quence
pal·in·gen·e·sis
pal·i·nop·sia
pal·i·phra·sia
pal·i·sade
  lay·er
pal·la·di·um
pall·an·es·the·sia
pal·les·cense
pall·es·the·sia
pall·es·thet·ic
  sen·si·bil·i·ty
pal·li·al
pal·li·ate
pal·li·a·tive
  treat·ment
pal·li·dal
  syn·drome
pal·li·dec·to·my
pal·li·do·a·myg·da·lot·o·my
pal·li·do·an·sot·o·my
pal·li·dot·o·my
pal·li·dum
pal·li·um
pal·lor
  ca·chec·tic p.
palm
  liv·er p.
palm
  grasp
  wax
pal·ma
pal·mae
pal·mar
  ap·o·neu·ro·sis
  crease
  fas·cia
  fi·bro·ma·to·sis
  flex·ion
  lig·a·ments
  re·flex
  space
  syph·i·lid
pal·mar car·po·met·a·car·pal
  lig·a·ments
pal·mar dig·i·tal
  veins
pal·mar in·ter·os·se·ous
  ar·tery
  mus·cle
pal·mar·is
pal·mar met·a·car·pal
  ar·tery
  lig·a·ments
  veins

pal·mar ra·di·o·car·pal
  lig·a·ment
pal·mar ul·no·car·pal
  lig·a·ment
pal·mate
  folds
palm-chin
  re·flex
pal·mel·lin
Palmer ac·id
  test for pep·tic ul·cer
pal·mi
palm·ic
pal·min
  test
pal·mi·tal·de·hyde
pal·mi·tate
pal·mit·ic ac·id
pal·mi·tin
  test
pal·mit·o·le·ic ac·id
pal·mi·tyl al·co·hol
pal·mod·ic
pal·mo·men·tal
  re·flex
pal·mo·plan·tar
  ker·a·to·der·ma
pal·mos·co·py
pal·mus
pal·pa·ble
  rale
pal·pate
pal·pa·tion
  light-touch p.
pal·pa·to·per·cus·sion
pal·pa·to·ry
  per·cus·sion
pal·pe·bra
  p. III
  p. ter·tia
pal·pe·brae
pal·pe·bral
  ar·ter·ies
  con·junc·ti·va
  fis·sure
  glands
  part
  ra·phe
pal·pe·bra·lis
pal·pe·brate
pal·pe·bra·tion
pal·pe·bro·na·sal
  fold
pal·pi·ta·tio cor·dis
pal·pi·ta·tion
pal·sy
  Bell's p.
  birth p.

brach·i·al birth p.
bul·bar p.
ce·re·bral p.
craft p.
creep·ing p.
crutch p.
Erb's p.
fa·cial p.
Féréol-Graux p.
lead p.
night p.
pos·ti·cus p.
pres·sure p.
pro·gress·ive su·pra·nu·cle·
ar p.
scriv·en·er's p.
shak·ing p.
trem·bling p.
wast·ing p.
pal·u·dal
fe·ver
pam·a·brom
pam·a·quine
pam·o·ate
pam·pin·i·form
body
plex·us
pam·pin·o·cele
pan·a·cea
pan·ac·i·nar
em·phy·se·ma
pan·ag·glu·ti·na·ble
pan·ag·glu·ti·nins
pan·an·gi·i·tis
pan·ar·ter·i·tis
pan·ar·thri·tis
pan·at·ro·phy
pan·blas·tic
pan·cake
kid·ney
pan·car·di·tis
pan·cer·vi·cal
smear
Pancoast
syn·drome
tu·mor
Pancoast's
su·ture
pan·co·lec·to·my
pan·cre·as
an·nu·lar p.
Aselli's p.
p. di·vi·sum
dor·sal p.
less·er p.
p. mi·nus
small p.
un·ci·form p.

un·ci·nate p.
ven·tral p.
Willis' p.
Winslow's p.
pan·cre·a·ta
pan·cre·a·tal·gia
pan·cre·a·tec·to·my
pan·cre·at·em·phrax·is
pan·cre·at·ic
cal·cu·lus
chol·era
col·ic
de·ox·y·ri·bo·nu·cle·ase
di·a·be·tes
di·ges·tion
di·ver·tic·u·la
dor·nase
duct
en·ceph·a·lop·a·thy
in·fan·ti·lism
is·lands
is·lets
juice
li·thi·a·sis
notch
plex·us
RNase
sphinc·ter
ste·a·tor·rhea
veins
pan·cre·at·ic hy·per·gly·ce·mic
hor·mone
pan·cre·at·ic lymph
nodes
pan·cre·at·i·co·du·o·de·nal
trans·plan·ta·tion
veins
pan·cre·at·i·co·du·o·de·nal
lymph
nodes
pan·cre·at·i·co·en·ter·ic
re·cess
pan·cre·at·i·co·splen·ic lymph
nodes
pan·cre·a·tin
pan·cre·a·ti·tis
acute hem·or·rhag·ic p.
pan·cre·at·o·cho·le·cys·tos·to·
my
pan·cre·at·o·du·o·de·nec·to·my
pan·cre·at·o·du·o·de·nos·to·my
pan·cre·at·o·gas·tros·to·my
pan·cre·a·to·gen·ic
pan·cre·a·tog·en·ous
di·ar·rhea
pan·cre·a·tog·ra·phy
pan·cre·a·to·je·ju·nos·to·my
pan·cre·at·o·lith

pan·cre·at·o·li·thec·to·my
pan·cre·at·o·li·thi·a·sis
pan·cre·at·o·li·thot·o·my
pan·cre·a·tol·y·sis
pan·cre·a·to·lyt·ic
pan·cre·a·to·meg·a·ly
pan·cre·at·o·my
pan·cre·a·top·a·thy
pan·cre·a·to·pep·ti·dase E
pan·cre·a·tot·o·my
pan·cre·a·tro·pic
pan·cre·ec·to·my
pan·cre·li·pase
pan·cre·o·lith
pan·cre·op·a·thy
pan·cre·o·priv·ic
pan·cre·o·zy·min
pan·cre·o·zy·min-se·cre·tin
   test
pan·cu·ro·ni·um bro·mide
pan·cy·to·pe·nia
   con·gen·i·tal p.
   Fanconi's p.
   trop·i·cal ca·nine p.
pan·dem·ic
pan·de·mic·i·ty
pan·dic·u·la·tion
Pan·dy's
   re·ac·tion
   test
pan·en·ceph·a·li·tis
   nod·u·lar p.
   sub·a·cute scle·ros·ing p.
pan·en·do·scope
pan·es·the·sia
Paneth's gran·u·lar
   cells
pang
   breast p.
pan·glos·sia
pan·hi·dro·sis
pan·hy·drom·e·ter
pan·hy·per·e·mia
pan·hy·po·pi·tu·i·tar·ism
pan·ic
   ho·mo·sex·u·al p.
pan·ic
   at·tack
   dis·or·der
pan·i·dro·sis
pan·im·mu·ni·ty
pan·leu·ko·pe·nia
   vi·rus of cats
pan·lob·u·lar
   em·phy·se·ma
pan·mix·is
pan·my·e·loph·thi·sis
pan·my·e·lo·sis

Panner's
   dis·ease
pan·neu·ri·tis
   p. en·de·mi·ca
pan·ni
pan·nic·u·lar
   her·nia
pan·nic·u·lec·to·my
pan·nic·u·li
pan·nic·u·li·tis
   cy·to·phag·ic p.
   nod·u·lar non·sup·pur·a·tive
   p.
   sub·a·cute mi·gra·to·ry p.
pan·nic·u·lus
   p. car·no·sus
pan·nic·u·lus car·no·sus
   mus·cle
pan·nus
   cor·ne·al p.
   p. cras·sus
   phlyc·ten·u·lar p.
   p. sic·cus
   p. ten·u·is
   tra·chom·a·tous p.
pan·od·ic
pan·oph·thal·mia
pan·oph·thal·mi·tis
pan·op·tic
   stain
pan·o·ram·ic
   roent·gen·o·gram
pan·o·ram·ic ro·tat·ing
   ma·chine
pan·o·ram·ic x-ray
   film
pan·o·the·nate
   p. syn·the·tase
pan·o·ti·tis
pan·pho·bia
pan·ple·gia
Pansch's
   fis·sure
pan·scle·ro·sis
pan·sin·u·i·tis
pan·si·nu·si·tis
pan·sper·ma·tism
pan·sper·mia
pan·spor·o·blast
pan·spo·ro·blas·tic
pan·sys·tol·ic
   mur·mur
pant
pan·ta·chro·mat·ic
pan·tal·gia
pan·ta·loon
   em·bo·lism
pan·ta·mor·phia

pan·ta·mor·phic
pan·tan·en·ce·pha·lia
pan·tan·en·ceph·a·ly
pan·tan·ky·lo·bleph·a·ron
pan·ta·pho·bia
pan·ta·tro·phia
pan·tat·ro·phy
pan·te·the·ine
  p. ki·nase
pan·te·thine
pan·the·nol
pan·thod·ic
pan·to·ate
pan·to·ate-ac·ti·vat·ing
  en·zyme
pan·to·graph
pan·to·ic ac·id
pan·to·mo·gram
pan·to·mo·graph
pan·to·mog·ra·phy
pan·to·mor·phia
pan·to·mor·phic
pan·to·nine
pan·to·scop·ic
  spec·ta·cles
pan·to·then·ic ac·id
  unit
pan·to·then·yl
  p. al·co·hol
pan·to·yl
pan·to·yl·tau·rine
pan·tro·pic
  vi·rus
Panum's
  ar·ea
pan·zer·herz
PAP
  tech·nique
Pap
  test
pa·pa·in
pa·pa·in·ase
Papanicolaou
  ex·am·i·na·tion
  smear
  stain
Papanicolaou smear
  test
Pa·pav·er
pa·pav·er·e·tum
pa·pav·er·ine
pa·paw
pa·pa·ya
pap·a·yo·tin
pa·per
  ar·tic·u·lat·ing p.
  Con·go red p.

fil·ter p.
oc·clud·ing p.
pa·per
  chro·ma·tog·ra·phy
  plate
pa·per mill work·er's
  dis·ease
Papez
  cir·cuit
pa·pil·la
  acous·tic p.
  Bergmeister's p.
  bile p.
  p. of breast
  cir·cum·val·late p.
  cla·vate pa·pil·lae
  con·ic pa·pil·lae
  pa·pil·lae of co·ri·um
  den·ti·nal p.
  der·mal pa·pil·lae
  fi·li·form pa·pil·lae
  fo·li·ate pa·pil·lae
  fun·gi·form pa·pil·lae
  hair p.
  in·ci·sive p.
  in·ter·den·tal p.
  in·ter·prox·i·mal p.
  lac·ri·mal p.
  len·tic·u·lar pa·pil·lae
  lin·gual p.
  ma·jor du·o·de·nal p.
  mi·nor du·o·de·nal p.
  nerve p.
  p. ner·vi op·ti·ci
  op·tic p.
  pal·a·tine p.
  pa·rot·id p.
  p. pi·li
  re·nal p.
  ret·ro·cus·pid p.
  tac·tile p.
  ure·thral p.
  p. ure·thra·lis
  val·late p.
  vas·cu·lar pa·pil·lae
pa·pil·lae
pap·il·lary
  ad·e·no·car·ci·no·ma
  ad·e·no·ma of large in·tes·
    tine
  car·ci·no·ma
  cyst·ad·e·no·ma lym·pho·
    ma·to·sum
  ducts
  ec·ta·sia
  fo·ram·i·na of kid·ney
  hi·drad·e·no·ma
  lay·er

pap·il·lary *(continued)*
  mus·cle
  pro·cess
  sta·sis
  tu·mor
pap·il·lary cys·tic
  ad·e·no·ma
pap·il·lary mus·cle
  dys·func·tion
  syn·drome
pap·il·late
pap·il·lec·to·my
pa·pil·le·de·ma
pap·il·lif·er·ous
pa·pil·li·form
pap·il·li·tis
  nec·ro·tiz·ing p.
pap·il·lo·ad·e·no·cys·to·ma
pap·il·lo·car·ci·no·ma
pap·il·lo·ma
  p. acu·mi·na·tum
  ba·sal cell p.
  p. ca·na·li·cu·lum
  ca·nine oral p.
  p. dif·fu·sum
  duct p.
  p. du·rum
  fi·bro·ep·i·the·li·al p.
  hard p.
  Hopmann's p.
  in·fec·tious p. of cat·tle
  p. in·gui·na·le tro·pi·cum
  in·tra·cys·tic p.
  in·tra·duc·tal p.
  in·vert·ed p.
  p. mol·le
  p. neu·ro·pa·thi·cum
  p. neu·ro·ti·cum
  soft p.
  tran·si·tion·al cell p.
  p. ve·ne·re·um
  vil·lous p.
  zy·mot·ic p.
pap·il·lo·ma·to·sis
  con·flu·ent and re·tic·u·late p.
  flor·id oral p.
  ju·ve·nile p.
  la·ryn·ge·al p.
  pal·a·tal p.
  sub·a·re·o·lar duct p.
pap·il·lo·ma·tous
Pa·pil·lo·ma·vi·rus
Papillon-Léage and Psaume
  syn·drome
Papillon-Lefèvre
  syn·drome
pap·il·lo·ret·i·ni·tis

pap·il·lot·o·my
pa·pil·lu·la
pa·pil·lu·lae
Pa·po·va·vir·i·dae
pa·po·va·vi·rus
pap·pa·ta·ci
  fe·ver
pap·pa·ta·ci fe·ver
  vi·rus·es
Pappenheimer
  bod·ies
Pappenheim's
  stain
pap·pose
pap·pous
pap·pus
pap·u·la
pap·u·lae
pap·u·lar
  ac·ro·der·ma·ti·tis of child·hood
  der·ma·ti·tis of preg·nan·cy
  fe·ver
  mu·ci·no·sis
  scrof·u·lo·der·ma
  syph·i·lid
  tu·ber·cu·lid
  ur·ti·car·ia
pap·u·lar sto·ma·ti·tis
  vi·rus of cat·tle
pap·u·la·tion
pap·ule
  Cel·sus' p.'s
  fol·lic·u·lar p.
  moist p.
  mu·cous p.
  pi·e·zo·gen·ic ped·al p.
  split p.'s
pap·u·lif·er·ous
pap·u·lo·er·y·them·a·tous
pap·u·lo·ne·crot·ic
  tu·ber·cu·lid
pap·u·lo·pus·tu·lar
pap·u·lo·pus·tule
pa·pu·lo·sis
  bow·en·oid p.
  lym·pho·ma·toid p.
  ma·lig·nant atroph·ic p.
pap·u·lo·squa·mous
  syph·i·lid
pap·u·lo·ves·i·cle
pap·u·lo·ve·sic·u·lar
pap·y·ra·ceous
  plate
  scars
para
para-aor·tic
  bod·ies

par·a-ap·pen·di·ci·tis
par·a·bal·lism
par·a·ban·ic ac·id
par·a·ba·sal
    body
    fil·a·ment
par·a·bi·o·sis
par·a·bi·ot·ic
    flap
par·a·blep·sia
pa·rab·o·loid
    con·dens·er
par·a·bra·chi·al
    nu·clei
par·a·bu·lia
par·ac·an·tho·ma
par·ac·an·tho·sis
par·a·car·ci·nom·a·tous
    en·ceph·a·lo·my·e·lop·a·thy
    my·e·lop·a·thy
par·a·car·mine
    stain
par·a·ca·se·in
par·a·cel·si·an
    meth·od
par·a·ce·nes·the·sia
par·a·cen·te·sis
par·a·cen·tet·ic
par·a·cen·tral
    ar·tery
    fis·sure
    lob·ule
    nu·cle·us of thal·a·mus
    sco·to·ma
par·a·cen·tric
    in·ver·sion
par·a·cer·vi·cal
par·a·cer·vi·cal block
    an·es·the·sia
par·a·cer·vix
par·ac·e·tal·de·hyde
par·a·cet·a·mol
par·a·chlo·ro·phe·nol
par·a·chol·er·a
par·a·chor·dal
    car·ti·lage
    plate
par·a·chroia
par·a·chro·ma
par·a·chro·ma·to·sis
par·a·chute
    de·for·mi·ty
    re·flex
par·a·chute mi·tral
    valve
par·a·chy·mo·sin
par·a·ci·ne·sia
par·a·ci·ne·sis

par·ac·ma·sis
par·ac·mas·tic
par·ac·me
par·a·coc·cid·i·o·i·dal
    gran·u·lo·ma
Par·a·coc·cid·i·oi·des bra·sil·i·
    en·sis
par·a·coc·cid·i·oi·din
par·a·coc·cid·i·oi·do·my·co·sis
par·a·col·ic
    re·cess·es
par·a·co·li·tis
par·a·co·lon
    ba·cil·lus
par·a·col·pi·tis
par·a·col·pi·um
par·a·cone
par·a·co·nid
par·a·cor·tex
par·a·cou·sis
par·a·crine
par·a·cu·sia
par·a·cu·sis
    false p.
    p. lo·ci
    Willis' p.
par·a·cy·clic
    o·vu·la·tion
par·a·cy·e·sis
par·a·cys·tic
    pouch
par·a·cys·ti·tis
par·a·cys·ti·um
par·a·cy·tic
par·ad·e·ni·tis
par·a·den·tal
par·a·den·ti·um
par·a·did·y·mal
par·a·did·y·mi·des
par·a·did·y·mis
par·a·dip·sia
par·a·dox
    Weber's p.
par·a·dox·i·cal
    con·trac·tion
    em·bo·lism
    in·con·ti·nence
    move·ment of eye·lids
    pulse
    pu·pil
    re·flex
    res·pi·ra·tion
    sleep
par·a·dox·i·cal di·a·phragm
    phe·nom·e·non
par·a·dox·i·cal ex·ten·sor
    re·flex

par·a·dox·i·cal flex·or
　re·flex
par·a·dox·i·cal pa·tel·lar
　re·flex
par·a·dox·i·cal pu·pil·lary
　phe·nom·e·non
　re·flex
par·a·dox·i·cal tri·ceps
　re·flex
par·a·du·o·de·nal
　fold
　fos·sa
　re·cess
par·a·dys·en·tery
　ba·cil·lus
par·a-e·qui·lib·ri·um
par·a·e·soph·a·ge·al
　her·nia
par·a·es·the·sia
par·af·fin
　chlo·ri·nat·ed p.
　hard p.
　liq·uid p.
　white soft p.
　yel·low soft p.
par·af·fin
　can·cer
　tu·mor
　wax
par·af·fi·no·ma
Par·a·fi·lar·ia mul·ti·pa·pil·lo·
　sa
par·a·fla·gel·la
par·a·flag·el·late
par·a·fla·gel·lum
par·a·fol·lic·u·lar
　cells
par·a·for·mal·de·hyde
par·a·fre·nal
　ab·scess
par·a·fuch·sin
par·a·gam·ma·cism
par·a·gan·glia
par·a·gan·gli·o·ma
　non·chro·maf·fin p.
par·a·gan·gli·on
par·a·gan·gli·on·ic
　cells
par·a·gene
par·a·gen·i·tal
　tu·bules
par·a·geu·sia
par·a·geu·sic
par·a·glen·oid
　groove
　sul·cus
pa·rag·na·thus
par·ag·no·men

par·a·gon·i·mi·a·sis
Par·a·gon·i·mus
　P. kel·li·cot·ti
　P. ring·eri
　P. wes·ter·mani
par·a·gon·or·rhe·al
par·a·gram·ma·tism
par·a·graph·ia
Par·a·guay
　tea
par·a·he·mo·phil·ia
par·a·he·pat·ic
par·a·hi·dro·sis
par·a·hip·po·cam·pal
　gy·rus
par·a·hor·mone
par·a·hyp·no·sis
par·a·hy·poph·y·sis
para I
para II
par·a·in·flu·en·za
　vi·rus·es
par·a·je·ju·nal
　fos·sa
par·a·kap·pa·cism
par·a·ker·a·to·sis
　p. os·tra·cea
　por·cine p.
　p. pso·ri·a·si·for·mis
　p. pus·tu·lo·sa
　p. scu·tu·la·ris
　p. va·ri·e·ga·ta
par·a·ki·ne·sia
par·a·ki·ne·sis
par·a·la·lia
　p. li·te·ra·lis
par·a·lamb·da·cism
par·al·de·hyde
par·a·lep·ro·sis
par·a·lep·sy
par·a·lex·ia
par·al·ge·sia
par·al·gia
par·a·lip·o·pho·bia
par·al·lac·tic
par·al·lax
　bin·oc·u·lar p.
　het·er·on·y·mous p.
　ho·mon·y·mous p.
　ster·e·o·scop·ic p.
　ver·ti·cal p.
par·al·lax
　meth·od
　test
par·al·lel
　at·tach·ment
　rays
par·al·lel·ism

par·al·lel·om·e·ter
par·al·ler·gic
par·a·lo·gia
 the·mat·ic p.
pa·ral·o·gism
pa·ral·o·gy
par·a·lu·te·al
 cell
pa·ral·y·ses
pa·ral·y·sis
 acute as·cend·ing p.
 acute atroph·ic p.
 p. ag·i·tans
 as·cend·ing p.
 Brown-Séquard's p.
 bul·bar p.
 cen·tral p.
 Chastek p.
 com·pres·sion p.
 con·ju·gate p.
 crossed p.
 crutch p.
 de·cu·bi·tus p.
 diph·the·rit·ic p.
 div·er's p.
 Duchenne-Erb p.
 Duchenne's p.
 Erb's p.
 Erb's spi·nal p.
 fa·cial p.
 fa·mil·i·al pe·ri·od·ic p.
 fau·cial p.
 fowl p.
 gin·ger p.
 glob·al p.
 glos·so·la·bi·o·la·ryn·ge·al
  p.
 glos·so·la·bi·o·pha·ryn·ge·al
  p.
 Gubler's p.
 hy·per·ka·le·mic pe·ri·od·ic
  p.
 hy·po·ka·le·mic pe·ri·od·ic
  p.
 im·mu·no·log·i·cal p.
 in·fec·tious bul·bar p.
 jake p.
 Klumpke's p.
 Kussmaul-Lan·dry p.
 la·bi·al p.
 lamb·ing p.
 Landry's p.
 lead p.
 mi·met·ic p.
 mixed p.
 mo·tor p.
 mus·cu·lo·spi·ral p.
 my·o·gen·ic p.

 nor·mo·ka·le·mic pe·ri·od·
  ic p.
 ob·stet·ri·cal p.
 oc·u·lar p.
 par·tu·ri·ent p.
 pe·ri·od·ic p.
 post·diph·the·rit·ic p.
 pos·ti·cus p.
 Pott's p.
 pres·sure p.
 pro·gress·ive bul·bar p.
 pseu·do·bul·bar p.
 pseu·do·hy·per·tro·phic
  mus·cu·lar p.
 sen·so·ry p.
 sleep p.
 so·di·um-re·spon·sive pe·ri·
  od·ic p.
 spas·tic spi·nal p.
 spi·nal p.
 su·pra·nu·cle·ar p.
 tick p.
 Todd's p.
 Todd's post·ep·i·lep·tic p.
 va·so·mo·tor p.
 wast·ing p.
 Zenker's p.
pa·ra·lys·sa
par·a·lyt·ic
 cho·rea
 de·men·tia
 ec·tro·pi·on
 il·e·us
 mi·o·sis
 my·dri·a·sis
 my·o·glo·bi·nu·ria
 ra·bies
 sco·li·o·sis
 stra·bis·mus
par·a·ly·zant
par·a·lyze
par·a·lyz·ing
 ver·ti·go
par·a·mag·net·ic
par·a·mag·ne·tism
par·a·mam·ma·ry lymph
 nodes
par·a·mas·ti·gote
par·a·mas·toid
 pro·cess
Par·a·me·ci·um
par·a·me·di·an
 in·ci·sion
par·a·med·ic
par·a·med·i·cal
par·a·me·nia
par·a·me·si·al

par·a·mes·o·neph·ric
  duct
pa·ram·e·ter
par·a·meth·a·di·one
par·a·meth·a·sone
  p. ac·e·tate
par·a·me·tria
par·a·me·tri·al
par·a·met·ric
  ab·scess
par·a·me·tris·mus
par·a·me·trit·ic
  ab·scess
par·a·me·tri·tis
par·a·me·tri·um
par·a·mim·ia
par·am·ne·sia
Par·a·moe·ba
par·a·mo·lar
par·a·mor·phia
par·a·mor·phic
par·a·mor·phine
Par·am·phis·to·mat·i·dae
par·am·phis·to·mi·a·sis
Par·am·phis·to·mum
par·a·mu·sia
par·am·y·loi·do·sis
par·a·my·oc·lo·nus
par·a·my·o·to·nia
  atax·ic p.
  p. con·gen·i·ta
  con·gen·i·tal p.
  symp·to·mat·ic p.
par·a·my·ot·o·nus
Par·a·myx·o·vir·i·dae
Par·a·myx·o·vi·rus
par·an·al·ge·sia
par·a·na·sal
  si·nus·es
par·a·ne·o·pla·sia
par·a·ne·o·plas·tic
  ac·ro·ker·a·to·sis
  syn·drome
par·a·neph·ric
  ab·scess
  body
par·a·neph·roi
par·a·neph·ros
par·an·es·the·sia
par·a·neu·ral
  in·fil·tra·tion
par·a·neu·rone
pa·ran·gi
par·a·noia
  acute hal·lu·ci·na·to·ry p.
  li·ti·gious p.
  p. ori·gi·na·ria
  p. que·ru·lans

par·a·noi·ac
par·a·noid
  per·son·al·i·ty
  schiz·o·phre·nia
par·a·no·mia
par·a·nu·cle·ar
  body
par·a·nu·cle·ate
par·a·nu·cle·o·lus
par·a·nu·cle·us
par·a·om·phal·ic
par·a·op·er·a·tive
par·a·o·ral
par·a·o·var·i·an
par·a·ox·on
par·a·pan·cre·at·ic
par·a·pa·re·sis
par·a·pa·ret·ic
par·a·pe·de·sis
par·a·per·i·to·ne·al
  her·nia
  ne·phrec·to·my
par·a·pes·tis
par·a·pha·ryn·ge·al
  space
par·a·pha·sia
  the·mat·ic p.
par·a·pha·sic
pa·ra·phia
par·a·phil·ia
par·a·phi·mo·sis
  p. pal·pe·brae
par·a·pho·nia
pa·raph·o·ra
par·a·phra·sia
par·a·phys·e·al
pa·raph·y·ses
par·a·phys·i·al
  cysts
pa·raph·y·sis
par·a·pin·e·al
par·a·plasm
par·a·plas·tic
par·a·plec·tic
par·a·ple·gia
  atax·ic p.
  con·gen·i·tal spas·tic p.
  p. do·lo·ro·sa
  p. in ex·ten·sion
  p. in flex·ion
  in·fan·tile spas·tic p.
  pain·ful p.
  Pott's p.
  se·nile p.
  spas·tic p.
  su·pe·ri·or p.
  tet·a·noid p.
par·a·ple·gic

par·ap·o·plexy
Par·a·pox·vi·rus
par·a·prax·ia
par·a·proc·tia
par·a·proc·ti·tis
par·a·proc·ti·um
par·a·pros·ta·ti·tis
par·a·pro·tein
par·a·pro·tein·e·mia
pa·rap·sia
par·a·pso·ri·a·sis
   p. en plaque
   p. gut·ta·ta
   p. li·che·noi·des
   p. li·che·noi·des et va·ri·o·
   li·for·mis acu·ta
   p. va·ri·o·li·for·mis
par·a·psy·chol·o·gy
par·a·quat
par·a·ra·ma
par·a·rec·tal
   fos·sa
   pouch
par·a·rec·tal lymph
   nodes
par·a·re·flex·ia
par·a·re·nal
par·a·rho·ta·cism
par·a·ro·san·i·lin
par·ar·rhyth·mia
par·a·sac·cu·lar
   her·nia
par·a·sac·ral
par·a·sag·it·tal
   plane
par·a·sal·pin·gi·tis
Par·as·ca·ris equo·rum
par·a·scar·la·ti·na
par·a·se·cre·tion
par·a·sep·tal
   car·ti·lage
   em·phy·se·ma
par·a·sex·u·al·i·ty
par·a·sig·ma·tism
par·a·si·noi·dal
   si·nus·es
par·a·site
   au·tis·tic p.
   au·toch·thon·ous p.
   com·men·sal p.
   eu·rox·e·nous p.
   fac·ul·ta·tive p.
   het·er·o·ge·net·ic p.
   het·er·ox·e·nous p.
   in·ci·den·tal p.
   in·qui·line p.
   ma·lig·nant ter·tian ma·lar·
   i·al p.

ob·li·gate p.
quar·tan p.
spe·cif·ic p.
sten·ox·ous p.
tem·po·rary p.
ter·tian p.
par·a·site-host
   ec·o·sys·tem
par·a·si·te·mia
par·a·sit·ic
   chy·lo·cele
   cyst
   dis·ease
   gran·u·lo·ma
   he·mop·ty·sis
   lei·o·my·o·ma
   mel·a·no·der·ma
   oti·tis
   thy·roid·i·tis
   twin
par·a·sit·i·ci·dal
par·a·sit·i·cide
par·a·sit·ism
   mul·ti·ple p.
par·a·si·tize
par·a·si·to·ce·nose
par·a·si·to·gen·e·sis
par·a·si·to·gen·ic
par·a·si·toid
par·a·si·tol·o·gist
par·a·si·tol·o·gy
par·a·si·tome
par·a·si·to·pho·bia
par·a·si·toph·or·ous
   vac·u·ole
par·a·sit·o·sis
par·a·si·to·tro·pic
par·a·si·tot·ro·pism
par·a·si·tot·ro·py
par·a·sol
   in·ser·tion
par·a·som·nia
par·a·spa·dia
par·a·spa·di·as
par·a·sta·sis
par·a·ster·nal
   her·nia
   line
par·a·ster·nal lymph
   nodes
par·a·stri·ate
   ar·ea
   cor·tex
par·a·stru·ma
par·a·sym·pa·thet·ic
   gan·glia
   nerve

par·a·sym·pa·thet·ic
(continued)
  part
    root of cil·i·ary gan·gli·on
par·a·sym·pa·thet·ic ner·vous
  sys·tem
par·a·sym·pa·tho·lyt·ic
par·a·sym·pa·tho·mi·met·ic
par·a·sym·pa·tho·par·a·lyt·ic
par·a·sym·pa·tho·to·nia
par·a·sy·nan·che
par·a·sy·nap·sis
par·a·sy·no·vi·tis
par·a·syph·i·lis
par·a·syph·i·lit·ic
par·a·syph·i·lo·sis
par·a·sys·to·le
par·a·sys·tol·ic
  beat
par·a·tax·ia
par·a·tax·ic
  dis·tor·tion
par·a·tax·is
par·a·te·ne·sis
par·a·ten·ic
  host
par·a·ten·on
par·a·ter·mi·nal
  body
  gy·rus
par·a·thi·on
par·a·thor·mone
par·a·thy·mia
par·a·thy·rin
par·a·thy·roid
  gland
  hor·mone
  in·suf·fi·cien·cy
  os·te·o·sis
  tet·a·ny
par·a·thy·roid·ec·to·my
par·a·thy·ro·pri·val
  tet·a·ny
par·a·thy·ro·tro·phic
par·a·thy·ro·tro·pic
par·a·tra·che·al lymph
  node
par·a·tri·cho·sis
par·a·trip·sis
par·a·trip·tic
par·a·tro·phic
par·a·tu·ber·cu·lous
  lym·phad·e·ni·tis
par·a·typh·li·tis
par·a·ty·phoid
  ba·cil·lus
  fe·ver

par·a·um·bil·i·cal
  veins
par·a·u·re·thral
  ducts
  glands
par·a·u·ter·ine lymph
  nodes
par·a·vac·cin·ia
  vi·rus
par·a·vag·i·nal
  hys·ter·ec·to·my
par·a·vag·i·nal lymph
  nodes
par·a·vag·i·ni·tis
par·a·val·vu·lar
par·a·ve·nous
par·a·ven·tric·u·lar
  nu·cle·us
par·a·ver·te·bral
  an·es·the·sia
  gan·glia
  line
  tri·an·gle
par·a·ves·i·cal
  fos·sa
  pouch
par·a·ves·i·cal lymph
  nodes
par·ax·i·al
  mes·o·derm
  rays
par·ax·on
Par·a·zoa
par·a·zo·on
parch·ment
  heart
  skin
parch·ment crack·ling
par·ec·ta·sia
par·ec·ta·sis
par·ec·tro·pia
par·e·gor·ic
pa·rei·ra
par·e·lec·tro·nom·ic
par·en·ce·pha·lia
par·en·ceph·a·li·tis
par·en·ceph·a·lo·cele
par·en·ceph·a·lous
pa·ren·chy·ma
pa·ren·chy·mal
  cell
pa·ren·chy·ma·ti·tis
par·en·chym·a·tous
  cell of cor·pus pi·ne·a·le
  de·gen·er·a·tion
  goi·ter
  hem·or·rhage
  ker·a·ti·tis

mas·ti·tis
neu·ri·tis
ton·sil·li·tis
par·ent
  cell
  cyst
pa·ren·tal
  gen·er·a·tion
  re·jec·tion
par·en·ter·al
  ab·sorp·tion
  al·i·men·ta·tion
  hy·per·al·i·men·ta·tion
  ther·a·py
par·en·ter·ic
  fe·ver
par·ep·i·cele
par·ep·i·did·y·mis
par·ep·i·thy·mia
par·e·re·thi·sis
par·er·ga·sia
Paré's
  su·ture
pa·re·sis
  par·tu·ri·ent p.
par·es·the·sia
  Berger's p.
par·es·thet·ic
pa·ret·ic
  im·po·tence
pa·reu·nia
par·gy·line hy·dro·chlo·ride
par·i·dro·sis
par·i·es
pa·ri·e·tal
  an·gle
  ar·ter·ies
  bone
  cell
  em·i·nence
  eye
  fis·tu·la
  fo·ra·men
  her·nia
  lay·er
  lobe
  mar·gin
  nodes
  notch
  plate
  pleu·ra
  re·gion
  throm·bus
  tu·ber
  veins
  wall
pa·ri·e·tal em·is·sary
  vein

pa·ri·e·tes
pa·ri·e·tis
pa·ri·e·to·fron·tal
pa·ri·e·tog·ra·phy
pa·ri·e·to·mas·toid
  su·ture
pa·ri·e·to-oc·cip·i·tal
  ar·tery
  fis·sure
  sul·cus
pa·ri·e·to·pon·tine
  tract
pa·ri·e·to·sphe·noid
pa·ri·e·to·splanch·nic
pa·ri·e·to·squa·mo·sal
pa·ri·e·to·tem·po·ral
pa·ri·e·to·vis·cer·al
Parinaud's
  con·junc·ti·vi·tis
  oph·thal·mo·ple·gia
  syn·drome
Parinaud's oc·u·lo·glan·du·lar
  syn·drome
Par·is
  line
Par·is green
Par·is yel·low
par·i·ty
Parker-Kerr
  su·ture
par·kin·so·ni·an
par·kin·son·ism
Parkinson's
  dis·ease
  fa·ci·es
Park's
  an·eu·rysm
Park-Williams
  ba·cil·lus
  fix·a·tive
par·oc·cip·i·tal
  pro·cess
par·o·don·ti·tis
pa·ro·don·ti·um
par·o·dyn·ia
pa·role
par·ol·fac·to·ry
  ar·ea
par·ol·i·vary
par·o·mo·my·cin sul·fate
par·om·pha·lo·cele
Parona's
  space
par·o·nei·ria
  p. sa·lax
par·o·ni·ria
par·o·nych·ia
par·o·nych·i·al

par·o·oph·o·rit·ic
cyst
par·o·oph·o·ri·tis
par·o·öph·o·ron
par·oph·thal·mia
par·op·sia
par·op·sis
par·or·chid·i·um
par·or·chis
par·o·rex·ia
par·os·mia
par·os·phre·sia
par·os·te·al
fas·ci·i·tis
par·os·te·i·tis
par·os·te·o·sis
par·os·ti·tis
par·os·to·sis
pa·rot·ic
pa·rot·id
ab·scess
bu·bo
duct
fas·cia
gland
notch
pa·pil·la
plex·us
re·cess
veins
pa·rot·i·dec·to·my
pa·rot·i·di·tis
ep·i·dem·ic p.
post·op·er·a·tive p.
punc·tate p.
pa·ro·ti·do·au·ri·cu·la·ris
par·o·tin
par·o·ti·tis
par·ous
par·o·var·i·an
par·o·var·i·ot·o·my
par·o·va·ri·tis
par·o·var·i·um
par·ox·y·pro·pi·one
par·ox·ysm
par·ox·ys·mal
sleep
tach·y·car·dia
par·ox·ys·mal ce·re·bral
dys·rhyth·mia
par·ox·ys·mal noc·tur·nal
dysp·nea
he·mo·glo·bi·nu·ria
par·ri·cide
par·rot
dis·ease
fe·ver
jaw

mouth
vi·rus
par·rot-beak
nail
Parrot's
dis·ease
par·ry
frac·ture
Parry's
dis·ease
pars
p. amor·pha
p. bas·i·la·ris pon·tis
p. car·ti·la·gi·nea sep·ti na·
si
p. ca·ver·no·sa
p. ce·ca ret·i·nae
p. cys·ti·ca
p. en·do·cri·na pan·cre·a·tis
p. ex·o·cri·na pan·cre·a·tis
p. fron·ta·lis cor·po·ris cal·
lo·si
par·tes gen·i·ta·les fe·mi·
ni·nae ex·ter·nae
par·tes gen·i·ta·les mas·cu·
li·nae ex·ter·nae
p. gran·u·lo·sa
p. he·pat·i·ca
p. hor·i·zon·ta·lis
p. in·fun·di·bu·la·ris
p. in·ter·me·dia com·mis·
su·ra
p. mas·toi·dea
p. ner·vo·sa hy·po·phys·e·
os
p. oc·ci·pi·ta·lis cor·po·ris
cal·lo·si
p. oper·cu·la·ris
p. or·bi·ta·lis
p. or·bi·ta·lis glan·du·lae
la·cri·ma·lis
p. or·bi·ta·lis mus·cu·li or·
bi·cu·la·ris oc·u·li
p. or·bi·ta·lis ner·vi op·ti·
ci
p. or·bi·ta·lis os·sis fron·
ta·lis
p. pel·vi·ca
p. pel·vi·ca ure·te·ris
p. per·i·phe·ri·ca
p. per·pen·di·cu·la·ris
p. phal·li·ca
p. pha·ryn·gea hy·po·phys·
e·os
p. pla·na
p. sel·la·ris
p. tec·ta
p. tec·ta du·o·de·ni

p. tec·ta pan·cre·a·tis
p. tec·ta re·na·lis
p. tec·ta ure·te·ra·lis
p. tho·ra·ci·ca
p. tho·ra·ci·ca aor·tae
p. tho·ra·ci·ca duc·tus tho·ra·ci·ci
p. tho·ra·ci·ca esoph·a·gi
p. tho·ra·ci·ca me·dul·lae spi·na·lis
p. tri·an·gu·la·ris

pars-pla·ni·tis

part

ab·dom·i·nal p.
alar p.
al·ve·o·lar p. of man·di·ble
an·te·ri·or p.
an·te·ri·or p. of pons
an·te·ri·or tib·i·o·ta·lar p.
as·cend·ing p.
as·cend·ing p. of aor·ta
au·to·nom·ic p.
ba·sal p. of oc·cip·i·tal bone
ba·sal p. of pul·mo·nary ar·tery
bas·i·lar p. of pons
bony p. of au·di·to·ry tube
bony p. of na·sal sep·tum
buc·co·pha·ryn·ge·al p.
car·di·ac p. of stom·ach
car·ti·lag·i·nous p. of au·di·to·ry tube
car·ti·lag·i·nous p. of skel·e·tal sys·tem
cav·ern·ous p. of in·ter·nal ca·rot·id ar·tery
cer·a·to·pha·ryn·ge·al p.
ce·re·bral p. of in·ter·nal ca·rot·id ar·tery
cer·vi·cal p.
cer·vi·cal p. of esoph·a·gus
cer·vi·cal p. of in·ter·nal ca·rot·id ar·tery
cer·vi·cal p. of spi·nal cord
cer·vi·cal p. of tho·rac·ic duct
chon·dro·pha·ryn·ge·al p.
cil·i·ary p. of ret·i·na
cla·vic·u·lar p.
coc·cyg·e·al p. of spi·nal cord
co·chle·ar p. of ves·tib·u·lo·co·chle·ar nerve
con·vo·lut·ed p. of kid·ney lob·ule
cor·ne·o·scler·al p.
cor·ti·cal p.

cos·tal p. of di·a·phragm
cri·co·pha·ryn·ge·al p.
cru·ci·form p. of fi·brous sheath
cu·pu·lar p.
cu·pu·late p.
deep p.
de·scend·ing p.
dis·tal p. of an·te·ri·or lobe of hy·poph·y·sis
dor·sal p. of pons
flac·cid p. of tym·pan·ic mem·brane
glos·so·pha·ryn·ge·al p.
hid·den p.
hor·i·zon·tal p.
p.'s of hu·man body
in·fe·ri·or p.
in·fe·ri·or p. of ves·tib·u·lo·co·chle·ar nerve
in·fra·cla·vic·u·lar p. of brach·i·al plex·us
in·fra·lo·bar p.
in·fra·seg·men·tal p.
in·fun·dib·u·lar p. of an·te·ri·or lobe of hy·poph·y·sis
in·su·lar p.
in·ter·car·ti·lag·i·nous p. of glot·tic open·ing
in·ter·me·di·ate p.
in·ter·mem·bra·nous p. of glot·tic open·ing
in·ter·seg·men·tal p.
in·tra·ca·nic·u·lar p. of op·tic nerve
in·tra·cra·ni·al p.
in·tra·lam·i·nar p. of op·tic nerve
in·tra·lo·bar p.
in·tra·oc·u·lar p. of op·tic nerve
in·tra·seg·men·tal p.
irid·i·al p. of ret·i·na
la·bi·al p.
la·ryn·ge·al p. of phar·ynx
lat·er·al p.
lum·bar p.
lum·bar p. of di·a·phragm
lum·bar p. of spi·nal cord
mar·gi·nal p.
mas·toid p.
me·di·al p.
me·di·as·ti·nal p.
mem·bra·nous p.
mem·bra·nous p. of male ure·thra
mem·bra·nous p. of na·sal sep·tum

part *(continued)*
my·lo·pha·ryn·ge·al p.
na·sal p.
na·sal p. of phar·ynx
ob·lique p.
op·tic p. of ret·i·na
oral p. of phar·ynx
or·bi·tal p.
or·bi·tal p. of op·tic nerve
os·se·ous p. of skel·e·tal
sys·tem
pal·pe·bral p.
par·a·sym·pa·thet·ic p.
pel·vic p.
pet·rous p.
p. pet·rous of in·ter·nal ca·
rot·id ar·tery
p. pet·rous of tem·po·ral
bone
post·com·mu·ni·cal p.
pos·te·ri·or p.
pos·te·ri·or tib·i·o·ta·lar p.
post·lam·i·nar p. of op·tic
nerve
post·sul·cal p.
pre·com·mu·ni·cal p.
pre·lam·i·nar p. of op·tic
nerve
pre·sul·cal p.
pter·y·go·pha·ryn·ge·al p.
py·lor·ic p. of stom·ach
quad·rate p.
right p.
sa·cral p. of spi·nal cord
soft p.'s
sphe·noi·dal p.
spi·nal p. of ac·ces·so·ry
nerve
spon·gi·ose p. of the male
ure·thra
ster·nal p. of di·a·phragm
ster·no·cos·tal p.
straight p.
sub·cu·ta·ne·ous p.
su·per·fi·cial p.
su·pe·ri·or p.
su·pe·ri·or p. of ves·tib·u·
lo·co·chle·ar nerve
su·pra·cla·vic·u·lar p. of
brach·i·al plex·us
sym·pa·thet·ic p.
tense p. of the tym·pan·ic
mem·brane
ter·mi·nal p.
tho·rac·ic p.
tho·rac·ic p. of aor·ta
tho·rac·ic p. of esoph·a·gus
tho·rac·ic p. of spi·nal cord

tho·rac·ic p. of tho·rac·ic
duct
thy·ro·pha·ryn·ge·al p.
tib·i·o·cal·ca·ne·al p.
tib·i·o·na·vic·u·lar p.
trans·verse p.
tym·pan·ic p. of tem·po·ral
bone
um·bil·i·cal p.
uter·ine p.
uve·al p.
va·gal p. of ac·ces·so·ry
nerve
ven·tral p. of the pons
ver·te·bral p.
ver·te·bral p. of di·a·
phragm
ves·tib·u·lar p. of ves·tib·
u·lo·co·chle·ar nerve
par·tes
par·the·no·gen·e·sis
par·the·no·pho·bia
par·tial
ag·glu·ti·nin
an·en·ceph·a·ly
an·eu·ploi·dy
an·o·don·tia
an·ti·gen
cys·tec·to·my
den·ture
den·ture, dis·tal ex·ten·sion
en·ter·o·cele
ep·i·lep·sy
groups
lip·o·at·ro·phy
pres·sure
scle·rec·ta·sia
sei·zure
vol·ume
par·tial adre·no·cor·ti·cal
in·suf·fi·cien·cy
par·tial den·ture
im·pres·sion
re·ten·tion
par·tial il·e·al
by·pass
par·tial-thick·ness
burn
flap
graft
par·tial throm·bo·plas·tin
time
par·tic·i·pant
ob·ser·ver
par·ti·cle
al·pha p.
be·ta p.
chro·ma·tin p.'s

Dane p.'s
el·e·men·ta·ry p.
kap·pa p.'s
Zimmermann's el·e·men·ta·ry p.
par·tic·u·late
par·ti·tion
chro·ma·tog·ra·phy
co·ef·fi·cient
par·tu·ri·ent
ca·nal
pa·ral·y·sis
pa·re·sis
par·tu·ri·fa·cient
par·tu·ri·om·e·ter
par·tu·ri·tion
pa·ru·li·des
pa·ru·lis
par·um·bil·i·cal
par·u·re·sis
par·val·bu·min
par·vi·cel·lu·lar
par·vi·loc·u·lar
cyst
Par·vo·bac·te·ri·a·ce·ae
par·vo·line
Par·vo·vir·i·dae
Par·vo·vi·rus
par·vule
par·vus
PAS
stain
pas·cal
Pascal's
law
Pascheff's
con·junc·ti·vi·tis
Paschen
bod·ies
pas·i·ni·a·zide
pas·pal·ism
pas·sage
na·so·pha·ryn·ge·al p.
Pas·sal·u·rus am·big·u·us
Passavant's
bar
cush·ion
pad
ridge
pas·si·flo·ra
pas·sion
pas·sion·al
at·ti·tudes
pas·sive
ag·glu·ti·na·tion
an·a·phy·lax·is
clot
con·ges·tion

duc·tion
erup·tion
he·mag·glu·ti·na·tion
hy·per·e·mia
im·mu·ni·ty
im·mu·ni·za·tion
in·con·ti·nence
in·ter·val
learn·ing
me·di·um
move·ment
pro·phy·lax·is
trans·fer·ence
trem·or
va·so·con·stric·tion
va·so·di·la·tion
pas·sive-ag·gres·sive
be·hav·ior
per·son·al·i·ty
pas·sive cu·ta·ne·ous
an·a·phy·lax·is
pas·sive cu·ta·ne·ous an·a·phy·lac·tic
re·ac·tion
pas·siv·ism
pas·siv·i·ty
pas·ta
pas·tae
paste
der·mat·o·log·ic p.
de·sen·si·tiz·ing p.
past·er
pas·tern
Pasteur
vac·cine
Pas·teu·rel·la
P. anat·i·pes·ti·fer
P. hae·mo·ly·ti·ca
P. mul·to·ci·da
P. no·vi·ci·da
P. pes·tis
P. pfaf·fii
P. pseu·do·tu·ber·cu·lo·sis
P. sep·ti·cae·mi·ae
P. tu·la·ren·sis
pas·teu·rel·la
pas·teu·rel·lae
pas·teur·el·lo·sis
pas·teur·i·za·tion
pas·teur·ize
pas·teur·iz·er
Pasteur's
ef·fect
Pastia's
sign
pas·til
ra·di·om·e·ter

pas·til
  Sabouraud's p.'s
pas·tille
pas·to·ral
  coun·sel·ing
past-point·ing
pa·ta·gia
pa·ta·gi·um
  cer·vi·cal p.
Patau's
  syn·drome
patch
  test
patch
  but·ter·fly p.
  cot·ton-wool p.'s
  her·ald p.
  Hutchinson's p.
  moth p.
  mu·cous p.
  opal·ine p.
  Peyer's p.'s
  salm·on p.
  sha·green p.
  smok·er's p.'s
  sol·dier's p.'s
pat·e·fac·tion
Patein's
  al·bu·min
pa·tel·la
  float·ing p.
  slip·ping p.
pa·tel·lae
pa·tel·lal·gia
pa·tel·lar
  fos·sa of vit·re·ous
  lig·a·ment
  net·work
  re·flex
  sur·face of fe·mur
pa·tel·lar ten·don
  re·flex
pat·el·lec·to·my
pa·tel·li·form
pa·tel·lo-ad·duc·tor
  re·flex
pat·el·lom·e·ter
pa·ten·cy
  probe p.
pa·tent
  duc·tus ar·te·ri·o·sus
  med·i·cine
pa·tent blue V
Paterson-Kelly
  syn·drome
path
  con·dyle p.
  gen·er·at·ed oc·clu·sal p.

  in·ci·sal p.
  p. of in·ser·tion
  milled-in p.'s
  oc·clu·sal p.
pa·the·ma
pa·the·mat·ic
  apha·sia
path·er·ga·sia
path·er·gy
pa·thet·ic
  nerve
path·find·er
path·ic
path·o·am·ine
path·o·bi·ol·o·gy
path·o·clis·is
path·o·crin·ia
path·o·dix·ia
path·o·don·tia
path·o·for·mic
path·o·gen
  be·hav·ior·al p.
  op·por·tun·is·tic p.
path·o·gen·e·sis
  drug p.
path·o·ge·net·ic
path·o·gen·ic
  oc·clu·sion
path·o·ge·nic·i·ty
pa·thog·e·ny
path·og·no·mon·ic
  symp·tom
path·og·no·my
path·og·nos·tic
pa·thog·ra·phy
path·o·le·sia
path·o·log·ic
  ab·sorp·tion
  amen·or·rhea
  am·pu·ta·tion
  cal·ci·fi·ca·tion
  di·ag·no·sis
  frac·ture
  gly·cos·ur·ia
  his·tol·o·gy
  my·o·pia
  phys·i·ol·o·gy
  ri·gid·i·ty
  sphinc·ter
path·o·log·i·cal
  anat·o·my
path·o·log·ic re·trac·tion
  ring
pa·thol·o·gist
pa·thol·o·gy
  an·a·tom·i·cal p.
  cel·lu·lar p.
  clin·i·cal p.

com·par·a·tive p.
den·tal p.
func·tion·al p.
hu·mor·al p.
med·i·cal p.
mo·lec·u·lar p.
oral p.
speech p.
sur·gi·cal p.
path·o·met·ric
pa·thom·e·try
path·o·mi·me·sis
path·o·mim·ic·ry
path·o·mi·o·sis
path·o·mor·phism
path·o·no·mia
pa·thon·o·my
path·o·pho·bia
path·o·phys·i·ol·o·gy
path·o·poi·e·sis
pa·tho·sis
pa·thot·ro·pism
path·way
au·di·to·ry p.
Embden-Meyerhof p.
Embden-Meyerhof-Parnas p.
pen·tose phos·phate p.
phos·pho·glu·co·nate p.
pa·tient
tar·get p.
Patois
vi·rus
pat·ri·cide
Patrick's
test
pat·ri·lin·e·al
pat·ten
pat·tern
bal·le·ri·na-foot p.
hour·glass p.
ju·ve·nile p.
oc·clu·sal p.
wax p.
pat·terned
al·o·pe·cia
pat·tern sen·si·tive
ep·i·lep·sy
pat·u·lin
pat·u·lous
pau·ci·bac·il·lary
pau·ci·sy·nap·tic
Pauling-Corey
he·lix
Pauling's
the·o·ry
Pauli's
prin·ci·ple

Paul's
re·ac·tion
test
paunch
pause
ap·ne·ic p.
com·pen·sa·to·ry p.
post·ex·tra·sys·tol·ic p.
pre·au·to·mat·ic p.
res·pi·ra·to·ry p.
si·nus p.
Pautrier's
ab·scess
mi·cro·ab·scess
Pauzat's
dis·ease
pave·ment
ep·i·the·li·um
pa·vex
Pavlov
meth·od
pouch
stom·ach
pav·lov·i·an
con·di·tion·ing
Pavlov's
re·flex
pav·or noc·tur·nus
Pavy's
dis·ease
paw·paw
Paxton's
dis·ease
Payne
op·er·a·tion
Payr's
clamp
mem·brane
sign
PBI
test
P-con·gen·i·ta·le
P-dex·tro·car·di·a·le
peach ker·nel oil
peak
mag·ni·tude
pea·nut oil
pearl
Elschnig p.'s
enam·el p.
ep·i·the·li·al p.
Epstein's p.'s
gouty p.
ker·a·tin p.
Laënnec's p.'s
squa·mous p.
pearl
cyst

pearl *(continued)*
  moss
  tu·mor
pearl-ash
pearl-work·er's
  dis·ease
pear-shaped
  ar·ea
peat
  moss
peau d'oran·ge
pec·cant
  hu·mors
pec·ca·ti·pho·bia
pe·cil·o·cin
peck·ing
  or·der
Pecquet's
  cis·tern
  duct
  res·er·voir
pec·tase
pec·ten
  anal p.
  p. pu·bis
pec·ten
  band
pec·ten·i·tis
pec·ten·o·sis
pec·tic
pec·tic ac·id
pec·tin
  sug·ar
pec·tin·ase
pec·ti·nate
  fi·bers
  lig·a·ment of ir·i·do·cor·ne·
    al an·gle
  lig·a·ment of iris
  line
  mus·cles
  zone
pec·tin·e·al
  lig·a·ment
  line
  line of pu·bis
  mus·cle
pec·tin·es·ter·ase
pec·ti·ne·us
pec·tin·ic ac·ids
pec·tin·i·form
  sep·tum
pec·ti·za·tion
pec·to·ra
pec·to·ral
  fas·cia
  glands
  re·flex

  re·gion
  re·gions
  ridge
  veins
pec·to·ral·gia
pec·to·ral lymph
  nodes
pec·to·ril·o·quy
  aphon·ic p.
  whis·pered p.
  whis·per·ing p.
pec·to·ris
pec·to·roph·o·ny
pec·tose
pec·tous
pec·tus
  p. ca·ri·na·tum
  p. ex·ca·va·tum
  p. re·cur·va·tum
ped·al
  sys·tem
pe·da·tro·phia
pe·dat·ro·phy
ped·er·ast
ped·er·as·ty
Pedersen's
  spec·u·lum
pe·des
pe·de·sis
pe·di·at·ric
  den·tis·try
pe·di·a·tric·ian
pe·di·at·rics
pe·di·at·rist
ped·i·at·ry
ped·i·cel
ped·i·cel·late
ped·i·cel·la·tion
ped·i·cle
  p. of arch of ver·te·bra
  Filatov-Gillies tubed p.
ped·i·cle
  flap
  graft
pe·dic·ter·us
pe·dic·u·lar
pe·dic·u·late
pe·dic·u·la·tion
pe·dic·u·li
pe·dic·u·li·cide
Pe·dic·u·loi·des ven·tri·co·sus
pe·dic·u·lo·pho·bia
pe·dic·u·lo·sis
  p. ca·pi·tis
  p. cor·po·ris
  p. pal·pe·bra·rum
  p. pu·bis

p. ves·ti·men·ti
p. ves·ti·men·to·rum
pe·dic·u·lous
bleph·a·ri·tis
Pe·dic·u·lus
pe·dic·u·lus
ped·i·cure
ped·i·gree
anal·y·sis
ped·i·lu·vi·um
ped·i·o·nal·gia
ped·i·o·neu·ral·gia
pe·di·o·pho·bia
ped·i·pha·lanx
pe·dis
pe·do·don·tia
pe·do·don·tics
pe·do·don·tist
ped·o·dy·na·mom·e·ter
pe·do·gen·e·sis
ped·o·gram
ped·o·graph
pe·dog·ra·phy
pe·dol·o·gist
pe·dol·o·gy
pe·dom·e·ter
pe·do·mor·phism
pe·do·phil·ia
pe·do·phil·ic
Pe·do·vir·i·dae
pe·dun·cle
ce·re·bral p.
p. of cor·pus cal·lo·sum
p. of floc·cu·lus
in·fe·ri·or cer·e·bel·lar p.
in·fe·ri·or tha·lam·ic p.
lat·er·al tha·lam·ic p.
p. of mam·il·lary body
mid·dle cer·e·bel·lar p.
ol·fac·to·ry p.
su·pe·ri·or cer·e·bel·lar p.
ven·tral tha·lam·ic p.
pe·dun·cu·lar
an·sa
loop
veins
pe·dun·cu·late
pe·dun·cu·lat·ed
hy·da·tid
pol·yp
pe·dun·cu·li
pe·dun·cu·lot·o·my
pe·dun·cu·lus
p. of pin·e·al body
p. thal·a·mi la·te·ra·lis
p. thal·a·mi ven·tra·lis
p. vi·tel·li·nus
peel·ing

pee·nash
peg
re·te p.'s
peg-and-sock·et
ar·tic·u·la·tion
joint
pegged
tooth
pe·jor·ism
pe·lade
pel·age
pel·ar·gon·ic ac·id
Pel-Ebstein
dis·ease
fe·ver
Pelger-Huët nu·cle·ar
anom·a·ly
pe·lid·no·ma
pe·li·o·ma
pe·li·o·sis
p. hep·a·tis
pe·li·o·sis
hep·a·ti·tis
Pelizaeus-Merzbacher
dis·ease
pel·lag·ra
in·fan·tile p.
sec·on·dary p.
p. sine p.
pel·lag·ra-pre·vent·ing (P-P)
fac·tor
pel·lag·roid
pel·lag·rous
Pellegrini's
dis·ease
Pellegrini-Stieda
dis·ease
pel·let
im·plan·ta·tion
pel·li·cle
ac·quired p.
brown p.
pel·lic·u·lar
pel·lic·u·lous
Pellizzi's
syn·drome
pe·llo·te
pel·lu·cid
zone
pel·ma
pel·mat·ic
pel·mat·o·gram
pe·lop·a·thy
pel·o·ther·a·py
pelt
pel·ta
pel·ta·tion
pel·ves

pel·vic
 ab·scess
 ax·is
 brim
 ca·nal
 cav·i·ty
 cel·lu·li·tis
 di·a·phragm
 ex·en·ter·a·tion
 gan·glia
 gir·dle
 he·ma·to·cele
 in·dex
 in·let
 kid·ney
 limb
 out·let
 part
 per·i·to·ni·tis
 plane of great·est di·men·sions
 plane of in·let
 plane of least di·men·sions
 plane of out·let
 plex·us
 pole
 pre·sen·ta·tion
 prom·on·to·ry
 sur·face of sa·crum
 ver·sion
pel·vic di·rec·tion
pel·vi·ceph·a·log·ra·phy
pel·vi·ceph·a·lom·e·try
pel·vic in·flam·ma·to·ry
 dis·ease
pel·vic splanch·nic
 nerves
pel·vi·fix·a·tion
pel·vi·graph
pel·vi·li·thot·o·my
pel·vim·e·ter
pel·vim·e·try
 man·u·al p.
 pla·no·graph·ic p.
 ster·e·o·scop·ic p.
pel·vi·o·li·thot·o·my
pel·vi·o·per·i·to·ni·tis
pel·vi·o·plas·ty
pel·vi·os·co·py
pel·vi·ot·o·my
pel·vi·per·i·to·ni·tis
pel·vi·rec·tal
 sphinc·ter
pel·vis
 an·droid p.
 an·thro·poid p.
 as·sim·i·la·tion p.
 beaked p.

brach·y·pel·lic p.
caou·tchouc p.
con·tract·ed p.
cor·date p.
cor·di·form p.
Deventer's p.
dol·i·cho·pel·lic p.
dwarf p.
false p.
flat p.
fro·zen p.
fun·nel-shaped p.
p. of gall·blad·der
gy·ne·coid p.
hard·ened p.
heart-shaped p.
in·vert·ed p.
p. jus·to ma·jor
p. jus·to mi·nor
ju·ve·nile p.
ky·pho·sco·li·ot·ic p.
ky·phot·ic p.
large p.
lon·gi·tu·di·nal oval p.
lor·dot·ic p.
mas·cu·line p.
me·sat·i·pel·lic p.
Nägele's p.
p. na·na
p. ob·tec·ta
os·te·o·ma·lac·ic p.
Otto p.
p. pla·na
plat·y·pel·lic p.
plat·y·pel·loid p.
Prague p.
pseu·do-os·te·o·ma·la·cic p.
ra·chit·ic p.
re·nal p.
ren·i·form p.
Robert's p.
Rokitansky's p.
ros·trate p.
round p.
rub·ber p.
sco·li·ot·ic p.
small p.
spi·der p.
split p.
spon·dy·lo·lis·thet·ic p.
p. spu·ria
trans·verse oval p.
true p.
p. ve·ra
pel·vi·sa·cral
pel·vi·scope
pel·vi·therm
pel·vit·o·my

pel·vi·u·re·ter·og·ra·phy
pel·vi·ver·te·bral
  an·gle
pel·vo·ceph·a·log·ra·phy
pel·vo·fem·o·ral mus·cu·lar
  dys·tro·phy
pel·vos·co·py
pel·vo·spon·dy·li·tis os·sif·i·
  cans
pem·o·line
pem·phi·goid
  be·nign mu·co·sal p.
  bul·lous p.
  cic·a·tri·cial p.
  oc·u·lar p.
pem·phi·goid
  syph·i·lid
pem·phi·gus
  p. acu·tus
  Bra·zil·ian p.
  p. con·ta·gi·o·sus
  p. crou·po·sus
  p. dip·the·ri·ti·cus
  p. er·y·the·ma·to·sus
  fa·mil·i·al be·nign chron·ic
    p.
  p. fo·li·a·ceus
  p. gan·gre·no·sus
  p. lep·ro·sus
  p. ve·ge·tans
  p. vul·ga·ris
pem·pi·dine
pen
  grasp
pen·cil
  ten·der·ness
pen·del·luft
Pendred's
  syn·drome
pen·du·lar
  move·ment
  nys·tag·mus
pen·du·lous
  ab·do·men
  heart
  pal·ate
pen·du·lum
  rhythm
pe·nec·to·my
pen·e·trance
pen·e·trant
  gene
pen·e·trate
pen·e·trat·ing
  ker·a·to·plas·ty
  ul·cer
  wound
pen·e·tra·tion

pen·e·trom·e·ter
pe·ni·al
pe·ni·a·pho·bia
pen·i·cil·la·mine
pen·i·cil·la·nate
pen·i·cil·lan·ic ac·id
pen·i·cil·lar·y
pen·i·cil·late
pe·ni·cil·li
pen·i·cil·lic ac·id
pen·i·cil·lin
  alu·mi·num p.
  p. B
  buff·ered crys·tal·line p. G
  chlo·ro·pro·caine p. O
  p. G
  p. G ben·za·thine
  p. G hy·dra·bam·ine
  p. G po·tas·si·um
  p. G pro·caine
  p. G so·di·um
  p. N
  p. O
  p. phe·nox·y·meth·yl
  p. V
  p. V ben·za·thine
  p. V hy·dra·bam·ine
pen·i·cil·li·nase
pen·i·cil·li·nate
pen·i·cil·lin G
  po·tas·si·um
Pen·i·cil·li·um
pen·i·cil·lo·ic ac·id
pen·i·cil·lo·yl pol·y·ly·sine
pen·i·cil·lus
pe·nile
  fi·bro·ma·to·sis
  im·plant
  ra·phe
  ure·thra
pe·nil·lic ac·ids
pen·in
pe·nis
  bi·fid p.
  clubbed p.
  dou·ble p.
  p. fe·mi·ne·us
  p. lu·na·tus
  p. mu·li·e·bris
  p. pal·ma·tus
  webbed p.
pe·nis
  bone
  en·vy
  spines
  thorns
pe·nis·chi·sis
pe·ni·tis

pen·nate
   mus·cle
pen·ni·form
pen·ny·roy·al
pe·no·scro·tal
   hy·po·spa·di·as
pe·not·o·my
Penrose
   drain
pen·sion
   neu·ro·sis
pen·ta·ba·sic
pen·tad
pen·ta·dac·tyl
pen·ta·dac·tyle
pen·ta·e·ryth·ri·tol
pen·ta·gas·trin
   test
pen·tal·o·gy
   p. of Fallot
pen·ta·mer
pen·ta·me·tho·ni·um bro·mide
pen·tam·i·dine is·e·thi·o·nate
pen·ta·no·ic ac·id
pen·ta·pip·er·ide fu·ma·rate
pen·ta·pi·per·i·um meth·yl·sul·fate
pen·ta·quine
Pen·tas·to·ma
pen·ta·sto·mi·a·sis
Pen·ta·stom·i·da
pent·a·tom·ic
Pen·ta·trich·o·mon·as
pen·ta·va·lent
pen·ta·va·lent gas gan·grene
   an·ti·tox·in
pen·taz·o·cine
pen·te·tate tri·so·di·um cal·ci·um
pen·tet·ic ac·id
pen·thi·e·nate bro·mide
pen·tif·yl·line
pen·ti·tol
pen·to·bar·bi·tal
pen·to·lin·i·um tar·trate
pen·ton
   an·ti·gen
pen·to·san
pen·tose
   p. nu·cle·o·tide
pen·tose nu·cle·ic ac·id
pen·tose phos·phate
   path·way
pen·to·su·ria
   al·i·men·ta·ry p.
   es·sen·tial p.
   pri·mary p.
pen·tox·ide

pen·tox·if·yl·line
pen·tu·lose
pen·tyl
pen·ty·lene·tet·ra·zol
pe·o·til·lo·ma·nia
pep
   pills
pep·lo·mer
pep·los
Pepper
   syn·drome
pep·per·mint
   p. cam·phor
   p. oil
pep·per and salt
   fun·dus
pep·sic
pep·sin
pep·sin A
pep·si·nate
pep·si·nif·er·ous
pep·sin·o·gen
pep·sin·og·e·nous
pep·si·nu·ria
pep·tic
   cell
   di·ges·tion
   esoph·a·gi·tis
   gland
   ul·cer
pep·ti·dase
pep·ti·dase P
pep·tide
   adre·no·cor·ti·co·tro·pic p.
   brad·y·ki·nin-po·ten·ti·at·ing p.
   het·er·o·mer·ic p.
   p. hy·dro·lase
   phen·yl·thi·o·car·bam·o·yl p.
   PTC p.
   S p.
   sig·ma p.
   p. syn·the·tase
pep·tide
   bond
pep·ti·der·gic
pep·ti·do·gly·can
pep·ti·doid
pep·ti·do·lyt·ic
pep·ti·dyl di·pep·ti·dase A
pep·ti·za·tion
Pep·to·coc·ca·ce·ae
Pep·to·coc·cus
   P. ac·ti·vus
   P. aer·o·genes
   P. an·aer·o·bi·us
   P. asac·cha·ro·lyt·i·cus

P. con·stel·la·tus
P. ni·ger
pep·to·crin·ine
pep·to·gen·ic
pep·tog·e·nous
pep·tol·y·sis
pep·to·lyt·ic
pep·tone
pep·ton·ic
pep·to·ni·za·tion
pep·to·nized
  iron
Pep·to·strep·to·coc·cus
P. an·aer·o·bi·us
P. evo·lu·tus
P. foe·ti·dus
P. in·ter·me·di·us
P. lan·ce·o·la·tus
P. mag·nus
P. micros
P. mor·bil·lo·rum
P. pa·le·o·pneu·mo·ni·ae
P. par·vu·lus
P. pla·ga·rum·bel·li
P. pro·duc·tus
P. pu·tri·dus
per·a·ceph·a·lus
per·ac·e·tate
per·a·ce·tic ac·id
per·ac·id
per·a·cute
per·am·bu·lat·ing
  ul·cer
per an·um
per·ar·tic·u·la·tion
per·a·to·dyn·ia
per·ax·il·lary
per·a·zine
per·bor·ic ac·id
per·cen·tile
per·cept
  anal·y·sis
per·cep·tion
  con·scious p.
  depth p.
  ex·tra·sen·so·ry p.
  fa·cial p.
  si·mul·ta·ne·ous p.
per·cep·tive
  deaf·ness
per·cep·tiv·i·ty
per·cep·to·ri·um
per·cep·tu·al
  ex·pan·sion
per·chlor·ic ac·id
per·chlo·ride
per·co·la·tion
per·co·la·tor

per·co·morph oil
per con·tig·u·um
per con·tin·u·um
per·cuss
per·cus·sion
  aus·cul·ta·to·ry p.
  bi·man·u·al p.
  cla·vic·u·lar p.
  deep p.
  di·rect p.
  fin·ger p.
  im·me·di·ate p.
  me·di·ate p.
  pal·pa·to·ry p.
  thresh·old p.
per·cus·sion
  sound
  wave
per·cus·sor
per·cu·ta·ne·ous
  chol·an·gi·og·ra·phy
  stim·u·la·tion
per·cu·ta·ne·ous ra·di·o·fre·quen·cy
  gan·gli·ol·y·sis
per·cu·ta·ne·ous trans·lu·mi·nal
  an·gi·o·plas·ty
per·en·ceph·a·ly
Perez
  re·flex
Perez'
  sign
per·fect
  fun·gus
  stage
  state
per·fec·tion·ism
per·fla·tion
per·fo·rans
per·fo·rat·ed
  lay·er of scle·ra
  space
  ul·cer
per·fo·rat·ing
  ab·scess
  ar·ter·ies
  ar·ter·ies of foot
  ar·ter·ies of hand
  ar·ter·ies of in·ter·nal
    mam·ma·ry
  ar·tery of per·o·ne·al
    fi·bers
  fol·lic·u·li·tis
  ker·a·to·plas·ty
  ul·cer of foot
  veins
  wound

per·fo·ra·tion
  Bezold's p.
per·fo·ra·tor
per·fo·ra·to·ri·um
per·form·ance
  test
per·for·mic ac·id
  re·ac·tion
per·frig·er·a·tion
per·fus·ate
per·fuse
per·fu·sion
  re·gion·al p.
per·fu·sion
  can·nu·la
per·go·lide mes·y·late
per·hex·il·ine ma·le·ate
per·hy·drase
  milk
per·i·ac·i·nal
per·i·ac·i·nous
per·i·ad·e·ni·tis
  p. mu·co·sa ne·cro·ti·ca re·
  cur·rens
per·i·al·ve·o·lar
  wir·ing
per·i·a·nal
per·i·a·nal odor·if·er·ous
  glands
per·i·an·gi·o·cho·li·tis
per·i·an·gi·tis
per·i·a·or·tic
per·i·a·or·ti·tis
per·i·a·pex
per·i·ap·i·cal
  ab·scess
  cu·ret·tage
  cyst
  gran·u·lo·ma
  os·te·o·fi·bro·sis
  ra·di·o·graph
  roent·gen·o·gram
  tis·sue
per·i·ap·i·cal ce·ment·al
  dys·pla·sia
per·i·ap·pen·di·ce·al
  ab·scess
per·i·ap·pen·di·ci·tis
  p. de·cid·u·a·lis
per·i·ap·pen·dic·u·lar
per·i·ar·te·ri·al
  pad
  plex·us
  sym·pa·thec·to·my
per·i·ar·te·ri·tis
  p. no·do·sa
per·i·ar·thric
per·i·ar·thri·tis

per·i·ar·tic·u·lar
  ab·scess
per·i·a·tri·al
per·i·au·ric·u·lar
per·i·ax·i·al
per·i·ax·il·lary
per·i·ax·o·nal
per·i·blast
per·i·bron·chi·al
per·i·bron·chi·o·lar
per·i·bron·chi·o·li·tis
per·i·bron·chi·tis
per·i·buc·cal
per·i·bul·bar
per·i·bur·sal
per·i·cal·lo·sal
  ar·tery
per·i·can·a·lic·u·lar
  fi·bro·ad·e·no·ma
per·i·cap·il·lary
  cell
per·i·car·dec·to·my
per·i·car·dia
per·i·car·di·ac
per·i·car·di·a·co·phren·ic
  ar·tery
  veins
per·i·car·di·al
  cav·i·ty
  de·com·pres·sion
  frem·i·tus
  knock
  mur·mur
  pleu·ra
  pou·drage
  re·flex
  rub
  veins
  vil·li
per·i·car·di·al fric·tion
  rub
  sound
per·i·car·di·cen·te·sis
per·i·car·di·ec·to·my
per·i·car·di·o·cen·te·sis
per·i·car·di·o·per·i·to·ne·al
  ca·nal
per·i·car·di·o·phren·ic
per·i·car·di·o·pleur·al
  fold
  mem·brane
per·i·car·di·or·rha·phy
per·i·car·di·os·to·my
per·i·car·di·ot·o·my
per·i·car·dit·ic
per·i·car·di·tis
  ad·he·sive p.
  chron·ic con·stric·tive p.

fi·brin·ous p.
in·ter·nal ad·he·sive p.
p. ob·li·te·r·ans
rheu·mat·ic p.
p. sic·ca
ure·mic p.
p. vil·lo·sa
per·i·car·di·um
ad·her·ent p.
bread-and-but·ter p.
shag·gy p.
per·i·car·di·um fi·bro·sum
per·i·car·di·um se·ro·sum
per·i·car·dot·o·my
per·i·ce·cal
per·i·cel·lu·lar
per·i·ce·men·tal
ab·scess
at·tach·ment
per·i·ce·men·ti·tis
per·i·cen·tral
fi·bro·sis
sco·to·ma
per·i·cen·tric
in·ver·sion
per·i·cha·reia
per·i·cho·lan·gi·tis
per·i·chon·dral
bone
per·i·chon·dri·al
per·i·chon·dri·tis
per·i·ster·nal p.
re·laps·ing p.
per·i·chon·dri·um
per·i·chord
per·i·chor·dal
per·i·cho·roid
space
per·i·cho·roi·dal
per·i·chrome
per·i·claus·tral
lam·i·na
per·i·col·ic
per·i·col·ic mem·brane
syn·drome
per·i·co·li·tis
p. dex·tra
p. si·nis·tra
per·i·co·lon·i·tis
per·i·col·pi·tis
per·i·con·chal
sul·cus
per·i·cor·ne·al
per·i·cor·o·nal
ab·scess
flap
per·i·cor·o·ni·tis

per·i·cor·pus·cu·lar
syn·apse
per·i·cra·ni·al
per·i·cra·ni·tis
per·i·cra·ni·um
per·i·cy·a·zine
per·i·cys·tic
per·i·cys·ti·tis
per·i·cys·ti·um
per·i·cyte
cap·il·lary p.
per·i·cy·ti·al
per·i·cyt·ic
ven·ules
per·i·dec·to·my
per·i·dens
per·i·den·tal
lig·a·ment
mem·brane
per·i·den·ti·tis
per·i·den·ti·um
per·i·derm
per·i·der·ma
per·i·der·mal
per·i·der·mic
per·i·des·mic
per·i·des·mi·tis
per·i·des·mi·um
per·i·did·y·mis
per·i·did·y·mi·tis
pe·rid·i·um
per·i·di·ver·tic·u·li·tis
per·i·du·o·de·ni·tis
per·i·du·ral
an·es·the·sia
per·i·en·ceph·a·li·tis
per·i·en·ter·ic
per·i·en·ter·i·tis
per·i·e·pen·dy·mal
per·i·e·soph·a·ge·al
per·i·e·soph·a·gi·tis
per·i·fo·cal
per·i·fol·lic·u·lar
per·i·fol·lic·u·li·tis
p. ab·sce·dens et suf·fo·di·ens
su·per·fi·cial pus·tu·lar p.
per·i·fuse
per·i·fu·sion
per·i·gan·gli·on·ic
per·i·gas·tric
per·i·gas·tri·tis
per·i·gem·mal
per·i·glan·du·li·tis
per·i·glot·tic
per·i·glot·tis
per·i·he·pat·ic
per·i·hep·a·ti·tis

per·i·her·ni·al
peri-im·plan·to·cla·sia
peri-in·farc·tion
   block
per·i·je·ju·ni·tis
per·i·kar·ya
per·i·kar·y·on
per·i·ke·rat·ic
per·i·ky·ma
per·i·ky·ma·ta
per·i·lab·y·rin·thi·tis
per·i·la·ryn·ge·al
per·i·lar·yn·gi·tis
per·i·len·tic·u·lar
per·i·lig·a·men·tous
per·i·lim·bal suc·tion
   cup
per·i·lymph
per·i·lym·pha
per·i·lym·phan·gi·al
per·i·lym·phan·gi·tis
per·i·lym·phat·ic
   duct
   space
per·i·men·in·gi·tis
pe·rim·e·ter
   arc p.
   Goldmann p.
   pro·jec·tion p.
   Tü·bing·er p.
per·i·me·tria
per·i·met·ric
per·i·me·trit·ic
per·i·me·tri·tis
per·i·me·tri·um
pe·rim·e·try
   com·put·ed p.
   flick·er p.
   ki·net·ic p.
   me·sop·ic p.
   ob·jec·tive p.
   quan·ti·ta·tive p.
   sco·top·ic p.
   stat·ic p.
per·i·mus·cu·lar
   fi·bro·sis
per·i·my·e·lis
per·i·my·e·li·tis
per·i·my·o·en·do·car·di·tis
per·i·my·o·si·tis
per·i·my·sia
per·i·my·si·al
per·i·my·si·i·tis
per·i·my·si·tis
per·i·my·si·um
   p. ex·ter·num
   p. in·ter·num

per·i·na·tal
   death
   med·i·cine
per·i·na·tal mor·tal·i·ty
   rate
per·i·nate
per·i·na·tol·o·gist
per·i·na·tol·o·gy
per·i·nea
per·i·ne·al
   ar·tery
   body
   flex·ure of rec·tum
   her·nia
   hy·po·spa·di·as
   li·thot·o·my
   mem·brane
   mus·cles
   nerves
   ra·phe
   re·gion
   sec·tion
   spac·es
   ure·thros·to·my
   ure·throt·o·my
per·i·ne·o·cele
per·i·ne·om·e·ter
per·i·ne·o·plas·ty
per·i·ne·or·rha·phy
per·i·ne·o·scro·tal
per·i·ne·os·to·my
per·i·ne·o·syn·the·sis
per·i·ne·ot·o·my
per·i·ne·o·vag·i·nal
   fis·tu·la
per·i·neph·ria
per·i·neph·ri·al
per·i·neph·ric
   ab·scess
per·i·neph·ri·tis
per·i·neph·ri·um
per·i·ne·um
   wa·ter·ing-can p.
per·i·neu·ral
   an·es·the·sia
   in·fil·tra·tion
per·i·neu·ria
per·i·neu·ri·al
per·i·neu·ri·tis
per·i·neu·ri·um
per·i·neu·ro·nal
   sat·el·lite
per·i·nu·cle·ar
   cat·a·ract
   space
per·i·oc·u·lar
pe·ri·od
   ab·so·lute re·frac·to·ry p.

crit·i·cal p.
eclipse p.
ef·fec·tive re·frac·to·ry p.
ejec·tion p.
ex·trin·sic in·cu·ba·tion p.
fer·tile p.
func·tion·al re·frac·to·ry p.
in·cu·ba·tion p.
in·duc·tion p.
in·ter·sys·tol·ic p.
in·tra·par·tum p.
iso·e·lec·tric p.
iso·met·ric p.
iso·met·ric p. of car·di·ac
  cy·cle
la·ten·cy p.
la·tent p.
mas·ti·ca·to·ry si·lent p.
men·stru·al p.
missed p.
mi·tot·ic p.
oe·di·pal p.
pre·e·jec·tion p.
pre·pa·tent p.
pu·er·per·al p.
pulse p.
re·frac·to·ry p.
re·frac·to·ry p. of elec·tron·
  ic pace·mak·er
rel·a·tive re·frac·to·ry p.
safe p.
si·lent p.
syn·the·sis p.
to·tal re·frac·to·ry p.
vul·ner·a·ble p.
vul·ner·a·ble p. of heart
Wenckebach p.
per·i·o·date
pe·ri·od·ic
  ar·thral·gia
  cat·a·to·nia
  dis·ease
  ede·ma
  fil·a·ri·a·sis
  law
  neu·tro·pe·nia
  oph·thal·mia
  pa·ral·y·sis
  per·i·to·ni·tis
  pol·y·ser·o·si·tis
  sys·tem
pe·ri·od·ic ac·id
pe·ri·od·ic ac·id-Schiff
  stain
per·i·o·dic·i·ty
  di·ur·nal p.
  fi·lar·i·al p.
  lu·nar p.

ma·lar·i·al p.
noc·tur·nal p.
sub·pe·ri·od·ic p.
pe·ri·od·ic mi·grain·ous
  neu·ral·gia
per·i·o·don·tal
  ab·scess
  an·es·the·sia
  at·ro·phy
  file
  lig·a·ment
  mem·brane
  pock·et
  probe
Per·i·o·don·tal Dis·ease In·dex
Per·i·o·don·tal In·dex
per·i·o·don·tal lig·a·ment
  fi·bers
per·i·o·don·tia
per·i·o·don·tics
per·i·o·don·tist
per·i·o·don·ti·tis
  ap·i·cal p.
  p. com·plex
  ju·ve·nile p.
  p. sim·plex
  sup·pu·ra·tive p.
per·i·o·don·ti·um
per·i·o·don·to·cla·sia
per·i·o·don·tol·y·sis
per·i·o·don·to·sis
per·i·om·phal·ic
per·i·o·nych·ia
per·i·o·nych·i·um
per·i·on·yx
per·i·o·nyx·is
per·i·o·o·pho·ri·tis
per·i·o·o·pho·ro·sal·pin·gi·tis
per·i·op·er·a·tive
per·i·oph·thal·mic
per·i·oph·thal·mi·tis
per·i·o·ple
per·i·op·lic
  band
per·i·o·ral
per·i·or·bit
pe·ri·or·bi·ta
per·i·or·bi·tal
  mem·brane
per·i·or·chi·tis
  p. hem·or·rha·gi·ca
per·i·or·i·fi·cial
  len·tig·i·no·sis
per·i·ost
pe·ri·os·tea
per·i·os·te·al
  bone
  bud

per·i·os·te·al *(continued)*
  chon·dro·ma
  el·e·va·tor
  gan·gli·on
  graft
  im·plan·ta·tion
  re·flex
  sar·co·ma
per·i·os·te·i·tis
per·i·os·te·o·ma
per·i·os·te·o·med·ul·li·tis
per·i·os·te·o·my·e·li·tis
per·i·os·te·op·a·thy
per·i·os·te·o·phyte
per·i·os·te·o·plas·tic
  am·pu·ta·tion
per·i·os·te·o·sis
per·i·os·te·o·tome
per·i·os·te·ot·o·my
per·i·os·te·ous
per·i·os·te·um
  al·ve·o·lar p.
  p. al·ve·o·la·re
  p. cra·nii
per·i·os·ti·tis
  or·bi·tal p.
per·i·os·to·ma
per·i·os·to·ses
per·i·os·to·sis
per·i·os·tos·te·i·tis
per·i·os·to·tome
per·i·os·tot·o·my
per·i·o·tic
  bone
  car·ti·lage
per·i·o·va·ri·tis
per·i·o·vu·lar
per·i·pach·y·men·in·gi·tis
per·i·pan·cre·a·ti·tis
per·i·pap·il·lary
per·i·pa·tet·ic
per·i·pe·ni·al
per·i·pha·ryn·ge·al
  space
pe·riph·er·ad
pe·riph·e·ral
  an·eu·rysm
  ap·nea
  cat·a·ract
  che·mo·re·cep·tor
  dys·os·to·sis
  glare
  ir·i·dec·to·my
  re·sis·tance
  sco·to·ma
  seal
  ta·bes
  vi·sion

pe·riph·e·ral an·te·ri·or
  syn·ech·ia
pe·ri·phe·ra·lis
pe·riph·e·ral ner·vous
  sys·tem
pe·riph·e·ral os·si·fy·ing
  fi·bro·ma
pe·riph·e·ro·cen·tral
pe·riph·e·ry
per·i·phle·bit·ic
per·i·phle·bi·tis
Per·i·pla·ne·ta
pe·rip·lo·cin
per·i·po·lar
  cell
per·i·po·le·sis
per·i·po·ri·tis
per·i·por·tal
  space of Mall
per·i·proc·tic
per·i·proc·ti·tis
per·i·pros·tat·ic
per·i·pros·ta·ti·tis
per·i·py·le·phle·bi·tis
per·i·py·lic
per·i·py·lor·ic
per·i·rec·tal
  ab·scess
per·i·rec·ti·tis
per·i·re·nal
  fas·cia
  in·suf·fla·tion
per·i·rhi·nal
per·i·rhi·zo·cla·sia
per·i·sal·pin·gi·tis
per·i·sal·pin·go-ova·ri·tis
per·i·sal·pinx
per·i·scop·ic
  lens
  me·nis·cus
per·i·sig·moi·di·tis
per·i·sin·u·ous
per·i·si·nu·soi·dal
  space
per·i·sper·ma·ti·tis
  p. se·ro·sa
per·i·splanch·nic
per·i·splanch·ni·tis
per·i·splen·ic
per·i·sple·ni·tis
per·i·spon·dyl·ic
per·i·spon·dy·li·tis
pe·ris·so·dac·tyl
pe·ris·so·dac·ty·lous
per·i·stal·sis
  mass p.
  re·versed p.
per·i·stal·tic

per·i·staph·y·li·tis
pe·ris·ta·sis
per·i·stat·ic
   hy·per·e·mia
per·i·ster·nal
   per·i·chon·dri·tis
pe·ris·to·le
per·i·stol·ic
pe·ris·to·ma
per·i·sto·mal
per·i·sto·ma·tous
per·i·stome
per·i·ston
per·i·stri·ate
   ar·ea
   cor·tex
per·i·stru·mous
per·i·syn·o·vi·al
per·i·sys·to·le
per·i·sys·tol·ic
per·i·tar·sal
   net·work
per·i·tec·to·my
pe·ri·ten·di·nea
pe·ri·ten·di·ne·um
per·i·ten·di·ni·tis
   p. cal·car·ea
   p. se·ro·sa
per·i·ten·on
per·i·ten·on·ti·tis
per·i·the·cia
per·i·the·ci·um
per·i·the·lia
per·i·the·li·al
   cell
per·i·the·li·o·ma
per·i·the·li·um
   Eberth's p.
per·i·tho·rac·ic
per·i·thy·roi·di·tis
pe·rit·o·mist
pe·rit·o·my
pe·ri·to·nea
per·i·to·ne·al
   but·ton
   cav·i·ty
   di·al·y·sis
   fos·sas
   trans·fu·sion
   vil·li
per·i·to·ne·al·gia
per·i·to·ne·o·cen·te·sis
per·i·to·ne·oc·ly·sis
per·i·to·ne·op·a·thy
per·i·to·ne·o·per·i·car·di·al
per·i·to·ne·o·pexy
per·i·to·ne·o·plas·ty
per·i·to·ne·o·scope

per·i·to·ne·os·co·py
per·i·to·ne·ot·o·my
per·i·to·ne·o·ve·nous
   shunt
per·i·to·ne·um
per·i·to·nism
per·i·to·ni·tis
   ad·he·sive p.
   be·nign par·ox·ys·mal p.
   bile p.
   chem·i·cal p.
   chyle p.
   cir·cum·scribed p.
   p. de·for·mans
   di·a·phrag·mat·ic p.
   dif·fuse p.
   p. en·cap·su·lans
   fe·line in·fec·tious p.
   fi·bro·ca·se·ous p.
   gas p.
   gen·er·al p.
   lo·cal·ized p.
   me·co·ni·um p.
   pel·vic p.
   pe·ri·od·ic p.
   pro·duc·tive p.
   tu·ber·cu·lous p.
per·i·ton·sil·lar
   ab·scess
per·i·ton·sil·li·tis
per·i·tra·che·al
   glands
pe·rit·ri·chal
pe·rit·ri·chate
per·i·trich·ic
Per·i·trich·i·da
pe·rit·ri·chous
per·i·tro·chan·ter·ic
per·i·tu·bu·lar
   den·tin
   zone
per·i·tu·bu·lar con·trac·tile
   cells
per·i·typh·lic
per·i·um·bil·i·cal
per·i·un·gual
   fi·bro·ma
per·i·u·re·ter·al
   ab·scess
per·i·u·re·ter·ic
per·i·u·re·ter·i·tis
   p. plas·ti·ca
per·i·u·re·thral
   ab·scess
per·i·u·re·thri·tis
per·i·u·ter·ine
per·i·u·vu·lar
per·i·vag·i·ni·tis

per·i·vas·cu·lar
cuffs
per·i·vas·cu·lar fi·brous
cap·sule
per·i·vas·cu·li·tis
per·i·ve·nous
per·i·ven·tric·u·lar
fi·bers
per·i·ver·te·bral
per·i·ves·i·cal
per·i·vis·cer·al
cav·i·ty
per·i·vis·cer·i·tis
per·i·vi·tel·line
space
per·i·win·kle
per·kin·ism
per·lèche
Perlia's
nu·cle·us
per·lin·gual
Perls'
test
Perls' Prus·sian blue
stain
per·ma·nent
cal·lus
car·ti·lage
res·to·ra·tion
stric·ture
tooth
per·ma·nent dom·i·nant
idea
per·ma·nent ped·i·cle
flap
per·man·ga·nate
per·man·gan·ic ac·id
per·me·a·bil·i·ty
the·o·ry of nar·co·sis
vi·ta·min
per·me·a·ble
per·me·ant
per·me·ase
per·me·ate
per·me·a·tion
per·na
dis·ease
per·nic·i·o·si·form
per·ni·cious
ane·mia
ma·lar·ia
vom·it·ing
per·ni·cious ane·mia type
met·a·ru·bri·cyte
pro·ru·bri·cyte
ru·bri·blast
per·ni·o·sis
pe·ro·bra·chi·us

pe·ro·ceph·a·lus
pe·ro·chi·rus
pe·ro·dac·tyl·ia
pe·ro·dac·ty·ly
per·o·gen
pe·ro·me·lia
pe·rom·e·ly
per·o·ne
per·o·ne·al
ar·tery
bone
node
phe·nom·e·non
pul·ley
veins
per·o·ne·al com·mu·ni·cat·ing
nerve
per·o·ne·al mus·cu·lar
at·ro·phy
per·o·ne·o·tib·i·al
pe·ro·pus
per·o·ral
per os
pe·ro·sis
pe·ro·splanch·nia
per·os·se·ous
per·ox·i·dase
re·ac·tion
stain
per·ox·i·das·es
horse·rad·ish p.
per·ox·ide
per·ox·i·some
per·ox·y·a·ce·tic ac·id
per·ox·y·a·ce·tyl ni·trate
per·oxy ac·id
per·ox·y·for·mic ac·id
per·ox·yl
per·pen·dic·u·lar
fas·cic·u·lus
plate
per·pet·u·al·ly grow·ing
tooth
per·phe·na·zine
per pri·mam
per rec·tum
per·salt
per sal·tum
per·se·cu·tion
com·plex
per·se·cu·to·ry
de·lu·sion
per·sev·er·a·tion
Per·sian re·laps·ing
fe·ver
per·sic oil
per·sis·tence
mi·cro·bi·al p.

per·sis·tent
  clo·a·ca
  trem·or
  trun·cus ar·te·ri·o·sus
per·sis·tent an·te·ri·or hy·per·
  plas·tic pri·mary
  vit·re·ous
per·sis·tent atri·o·ven·tric·u·lar
  ca·nal
per·sis·tent chron·ic
  hep·a·ti·tis
per·sis·tent·ly grow·ing
  tooth
per·sis·tent pos·te·ri·or hy·per·
  plas·tic pri·mary
  vit·re·ous
per·sist·er
per·so·na
per·son·al
  equa·tion
  mo·ti·va·tion
  space
per·son·al growth
  lab·o·ra·tory
per·son·al·i·ty
  dis·or·der
  for·ma·tion
  in·te·gra·tion
  in·ven·to·ry
  pro·file
  test
per·son·al·i·ty
  al·lo·tro·pic p.
  an·ti·so·cial p.
  au·thor·i·tar·i·an p.
  avoid·ant p.
  ba·sic p.
  bor·der·line p.
  com·pul·sive p.
  cy·clo·thy·mic p.
  de·pen·dent p.
  du·al p.
  his·tri·on·ic p.
  hys·ter·i·cal p.
  in·ad·e·quate p.
  mas·och·is·tic p.
  mul·ti·ple p.
  par·a·noid p.
  pas·sive-ag·gres·sive p.
  psy·cho·path·ic p.
  schiz·oid p.
  schiz·o·typ·i·cal p.
  shut-in p.
  syn·ton·ic p.
  type A p.
  type B p.
per·son-years

pers·pi·ra·tion
  in·sen·si·ble p.
  sen·si·ble p.
per·spi·ra·to·ry
  glands
per·stil·la·tion
per·sua·sion
per·sul·fate
per·sul·fide
per·sul·fu·ric ac·id
Perthes
  dis·ease
Perthes'
  test
Pertik's
  di·ver·tic·u·lum
per·tro·chan·ter·ic
  frac·ture
per tu·bam
per·tus·sis
  im·mu·no·glob·u·lin
  vac·cine
per·tus·sis im·mune
  glob·u·lin
Pe·ru·vi·an
  bark
  ta·ran·tu·la
  wart
Pe·ru·vi·an bark
per·vap·o·ra·tion
per·va·sive de·vel·op·men·tal
  dis·or·der
per·ve·nous
  pace·mak·er
per·ver·sion
  pol·y·mor·phous p.
  sex·u·al p.
per·vert
per·vert·ed
  nys·tag·mus
per·vert·ed
per·vert·ed oc·u·lar
  move·ment
per vi·as na·tu·ra·les
per·vi·gi·li·um
per·vi·ous
pes
  p. ab·duc·tus
  p. ad·duc·tus
  p. an·se·ri·nus
  p. cav·us
  p. equi·no·val·gus
  p. equi·no·var·us
  p. fe·bri·ci·tans
  p. gi·gas
  p. pe·dun·cu·li
  p. pla·nus
  p. pro·na·tus

pes *(continued)*
  p. val·gus
  p. var·us
pes·sa·ry
  di·a·phragm p.
  Dumontpallier's p.
  Gariel's p.
  Hodge's p.
  Mayer's p.
  Menge's p.
  ring p.
pes·sa·ry
  cell
  cor·pus·cle
pes·si·mism
  ther·a·peu·tic p.
pest
  fowl p.
  swine p.
pes·ti·ce·mia
pes·ti·cide
pes·tif·er·ous
pes·ti·lence
pes·ti·len·tial
pes·tis
  p. am·bu·lans
  p. ful·mi·nans
  p. ma·jor
  p. mi·nor
  p. si·de·rans
pes·ti·vi·rus
pes·tle
pe·te·chia
pe·te·chi·ae
  Tardieu's pe·te·chi·ae
pe·te·chi·al
  an·gi·o·mas
  fe·ver
  hem·or·rhage
pe·te·chi·a·sis
Peters'
  anom·a·ly
  ovum
Petersen's
  bag
pet·i·o·late
pet·i·o·lat·ed
pet·i·ole
pet·i·oled
pe·ti·o·lus
pe·tit
  mal
pe·tit mal
  ep·i·lep·sy
Petit's
  ap·o·neu·ro·sis
  ca·nals
  her·nia

her·ni·ot·o·my
lig·a·ment
si·nus
Petit's lum·bar
  tri·an·gle
Petri
  dish
pet·ri·fac·tion
pé·tris·sage
pet·roc·cip·i·tal
pe·tro·la·tum
  heavy liq·uid p.
  hy·dro·phil·ic p.
  light liq·uid p.
  white p.
pe·tro·le·um
  p. ben·zin
  p. ether
  liq·uid p.
pe·tro·le·um jel·ly
pet·ro·mas·toid
pet·ro-oc·cip·i·tal
  fis·sure
  joint
pet·ro·pha·ryn·ge·us
pe·tro·sa
pe·tro·sae
pe·tro·sal
  bone
  fo·ra·men
  fos·sa
  gan·gli·on
  im·pres·sion of the pal·li·
    um
  si·nus
  vein
pe·tro·sal·pin·go·sta·phy·li·nus
pet·ro·si·tis
pet·ro·so·mas·toid
pet·ro·sphe·noid
pet·ro·sphe·noid·al
  syn·drome
pet·ro·squa·mo·sal
pet·ro·squa·mous
  fis·sure
  su·ture
pe·tro·sta·phy·li·nus
pet·ro·tym·pan·ic
  fis·sure
pet·rous
  bone
  gan·gli·on
  part
  pyr·a·mid
pet·rou·si·tis
Pette-Döring
  dis·ease

Peutz-Jeghers
syn·drome
Peutz's
syn·drome
pex·in
pex·in·o·gen
pex·is
Peyer's
glands
patch·es
pe·yo·te
pe·yo·tl
Peyronie's
dis·ease
Peyrot's
tho·rax
Pezzer
cath·e·ter
Pfannenstiel's
in·ci·sion
Pfaundler-Hurler
syn·drome
Pfeiffer
syn·drome
Pfeif·fer·el·la
Pfeiffer's
ba·cil·lus
phe·nom·e·non
Pfeiffer's blood
agar
Pflüger's
law
Pfuhl's
sign
pH
scale
pH
crit·i·cal p.
op·ti·mum p.
phac·o·an·a·phy·lac·tic
uve·i·tis
phac·o·an·a·phy·lax·is
phac·o·cele
phac·o·cyst
phac·o·cys·tec·to·my
phac·o·don·e·sis
phac·o·e·mul·si·fi·ca·tion
phac·o·er·y·sis
phac·o·frag·men·ta·tion
phac·o·gen·ic
glau·co·ma
uve·i·tis
pha·coid
pha·col·y·sis
pha·co·lyt·ic
glau·co·ma
pha·co·ma
pha·co·ma·la·cia

phac·o·ma·to·sis
phac·o·met·a·cho·re·sis
pha·com·e·ter
phac·o·mor·phic
glau·co·ma
phac·o·scope
Phae·ni·cia ser·i·ca·ta
phae·o·hy·pho·my·co·sis
phae·o·my·cot·ic
cyst
phage
de·fec·tive p.
phag·e·de·na
p. gan·gre·no·sa
p. no·so·co·mi·a·lis
slough·ing p.
p. tro·pi·ca
phag·e·den·ic
ul·cer
phag·o·cyte
phag·o·cyt·ic
in·dex
pneu·mo·no·cyte
phag·o·cy·tin
phag·o·cy·tize
phag·o·cy·to·blast
phag·o·cy·tol·y·sis
phag·o·cy·to·lyt·ic
phag·o·cy·tose
phag·o·cy·to·sis
in·duced p.
spon·ta·ne·ous p.
phag·o·dy·na·mom·e·ter
pha·gol·y·sis
phag·o·ly·so·some
phag·o·lyt·ic
phag·o·ma·nia
phag·o·pho·bia
phag·o·some
phag·o·type
pha·kic
eye
pha·ko·ma
phak·o·ma·to·sis
phal·a·cro·sis
pha·lan·ge·al
cells
joints
phal·an·gec·to·my
pha·lan·ges
pha·lan·gis
pha·lanx
tufted p.
un·gual p.
phal·lal·gia
phal·lec·to·my
phalli

phal·lic
  phase
  tu·ber·cle
phal·li·cism
phal·li·form
phal·lism
phal·li·tis
phal·lo·camp·sis
phal·lo·cryp·sis
phal·lo·dyn·ia
phal·loid
phal·loi·din
phal·lol·y·sin
phal·lon·cus
phal·lo·plas·ty
phal·lor·rha·gia
phal·lor·rhea
phal·lot·o·my
phal·lus
phan·er·o·gen·ic
phan·er·o·ma·nia
phan·er·o·scope
phan·er·o·sis
  fat·ty p.
phan·er·o·zo·ite
phan·quone
phan·ta·sia
phan·tasm
phan·tas·ma·go·ria
phan·tas·ma·to·mo·ria
phan·tas·mol·o·gy
phan·tas·mo·sco·pia
phan·tas·mos·co·py
phan·tom
  Schultze's p.
phan·tom
  an·eu·rysm
  cor·pus·cle
  limb
  preg·nan·cy
  tu·mor
phan·tom·ize
phan·tom limb
  pain
phar·ma·cal
phar·ma·ceu·tic
phar·ma·ceu·ti·cal
  chem·is·try
phar·ma·ceu·tics
phar·ma·ceu·tist
phar·ma·cist
phar·ma·co·chem·is·try
phar·ma·co·di·ag·no·sis
phar·ma·co·dy·nam·ic
phar·ma·co·dy·nam·ics
phar·ma·co·en·do·cri·nol·o·gy
phar·ma·co·ge·net·ics
phar·ma·cog·no·sist

phar·ma·cog·no·sy
phar·ma·cog·ra·phy
phar·ma·co·ki·net·ic
phar·ma·co·ki·net·ics
phar·ma·co·log·ic
  me·di·a·tors of an·a·phy·
    lax·is
phar·ma·co·log·i·cal
phar·ma·col·o·gist
  clin·i·cal p.
phar·ma·col·o·gy
  bi·o·chem·i·cal p.
  clin·i·cal p.
  ma·rine p.
phar·ma·co·ma·nia
phar·ma·co·pe·dia
phar·ma·co·pe·dics
Phar·ma·co·pe·ia
phar·ma·co·pe·ial
  gel
phar·ma·co·phi·lia
phar·ma·co·pho·bia
Phar·ma·co·poe·ia
phar·ma·co·psy·cho·sis
phar·ma·co·ther·a·py
phar·ma·cy
  clin·i·cal p.
phar·yn·gal·gia
pha·ryn·ge·al
  an·es·the·sia
  arch·es
  bur·sa
  cal·cu·lus
  ca·nal
  fis·tu·la
  flap
  glands
  grooves
  hy·poph·y·sis
  isth·mus
  mem·branes
  open·ing of au·di·to·ry tube
  open·ing of eu·sta·chi·an
    tube
  pi·tu·i·tary
  plex·us
  pouch·es
  re·cess
  re·flex
  space
  ton·sil
  tu·ber·cle
  veins
pha·ryn·ge·al pouch
  syn·drome
phar·yn·gec·to·my
phar·yn·gem·phrax·is
pha·ryn·ges

pha·ryn·ge·us
pha·ryn·gis
phar·yn·gis·mus
phar·yn·git·ic
phar·yn·gi·tis
   acute lym·pho·nod·u·lar p.
   atroph·ic p.
   croup·ous p.
   fol·lic·u·lar p.
   gan·gre·nous p.
   glan·du·lar p.
   gran·u·lar p.
   p. her·pe·ti·ca
   p. hy·per·tro·phi·ca la·te·
     ra·lis
   mem·bra·nous p.
   p. sic·ca
   ul·cer·a·tive p.
   ul·cer·o·mem·bra·nous p.
pha·ryn·go·bas·i·lar
   fas·cia
pha·ryn·go·bran·chi·al
   ducts
pha·ryn·go·cele
pha·ryn·go·con·junc·ti·val
   fe·ver
pha·ryn·go·con·junc·ti·val fe·
  ver
   vi·rus
pha·ryn·go·dyn·ia
pha·ryn·go·ep·i·glot·tic
   fold
pha·ryn·go·ep·i·glot·tid·e·an
pha·ryn·go·e·soph·a·ge·al
   cush·ions
   di·ver·tic·u·lum
   pads
pha·ryn·go·e·soph·a·go·plas·ty
pha·ryn·go·glos·sal
pha·ryn·go·glos·sus
pha·ryn·go·ker·a·to·sis
pha·ryn·go·la·ryn·ge·al
pha·ryn·go·lar·yn·gi·tis
pha·ryn·go·lith
phar·yn·gol·o·gy
pha·ryn·go·max·il·lary
   space
pha·ryn·go·my·co·sis
pha·ryn·go·na·sal
   cav·i·ty
pha·ryn·go-oral
pha·ryn·go·pal·a·tine
   arch
pha·ryn·go·pa·la·ti·nus
pha·ryn·go·path·ia
phar·yn·gop·a·thy
pha·ryn·go·pe·ris·to·le
pha·ryn·go·plas·ty

pha·ryn·go·ple·gia
pha·ryn·go·rhi·ni·tis
pha·ryn·go·rhi·nos·co·py
pha·ryn·go·scle·ro·ma
pha·ryn·go·scope
phar·yn·gos·co·py
pha·ryn·go·spasm
pha·ryn·go·sta·phy·li·nus
pha·ryn·go·ste·no·sis
phar·yn·got·o·my
pha·ryn·go·ton·sil·li·tis
pha·ryn·go·tym·pan·ic
   groove
   tube
pha·ryn·go·ty·phoid
pha·ryn·go·xe·ro·sis
phar·ynx
   la·ryn·ge·al p.
   na·sal p.
   oral p.
phase
   anal p.
   aque·ous p.
   cis p.
   con·tin·u·ous p.
   cou·pling p.
   dis·con·tin·u·ous p.
   dis·persed p.
   dis·per·sion p.
   eclipse p.
   erup·tive p.
   ex·ter·nal p.
   gen·i·tal p.
   in·ter·nal p.
   lag p.
   la·ten·cy p.
   log·a·rith·mic p.
   lu·te·al p.
   mei·ot·ic p.
   neg·a·tive p.
   oe·di·pal p.
   oral p.
   phal·lic p.
   pos·i·tive p.
   post·mei·ot·ic p.
   post·re·duc·tion p.
   pre·gen·i·tal p.
   pre·mei·ot·ic p.
   pre-oed·i·pal p.
   pre·re·duc·tion p.
   ra·di·al growth p.
   re·duc·tion p.
   S p.
   short lu·te·al p.
   sta·tion·ary p.
   su·per·nor·mal re·cov·ery p.
   syn·ap·tic p.
   trans p.

phase *(continued)*
   ver·ti·cal growth p.
   vul·ner·a·ble p.
in phase
phase
   mi·cro·scope
   rule
phase-con·trast
   mi·cro·scope
phase I
   block
phase II
   block
pha·sic
   re·flex
pha·sic si·nus
   ar·rhyth·mia
phas·mid
Phas·mid·ia
phas·mo·pho·bia
phat·nor·rha·gia
PHC
   syn·drome
P-H con·duc·tion
   time
Phem·is·ter
   graft
phen·a·caine hy·dro·chlo·ride
phen·ac·e·mide
phen·ac·e·tin
phen·ac·e·tur·ic ac·id
phen·ac·ri·dane chlo·ride
phen·a·cy·cla·mine
phen·a·dox·one hy·dro·chlo·ride
phen·a·gly·co·dol
phen·an·threne
   nu·cle·us
phen·ar·sen·a·mine
phen·ar·sone sulf·ox·y·late
phe·nate
phen·az·a·cil·lin
phe·naz·o·cine
phen·az·o·line hy·dro·chlo·ride
phen·az·o·pyr·i·dine hy·dro·
   chlo·ride
phen·cy·cli·dine
phen·di·me·tra·zine tar·trate
phen·el·zine sul·fate
phe·net·a·mine
phen·e·thar·bi·tal
phe·neth·i·cil·lin po·tas·si·um
phen·eth·yl al·co·hol
phe·net·sal
phe·net·u·ride
phen·for·min hy·dro·chlo·ride
phen·glu·tar·i·mide hy·dro·
   chlo·ride
phen·go·pho·bia

phe·nic ac·id
phen·i·car·ba·zide
phe·nin·da·mine tar·trate
phen·in·di·one
phen·ir·a·mine ma·le·ate
phen·meth·y·lol
phen·met·ra·zine hy·dro·chlo·
   ride
phe·no·bar·bi·tal
phe·no·bu·ti·o·dil
phe·no·copy
phe·no·de·vi·ant
phe·no·din
phe·nol
   cam·phor·at·ed p.
   liq·ue·fied p.
   p. ox·i·dase
phe·nol
   co·ef·fi·cient
phe·no·lase
phe·no·lat·ed
phe·nol·e·mia
phe·nol·o·gy
phe·nol·phthal·e·in
phe·nol red
phe·nol·sul·fon·phthal·e·in
   test
phe·nol·u·ria
phe·nom·e·na
phe·nom·e·nol·o·gy
phe·nom·e·non
   ad·he·sion p.
   AFORMED p.
   Anrep p.
   aque·ous in·flux p.
   Arias-Stella p.
   arm p.
   Arthus p.
   Ascher's aque·ous in·flux p.
   Aschner's p.
   Ashley's p.
   Ashman's p.
   Aubert's p.
   au·to·scop·ic p.
   Babinski's p.
   Bell's p.
   Bom·bay p.
   Bordet-Gengou p.
   break·a·way p.
   break·off p.
   Brücke-Bartley p.
   Capgras' p.
   cer·vi·co·lum·bar p.
   cog·wheel p.
   con·stan·cy p.
   crossed phren·ic p.
   Cushing p.
   Danysz p.

dawn p.
Debré p.
de·clamp·ing p.
dé·jà vu p.
Dejerine-Lichtheim p.
Dejerine's hand p.
Denys-Leclef p.
d'Herelle p.
di·a·phragm p.
dip p.
Donath-Landsteiner p.
Doppler p.
Duckworth's p.
Ehret's p.
Ehrlich's p.
eryth·ro·cyte ad·her·ence p.
es·cape p.
fa·ci·a·lis p.
fin·ger p.
Friedreich's p.
Galassi's pu·pil·lary p.
Gallavardin's p.
gap p.
Gärtner's vein p.
gen·er·al·ized Shwartzman
  p.
Gengou p.
ge·stalt p.
Goldblatt p.
Grasset-Gaussel p.
Grasset's p.
Gunn p.
Hamburger's p.
Hill's p.
hip p.
hip-flex·ion p.
Hoffmann's p.
Houssay p.
hunt·ing p.
Hunt's par·a·dox·i·cal p.
im·mune ad·her·ence p.
jaw-wink·ing p.
Jod-Basedow p.
knee p.
Köbner's p.
Koch's p.
Kohnstamm's p.
Kühne's p.
LE p.
leg p.
Leichtenstern's p.
Litten's p.
Lucio's lep·ro·sy p.
Marcus Gunn p.
mis·di·rec·tion p.
Mitzuo's p.
Negro's p.
no re·flow p.

on-off p.
or·bi·cu·la·ris p.
par·a·dox·i·cal di·a·phragm
  p.
par·a·dox·i·cal pu·pil·lary
  p.
per·o·ne·al p.
Pfeiffer's p.
phi p.
phren·ic p.
Pool's p.
pseu·do-Graefe's p.
psi p.
Purkinje's p.
quel·lung p.
ra·di·al p.
Raynaud's p.
re·bound p.
re·clot·ting p.
red cell ad·her·ence p.
re·en·try p.
re·lease p.
Ritter-Rollet p.
R-on-T p.
Rust's p.
Sanarelli p.
Sanarelli-Shwartzman p.
Schellong-Strisower p.
Schiff-Sherrington p.
Schüller's p.
Schultz-Charlton p.
Sherrington p.
shot-silk p.
Shwartzman p.
Somogyi p.
Soret's p.
Splendore-Hoeppli p.
stair·case p.
steal p.
Strassman's p.
Strümpell's p.
sym·bi·ot·ic fer·men·ta·tion
  p.
Theobald Smith's p.
tib·i·al p.
toe p.
tongue p.
Tournay's p.
Twort p.
Twort-d'Herelle p.
Tyndall p.
Wenckebach p.
Westphal-Piltz p.
Westphal's p.
Wever-Bray p.
phe·no·per·i·dine
phe·no·thi·a·zine
phe·no·type

phe·no·typ·ic
mix·ing
val·ue
phen·ox·a·zine
phen·ox·a·zone
phe·nox·y·ben·za·mine hy·dro·chlo·ride
phe·nox·y·meth·yl·pen·i·cil·lin
phe·no·zy·gous
phen·pen·ter·mine tar·trate
phen·pro·ba·mate
phen·pro·cou·mon
phen·pro·pi·o·nate
phen·sux·i·mide
phen·ter·mine
phen·tol·a·mine
test
phen·tol·a·mine hy·dro·chlo·ride
phen·tol·a·mine mes·y·late
phen·yl
p. al·co·hol
p. ami·no·sa·lic·y·late
p. sa·lic·y·late
phen·yl·a·ce·tic ac·id
phen·yl·a·ce·tur·ic ac·id
phen·yl·a·ce·tyl·u·rea
phen·yl·a·cryl·ic ac·id
phen·yl·al·a·nin·ase
phen·yl·al·a·nine
phen·yl·al·a·nyl
chain
phen·yl·a·mine
phen·yl·ben·zene
phen·yl·bu·ta·zone
phen·yl·car·bi·nol
phen·yl·eph·rine hy·dro·chlo·ride
phen·yl·eth·yl al·co·hol
phen·yl·eth·yl·bar·bi·tur·ic ac·id
phen·yl·eth·yl·mal·o·nyl·u·rea
phen·yl·gly·col·ic ac·id
phen·yl·in·dane·di·one
phen·yl·i·so·thi·o·cy·a·nate
phen·yl·ke·to·nu·ria
phen·yl·lac·tic ac·id
phen·yl·mer·cu·ric ac·e·tate
phen·yl·mer·cu·ric ni·trate
phen·yl·pip·er·one
phen·yl·pro·pa·nol·a·mine
phe·nyl·py·ru·vic
amen·tia
phen·yl·thi·o·car·ba·mide
phen·yl·thi·o·car·bam·o·yl
pep·tide
pro·tein
phen·yl·thi·o·hy·dan·to·in

phen·yl·thi·o·u·rea
phen·yl·to·lox·a·mine
phen·yl·tri·meth·yl·am·mo·ni·um
phen·y·ram·i·dol hy·dro·chlo·ride
phen·yt·o·in
phe·o·chrome
cell
phe·o·chro·mo·blast
phe·o·chro·mo·blas·to·ma
phe·o·chro·mo·cyte
phe·o·chro·mo·cy·to·ma
phe·o·mel·a·nin
phe·o·mel·a·no·gen·e·sis
phe·o·mel·a·no·some
phe·o·phor·bide
phe·o·phor·bin
phe·o·phy·tin
phe·re·sis
pher·o·mones
phi
phe·nom·e·non
phi·al
phi·a·lide
phi·a·lo·co·nid·ia
phi·a·lo·co·nid·i·um
Phi·a·loph·o·ra
Phi·a·lo·phore-type
co·nid·i·o·phore
Phil·a·del·phia
chro·mo·some
cock·tail
phil·an·throp·ic
hos·pi·tal
phil·i·a·ter
Philippe's
tri·an·gle
Philip's
glands
Phillips'
cath·e·ter
Phillipson's
re·flex
phi·lo·mi·me·sia
Phil·o·pia ca·sei
phil·o·pro·gen·i·tive
phil·tra
phil·trum
phi·mo·ses
phi·mo·sis
p. va·gi·na·lis
phi·mot·ic
phle·bal·gia
phleb·ar·ter·i·ec·ta·sia
phleb·ec·ta·sia
phle·bec·to·my
phle·bec·to·pia

phle·bec·to·py
phleb·em·phrax·is
phleb·eu·rysm
phle·bis·mus
phle·bit·ic
phle·bi·tis
    ad·he·sive p.
    p. no·du·la·ris ne·cro·ti·
     sans
    pu·er·per·al p.
    sep·tic p.
    si·nus p.
phleb·o·cly·sis
    drip p.
phleb·o·dy·nam·ics
phleb·o·gram
phleb·o·graph
phle·bog·ra·phy
phleb·oid
phleb·o·lite
phleb·o·lith
phleb·o·li·thi·a·sis
phle·bol·o·gy
phle·bo·ma·nom·e·ter
phleb·o·me·tri·tis
phleb·o·my·o·ma·to·sis
phleb·o·phle·bos·to·my
phleb·o·plas·ty
phleb·or·rha·gia
phle·bor·rha·phy
phleb·or·rhex·is
phleb·o·scle·ro·sis
phle·bos·ta·sis
phleb·o·ste·no·sis
phleb·o·strep·sis
phleb·o·throm·bo·sis
phle·bot·o·mine
phle·bot·o·mist
Phle·bot·o·mus
    P. ar·gen·ti·pes
    P. chin·en·sis
    P. fla·vis·cu·tel·la·tus
    P. lon·gi·pal·pis
    P. ma·jor
    P. no·gu·chi
    P. or·i·en·ta·lis
    P. pa·pa·ta·si·i
    P. per·ni·ci·o·sus
    P. ser·genti
    P. ver·ru·ca·rum
phle·bot·o·mus
    fe·ver
phle·bot·o·mus fe·ver
    vi·rus·es
phle·bot·o·my
    blood·less p.
Phleb·o·vi·rus
phlegm

phleg·ma·sia
    p. al·ba do·lens
    cel·lu·lit·ic p.
    p. ce·ru·lea do·lens
    p. do·lens
    p. ma·la·ba·ri·ca
    throm·bot·ic p.
phleg·mat·ic
phleg·mon
    dif·fuse p.
    em·phy·sem·a·tous p.
    gas p.
phleg·mon·ous
    ab·scess
    cel·lu·li·tis
    en·ter·i·tis
    er·y·sip·e·las
    gas·tri·tis
    mas·ti·tis
    ul·cer
phlo·go·cyte
phlo·go·cy·to·sis
phlo·go·gen·ic
phlo·gog·e·nous
phlo·go·sin
phlo·go·ther·a·py
phlo·rid·zin
    di·a·be·tes
    gly·cos·ur·ia
phlo·ri·zin
    gly·cos·ur·ia
phlor·o·glu·cin
phlor·o·glu·cin·ol
phlor·o·glu·col
phlox·ine
phlyc·te·na
phlyc·te·nae
phlyc·te·nar
phlyc·te·noid
phlyc·te·no·sis
phlyc·te·nous
phlyc·ten·u·la
phlyc·ten·u·lae
phlyc·ten·u·lar
    con·junc·ti·vi·tis
    ker·a·ti·tis
    oph·thal·mia
    pan·nus
phlyc·ten·ule
phlyc·ten·u·lo·sis
PhNCS
    pro·tein
pho·ban·thro·py
pho·bia
pho·bic
pho·bo·pho·bia
pho·co·me·lia

781

pho·co·me·lic
dwarf·ism
pho·com·e·ly
phol·co·dine
phol·e·drine
Pho·ma
pho·nac·o·scope
pho·na·cos·co·py
pho·nal
phon·as·the·nia
pho·na·tion
pho·na·tory
phon·au·to·graph
pho·neme
pho·ne·mic
re·gres·sion
pho·nen·do·scope
pho·net·ic
pho·net·ics
pho·ni·at·rics
phon·ic
spasm
pho·nism
pho·no·an·gi·og·ra·phy
pho·no·car·di·o·gram
pho·no·car·di·o·graph
lin·e·ar p.
log·a·rith·mic p.
spec·tral p.
steth·o·scop·ic p.
pho·no·car·di·og·ra·phy
pho·no·cath·e·ter
pho·no·gram
pho·nol·o·gy
pho·no·ma·nia
pho·nom·e·ter
pho·no·my·oc·lo·nus
pho·no·my·og·ra·phy
pho·nop·a·thy
pho·no·pho·bia
pho·no·phore
pho·no·pho·tog·ra·phy
pho·nop·sia
pho·no·re·cep·tor
pho·no·re·no·gram
pho·no·scope
pho·nos·co·py
phor·bide
phor·bin
phor·bol
pho·re·sis
phor·e·sy
phor·ia
Phor·mia re·gi·na
pho·rom·e·ter
pho·ro-op·tom·e·ter
pho·rop·ter
phor·o·scope

phor·o·zo·on
phos·gene
phos·pha·gen
phos·pha·gen·ic
phos·pham·ic ac·id
phos·pham·i·dase
phos·pha·stat
phos·pha·tase
ac·id p.
al·ka·line p.
phos·pha·tase
unit
phos·phate
di·a·be·tes
tet·a·ny
phos·phate
bone p.
cy·clic p.
di·hy·dro·gen p.
di·so·di·um p.
en·er·gy-rich p.'s
high en·er·gy p.'s
mon·o·po·tas·si·um p.
mon·o·so·di·um p.
nor·mal p.
or·gan·ic p.
tri·ple p.
phos·phate ace·tyl·trans·fer·ase
phos·phat·ed
phos·pha·te·mia
phos·phat·ic
phos·pha·ti·dal
phos·pha·ti·dase
phos·pha·ti·date
phos·pha·tide
phos·pha·tid·ic ac·id
phos·pha·ti·do·lip·ase
phos·pha·ti·dyl
phos·pha·ti·dyl·cho·line
phos·pha·ti·dyl·eth·a·nol·a·mine
phos·phat·i·dyl·glyc·er·ol
phos·pha·ti·dyl·in·o·si·tol
phos·pha·ti·dyl·ser·ine
phos·pha·tu·ria
phos·phene
ac·com·mo·da·tion p.
phos·phide
phos·phine
phos·phite
phos·pho·ac·y·lase
phos·pho·am·i·dase
phos·pho·am·ides
phos·pho·ar·gi·nine
phos·pho·cho·line
phos·pho·cre·a·tine
phos·pho·di·es·ter
p. hy·dro·las·es

phos·pho·di·es·ter·as·es
 spleen p.
phos·pho·dis·mu·tase
phos·pho·e·nol·pyr·u·vic ac·id
phos·pho·ga·lac·to·i·som·er·ase
phos·pho·glu·co·ki·nase
phos·pho·glu·co·mu·tase
phos·pho·glu·co·nate
 path·way
phos·pho·glu·co·nate de·hy·dro·
 gen·ase
phos·pho·glyc·er·ac·e·tals
phos·pho·glyc·er·ate ki·nase
phos·pho·gly·cer·ic ac·id
phos·pho·glyc·er·ides
phos·pho·glyc·er·o·mu·tase
phos·pho·hex·o·ki·nase
phos·pho·hex·o·mu·tase
phos·pho·hex·ose isom·er·ase
 de·fi·cien·cy
phos·pho·hy·dro·las·es
phos·pho·in·o·si·tide
phos·pho·ki·nase
phos·pho·li·pase
 p. B
 p. C
 p. D
phos·pho·lip·id
phos·pho·mu·tase
phos·pho·ne·cro·sis
phos·pho·ni·um
phos·pho·pen·tose isom·er·ase
phos·pho·pro·tein
phos·pho·py·ru·vate hy·dra·tase
phos·phor
phos·phor·at·ed
phos·pho·res·cence
phos·pho·res·cent
phos·phor·hi·dro·sis
phos·pho·ri·bo·i·som·er·ase
phos·pho·ri·bo·syl·gly·cine·a·
 mide syn·the·tase
phos·pho·ri·bo·syl·trans·fer·ase
phos·pho·ri·bu·lo·ki·nase
phos·pho·ri·bu·lose ep·i·mer·
 ase
phos·phor·ic ac·id
 cy·clic p. a.
 di·lute p. a.
 gla·cial p. a.
phos·phor·i·dro·sis
phos·phor·ism
phos·phor·ized
phos·phor·o·clas·tic
 cleav·age
 re·ac·tion
phos·pho·rol·y·sis
phos·pho·rous

phos·pho·rous ac·id
phos·phor·u·ria
phos·pho·rus
 amor·phous p.
 p. pen·tox·ide
 red p.
phos·pho·ryl
phos·pho·ryl·ase
 p. *a*
 p. *b*
 p. phos·pha·tase
phos·pho·ryl·ase-rup·tur·ing
 en·zyme
phos·pho·ryl·as·es
 nu·cle·o·side p.
phos·pho·ryl·a·tion
 ox·i·da·tive p.
phos·pho·ryl·cho·line
phos·pho·ryl·eth·a·nol·a·mine
 glyc·er·ide·trans·fer·ase
phos·pho·sphin·go·sides
phos·pho·sug·ar
phos·pho·trans·a·cet·y·lase
phos·pho·trans·fer·as·es
phos·pho·tri·ose isom·er·ase
phos·pho·tung·stic ac·id
 he·ma·tox·y·lin
 stain
phos·phu·ret·ed
 hy·dro·gen
phos·phu·ria
phos·vi·tin
phot
pho·tal·gia
pho·tau·gi·a·pho·bia
pho·tech·ic
 ef·fect
pho·techy
pho·te·ryth·rous
pho·tes·the·sia
pho·tic
 driv·ing
 stim·u·la·tion
pho·tism
pho·to
 ret·i·nop·a·thy
pho·to·ac·tin·ic
pho·to·al·ler·gic
 sen·si·tiv·i·ty
pho·to·al·ler·gy
pho·to·au·to·troph
pho·to·au·to·tro·phic
pho·to·bac·te·ria
Pho·to·bac·te·ri·um
 P. har·veyi
 P. phos·pho·re·um
pho·to·bac·te·ri·um
pho·to·bi·ol·o·gy

pho·to·bi·ot·ic
pho·to·cat·a·lyst
pho·to·cep·tor
pho·to·chem·i·cal
pho·to·chem·is·try
pho·to·che·mo·ther·a·py
pho·to·chro·mic
  lens
  spec·ta·cles
pho·to·chro·mo·gens
pho·to·co·ag·u·la·tion
pho·to·co·ag·u·la·tor
  la·ser p.
  xe·non-arc p.
pho·to·der·ma·ti·tis
pho·to·dis·tri·bu·tion
pho·tod·ro·my
pho·to·dy·nam·ic
  sen·si·ti·za·tion
pho·to·dyn·ia
pho·to·dys·pho·ria
pho·to·e·lec·tric
  ef·fect
pho·to·e·lec·trom·e·ter
pho·to·e·lec·tron
pho·to·er·y·the·ma
pho·to·es·thet·ic
pho·to·flu·o·rog·ra·phy
pho·to·gas·tro·scope
pho·to·gen
pho·to·gen·e·sis
pho·to·gen·ic
  ep·i·lep·sy
pho·tog·e·nous
pho·to·he·mo·ta·chom·e·ter
pho·to·het·er·o·troph
pho·to·het·er·o·tro·phic
pho·to·in·ac·ti·va·tion
pho·to·ki·ne·sis
pho·to·ki·net·ic
pho·to·ki·net·ics
pho·to·ky·mo·graph
pho·tol·o·gy
pho·to·lu·mi·nes·cent
pho·to·ly·ase
pho·tol·y·sis
pho·to·lyte
pho·to·lyt·ic
pho·to·mac·rog·ra·phy
pho·to·ma·nia
pho·tom·e·ter
  flame p.
  flick·er p.
pho·tom·e·try
pho·to·mi·cro·graph
pho·to·mi·crog·ra·phy
pho·to·mul·ti·pli·er
  tube

pho·to·my·oc·lo·nus
  he·red·i·tary p.
pho·ton
  den·si·ty
pho·ton·cia
pho·ton·o·sus
pho·to-patch
  test
pho·top·a·thy
pho·to·per·cep·tive
pho·to·pe·ri·od·ism
pho·to·pho·bia
pho·to·pho·bic
pho·to·phore
pho·to·phos·pho·ry·la·tion
pho·toph·thal·mia
pho·to·pia
pho·top·ic
  ad·ap·ta·tion
  eye
  vi·sion
pho·top·sia
pho·top·sin
pho·top·sy
pho·to·ptar·mo·sis
pho·top·tom·e·try
pho·to·ra·di·a·tion
  ther·a·py
pho·to·re·ac·tion
pho·to·re·ac·ti·vat·ing
  en·zyme
pho·to·re·ac·ti·va·tion
pho·to·re·cep·tive
pho·to·re·cep·tor
  cells
pho·to·ret·i·ni·tis
pho·to·ret·i·nop·a·thy
pho·to·scan
pho·to·sen·si·ti·za·tion
pho·to·sen·sor
  oc·u·log·ra·phy
pho·to·sta·ble
pho·to·steth·o·scope
pho·to·stress
  test
pho·to·syn·the·sis
pho·to·tax·is
pho·to·ther·a·py
pho·to·ther·mal
pho·tot·o·nus
pho·to·tox·ic
  sen·si·tiv·i·ty
pho·to·tox·is
pho·tot·ro·pism
pho·tu·ria
phrag·mo·plast
phren
phre·nal·gia

phre·nec·to·my
phren·em·phrax·is
phre·net·ic
phren·ic
    gan·glia
    nerve
    phe·nom·e·non
    plex·us
    veins
    wave
phren·i·cec·to·my
phren·i·cla·sia
phren·i·co·col·ic
    lig·a·ment
phren·i·co·cos·tal
    si·nus
phren·i·co·ex·er·e·sis
phren·i·co·li·e·nal
    lig·a·ment
phren·i·co·me·di·as·ti·nal
    re·cess
phren·i·co·neu·rec·to·my
phren·i·co·pleur·al
    fas·cia
phren·i·co·splen·ic
    lig·a·ment
phren·i·cot·o·my
phren·i·co·trip·sy
phren·ic pres·sure
    test
phren·o·car·dia
phren·o·col·ic
phren·o·col·o·pexy
phren·o·gas·tric
    lig·a·ment
phren·o·glot·tic
phren·o·graph
phren·o·he·pat·ic
phre·nol·o·gist
phre·nol·o·gy
phre·no·per·i·car·di·al
    an·gle
phren·o·ple·gia
phren·op·to·sia
phren·o·sin
phren·o·sin·ic ac·id
phren·o·spasm
phren·o·splen·ic
    lig·a·ment
phren·o·tro·pic
phric·to·path·ic
phryg·i·an
    cap
phryn·o·der·ma
phry·nol·y·sin
pH-stat
phthal·ein
    test

phthal·ic ac·id
phthal·o·yl
phthal·yl
phthal·yl·sul·fa·cet·a·mide
phthal·yl·sul·fa·thi·a·zole
phthin·oid
    chest
phthi·ri·o·pho·bia
Phthi·rus
phthis·ic
phthis·i·cal
phthi·sis
    an·eu·rys·mal p.
    p. bul·bi
    es·sen·tial p. bul·bi
    mar·ble cut·ters' p.
phy·co·bil·ins
phy·co·chrome
phy·co·cy·a·nin
phy·co·e·ryth·rin
Phy·co·my·ce·tes
phy·co·my·ce·to·sis
phy·co·my·co·sis
phy·go·ga·lac·tic
phy·la
phy·lac·a·gog·ic
phy·lax·is
phy·let·ic
phyl·lo·chro·ma·nol
phyl·lo·chro·me·nol
phyl·lode
phyl·lodes
    tu·mor
phyl·lo·er·y·thrin
phyl·lo·por·phy·rin
phyl·lo·pyr·role
phyl·lo·qui·none
    p. re·duc·tase
phyl·lo·qui·none K
phy·lo·a·nal·y·sis
phy·lo·gen·e·sis
phy·lo·ge·net·ic
phy·lo·gen·ic
phy·log·e·ny
phy·lum
phy·ma
phy·ma·toid
phy·ma·tor·rhy·sin
phy·ma·to·sis
Phy·sa
phys·a·lif·er·ous
phy·sal·i·form
phy·sal·i·phore
phys·a·liph·or·ous
    cell
phys·a·lis
Phy·sa·lop·tera
phy·sa·lop·ter·i·a·sis

phys·e·al
phys·i·at·rics
phys·i·a·trist
phys·i·a·try
phys·ic
phys·i·cal
   age
   al·ler·gy
   an·thro·pol·o·gy
   di·ag·no·sis
   elas·tic·i·ty of mus·cle
   ex·am·i·na·tion
   fit·ness
   half-life
   med·i·cine
   sign
   ther·a·py
phys·i·cal mix·ture
phy·si·cian
   os·te·o·path·ic p.
phy·si·cian as·sis·tant
Physick's
   pouch·es
phys·i·co·chem·i·cal
phys·ics
phys·i·o·gen·ic
phys·i·og·no·my
phys·i·og·no·sis
phys·i·o·log·ic
   age
   al·bu·min·ur·ia
   amen·or·rhea
   ane·mia
   an·ti·dote
   con·ges·tion
   cup
   dwarf·ism
   elas·tic·i·ty of mus·cle
   equi·lib·ri·um
   ex·ca·va·tion
   hy·per·tro·phy
   ic·ter·us
   in·com·pat·i·bil·i·ty
   jaun·dice
   leu·ko·cy·to·sis
   oc·clu·sion
   scle·ro·sis
   sco·to·ma
   unit
phys·i·o·log·i·cal
   anat·o·my
   chem·is·try
   drives
   ho·me·o·sta·sis
   sa·line
   sphinc·ter
phys·i·o·log·i·cal·ly bal·anced
   oc·clu·sion

phys·i·o·log·ic dead
   space
phys·i·o·log·i·co·an·a·tom·i·cal
phys·i·o·log·ic rest
   po·si·tion
phys·i·o·log·ic re·trac·tion
   ring
phys·i·ol·o·gist
phys·i·ol·o·gy
   com·par·a·tive p.
   de·vel·op·men·tal p.
   gen·er·al p.
   hom·i·nal p.
   path·o·log·ic p.
phys·i·o·med·i·cal
phys·i·o·path·o·log·ic
phys·i·o·pa·thol·o·gy
phys·i·o·psy·chic
phys·i·o·py·rex·ia
phys·i·o·ther·a·peu·tic
phys·i·o·ther·a·pist
phys·i·o·ther·a·py
   oral p.
phy·sique
phy·sis
phy·so·cele
Phy·so·ceph·a·lus sex·a·la·tus
phy·so·ceph·a·ly
phy·so·me·tra
Phy·sop·sis
phy·so·py·o·sal·pinx
phy·so·stig·ma
phy·so·stig·mine
   p. sa·lic·y·late
phy·tan·ate
phy·tan·ic ac·id
phy·tate
phy·tic ac·id
phy·tin
phy·to·ag·glu·ti·nin
phy·to·be·zoar
phy·to·chem·is·try
phy·to·cho·les·ter·ol
phy·to·der·ma·ti·tis
Phy·to·fla·gel·la·ta
phy·to·flu·ene
phy·to·hem·ag·glu·ti·nin
phy·toid
phy·tol
phy·to·lec·tin
Phy·to·mas·ti·gi·na
Phy·to·mas·ti·go·pho·ras·i·da
Phy·to·mas·ti·goph·o·rea
phy·to·men·a·di·one
phy·to·mi·to·gen
phy·to·na·di·one
phy·to·nu·cle·ic ac·id
phy·toph·a·gous

phy·to·phlyc·to·der·ma·ti·tis
phy·to·pho·to·der·ma·ti·tis
phy·to·pneu·mo·co·ni·o·sis
phy·to·por·phy·rin
phy·to·sphin·go·sine
phy·to·ste·a·rin
phy·to·ster·in
phy·to·ste·rol
Phy·to·tox·ic
phy·to·tox·in
phy·to·trich·o·be·zoar
phy·tyl
phy·tyl al·co·hol
pia-a·rach·ni·tis
pia-a·rach·noid
pi·al
   fun·nel
pi·al-gli·al
   mem·brane
pia mat·er
pia mat·er en·ceph·a·li
pia mat·er spi·na·lis
pi·an
   p. bois
   hem·or·rhag·ic p.
pi·a·nist's
   cramp
pi·a·no-play·er's
   cramp
pi·a·rach·noid
pi·blok·to
pi·blok·tog
pi·ca
Picchini's
   syn·drome
Pick
   cell
pick·ling
Pick's
   at·ro·phy
   bod·ies
   bun·dle
   dis·ease
   syn·drome
Pick's tu·bu·lar
   ad·e·no·ma
Pick·wick·i·an
   syn·drome
pi·co·gram
pi·co·lin·ic ac·id
pi·co·li·nur·ic ac·id
pi·com·e·ter
pi cone
   mon·o·chro·ma·sy
Pi·cor·na·vir·i·dae
pi·cor·na·vi·rus
pic·ram·ic ac·id
Pic·ras·ma

pic·rate
pic·ric ac·id
pic·ro·car·mine
   stain
pic·ro·for·mol
   fix·a·tive
pic·ro-Mallory tri·chrome
   stain
pic·ro·ni·gro·sin
   stain
pic·ro·tox·in
pic·ro·tox·in·in
pic·ryl
pic·to·graph
pic·ture
   el·e·ment
pie·bald
   eye·lash
   skin
pie·bald·ism
pie·bald·ness
piece
   end p.
   Fab p.
   Fc p.
   mid·dle p.
   prin·ci·pal p.
pie·dra
   black p.
   p. nos·tras
   white p.
Pi·e·dra·ia
pieds ter·mi·naux
Pierre Robin
   syn·drome
pi·e·ses·the·sia
pi·e·sim·e·ter
   Hales' p.
pi·e·sis
pi·e·som·e·ter
pi·e·zo·chem·is·try
pi·e·zo·e·lec·tric
pi·e·zo·e·lec·tric·i·ty
pi·e·zo·gen·ic
pi·e·zo·gen·ic ped·al
   pap·ule
pi·e·zom·e·ter
pig
   skin
pig·bel
pi·geon
   breast
pi·geon's
   milk
pig·ment
   cell
   cells of iris
   cell of skin

pig·ment *(continued)*
  cells of ret·i·na
  ep·i·the·li·op·a·thy
  ep·i·the·li·um
  in·du·ra·tion of the lung
pig·ment
  bile p.'s
  for·ma·lin p.
  he·ma·tog·e·nous p.
  he·pa·tog·e·nous p.
  ma·lar·i·al p.
  mel·a·not·ic p.
  res·pi·ra·to·ry p.'s
  vi·su·al p.'s
  wear-and-tear p.
pig·men·tary
  cir·rho·sis
  glau·co·ma
  ret·i·nop·a·thy
  syph·i·lid
pig·men·ta·tion
  ar·se·nic p.
  ex·og·e·nous p.
pig·ment·ed
  am·e·lo·blas·to·ma
  der·mat·o·fi·bro·sar·co·ma
   pro·tu·ber·ans
  epu·lis
  lay·er of cil·i·ary body
  lay·er of iris
  lay·er of ret·i·na
pig·ment·ed hair ep·i·der·mal
  ne·vus
pig·ment·ed ke·rat·ic
  pre·cip·i·tates
pig·ment·ed pur·pu·ric li·chen·
  oid
  der·ma·to·sis
pig·ment·ed vil·lo·nod·u·lar
  syn·o·vi·tis
pig·men·to·ly·sin
pig·men·tum ni·grum
pig·my
Pignet's
  for·mu·la
pi·lar
  cyst
  tu·mor of scalp
pi·la·ry
pile
  sen·ti·nel p.
  ther·mo·e·lec·tric p.
pi·le·ous
  gland
piles
pi·le·us
pi·li

pi·lif·er·ous
  cyst
pi·li·mic·tion
pill
  bread p.
  pep p.'s
pil·lar
  an·te·ri·or p. of fau·ces
  an·te·ri·or p. of for·nix
  Corti's p.'s
  p.'s of fau·ces
  p.'s of for·nix
  p. of iris
  pos·te·ri·or p. of fau·ces
  pos·te·ri·or p. of for·nix
pil·lar
  cells
  cells of Corti
pil·let
pill-roll·ing
pi·lo·be·zoar
pi·lo·car·pine
pi·lo·cys·tic
pi·lo·e·rec·tion
pi·loid
  as·tro·cy·to·ma
  gli·o·sis
pi·lo·jec·tion
pi·lo·ma·trix·o·ma
pi·lo·mo·tor
  fi·bers
  re·flex
pi·lon
  frac·ture
pi·lo·ni·dal
  cyst
  fis·tu·la
  si·nus
pi·lose
pi·lo·se·ba·ceous
pi·lo·sis
Piltz
  sign
pil·u·la
pil·u·lae
pil·u·lar
  mass
pil·ule
pi·lus
  pi·li an·nu·la·ti
  pi·li cu·ni·cu·la·ti
  F pi·li
  I pi·li
  pi·li in·car·na·ti
  pi·li mul·ti·ge·mi·ni
  R pi·li
  pi·li tor·ti
pi·mar·i·cin

pi·mel·ic ac·id
pim·e·lo·pter·y·gi·um
pim·e·lor·rhea
pim·e·lor·thop·nea
pi·men·ta
    p. oil
pi·men·to
pim·in·o·dine
pim·o·zide
pim·ple
pin
    Steinmann p.
pin
    amal·gam
    im·plant
pin·a·cy·a·nol
Pinard's
    ma·neu·ver
pince·ment
pin·cer
    nail
pinch
    graft
Pindborg
    tu·mor
pin·do·lol
pine
    p.-nee·dle oil
    p. oil
    p. tar
    white p.
pin·e·al
    body
    cells
    cyst
    eye
    gland
    ha·ben·u·la
    re·cess
    stalk
pin·e·al·ec·to·my
pin·e·a·lo·cyte
pin·e·a·lo·ma
    ec·top·ic p.
    ex·tra·pin·e·al p.
pin·e·a·lop·a·thy
pine·ap·ple
Pinel's
    sys·tem
pin·e·o·blas·to·ma
ping-pong
    bone
    frac·ture
    gaze
    mech·a·nism
pin·guec·u·la
pin·guic·u·la

pin·hole
    pu·pil
pin·i·form
pink
    dis·ease
    eye
pink·eye
pin·ledge
pin·na
    p. na·si
pin·nae
pin·nal
pin·ni·ped
pin·o·cyte
pin·o·cy·to·sis
pin·o·cy·tot·ic
    ves·i·cle
pin·o·some
Pins'
    sign
    syn·drome
pint
pin·ta
pin·tids
pin·toid
pi·nus
pin·worm
    vag·i·ni·tis
pi·o·ep·i·the·li·um
Pi·oph·i·la ca·sei
pi·or·thop·nea
PIP
    joints
pi·pam·a·zine
pi·pam·per·one
pi·paz·e·thate
pipe
    bone
pip·e·co·lic ac·id
pip·e·co·lin·ic ac·id
pi·pen·zo·late meth·yl·bro·mide
pip·er
pi·per·a·cet·a·zine
pi·per·a·cil·lin so·di·um
pi·per·a·zine
    p. ad·i·pate
    p. cal·ci·um ed·e·tate
    p. cit·rate
    p. es·trone sul·fate
pi·per·i·dine
pi·per·i·do·late hy·dro·chlo·ride
pi·per·o·caine hy·dro·chlo·ride
pi·per·ox·an hy·dro·chlo·ride
Piper's
    for·ceps
pipe-smok·er's
    can·cer

pipe·stem
  ar·ter·ies
  fi·bro·sis
pi·pet
pi·pette
pip·o·bro·man
pi·po·sul·fan
pi·pra·drol hy·dro·chlo·ride
pi·prin·hy·dri·nate
pip·syl
pi·qûre
  di·a·be·tes
pir·bu·ter·ol
Pi·re·nel·la
Pirie's
  bone
pir·i·form
  ar·ea
  cor·tex
  fos·sa
  mus·cle
  open·ing
  re·cess
  si·nus
pir·i·ni·tra·mide
Pirogoff's
  am·pu·ta·tion
  an·gle
  tri·an·gle
pir·o·men
Pi·ro·plas·ma
Pi·ro·plas·mi·da
pir·o·plas·mo·sis
pir·ox·i·cam ol·a·mine
pir·pro·fen
Pirquet's
  re·ac·tion
  test
Pis·ces
pis·ci·form
  cat·a·ract
pis·i·form
  bone
pi·so·ha·mate
  lig·a·ment
pi·so·met·a·car·pal
  lig·a·ment
pi·so·tri·que·tral
  joint
pis·oun·ci·form
  lig·a·ment
pis·oun·ci·nate
  lig·a·ment
pis·tol-shot fem·o·ral
  sound
pis·ton
  pulse

pit
  car·ies
pit
  anal p.
  ar·tic·u·lar p. of head of
    ra·di·us
  au·di·to·ry p.'s
  buc·cal p.
  cen·tral p.
  cos·tal p. of trans·verse
    pro·cess
  p. for dens of at·las
  gas·tric p.
  gran·u·lar p.'s
  p. of head of fe·mur
  in·fe·ri·or ar·tic·u·lar p. of
    at·las
  in·fe·ri·or cos·tal p.
  iris p.'s
  lens p.'s
  Mantoux p.
  nail p.'s
  na·sal p.'s
  ob·long p. of ar·y·te·noid
    car·ti·lage
  ol·fac·to·ry p.'s
  post·na·tal p. of the new·
    born
  prim·i·tive p.
  pter·y·goid p.
  p. of stom·ach
  sub·lin·gual p.
  su·pe·ri·or ar·tic·u·lar p. of
    at·las
  su·pe·ri·or cos·tal p.
  su·pra·me·a·tal p.
  tri·an·gu·lar p. of ar·y·te·
    noid car·ti·lage
  troch·le·ar p.
pitch
  Bur·gun·dy p.
  liq·uid p.
  white p.
pitch
  poi·son·ing
  wart
pitch·blende
pitch-work·er's
  can·cer
pit and fis·sure
  car·ies
pith
pith·e·coid
pith·ode
Pitkin
  sy·ringe
Pitot
  tube

Pitres'
  ar·ea
  sign
pit·ted
  ker·a·tol·y·sis
pit·ting
  ede·ma
pit·ting
Pitts·burgh
  pneu·mo·nia
Pitts·burgh pneu·mo·nia
  agent
pi·tu·i·cyte
pi·tu·i·cy·to·ma
pi·tu·i·ta
pi·tu·i·tar·ism
pi·tu·i·ta·ri·um
pi·tu·i·tary
  an·te·ri·or p.
  des·ic·cat·ed p.
  pha·ryn·ge·al p.
  pos·te·ri·or p.
pi·tu·i·tary
  ad·a·man·ti·no·ma
  ad·e·no·ma
  ap·o·plexy
  ba·so·phil·ia
  ba·soph·i·lism
  ca·chex·ia
  di·ver·tic·u·lum
  dwarf·ism
  fos·sa
  gi·gan·tism
  gland
  in·fan·ti·lism
  mem·brane
  myx·e·de·ma
  stalk
pi·tu·i·tary go·nad·o·tro·pic
  hor·mone
pi·tu·i·tary growth
  hor·mone
pi·tu·i·tary stalk
  sec·tion
pi·tu·i·tous
pit·y·ri·a·sic
pit·y·ri·a·sis
  p. al·ba
  p. al·ba atroph·i·cans
  p. am·i·an·ta·cea
  p. ca·pi·tis
  p. cir·ci·na·ta
  p. fur·fu·ra·cea
  p. li·che·noi·des
  p. li·che·noi·des et va·ri·o·
   li·for·mis acu·ta
  p. lin·guae
  p. ma·cu·la·ta

  p. nig·ra
  p. ro·sea
  p. ru·bra
  p. ru·bra pi·la·ris
  p. sic·ca
  p. ver·si·col·or
pit·y·roid
Pit·y·ro·spo·rum
  P. or·bic·u·la·re
  P. ova·le
piv·a·late
piv·ot
  ad·just·a·ble oc·clu·sal p.
  oc·clu·sal p.
piv·ot
  joint
piv·ot shift
  test
pix·el
P-J
  in·ter·val
place
  the·o·ry
pla·ce·bo
pla·cen·ta
  ac·ces·so·ry p.
  p. ac·cre·ta
  p. ac·cre·ta ve·ra
  ad·her·ent p.
  an·nu·lar p.
  bat·tle·dore p.
  bi·dis·coi·dal p.
  p. bi·lo·ba
  p. bi·par·ti·ta
  cen·tral p. pre·via
  cho·ri·o·al·lan·to·ic p.
  cho·ri·o·am·ni·on·ic p.
  cho·ri·o·vi·tel·line p.
  p. cir·cum·val·la·ta
  cot·y·le·don·ary p.
  de·cid·u·ate p.
  di·cho·ri·on·ic di·am·ni·ot·
   ic p.
  p. dif·fu·sa
  p. di·mi·di·a·ta
  dis·perse p.
  p. du·plex
  en·do·the·li·o·cho·ri·al p.
  en·do·the·li·o-en·do·the·li·al
   p.
  ep·i·the·li·o·cho·ri·al p.
  p. ex·tra·cho·ra·les
  p. fe·nes·tra·ta
  fe·tal p.
  p. fe·ta·lis
  he·mo·cho·ri·al p.
  he·mo·en·do·the·li·al p.
  horse·shoe p.

pla·cen·ta *(continued)*
 in·car·cer·at·ed p.
 p. in·cre·ta
 lab·y·rin·thine p.
 p. mar·gi·na·ta
 ma·ter·nal p.
 p. mem·bra·na·cea
 mon·o·cho·ri·on·ic di·am·
  ni·ot·ic p.
 mon·o·cho·ri·on·ic mon·o·
  am·ni·ot·ic p.
 p. mul·ti·lo·ba
 non·de·cid·u·ous p.
 p. pan·du·ra·for·mis
 p. per·cre·ta
 p. pre·via
 p. pre·via cen·tra·lis
 p. pre·via mar·gi·na·lis
 p. pre·via par·ti·a·lis
 p. re·flexa
 p. re·ni·for·mis
 re·tained p.
 Schultze's p.
 p. spu·ria
 suc·cen·tu·ri·ate p.
 su·per·nu·mer·ary p.
 syn·des·mo·cho·ri·al p.
 to·tal p. pre·via
 p. tri·lo·ba
 p. tri·par·ti·ta
 p. tri·plex
 twin p.
 p. ute·ri·na
 p. ve·la·men·to·sa
 vil·lous p.
 zo·na·ry p.
pla·cen·ta
 pro·tein
pla·cen·tal
 bar·ri·er
 cir·cu·la·tion
 dys·to·cia
 lobe
 mem·brane
 plas·mo·di·um
 pol·yp
 pre·sen·ta·tion
 sep·ta
 sign
 souf·fle
 throm·bo·sis
pla·cen·tal dys·func·tion
 syn·drome
pla·cen·tal growth
 hor·mone
Pla·cen·ta·lia
pla·cen·tal par·a·sit·ic
 twin

pla·cen·tal stage
pla·cen·tal sul·fa·tase
 de·fi·cien·cy
pla·cen·ta·scan
plac·en·ta·tion
plac·en·ti·tis
plac·en·tog·ra·phy
 in·di·rect p.
plac·en·to·ma
pla·cen·to·ther·a·py
Placido's
 disk
plac·ode
 au·di·to·ry p.'s
 ep·i·bran·chi·al p.'s
 lens p.'s
 na·sal p.'s
 ol·fac·to·ry p.'s
 op·tic p.'s
 otic p.'s
plad·a·ro·ma
plad·a·ro·sis
pla·fond
pla·gi·o·ce·phal·ic
pla·gi·o·ceph·a·lism
pla·gi·o·ceph·a·lous
pla·gi·o·ceph·a·ly
plague
 am·bu·lant p.
 am·bu·la·to·ry p.
 black p.
 bu·bon·ic p.
 cat·tle p.
 duck p.
 fowl p.
 glan·du·lar p.
 hem·or·rhag·ic p.
 lar·val p.
 Pah·vant Val·ley p.
 pneu·mon·ic p.
 rab·bit p.
 sep·ti·ce·mic p.
 syl·vat·ic p.
plague
 ba·cil·lus
 pneu·mo·nia
 vac·cine
plain
 film
plak·al·bu·min
pla·kins
pla·na
plan·chet
Planck's
 con·stant
 the·o·ry
plane
 joint

su·ture
wart
plane
  Addison's clin·i·cal p.'s
  Aeby's p.
  au·ric·u·lo-in·fra·or·bit·al p.
  ax·i·o·la·bi·o·lin·gual p.
  ax·i·o·me·si·o·dis·tal p.
  bite p.
  Bolton p.
  Bolton-Broadbent p.
  Bolton-na·si·on p.
  Broca's vi·su·al p.
  Camper's p.
  can·tho·me·a·tal p.
  cor·o·nal p.
  da·tum p.
  Daubenton's p.
  equa·to·ri·al p.
  eye-ear p.
  fa·cial p.
  first par·al·lel pel·vic p.
  fourth par·al·lel pel·vic p.
  Frankfort p.
  Frankfort hor·i·zon·tal p.
  fron·tal p.
  guide p.
  hor·i·zon·tal p.
  p. of in·ci·dence
  in·fra·or·bi·to·me·a·tal p.
  p. of in·let
  in·ter·spi·nal p.
  in·ter·tu·ber·cu·lar p.
  la·bi·o·lin·gual p.
  p. of least pel·vic di·men·
    sions
  mean foun·da·tion p.
  Meckel's p.
  me·di·an p.
  p. of mid·pel·vis
  mid·sag·it·tal p.
  Morton's p.
  na·si·on-post·con·dy·lar p.
  no·dal p.
  nu·chal p.
  oc·cip·i·tal p.
  oc·clu·sal p.
  p. of oc·clu·sion
  or·bi·tal p.
  p. of out·let
  par·a·sag·it·tal p.
  p. of pel·vic ca·nal
  pel·vic p. of great·est di·
    men·sions
  pel·vic p. of in·let
  pel·vic p. of least di·men·
    sions
  pel·vic p. of out·let

pop·lit·e·al p. of fe·mur
prin·ci·pal p.
p.'s of ref·er·ence
p. of re·gard
sag·it·tal p.
sec·ond par·al·lel pel·vic p.
spec·ta·cle p.
ster·nal p.
sub·cos·tal p.
su·pra·crest·al p.
su·pra·or·bi·to·me·a·tal p.
su·pra·ster·nal p.
tem·po·ral p.
third par·al·lel pel·vic p.
tooth p.
trans·py·lor·ic p.
trans·verse p.
wide p.
pla·nig·ra·phy
pla·nim·e·ter
plan·ing
plan·i·tho·rax
plank·ter
plank·ton
plank·ton·ic
pla·no·cel·lu·lar
pla·no·con·cave
  lens
pla·no·con·vex
  lens
pla·no·graph·ic
  pel·vim·e·try
pla·nog·ra·phy
plan·o·ma·nia
Pla·nor·bis
plan·o·top·o·ki·ne·sia
pla·no·val·gus
plant
  ag·glu·ti·nin
  an·ti·tox·in
  ca·sein
  der·ma·ti·tis
  in·di·can
  RNase
  tox·in
  vi·rus·es
plan·ta
plan·tae
plan·ta·go
  p. ova·ta coat·ing
  p. seed
plan·tal·gia
plan·tar
  ap·o·neu·ro·sis
  arch
  cush·ion
  fas·cia
  fi·bro·ma·to·sis

plan·tar *(continued)*
flex·ion
lig·a·ments
mus·cle
re·flex
space
syph·i·lid
wart
plan·tar cal·ca·ne·o·cu·boid
lig·a·ment
plan·tar cal·ca·ne·o·na·vic·u·lar
lig·a·ment
plan·tar cu·boi·de·o·na·vic·u·lar
lig·a·ment
plan·tar cu·ne·o·cu·boid
lig·a·ment
plan·tar cu·ne·o·na·vic·u·lar
lig·a·ments
plan·tar dig·i·tal
veins
plan·tar in·ter·os·se·ous
mus·cle
plan·tar·is
plan·tar met·a·tar·sal
ar·tery
lig·a·ments
veins
plan·tar mus·cle
re·flex
plan·tar quad·rate
mus·cle
plan·tar ve·nous
arch
net·work
plan·ti·grade
plan·u·la
in·vag·i·nate p.
plan·u·lae
pla·num
p. oc·ci·pi·ta·le
p. or·bi·ta·le
p. pop·li·te·um
p. sem·i·lu·na·tum
p. sphe·noi·da·le
p. ster·na·le
p. tem·po·ra·le
pla·nu·ria
plaque
ath·er·om·a·tous p.
bac·te·ri·al p.
den·tal p.
Hollenhorst p.'s
mu·ci·nous p.
mu·cous p.
neu·rit·ic p.
se·nile p.
Plaque In·dex

plasm
plas·ma
an·ti·he·mo·phil·ic p.
an·ti·he·mo·phil·ic p. hu·man
blood p.
fresh fro·zen p.
p. hy·drol·y·sate
p. ma·ri·num
mus·cle p.
nor·mal hu·man p.
salt·ed p.
plas·ma
cell
fac·tor X
fi·bro·nec·tin
lay·er
mem·brane
pro·teins
scal·pel
stain
sub·sti·tute
ther·a·py
plas·ma ac·cel·er·a·tor
glob·u·lin
plas·ma·blast
plas·ma cell
bal·a·ni·tis
hep·a·ti·tis
leu·ke·mia
mas·ti·tis
my·e·lo·ma
plas·ma·crit
test
plas·ma·cyte
plas·ma·cy·to·blast
plas·ma·cy·to·ma
plas·ma·cy·to·sis
plas·ma ex·pand·er
plas·ma·gene
plas·ma io·do·pro·tein
dis·or·der
plas·mal
re·ac·tion
plas·ma la·bile
fac·tor
plas·ma·lem·ma
plas·mal·o·gens
plas·mals
plas·ma·phe·re·sis
plas·ma·phe·ret·ic
plas·ma re·nin
ac·tiv·i·ty
plas·ma throm·bo·plas·tin
an·te·ced·ent
com·po·nent
fac·tor
fac·tor B

plas·mat·ic
  stain
plas·ma·tog·a·my
plas·men·ic ac·id
plas·mic
  stain
plas·mid
  bac·te·ri·o·cin·o·gen·ic p.'s
  con·ju·ga·tive p.
  F p.
  Fp.
  in·fec·tious p.
  non·con·ju·ga·tive p.
  R p.'s
  re·sis·tance p.'s
  trans·mis·si·ble p.
plas·min
plas·min·o·gen
  ac·ti·va·tor
plas·min·o·ki·nase
plas·min·o·plas·tin
plas·min pro·throm·bins con·ver·sion
  fac·tor
plas·mo·cyt·ic
  leu·ke·moid re·ac·tion
plas·mo·dia
plas·mo·di·al
  troph·o·blast
plas·mo·di·o·tro·pho·blast
Plas·mo·di·um
  P. ae·thi·o·pi·cum
  P. berg·hei
  P. bra·zi·li·a·num
  P. ca·the·me·ri·um
  P. cyn·o·mol·gi
  P. du·rae
  P. fal·cip·a·rum
  P. gal·li·na·ceum
  P. jux·ta·nu·cle·a·re
  P. know·le·si
  P. ko·chi
  P. ma·lar·i·ae
  P. ova·le
  P. re·lic·tum
  P. vi·vax
plas·mo·di·um
  pla·cen·tal p.
Plas·mo·dro·ma·ta
plas·mog·a·my
plas·mo·gen
plas·mo·ki·nin
plas·mo·lem·ma
plas·mol·y·sis
plas·mo·lyt·ic
plas·mo·lyze
plas·mon
plas·mor·rhex·is

plas·mos·chi·sis
plas·mo·sin
plas·mo·some
plas·mot·o·my
plas·mo·tro·pic
plas·mot·ro·pism
plas·mo·type
plas·mo·zyme
plas·tein
plas·ter
  ban·dage
  splint
plas·ter
  p. of Par·is
plas·ter of Par·is
  dis·ease
plas·tic
  anat·o·my
  bron·chi·tis
  cor·pus·cle
  cy·cli·tis
  in·du·ra·tion
  iri·tis
  lymph
  mo·tor
  op·er·a·tion
  pleu·ri·sy
  sur·gery
  teeth
plas·tic
  Bingham p.
  mod·el·ing p.
plas·tic·i·ty
plas·tic res·to·ra·tion
  ma·te·ri·al
plas·tic sec·tion
  stain
plas·tid
  blood p.
plas·tog·a·my
plas·to·quin·one
plas·tron
plas·ty
plate
  alar p. of neu·ral tube
  anal p.
  ax·i·al p.
  ba·sal p. of neu·ral tube
  base p.
  blood p.
  bone p.
  but·tress p.
  car·di·o·gen·ic p.
  cho·ri·on·ic p.
  clo·a·cal p.
  crib·ri·form p. of eth·moid bone
  cu·tis p.

plate *(continued)*

dor·sal p. of neu·ral tube

end p.

ep·i·phys·i·al p.

equa·to·ri·al p.

eth·mo·vo·mer·ine p.

flat p.

floor p.

foot p.

fron·tal p.

hor·i·zon·tal p. of pal·a·tine bone

Kühne's p.

Lane's p.'s

lat·er·al p.

lat·er·al p. of pter·y·goid pro·cess

left p. of thy·roid car·ti·lage

lin·gual p.

me·di·al p. of pter·y·goid pro·cess

med·ul·lary p.

p. of mo·di·o·lus

mo·tor p.

mus·cle p.

nail p.

neu·ral p.

neu·tral·i·za·tion p.

no·to·chor·dal p.

oral p.

or·bi·tal p.

pal·a·tal p.

pa·per p.

pap·y·ra·ceous p.

par·a·chor·dal p.

pa·ri·e·tal p.

per·pen·dic·u·lar p.

po·lar p.'s

pre·chor·dal p.

pro·chor·dal p.

pter·y·goid p.'s

quad·ri·gem·i·nal p.

right p. of thy·roid car·ti·lage

roof p.

sec·on·dary spi·ral p.

seg·men·tal p.

sieve p.

sole p.

spi·ral p.

suc·tion p.

tar·sal p.'s

ter·mi·nal p.

tym·pan·ic p.

ure·thral p.

ven·tral p.

ven·tral p. of neu·ral tube

ver·ti·cal p.

vis·cer·al p.

wing p.

plate

throm·bo·sis

pla·teau

ven·tric·u·lar p.

pla·teau

iris

pulse

Plateau-Talbot

law

plate·let

ac·to·my·o·sin

co·fac·tor

co·fac·tor II

throm·bo·sis

plate·let-ac·ti·vat·ing

fac·tor

plate·let-ag·gre·gat·ing

fac·tor

plate·let ag·gre·ga·tion

test

plate·let-de·rived growth

fac·tor

plate·let·phe·re·sis

plate·let tis·sue

fac·tor

plat·ing

com·pres·sion p.

pla·tin·ic

plat·i·nous

plat·i·num

plat·i·num black

plat·i·num foil

plat·i·num group

plat·y·ba·sia

plat·y·ceph·a·ly

plat·yc·ne·mia

plat·yc·ne·mic

plat·yc·ne·mism

plat·y·cra·nia

plat·y·cyte

plat·y·glos·sal

plat·y·hel·minth

Plat·y·hel·min·thes

plat·y·hi·er·ic

plat·y·me·ric

plat·y·mor·phia

plat·y·o·pia

plat·y·op·ic

plat·y·pel·lic

pel·vis

plat·y·pel·loid

pel·vis

pla·typ·nea

plat·yr·rhine

plat·yr·rhi·ny

pla·tys·ma
pla·tys·mas
pla·tys·ma·ta
plat·y·spon·dyl·ia
plat·y·spon·dyl·i·sis
pla·tys·ten·ceph·a·ly
Plaut's
  ba·cil·lus
play
  ther·a·py
Pleasure
  curve
plea·sure
  prin·ci·ple
plec·trid·i·um
pled·get
plei·o·tro·pia
plei·o·tro·pic
  gene
plei·ot·ro·py
ple·o·chro·ic
ple·och·ro·ism
ple·o·chro·mat·ic
ple·o·chro·ma·tism
ple·o·cy·to·sis
ple·o·mas·tia
ple·o·ma·zia
ple·o·mor·phic
  ad·e·no·ma
  li·po·ma
ple·o·mor·phism
ple·o·mor·phous
ple·o·nasm
ple·o·nec·tic
ple·o·nex·ia
ple·on·os·te·o·sis
  Leris p.
ple·op·tics
ple·op·to·phor
ple·ro·cer·coid
ple·si·o·mor·phic
ple·si·o·mor·phism
ple·si·o·mor·phous
ples·ses·the·sia
ples·sim·e·ter
ples·si·met·ric
ples·sor
pleth·o·ra
pleth·o·ric
ple·thys·mo·graph
  body p.
  pres·sure p.
  vol·ume-dis·place·ment p.
ple·thys·mo·graph·ic
  gog·gle
pleth·ys·mog·ra·phy
  im·ped·ance p.
  ve·nous oc·clu·sion p.

pleth·ys·mom·e·try
pleu·ra
  cer·vi·cal p.
  di·a·phrag·mat·ic p.
  pa·ri·e·tal p.
  p. pe·ri·car·di·a·ca
  per·i·car·di·al p.
  p. phre·ni·ca
  vis·cer·al p.
  p. vis·ce·ra·lis
pleu·ra·cen·te·sis
pleu·rae
pleu·ral
  cal·cu·lus
  cav·i·ty
  flu·id
  frem·i·tus
  pou·drage
  pres·sure
  re·cess·es
  si·nus·es
  space
  vil·li
pleu·ral·gia
pleur·a·poph·y·sis
pleur·ec·to·my
pleu·ri·sy
  ad·he·sive p.
  be·nign dry p.
  cos·tal p.
  di·a·phrag·mat·ic p.
  dry p.
  en·cyst·ed p.
  ep·i·dem·ic be·nign dry p.
  ep·i·dem·ic di·a·phrag·mat·ic p.
  fi·brin·ous p.
  hem·or·rhag·ic p.
  in·ter·lob·u·lar p.
  plas·tic p.
  pro·duc·tive p.
  pro·lif·er·at·ing p.
  pul·mo·nary p.
  pu·ru·lent p.
  sac·cu·lat·ed p.
  se·ro·fi·brin·ous p.
  se·rous p.
  sup·pu·ra·tive p.
  ty·phoid p.
  vis·cer·al p.
  wet p.
  p. with ef·fu·sion
pleu·rit·ic
  rub
pleu·ri·tis
pleur·i·tog·e·nous
pleu·ro·cele
pleu·ro·cen·te·sis

pleu·ro·cen·trum
pleu·roc·ly·sis
pleu·rod·e·sis
pleu·ro·dyn·ia
   ep·i·dem·ic p.
pleu·ro·e·soph·a·ge·al
   line
   mus·cle
pleu·ro·gen·ic
pleu·rog·e·nous
pleu·rog·ra·phy
pleu·ro·hep·a·ti·tis
pleu·ro·lith
pleu·rol·y·sis
pleu·ro·per·i·car·di·al
   ca·nals
   hi·a·tus
   mem·brane
   mur·mur
pleu·ro·per·i·car·di·tis
pleu·ro·per·i·to·ne·al
   ca·nal
   cav·i·ty
   fold
   hi·a·tus
   mem·brane
pleu·ro·pneu·mo·nia
   con·ta·gious bo·vine p.
   con·ta·gious cap·rine p.
pleu·ro·pneu·mo·nia-like
   or·ga·nisms
pleu·ro·pul·mo·nary
pleu·ror·rhea
pleu·ro·thot·o·nos
pleu·ro·thot·o·nus
pleu·rot·o·my
pleu·ro·ty·phoid
pleu·ro·vis·cer·al
plex·al
plex·ect·o·my
plex·i·form
   lay·er
   lay·er of ce·re·bral cor·tex
   lay·ers of ret·i·na
   neu·ro·fi·bro·ma
   neu·ro·ma
plex·im·e·ter
plex·i·tis
plex·o·gen·ic
plex·o·gen·ic pul·mo·nary
   ar·te·ri·op·a·thy
plex·om·e·ter
plex·or
plex·us
plex·us
   ab·dom·i·nal aor·tic p.
   an·nu·lar p.
   p. an·nu·la·ris

   p. of an·te·ri·or ce·re·bral
   ar·tery
an·te·ri·or cor·o·nary p.
aor·tic p.
   p. aor·ti·cus
   p. ar·te·ri·ae ce·re·bri an·
   te·ri·o·ris
   p. ar·te·ri·ae ce·re·bri me·
   di·ae
   p. ar·te·ri·ae cho·roi·de·ae
as·cend·ing pha·ryn·ge·al p.
Auerbach's p.
   p. au·ric·u·la·ris pos·te·ri·
   or
au·to·nom·ic plex·us·es
   p. ax·il·la·ris
ax·il·lary p.
bas·i·lar p.
Batson's p.
brach·i·al p.
car·di·ac p.
   p. car·di·a·cus pro·fun·dus
   p. car·di·a·cus su·per·fi·ci·
   a·lis
   p. ca·ro·ti·cus in·ter·nus
   p. ca·ver·no·sus
cav·ern·ous p.
cav·ern·ous p. of clit·o·ris
cav·ern·ous p. of con·chae
cav·ern·ous p. of pe·nis
ce·li·ac p.
   p. ce·li·a·cus
cer·vi·cal p.
cho·roid p.
   p. of cho·roid ar·tery
cho·roid p. of fourth ven·
   tri·cle
cho·roid p. of lat·er·al ven·
   tri·cle
cho·roid p. of third ven·tri·
   cle
cil·i·ary gan·gli·on·ic p.
coc·cyg·eal p.
com·mon ca·rot·id p.
   p. co·ro·na·ri·us cor·dis
cor·o·nary p.
Cruveilhier's p.
deep car·di·ac p.
def·er·en·tial p.
en·ter·ic p.
esoph·a·ge·al p.
Exner's p.
ex·ter·nal ca·rot·id p.
ex·ter·nal il·i·ac p.
ex·ter·nal max·il·lary p.
fa·cial p.
fem·o·ral p.
   p. gan·gli·o·sus cil·i·ar·is

gas·tric plex·us·es of au·to·
  nom·ic sys·tem
p. gu·lae
Haller's p.
Heller's p.
hem·or·rhoi·dal p.
he·pa·tic p.
il·i·ac p.
p. il·i·a·cus ex·ter·nus
in·fe·ri·or den·tal p.
in·fe·ri·or hem·or·rhoi·dal
  plex·us·es
in·fe·ri·or hy·po·gas·tric p.
in·fe·ri·or mes·en·ter·ic p.
in·fe·ri·or rec·tal plex·us·es
in·fe·ri·or thy·roid p.
in·fe·ri·or ves·i·cal p.
in·gui·nal p.
p. in·gui·na·lis
in·ter·mes·en·ter·ic p.
in·ter·nal ca·rot·id p.
in·ter·nal ca·rot·id ve·nous
  p.
in·ter·nal mam·ma·ry p.
in·ter·nal max·il·lary p.
in·ter·nal tho·rac·ic p.
is·chi·ad·ic p.
Jacobson's p.
Jacques' p.
jug·u·lar p.
p. ju·gu·la·ris
Leber's p.
lin·gual p.
p. lin·gua·lis
p. lum·ba·lis
lum·bar p.
lum·bo·sa·cral p.
lym·phat·ic p.
p. mam·ma·ri·us
p. mam·ma·ri·us in·ter·nus
mam·ma·ry p.
p. max·il·la·ris ex·ter·nus
p. max·il·la·ris in·ter·nus
max·il·lary p.
Meissner's p.
me·nin·ge·al p.
p. men·in·ge·us
p. of mid·dle ce·re·bral ar·
  tery
mid·dle hem·or·rhoi·dal
  plex·us·es
mid·dle rec·tal plex·us·es
mid·dle sa·cral p.
my·en·ter·ic p.
nerve p.
p. ner·vo·sus
oc·cip·i·tal p.
p. oc·ci·pi·ta·lis

oph·thal·mic p.
p. oph·thal·mi·cus
ovar·i·an p.
pam·pin·i·form p.
pan·cre·at·ic p.
pa·rot·id p.
pel·vic p.
per·i·ar·te·ri·al p.
pha·ryn·ge·al p.
p. pha·ryn·ge·us as·cen·dens
phren·ic p.
p. phre·ni·cus
pop·lit·e·al p.
p. pop·li·te·us
pos·te·ri·or au·ric·u·lar p.
pos·te·ri·or cor·o·nary p.
pros·tat·ic p.
pros·tat·i·co·ves·i·cal p.
p. pros·tat·i·co·ve·si·ca·lis
pros·tat·ic ve·nous p.
pter·y·goid p.
p. pu·den·da·lis
p. pu·den·dus ner·vo·sus
pul·mo·nary p.
Quénu's hem·or·rhoi·dal p.
Ranvier's p.
rec·tal plex·us·es
rec·tal ve·nous p.
Remak's p.
re·nal p.
sa·cral p.
p. sa·cra·lis me·di·us
sa·cral ve·nous p.
Sappey's p.
sci·at·ic p.
so·lar p.
sper·mat·ic p.
p. of spi·nal nerves
splen·ic p.
Stensen's p.
stro·ma p.
sub·cla·vi·an p.
sub·mu·co·sal p.
sub·oc·cip·i·tal ve·nous p.
sub·se·rous p.
su·per·fi·cial car·di·ac p.
su·per·fi·cial tem·po·ral p.
su·pe·ri·or den·tal p.
su·pe·ri·or hem·or·rhoi·dal
  p.
su·pe·ri·or hy·po·gas·tric p.
su·pe·ri·or mes·en·ter·ic p.
su·pe·ri·or rec·tal p.
su·pe·ri·or thy·roid p.
su·pra·re·nal p.
sym·pa·thet·ic plex·us·es
p. tem·po·ra·lis su·per·fi·
  ci·a·lis

plex·us *(continued)*
  tes·tic·u·lar p.
  tho·rac·ic aor·tic p.
  p. thy·roi·de·us in·fe·ri·or
  p. thy·roi·de·us su·pe·ri·or
  tym·pan·ic p.
  ure·ter·ic p.
  uter·ine ve·nous p.
  uter·o·vag·i·nal p.
  vag·i·nal ve·nous p.
  vas·cu·lar p.
  ve·nous p.
  ve·nous p. of blad·der
  ve·nous p. of fo·ra·men
   ova·le
  ve·nous p. of hy·po·glos·sal
   ca·nal
  ver·te·bral p.
  ver·te·bral ve·nous p.
  ves·i·cal p.
  p. ve·si·ca·lis in·fe·ri·or
  Walther's p.
plex·us·es
pli·ca
  pli·cae adi·po·sae
  p. am·pul·la·ris
  p. ax·il·la·ris
  p. cho·roi·dea
  p. ep·i·gas·tri·ca
  p. ep·i·glot·ti·ca
  p. gu·ber·na·trix
  p. hy·po·gas·tri·ca
  p. in·gui·na·lis
  p. in·ter·dig·i·tal·is
  p. lu·na·ta
  p. mem·bra·nae tym·pa·ni
  pli·cae rec·ti
  p. rec·to·va·gi·na·lis
  p. sem·i·lu·na·ris con·junc·
   ti·vae
  p. sig·moi·dea
  p. syn·o·vi·a·lis pa·tel·la·ris
  p. tu·bo·pa·la·ti·na
  p. um·bi·li·ca·lis me·dia
  p. ura·chi
  p. ure·te·ri·ca
  p. ute·ro·ve·si·ca·lis
  p. ven·tric·u·lar·is
  p. ve·si·co·u·te·ri·na
  p. ves·tib·u·li
pli·cae
pli·cate
pli·ca·tion
pli·cot·o·my
Plimmer's
  bod·ies
ploi·dy
plom·bage

plo·sive
Plotz
  ba·cil·lus
plug
  Dittrich's p.'s
  ep·i·the·li·al p.
  lam·i·nat·ed ep·i·the·li·al
   p.
  mu·cous p.
  Traube's p.'s
  vag·i·nal p.
plug·ger
  au·to·mat·ic p.
  back-ac·tion p.
  foot p.
  root ca·nal p.
plug·ging
  in·stru·ment
plum·ba·go
plum·bic
plum·bism
plum·bum
Plummer's
  bag
  di·la·tor
  dis·ease
Plummer-Vinson
  syn·drome
plu·mose
plu·ral
  preg·nan·cy
plu·ri·cau·sal
plu·ri·glan·du·lar
  ad·e·no·ma·to·sis
plu·ri·loc·u·lar
plu·ri·nu·cle·ar
plu·rip·o·tent
  cells
plu·ri·po·ten·tial
plu·ri·re·sis·tant
plus
  lens
  strand
plu·to·ma·nia
plu·to·nism
plu·to·ni·um
PMA
  in·dex
P-mit·ra·le
pne·o·car·di·ac
  re·flex
pne·o·dy·nam·ics
pne·om·e·ter
pne·om·e·try
pne·o·pne·ic
  re·flex
pne·o·scope
pneu·marth·ro·gram

pneu·marth·rog·ra·phy
pneu·mar·thro·sis
pneu·mat·ic
  bone
  cab·i·net
  space
  to·nom·e·ter
pneu·mat·ics
pneu·mat·ic tire
  in·ju·ry
pneu·ma·ti·nu·ria
pneu·ma·ti·za·tion
pneu·ma·tized
pneu·ma·to·car·dia
pneu·ma·to·cele
  ex·tra·cra·ni·al p.
  in·tra·cra·ni·al p.
pneu·ma·to·en·ter·ic
  re·cess
pneu·ma·to·he·mia
pneu·ma·tol·o·gy
pneu·ma·tom·e·ter
pneu·ma·tor·rha·chis
pneu·ma·to·scope
pneu·ma·to·sis
  p. cys·toi·des in·tes·ti·na·lis
pneu·ma·to·thor·ax
pneu·ma·tu·ria
pneu·ma·type
pneu·mec·to·my
pneu·mo·an·gi·og·ra·phy
pneu·mo·ar·throg·ra·phy
pneu·mo·ba·cil·lus
pneu·mo·bul·bar
pneu·mo·car·di·al
pneu·mo·cele
  ex·tra·cra·ni·al p.
  in·tra·cra·ni·al p.
pneu·mo·cen·te·sis
pneu·mo·ceph·a·lus
pneu·mo·cho·le·cys·ti·tis
pneu·mo·coc·cal
  pneu·mo·nia
  pol·y·sac·char·ide
  vac·cine
pneu·mo·coc·ce·mia
pneu·mo·coc·ci
pneu·mo·coc·ci·dal
pneu·mo·coc·col·y·sis
pneu·mo·coc·co·sis
pneu·mo·coc·co·su·ria
pneu·mo·coc·cus
  Fraenkel's p.
  Fraenkel-Weichselbaum p.
pneu·mo·coc·cus
  ul·cer
pneu·mo·co·lon
pneu·mo·co·ni·o·ses

pneu·mo·co·ni·o·sis
  baux·ite p.
pneu·mo·cra·ni·um
pneu·mo·cys·ti·a·sis
Pneu·mo·cys·tis ca·ri·nii
pneu·mo·cys·tog·ra·phy
pneu·mo·cys·to·sis
pneu·mo·cyte
pneu·mo·der·ma
pneu·mo·dy·nam·ics
pneu·mo·em·py·e·ma
pneu·mo·en·ceph·a·lo·gram
pneu·mo·en·ceph·a·log·ra·phy
pneu·mo·en·ter·ic
  re·cess
pneu·mo·gas·tric
  nerve
pneu·mo·gas·trog·ra·phy
pneu·mo·gen·ic
  os·te·o·ar·throp·a·thy
pneu·mo·gram
pneu·mo·graph
pneu·mog·ra·phy
pneu·mo·he·mia
pneu·mo·he·mo·per·i·car·di·um
pneu·mo·he·mo·thor·ax
pneu·mo·hy·dro·me·tra
pneu·mo·hy·dro·per·i·car·di·um
pneu·mo·hy·dro·per·i·to·ne·um
pneu·mo·hy·dro·thor·ax
pneu·mo·hy·po·der·ma
pneu·mo·lith
pneu·mo·li·thi·a·sis
pneu·mol·o·gy
pneu·mol·y·sis
pneu·mo·ma·la·cia
pneu·mo·mas·sage
pneu·mo·me·di·as·ti·num
pneu·mo·mel·a·no·sis
pneu·mom·e·ter
pneu·mom·e·try
pneu·mo·my·co·sis
pneu·mo·my·e·log·ra·phy
pneu·mo·nec·to·my
pneu·mo·nia
  acute in·ter·sti·tial p.
  an·thrax p.
  apex p.
  ap·i·cal p.
  as·pi·ra·tion p.
  atyp·i·cal p.
  bron·chi·al p.
  ca·se·ous p.
  cen·tral p.
  chem·i·cal p.
  con·gen·i·tal p.
  con·tu·sion p.
  core p.

pneu·mo·nia *(continued)*
de·glu·ti·tion p.
des·qua·ma·tive in·ter·sti·tial p.
p. dis·se·cans
dou·ble p.
Eaton agent p.
em·bol·ic p.
eo·sin·o·phil·ic p.
Friedländer's p.
gan·gre·nous p.
gi·ant cell p.
Hecht's p.
hy·po·stat·ic p.
in·flu·en·zal p.
p. in·ter·lo·bu·la·ris pu·ru·len·ta
in·ter·sti·tial gi·ant cell p.
in·ter·sti·tial plas·ma cell p.
in·tra·u·ter·ine p.
lip·id p.
lip·oid p.
lo·bar p.
met·a·stat·ic p.
mi·gra·to·ry p.
mon·i·li·a·sis p.
my·co·plas·mal p.
my·co·plas·ma p. of pigs
oil p.
or·ga·nized p.
Pitts·burgh p.
plague p.
pneu·mo·coc·cal p.
post·op·er·a·tive p.
pri·mary atyp·i·cal p.
rheu·mat·ic p.
sep·tic p.
staph·y·lo·coc·cal p.
strep·to·coc·cal p.
sup·pu·ra·tive p.
ter·mi·nal p.
trau·mat·ic p.
tu·la·re·mic p.
ty·phoid p.
un·re·solved p.
ure·mic p.
vi·rus p. of pigs
wan·der·ing p.
wool-sor·ters' p.
pneu·mo·nia
vi·rus of mice
pneu·mon·ic
plague
pneu·mo·ni·tis
fe·line p.
hy·per·sen·si·tiv·i·ty p.
ure·mic p.
pneu·mo·no·cele

pneu·mo·no·cen·te·sis
pneu·mo·no·coc·cal
pneu·mo·no·coc·cus
pneu·mo·no·co·ni·o·sis
pneu·mo·no·cyte
gran·u·lar p.'s
phag·o·cyt·ic p.
pneu·mo·no·mel·a·no·sis
pneu·mo·no·mon·i·li·a·sis
pneu·mo·no·my·co·sis
pneu·mo·no·pexy
pneu·mo·nor·rha·phy
pneu·mo·not·o·my
Pneu·mo·nys·sus si·mi·co·la
pneu·mo-or·bi·tog·ra·phy
pneu·mo·per·i·car·di·um
pneu·mo·per·i·to·ne·um
pneu·mo·per·i·to·ni·tis
pneu·mo·pexy
pneu·mo·pha·gia
pneu·mo·pleu·ri·tis
pneu·mo·py·e·log·ra·phy
pneu·mo·py·o·thor·ax
pneu·mo·ra·di·og·ra·phy
pneu·mo·re·sec·tion
pneu·mo·ret·ro·per·i·to·ne·um
pneu·mo·roent·gen·og·ra·phy
pneu·mor·rha·chis
pneu·mo·scope
pneu·mo·ser·o·thor·ax
pneu·mo·sil·i·co·sis
pneu·mo·tach·o·gram
pneu·mo·tach·o·graph
Fleisch p.
Silverman-Lilly p.
pneu·mo·ta·chom·e·ter
pneu·mo·tax·ic
lo·cal·i·za·tion
pneu·mo·ther·mo·mas·sage
pneu·mo·thor·ax
ar·ti·fi·cial p.
ex·tra·pleu·ral p.
open p.
p. sim·plex
spon·ta·ne·ous p.
ten·sion p.
ther·a·peu·tic p.
val·vu·lar p.
pneu·mot·o·my
pneu·mo·ven·tri·cle
Pneu·mo·vi·rus
pneu·sis
pni·go·pho·bia
PNP
syn·drome
P/O
ra·ti·o
pock

pock·et
  gin·gi·val p.
  in·fra·bony p.
  in·tra·bony p.
  per·i·o·don·tal p.
  Rathke's p.
  Seessel's p.
  sub·crest·al p.
  Tröltsch's p.'s
pock·et·ed
  cal·cu·lus
pock·mark
po·cu·lum
  p. di·og·e·nis
po·dag·ra
po·dag·ral
po·dag·ric
po·dag·rous
po·dal·gia
po·dal·ic
  ex·trac·tion
  ver·sion
pod·ar·thri·tis
pod·e·de·ma
po·di·a·tric
  med·i·cine
po·di·a·trist
po·di·a·try
po·dis·mus
po·di·tis
  tour·ni·quet p.
pod·o·bro·mi·dro·sis
pod·o·cyte
pod·o·derm
pod·o·der·ma·ti·tis
pod·o·dy·na·mom·e·ter
pod·o·dyn·ia
pod·o·gram
pod·o·graph
pod·o·lite
po·dol·o·gist
po·dol·o·gy
pod·o·mech·a·no·ther·a·py
po·dom·e·ter
pod·o·phyl·lin
pod·o·phyl·lo·tox·in
pod·o·phyl·lum
  In·di·an p.
pod·o·phyl·lum
  res·in
pod·o·spasm
pod·o·spas·mus
POEMS
  syn·drome
po·go·ni·a·sis
po·go·ni·on
Po·go·no·myr·mex
poi·ki·lo·blast

poi·ki·lo·cyte
poi·ki·lo·cy·the·mia
poi·ki·lo·cy·to·sis
poi·ki·lo·den·to·sis
poi·ki·lo·der·ma
  p. atroph·i·cans and cat·a·ract
  p. atroph·i·cans vas·cu·la·re
  p. of Civatte
  p. con·gen·i·ta·le
poi·ki·lo·therm
poi·ki·lo·ther·mal
poi·ki·lo·ther·mic
poi·ki·lo·ther·mism
poi·ki·lo·ther·mous
poi·ki·lo·ther·my
poi·ki·lo·throm·bo·cyte
poi·ki·lo·thy·mia
point
  p. A
  ab·sor·bent p.'s
  al·ve·o·lar p.
  an·te·ri·or fo·cal p.
  apoph·y·sary p.
  ap·o·phys·i·al p.
  au·ric·u·lar p.
  ax·i·al p.
  p. B
  boil·ing p.
  Bolton p.
  Capuron's p.'s
  car·di·nal p.'s
  cen·tral-bear·ing p.
  Clado's p.
  cold-rig·or p.
  con·gru·ent p.'s
  con·ju·gate p.
  con·tact p.
  p.'s of con·ver·gence
  cra·ni·o·met·ric p.'s
  crit·i·cal p.
  dew p.
  p. of el·bow
  end p.
  far p.
  p. of fix·a·tion
  flash p.
  fo·cal p.
  freez·ing p.
  fus·ing p.
  Guéneau de Mussy's p.
  gut·ta-per·cha p.'s
  Hallé's p.
  heat-ri·gor p.
  in·ci·dent p.
  in·ci·sal p.
  iso·e·lec·tric p.
  iso·i·on·ic p.

point *(continued)*
  isos·best·ic p.
  J p.
  ju·gal p.
  low·er al·ve·o·lar p.
  ma·lar p.
  p. of max·i·mal im·pulse
  max·i·mum oc·cip·i·tal p.
  Mayo-Robson's p.
  McBurney's p.
  me·di·an man·dib·u·lar p.
  melt·ing p.
  men·tal p.
  me·top·ic p.
  mo·tor p.
  Munro's p.
  na·sal p.
  near p.
  neu·tral p.
  no·dal p.
  oc·cip·i·tal p.
  p. of os·si·fi·ca·tion
  pain·ful p.
  pos·te·ri·or fo·cal p.
  pow·er p.
  pre·au·ric·u·lar p.
  pres·sure p.
  pri·mary p. of os·si·fi·ca·tion
  prin·ci·pal p.
  p. of prox·i·mal con·tact
  p. of re·gard
  re·ten·tion p.
  sec·on·dary p. of os·si·fi·ca·tion
  sil·ver p.
  spi·nal p.
  sub·na·sal p.
  Sudeck's crit·i·cal p.
  su·pra-au·ric·u·lar p.
  su·pra·na·sal p.
  su·pra·or·bit·al p.
  syl·vi·an p.
  ten·der p.'s
  trig·ger p.
  Trousseau's p.
  Valleix's p.'s
  Weber's p.
  zy·go·max·il·lary p.
point
  an·gle
  de·le·tion
  ep·i·dem·ic
  mu·ta·tion
poin·ted
  con·dy·lo·ma
  wart
poin·til·lage

point·ing
point source
point sys·tem
  test types
Poirier's
  gland
  line
poise
Poiseuille's
  law
  space
Poiseuille's vis·cos·i·ty
  co·ef·fi·cient
poi·son
  ac·rid p.
  ar·row p.
  fish p.
  fu·gu p.
poi·son·ing
  ack·ee p.
  acute lead p.
  acute mer·cu·ry p.
  bac·te·ri·al food p.
  blood p.
  brack·en p.
  car·bon di·sul·fide p.
  car·bon mon·ox·ide p.
  chron·ic lead p.
  chron·ic mer·cu·ry p.
  clay pi·geon p.
  cro·ta·lar·ia p.
  cy·a·nide p.
  Da·tu·ra p.
  djen·kol p.
  fes·cue p.
  food p.
  lead p.
  lech·e·guil·la p.
  mer·cu·ry p.
  mush·room p.
  ox·y·gen p.
  pitch p.
  salm·on p.
  Sal·mo·nel·la food p.
  salt p.
  scom·broid p.
  se·le·ni·um p.
  sil·ver p.
  Sta·phy·lo·coc·cus food p.
  sweet clo·ver p.
  sys·tem·ic p.
  tet·ra·eth·yl p.
  thal·li·um p.
  tur·pen·tine p.
  wheat pas·ture p.
poi·son ivy
poi·son oak
poi·son·ous

poi·son su·mac
Poisson
  dis·tri·bu·tion
Poisson-Pearson
  for·mu·la
pok·er
  back
  spine
poke·weed
  mi·to·gen
po·lar
  ane·mia
  body
  cat·a·ract
  cell
  com·pound
  glob·ule
  hy·po·gen·e·sis
  plates
  pre·sen·ta·tion
  ring
  sol·vents
  star
  zone
po·lar·im·e·ter
po·lar·im·e·try
po·lar·i·scope
po·lar·i·scop·ic
po·lar·is·co·py
po·lar·i·ty
po·lar·i·za·tion
po·lar·ize
po·lar·ized
  light
po·la·riz·er
po·lar·iz·ing
  mi·cro·scope
po·lar·og·ra·phy
pol·dine meth·yl·sul·fate
pole
  abap·i·cal p.
  an·i·mal p.
  an·te·ri·or p. of eye·ball
  an·te·ri·or p. of lens
  ce·phal·ic p.
  fron·tal p.
  ger·mi·nal p.
  in·fe·ri·or p.
  lat·er·al p.
  me·di·al p.
  oc·cip·i·tal p.
  pel·vic p.
  pos·te·ri·or p. of eye·ball
  pos·te·ri·or p. of lens
  su·pe·ri·or p.
  tem·po·ral p.
  veg·e·tal p.

veg·e·ta·tive p.
  vi·tel·line p.
pole
  li·ga·tion
Polenské
  num·ber
po·li
po·lice·man
po·lio
  French p.
po·li·o·clas·tic
po·li·o·dys·tro·phia
  p. ce·re·bri pro·gres·si·va
    in·fan·ta·lis
po·li·o·dys·tro·phy
  pro·gress·ive ce·re·bral p.
po·li·o·en·ceph·a·li·tis
  p. in·fec·ti·va
  in·fe·ri·or p.
  su·pe·ri·or p.
  su·pe·ri·or hem·or·rhag·ic
    p.
po·li·o·en·ceph·a·lo·me·nin·go·
  my·e·li·tis
po·li·o·en·ceph·a·lo·my·e·li·tis
po·li·o·en·ceph·a·lop·a·thy
po·li·o·my·el·en·ceph·a·li·tis
po·li·o·my·e·li·tis
  acute an·te·ri·or p.
  acute bul·bar p.
  chron·ic an·te·ri·or p.
  mouse p.
po·li·o·my·e·li·tis
  im·mu·no·glob·u·lin
  vac·cines
  vi·rus
po·li·o·my·e·li·tis im·mune
  glob·u·lin (hu·man)
po·li·o·my·e·lo·en·ceph·a·li·tis
po·li·o·my·e·lop·a·thy
po·li·o·sis
po·li·o·vi·rus
  vac·cines
po·li·o·vi·rus hom·i·nis
pol·ish·ing
  brush
pol·ish·ing
Politzer
  bag
  meth·od
pol·itz·er·i·za·tion
  neg·a·tive p.
Politzer's lu·mi·nous
  cone
pol·ka
  fe·ver
pol·kis·sen of Zimmermann

poll
  evil
pol·la·ki·dip·sia
pol·la·ki·u·ria
pol·len
  an·ti·gen
  ex·tract
pol·le·no·sis
pol·lex
  p. pe·dis
pol·li·ces
pol·li·cis
pol·li·ci·za·tion
pol·li·no·sis
pol·lo·dic
pol·lu·tant
pol·lu·tion
  air p.
  noise p.
po·lo·cyte
po·lo·ni·um
pol·ox·a·lene
pol·ox·al·kol
pol·ster
po·lus
  po·li li·e·na·lis in·fe·ri·or
    et su·pe·ri·or
  po·li re·na·lis in·fe·ri·or et
    su·pe·ri·or
poly
Pólya
  gas·trec·to·my
pol·y·ac·id
pol·y·ad·e·ni·tis
  p. ma·lig·na
pol·y·ad·e·nop·a·thy
pol·y·ad·e·no·sis
pol·y·ad·e·nous
pol·y·al·co·hol
pol·y(al·co·hol)
pol·y·al·lel·ism
pol·y·a·mine
pol·y(amine)
pol·y·a·mine-meth·yl·ene
  res·in
pol·y(ami·no ac·ids)
pol·y·an·gi·i·tis
pol·y·an·i·on
pol·y·ar·ter·i·tis
  p. no·do·sa
pol·y·ar·thric
pol·y·ar·thri·tis
  p. chron·i·ca
  p. chron·i·ca vil·lo·sa
  ep·i·dem·ic p.
  p. rheu·ma·ti·ca acu·ta
  ver·te·bral p.
pol·y·ar·tic·u·lar

Pólya's
  op·er·a·tion
pol·y·a·vi·ta·min·o·sis
pol·y·ax·i·al
  joint
pol·y·ba·sic
  ac·id
pol·y·blast
pol·y·blen·nia
pol·y·car·bo·phil
pol·y·car·box·y·late
  ce·ment
pol·y·car·dia
pol·y·cen·tric
pol·y·chei·ria
pol·y·chi·ria
pol·y·chlo·rin·at·ed
  bi·phen·yl
pol·y·chon·dri·tis
  chron·ic atroph·ic p.
  re·laps·ing p.
pol·y·chro·ma·sia
pol·y·chro·mat·ic
  cell
pol·y·chro·mat·o·cyte
pol·y·chro·ma·to·phil
  cell
pol·y·chro·ma·to·phile
pol·y·chro·ma·to·phil·ia
pol·y·chro·ma·to·phil·ic
pol·y·chro·ma·to·sis
pol·y·chrome
  meth·yl·ene blue
pol·y·chro·me·mia
pol·y·chro·mia
pol·y·chro·mo·phil
pol·y·chro·mo·phil·ia
pol·y·chy·lia
pol·y·cin·e·ma·to·som·nog·ra·
  phy
pol·y·clin·ic
pol·y·clo·nal
pol·y·clo·nia
pol·y·co·ria
pol·y·crot·ic
po·lyc·ro·tism
pol·y·cy·e·sis
pol·y·cys·tic
  dis·ease of kid·neys
  kid·ney
  liv·er
  ova·ry
pol·y·cys·tic liv·er
  dis·ease
pol·y·cys·tic ova·ry
  syn·drome
pol·y·cy·the·mia
  com·pen·sa·to·ry p.

p. hy·per·to·ni·ca
rel·a·tive p.
p. ru·bra
p. ru·bra ve·ra
p. ve·ra
pol·y·dac·tyl·ia
pol·y·dac·tyl·ism
pol·y·dac·tyl·ous
pol·y·dac·ty·ly
pol·y·den·tia
pol·y·dip·sia
hys·ter·i·cal p.
psy·cho·gen·ic p.
psy·cho·gen·ic noc·tur·nal p.
pol·y·dis·per·soid
pol·y·dys·pla·sia
pol·y·dys·tro·phia
pol·y·dys·tro·phic
dwarf·ism
pol·y·dys·tro·phy
pol·y·em·bry·o·ny
pol·y·en·do·crine de·fi·cien·cy
syn·drome
pol·y·ene
pol·y·e·nic ac·ids
pol·y·e·no·ic ac·ids
pol·y·er·gic
pol·y·es·ter
res·in
pol·y·es·the·sia
pol·y·es·tra·di·ol phos·phate
pol·y·es·trous
pol·y·eth·y·lene gly·cols
pol·y·fruc·tose
pol·y·ga·lac·tia
pol·y·ga·lac·tu·ro·nase
pol·y·gan·gli·on·ic
pol·y·gene
pol·y·gen·ic
in·her·i·tance
pol·y·glan·du·lar
pol·y·glan·du·lar de·fi·cien·cy
syn·drome
pol·y·glu·ta·mate
poly(gly·col·ic ac·id)
pol·y·gna·thus
pol·y·graph
Mackenzie's p.
pol·y·gy·ria
pol·y·he·dral
pol·y·hex·os·es
pol·y·hi·dro·sis
pol·y·hy·brid
pol·y·hy·dram·ni·os
pol·y·hy·dric
pol·y·hy·per·men·or·rhea
pol·y·hy·po·men·or·rhea

pol·y·i·dro·sis
pol·y·kar·y·o·cyte
pol·y·lep·tic
fe·ver
pol·y·lo·gia
pol·y·mas·tia
pol·y·mas·ti·gote
pol·y·ma·zia
pol·y·me·lia
pol·y·men·or·rhea
pol·y·mer
cross-linked p.
pol·y·mer·ase
pol·y·mer fume
fe·ver
pol·y·me·ria
pol·y·mer·ic
po·lym·er·id
po·lym·er·i·za·tion
po·lym·er·ize
pol·y·met·a·car·pa·lia
pol·y·met·a·car·pa·lism
pol·y·met·a·tar·sa·lia
pol·y·met·a·tar·sa·lism
pol·y·mi·cro·lip·o·ma·to·sis
po·lym·i·tus
pol·y·morph
pol·y·mor·phic
re·tic·u·lo·sis
pol·y·mor·phic light
erup·tion
pol·y·mor·phic su·per·fi·cial
ker·a·ti·tis
pol·y·mor·phism
bal·anced p.
DNA p.
frag·ment length p.
ge·net·ic p.
lip·o·pro·tein p.
re·stric·tion length p.
re·stric·tion-site p.
pol·y·mor·pho·cel·lu·lar
pol·y·mor·pho·cyt·ic
leu·ke·mia
pol·y·mor·pho·nu·cle·ar
leu·ko·cyte
pol·y·mor·phous
lay·er
per·ver·sion
pol·y·my·al·gia
p. ar·te·ri·ti·ca
p. rheu·ma·ti·ca
pol·y·my·oc·lo·nus
pol·y·my·o·si·tis
pol·y·myx·in
p. B sul·fate
pol·y·ne·sic
pol·y·neu·ral

pol·y·neu·ral·gia
pol·y·neu·rit·ic
  psy·cho·sis
pol·y·neu·ri·tis
  acute id·i·o·path·ic p.
  chron·ic fa·mil·i·al p.
  eryth·re·de·ma p.
  in·fec·tious p.
pol·y·neu·ro·ni·tis
pol·y·neu·rop·a·thy
  buck·thorn p.
  nu·trit·ion·al p.
  ure·mic p.
pol·y·nox·y·lin
pol·y·nu·cle·ar
  leu·ko·cyte
pol·y·nu·cle·ate
pol·y·nu·cle·o·sis
pol·y·nu·cle·o·ti·das·es
pol·y·nu·cle·o·tide
  p. phos·pho·ryl·ase
pol·y·o·don·tia
pol·y·ol
  p. de·hy·dro·gen·as·es
pol·y·o·ma
  vi·rus
Pol·y·o·ma·vi·rus
pol·y·on·cho·sis
pol·y·on·co·sis
  cu·ta·ne·o·man·dib·u·lar p.
pol·y·o·nych·ia
pol·y·o·pia
pol·y·op·sia
pol·y·or·chid·ism
pol·y·or·chism
pol·y·os·tot·ic
pol·y·os·tot·ic fi·brous
  dys·pla·sia
pol·y·o·tia
pol·y·ov·u·lar
pol·y·ov·u·lar ovar·i·an
  fol·li·cle
pol·y·ov·u·la·tory
pol·yp
  ad·e·nom·a·tous p.
  bleed·ing p.
  bron·chi·al p.
  car·di·ac p.
  cel·lu·lar p.
  cho·a·nal p.
  cys·tic p.
  den·tal p.
  fi·brin·ous p.
  fi·brous p.
  fleshy p.
  ge·lat·i·nous p.
  Hopmann's p.
  hy·da·tid p.

hy·per·plas·tic p.
in·flam·ma·to·ry p.
ju·ve·nile p.
la·ryn·ge·al p.
li·po·ma·tous p.
lym·phoid p.
met·a·plas·tic p.
mu·cous p.
my·o·ma·tous p.
na·sal p.
os·se·ous p.
pe·dun·cu·lat·ed p.
pla·cen·tal p.
pulp p.
re·gen·er·a·tive p.
re·ten·tion p.
ses·sile p.
tooth p.
vas·cu·lar p.
pol·y·pap·il·lo·ma
pol·y·path·ia
pol·y·pec·to·my
pol·y·pep·tide
  gas·tric in·hib·i·to·ry p.
  va·so·ac·tive in·tes·ti·nal p.
pol·y·pha·gia
pol·y·pha·lan·gism
pol·y·phal·lic
pol·y·phar·ma·cy
pol·y·phen·ic
  gene
pol·y·phe·nol ox·i·dase
pol·y·pho·bia
pol·y·phos·phor·y·lase
pol·y·phra·sia
pol·y·phy·let·ic
  the·o·ry
pol·y·phy·le·tism
pol·y·phy·o·dont
po·ly·pi
pol·yp·i·form
pol·y·plas·mia
pol·y·plast
pol·y·plas·tic
Pol·y·plax
pol·y·ple·gia
pol·yp·loid
pol·y·ploi·dy
pol·yp·nea
pol·y·po·dia
pol·yp·oid
  ad·e·no·ma
po·lyp·or·ous
Pol·y·po·rus
pol·y·po·sia
pol·yp·o·sis
  p. co·li

fa·mil·i·al in·tes·ti·nal p.
mul·ti·ple in·tes·ti·nal p.
po·lyp·o·tome
pol·yp·o·trite
pol·y·pous
en·do·car·di·tis
gas·tri·tis
pol·y·prag·ma·sy
pol·yp·tych·i·al
pol·y·pus
pol·y·ra·dic·u·li·tis
pol·y·ra·dic·u·lo·my·op·a·thy
pol·y·ra·dic·u·lo·neu·rop·a·thy
pol·y·ra·dic·u·lop·a·thy
pol·y·ri·bo·nu·cle·o·tide nu·cle·
o·tid·yl trans·fer·ase
pol·y·ri·bo·somes
pol·yr·rhea
pol·y·sac·char·ide
pneu·mo·coc·cal p.
spe·cif·ic sol·u·ble p.
pol·y·sce·lia
pol·y·scope
pol·y·ser·o·si·tis
fa·mil·i·al par·ox·ys·mal p.
fa·mil·i·al re·cur·rent p.
pe·ri·od·ic p.
pol·y·si·nu·si·tis
pol·y·somes
pol·y·so·mia
pol·y·so·mic
pol·y·som·no·gram
pol·y·som·nog·ra·phy
pol·y·so·my
pol·y·sper·mia
pol·y·sper·mism
pol·y·sper·my
pol·y·sple·nia
syn·drome
pol·y·ster·ax·ic
pol·y·stich·ia
pol·y·sul·fide rub·ber
pol·y·sus·pen·soid
pol·y·sym·brach·y·dac·ty·ly
pol·y·syn·ap·tic
pol·y·syn·dac·ty·ly
pol·y·ten·di·ni·tis
pol·y·tene
chro·mo·some
pol·y·the·lia
pol·y·thi·a·zide
po·lyt·o·cous
pol·y·to·mog·ra·phy
pol·y·trich·ia
pol·y·tri·cho·sis
pol·y·un·guia
pol·y·u·ria
test

pol·y·va·lent
al·ler·gy
an·ti·se·rum
se·rum
vac·cine
pol·y·vi·done
pol·y·vi·nyl
pol·y·vi·nyl al·co·hol
pol·y·vi·nyl chlo·ride
pol·y·vi·nyl pyr·rol·i·done
pol·y·vi·nyl pyr·rol·i·done-io·
dine com·plex
pol·y·zo·ic
pol·y·zy·got·ic
twins
po·made
ac·ne
po·ma·tum
pome·gran·ate
Pomeroy's
op·er·a·tion
Pompe's
dis·ease
pom·pho·lyx
pom·phus
Pon·ceau de xy·li·dine
pond
frac·ture
pon·der·al
in·dex
Ponfick's
shad·ow
po·no·graph
po·no·pal·mo·sis
po·no·pho·bia
po·nos
pons
p. ce·re·bel·li
p. hep·a·tis
p. va·ro·lii
pon·tes
pon·tic
pon·ti·cu·lus
p. hep·a·tis
p. na·si
p. pro·mon·to·rii
pon·tile
ap·o·plexy
pon·tine
an·gle
ar·ter·ies
cis·tern
flex·ure
hem·or·rhage
nu·clei
veins
pon·tine an·gle
tu·mor

pon·tine gray
  mat·ter
pon·to·cer·e·bel·lar
  re·cess
pon·to·med·ul·lary
  groove
pool
  ab·dom·i·nal p.
  gene p.
  met·a·bol·ic p.
  vag·i·nal p.
pooled
  se·rum
pooled blood
  se·rum
Pool's
  phe·nom·e·non
Pool-Schlesinger
  sign
poor·ly dif·fer·en·ti·at·ed lym·pho·cyt·ic
  lym·pho·ma
pop·lar
pop·les
pop·lit·e·al
  ar·tery
  fas·cia
  fos·sa
  groove
  line
  mus·cle
  notch
  plane of fe·mur
  plex·us
  re·gion
  space
  sur·face of fe·mur
  vein
pop·lit·e·al com·mu·ni·cat·ing
  nerve
pop·lit·e·al en·trap·ment
  syn·drome
pop·lit·e·al lymph
  nodes
pop·li·te·us
pop·py
  p. oil
pop·u·la·tion
  ge·net·ics
por·ce·lain
  in·lay
por·cine
  ad·e·no·vi·rus·es
  ame·lia
  graft
  par·a·ker·a·to·sis
  valve

por·cine he·mag·glu·ti·nat·ing en·ceph·a·li·tis
  vi·rus
por·cine trans·mis·si·ble gas·tro·en·ter·i·tis
por·cu·pine
  skin
pore
  au·di·to·ry p.
  di·lat·ed p.
  ex·ter·nal acous·tic p.
  ex·ter·nal au·di·to·ry p.
  gus·ta·to·ry p.
  in·ter·al·ve·o·lar p.'s
  in·ter·nal acous·tic p.
  Kohn's p.'s
  nu·cle·ar p.
  slit p.'s
  sweat p.
  taste p.
por·en·ce·pha·lia
por·en·ce·phal·ic
por·en·ceph·a·li·tis
por·en·ceph·a·lous
por·en·ceph·a·ly
Porges
  meth·od
Porges-Meier
  test
po·ri
po·ria
Po·rif·era
por·i·o·ma·nia
por·i·on
por·no·lag·nia
po·ro·cele
po·ro·ceph·a·li·a·sis
Po·ro·ce·phal·i·dae
po·ro·ceph·a·lo·sis
Po·ro·ceph·a·lus
  P. ar·mil·la·tus
po·ro·co·nid·i·um
po·ro·ker·a·to·sis
  ac·tin·ic p.
po·ro·ma
  ec·crine p.
po·ro·ses
po·ro·sis
  ce·re·bral p.
po·ros·i·ty
por·o·spore
po·rot·ic
po·rot·o·my
po·rous
por·phin
por·phine
por·pho·bi·lin

por·pho·bi·lin·o·gen
  p. syn·thase
por·phyr·ia
  acute p.
  acute in·ter·mit·tent p.
  bo·vine p.
  con·gen·i·tal eryth·ro·poi·
    et·ic p.
  p. cu·ta·nea tar·da
  eryth·ro·he·pat·ic p.
  eryth·ro·poi·et·ic p.
  he·pa·tic p.
  in·ter·mit·tent acute p.
  o·vu·lo·cy·clic p.
  South Af·ri·can type p.
  squir·rel p.
  swine p.
  symp·to·mat·ic p.
  var·ie·gate p.
por·phy·rin
por·phy·rin·o·gens
por·phy·rins
por·phy·ri·nu·ria
por·phy·ri·za·tion
por·phy·ru·ria
por·ri·go
  p. de·cal·vans
  p. fa·vo·sa
  p. fur·fu·rans
  p. lar·va·lis
  p. lu·pi·no·sa
  p. scu·tu·la·ta
Porro
  hys·ter·ec·to·my
  op·er·a·tion
por·rop·sia
por·ta
  p. li·e·nis
  p. pul·mo·nis
  p. re·nis
por·ta·ca·val
  shunt
por·tae
por·tal
  an·te·ri·or in·tes·ti·nal p.
  in·tes·ti·nal p.'s
  pos·te·ri·or in·tes·ti·nal p.
por·tal
  ca·nals
  cir·cu·la·tion
  cir·rho·sis
  fis·sure
  hy·per·ten·sion
  lob·ule of liv·er
  py·e·mia
  sys·tem
  vein

por·tal-sys·tem·ic
  en·ceph·a·lop·a·thy
por·ta·sys·tem·ic
  shunt
Porter's
  fas·cia
Porter-Silber
  chro·mo·gens
  re·ac·tion
Porter-Silber chro·mo·gens
  test
por·tio
  p. in·ter·me·dia
  p. ma·jor ner·vi tri·gem·i·
    ni
  p. mi·nor ner·vi tri·gem·i·
    ni
por·ti·o·nes
por·ti·plex·us
por·to·bil·i·o·ar·te·ri·al
por·to·en·ter·os·to·my
por·to·gram
por·tog·ra·phy
por·to·sys·tem·ic
por·to·ve·nog·ra·phy
Por·tu·guese-A·zor·e·an
  dis·ease
port-wine
  mark
  stain
po·rus
  p. cro·ta·phy·ti·co·buc·ci·
    na·to·ri·us
  p. op·ti·cus
Posadas
  dis·ease
po·si·tion
  ag·no·sia
  ef·fect
  sense
po·si·tion
  an·a·tom·i·cal p.
  Bozeman's p.
  Casselberry p.
  cen·tric p.
  con·dy·lar hinge p.
  dor·sal p.
  dor·so·sa·cral p.
  ec·cen·tric p.
  elec·tri·cal heart p.
  Elliot's p.
  English p.
  flank p.
  Fowler's p.
  fron·to·an·te·ri·or p.
  fron·to·pos·te·ri·or p.
  fron·to·trans·verse p.
  gen·u·cu·bi·tal p.

po·si·tion *(continued)*
  gen·u·pec·to·ral p.
  heart p.
  hinge p.
  in·ter·cus·pal p.
  knee-chest p.
  knee-el·bow p.
  lat·er·al re·cum·bent p.
  leap·frog p.
  left fron·to·an·te·ri·or
  left fron·to·pos·te·ri·or
  left fron·to·trans·verse
  left men·to·an·te·ri·or
  left men·to·pos·te·ri·or
  left men·to·trans·verse
  left oc·cip·i·to·an·te·ri·or
  left oc·cip·i·to·pos·te·ri·or
  left oc·cip·i·to·trans·verse
  left sa·cro·an·te·ri·or
  left sa·cro·pos·te·ri·or
  left sa·cro·trans·verse
  li·thot·o·my p.
  man·dib·u·lar hinge p.
  Mayo-Robson's p.
  men·to·an·te·ri·or p.
  men·to·pos·te·ri·or p.
  men·to·trans·verse p.
  Noble's p.
  ob·stet·ric p.
  oc·cip·i·to·an·te·ri·or p.
  oc·cip·i·to·pos·te·ri·or p.
  oc·cip·i·to·trans·verse p.
  oc·clu·sal p.
  phys·i·o·log·ic rest p.
  pos·tur·al p.
  pos·tur·al rest·ing p.
  prone p.
  pro·tru·sive p.
  rest p.
  right fron·to·an·te·ri·or
  right fron·to·pos·te·ri·or
  right fron·to·trans·verse
  right men·to·an·te·ri·or
  right men·to·pos·te·ri·or
  right men·to·trans·verse
  right oc·cip·i·to·an·te·ri·or
  right oc·cip·i·to·pos·te·ri·or
  right oc·cip·i·to·trans·verse
  right sa·cro·an·te·ri·or
  right sa·cro·pos·te·ri·or
  right sa·cro·trans·verse
  Rose's p.
  sa·cro·an·te·ri·or p.
  sa·cro·pos·te·ri·or p.
  sa·cro·trans·verse p.
  Scultetus' p.
  sem·i·prone p.
  Simon's p.
  Sims' p.
  su·pine p.
  ter·mi·nal hinge p.
  Trendelenburg's p.
  Valentine's p.
  Walcher p.
po·si·tion·al
  nys·tag·mus
po·si·tion·er
pos·i·tive
  false p.
pos·i·tive
  ac·com·mo·da·tion
  af·ter·im·age
  an·er·gy
  cat·a·lyst
  chro·not·ro·pism
  con·ver·gence
  elec·trode
  elec·tron
  elec·tro·tax·is
  feed·back
  me·nis·cus
  phase
  rays
  sco·to·ma
  stain
  tax·is
  ther·mo·tax·is
  trans·fer·ence
  va·lence
pos·i·tive che·mo·tax·is
pos·i·tive cy·to·tax·is
pos·i·tive end-ex·pi·ra·to·ry
  pres·sure
pos·i·tive G
pos·i·tive hy·drot·ro·pism
pos·i·tive leu·ko·cy·to·tax·ia
pos·i·tive·ly
  bath·mo·tro·pic
  dro·mo·tro·pic
  in·o·tro·pic
pos·i·tive-neg·a·tive pres·sure
  breath·ing
pos·i·tive neu·tro·tax·is
pos·i·tive p
pos·i·tive pho·tod·ro·my
pos·i·tive pho·to·tax·is
pos·i·tive pho·tot·ro·pism
pos·i·tive re·in·forc·er
pos·i·tive ster·e·ot·ro·pism
pos·i·tive sup·port·ing
  re·ac·tions
pos·i·tive tro·pism
pos·i·tron
pos·i·tron emis·sion
  to·mog·ra·phy
po·so·log·ic

po·sol·o·gy
post
  dam
  im·plant
post·ac·e·tab·u·lar
post·ad·o·les·cence
post·a·dre·nal·ec·to·my
  syn·drome
post·age stamp
  grafts
post·a·nal
  gut
post·an·es·thet·ic
post·ap·o·plec·tic
post·ax·i·al
post·ax·il·lary
  line
post·ba·sic
  stare
post·bra·chi·al
post·cap·il·lary
  ven·ules
post·car·di·nal
post·car·di·ot·o·my
  syn·drome
post·ca·va
post·ca·val
post·cen·tral
  ar·ea
  ar·tery
  fis·sure
  gy·rus
  sul·cus
post·cho·le·cys·tec·to·my
  syn·drome
post·chrom·ing
post·ci·bal
post·cla·vic·u·lar
post·clo·a·cal
  gut
post·co·i·tal
post·co·i·tus
post·com·mis·sur·ot·o·my
  syn·drome
post·com·mu·ni·cal
  part
post·con·cus·sion
  neu·ro·sis
  syn·drome
post·cor·dial
post·cos·tal
  anas·to·mo·sis
post·crown
post·cu·bi·tal
post dam
  ar·ea
post·dam
post·di·a·stol·ic

post·di·crot·ic
post·diph·the·rit·ic
  pa·ral·y·sis
post·dor·mi·tal
post·dor·mi·tum
post·drive
  de·pres·sion
post·duc·tal
post·en·ceph·a·lit·ic
post·ep·i·lep·tic
pos·te·ri·or
  arch of at·las
  asyn·cli·tism
  bor·der of pet·rous part of
    tem·po·ral bone
  cells
  cham·ber of eye
  cho·roid·i·tis
  col·umn of spi·nal cord
  cord of brach·i·al plex·us
  cusp
  em·bry·o·tox·on
  ex·trem·i·ty
  fon·ta·nel
  fu·nic·u·lus
  horn
  lay·er of rec·tus ab·do·mi·
    nis sheath
  lig·a·ment of head of fib·u·
    la
  lig·a·ment of in·cus
  lig·a·ment of knee
  limb of in·ter·nal cap·sule
  limb of sta·pes
  lip
  lobe of hy·poph·y·sis
  mar·gin
  na·ris
  ne·phrec·to·my
  notch of cer·e·bel·lum
  oc·clu·sion
  part
  pil·lar of fau·ces
  pil·lar of for·nix
  pi·tu·i·tary
  pole of eye·ball
  pole of lens
  pro·cess of sep·tal car·ti·
    lage
  pyr·a·mid of the me·dul·la
  ra·chis·chi·sis
  re·cess of tym·pan·ic mem·
    brane
  re·gion of fore·arm
  re·gion of neck
  rhi·nos·co·py
  rhi·zot·o·my
  root

pos·te·ri·or *(continued)*
scle·ri·tis
scle·ro·sis
scle·rot·o·my
seg·ment
staph·y·lo·ma
sur·face
sur·face of eye·lids
sur·face of pet·rous part
sym·bleph·a·ron
syn·ech·ia
teeth
tri·an·gle of neck
tu·ber·cle of at·las
tu·ber·cle of cer·vi·cal ver·
te·brae
ure·thri·tis
uve·i·tis
vag·i·nis·mus
vein of left ven·tri·cle
vein of sep·tum pel·lu·ci·
dum
vit·rec·to·my
wall of mid·dle ear
wall of stom·ach
wall of va·gi·na
pos·te·ri·or al·ve·o·lar
ar·tery
pos·te·ri·or am·pul·lar
nerve
pos·te·ri·or an·te·brach·i·al
nerve
pos·te·ri·or an·te·ri·or jug·u·
lar
vein
pos·te·ri·or ar·tic·u·lar
sur·face of dens
pos·te·ri·or at·lan·to-oc·cip·i·
tal
mem·brane
pos·te·ri·or au·ric·u·lar
ar·tery
groove
mus·cle
nerve
plex·us
vein
pos·te·ri·or ax·il·lary
line
pos·te·ri·or ba·sal
seg·ment
pos·te·ri·or cal·ca·ne·al ar·tic·
u·lar
sur·face
pos·te·ri·or car·di·nal
veins
pos·te·ri·or car·pal
re·gion

pos·te·ri·or ce·cal
ar·tery
pos·te·ri·or cen·tral
con·vo·lu·tion
gy·rus
pos·te·ri·or ce·re·bral
ar·tery
com·mis·sure
pos·te·ri·or cer·vi·cal in·ter·
trans·verse
mus·cles
pos·te·ri·or cho·roi·dal
ar·tery
pos·te·ri·or cir·cum·flex hu·
mer·al
ar·tery
pos·te·ri·or col·umn
cor·dot·o·my
pos·te·ri·or com·mu·ni·cat·ing
ar·tery
pos·te·ri·or con·dy·loid
fo·ra·men
pos·te·ri·or con·junc·ti·val
ar·tery
pos·te·ri·or cor·o·nary
plex·us
pos·te·ri·or cos·to·trans·verse
lig·a·ment
pos·te·ri·or cra·ni·al
fos·sa
pos·te·ri·or cri·co·ar·y·te·noid
lig·a·ment
mus·cle
pos·te·ri·or cru·ci·ate
lig·a·ment
pos·te·ri·or cu·bi·tal
re·gion
pos·te·ri·or cu·ta·ne·ous
nerve of arm
nerve of fore·arm
nerve of thigh
pos·te·ri·or den·tal
ar·tery
pos·te·ri·or de·scend·ing
ar·tery
pos·te·ri·or elas·tic
lay·er
pos·te·ri·or eth·moi·dal
ar·tery
nerve
pos·te·ri·or fa·cial
vein
pos·te·ri·or fo·cal
point
pos·te·ri·or hy·po·tha·lam·ic
nu·cle·us

pos·te·ri·or in·fe·ri·or cer·e·bel·lar
ar·tery
pos·te·ri·or in·fe·ri·or cer·e·bel·lar ar·tery
syn·drome
pos·te·ri·or in·fe·ri·or il·i·ac
spine
pos·te·ri·or in·ter·con·dy·lar
ar·ea
pos·te·ri·or in·ter·cos·tal
ar·tery
veins
pos·te·ri·or in·ter·me·di·ate
groove
pos·te·ri·or in·ter·os·se·ous
ar·tery
nerve
pos·te·ri·or in·ter·ven·tric·u·lar
ar·tery
groove
pos·te·ri·or in·tes·ti·nal
por·tal
pos·te·ri·or in·tra·oc·cip·i·tal
joint
pos·te·ri·or la·bi·al
ar·ter·ies
com·mis·sure
nerves
veins
pos·te·ri·or lac·ri·mal
crest
pos·te·ri·or lat·er·al na·sal
ar·ter·ies
pos·te·ri·or lim·it·ing
lay·er of cor·nea
pos·te·ri·or lon·gi·tu·di·nal
bun·dle
lig·a·ment
pos·te·ri·or lu·nate
lob·ule
pos·te·ri·or mar·gi·nal
vein
pos·te·ri·or me·di·al
nu·cle·us of thal·a·mus
pos·te·ri·or me·di·an
fis·sure of the me·dul·la ob·lon·ga·ta
fis·sure of spi·nal cord
line
sul·cus of me·dul·la ob·lon·ga·ta
sul·cus of spi·nal cord
pos·te·ri·or me·di·as·ti·nal lymph
nodes
pos·te·ri·or med·ul·lary
ve·lum

pos·te·ri·or me·nin·ge·al
ar·tery
pos·te·ri·or me·nis·co·fem·o·ral
lig·a·ment
pos·te·ri·or my·o·car·di·al
in·farc·tion
pos·te·ri·or na·sal
spine
pos·te·ri·or oc·cip·i·to·ax·i·al
lig·a·ment
pos·te·ri·or pal·a·tal
seal
pos·te·ri·or pal·a·tal seal
ar·ea
pos·te·ri·or pal·a·tine
arch
fo·ra·men
spine
pos·te·ri·or pan·cre·at·i·co·du·o·de·nal
ar·tery
pos·te·ri·or pa·ri·e·tal
ar·tery
pos·te·ri·or par·ol·fac·to·ry
sul·cus
pos·te·ri·or pa·rot·id
veins
pos·te·ri·or pel·vic
ex·en·ter·a·tion
pos·te·ri·or per·fo·rat·ed
sub·stance
pos·te·ri·or per·i·cal·lo·sal
vein
pos·te·ri·or per·i·ven·tric·u·lar
nu·cle·us
pos·te·ri·or per·o·ne·al
ar·ter·ies
pos·te·ri·or pri·mary
di·vi·sion
pos·te·ri·or sa·cro·il·i·ac
lig·a·ments
pos·te·ri·or sa·cro·sci·at·ic
lig·a·ment
pos·te·ri·or sag·it·tal
di·am·e·ter
pos·te·ri·or sca·lene
mus·cle
pos·te·ri·or scap·u·lar
nerve
pos·te·ri·or scro·tal
nerves
veins
pos·te·ri·or sem·i·cir·cu·lar
ca·nals
pos·te·ri·or sep·tal
ar·tery of nose

pos·te·ri·or spi·nal
  ar·tery
  scle·ro·sis
pos·te·ri·or spi·no·cer·e·bel·lar
  tract
pos·te·ri·or ster·no·cla·vic·u·lar
  lig·a·ment
pos·te·ri·or sub·cap·su·lar
  cat·a·ract
pos·te·ri·or su·pe·ri·or al·ve·o·
  lar
  ar·tery
pos·te·ri·or su·pe·ri·or il·i·ac
  spine
pos·te·ri·or su·pra·cla·vic·u·lar
  nerve
pos·te·ri·or ta·lo·fib·u·lar
  lig·a·ment
pos·te·ri·or ta·lo·tib·i·al
  lig·a·ment
pos·te·ri·or tem·po·ral
  ar·tery
pos·te·ri·or tho·rac·ic
  nerve
pos·te·ri·or tib·i·al
  ar·tery
  mus·cle
  node
  veins
pos·te·ri·or tib·i·al re·cur·rent
  ar·tery
pos·te·ri·or tib·i·o·fib·u·lar
  lig·a·ment
pos·te·ri·or tib·i·o·ta·lar
  part
pos·te·ri·or tooth
  form
pos·te·ri·or tym·pan·ic
  ar·tery
pos·te·ri·or ure·thral
  valves
pos·te·ri·or vag·i·nal
  her·nia
pos·te·ri·us
pos·ter·o·an·te·ri·or
pos·ter·o·clu·sion
pos·ter·o·ex·ter·nal
pos·ter·o·in·ter·nal
pos·ter·o·lat·er·al
  fis·sure
  fon·ta·nel
  groove
  sul·cus
pos·ter·o·lat·er·al cen·tral
  ar·ter·ies
pos·ter·o·me·di·al
pos·ter·o·me·di·al cen·tral
  ar·ter·ies

pos·ter·o·me·di·an
pos·ter·o·pa·ri·e·tal
pos·ter·o·su·pe·ri·or
pos·ter·o·tem·po·ral
post·e·rup·tion
  cu·ti·cle
post·e·soph·a·ge·al
post·es·trum
post·es·trus
post·ex·tra·sys·tol·ic
  pause
post·ex·tra·sys·tol·ic T
  wave
post·feb·rile
post·gan·gli·on·ic
post·gan·gli·on·ic mo·tor
  neu·ron
post·gas·trec·to·my
  syn·drome
post·gle·noid
  fo·ra·men
post·hem·i·ple·gic
  ath·e·to·sis
  cho·rea
post·hem·or·rha·gic
  ane·mia
post·he·pat·ic
post·hep·a·tit·ic
  cir·rho·sis
pos·thet·o·my
pos·thi·o·plas·ty
post·hip·po·cam·pal
  fis·sure
pos·thi·tis
pos·tho·lith
post·hy·oid
post·hyp·not·ic
  am·ne·sia
  psy·cho·sis
  sug·ges·tion
post·hy·po·gly·ce·mic
  hy·per·gly·ce·mia
post·ic·tal
pos·ti·cus
  pal·sy
  pa·ral·y·sis
post·in·fec·tious
  bra·dy·car·dia
  psy·cho·sis
post·in·flu·en·zal
post·is·chi·al
post-ka·la azar der·mal
  leish·man·oid
post·lam·i·nar
  part of op·tic nerve
post·lin·gual
  deaf·ness
  fis·sure

post·lu·nate
  fis·sure
post·ma·lar·i·al
post·mas·toid
post·ma·ture
post·ma·tur·i·ty
  syn·drome
post·me·di·an
post·me·di·as·ti·nal
post·me·di·as·ti·num
post·mei·ot·ic
  phase
post·men·in·git·ic
  hy·dro·ceph·a·lus
post·men·o·pau·sal
  at·ro·phy
post·min·i·mus
post·mor·tem
  clot
  de·liv·ery
  ex·am·i·na·tion
  hy·pos·ta·sis
  li·ve·do
  li·vid·i·ty
  pus·tule
  ri·gid·i·ty
  sug·gil·la·tion
  throm·bus
  tu·ber·cle
  wart
post·my·o·car·di·al in·farc·tion
  syn·drome
post·na·ri·al
post·na·ris
post·na·sal
  drip
post·na·tal
  life
  pit of the new·born
post·ne·crot·ic
  cir·rho·sis
post·neu·rit·ic
post·nor·mal
  oc·clu·sion
post·oc·u·lar
post·op·er·a·tive
  pa·rot·i·di·tis
  pneu·mo·nia
  tet·a·ny
post·op·er·a·tive pres·sure
  al·o·pe·cia
post·o·ral
  arch·es
post·or·bi·tal
post·pal·a·tal
  seal
post·pal·a·tal seal
  ar·ea

post·pal·a·tine
post·par·a·lyt·ic
post·par·tum
  al·o·pe·cia
  amen·or·rhea
  car·di·o·my·op·a·thy
  es·trus
  hem·or·rhage
  hy·per·ten·sion
  psy·cho·sis
  tet·a·nus
post·par·tum pi·tu·i·tary ne·cro·sis
  syn·drome
post·par·tu·ri·ent
  he·mo·glo·bi·nu·ria
post·per·fu·sion
  lung
post·per·i·car·di·ot·o·my
  syn·drome
post·pha·ryn·ge·al
  space
post·phle·bit·ic
  syn·drome
post·pneu·mon·ic
post·pran·di·al
  li·pe·mia
post·pri·mary
  tu·ber·cu·lo·sis
post·pu·ber·al
post·pu·ber·tal
post·pu·ber·ty
post·pu·bes·cent
post·pyk·not·ic
post·py·lor·ic
  sphinc·ter
post·py·ram·i·dal
  fis·sure
post·re·duc·tion
  phase
post·re·nal
  al·bu·min·ur·ia
post·rhi·nal
  fis·sure
post·ro·lan·dic
post·ru·bel·la
  syn·drome
post·sa·cral
post·scap·u·lar
post·scar·la·ti·nal
post·sphe·noid
  bone
post·sphyg·mic
  in·ter·val
post·splen·ic
post·sul·cal
  part

post·syn·ap·tic
 mem·brane
post·tar·sal
post·tec·ta
post-term
 in·fant
post·tib·i·al
post·trans·verse
post·trau·mat·ic
 de·lir·i·um
 de·men·tia
 ep·i·lep·sy
 hy·dro·ceph·a·lus
 neu·ro·sis
 os·te·o·po·ro·sis
 psy·cho·sis
 syn·drome
post·trau·mat·ic ar·te·ri·al
 throm·bo·sis
post·trau·mat·ic lep·to·me·nin·ge·al
 cyst
post·trau·mat·ic neck
 syn·drome
post·trau·mat·ic stress
 dis·or·der
 syn·drome
post·trau·mat·ic ve·nous
 throm·bo·sis
post·tre·mat·ic
post·tus·sis
post·tus·sis suc·tion
 sound
post·tus·sive
 suc·tion
post·ty·phoid
pos·tu·late
 Ampère's p.
 Avogadro's p.
 Ehrlich's p.
 Koch's p.'s
pos·tur·al
 al·bu·min·ur·ia
 con·trac·tion
 drain·age
 hy·po·ten·sion
 is·che·mia
 my·o·neu·ral·gia
 po·si·tion
 pro·tein·u·ria
 re·flex
 set
 syn·co·pe
 trem·or
 ver·sion
 ver·ti·go
pos·tur·al rest·ing
 po·si·tion

pos·ture
 sense
pos·ture
 Stern's p.
post·u·ter·ine
post·vac·ci·nal
 en·ceph·a·li·tis
post·val·var
post·val·vu·lar
po·ta·ble
 wa·ter
Potain's
 sign
pot·a·mo·pho·bia
pot·ash
 caus·tic p.
 sul·fu·rat·ed p.
po·tas·sic
po·tas·si·o·cu·pric
po·tas·si·o·mer·cu·ric
po·tas·si·um
 p. ac·e·tate
 p. ac·id tar·trate
 p. al·um
 p. ami·no·sa·lic·y·late
 p. an·ti·mo·nyl tar·trate
 p. atrac·ty·late
 p. bi·car·bon·ate
 p. bi·chro·mate
 p. bi·tar·trate
 p. bro·mide
 p. chlo·rate
 p. chlo·ride
 p. cit·rate
 p. cy·a·nide
 di·ba·sic p. phos·phate
 p. di·chro·mate
 ef·fer·ves·cent p. cit·rate
 p. fer·ro·cy·a·nide
 p. glu·co·nate
 p. guai·a·col·sul·fo·nate
 p. hy·drox·ide
 p. hy·po·phos·phite
 p. io·date
 p. io·dide
 p. met·a·phos·phate
 mon·o·ba·sic p. phos·phate
 p. ni·trate
 pen·i·cil·lin G p.
 p. per·chlo·rate
 p. per·man·ga·nate
 p. phos·phate
 p. rho·da·nate
 p. so·di·um tar·trate
 p. sor·bate
 p. suc·ci·nate
 p. sul·fate
 p. sul·fo·cy·a·nate

p. tar·trate
p. thi·o·cy·a·nate
po·tas·si·um
in·hi·bi·tion
po·ta·to
nose
tu·mor of neck
po·ta·to dex·trose
agar
po·ten·cy
sex·u·al p.
po·tent
po·ten·tial
ac·tion p.
af·ter-p.
bi·o·e·lec·tric p.
bi·ot·ic p.
brain p.
de·mar·ca·tion p.
ear·ly re·cep·tor p.
e·voked p.
ex·cit·a·to·ry post·syn·ap·tic
p.
ex·treme so·ma·to·sen·so·ry
e·voked p.
gen·er·a·tor p.
in·hib·i·to·ry post·syn·ap·tic
p.
in·ju·ry p.
mem·brane p.
my·o·gen·ic p.
os·cil·la·to·ry p.
Ottoson p.
re·dox p.
S p.
spike p.
ther·mo·dy·nam·ic p.
trans·mem·brane p.
vi·su·al e·voked p.
ze·ta p.
zo·o·not·ic p.
po·ten·tial
en·er·gy
po·ten·ti·a·tion
po·ten·ti·a·tor
po·ten·ti·om·e·ter
po·ten·ti·o·met·ric
ti·tra·tion
po·tion
Po·to·mac horse
fe·ver
Potter's
dis·ease
fa·ci·es
syn·drome
ver·sion
Potts'
anas·to·mo·sis

clamp
op·er·a·tion
Pott's
ab·scess
an·eu·rysm
cur·va·ture
dis·ease
frac·ture
gan·grene
pa·ral·y·sis
par·a·ple·gia
Pott's puffy
tu·mor
pouch
an·tral p.
bran·chi·al p.'s
Broca's p.
ce·lom·ic p.'s
Denis Browne's p.
Douglas' p.
en·do·der·mal p.'s
gut·tur·al p.
Hartmann's p.
Heidenhain p.
he·pa·to·re·nal p.
hy·po·phy·se·al p.
Kock p.
la·ryn·ge·al p.
Morison's p.
par·a·cys·tic p.
par·a·rec·tal p.
par·a·ves·i·cal p.
Pavlov p.
pha·ryn·ge·al p.'s
Physick's p.'s
Prussak's p.
Rathke's p.
rec·to·u·ter·ine p.
rec·to·vag·i·no·u·ter·ine p.
rec·to·ves·i·cal p.
Seessel's p.
su·per·fi·cial in·gui·nal p.
ul·ti·mo·bran·chi·al p.
uter·o·ves·i·cal p.
ves·i·co·u·ter·ine p.
Willis' p.
pou·drage
per·i·car·di·al p.
pleu·ral p.
poul·tice
poul·try han·dler's
dis·ease
poul·try·man's
itch
pound
pound·al

Poupart's
  lig·a·ment
  line
po·vi·done
po·vi·done-io·dine
Pow·as·san
  en·ceph·a·li·tis
  vi·rus
pow·der
  bleach·ing p.
pow·dered
  gold
  ip·e·cac
  opi·um
  stom·ach
pow·er
  fail·ure
  point
pow·er
  back ver·tex p.
  equiv·a·lent p.
  re·solv·ing p.
pox
  Kaf·fir p.
Pox·vir·i·dae
pox·vi·rus
  p. of·fi·ci·na·lis
Pozzi's
  mus·cle
P and P
  test
P-P
  in·ter·val
P-pul·mo·na·le
P-Q
  in·ter·val
PR
  en·zyme
P-R
  in·ter·val
  seg·ment
prac·ti·cal
  anat·o·my
  units
prac·tice
  ex·tra·mu·ral p.
  group p.
  in·tra·mu·ral p.
prac·ti·tion·er
prac·to·lol
Prader-Willi
  syn·drome
prag·mat·ag·no·sia
prag·mat·am·ne·sia
prag·mat·ics
prag·ma·tism

Prague
  ma·neu·ver
  pel·vis
prai·rie
  con·junc·ti·vi·tis
  itch
pral·i·dox·ime chlo·ride
pra·mox·ine hy·dro·chlo·ride
pran·di·al
pra·se·o·dym·i·um
Pratt's
  symp·tom
Prausnitz-Küstner
  an·ti·body
  re·ac·tion
prax·i·ol·o·gy
prax·is
pra·ze·pam
pra·zi·quan·tel
pra·zo·sin hy·dro·chlo·ride
pre·ag·o·nal
pre·al·bu·min
  thy·rox·ine-bind·ing p.
pre·a·nal
pre·an·es·thet·ic
  med·i·ca·tion
pre·an·ti·sep·tic
pre·a·or·tic
pre·a·sep·tic
pre·a·tax·ic
pre·au·ric·u·lar
  groove
  point
  sul·cus
pre·au·ric·u·lar sub·fas·cial pa·rot·id lymph
  nodes
pre·au·to·mat·ic
  pause
pre·ax·i·al
pre·ax·il·lary
  line
pre·can·cer
pre·can·cer·ous
  le·sion
  mel·a·no·sis of Dubreuilh
pre·cap·il·lary
  anas·to·mo·sis
pre·car·di·ac
pre·car·di·nal
pre·car·ti·lage
pre·ca·va
pre·ce·cal lymph
  nodes
pre·cen·tral
  ar·ea
  ar·tery

gy·rus
sul·cus
pre·cen·tral cer·e·bel·lar
vein
pre·cer·vi·cal
si·nus
pre·chi·as·mat·ic
sul·cus
pre·chor·dal
plate
pre·chrom·ing
pre·cip·i·ta·ble
pre·cip·i·tant
pre·cip·i·tate
ke·rat·ic p.'s
mut·ton-fat ke·rat·ic p.'s
pig·ment·ed ke·rat·ic p.'s
red p.
sweet p.
white mer·cu·ric p.
yel·low p.
pre·cip·i·tate
la·bor
pre·cip·i·tat·ed
cal·ci·um car·bon·ate
sul·fur
pre·cip·i·tat·ing
an·ti·body
pre·cip·i·ta·tion
test
pre·cip·i·ta·tion
dou·ble an·ti·body p.
im·mune p.
pre·cip·i·tin
re·ac·tion
test
pre·cip·i·tin·o·gen
pre·cip·i·tin·o·ge·noid
pre·cip·i·to·gen
pre·cip·i·toid
pre·cip·i·to·phore
pre·ci·sion
at·tach·ment
rest
pre·clin·i·cal
pre·co·cious
pseu·do·pu·ber·ty
pu·ber·ty
pre·coc·i·ty
pre·cog·ni·tion
pre·col·lag·e·nous
fi·bers
pre·com·mis·sur·al
bun·dle
sep·tum
pre·com·mis·sur·al sep·tal
ar·ea

pre·com·mu·ni·cal
part
pre·con·cep·tu·al
stage
pre·con·scious
pre·con·vul·sive
pre·cor·dia
pre·cor·di·al
leads
pre·cor·di·al catch
syn·drome
pre·cor·di·al·gia
pre·cor·di·um
pre·cor·ne·al
film
pre·cos·tal
anas·to·mo·sis
pre·crit·i·cal
pre·cu·ne·al
ar·tery
pre·cu·ne·ate
pre·cu·ne·us
pre·cur·sor
pre·cur·so·ry
car·ti·lage
pre·de·cid·u·al
pre·den·tin
pre·di·a·be·tes
pre·di·as·to·le
pre·di·a·stol·ic
pre·di·crot·ic
pre·dic·tive
va·lid·i·ty
val·ue
pre·di·ges·tion
pre·dis·pose
pre·dis·pos·ing
cause
pre·dis·po·si·tion
pred·nis·o·lone
p. ac·e·tate
p. bu·tyl·ac·e·tate
p. so·di·um phos·phate
p. suc·ci·nate
p. teb·u·tate
pred·ni·sone
pred·nyl·i·dene
pre·dor·mi·tal
pre·dor·mi·tum
pre·dor·sal
bun·dle
pre·duc·tal
pre·e·clamp·sia
su·per·im·posed p.
pre·e·jec·tion
pe·ri·od
preen
gland

pre·ep·i·glot·tic
pre·e·rup·tive
pre·ex·ci·ta·tion
  syn·drome
pre·ex·trac·tion
  rec·ord
pre·for·ma·tion
pre·fron·tal
  ar·ea
  cor·tex
  leu·kot·o·my
  lo·bot·o·my
  veins
pre·gan·gli·on·ic
pre·gan·gli·on·ic mo·tor
  neu·ron
pre·gen·i·tal
  or·ga·ni·za·tion
  phase
preg·nan·cy
  cells
  di·a·be·tes
  dis·ease of sheep
  lu·te·o·ma
  tu·mor
preg·nan·cy
  ab·dom·i·nal p.
  abort·ed ec·top·ic p.
  am·pul·lar p.
  bi·gem·i·nal p.
  cer·vi·cal p.
  com·bined p.
  com·pound p.
  cor·nu·al p.
  ec·top·ic p.
  ex·tra·am·ni·ot·ic p.
  ex·tra·cho·ri·al p.
  ex·tra·mem·bra·nous p.
  ex·tra·u·ter·ine p.
  fal·lo·pi·an p.
  false p.
  het·er·o·top·ic p.
  hy·da·tid p.
  in·ter·sti·tial p.
  in·tra·lig·a·men·ta·ry p.
  in·tra·mu·ral p.
  in·tra·per·i·to·ne·al p.
  mes·o·met·ric p.
  mo·lar p.
  mul·ti·ple p.
  mu·ral p.
  ovar·i·an p.
  ovar·i·o·ab·dom·i·nal p.
  phan·tom p.
  plu·ral p.
  sec·on·dary ab·dom·i·nal p.
  spu·ri·ous p.
  tub·al p.

  tu·bo·ab·dom·i·nal p.
  tu·bo·o·var·i·an p.
  tu·bo·u·ter·ine p.
  twin p.
  uter·ine p.
  uter·o·ab·dom·i·nal p.
preg·nane
preg·nane·di·ol
preg·nane·di·one
preg·nane·tri·ol
preg·nant
preg·nant mare's se·rum
  go·nad·o·tro·pin
preg·nene
preg·nen·in·o·lone
preg·nen·o·lone
  p. suc·ci·nate
pre·gra·nu·lo·sa
  cells
pre·hal·lux
pre·hel·i·cine
pre·he·ma·ta·min·ic ac·id
pre·hem·i·ple·gic
pre·hen·sile
pre·hen·sion
pre·hor·mone
pre·hy·oid
  gland
pre·ic·tal
pre·in·duc·tion
pre·in·farc·tion
  syn·drome
pre·in·ter·pa·ri·e·tal
  bone
Preisz-Nocard
  ba·cil·lus
pre·lac·ri·mal
pre·lam·i·nar
  part of op·tic nerve
pre·la·ryn·ge·al
pre·la·ryn·ge·al lymph
  nodes
pre·lep·to·tene
pre·lim·bic
pre·lim·i·nary
  im·pres·sion
pre·lin·gual
  deaf·ness
pre·load
  ven·tric·u·lar p.
pre·log·i·cal
  mind
  think·ing
pre·ma·lig·nant
pre·mam·ma·ry
  ab·scess
pre·ma·ni·a·cal

pre·ma·ture
  al·o·pe·cia
  beat
  birth
  con·tact
  con·trac·tion
  de·liv·ery
  ejac·u·la·tion
  la·bor
  sys·to·le
pre·ma·ture se·nil·i·ty
  syn·drome
pre·ma·tu·ri·ty
  my·o·pia
pre·max·il·la
pre·max·il·lary
  bone
  su·ture
pre·med·i·ca·tion
pre·mei·ot·ic
  phase
pre·mel·a·no·some
pre·men·stru·al
  ede·ma
  syn·drome
  ten·sion
pre·men·stru·al sal·i·vary
  syn·drome
pre·men·stru·al ten·sion
  syn·drome
pre·men·stru·um
pre·mo·lar
  tooth
pre·mon·o·cyte
pre·mor·bid
pre·mo·tor
  ar·ea
  cor·tex
  syn·drome
pre·mu·ni·tion
pre·mu·ni·tive
pre·my·e·lo·blast
pre·my·e·lo·cyte
pre·na·res
pre·na·ris
pre·na·tal
  di·ag·no·sis
  life
  screen·ing
pre·ne·o·plas·tic
pre·nod·u·lar
  fis·sure
Prentice's
  rule
pren·yl
pre·nyl·a·mine
pre·oc·cip·i·tal
  notch

pre-oed·i·pal
  phase
pre·op·er·a·tive
  rec·ord
pre·op·tic
  ar·ea
  re·gion
pre·o·ral
  gut
pre·os·te·o·blast
pre·ox·y·gen·a·tion
pre·pal·a·tal
pre·pap·il·lary
  sphinc·ter
pre·par·a·lyt·ic
prep·a·ra·tion
  cav·i·ty p.
  cor·ro·sion p.
  cy·to·log·ic fil·ter p.
  heart-lung p.
pre·pared
  chalk
  ip·e·cac·u·a·nha
  su·et
pre·pared mut·ton
  tal·low
pre·pa·tel·lar
  bur·sa
  bur·si·tis
pre·pa·tent
  pe·ri·od
pre·per·i·car·di·ac lymph
  nodes
pre·per·i·to·ne·al
pre·phe·nic ac·id
pre·pir·i·form
  gy·rus
pre·pla·cen·tal
pre·po·ten·tial
pre·psy·chot·ic
pre·pu·ber·al
pre·pu·ber·tal
pre·pu·bes·cent
pre·puce
pre·pu·tia
pre·pu·ti·al
  cal·cu·lus
  glands
  ring
  sac
pre·pu·ti·ot·o·my
pre·pu·ti·um
pre·py·lor·ic
  sphinc·ter
  vein
pre·py·ram·i·dal
  tract

pre·rec·tal
  li·thot·o·my
pre·re·duced
pre·re·duc·tion
  phase
pre·re·nal
  al·bu·min·ur·ia
  az·o·te·mia
pre·re·pro·duc·tive
pre·ret·i·nal
pre·ru·bral
  field
  nu·cle·us
pre·sa·cral
  an·es·the·sia
  nerve
  neu·rec·to·my
  sym·pa·thec·to·my
pres·by·a·cou·sia
pres·by·a·cu·sia
pres·by·a·cu·sis
pres·by·at·rics
pres·by·cu·sis
pres·by·o·pia
pres·by·op·ic
pre·scribe
pre·scrip·tion
  shot·gun p.
pre·se·nile
  de·men·tia
pre·se·nile spon·ta·ne·ous
  gan·grene
pre·se·nil·i·ty
pre·se·ni·um
pre·sent
pre·sen·ta·tion
  acro·mi·on p.
  breech p.
  brow p.
  ce·phal·ic p.
  face p.
  foot p.
  foot·ling p.
  frank breech p.
  full breech p.
  head p.
  in·com·plete foot p.
  in·com·plete knee p.
  knee p.
  pel·vic p.
  pla·cen·tal p.
  po·lar p.
  shoul·der p.
  sin·cip·i·tal p.
  trans·verse p.
  ver·tex p.
pre·ser·va·tive

pre·so·mite
  em·bryo
pre·sphe·noid
  bone
pre·sphyg·mic
  in·ter·val
pre·spi·nal
pre·splen·ic
  fold
pre·spon·dy·lo·lis·the·sis
pres·sor
  amine
  base
  fi·bers
  nerve
  sub·stance
pres·so·re·cep·tive
  mech·a·nism
pres·so·re·cep·tor
  nerve
  re·flex
  sys·tem
pres·so·sen·si·tive
pres·so·sen·si·tiv·i·ty
  re·flex·o·gen·ic p.
pres·sure
  ab·dom·i·nal p.
  at·mo·spher·ic p.
  back p.
  bar·o·met·ric p.
  bit·ing p.
  blood p.
  cen·tral ve·nous p.
  cer·e·bro·spi·nal p.
  con·tin·u·ous pos·i·tive air·
    way p.
  crit·i·cal p.
  de·tru·sor p.
  di·a·stol·ic p.
  dif·fer·en·tial blood p.
  Donders' p.
  ef·fec·tive os·mot·ic p.
  gauge p.
  hy·dro·stat·ic p.
  in·tra·cra·ni·al p.
  in·tra·oc·u·lar p.
  neg·a·tive p.
  neg·a·tive end-ex·pi·ra·to·ry
    p.
  oc·clu·sal p.
  on·cot·ic p.
  os·mot·ic p.
  par·tial p.
  pleu·ral p.
  pos·i·tive end-ex·pi·ra·to·ry
    p.
  pul·mo·nary p.

pul·mo·nary cap·il·lary
  wedge p.
pulp p.
pulse p.
se·lec·tion p.
so·lu·tion p.
stan·dard p.
sys·tol·ic p.
trans·mu·ral p.
trans·pul·mo·nary p.
trans·tho·rac·ic p.
va·por p.
ven·tric·u·lar fill·ing p.
wedge p.
ze·ro end-ex·pi·ra·to·ry p.
pres·sure
  am·au·ro·sis
  an·es·the·sia
  at·ro·phy
  col·lapse
  dress·ing
  epiph·y·sis
  gan·grene
  pal·sy
  pa·ral·y·sis
  ple·thys·mo·graph
  point
  re·ver·sal
  sense
  sore
  sta·sis
pres·sure-con·trolled
  res·pi·ra·tor
pres·sure-vol·ume
  in·dex
pre·ster·nal
  notch
  re·gion
pre·ster·num
pre·stri·ate
  ar·ea
pre·sul·cal
  part
pre·sumed oc·u·lar
  his·to·plas·mo·sis
pre·sump·tive
  re·gion
pre·sup·pu·ra·tive
pre·syn·ap·tic
  mem·brane
pre·sys·to·le
pre·sys·tol·ic
  gal·lop
  mur·mur
  thrill
pre·tar·sal
pre·tec·ta

pre·tec·tal
  ar·ea
  re·gion
pre·tec·tum
pre·term
  in·fant
pre·thy·roid
pre·thy·roi·de·al
pre·thy·roi·de·an
pre·tib·i·al
  fe·ver
  myx·e·de·ma
pre·tra·che·al
  fas·cia
  lay·er
pre·tra·che·al lymph
  nodes
pre·tre·mat·ic
pre·tym·pan·ic
prev·a·lence
pre·ven·tive
  den·tis·try
  dose
  med·i·cine
  treat·ment
pre·ver·te·bral
  fas·cia
  gan·glia
  lay·er
pre·ver·te·bral lymph
  nodes
pre·ves·i·cal
pre·vil·lous
  cho·ri·on
  em·bryo
pre·vi·us
pre·zone
pri·a·pism
pri·a·pi·tis
pri·a·pus
Pribnow
  box
Price-Jones
  curve
prick·le
  cell
prick·le cell
  lay·er
prick·ly
  heat
pril·o·caine hy·dro·chlo·ride
pri·ma·clone
pri·ma·cy
  gen·i·tal p.
  oral p.
pri·mal
  re·pres·sion
pri·mal scene

pri·ma·quine
 sen·si·tiv·i·ty
pri·ma·quine phos·phate
pri·mary
 ad·he·sion
 aer·o·don·tal·gia
 agam·ma·glob·u·lin·e·mia
 al·co·hol
 al·do·ste·ron·ism
 amen·or·rhea
 am·pu·ta·tion
 am·y·loi·do·sis
 an·es·thet·ic
 an·oph·thal·mia
 at·el·ec·ta·sis
 bron·chus
 bu·bo
 bu·tyl al·co·hol
 car·ci·no·ma
 car·di·o·my·op·a·thy
 car·ies
 ce·men·tum
 cen·ter of os·si·fi·ca·tion
 cho·a·na
 coc·cid·i·oi·do·my·co·sis
 col·or
 com·plex
 con·stric·tion
 de·men·tia
 den·tin
 den·ti·tion
 de·vi·a·tion
 di·ges·tion
 dis·ease
 drives
 dys·men·or·rhea
 fis·sure of the cer·e·bel·lum
 gain
 he·mo·chro·ma·to·sis
 hem·or·rhage
 hy·dro·ceph·a·lus
 hy·per·ox·al·u·ria and ox·
  a·lo·sis
 hy·per·par·a·thy·roid·ism
 hy·per·ten·sion
 hy·per·thy·roid·ism
 hy·po·gam·ma·glob·u·lin·e·
  mia
 hy·po·go·nad·ism
 im·pres·sion
 ir·ri·tant
 lymph·e·de·ma
 ly·so·somes
 mes·o·derm
 met·he·mo·glo·bi·ne·mia
 nar·cis·sism
 neur·as·the·nia
 nod·ule

 non·dis·junc·tion
 oo·cyte
 or·ga·niz·er
 pal·ate
 pen·to·su·ria
 point of os·si·fi·ca·tion
 pro·cess
 pro·te·ose
 py·o·der·ma
 rays
 re·ac·tion
 re·in·force·ment
 re·jec·tion
 screw-worm
 sen·sa·tion
 se·ques·trum
 shock
 so·di·um phos·phate
 sper·ma·to·cyte
 syph·i·lis
 tooth
 tu·ber·cu·lo·sis
 un·ion
 vil·lus
 vit·re·ous
pri·mary adre·no·cor·ti·cal
 in·suf·fi·cien·cy
pri·mary ame·bic
 me·nin·go·en·ceph·a·li·tis
pri·mary am·ide
pri·mary amine
pri·mary atyp·i·cal
 pneu·mo·nia
pri·mary bil·i·ary
 cir·rho·sis
pri·mary brain
 ves·i·cle
pri·mary den·tal
 lam·i·na
pri·mary dried
 yeast
pri·mary egg
 mem·brane
pri·mary em·bry·on·ic
 cell
pri·mary eryth·ro·blas·tic
 ane·mia
pri·mary ex·tra·pul·mo·nary
 coc·cid·i·oi·do·my·co·sis
pri·mary gen·er·al·ized
 ep·i·lep·sy
pri·mary her·pet·ic
 sto·ma·ti·tis
pri·mary id·i·o·path·ic mac·u·
 lar
 at·ro·phy
pri·mary im·mune
 re·sponse

pri·mary in·ter·a·tri·al
  fo·ra·men
pri·mary ir·ri·tant
  der·ma·ti·tis
pri·mary la·bi·al
  groove
pri·mary mac·u·lar
  at·ro·phy of skin
pri·mary med·i·cal
  care
pri·mary my·e·loid
  met·a·pla·sia
pri·mary neu·ro·nal
  de·gen·er·a·tion
pri·mary ovar·i·an
  fol·li·cle
pri·mary pig·men·tary
  de·gen·er·a·tion of ret·i·na
pri·mary pro·gress·ive cer·e·
  bel·lar
  de·gen·er·a·tion
pri·mary pul·mo·nary
  lob·ule
pri·mary re·frac·to·ry
  ane·mia
pri·mary re·nal
  cal·cu·lus
pri·mary re·nal tu·bu·lar
  ac·i·do·sis
pri·mary scle·ros·ing
  chol·an·gi·tis
pri·mary se·nile
  de·men·tia
pri·mary sex
  char·ac·ters
pri·mary skin
  graft
pri·mary uter·ine
  in·er·tia
pri·mary vi·su·al
  ar·ea
  cor·tex
pri·mate
Pri·ma·tes
pri·mer·ite
pri·mi·done
pri·mi·grav·i·da
pri·mip·a·ra
pri·mi·par·i·ty
pri·mip·a·rous
pri·mite
prim·i·tive
  aor·ta
  cho·a·na
  cho·ri·on
  fur·row
  groove
  knot

node
palate
pit
ridge
streak
prim·i·tive cos·tal
  arch·es
prim·i·tive per·i·vis·cer·al
  cav·i·ty
prim·i·tive re·tic·u·lar
  cell
pri·mor·dia
pri·mor·di·al
  car·ti·lage
  cell
  cyst
  dwarf·ism
  gi·gan·tism
  kid·ney
pri·mor·di·al germ
  cell
pri·mor·di·al ovar·i·an
  fol·li·cle
pri·mor·di·um
prim·u·la
pri·mu·lin
pri·mus
prin·ceps
  p. cer·vi·cis
  p. pol·li·cis
prin·ceps cer·vi·cis
  ar·tery
Prin·ceteau's
  tu·ber·cle
prin·ci·pal
  ar·tery of thumb
  fo·cus
  is·lets
  piece
  plane
  point
prin·ci·pal op·tic
  ax·is
prin·ci·pes
prin·ci·ple
  ac·tive p.
  an·ti·a·ne·mic p.
  az·y·gos vein p.
  Bernoulli's p.
  clo·sure p.
  con·sis·ten·cy p.
  Fick p.
  fol·li·cle-stim·u·lat·ing p.
  found·er p.
  hem·a·tin·ic p.
  p. of in·er·tia
  Le Chatelier's p.
  low flow p.

prin·ci·ple *(continued)*
  lu·te·i·niz·ing p.
  mel·a·no·phore-ex·pand·ing
    p.
  nir·va·na p.
  or·gan·ic p.
  pain p.
  pain-plea·sure p.
  Pauli's p.
  plea·sure p.
  prox·i·mate p.
  re·al·i·ty p.
  rep·e·ti·tion-com·pul·sion p.
  ul·ti·mate p.
Pringle's
  dis·ease
Prinzmetal's
  an·gi·na
pri·on
prism
  enam·el p.'s
  Fresnel p.
  Nicol p.
  Risley's ro·ta·ry p.
prism
  di·op·ter
pris·ma
  pris·ma·ta ad·a·man·ti·na
pris·ma·ta
pris·mat·ic
prism bar
prism ver·gence
  test
pri·va·cy
pri·vate
  an·ti·gens
  hos·pi·tal
pri·vate du·ty
  nurse
priv·et
  cough
priv·i·leged
  site
pro·ac·cel·er·in
pro·ac·ro·so·mal
  gran·ules
pro·ac·tin·i·um
pro·ac·ti·va·tor
pro·ac·tive
  in·hi·bi·tion
pro·al
pro·am·ni·on
pro·at·las
prob·a·bil·i·ty
  curve
pro·bac·te·ri·o·phage
  de·fec·tive p.
pro·band

pro·bang
probe
  Anel's p.
  Bowman's p.
  nu·cle·ic ac·id p.
  per·i·o·don·tal p.
  ra·di·o·ac·tive p.
  ver·te·brat·ed p.
  vi·ral p.
probe
  gor·get
  pa·ten·cy
  sy·ringe
pro·ben·e·cid
pro·bil·i·fus·cins
pro·bi·o·sis
pro·bi·ot·ic
prob·lem
prob·lem-o·ri·ent·ed
  rec·ord
pro·bos·ci·des
pro·bos·cis
pro·bos·ci·ses
Probst·y·may·ria vi·vip·a·ra
pro·bu·col
pro·cain·a·mide hy·dro·chlo·
  ride
pro·caine hy·dro·chlo·ride
pro·cap·sid
pro·car·ba·zine hy·dro·chlo·ride
pro·car·box·y·pep·ti·dase
Pro·car·y·o·tae
pro·car·y·ote
pro·car·y·ot·ic
pro·cat·arc·tic
pro·cat·arx·is
pro·ce·dure
  Adson's p.
  com·man·do p.
  Eloesser p.
  en·do·rec·tal pull-through p.
  Ewart's p.
  Fontan p.
  Girdlestone p.
  Mustard p.
  Noble-Collip p.
  Puestow p.
  push-back p.
  Putti-Platt p.
  Rastelli p.
  shelf p.
  Stanley Way p.
  Sugiura p.
  Thal p.
  Vineberg p.
  V-Y p.
  W p.
  Z p.

pro·ce·lia
pro·ce·lous
pro·cen·tri·ole
  or·ga·niz·er
pro·ce·phal·ic
pro·cer·coid
pro·ce·rus
  mus·cle
pro·cess
  schiz·o·phre·nia
pro·cess
  ·A.B.C. p.
  ac·ces·so·ry p.
  acro·mi·al p.
  agene p.
  alar p.
  al·ve·o·lar p.
  an·te·ri·or p. of mal·le·us
  ap·i·cal p.
  ar·tic·u·lar p.
  as·cend·ing p.
  au·di·to·ry p.
  ax·o·nal p.
  bas·i·lar p.
  Budde p.
  Burns' fal·ci·form p.
  cal·ca·ne·al p. of cu·boid
    bone
  cau·date p.
  cil·i·ary p.
  Civinini's p.
  cli·noid p.
  co·chle·ar·i·form p.
  com·plex learn·ing p.'s
  con·dy·lar p.
  con·dy·loid p.
  co·noid p.
  cor·a·coid p.
  cor·o·noid p.
  cos·tal p.
  Deiters' p.
  den·drit·ic p.
  den·tal p.
  en·si·form p.
  eth·moi·dal p.
  fal·ci·form p.
  fol·li·an p.
  Folli's p.
  foot p.
  fron·tal p.
  fron·to·na·sal p.
  fron·to·sphe·noi·dal p.
  fu·nic·u·lar p.
  glob·u·lar p.
  ham·u·lar p. of lac·ri·mal
    bone
  ham·u·lar p. of sphe·noid
    bone

  head p.
  in·tra·jug·u·lar p.
  jug·u·lar p.
  lac·ri·mal p.
  lat·er·al p. of cal·ca·ne·al
    tu·ber·os·i·ty
  lat·er·al p. of mal·le·us
  lat·er·al na·sal p.
  lat·er·al p. of ta·lus
  Lenhossék's p.'s
  len·tic·u·lar p. of in·cus
  long p. of mal·le·us
  ma·lar p.
  mam·il·lary p.
  man·dib·u·lar p.
  mas·toid p.
  max·il·lary p.
  max·il·lary p. of em·bryo
  me·di·al p. of cal·ca·ne·al
    tu·ber·os·i·ty
  me·di·al na·sal p.
  men·tal p.
  mus·cu·lar p. of ar·y·te·
    noid car·ti·lage
  na·sal p.
  no·to·chor·dal p.
  odon·to·blas·tic p.
  odon·toid p.
  odon·toid p. of ep·i·stro·
    phe·us
  olec·ra·non p.
  or·bic·u·lar p.
  or·bi·tal p.
  pack·ing p.
  pal·a·tal p.'s
  pal·a·tine p.
  pap·il·lary p.
  par·a·mas·toid p.
  par·oc·cip·i·tal p.
  pos·te·ri·or p. of sep·tal
    car·ti·lage
  pri·mary p.
  pro·gress·ive p.'s
  pter·y·goid p.
  pter·y·go·spi·nous p.
  py·ram·i·dal p.
  Rau's p.
  Ravius' p.
  sec·on·dary p.
  sheath p. of sphe·noid bone
  short p. of mal·le·us
  slen·der p. of mal·le·us
  sphe·noid p.
  sphe·noid p. of sep·tal car·
    ti·lage
  spi·nous p.
  spi·nous p. of tib·ia
  Stieda's p.

pro·cess *(continued)*
  sty·loid p. of fib·u·la
  sty·loid p. of ra·di·us
  sty·loid p. of tem·po·ral bone
  sty·loid p. of third met·a·car·pal bone
  sty·loid p. of ul·na
  su·pe·ri·or ar·tic·u·lar p. of sa·crum
  su·pra·con·dy·lar p.
  su·pra·ep·i·con·dy·lar p.
  tem·po·ral p.
  Tomes' p.'s
  trans·verse p.
  troch·le·ar p.
  un·ci·nate p. of eth·moid bone
  un·ci·nate p. of pan·cre·as
  vag·i·nal p.
  vag·i·nal p. of per·i·to·ne·um
  vag·i·nal p. of tes·tis
  ver·mi·form p.
  vo·cal p.
  xi·phoid p.
  zy·go·mat·ic p.
pro·ces·sus
  p. as·cen·dens
  p. bre·vis
  p. fer·reini
  p. grac·i·lis
  p. ra·vii
  p. ret·ro·man·di·bu·la·ris
  p. troch·le·ar·is
  p. va·gi·na·lis pe·ri·to·nei
  p. ver·mi·for·mis
pro·ces·sus
pro·chei·lia
pro·chei·lon
pro·chi·lia
pro·chi·lon
pro·chlor·per·a·zine
pro·chon·dral
pro·chor·dal plate
pro·chy·mo·sin
pro·ci·den·tia
  p. uter·i
pro·col·la·gen
pro·con·ver·tin
pro·cre·ate
pro·cre·a·tion
pro·cre·a·tive
proc·tag·ra
proc·tal·gia
  p. fu·gax

proc·ta·tre·sia
proc·tec·ta·sia
proc·tec·to·my
proc·ten·clei·sis
proc·ten·cli·sis
proc·teu·ryn·ter
proc·ti·tis
  chron·ic ul·cer·a·tive p.
  ep·i·dem·ic gan·gre·nous p.
  id·i·o·path·ic p.
proc·to·cele
proc·to·cly·sis
proc·to·coc·cy·pexy
proc·to·co·lec·to·my
proc·to·co·li·tis
proc·to·co·lo·nos·co·py
proc·to·col·po·plas·ty
proc·to·cys·to·cele
proc·to·cys·to·plas·ty
proc·to·cys·tot·o·my
proc·to·dea
proc·to·de·al
proc·to·de·um
proc·to·dyn·ia
proc·to·el·y·tro·plas·ty
proc·to·log·ic
proc·tol·o·gist
proc·tol·o·gy
proc·to·pa·ral·y·sis
proc·to·per·i·ne·o·plas·ty
proc·to·per·i·ne·or·rha·phy
proc·to·pexy
proc·to·pho·bia
proc·to·plas·ty
proc·to·ple·gia
proc·to·pol·y·pus
proc·top·to·sia
proc·top·to·sis
proc·tor·rha·gia
proc·tor·rha·phy
proc·tor·rhea
proc·to·scope
  Tuttle's p.
proc·tos·co·py
proc·to·sig·moi·dec·to·my
proc·to·sig·moi·di·tis
proc·to·sig·moi·dos·co·py
proc·to·spasm
proc·tos·ta·sis
proc·to·stat
proc·to·ste·no·sis
proc·tos·to·my
proc·to·tome
proc·tot·o·my
proc·to·tre·sia
proc·to·val·vot·o·my
pro·cum·bent

pro·cur·sive
  cho·rea
  ep·i·lep·sy
pro·cur·va·tion
pro·cy·cli·dine hy·dro·chlo·ride
pro·cy·cli·dine meth·o·chlo·ride
pro·dro·mal
  stage
pro·drome
prod·ro·mi
pro·dro·mic
  sign
pro·dro·mous
prod·ro·mus
pro·drug
pro·duct
  cleav·age p.
  dou·ble p.
  fi·brin/fi·brin·o·gen deg·ra·
    da·tion p.'s
  fis·sion p.
  or·phan p.'s
  spall·a·tion p.
  sub·sti·tu·tion p.
pro·duc·tive
  in·flam·ma·tion
  per·i·to·ni·tis
  pleu·ri·sy
pro·duct-mo·ment
  cor·re·la·tion
pro·e·mi·al
pro·en·ceph·a·lon
pro·en·keph·a·lin
pro·en·zyme
pro·e·ryth·ro·blast
pro·e·ryth·ro·cyte
pro·es·tro·gen
pro·es·trum
pro·es·trus
pro·fen·a·mine hy·dro·chlo·ride
pro·fer·ment
pro·fes·sion·al
  neu·ro·sis
  spasm
Profeta's
  law
pro·fi·bri·nol·y·sin
Profichet's
  dis·ease
pro·file
  rec·ord
pro·file
  bi·o·chem·i·cal p.
  fa·cial p.
  per·son·al·i·ty p.
  test p.
  ure·thral pres·sure p.
pro·fi·lom·e·ter

pro·fla·vine (hem·i)sul·fate
pro·fon·dom·e·ter
pro·for·mi·phen
pro·found
  hy·po·ther·mia
pro·fun·da
pro·fun·dus
pro·gas·trin
pro·ge·nia
pro·ge·ni·ta·lis
pro·gen·i·tor
prog·e·ny
pro·ge·ria
  p. with cat·a·ract
  p. with mi·croph·thal·mia
pro·ger·oid
pro·ges·ta·tion·al
  hor·mone
pro·ges·ter·one
  unit
pro·ges·tin
pro·ges·to·gen
pro·glos·sis
pro·glot·tid
pro·glot·ti·des
pro·glot·tis
prog·nath·ic
prog·na·thism
  bas·i·lar p.
prog·na·thous
prog·nose
prog·no·sis
  den·ture p.
prog·nos·tic
prog·nos·ti·cate
prog·nos·ti·cian
pro·gon·o·ma
  p. of jaw
  mel·a·not·ic p.
pro·gran·u·lo·cyte
pro·gress
pro·gress·ive
  cat·a·ract
  cleav·age
  hy·po·cy·the·mia
  lip·o·dys·tro·phy
  pro·cess·es
  stain·ing
  vac·cin·ia
pro·gress·ive bac·te·ri·al syn·
  er·gis·tic
  gan·grene
pro·gress·ive bul·bar
  pa·ral·y·sis
pro·gress·ive cer·e·bel·lar
  trem·or
pro·gress·ive ce·re·bral
  po·li·o·dys·tro·phy

831

pro·gress·ive cho·roi·dal
  at·ro·phy
pro·gress·ive em·phy·sem·a·tous
  ne·cro·sis
pro·gress·ive lin·gual
  hem·i·at·ro·phy
pro·gress·ive mul·ti·fo·cal
  leu·ko·en·ceph·a·lop·a·thy
pro·gress·ive mus·cu·lar
  at·ro·phy
  dys·tro·phy
pro·gress·ive pig·men·tary
  der·ma·to·sis
pro·gress·ive pneu·mo·nia
  vi·rus
pro·gress·ive spi·nal
  amy·ot·ro·phy
pro·gress·ive sub·cor·ti·cal
  en·ceph·a·lop·a·thy
pro·gress·ive su·pra·nu·cle·ar
  pal·sy
pro·gress·ive sys·tem·ic
  scle·ro·sis
pro·gress·ive ta·pe·to·cho·roi·dal
  dys·tro·phy
pro·gress·ive tor·sion
  spasm
pro·gua·nil hy·dro·chlo·ride
pro·hor·mone
pro·in·su·lin
pro·i·o·sys·to·le
pro·i·o·sys·tol·ia
pro·jec·tile
  vom·it·ing
pro·jec·tion
  fi·bers
  pe·rim·e·ter
  sys·tem
pro·jec·tion
  ax·i·al p.
  base p.
  Caldwell p.
  enam·el p.
  er·ro·ne·ous p.
  false p.
  Stenvers p.
  Towne p.
  vi·su·al p.
pro·jec·tive
  test
Pro·kar·y·o·tae
pro·kar·y·ote
pro·kar·y·ot·ic
pro·la·bi·al
pro·la·bi·um

pro·lac·tin
  cell
  unit
pro·lac·tin in·hib·it·ing
  fac·tor
  hor·mone
pro·lac·ti·no·ma
pro·lac·tin-pro·duc·ing
  ad·e·no·ma
pro·lac·tin re·leas·ing
  fac·tor
  hor·mone
pro·lac·to·lib·er·in
pro·lac·to·stat·in
pro·lam·ines
pro·lapse
  p. of the cor·pus lu·te·um
  first de·gree p.
  mi·tral valve p.
  Morgagni's p.
  sec·ond de·gree p.
  third de·gree p.
  p. of um·bil·i·cal cord
  p. of the uter·us
pro·lep·sis
pro·lep·tic
pro·leu·ko·cyte
pro·li·dase
pro·lif·er·ate
pro·lif·er·at·ing
  end·ar·te·ri·tis
  pleu·ri·sy
pro·lif·er·at·ing sys·tem·a·tized
  an·gi·o·en·do·the·li·o·ma·to·sis
pro·lif·er·at·ing trich·o·lem·mal
  cyst
pro·lif·er·a·tion
  cyst
  ther·a·py
pro·lif·er·a·tion
  dif·fuse mes·an·gi·al p.
  gin·gi·val p.
pro·lif·er·a·tive
  ar·thri·tis
  bron·chi·ol·i·tis
  cho·roid·i·tis
  cyst
  der·ma·ti·tis
  fas·ci·i·tis
  gin·gi·vi·tis
  glo·mer·u·lo·ne·phri·tis
  in·flam·ma·tion
  in·ti·mi·tis
  my·o·si·tis
  ret·i·nop·a·thy
pro·lif·er·ous
  cyst

pro·lif·ic
pro·lig·er·ous
   disk
   mem·brane
pro·li·nase
pro·line
   p. ami·no·pep·ti·dase
   p. de·hy·dro·gen·ase
   p. di·pep·ti·dase
   p. im·i·no·pep·ti·dase
   p. ox·i·dase
   p. rac·e·mase
D-pro·line re·duc·tase
pro·longed ac·tion
   tab·let
pro·lyl
   p. di·pep·ti·dase
pro·lyl·gly·cine di·pep·ti·dase
pro·mas·ti·gote
pro·ma·zine hy·dro·chlo·ride
pro·meg·a·lo·blast
pro·met·a·phase
   band·ing
pro·meth·a·zine hy·dro·chlo·ride
pro·meth·a·zine the·o·clate
pro·meth·es·trol di·pro·pi·o·nate
pro·me·thi·um
prom·i·nence
   Ammon's p.
   ca·nine p.
   car·di·ac p.
   p. of fa·cial ca·nal
   fore·brain p.
   he·pa·tic p.
   hy·po·the·nar p.
   la·ryn·ge·al p.
   p. of lat·er·al sem·i·cir·cu·lar ca·nal
   mal·le·ar p.
   spi·ral p.
   sty·loid p.
   the·nar p.
pro·mi·nens
prom·i·nent
   heel
prom·i·nen·tia
prom·i·nen·ti·ae
pro·mon·o·cyte
prom·on·to·ria
prom·on·to·ri·um
   p. ca·vi tym·pa·ni
   p. os·sis sa·cri
prom·on·to·ry
   pel·vic p.
   p. of the sa·crum
   tym·pan·ic p.

prom·on·to·ry lymph
   nodes
pro·mot·er
pro·mot·ing
   agent
pro·mo·tion
prompt in·su·lin zinc
   sus·pen·sion
pro·my·e·lo·cyte
pro·na·si·on
pro·nate
pro·na·tion
   p. of foot
   p. of fore·arm
pro·na·tis
pro·na·tor
   re·flex
   ridge
prone
   po·si·tion
pro·neph·ric
   duct
   tu·bule
pro·neph·roi
pro·neph·ros
pro·neth·a·lol hy·dro·chlo·ride
pro·no·grade
pro·nom·e·ter
pro·nor·mo·blast
pro·nu·clei
pro·nu·cle·us
proof
   spir·it
pro·o·tic
pro·pa·di·ene
prop·a·gate
prop·a·gat·ed
   throm·bus
prop·a·ga·tion
prop·a·ga·tive
pro·pal·i·nal
pro·pam·i·dine
pro·pane
pro·pane·di·o·ic ac·id
pro·pan·i·did
pro·pa·no·ic ac·id
pro·pa·nol
pro·pan·o·lol
pro·pa·no·yl
pro·pan·the·line bro·mide
pro·par·a·caine hy·dro·chlo·ride
pro·pa·tyl ni·trate
pro·pene
pro·pent·dy·o·pents
pro·pe·nyl
pro·pep·sin
pro·pep·tone

prop·er
  fas·cic·u·li
  lig·a·ment of ova·ry
  sub·stance
pro·per·din
  fac·tor A
  fac·tor B
  fac·tor D
  fac·tor E
  sys·tem
prop·er he·pa·tic
  ar·tery
pro·per·i·to·ne·al
pro·per·i·to·ne·al in·gui·nal
  her·nia
prop·er pal·mar dig·i·tal
  ar·tery
  nerves
prop·er plan·tar dig·i·tal
  ar·tery
  nerves
pro·phage
  de·fec·tive p.
pro·phase
pro·phen·py·rid·a·mine ma·le·ate
pro·phlo·gis·tic
pro·phy·lac·tic
  mem·brane
  odon·tot·o·my
  treat·ment
pro·phy·lax·es
pro·phy·lax·is
  ac·tive p.
  chem·i·cal p.
  den·tal p.
  pas·sive p.
pro·pi·cil·lin
pro·pi·o·lac·tone
pro·pi·o·ma·zine
pro·pi·o·nate
Pro·pi·on·i·bac·te·ri·um
  P. ac·nes
  P. freu·den·rei·chii
  P. jen·se·nii
pro·pi·on·ic ac·id
pro·pi·on·ic·ac·i·de·mia
pro·pi·o·nyl
pro·pit·o·caine hy·dro·chlo·ride
pro·pla·sia
pro·plas·ma·cyte
pro·plex·us
pro·por·tion·al
  count·er
  lim·it
pro·por·tion·ate
  in·fan·ti·lism
pro·po·si·ti

pro·pos·i·tus
pro·pox·y·caine hy·dro·chlo·ride
pro·pox·y·phene hy·dro·chlo·ride
pro·pox·y·phene nap·syl·ate
pro·pran·o·lol hy·dro·chlo·ride
pro·pri·e·tary
  hos·pi·tal
  med·i·cine
pro·pri·e·tary name
pro·pri·o·cep·tive
  mech·a·nism
  re·flex·es
  sen·si·bil·i·ty
pro·pri·o·cep·tive-oc·u·lo·ceph·al·ic
  re·flex
pro·pri·o·cep·tor
pro·pri·o·spi·nal
prop·tom·e·ter
prop·to·sis
prop·tot·ic
pro·pul·sion
pro·pyl
  p. al·co·hol
  p. gal·late
  p. hy·drox·y·ben·zo·ate
pro·pyl·car·bi·nol
pro·py·lene
  p. gly·col
pro·pyl·hex·e·drine
pro·pyl·i·o·done
pro·pyl·par·a·ben
pro·pyl·thi·o·ur·a·cil
pro·py·ro·ma·zine
pro re na·ta
pro·ren·nin
pror·sad
pro·ru·bri·cyte
  per·ni·cious ane·mia type p.
pro·scil·lar·i·din
pro·sco·lex
pro·se·cre·tin
pro·se·cre·tion
  gran·ules
pro·sect
pro·sec·tor
pro·sec·to·ri·um
pro·sec·tor's
  tu·ber·cle
  wart
pros·en·ceph·a·lon
pro·se·rum pro·throm·bin con·ver·sion
  ac·cel·er·a·tor
pros·o·dem·ic
pros·o·pag·no·sia
pro·sop·a·gus

pros·o·pal·gia
pros·o·pal·gic
pros·o·pec·ta·sia
pros·o·pla·sia
pros·o·po·a·nos·chi·sis
pros·o·po·di·ple·gia
pros·o·po·neu·ral·gia
pros·o·pop·a·gus
pros·o·po·ple·gia
pros·o·po·ple·gic
pros·o·pos·chi·sis
pros·o·po·spasm
pros·o·po·thor·a·cop·a·gus
pro·sper·mia
pros·ta·cy·clin
pros·ta·glan·din
pros·ta·no·ic ac·id
pros·ta·ta
pros·ta·tal·gia
pros·tate
    fe·male p.
pros·tate
    gland
pros·ta·tec·to·my
pros·tat·ic
    ad·e·no·ma
    cal·cu·lus
    cath·e·ter
    ducts
    duc·tules
    flu·id
    mas·sage
    plex·us
    si·nus
    ure·thra
    utri·cle
pros·tat·i·co·ves·i·cal
    plex·us
pros·tat·ic ve·nous
    plex·us
pros·ta·tism
pros·ta·tit·ic
pros·ta·ti·tis
pros·ta·to·cys·ti·tis
pros·ta·to·cys·tot·o·my
pros·ta·to·dyn·ia
pros·tat·o·lith
pros·ta·to·li·thot·o·my
pros·ta·to·meg·a·ly
pros·tat·o·my
pros·ta·tor·rhea
pros·ta·to·sem·i·nal ve·sic·u·
    lec·to·my
pros·ta·tot·o·my
pros·ta·to·ve·sic·u·lec·to·my
pros·ta·to·ve·sic·u·li·tis
pros·ter·na·tion
pros·the·on

pros·the·ses
pros·the·sis
    car·di·ac valve p.
    co·chle·ar p.
    de·fin·i·tive p.
    den·tal p.
    hy·brid p.
    man·dib·u·lar guide p.
    oc·u·lar p.
    pro·vi·sion·al p.
    sur·gi·cal p.
pros·thet·ic
    den·tis·try
    group
pros·thet·ics
    den·tal p.
    max·il·lo·fa·cial p.
pros·the·tist
pros·the·to·phac·os
pros·thi·on
pros·tho·don·tia
pros·tho·don·tics
pros·tho·don·tist
Pros·tho·gon·i·mus ma·cror·
    chis
pros·tho·ker·a·to·plas·ty
pro·sto·mi·al
    mes·o·derm
pros·tra·tion
    heat p.
prot·ac·tin·i·um
pro·tal·bu·mose
pro·tam·i·nase
prot·a·mine
    p. sul·fate
prot·a·mine zinc
    in·su·lin
pro·ta·nom·a·ly
pro·ta·no·pia
pro·te·an
pro·te·ase
pro·tec·tion
    test
pro·tec·tive
    block
    col·loid
    pro·tein
    spec·ta·cles
    zone
pro·tec·tive la·ryn·ge·al
    re·flex
pro·te·id
pro·tein
    ac·yl car·ri·er p.
    an·ti·vi·ral p.
    au·tol·o·gous p.
    Bence Jones p.
    p. C

pro·tein *(continued)*
   cAMP re·cep·tor p.
   ca·tab·o·lite (gene) ac·ti·va·tor p.
   com·pound p.
   con·ju·gat·ed p.
   cor·ti·co·ste·roid-bind·ing p.
   C-re·ac·tive p.
   de·na·tured p.
   de·rived p.
   fi·brous p.
   for·eign p.
   glob·u·lar p.
   het·er·ol·o·gous p.
   im·mune p.
   M p.
   mon·o·clo·nal p.
   my·e·lo·blas·tic p.
   na·tive p.
   non·spe·cif·ic p.
   phen·yl·thi·o·car·bam·o·yl p.
   PhNCS p.
   pla·cen·ta p.
   plas·ma p.'s
   pro·tec·tive p.
   PTC p.
   pu·ri·fied pla·cen·tal p.
   re·cep·tor p.
   S p.
   p. S
   sim·ple p.
   strong sil·ver p.
   Tamm-Horsfall p.
   thy·rox·ine-bind·ing p.
   whey p.
pro·tein
   fac·tor
   fe·ver
   me·tab·o·lism
   shock
   syn·the·sis
pro·tein·a·ceous
pro·tein·as·es
pro·tein-bound
   io·dine
pro·tein-bound io·dine
   test
pro·tein hy·drol·y·sate
pro·tein-los·ing
   en·ter·op·a·thy
pro·tein·o·sis
   lip·id p.
   pul·mo·nary al·ve·o·lar p.
pro·tein shock
   ther·a·py
pro·tein·u·ria
   Bence Jones p.

   ges·ta·tion·al p.
   iso·lat·ed p.
   non·iso·lat·ed p.
   or·tho·stat·ic p.
   pos·tur·al p.
pro·ten·si·ty
pro·te·o·clas·tic
pro·te·o·gly·cans
pro·te·o·hor·mone
pro·te·o·lip·ids
pro·te·ol·y·sis
pro·te·o·lyt·ic
pro·te·o·met·a·bol·ic
pro·te·o·me·tab·o·lism
Pro·te·o·myx·id·ia
pro·te·o·pec·tic
pro·te·o·pep·sis
pro·te·o·pex·ic
pro·te·o·pex·is
pro·te·ose
   pri·mary p.
   sec·on·dary p.
Pro·teus
   P. in·con·stans
   P. mi·ra·bi·lis
   P. mor·ga·nii
   P. rett·geri
   P. vul·ga·ris
pro·thi·pen·dyl
pro·tho·rac·ic
   glands
pro·throm·base
pro·throm·bin
   ac·cel·er·a·tor
   test
   time
pro·throm·bin·ase
pro·throm·bi·no·gen
pro·throm·bi·no·pe·nia
pro·throm·bin and pro·con·ver·tin
   test
pro·throm·bo·ki·nase
pro·thy·mia
pro·tide
pro·ti·o·dide
pro·ti·re·lin
pro·tist
Pro·tis·ta
pro·tis·tol·o·gist
pro·tis·tol·o·gy
pro·ti·um
pro·to·ac·tin·i·um
pro·to·al·bu·mose
pro·tobe
pro·to·bi·ol·o·gy
pro·to·cat·e·chu·ic ac·id
pro·to·chlo·ride

pro·to·chor·dal
   knot
pro·to·col
pro·to·cone
pro·to·co·nid
pro·to·cop·ro·por·phyr·ia
   p. he·re·di·ta·ria
Pro·toc·tis·ta
pro·to·derm
pro·to·di·a·stol·ic
   gal·lop
pro·to·du·o·de·num
pro·to·e·ryth·ro·cyte
pro·to·fil·a·ment
pro·to·gen
pro·to·gen A
pro·to·glob·u·lose
pro·to·gon·o·plasm
pro·to·heme
pro·to·i·o·dide
pro·to·ky·lol hy·dro·chlo·ride
pro·to·leu·ko·cyte
pro·tol·y·sate
pro·tom·e·rite
pro·to·me·tro·cyte
pro·ton
pro·to·neu·ron
pro·to-on·co·gene
pro·to·path·ic
   sen·si·bil·i·ty
pro·to·pec·tin
pro·to·pi·an·o·ma
pro·to·plasm
   to·ti·po·ten·tial p.
pro·to·plas·mat·ic
pro·to·plas·mic
   as·tro·cyte
   as·tro·cy·to·ma
   move·ment
pro·to·plas·mol·y·sis
pro·to·plast
pro·to·por·phyr·ia
   eryth·ro·poi·et·ic p.
pro·to·por·phy·rin type III
pro·to·pro·te·ose
pro·to·salt
pro·to·spasm
pro·to·spore
Pro·to·stron·gy·lus ru·fes·cens
pro·to·sul·fate
pro·to·syph·i·lis
pro·to·tax·ic
Pro·to·the·ca
pro·to·the·co·sis
pro·to·tox·in
pro·to·tox·oid
pro·to·troph

pro·to·tro·phic
   strains
pro·to·type
pro·to·ver·a·trine A and B
pro·to·ver·te·bra
pro·to·ver·te·bral
prot·ox·ide
Pro·to·zoa
pro·to·zoa
pro·to·zo·al
pro·to·zo·an
   cyst
pro·to·zo·i·a·sis
pro·to·zo·i·cide
pro·to·zo·ol·o·gist
pro·to·zo·ol·o·gy
pro·to·zo·on
pro·to·zo·o·phage
pro·trac·tion
   man·dib·u·lar p.
   max·il·lary p.
pro·trac·tor
pro·trip·ty·line hy·dro·chlo·ride
pro·trude
pro·trud·ed
   disk
pro·trud·ing
   teeth
pro·tru·sio ac·e·tab·u·li
pro·tru·sion
   bi·max·il·lary p.
   bi·max·il·lary den·to·al·ve·
      o·lar p.
   dou·ble p.
pro·tru·sive
   ex·cur·sion
   oc·clu·sion
   po·si·tion
   rec·ord
   re·la·tion
pro·tru·sive in·ter·oc·clu·sal
   rec·ord
pro·tru·sive jaw
   re·la·tion
pro·tryp·sin
pro·tu·ber·ance
   Bichat's p.
   ex·ter·nal oc·cip·i·tal p.
   in·ter·nal oc·cip·i·tal p.
   men·tal p.
pro·tu·ber·ant
   ab·do·men
pro·tu·be·ran·tia
   p. la·ryn·gea
proud
   flesh

Proust's
  law
  space
pro·ven·tri·cu·lus
pro·ver·te·bra
Pro·vi·den·cia
  P. al·ca·li·fa·ci·ens
  P. stu·ar·tii
pro·vi·rus
pro·vi·sion·al
  cal·lus
  cor·tex
  den·ture
  lig·a·ture
  pros·the·sis
pro·vi·ta·min
  p. A
prov·o·ca·tion
  ty·phoid
pro·voc·a·tive
  test
pro·voc·a·tive Wassermann
  test
Prowazek
  bod·ies
Prowazek-Greeff
  bod·ies
Pro·wa·ze·kia
prox·em·ics
prox·i·mad
prox·i·mal
  car·ies
  cen·tri·ole
  con·tact
  sep·tum
prox·i·mal fem·o·ral fo·cal
  de·fi·cien·cy
prox·i·mal in·ter·pha·lan·ge·al
  joints
prox·i·ma·lis
prox·i·mal ra·di·o·ul·nar
  ar·tic·u·la·tion
prox·i·mal spi·ral
  sep·tum
prox·i·mate
  cause
  con·tact
  prin·ci·ple
prox·i·mo·a·tax·ia
prox·i·mo·buc·cal
prox·i·mo·la·bi·al
prox·i·mo·lin·gual
prox·y·met·a·caine hy·dro·chlo·
  ride
pro·za·pine
pro·zone
  re·ac·tion
pro·zy·go·sis

prune
  bel·ly
prune bel·ly
  syn·drome
prune-juice
  ex·pec·to·ra·tion
  spu·tum
Pru·nus
  P. ser·o·ti·na
  P. vir·gi·ni·ana
pru·rig·i·nous
pru·ri·go
  p. aes·ti·va·lis
  p. ag·ria
  Besnier's p.
  p. fe·rox
  p. ges·ta·tio·nis
  Hebra's p.
  p. in·fan·ti·lis
  p. mi·tis
  p. no·du·la·ris
  p. sim·plex
  sum·mer p.
pru·rit·ic
pru·ri·tus
  p. aes·ti·va·lis
  p. ani
  aq·ua·gen·ic p.
  p. bal·nea
  bath p.
  es·sen·tial p.
  p. hi·e·ma·lis
  se·nile p.
  p. se·ni·lis
  symp·to·mat·ic p.
  p. vul·vae
Prussak's
  fi·bers
  pouch
  space
Prus·sian blue
  stain
prus·si·ate
prus·sic ac·id
psal·ter·ia
psal·ter·i·al
  cord
psal·ter·i·um
psam·mo·car·ci·no·ma
psam·mo·ma
  Virchow's p.
psam·mo·ma
  bod·ies
psam·mo·ma·tous
  me·nin·gi·o·ma
psam·mous
pse·la·phe·sia
pse·laph·e·sis

psel·lism
pseud·ac·ro·meg·a·ly
pseud·a·graph·ia
pseud·al·bu·min·u·ria
Pseud·al·les·che·ria boy·dii
pseud·al·les·che·ri·a·sis
Pseu·dam·phis·to·mum
pseud·an·gi·na
pseud·an·ky·lo·sis
pseud·aph·ia
pseud·ar·thro·sis
pseu·del·minth
pseud·es·the·sia
pseu·di·no·ma
pseudo-
    hem·i·a·nop·sia
pseu·do·ac·an·tho·sis ni·gri·
  cans
pseu·do·a·ceph·a·lus
pseu·do·a·chon·dro·pla·sia
pseu·do··a·chon·dro·plas·tic
   spon·dy·lo·ep·i·phys·i·al
   dys·pla·sia
pseu·do·ag·glu·ti·na·tion
pseu·do·a·gram·ma·tism
pseu·do·a·graph·ia
pseu·do-ai·nhum
pseu·do·al·bu·mi·nu·ria
pseu·do·al·lele
pseu·do·al·lel·ic
pseu·do·al·lel·ism
pseu·do-al·o·pe·cia ar·e·a·ta
pseu·do·an·a·phy·lac·tic
pseu·do·an·a·phy·lax·is
pseu·do·a·ne·mia
pseu·do·an·eu·rysm
pseu·do·an·gi·na
pseu·do·an·gi·o·sar·co·ma
   Masson's p.
pseu·do·an·o·don·tia
pseu·do·ap·o·plexy
pseu·do·ap·pen·di·ci·tis
pseu·do·a·prax·ia
pseu·do·ar·thro·sis
pseu·do·a·tax·ia
pseu·do·au·then·tic·i·ty
pseu·do·ba·cil·lus
pseu·do·bac·te·ri·um
pseu·do·blep·sia
pseu·do·blep·sis
pseu·do·bul·bar
   pa·ral·y·sis
pseu·do·car·ci·nom·a·tous
   hy·per·pla·sia
pseu·do·car·ti·lage
pseu·do·car·ti·lag·i·nous
pseu·do·cast
pseu·do·cele

pseu·do·ce·lom
pseu·do·ceph·a·lo·cele
pseu·do·chan·cre
pseu·do·cho·lin·es·ter·ase
   atyp·i·cal p.
   typ·i·cal p.
pseu·do·cho·lin·es·ter·ase
   de·fi·cien·cy
pseu·do·cho·rea
pseu·do·chro·mes·the·sia
pseu·do·chrom·hi·dro·sis
pseu·do·chro·mi·dro·sis
pseu·do·chy·lous
   as·ci·tes
pseu·do·cir·rho·sis
pseu·do·clo·nus
pseu·do·co·arc·ta·tion
pseu·do·col·loid
   p. of lips
pseu·do·col·lu·sion
pseu·do·co·ma
pseu·do·cow·pox
   vi·rus
pseu·do·cox·al·gia
pseu·do·cri·sis
pseu·do·croup
pseu·do·cryp·tor·chism
pseu·do·cu·mene
pseu·do·cu·mol
pseu·do·cy·e·sis
pseu·do·cyl·in·droid
pseu·do·cyst
pseu·do·de·cid·u·o·sis
pseu·do·de·men·tia
pseu·do·di·a·be·tes
pseu·do·di·a·stol·ic
pseu·do·dig·i·tox·in
pseu·do·diph·the·ria
pseu·do·dip·sia
pseu·do·di·ver·tic·u·lum
pseu·do·dys·en·tery
pseu·do·e·de·ma
pseu·do·e·phed·rine hy·dro·
   chlo·ride
pseu·do·ep·i·the·li·om·a·tous
   hy·per·pla·sia
pseu·do·er·y·sip·e·las
pseu·do·es·the·sia
pseu·do·ex·fo·li·a·tion
   p. of lens cap·sule
pseu·do·ex·fo·li·a·tive cap·su·
  lar
   glau·co·ma
pseu·do·fluc·tu·a·tion
pseu·do·fol·lic·u·li·tis
pseu·do·frac·ture
pseu·do·fruc·tose

pseu·do·fu·sion
  beat
pseu·do·gan·gli·on
pseu·do-Gaucher
  cell
pseu·do·gene
pseu·do·geu·ses·the·sia
pseu·do·geu·sia
pseu·do·glan·ders
pseu·do·glau·co·ma
pseu·do·gli·o·ma
pseu·do·glo·mer·u·lus
pseu·do·glu·co·sa·zone
pseu·do·gout
pseu·do-Graefe
  sign
pseu·do-Graefe's
  phe·nom·e·non
pseu·do·gy·ne·co·mas·tia
pseu·do·he·ma·tu·ria
pseu·do·he·mop·ty·sis
pseu·do·her·maph·ro·dite
pseu·do·her·maph·ro·dit·ism
  fe·male p.
  male p.
pseu·do·her·nia
pseu·do·het·er·o·to·pia
pseu·do·hy·dro·ceph·a·ly
pseu·do·hy·dro·ne·phro·sis
pseu·do·hy·per·par·a·thy·roid·
  ism
pseu·do·hy·per·tel·or·ism
pseu·do·hy·per·tro·phic
pseu·do·hy·per·tro·phic mus·cu·
  lar
  at·ro·phy
  dys·tro·phy
  pa·ral·y·sis
pseu·do·hy·per·tro·phy
pseu·do·hy·pha
pseu·do·hy·po·na·tre·mia
pseu·do·hy·po·par·a·thy·roid·
  ism
pseu·do·ic·ter·us
pseu·do·il·e·us
pseu·do·in·flu·en·za
pseu·do·in·tra·lig·a·men·tous
pseu·do·i·so·chro·mat·ic
pseu·do·jaun·dice
pseu·do·ker·a·tin
pseu·do·lep·ro·ma·tous
  leish·man·i·a·sis
pseu·do·li·po·ma
pseu·do·li·thi·a·sis
pseu·do·lob·ster-claw
  de·for·mi·ty
pseu·do·lo·gia
  p. phan·tas·ti·ca

pseu·do·lym·pho·cyte
pseu·do·lym·pho·cyt·ic cho·ri·
  o·men·in·gi·tis
  vi·rus
pseu·do·lym·pho·ma
  Spiegler-Fendt p.
pseu·do·ly·so·gen·ic
  strain
pseu·do·ly·sog·e·ny
pseu·do·ma·lig·nan·cy
pseu·do·mam·ma
pseu·do·ma·nia
pseu·do·mas·tur·ba·tion
pseu·do·mel·a·no·sis
pseu·do·mem·brane
pseu·do·mem·bra·nous
  bron·chi·tis
  co·li·tis
  con·junc·ti·vi·tis
  en·ter·i·tis
  en·ter·o·co·li·tis
  gas·tri·tis
  in·flam·ma·tion
  rhi·ni·tis
pseu·do·men·in·gi·tis
pseu·do·men·stru·a·tion
pseu·do·met·a·pla·sia
pseu·dom·ne·sia
pseu·do·mo·nad
Pseu·do·mo·nas
  P. ac·id·ov·o·rans
  P. ae·ru·gi·no·sa
  P. ce·pa·cia
  P. di·mi·nu·ta
  P. flu·o·res·cens
  P. mal·lei
  P. mal·to·phil·ia
  P. pseu·do·al·ca·lig·e·nes
  P. pseu·do·mal·lei
  P. pu·tre·fa·ciens
  P. py·o·cy·a·nea
  P. stut·zer·i
  P. ve·si·cu·la·re
pseu·do·morph
pseu·do·mu·ci·nous
  cyst
pseu·do·mus·cu·lar
  hy·per·tro·phy
pseu·do·my·ce·li·um
pseu·do·my·o·pia
pseu·do·myx·o·ma
  p. pe·ri·to·nei
pseu·do·nar·cot·ic
pseu·do·ne·o·plasm
pseu·do·neu·ri·tis
pseu·do·neu·ro·gen·ic
  blad·der
pseu·do·neu·ro·ma

pseu·do·neu·rot·ic
  schiz·o·phre·nia
pseu·do·nit
pseu·do·nys·tag·mus
pseu·do-os·te·o·ma·la·cia
pseu·do-os·te·o·ma·la·cic
  pel·vis
pseu·do·pap·il·le·de·ma
pseu·do·pa·ral·y·sis
  ar·thrit·ic gen·er·al p.
  con·gen·i·tal aton·ic p.
pseu·do·par·a·ple·gia
  Basedow's p.
pseu·do·par·a·site
pseu·do·pa·ren·chy·ma
pseu·do·pa·re·sis
pseu·do·pe·lade
pseu·do·per·i·car·di·tis
pseu·do·per·i·to·ni·tis
pseu·do·phac·os
pseu·do·pha·kia
pseu·do·pha·ko·do·ne·sis
pseu·do·phleg·mon
  Hamilton's p.
pseu·do·pho·tes·the·sia
pseu·do·phyl·lid
Pseu·do·phyl·lid·ea
pseu·do·plas·tic
  flu·id
pseu·do·plate·let
pseu·do·ple·gia
pseu·do·pock·et
pseu·do·pod
pseu·do·po·dia
pseu·do·po·di·um
pseu·do·pol·y·dys·tro·phy
pseu·do·pol·yp
pseu·do·por·phyr·ia
pseu·do·preg·nan·cy
pseu·do·prog·na·thism
pseu·do-pseu·do·hy·po·par·a·
  thy·roid·ism
pseu·dop·sia
pseu·do·pte·ryg·i·um
pseu·dop·to·sis
pseu·do·pu·ber·ty
  pre·co·cious p.
pseu·do·ra·bies
  vi·rus
pseu·do·re·ac·tion
pseu·do·rep·li·ca
pseu·do·ret·i·ni·tis pig·men·to·
  sa
pseu·do·rheu·ma·tism
pseu·do·rick·ets
pseu·do·ro·sette
pseu·do·ru·bel·la
pseu·do·sar·co·ma

pseu·do·sar·co·ma·tous
  fas·ci·i·tis
pseu·do·scar·la·ti·na
pseu·do·scle·ro·sis
  Westphal's p.
  Westphal-Strümpell p.
pseu·do·small·pox
pseu·dos·mia
Pseu·do·ster·ta·gia bul·lo·sa
pseu·dos·to·ma
pseu·do·stra·bis·mus
pseu·do·strat·i·fied
  ep·i·the·li·um
pseu·do·ta·bes
  pu·pil·lo·ton·ic p.
pseu·do·tha·lid·o·mide
  syn·drome
pseu·do·trich·i·ni·a·sis
pseu·do·trich·i·no·sis
pseu·do·trun·cus ar·te·ri·o·sus
pseu·do·tu·ber·cle
pseu·do·tu·ber·cu·lar
  yer·sin·i·o·sis
pseu·do·tu·ber·cu·lo·sis
pseu·do·tu·ber·cu·lous
  oph·thal·mia
pseu·do·tu·bu·lar
  de·gen·er·a·tion
pseu·do·tu·mor
  p. ce·re·bri
  in·flam·ma·to·ry p.
pseu·do-Tur·ner's
  syn·drome
pseu·do·u·ni·po·lar
  cell
  neu·ron
pseu·do·u·ri·dine
pseu·do·vac·u·ole
pseu·do·va·ri·o·la
pseu·do·ven·tri·cle
pseu·do·vi·ta·min
pseu·do·vom·it·ing
pseu·do·xan·tho·ma
  cell
pseu·do·xan·tho·ma elas·ti·cum
psi
  phe·nom·e·non
D-psi·cose
psi·lo·cin
Psil·o·cy·be
psi·lo·cy·bin
psi·lo·sis
psil·o·thin
psi·lot·ic
P-sin·is·tro·car·di·a·le
psit·ta·cine
psit·ta·co·sis
  vi·rus

psit·ta·co·sis in·clu·sion
  bod·ies
pso·as
  ab·scess
pso·mo·pha·gia
pso·moph·a·gy
pso·ra
psor·a·len
pso·rel·co·sis
psor·en·ter·i·tis
Psor·er·ga·tes
pso·ri·a·sic
pso·ri·a·si·form
pso·ri·a·sis
  p. an·nu·la·ris
  p. an·nu·la·ta
  p. ar·thro·pi·ca
  p. cir·ci·na·ta
  p. dif·fu·sa
  dif·fused p.
  p. dis·coi·dea
  gen·er·al·ized pus·tu·lar p.
    of Zambusch
  p. ge·o·gra·phi·ca
  p. gut·ta·ta
  p. gy·ra·ta
  p. in·ve·te·ra·ta
  p. num·mu·la·ris
  p. or·bi·cu·la·ris
  p. os·tre·a·cea
  p. punc·ta·ta
  pus·tu·lar p.
  p. ru·pi·oi·des
  p. spon·dy·li·ti·ca
  p. uni·ver·sa·lis
pso·ri·at·ic
  ar·thri·tis
pso·ric
pso·roid
pso·roph·thal·mia
Pso·rop·tes
pso·rop·tic
  ac·a·ri·a·sis
  mange
pso·rous
psy·cha·go·gy
psy·chal·ga·lia
psy·chal·gia
psy·cha·lia
psy·cha·nop·sia
psy·cha·tax·ia
psy·che
psy·che·del·ic
  ther·a·py
psy·chen·to·nia
psy·chi·at·ric
  no·sol·o·gy
psy·chi·at·rics

psy·chi·at·ric trend
psy·chi·a·trist
psy·chi·a·try
  an·a·lyt·ic p.
  com·mu·ni·ty p.
  con·trac·tu·al p.
  dy·nam·ic p.
  ex·is·ten·tial p.
  fo·ren·sic p.
  le·gal p.
  psy·cho·an·a·lyt·ic p.
  so·cial p.
psy·chic
  con·ta·gion
  de·ter·mi·nism
  en·er·gy
  force
  im·po·tence
  in·er·tia
  over·tone
  sei·zure
  tic
  trau·ma
psy·chi·cal
psy·chism
psy·cho·a·cous·tics
psy·cho·ac·tive
psy·cho·al·ler·gy
psy·cho·a·nal·y·sis
  ac·tive p.
  ad·le·ri·an p.
  freud·i·an p.
  jung·i·an p.
psy·cho·an·a·lyst
psy·cho·an·a·lyt·ic
  psy·chi·a·try
  psy·cho·ther·a·py
  sit·u·a·tion
  ther·a·py
psy·cho·au·di·to·ry
psy·cho·bi·ol·o·gy
psy·cho·car·di·ac
  re·flex
psy·cho·ca·thar·sis
psy·cho·chem·is·try
psy·cho·chrome
psy·cho·chro·mes·the·sia
psy·cho·di·ag·no·sis
Psy·chod·i·dae
psy·cho·dom·e·try
psy·cho·dra·ma
psy·cho·dy·nam·ics
psy·cho·en·do·cri·nol·o·gy
psy·cho·ex·plor·a·tion
psy·cho·gal·van·ic
  re·ac·tion
  re·flex
  re·sponse

psy·cho·gal·van·ic skin
  re·ac·tion
  re·flex
  re·sponse
psy·cho·gal·va·nom·e·ter
psy·cho·gen·der
psy·cho·gen·e·sis
psy·cho·ge·net·ic
psy·cho·gen·ic
  deaf·ness
  pain
  pol·y·dip·sia
  pur·pu·ra
  tor·ti·col·lis
  vom·it·ing
psy·cho·gen·ic noc·tur·nal
  pol·y·dip·sia
psy·cho·gen·ic noc·tur·nal pol·
  y·dip·sia
  syn·drome
psy·cho·gen·ic pain
  dis·or·der
psy·chog·e·ny
psy·cho·geu·sic
psy·cho·gog·ic
psy·cho·graph·ic
  dis·tur·banc·es
psy·chog·ra·phy
psy·cho·his·to·ry
psy·cho·ki·ne·sia
psy·cho·ki·ne·sis
psy·cho·kym
psy·cho·lag·ny
psy·cho·lep·sy
psy·cho·lin·guis·tics
psy·cho·log·ic
psy·cho·log·i·cal
  tests
psy·chol·o·gist
psy·chol·o·gy
  ad·le·ri·an p.
  an·a·lyt·i·cal p.
  at·om·is·tic p.
  be·hav·ior·al p.
  clin·i·cal p.
  cog·ni·tive p.
  com·mu·ni·ty p.
  com·par·a·tive p.
  con·sti·tu·tion·al p.
  coun·sel·ing p.
  crim·i·nal p.
  depth p.
  de·vel·op·men·tal p.
  dy·nam·ic p.
  ed·u·ca·tion·al p.
  en·vi·ron·men·tal p.
  ex·is·ten·tial p.
  ex·per·i·men·tal p.

fo·ren·sic p.
ge·net·ic p.
ge·stalt p.
ho·lis·tic p.
hu·man·is·tic p.
in·di·vid·u·al p.
in·dus·tri·al p.
med·i·cal p.
ob·jec·tive p.
sub·jec·tive p.
psy·cho·met·rics
psy·chom·e·try
psy·cho·mo·tor
  ep·i·lep·sy
  re·tar·da·tion
  sei·zure
  tests
psy·cho·neu·ro·sis
  p. mai·di·ca
psy·cho·neu·rot·ic
psy·cho·nom·ic
psy·chon·o·my
psy·cho·no·sol·o·gy
psy·cho·nox·ious
psy·cho·path
psy·cho·path·ic
  per·son·al·i·ty
psy·chop·a·thist
psy·cho·pa·thol·o·gist
psy·cho·pa·thol·o·gy
psy·chop·a·thy
psy·cho·phar·ma·ceu·ti·cals
psy·cho·phar·ma·col·o·gy
psy·cho·phys·i·cal
psy·cho·phys·ics
psy·cho·phys·i·o·log·ic
  dis·or·der
  man·i·fes·ta·tion
psy·cho·phys·i·ol·o·gy
psy·cho·pro·phy·lax·is
psy·cho·re·lax·a·tion
psy·cho·rhyth·mia
psy·chor·mic
psy·chor·rhea
psy·chor·rhyth·mia
psy·cho·sen·so·ri·al
psy·cho·sen·so·ry
  apha·sia
psy·cho·ses
psy·cho·sex·u·al
  de·vel·op·ment
  dys·func·tion
psy·cho·sine
psy·cho·sis
  af·fec·tive p.
  al·co·hol·ic psy·cho·ses
  am·nes·tic p.
  ar·te·ri·o·scle·rot·ic p.

843

psy·cho·sis *(continued)*
  Cheyne-Stokes p.
  cli·mac·ter·ic p.
  drug p.
  dys·mne·sic p.
  ex·haus·tion p.
  feb·rile p.
  ges·ta·tion·al p.
  hys·ter·i·cal p.
  ICU p.
  in·fec·tion-ex·haus·tion p.
  in·vo·lu·tion·al p.
  Korsakoff's p.
  man·ic-de·pres·sive p.
  pol·y·neu·rit·ic p.
  post·hyp·not·ic p.
  post·in·fec·tious p.
  post·par·tum p.
  post·trau·mat·ic p.
  pu·er·per·al p.
  schiz·o-af·fec·tive p.
  se·nile p.
  sit·u·a·tion·al p.
  tox·ic p.
  trau·mat·ic p.
  Win·di·go p.
  Wit·ti·go p.
psy·cho·so·cial
psy·cho·so·mat·ic
  dis·or·der
  med·i·cine
psy·cho·so·mi·met·ic
psy·cho·stim·u·lant
psy·cho·sur·gery
psy·cho·syn·the·sis
psy·cho·tech·nics
psy·cho·ther·a·peu·tic
psy·cho·ther·a·peu·tics
psy·cho·ther·a·pist
psy·cho·ther·a·py
  an·a·clit·ic p.
  au·ton·o·mous p.
  con·trac·tu·al p.
  di·rec·tive p.
  dy·ad·ic p.
  dy·nam·ic p.
  ex·is·ten·tial p.
  group p.
  het·er·on·o·mous p.
  hyp·not·ic p.
  in·ten·sive p.
  mar·a·thon group p.
  non·di·rec·tive p.
  psy·cho·an·a·lyt·ic p.
  re·con·struc·tive p.
  sug·ges·tive p.
  sup·port·ive p.
  trans·ac·tion·al p.

psy·chot·ic
  man·i·fes·ta·tion
psy·chot·o·gen
psy·chot·o·gen·ic
psy·chot·o·mi·met·ic
psy·cho·tro·pic
psy·chro·al·gia
psy·chro·es·the·sia
psy·chrom·e·ter
  sling p.
psy·chrom·e·try
psy·chro·phil
psy·chro·phile
psy·chro·phil·ic
psy·chro·pho·bia
psy·chro·phore
psyl·li·um hy·dro·phil·ic mu·cil·loid
PTA
  stain
ptar·mic
ptar·mus
PTC
  pep·tide
  pro·tein
pter·i·dine
pter·in
  p. de·am·i·nase
pter·i·on
pte·ro·ic ac·id
pter·op·ter·in
pter·o·yl·mon·o·glu·tam·ic ac·id
pter·o·yl·tri·glu·tam·ic ac·id
pte·ryg·i·um
  p. col·li
  p. un·guis
pte·ryg·i·um
  syn·drome
pter·y·goid
  ca·nal
  chest
  de·pres·sion
  fis·sure
  fos·sa
  ham·u·lus
  lam·i·nae
  nerve
  notch
  pit
  plates
  plex·us
  pro·cess
  ridge of sphe·noid bone
  tu·ber·cle
  tu·ber·os·i·ty
pter·y·go·man·dib·u·lar
  lig·a·ment

ra·phe
space
pte·ry·go·max·il·la·re
pter·y·go·max·il·lary
  fis·sure
  fos·sa
  notch
pter·y·go·pal·a·tine
  ca·nal
  fos·sa
  gan·gli·on
  groove
  nerves
pter·y·go·pha·ryn·ge·al
  part
pter·y·go·qua·drate
pter·y·go·spi·nal
  lig·a·ment
pter·y·go·spi·nous
  lig·a·ment
  pro·cess
pthi·ri·a·sis
  p. ca·pi·tis
  p. cor·po·ris
  p. pu·bis
Pthir·us
pti·lo·sis
pto·maine
pto·mai·ne·mia
pto·ma·tine
pto·mat·ro·pine
ptosed
pto·ses
pto·sis
  p. adi·po·sa
  p. sym·pa·the·ti·ca
pto·tic
  or·gan
pty·al·a·gogue
pty·a·lec·ta·sis
pty·a·lin
pty·a·lism
pty·a·lo·cele
pty·a·log·ra·phy
pty·a·lo·lith
pty·a·lo·li·thi·a·sis
pty·a·lo·li·thot·o·my
pty·cho·tis oil
pty·oc·ri·nous
pu·bar·che
pu·ber·al
pu·ber·tal
pu·ber·tas prae·cox
pu·ber·ty
  pre·co·cious p.
pu·bes
pu·bes·cence
pu·bes·cent

pu·bic
  an·gle
  arch
  ar·ter·ies
  bald·ness
  body
  bone
  crest
  ra·mi
  re·gion
  spine
  sym·phy·sis
  tu·ber·cle
pu·bi·ot·o·my
pu·bis
pub·lic
  an·ti·gens
  health
  hos·pi·tal
pub·lic health
  den·tis·try
  nurse
pu·bo·cap·su·lar
  lig·a·ment
pu·bo·coc·cy·ge·al
  mus·cle
pu·bo·fem·o·ral
  lig·a·ment
pu·bo·ma·de·sis
pu·bo·pros·tat·ic
  lig·a·ment
  mus·cle
pu·bo·rec·tal
  mus·cle
pu·bo·u·re·thral
  tri·an·gle
pu·bo·vag·i·nal
  mus·cle
pu·bo·ves·i·cal
  lig·a·ment
  mus·cle
Puchtler-Sweat
  stain for base·ment mem·
    branes
  stain for he·mo·glo·bin and
    he·mo·sid·er·in
Puchtler-Sweat stains
pud·ding
  opi·um
pud·dle
  sign
pu·den·da
pu·den·dal
  an·es·the·sia
  ca·nal
  cleav·age
  he·ma·to·cele
  her·nia

pu·den·dal *(continued)*
  nerve
  sac
  slit
  ul·cer
  veins
pu·den·dum
  p. mu·li·e·bre
pu·dic
  nerve
pu·er·ile
  res·pi·ra·tion
pu·er·pera
pu·er·per·ae
pu·er·per·al
  con·vul·sions
  ec·lamp·sia
  fe·ver
  he·mo·glo·bi·ne·mia
  he·mo·glo·bi·nu·ria
  mas·ti·tis
  mor·bid·i·ty
  pe·ri·od
  phle·bi·tis
  psy·cho·sis
  sep·sis
  sep·ti·ce·mia
  tet·a·nus
pu·er·per·ant
pu·er·pe·ria
pu·er·pe·ri·um
Puestow
  pro·ce·dure
puff
  veiled p.
puff·ball
Pu·lex
  P. che·o·pis
  P. fas·ci·a·tus
  P. ir·ri·tans
  P. pen·e·trans
  P. ser·ra·ti·ceps
pu·lic·i·cide
pu·li·cide
pul·ley
  p. of hu·mer·us
  mus·cu·lar p.
  per·o·ne·al p.
  p. of ta·lus
pul·lo·rum
  dis·ease
pul·lu·la·nase
pul·lu·late
pul·lu·la·tion
pul·mo
pul·mo·a·or·tic
pul·mo·lith
pul·mom·e·ter

pul·mom·e·try
pul·mo·nary
  ac·a·ri·a·sis
  ac·i·nus
  ad·e·no·ma·to·sis
  ad·e·no·ma·to·sis of sheep
  an·thrax
  arc
  ar·ea
  ar·tery
  as·per·gil·lo·sis
  atre·sia
  bul·la
  cir·cu·la·tion
  col·lapse
  cone
  co·nus
  dis·to·mi·a·sis
  ede·ma
  em·bo·lism
  em·phy·se·ma
  fis·tu·la
  glo·man·gi·o·sis
  ham·ar·to·ma
  heart
  he·mo·sid·er·o·sis
  hy·per·ten·sion
  hy·pos·ta·sis
  in·com·pe·tence
  in·suf·fi·cien·cy
  lig·a·ment
  mur·mur
  open·ing
  os·te·o·ar·throp·a·thy
  pleu·ri·sy
  plex·us
  pres·sure
  pulse
  ridg·es
  sa·lient
  ste·no·sis
  sul·cus
  sur·face of heart
  tran·spi·ra·tion
  trunk
  tu·ber·cu·lo·sis
  valve
  veins
  ven·ti·la·tion
pul·mo·nary al·ve·o·lar
  mi·cro·li·thi·a·sis
  pro·tein·o·sis
pul·mo·nary cap·il·lary wedge
  pres·sure
pul·mo·nary dys·ma·tu·ri·ty
  syn·drome
pul·mo·nary lymph
  nodes

pul·mo·nec·to·my
pul·mo·nes
pul·mon·ic
  in·com·pe·tence
  mur·mur
pul·mo·nis
pul·mo·ni·tis
pul·mo·no·cor·o·nary
  re·flex
pul·mo·tor
pulp
  cor·o·nal p.
  dead p.
  den·tal p.
  den·ti·nal p.
  dig·i·tal p.
  enam·el p.
  ex·posed p.
  p. of fin·ger
  mum·mi·fied p.
  ne·crot·ic p.
  non·vit·al p.
  pu·tres·cent p.
  ra·dic·u·lar p.
  red p.
  splen·ic p.
  tooth p.
  ver·te·bral p.
  vi·tal p.
  white p.
pulp
  ab·scess
  am·pu·ta·tion
  at·ro·phy
  cal·ci·fi·ca·tion
  cal·cu·lus
  ca·nal
  cav·i·ty
  cham·ber
  horn
  nod·ule
  pol·yp
  pres·sure
  stone
  test
pul·pa
  p. li·e·nis
pul·pal
  wall
pul·pal·gia
pulp·ar
  cell
pul·pa·tion
pulp·ec·to·my
pul·pi·fac·tion
pulp·i·form
pulp·i·fy

pul·pit
  spec·ta·cles
pulp·i·tis
  hy·per·plas·tic p.
  hy·per·tro·phic p.
  ir·re·vers·i·ble p.
  re·vers·i·ble p.
  sup·pu·ra·tive p.
pulp·less
  tooth
pulp·less
pulp·o·don·tia
pul·po·sus
pulp·ot·o·my
pulpy
pulpy kid·ney
  dis·ease
pul·sate
pul·sa·tile
pul·sat·ing
  em·py·e·ma
  me·tas·ta·ses
  neur·as·the·nia
pul·sa·tion
pul·sa·tor
pulse
  ab·dom·i·nal p.
  al·ter·nat·ing p.
  an·a·crot·ic p.
  an·a·di·crot·ic p.
  bi·gem·i·nal p.
  bis·fer·i·ous p.
  bul·bar p.
  can·non·ball p.
  cap·il·lary p.
  cat·a·crot·ic p.
  cat·a·di·crot·ic p.
  col·laps·ing p.
  cordy p.
  Corrigan's p.
  cou·pled p.
  di·crot·ic p.
  ent·op·tic p.
  fi·li·form p.
  gas·e·ous p.
  gut·tur·al p.
  hard p.
  in·ter·mit·tent p.
  jug·u·lar p.
  Kussmaul's par·a·dox·i·cal
    p.
  long p.
  mon·o·crot·ic p.
  mouse·tail p.
  mov·a·ble p.
  nail p.
  par·a·dox·i·cal p.
  pis·ton p.

pulse *(continued)*
  pla·teau p.
  pul·mo·nary p.
  quad·ri·gem·i·nal p.
  Quincke's p.
  res·pi·ra·to·ry p.
  re·versed par·a·dox·i·cal p.
  Riegel's p.
  soft p.
  tense p.
  thready p.
  tri·gem·i·nal p.
  trip·ham·mer p.
  un·du·lat·ing p.
  va·gus p.
  ve·nous p.
  ver·mic·u·lar p.
  wa·ter-ham·mer p.
  wiry p.
pulse
  curve
  def·i·cit
  du·ra·tion
  gen·er·a·tor
  pe·ri·od
  pres·sure
  rate
  ther·a·py
  wave
pulse·less
  dis·ease
pul·sel·lum
pul·sim·e·ter
pul·sion
  di·ver·tic·u·lum
pul·som·e·ter
pul·sus
  p. ab·do·mi·na·lis
  p. al·ter·nans
  p. an·a·di·cro·tus
  p. bi·gem·i·nus
  p. bis·fe·ri·ens
  p. cap·ri·sans
  p. cat·a·cro·tus
  p. ca·ta·di·cro·tus
  p. ce·ler
  p. ce·le·ri·mus
  p. cor·dis
  p. de·bil·is
  p. dif·fer·ens
  p. du·plex
  p. du·rus
  p. fi·li·for·mis
  p. flu·ens
  p. for·mi·cans
  p. for·tis
  p. fre·quens
  p. het·er·o·chro·ni·cus

  p. in·ae·qua·lis
  p. in·con·gru·ens
  p. in·fre·quens
  p. in·ter·ci·dens
  p. in·ter·cur·rens
  p. ir·reg·u·la·ris per·pe·tu·us
  p. mag·nus
  p. mol·lis
  p. mon·o·cro·tus
  p. my·ur·us
  p. par·a·dox·us
  p. par·vus
  p. quad·ri·ge·mi·nus
  p. ra·rus
  p. res·pi·ra·ti·o·ne in·ter·mit·tens
  p. tar·dus
  p. trem·u·lus
  p. tri·gem·i·nus
  p. va·cu·us
  p. ve·no·sus
pul·sus
  al·ter·nans
pul·ta·ceous
pul·ver·i·za·tion
pul·ver·ize
pul·ver·u·lent
pul·vi·nar
pul·vi·nate
pum·ice
pum·iced
  foot
pump
  fail·ure
  lung
pump
  breast p.
  Carrel-Lindbergh p.
  con·stant in·fu·sion p.
  den·tal p.
  in·tra-a·or·tic bal·loon p.
  jet ejec·tor p.
  sa·li·va p.
  so·di·um p.
  so·di·um-po·tas·si·um p.
  stom·ach p.
pump-ox·y·gen·a·tor
pu·na
punch
  bi·op·sy
  grafts
punch·drunk
  syn·drome
punc·ta
punc·ta·ta al·bes·cens
  ret·i·nop·a·thy

punc·tate
  ba·so·phil·ia
  cat·a·ract
  hem·or·rhage
  hy·a·lo·sis
  ker·a·ti·tis
  ker·a·to·der·ma
  pa·rot·i·di·tis
  ret·i·ni·tis
punc·ti
punc·ti·form
punc·tum
  p. ce·cum
  p. cox·a·le
  p. do·lo·ro·sum
  lac·ri·mal p.
  p. lu·te·um
  p. prox·i·mum
  p. re·mo·tum
  p. vas·cu·lo·sum
punc·ture
  Bernard's p.
  cis·ter·nal p.
  di·a·bet·ic p.
  lum·bar p.
  Quincke's p.
  spi·nal p.
  ster·nal p.
punc·ture
  di·a·be·tes
  wound
pun·gent
pu·pa
pu·pae
pu·pil
  Adie's p.
  am·au·rot·ic p.
  Argyll Robertson p.
  ar·ti·fi·cial p.
  bound·ing p.
  Bumke's p.
  cat·a·ton·ic p.
  cat's-eye p.
  cog·wheel p.
  fixed p.
  Gunn p.
  Holmes-Adie p.
  Horner's p.
  Hutchinson's p.
  key·hole p.
  Marcus Gunn p.
  neu·ro·ton·ic p.
  par·a·dox·i·cal p.
  pin·hole p.
  rig·id p.
  Robertson p.
  Saenger p.
  ton·ic p.

pu·pil·la
pu·pil·lae
pu·pil·lary
  ath·e·to·sis
  ax·is
  dis·tance
  mar·gin
  mem·brane
  re·flex
  zone
pu·pil·lary block
  glau·co·ma
pu·pil·lary-skin
  re·flex
pu·pil·log·ra·phy
pu·pil·lom·e·ter
pu·pil·lom·e·try
pu·pil·lo·mo·tor
pu·pil·lo·ple·gia
pu·pil·los·co·py
pu·pil·lo·sta·tom·e·ter
pu·pil·lo·ton·ic
  pseu·do·ta·bes
pu·pip·a·rous
pure
  ab·sence
  apha·si·as
  col·or
  cul·ture
  line
pure·bred
pure red cell
  ane·mia
  apla·sia
pure-tone
  au·di·om·e·ter
  au·di·om·e·try
pure tone
  au·di·o·gram
pur·ga·tion
pur·ga·tive
  sa·line p.
purge
purg·ing cas·sia
pu·ri·fied
  cot·ton
  ozo·ker·ite
  wa·ter
pu·ri·fied pla·cen·tal
  pro·tein
pu·ri·fied pro·tein de·riv·a·tive of
  tu·ber·cu·lin
pu·ri·form
pu·rine
  p.-nu·cle·o·side phos·pho·ryl·ase
  p. ri·bo·nu·cle·o·side

pu·rine
bod·ies
pu·ri·ne·mia
pu·rine-re·strict·ed
di·et
pu·ri·ty
ra·di·o·chem·i·cal p.
ra·di·o·i·so·to·pic p.
ra·di·o·nu·clid·ic p.
ra·di·o·phar·ma·ceu·ti·cal p.
Purkinje
con·duc·tion
im·ag·es
shift
sys·tem
Purkinje's
cells
cor·pus·cles
fi·bers
fig·ures
lay·er
net·work
phe·nom·e·non
Purkinje-Sanson
im·ag·es
Purmann's
meth·od
pu·ro·mu·cous
pu·ro·my·cin
pur·ple
vi·su·al p.
pur·pu·ra
acute vas·cu·lar p.
al·ler·gic p.
an·a·phy·lac·toid p.
p. an·gi·o·neu·ro·ti·ca
p. an·nu·la·ris tel·an·gi·ec·
to·des
fac·ti·tious p.
fi·bri·no·lyt·ic p.
p. ful·mi·nans
p. hem·or·rha·gi·ca
Henoch's p.
Henoch-Schönlein p.
hy·per·glob·u·lin·e·mic p.
id·i·o·path·ic throm·bo·cy·
to·pe·nic p.
im·mune throm·bo·cy·to·pe·
nic p.
iod·ic p.
p. io·di·ca
p. ner·vo·sa
non·throm·bo·cy·to·pe·nic
p.
psy·cho·gen·ic p.
p. pu·li·cans
p. pu·li·co·sa
p. rheu·ma·ti·ca

Schönlein's p.
p. se·ni·lis
p. sim·plex
p. symp·to·ma·ti·ca
throm·bo·cy·to·pe·nic p.
throm·bot·ic throm·bo·cy·
to·pe·nic p.
p. ur·ti·cans
Waldenström's p.
pur·pu·rea gly·co·sides A
pur·pu·rea gly·co·sides B
pur·pu·ric
pur·pu·rif·er·ous
pur·pu·rig·e·nous
pur·pu·rin
pur·pu·ri·nu·ria
pur·pu·rip·a·rous
purr
pursed lips
breath·ing
purse-string
in·stru·ment
su·ture
Purtscher's
dis·ease
pu·ru·lence
pu·ru·len·cy
pu·ru·lent
con·junc·ti·vi·tis
cy·cli·tis
en·ceph·a·li·tis
in·flam·ma·tion
oph·thal·mia
pleu·ri·sy
ret·i·ni·tis
rhi·ni·tis
syn·o·vi·tis
pu·ru·loid
pus
blue p.
cheesy p.
curdy p.
green p.
ichor·ous p.
laud·a·ble p.
sa·ni·ous p.
pus
ba·sin
cell
cor·pus·cle
tube
push-back
pro·ce·dure
pus·tu·lant
pus·tu·lar
bleph·a·ri·tis
mil·i·a·ria

pso·ri·a·sis
syph·i·lid
pus·tu·la·tion
pus·tule
  ma·lig·nant p.
  post·mor·tem p.
  spon·gi·form p. of Kogoj
pus·tu·li·form
pus·tu·lo·crus·ta·ceous
pus·tu·lo·sis
  p. pal·mar·is et plan·tar·is
  p. vac·ci·ni·for·mis acu·ta
pu·ta·men
Putnam-Dana
  syn·drome
pu·tre·fac·tion
pu·tre·fac·tive
pu·tre·fy
pu·tres·cence
pu·tres·cent
  pulp
pu·tres·cine
pu·trid
  bron·chi·tis
  throat
Putti-Platt
  op·er·a·tion
  pro·ce·dure
put·ty
  kid·ney
PVM
  vi·rus
py·ar·thro·sis
py·e·lec·ta·sia
py·e·lec·ta·sis
py·e·lit·ic
py·e·li·tis
py·e·lo·cal·i·ce·al
py·e·lo·cal·i·ec·ta·sis
py·e·lo·cal·y·ce·al
py·e·lo·cys·ti·tis
py·e·lo·flu·o·ros·co·py
py·el·o·gram
py·e·log·ra·phy
  an·te·grade p.
py·e·lo·li·thot·o·my
py·e·lo·lym·phat·ic
py·e·lo·ne·phrit·ic
  kid·ney
py·e·lo·ne·phri·tis
  acute p.
  as·cend·ing p.
  chron·ic p.
  con·ta·gious bo·vine p.
  xan·tho·gran·u·lo·ma·tous
    p.
py·e·lo·ne·phro·sis

py·e·lo·plas·ty
  Anderson-Hynes p.
  cap·su·lar flap p.
  Culp p.
  dis·joined p.
  dis·mem·bered p.
  Foley Y-plas·ty p.
  Scardino ver·ti·cal flap p.
py·e·lo·pli·ca·tion
py·e·los·co·py
py·e·los·to·my
py·e·lot·o·my
  ex·tend·ed p.
py·e·lo·u·re·ter·ec·ta·sis
py·e·lo·u·re·ter·og·ra·phy
py·e·lo·ve·nous
py·em·e·sis
py·e·mia
  cryp·to·gen·ic p.
  por·tal p.
py·e·mic
  ab·scess
  em·bo·lism
Py·e·mo·tes tri·ti·ci
py·en·ceph·a·lus
py·e·sis
py·gal
py·gal·gia
pyg·ma·li·on·ism
pyg·my
py·go·a·mor·phus
py·go·did·y·mus
py·gom·e·lus
py·gop·a·gus
pyk·nic
pyk·no·dys·os·to·sis
pyk·no·ep·i·lep·sy
pyk·no·lep·sy
pyk·no·mor·phous
pyk·no·phra·sia
pyk·no·sis
pyk·not·ic
py·la
py·lar
py·lem·phrax·is
py·le·phle·bec·ta·sia
py·le·phle·bec·ta·sis
py·le·phle·bi·tis
py·le·throm·bo·phle·bi·tis
py·le·throm·bo·sis
py·lic
py·lon
py·lo·ral·gia
py·lo·rec·to·my
py·lo·ri
py·lor·ic
  an·trum
  ar·tery

py·lor·ic *(continued)*
 ca·nal
 cap
 glands
 in·com·pe·tence
 in·suf·fi·cien·cy
 or·i·fice
 part of stom·ach
 sphinc·ter
 ste·no·sis
 valve
 vein
py·lor·ic lymph
 nodes
py·lo·ri·ste·no·sis
py·lo·ri·tis
py·lo·ro·di·o·sis
py·lo·ro·du·o·de·ni·tis
py·lo·ro·gas·trec·to·my
py·lo·ro·my·ot·o·my
py·lo·ro·plas·ty
 Finney p.
 Heineke-Mikulicz p.
 Jaboulay p.
py·lor·op·to·sia
py·lor·op·to·sis
py·lo·ro·spasm
py·lo·ro·ste·no·sis
py·lo·ros·to·my
py·lo·rot·o·my
py·lo·rus
Pym's
 fe·ver
py·o·cele
py·o·ce·lia
py·o·ceph·a·lus
 cir·cum·scribed p.
 ex·ter·nal p.
 in·ter·nal p.
py·o·che·zia
py·o·cin
py·o·coc·cus
py·o·col·po·cele
py·o·col·pos
py·o·cy·an·ic
py·o·cy·a·no·gen·ic
py·o·cy·a·nol·y·sin
py·o·cyst
py·o·cys·tis
py·o·cyte
py·o·der·ma
 chan·cri·form p.
 p. gan·gre·no·sum
 pri·mary p.
 sec·on·dary p.
 p. ve·ge·tans
py·o·der·ma·ti·tis
py·o·der·ma·to·sis

py·o·gen
py·o·gen·e·sis
py·o·ge·net·ic
py·o·gen·ic
 bac·te·ri·um
 fe·ver
 gran·u·lo·ma
 in·fec·tion
 mem·brane
 pach·y·men·in·gi·tis
 sal·pin·gi·tis
py·og·e·nous
py·o·he·mia
py·o·he·mo·tho·rax
py·oid
py·o·lab·y·rin·thi·tis
py·o·me·tra
py·o·me·tri·tis
py·o·my·o·si·tis
 trop·i·cal p.
py·o·ne·phri·tis
py·o·neph·ro·li·thi·a·sis
py·o·ne·phro·sis
pyo-ova·ri·um
py·o·per·i·car·di·tis
py·o·per·i·car·di·um
py·o·per·i·to·ne·um
py·o·per·i·to·ni·tis
py·oph·thal·mia
py·oph·thal·mi·tis
py·o·phy·so·me·tra
py·o·pneu·mo·cho·le·cys·ti·tis
py·o·pneu·mo·hep·a·ti·tis
py·o·pneu·mo·per·i·car·di·um
py·o·pneu·mo·per·i·to·ne·um
py·o·pneu·mo·per·i·to·ni·tis
py·o·pneu·mo·tho·rax
 sub·di·a·phrag·mat·ic p.
 sub·phren·ic p.
py·o·poi·e·sis
py·o·poi·et·ic
py·op·ty·sis
py·o·py·e·lec·ta·sis
py·or·rhea
py·o·sal·pin·gi·tis
py·o·sal·pin·go-ooph·o·ri·tis
py·o·sal·pin·go-oo·the·ci·tis
py·o·sal·pinx
py·o·se·mia
py·o·sep·ti·ce·mia
py·o·sis
 Manson's p.
 p. pal·mar·is
 p. tro·pi·ca
py·o·sper·mia
py·o·stat·ic
py·o·sto·ma·ti·tis
 p. ve·ge·tans

py·o·tho·rax
py·o·u·ra·chus
py·o·u·re·ter
py·o·xan·thin
py·o·xan·those
pyr·a·cin
pyr·a·mid
  an·te·ri·or p.
  cer·e·bel·lar p.
  Fer·rein's p.
  Lallouette's p.
  p. of light
  Malacarne's p.
  mal·pi·ghi·an p.
  p. of me·dul·la ob·lon·ga·ta
  med·ul·lary p.
  ol·fac·to·ry p.
  pet·rous p.
  pos·te·ri·or p. of the me·
    dul·la
  re·nal p.
  p. of thy·roid
  p. of tym·pa·num
  p. of ves·ti·bule
pyr·a·mid
  sign
py·ram·i·dal
  bone
  cat·a·ract
  cells
  de·cus·sa·tion
  em·i·nence
  fi·bers
  frac·ture
  lobe of thy·roid gland
  mus·cle
  mus·cle of au·ri·cle
  pro·cess
  ra·di·a·tion
  tract
  trac·tot·o·my
py·ram·i·dal cell
  lay·er
py·ra·mi·da·le
py·ra·mi·da·lis
py·ra·mi·des
py·ram·i·dot·o·my
  med·ul·lary p.
  spi·nal p.
pyr·a·min
pyr·a·mine
pyr·a·mis
  p. tym·pa·ni
py·ran
pyr·a·none
pyr·a·nose
py·ran·tel pam·o·ate

pyr·a·thi·a·zine hy·dro·chlo·
  ride
pyr·a·zin·a·mide
pyr·az·o·lone
py·rec·tic
py·re·ne·mia
Py·re·no·chae·ta ro·me·roi
py·re·noid
py·re·thrins
py·re·thro·lone
py·re·thrum
py·ret·ic
py·ret·o·gen
py·re·to·gen·e·sis
py·re·to·ge·net·ic
py·re·to·gen·ic
py·re·tog·e·nous
py·re·to·ther·a·py
py·rex·ia
py·rex·i·al
py·rex·i·o·pho·bia
pyr·i·ben·zyl meth·yl sul·fate
pyr·i·dine
pyr·i·dof·yl·line
pyr·i·do·stig·mine bro·mide
pyr·i·dox·al
  p. ki·nase
pyr·i·dox·a·mine
pyr·i·dox·a·mine-phos·phate ox·
  i·dase
pyr·i·dox·ine
pyr·i·dox·ol
pyr·i·dox·on·i·um (chlo·ride)
pyr·i·form
  ap·pa·ra·tus
pyr·i·form ap·er·ture
  wir·ing
py·ril·a·mine ma·le·ate
py·ri·meth·a·mine
py·rim·i·dine
  p. trans·fer·ase
pyr·i·thi·a·min
py·ro·bo·ric ac·id
py·ro·cal·cif·er·ol
py·ro·cat·e·chase
py·ro·cat·e·chin
py·ro·cat·e·chol
py·ro·gal·lic ac·id
py·ro·gal·lol
py·ro·gal·lol phthal·e·in
py·ro·gen
py·ro·gen·ic
py·ro·glob·u·lins
py·ro·lag·nia
py·ro·lig·ne·ous
  al·co·hol
  spir·it
  vin·e·gar

py·rol·y·sis
py·ro·ma·nia
py·ro·ma·ni·ac
py·ro·men
py·rom·e·ter
  re·sis·tance p.
py·rone
py·ro·nin
py·ro·nin B
py·ro·nin G
py·ro·ni·no·phil·ia
py·ro·nin Y
py·ro·pho·bia
py·ro·phos·pha·tase
  in·or·gan·ic p.
py·ro·phos·phate
py·ro·phos·pho·ki·nas·es
py·ro·phos·phor·ic ac·id
py·ro·phos·pho·ryl·as·es
py·ro·phos·pho·trans·fer·as·es
py·rop·to·thy·mia
py·ro·scope
py·ro·sis
py·ro·ther·a·py
py·rot·ic
py·ro·tox·in
pyr·o·val·er·one hy·dro·chlo·ride
pyr·ox·yl·ic
  spir·it
pyr·ox·y·lin
pyr·rhol
  cell
pyr·ro·bu·ta·mine phos·phate

pyr·rol
  cell
pyr·ro·lase
pyr·rol blue
pyr·role
  nu·cle·us
pyr·rol·i·dine
pyr·rol·i·done
pyr·ro·line
pyr·rol·ni·trin
py·ru·val·dox·ine
py·ru·vate
  p. car·box·yl·ase
  p. de·car·box·yl·ase
  p. de·hy·dro·gen·ase (cy·to·chrome)
  p. de·hy·dro·gen·ase (lip·o·am·ide)
  p. ki·nase
  p. ox·i·dase
py·ru·vate ki·nase
  de·fi·cien·cy
py·ru·vate ox·i·da·tion
  fac·tor
py·ru·vic ac·id
py·ru·vic al·de·hyde
py·ru·vic-mal·ic car·box·yl·ase
pyr·vin·i·um pam·o·ate
Pyth·i·um in·si·di·o·sum
py·tho·gen·e·sis
py·tho·gen·ic
py·thog·e·nous
py·u·ria

Q
an·gle
bands
disks
en·zyme
fe·ver
wave
Q-
band·ing
Q-band·ing
stain
Q-R
in·ter·val
Q-RB
in·ter·val
QRS
com·plex
in·ter·val
Q-T
in·ter·val
quack
med·i·cine
quack·ery
qua·der
qua·dran·gu·lar
car·ti·lage
lob·ule
mem·brane
ther·a·py
quad·rant
quad·rant·a·nop·sia
quad·ran·tic
hem·i·a·nop·sia
sco·to·ma
quad·rate
lig·a·ment
lobe
lob·ule
mus·cle
mus·cle of loins
mus·cle of sole
mus·cle of thigh
mus·cle of up·per lip
part
quad·rate pro·na·tor
mus·cle
quad·ra·tus fe·mo·ris
bur·sa
quad·ri·ba·sic

quad·ri·ceps
ar·tery of fe·mur
mus·cle of thigh
re·flex
quad·ri·ceps·plas·ty
quad·ri·cus·pid
quad·ri·dig·i·tate
quad·ri·gem·i·nal
bod·ies
plate
pulse
rhythm
quad·ri·ge·mi·num
quad·ri·ge·mi·nus
quad·ri·ge·mi·ny
quad·ri·pa·re·sis
qua·dri·pe·dal ex·ten·sor
re·flex
quad·ri·ple·gia
quad·ri·ple·gic
quad·ri·po·lar
quad·ri·sect
quad·ri·sec·tion
quad·ri·tu·ber·cu·lar
quad·ri·va·lent
quad·ru·ped
quad·ru·ple
am·pu·ta·tion
rhythm
quad·rup·let
quail bron·chi·tis
vi·rus
qua·lim·e·ter
qual·i·ta·tive
al·ter·a·tion
anal·y·sis
trait
qual·i·ty
con·trol
qual·i·ty con·trol
chart
quan·ta
quan·tim·e·ter
quan·ti·ta·tive
al·ter·a·tion
anal·y·sis
ge·net·ics
hy·per·tro·phy
pe·rim·e·try

Quant's
sign
quan·tum
lim·it
the·o·ry
Quar·an·fil
vi·rus
quar·an·tine
quart
quar·tan
dou·ble q.
tri·ple q.
quar·tan
fe·ver
ma·lar·ia
par·a·site
quar·ter
evil
quar·ter-crack
quar·ti·sect
quartz
glass
qua·si·dom·i·nance
qua·si·dom·i·nant
quas·sa·tion
quas·sia
qua·ter·na·ry
syph·i·lis
qua·ter·na·ry am·mo·ni·um ion
qua·ter·na·ry car·bon
at·om
Quatrefages'
an·gle
qua·ze·pam
que·brach·ine
que·bra·cho
Queckenstedt-Stookey
test
queen
quel·lung
phe·nom·e·non
re·ac·tion
test
quench·ing
flu·o·res·cence q.
Quénu-Muret
sign
Quénu's hem·or·rhoi·dal
plex·us
quer·ce·tin
quer·cus
quer·u·lent
ques·tion·naire
Holmes-Rahe q.
quick
quick cure
res·in
quick·en·ing

quick·lime
Quick's
meth·od
test
quick·sil·ver
qui·es·cent
qui·et
iri·tis
lung
qui·et hip
dis·ease
quilt·ed
su·ture
qui·na
quin·a·crine chro·mo·some band·ing
stain
quin·a·crine hy·dro·chlo·ride
quin·al·dic ac·id
quin·al·dine red
quin·al·din·ic ac·id
qui·na·qui·na
qui·nate
q. de·hy·dro·gen·ase
quince
Quincke's
dis·ease
ede·ma
pulse
punc·ture
sign
quin·es·tra·di·ol
quin·es·tra·dol
quin·eth·a·zone
quin·ges·ta·nol ac·e·tate
quin·hy·drone
elec·trode
quin·ic ac·id
quin·i·dine
qui·nine
q. bi·sul·fate
q. car·ba·cryc·lic res·in
q. eth·yl·car·bon·ate
q. sul·fate
q. and urea hy·dro·chlo·ride
q. ure·than
qui·nine car·ba·cryl·ic res·in
qui·nine car·ba·cryl·ic res·in
test
qui·nin·ism
Quinlan's
test
quin·o·cide hy·dro·chlo·ride
quin·ol
quin·o·line
quin·o·lin·ic ac·id
qui·nol·o·gy

quin·o·lones
qui·none
   q. re·duc·tase
qui·no·vose
Quinquaud's
   dis·ease
quin·que·dig·i·tate
quin·que·tu·ber·cu·lar
quin·que·va·lent
quin·qui·na
quin·sy
   lin·gual q.
quin·tan
   fe·ver

quin·tu·plet
quit·tor
quo·tid·i·an
   fe·ver
   ma·lar·ia
quo·tient
   achieve·ment q.
   Ayala's q.
   blood q.
   cog·ni·tive lat·er·al·i·ty q.
   growth q.
   in·tel·li·gence q.
   res·pi·ra·to·ry q.
   spi·nal q.

R

R
  an·ti·gen
  en·zyme
  fac·tors
  pi·li
  plas·mids
  wave
R-
  band·ing
rab·bet·ing
rab·bit
  fe·ver
  fi·bro·ma
  plague
  snuf·fles
rab·bit fi·bro·ma
  vi·rus
rab·bit myx·o·ma
  vi·rus
rab·bit·pox
  vi·rus
rab·id
ra·bies
  dumb r.
  fu·ri·ous r.
  par·a·lyt·ic r.
ra·bies
  im·mu·no·glob·u·lin
  vac·cine
  vac·cine, Flury strain egg-
    pas·sage
  vi·rus
  vi·rus, Flury strain
  vi·rus, Kelev strain
ra·bies im·mune
  glob·u·lin (hu·man)
ra·bi·form
rac·coon
  eyes
race
ra·ce·fem·ine
rac·e·mase
rac·e·mate
ra·ceme
ra·ce·mic
  cal·ci·um pan·to·then·ate
rac·e·mi·za·tion
rac·e·mose
  an·eu·rysm

  gland
  he·man·gi·o·ma
rac·e·phed·rine hy·dro·chlo·ride
ra·chi·al
ra·chi·cen·te·sis
rach·i·des
ra·chid·i·al
ra·chid·i·an
ra·chi·graph
ra·chil·y·sis
ra·chi·o·camp·sis
ra·chi·o·cen·te·sis
ra·chi·och·y·sis
ra·chi·om·e·ter
ra·chi·op·a·gus
ra·chi·op·a·thy
ra·chi·o·ple·gia
ra·chi·o·sco·li·o·sis
ra·chi·o·tome
ra·chi·ot·o·my
ra·chip·a·gus
ra·chis
ra·chis·chi·sis
  r. par·ti·a·lis
  pos·te·ri·or r.
  r. pos·te·ri·or
  r. to·ta·lis
ra·chis·es
ra·chit·ic
  pel·vis
  ro·sa·ry
  sco·li·o·sis
ra·chi·tis
  r. fe·ta·lis
  r. fe·ta·lis an·nu·la·ris
  r. fe·ta·lis mi·cro·mel·i·ca
  r. in·tra·u·te·ri·na
  r. tar·da
  r. ute·ri·na
ra·chi·tism
rach·i·to·gen·ic
ra·chi·tome
ra·chit·o·my
ra·cial
  mel·a·no·der·ma
rack·et
  am·pu·ta·tion
  nail
ra·co·ma

rac·quet
  hy·pha
ra·dar·ky·mog·ra·phy
ra·dec·to·my
Radford
  nom·o·gram
ra·di·a·bil·i·ty
ra·di·a·ble
ra·di·ad
ra·di·al
  ac·cel·er·a·tion
  ar·tery
  bor·der
  bur·sa
  em·i·nence of wrist
  fos·sa
  head
  im·mu·no·dif·fu·sion
  ker·a·tot·o·my
  nerve
  notch
  phe·nom·e·non
  re·flex
  scar
  veins
ra·di·al apla·sia-throm·bo·cy·to·pe·nia
  syn·drome
ra·di·al col·lat·er·al
  ar·tery
  lig·a·ment
  lig·a·ment of wrist
ra·di·al flex·or
  mus·cle of wrist
ra·di·al growth
  phase
ra·di·al in·dex
  ar·tery
ra·di·a·lis
ra·di·al re·cur·rent
  ar·tery
ra·di·al scle·ros·ing
  le·sion
ra·di·al sty·loid
  ten·do·vag·i·ni·tis
ra·di·an
ra·di·ant
  en·er·gy
  heat
ra·di·ate
  crown
  lay·er of tym·pan·ic mem·brane
  lig·a·ment of rib
  lig·a·ment of wrist
ra·di·ate ster·no·cos·tal
  lig·a·ments

ra·di·a·tio
  r. py·ra·mi·da·lis
ra·di·a·tion
  acous·tic r.
  an·ni·hi·la·tion r.
  back·ground r.
  be·ta r.
  Cerenkov r.
  r. of cor·pus cal·lo·sum
  cor·pus·cu·lar r.
  elec·tro·mag·net·ic r.
  ge·nic·u·lo·cal·ca·rine r.
  Gratiolet's r.
  het·er·o·ge·neous r.
  ho·mo·ge·neous r.
  ion·iz·ing r.
  K-r.
  L-r.
  oc·cip·i·to·tha·lam·ic r.
  op·tic r.
  py·ram·i·dal r.
  scat·tered r.
  Wernicke's r.
ra·di·a·tion
  ane·mia
  bi·ol·o·gy
  burn
  car·ies
  cat·a·ract
  chem·is·try
  chi·me·ra
  der·ma·to·sis
  my·e·lop·a·thy
  sick·ness
  ther·a·py
ra·di·a·ti·o·nes
rad·i·cal
  ac·id r.
  col·or r.
  free r.
rad·i·cal
  cys·tec·to·my
  hys·ter·ec·to·my
  mas·tec·to·my
  mas·toid·ec·to·my
  op·er·a·tion for her·nia
ra·di·ces
ra·di·cis
rad·i·cle
rad·i·cot·o·my
ra·dic·u·la
ra·dic·u·lal·gia
ra·dic·u·lar
  ab·scess
  ar·ter·ies
  cyst
  pulp
  syn·drome

ra·dic·u·lec·to·my
ra·dic·u·li·tis
  acute brach·i·al r.
ra·dic·u·lo·gang·li·o·ni·tis
ra·dic·u·lo·me·nin·go·my·e·li·tis
ra·dic·u·lo·my·e·lop·a·thy
ra·dic·u·lo·neu·rop·a·thy
ra·dic·u·lop·a·thy
ra·di·ec·to·my
ra·dif·er·ous
ra·dii
ra·di·o·ac·tive
  at·om
  con·stant
  cy·a·no·co·bal·a·min
  equi·lib·ri·um
  io·dine
  iso·tope
  probe
  thy·rox·ine
ra·di·o·ac·tive cow
ra·di·o·ac·tive io·dide up·take
  test
ra·di·o·ac·tiv·i·ty
  ar·ti·fi·cial r.
  in·duced r.
ra·di·o·al·ler·go·sor·bent
  test
ra·di·o·an·a·phy·lax·is
ra·di·o·au·to·gram
ra·di·o·au·tog·ra·phy
ra·di·o·bi·cip·i·tal
  re·flex
ra·di·o·bi·ol·o·gy
ra·di·o·cal·ci·um
ra·di·o·car·bon
ra·di·o·car·di·o·gram
ra·di·o·car·di·og·ra·phy
ra·di·o·car·pal
  ar·tic·u·la·tion
  joint
ra·di·o·chem·i·cal
  pu·ri·ty
ra·di·o·chem·is·try
ra·di·o·chlo·rine
ra·di·o·cin·e·ma·tog·ra·phy
ra·di·o·co·balt
ra·di·o·cur·a·ble
ra·di·ode
ra·di·o·dense
ra·di·o·den·si·ty
ra·di·o·der·ma·ti·tis
ra·di·o·di·ag·no·sis
ra·di·o·dig·i·tal
ra·di·o·e·lec·tro·phys·i·ol·o·gram

ra·di·o·e·lec·tro·phys·i·ol·o·graph
ra·di·o·e·lec·tro·phys·i·o·log·ra·phy
ra·di·o·el·e·ment
ra·di·o·ep·i·der·mi·tis
ra·di·o·ep·i·the·li·tis
ra·di·o·fre·quen·cy
ra·di·o·gal·li·um
ra·di·o·gen·e·sis
ra·di·o·gen·ic
ra·di·o·gen·ics
ra·di·o·gold col·loid
ra·di·o·gram
ra·di·o·graph
  bite·wing r.
  oc·clu·sal r.
  per·i·ap·i·cal r.
ra·di·og·ra·phy
  elec·tron r.
  mag·ni·fi·ca·tion r.
ra·di·o·hu·mer·al
ra·di·o·im·mu·ni·ty
ra·di·o·im·mu·no·as·say
ra·di·o·im·mu·no·dif·fu·sion
ra·di·o·im·mu·no·elec·tro·pho·re·sis
ra·di·o·im·mu·no·pre·cip·i·ta·tion
ra·di·o·io·din·at·ed
ra·di·o·io·din·at·ed se·rum
  al·bu·min
ra·di·o·i·o·dine
ra·di·o·i·ron
ra·di·o·i·so·tope
ra·di·o·i·so·to·pic
  pu·ri·ty
ra·di·o·la·beled
ra·di·o·lead
ra·di·o·le·sion
ra·di·o·li·gand
ra·di·o·log·ic
ra·di·o·log·i·cal
  anat·o·my
  sphinc·ter
ra·di·ol·o·gist
ra·di·ol·o·gy
ra·di·o·lu·cen·cy
ra·di·o·lu·cent
ra·di·o·lus
ra·di·om·e·ter
  pas·til r.
ra·di·o·mi·crom·e·ter
ra·di·o·mi·met·ic
ra·di·o·mus·cu·lar
ra·di·o·ne·cro·sis
ra·di·o·neu·ri·tis
ra·di·o·ni·tro·gen

ra·di·o·nu·clide
  an·gi·og·ra·phy
  cis·tern·og·ra·phy
  gen·er·a·tor
ra·di·o·nu·clid·ic
  pu·ri·ty
ra·di·o·pac·i·ty
ra·di·o·pal·mar
ra·di·o·paque
ra·di·o·pa·thol·o·gy
ra·di·o·pel·vim·e·try
ra·di·o·per·i·os·te·al
  re·flex
ra·di·o·phar·ma·ceu·ti·cal
  pu·ri·ty
ra·di·o·phar·ma·ceu·ti·cals
ra·di·o·pho·bia
ra·di·o·phos·pho·rus
ra·di·o·phy·lax·is
ra·di·o·pill
ra·di·o·po·tas·si·um
ra·di·o·prax·is
ra·di·o·re·ac·tion
ra·di·o·re·cep·tor
  as·say
ra·di·o·re·sis·tant
ra·di·os·co·py
ra·di·o·sen·si·tive
ra·di·o·sen·si·tiv·i·ty
ra·di·o·so·di·um
ra·di·o·ster·e·os·co·py
ra·di·o·stron·ti·um
ra·di·o·sul·fur
ra·di·o·tel·e·me·ter·ing
  cap·sule
ra·di·o·te·lem·e·try
ra·di·o·ther·a·peu·tic
ra·di·o·ther·a·peu·tics
ra·di·o·ther·a·pist
ra·di·o·ther·a·py
  man·tle r.
ra·di·o·ther·my
ra·di·o·thy·roid·ec·to·my
ra·di·o·thy·rox·in
ra·di·o·tox·e·mia
ra·di·o·trans·par·ent
ra·di·o·trop·ic
ra·di·o·ul·nar
  disk
  syn·des·mo·sis
ra·di·o·ul·nar ar·tic·u·lar
  disk
ra·di·sec·to·my
ra·di·um
  em·a·na·tion
ra·di·um-226
ra·di·um beam
  ther·a·py

ra·di·us
  r. fix·us
ra·dix
  r. ar·cus ver·te·brae
  r. bre·vis gan·glii cil·i·ar·is
  r. lon·ga gan·glii cil·i·ar·is
  r. ner·vi fa·ci·a·lis
  ra·di·ces ner·vi tri·gem·i·ni
  r. pi·li
ra·don
Raeder's par·a·tri·gem·i·nal
  syn·drome
raf·fi·nose
rage
  sham r.
rag-sort·er's
  dis·ease
Rahe
Rahn-Otis
  sam·ple
RAI
  test
Rail·li·e·ti·na
rail·li·e·ti·ni·a·sis
rail·road
  nys·tag·mus
rain·bow
  symp·tom
Rainey's
  cor·pus·cles
Raji
  cell
Raji cell ra·di·o·im·mune
  as·say
rale
  am·phor·ic r.
  at·e·lec·tat·ic r.
  bub·bling r.
  cav·ern·ous r.
  click·ing r.
  con·so·nat·ing r.
  crep·i·tant r.
  dry r.
  gur·gling r.
  gut·tur·al r.
  me·tal·lic r.
  moist r.
  mu·cous r.
  pal·pa·ble r.
  sib·i·lant r.
  Skoda's r.
  so·no·rous r.
  sub·crep·i·tant r.
  ve·sic·u·lar r.
  whis·tling r.
ra·mal

Raman
   ef·fect
   spec·trum
Rambourg's chro·mic ac·id-phos·pho·tung·stic ac·id
   stain
Rambourg's pe·ri·od·ic ac·id-chro·mic meth·en·a·mine-sil·ver
   stain
Rambourg's stains
ra·mex
ra·mi
Ra·mi·bac·te·ri·um
   R. ra·mo·sum
ram·i·cot·o·my
ram·i·fi·ca·tion
ram·i·fy
ram·i·sec·tion
ram·i·tis
ra·mose
ra·mous
ramp
Ramsay Hunt's
   syn·drome
Ramsden's
   oc·u·lar
Ramstedt
   op·er·a·tion
ram·u·li
ram·u·lus
ra·mus
   r. anas·to·mo·ti·cus
   r. an·te·ri·or la·te·ra·lis
   r. car·di·a·cus
   ra·mi ca·rot·i·co·tym·pa·ni·ci
   r. com·mu·ni·cans fib·u·la·ris
   ra·mi ep·i·plo·i·ci
   ra·mi in·ter·ven·tri·cu·la·res sep·ta·les
   is·chi·o·pu·bic r.
   r. pro·fun·dus ar·te·ri·ae trans·ver·sae col·li
   r. pro·fun·dus ar·te·ria sca·pu·la·ris de·scen·dens
   pu·bic ra·mi
   r. pu·bi·cus ar·te·ri·ae ep·i·gas·tri·cae in·fe·ri·o·ris
   ra·mi sep·ta·les
ra·my·cin
ran·cid
ran·cid·i·fy
ran·cid·i·ty
Randall stone
   for·ceps

ran·dom
   mat·ing
   sam·ple
   waves
ran·dom mat·ing
   equi·lib·ri·um
ran·dom pat·tern
   flap
Raney
   al·loy
   cat·a·lyst
Raney Nick·el
range
range of
   ac·com·mo·da·tion
   con·ver·gence
Ranikhet
   dis·ease
ra·nine
   ar·tery
   tu·mor
ra·ni·ti·dine
rank-dif·fer·ence
   cor·re·la·tion
Ranke's
   an·gle
   for·mu·la
Rankine
   scale
Rankin's
   clamp
Ransohoff's
   sign
ran·u·la
   r. pan·cre·a·ti·ca
ran·u·lar
Ranvier's
   cross·es
   disks
   node
   plex·us
   seg·ment
Raoult's
   law
rape
rape·seed oil
ra·pha·nia
ra·phe
   am·ni·ot·ic r.
   r. ano·coc·cy·gea
   ano·gen·i·tal r.
   r. cor·po·ris cal·losi
   lat·er·al pal·pe·bral r.
   r. lin·guae
   me·di·an lon·gi·tu·di·nal r. of tongue
   r. nu·clei
   pal·a·tine r.

ra·phe *(continued)*
  pal·pe·bral r.
  pe·nile r.
  per·i·ne·al r.
  pter·y·go·man·dib·u·lar r.
  r. ret·i·nae
  scro·tal r.
  Stilling's r.
ra·phe
  nu·clei
rap·id
  ca·ni·ti·es
  de·com·pres·sion
rap·id bi·plane
  an·gi·o·car·di·og·ra·phy
rap·id eye
  move·ments
rap·id eye move·ment
  sleep
rap·id·ly pro·gress·ive
  glo·mer·u·lo·ne·phri·tis
rap·id plas·ma re·a·gin
  test
Rapoport
  test
Rapoport-Luebering
  shunt
Rappaport
  clas·si·fi·ca·tion
rap·port
rap·ture of the deep
rare
  earths
rare earth
  el·e·ments
  met·al
rar·e·fac·tion
rar·e·fy
ra·sce·ta
rash
  am·mo·nia r.
  an·ti·tox·in r.
  as·ta·coid r.
  black cur·rant r.
  but·ter·fly r.
  cat·er·pil·lar r.
  crys·tal r.
  di·a·per r.
  drug r.
  heat r.
  hy·da·tid r.
  Murray Val·ley r.
  nap·kin r.
  net·tle r.
  se·rum r.
  sum·mer r.
  wild·fire r.
ra·sion

Rasmussen's
  an·eu·rysm
ras·pa·to·ry
rasp·ber·ry
  tongue
Rastelli
  pro·ce·dure
rat
  lep·ro·sy
rat
  al·bi·no r.'s
  Wistar r.'s
rat-bite
  fe·ver
rate
  con·stants
  me·ter
rate
  abor·tion r.
  at·tack r.
  ba·sal met·a·bol·ic r.
  base·line fe·tal heart r.
  birth r.
  case fa·tal·i·ty r.
  con·cor·dance r.
  crit·i·cal r.
  death r.
  eryth·ro·cyte sed·i·men·ta·tion r.
  fa·tal·i·ty r.
  fe·tal death r.
  fe·tal heart r.
  glo·mer·u·lar fil·tra·tion r.
  growth r.
  heart r.
  in·fant mor·tal·i·ty r.
  le·thal·i·ty r.
  ma·ter·nal death r.
  mi·tot·ic r.
  mor·bid·i·ty r.
  mor·tal·i·ty r.
  mu·ta·tion r.
  ne·o·na·tal mor·tal·i·ty r.
  per·i·na·tal mor·tal·i·ty r.
  pulse r.
  rep·e·ti·tion r.
  res·pi·ra·tion r.
  sed·i·men·ta·tion r.
  shear r.
  slew r.
  ste·roid met·a·bol·ic clear·ance r.
  ste·roid pro·duc·tion r.
  ste·roid se·cre·to·ry r.
  still·birth r.
  void·ing flow r.
rat-fish

Rathke's
bun·dles
di·ver·tic·u·lum
pock·et
pouch
Rathke's cleft
cyst
Rathke's pouch
tu·mor
ra·ti·o
scale
ra·ti·o
ab·so·lute ter·mi·nal in·ner·va·tion r.
ac·com·mo·da·tive con·ver·gence-ac·com·mo·da·tion r.
al·bu·min-glob·u·lin r.
ALT:AST r.
am·y·lase-cre·at·i·nine clear·ance r.
bod·y-weight r.
car·di·o·tho·rac·ic r.
r. of de·cayed and filled sur·fac·es
r. of de·cayed and filled teeth
ex·trac·tion r.
flux r.
func·tion·al ter·mi·nal in·ner·va·tion r.
hand r.
IRI/G r.
ke·to·gen·ic-an·ti·ke·to·gen·ic r.
lec·i·thin/sphin·go·my·e·lin r.
M:E r.
men·de·li·an r.
mo·lec·u·lar weight r.
nu·cle·ar-cy·to·plas·mic r.
nu·tri·tive r.
P/O r.
res·pi·ra·to·ry ex·change r.
seg·re·ga·tion r.
sex r.
ther·a·peu·tic r.
ven·ti·la·tion/per·fu·sion r.
ze·ta sed·i·men·ta·tion r.
ra·tion·al
for·mu·la
ther·a·py
ra·tion·al·i·za·tion
rat mite
der·ma·ti·tis
rats·bane
rat·tle·snake
Rat·tus

Rauber's
lay·er
Rau's
pro·cess
Rauscher's
vi·rus
Rau·wol·fia
Ravius
Ravius'
pro·cess
raw
score
ray
fun·gus
ther·a·peu·tics
ray
ac·tin·ic r.
al·pha r.
an·ode r.'s
Becquerel r.'s
be·ta r.
bor·der·line r.'s
Bucky's r.'s
cath·ode r.'s
chem·i·cal r.
cos·mic r.'s
di·rect r.'s
Dorno r.'s
dy·nam·ic r.'s
gam·ma r.'s
glass r.'s
grenz r.
H r.'s
hard r.'s
in·ci·dent r.
in·di·rect r.'s
in·fra·red r.
in·ter·me·di·ate r.'s
mar·gi·nal r.'s
med·ul·lary r.
mon·o·chro·mat·ic r.'s
Niewenglowski r.'s
par·al·lel r.'s
par·ax·i·al r.'s
pos·i·tive r.'s
pri·mary r.'s
re·flect·ed r.
roent·gen r.
sec·on·dary r.'s
soft r.'s
su·per·son·ic r.'s
tran·si·tion r.'s
ul·tra·son·ic r.'s
ul·tra·vi·o·let r.'s
W r.'s
x-r.
ray·age

Rayer's
dis·ease
Rayleigh
equa·tion
test
Raymond type of
ap·o·plexy
Raynaud's
dis·ease
phe·nom·e·non
syn·drome
R-band·ing
stain
re·act
re·ac·tance
re·ac·tant
acute phase r.'s
re·ac·tion
ac·cel·er·at·ed r.
ac·id r.
acute sit·u·a·tion·al r.
ad·verse r.
alarm r.
al·de·hyde r.
al·ka·line r.
al·ler·gic r.
am·pho·ter·ic r.
an·am·nes·tic r.
an·ti·gen-an·ti·body r.
anx·i·e·ty r.
Arias-Stella r.
arous·al r.
Arthus r.
Ascoli r.
as·so·ci·a·tive r.
Bence Jones r.
Berthelot r.
bi-bi r.
Bittorf's r.
bi·u·ret r.
Bloch's r.
Brunn r.
Burchard-Liebermann r.
Cannizzaro's r.
Carr-Price r.
cat·a·lat·ic r.
cat·a·stroph·ic r.
cell-me·di·at·ed r.
chain r.
Chantemesse r.
chol·era-red r.
chro·maf·fin r.
cir·cu·lar r.
co·carde r.
cock·ade r.
com·ple·ment-fix·a·tion r.
con·sen·su·al r.
con·sti·tu·tion·al r.

con·ver·sion r.
cross r.
cu·ta·ne·ous r.
cy·to·tox·ic r.
Dale r.
dark r.
de·cid·u·al r.
r. of de·gen·er·a·tion
de·layed r.
de·pot r.
der·mo·tu·ber·cu·lin r.
di·a·zo r.
dig·i·to·nin r.
Dische r.
dis·so·ci·a·tive r.
do·pa r.
dys·ton·ic r.
ear·ly r.
Ebbecke's r.
echo r.
Ehrlich r.
Ehrlich's benz·al·de·hyde r.
Ehrlich's di·a·zo r.
eo·sin·o·pe·nic r.
eryth·ro·phore r.
false-neg·a·tive r.
false-pos·i·tive r.
Fernandez r.
fer·ric chlo·ride r. of ep·i·
    neph·rine
Feulgen r.
first-or·der r.
fix·a·tion r.
floc·cu·la·tion r.
fo·cal r.
Folin's r.
Forssman r.
Forssman an·ti·gen-an·ti·
    body r.
Frei-Hoffman r.
fright r.
fuch·sin·o·phil r.
fur·fu·rol r.
gal·van·ic skin r.
gel dif·fu·sion r.'s
Gell and Coombs r.'s
ge·mis·to·cyt·ic r.
gen·er·al ad·ap·ta·tion r.
Gerhardt's r.
graft ver·sus host r.
group r.
Gruber's r.
Gruber-Widal r.
Günning's r.
har·le·quin r.
heel-tap r.
he·mo·clas·tic r.
Henle's r.

Herxheimer's r.
Hill r.
hunt·ing r.
hy·per·sen·si·tiv·i·ty r.
id r.
r. of iden·ti·ty
im·me·di·ate r.
im·mune r.
in·com·pat·i·ble blood
  trans·fu·sion r.
in·di·rect pu·pil·lary r.
in·tra·cu·ta·ne·ous r.
in·tra·der·mal r.
io·date r. of ep·i·neph·rine
io·dine r. of ep·i·neph·rine
ir·re·vers·i·ble r.
Jaffe r.
Jarisch-Herxheimer r.
Jolly's r.
late r.
length·en·ing r.
lep·ro·min r.
leu·ke·moid r.
lid clo·sure r.
lo·cal r.
lo·cal an·es·thet·ic r.
Loewenthal's r.
mag·net r.
Marchi's r.
Mazzotti r.
Millon r.
mi·o·stag·min r.
Mitsuda r.
mixed ag·glu·ti·na·tion r.
mixed lym·pho·cyte cul·ture
  r.
mon·o·mo·lec·u·lar r.
my·as·then·ic r.
Nadi r.
near r.
neg·a·tive sup·port·ing r.'s
Neufeld r.
neu·ro·ton·ic r.
neu·tral r.
nin·hy·drin r.
ni·tri·toid r.
r. of non·i·den·ti·ty
nu·cle·ar r.
ox·i·dase r.
ox·i·da·tion-re·duc·tion r.
pain r.
Pandy's r.
r. of par·tial iden·ti·ty
pas·sive cu·ta·ne·ous an·a·
  phy·lac·tic r.
Paul's r.
per·for·mic ac·id r.
per·ox·i·dase r.

phos·phor·o·clas·tic r.
Pirquet's r.
plas·mal r.
Porter-Silber r.
pos·i·tive sup·port·ing r.'s
Prausnitz-Küstner r.
pre·cip·i·tin r.
pri·mary r.
pro·zone r.
psy·cho·gal·van·ic r.
psy·cho·gal·van·ic skin r.
quel·lung r.
re·versed Prausnitz-Küstner
  r.
re·vers·i·ble r.
Sakaguchi r.
Schardinger r.
Schultz r.
Schultz-Charlton r.
Schultz-Dale r.
se·rum r.
short·en·ing r.
Shwartzman r.
skin r.
spe·cif·ic r.
star·tle r.
Straus r.
stress r.
sup·port·ing r.'s
symp·to·mat·ic r.
ther·mo·pre·cip·i·tin r.
Trep·o·ne·ma pal·li·dum
  im·mo·bi·li·za·tion r.
tri·ke·to·hy·drin·dene r.
uni·mo·lec·u·lar r.
vac·ci·noid r.
Voges-Proskauer r.
Wassermann r.
Weidel's r.
Weil-Felix r.
Weinberg's r.
Wernicke's r.
wheal-and-er·y·the·ma r.
wheal-and-flare r.
Widal's r.
Yorke's au·to·lyt·ic r.
ze·ro-or·der r.
Zimmermann r.
re·ac·tion
  cen·ter
  for·ma·tion
  time
re·ac·ti·vate
re·ac·ti·va·tion
re·ac·tive
  as·tro·cyte
  cell
  de·pres·sion

re·ac·tive *(continued)*
  hy·per·e·mia
  schiz·o·phre·nia
re·ac·tive per·fo·rat·ing
  col·lag·e·no·sis
re·ac·tiv·i·ty
read·ing
  frame
read·ing-frame-shift
  mu·ta·tion
read·through
re·a·gent
  Benedict-Hopkins-Cole r.
  bi·u·ret r.
  Cleland's r.
  di·a·zo r.
  Edlefsen's r.
  Edman's r.
  Ehrlich's di·a·zo r.
  Erdmann's r.
  Esbach's r.
  Exton r.
  Fehling's r.
  Fouchet's r.
  Froehde's r.
  Frohn's r.
  Girard's r.
  Günzberg's r.
  Hahn's ox·ine r.
  Hammarsten's r.
  Ilosvay r.
  Kasten's flu·o·res·cent Schiff
   r.'s
  Lloyd's r.
  Mandelin's r.
  Marme's r.
  Marquis' r.
  Mecke's r.
  Meyer's r.
  Millon's r.
  Nessler's r.
  Rosenthaler-Turk r.
  Sanger's r.
  Schaer's r.
  Scheibler's r.
  Schiff's r.
  Scott-Wilson r.
  Sulkowitch's r.
  Uffelmann's r.
  Wurster's r.
re·a·gin
  atop·ic r.
re·a·gin·ic
  an·ti·body
real
  fo·cus
  im·age

re·al·i·ty
  ad·ap·ta·tion
  prin·ci·ple
re·al·i·ty aware·ness
re·al·i·ty test·ing
real or·i·gin
real-time
  ul·tra·sound
ream·er
  en·gine r.
  in·tra·med·ul·lary r.
reap·er's
  oph·thal·mia
re·at·tach·ment
Réaumur
  scale
re·base
re·bound
  phe·nom·e·non
  ten·der·ness
re·breath·ing
  an·es·the·sia
  tech·nique
Rebuck skin win·dow
  tech·nique
re·cal·ci·fi·ca·tion
re·call
Récamier's
  op·er·a·tion
re·ca·nal·i·za·tion
re·ca·pi·tu·la·tion
  the·o·ry
re·ceiv·er
re·cep·tac·u·la
re·cep·tac·u·lum
  r. chy·li
  r. gan·glii pe·tro·si
  r. pec·que·ti
re·cep·tive
  apha·sia
re·cep·to·ma
re·cep·tor
  ad·re·ner·gic r.'s
  cho·lin·er·gic r.'s
  Fc r.
  opi·ate r.'s
  sen·so·ry r.'s
  stretch r.'s
re·cep·tor
  pro·tein
  site
re·cess
  an·te·ri·or r. of tym·pan·ic
   mem·brane
  ce·cal r.
  cer·e·bel·lo·pon·tine r.
  co·chle·ar r.
  cos·to·di·a·phrag·mat·ic r.

cos·to·me·di·as·ti·nal r.
du·o·de·no·je·ju·nal r.
el·lip·ti·cal r.
ep·i·tym·pan·ic r.
he·pa·to·en·ter·ic r.
he·pa·to·re·nal r.
Hyrtl's ep·i·tym·pan·ic r.
in·fe·ri·or du·o·de·nal r.
in·fe·ri·or il·e·o·ce·cal r.
in·fe·ri·or omen·tal r.
in·fun·dib·u·lar r.
in·ter·sig·moid r.
Jacquemet's r.
lat·er·al r. of fourth ven·tri·cle
mes·en·ter·i·co·pa·ri·e·tal r.
op·tic r.
pan·cre·at·i·co·en·ter·ic r.
par·a·col·ic r.'s
par·a·du·o·de·nal r.
pa·rot·id r.
pha·ryn·ge·al r.
phren·i·co·me·di·as·ti·nal r.
pin·e·al r.
pir·i·form r.
pleu·ral r.'s
pneu·ma·to·en·ter·ic r.
pneu·mo·en·ter·ic r.
pon·to·cer·e·bel·lar r.
pos·te·ri·or r. of tym·pan·ic mem·brane
Reichert's co·chle·ar r.
ret·ro·ce·cal r.
ret·ro·du·o·de·nal r.
Rosenmüller's r.
sac·ci·form r.
sphe·no·eth·moi·dal r.
spher·i·cal r.
splen·ic r.
sub·he·pat·ic r.
sub·phren·ic r.'s
sub·pop·lit·e·al r.
su·pe·ri·or du·o·de·nal r.
su·pe·ri·or il·e·o·ce·cal r.
su·pe·ri·or r. of less·er per·i·to·ne·al sac
su·pe·ri·or omen·tal r.
su·pe·ri·or r. of tym·pan·ic mem·brane
su·pra·pin·e·al r.
su·pra·ton·sil·lar r.
tri·an·gu·lar r.
Tröltsch's r.'s
tu·bo·tym·pan·ic r.
re·ces·sion
gin·gi·val r.
ten·don r.
re·ces·si·tiv·i·ty

re·ces·sive
char·ac·ter
gene
in·her·i·tance
trait
re·ces·sus
re·ces·sus
r. an·te·ri·or
r. in·fun·di·bu·li·for·mis
r. pa·ro·ti·de·us
r. pos·te·ri·or
r. sac·ci·for·mis
r. tri·an·gu·la·ris
re·cid·i·va·tion
re·cid·i·vism
re·cid·i·vist
rec·i·pe
re·cip·i·o·mo·tor
re·cip·ro·cal
an·chor·age
arm
beat
bi·gem·i·ny
forc·es
in·hi·bi·tion
in·ner·va·tion
rhythm
trans·fu·sion
trans·lo·ca·tion
re·cip·ro·cat·ing
rhythm
re·cip·ro·ca·tion
rec·i·proc·i·ty
law
Recklinghausen's
dis·ease
dis·ease of bone
tu·mor
rec·li·na·tion
re·clot·ting
phe·nom·e·non
rec·og·ni·tion
fac·tors
time
re·coil
at·om
wave
rec·ol·lec·tion
re·com·bi·nant
DNA
strain
re·com·bi·na·tion
frac·tion
re·com·bi·na·tion
ge·net·ic r.
re·con
re·con·sti·tu·tion

re·con·struc·tive
  mam·ma·plas·ty
  psy·cho·ther·a·py
  sur·gery
rec·ord
  base
  rim
rec·ord
  an·es·the·sia r.
  cen·tric in·ter·oc·clu·sal r.
  ec·cen·tric in·ter·oc·clu·sal r.
  face-bow r.
  func·tion·al chew-in r.
  hos·pi·tal r.
  in·ter·oc·clu·sal r.
  lat·er·al in·ter·oc·clu·sal r.
  max·il·lo·man·dib·u·lar r.
  med·i·cal r.
  oc·clud·ing cen·tric re·la·tion r.
  pre·ex·trac·tion r.
  pre·op·er·a·tive r.
  prob·lem-o·ri·ent·ed r.
  pro·file r.
  pro·tru·sive r.
  pro·tru·sive in·ter·oc·clu·sal r.
  ter·mi·nal jaw re·la·tion r.
  three-di·men·sion·al r.
re·cord·ing
  clin·i·cal r.
  depth r.
re·cov·ery
  creep r.
  spon·ta·ne·ous r.
  ul·tra·son·ic egg r.
re·cov·ery
  score
re·cov·ery room
rec·re·a·tion·al
  drug
re·cru·des·cence
re·cru·des·cent
  ty·phus
re·cru·des·cent ty·phus
  fe·ver
re·cruit·ing
  re·sponse
re·cruit·ment
rec·ta
rec·tal
  al·i·men·ta·tion
  an·es·the·sia
  col·umns
  folds
  plex·us·es
  re·flex

  shelf
  si·nus·es
  valves
  val·vot·o·my
rec·tal·gia
rec·tal ve·nous
  plex·us
rect·an·gu·lar
  am·pu·ta·tion
rec·tec·to·my
rec·ti·fied
  spir·it
  tar oil
  tur·pen·tine oil
rec·ti·fy
rec·ti·tis
rec·to·ab·dom·i·nal
rec·to·car·di·ac
  re·flex
rec·to·cele
rec·toc·ly·sis
rec·to·coc·cyg·e·al
  mus·cle
rec·to·coc·cy·pexy
rec·to·co·li·tis
rec·to·la·bi·al
  fis·tu·la
rec·to·la·ryn·ge·al
  re·flex
rec·to·per·i·ne·al
rec·to·per·i·ne·or·rha·phy
rec·to·pexy
rec·to·pho·bia
rec·to·plas·ty
rec·tor·rha·phy
rec·to·scope
rec·tos·co·py
rec·to·sig·moid
  sphinc·ter
rec·to·ste·no·sis
rec·tos·to·my
rec·to·tome
rec·tot·o·my
rec·to·u·re·thral
  fis·tu·la
  mus·cle
rec·to·u·ter·ine
  fold
  pouch
rec·to·vag·i·nal
  fis·tu·la
  fold
  sep·tum
rec·to·vag·i·no·u·ter·ine
  pouch
rec·to·ves·i·cal
  fas·cia
  fis·tu·la

fold
mus·cle
pouch
sep·tum
rec·to·ves·tib·u·lar
fis·tu·la
rec·to·vul·var
fis·tu·la
rec·tum
rec·tus
mus·cle of ab·do·men
mus·cle of thigh
re·cum·bent
re·cu·per·ate
re·cu·per·a·tion
re·cur·rence
risk
re·cur·rent
al·bu·min·ur·ia
ar·tery
car·ies
en·ceph·a·lop·a·thy
fe·ver
hy·po·py·on
nerve
stric·ture
re·cur·rent aph·thous
sto·ma·ti·tis
ul·cers
re·cur·rent cen·tral
ret·i·ni·tis
re·cur·rent cor·ne·al
ero·sion
re·cur·rent her·pet·ic
sto·ma·ti·tis
re·cur·rent in·ter·os·se·ous
ar·tery
re·cur·rent la·ryn·ge·al
nerve
re·cur·rent me·nin·ge·al
nerve
re·cur·rent scar·ring
aph·thae
re·cur·rent ul·cer·a·tive
sto·ma·ti·tis
re·cur·rent ul·nar
ar·tery
re·cur·ring dig·i·tal
fi·bro·mas of child·hood
re·cur·va·tion
red
at·ro·phy
cor·pus·cle
de·gen·er·a·tion
fe·ver
fe·ver of the Con·go
fi·bers
gum

half-moon
hep·a·ti·za·tion
in·du·ra·tion
in·farct
lead
mange
mus·cle
neu·ral·gia
nu·cle·us
phos·pho·rus
pre·cip·i·tate
pulp
re·flex
sweat
test
throm·bus
vi·sion
wine
red blood
cell
red bone
mar·row
red cell ad·her·ence
phe·nom·e·non
test
re·dia
re·di·ae
re·dif·fer·en·ti·a·tion
re·din·te·gra·tion
re·dox
elec·trode
in·di·ca·tor
po·ten·tial
sys·tem
red ox·ide of
lead
red pulp
cords
re·dresse·ment for·cé
re·dress·ment
re·duce
re·duced
eye
hem·a·tin
he·mo·glo·bin
re·duced enam·el
ep·i·the·li·um
re·duced glu·ta·thi·one
re·duced in·ter·arch
dis·tance
re·duc·i·ble
her·nia
re·duc·ing
di·et
en·zyme
sug·ar
valve
re·duc·tant

re·duc·tase
re·duc·tic ac·id
re·duc·tion
    r. of chro·mo·somes
    closed r. of frac·tures
    r. en mas·se
    open r. of frac·tures
    tu·ber·os·i·ty r.
re·duc·tion
    de·for·mi·ty
    di·vi·sion
    mam·ma·plas·ty
    nu·cle·us
    phase
re·du·pli·cat·ed
    cat·a·ract
re·du·pli·ca·tion
re·du·vi·id
Red·u·vi·i·dae
red·wa·ter
    fe·ver
Reed
    cells
reed in·stru·ment
    the·o·ry
Reed-Sternberg
    cells
reedy
    nail
reef·ing
    stom·ach r.
reel
    foot
re·en·act·ment
re·en·try
    phe·nom·e·non
    the·o·ry
Rees-Ecker
    flu·id
re·fec·tion
ref·er·ence
    elec·trode
    meth·od
    val·ues
re·ferred
    pain
    sen·sa·tion
Refetoff
    syn·drome
re·fine
re·flect
re·flect·ed
    col·ors
    light
    ray
re·flect·ing
    ret·i·no·scope

re·flec·tion
    co·ef·fi·cient
re·flec·tor
re·flex
    ab·dom·i·nal r.'s
    ab·dom·i·no·car·di·ac r.
    Abrams' heart r.
    ac·com·mo·da·tion r.
    Achil·les r.
    Achil·les ten·don r.
    acous·ti·co·pal·pe·bral r.
    ac·quired r.
    acro·mi·al r.
    ad·duc·tor r.
    al·lied r.'s
    anal r.
    an·kle r.
    an·tag·o·nis·tic r.'s
    aor·tic r.
    ap·o·neu·rot·ic r.
    Aschner-Dagnini r.
    Aschner's r.
    at·ti·tu·di·nal r.'s
    au·di·to·ry r.
    au·di·to·ry oc·u·lo·gy·ric r.
    au·ric·u·lar r.
    au·ric·u·lo·pal·pe·bral r.
    au·ric·u·lo·pres·sor r.
    au·ro·pal·pe·bral r.
    ax·on r.
    Babinski r.
    back of foot r.
    Bainbridge r.
    Barkman's r.
    ba·sal joint r.
    Bechterew-Mendel r.
    be·hav·ior r.
    Benedek's r.
    Bezold-Jarisch r.
    bi·ceps r.
    bi·ceps fe·mo·ris r.
    Bing's r.
    blad·der r.
    body right·ing r.'s
    bone r.
    bra·chi·o·ra·di·al r.
    Brain's r.
    breg·mo·car·di·ac r.
    Brissaud's r.
    bul·bo·cav·er·no·sus r.
    bul·bo·mim·ic r.
    Capps' r.
    car·di·ac de·pres·sor r.
    ca·rot·id si·nus r.
    ce·li·ac plex·us r.
    ce·phal·ic r.'s
    ceph·a·lo·pal·pe·bral r.
    cer·e·bro·pu·pil·lary r.

Chaddock r.
chain r.
chin r.
Chodzko's r.
cil·i·o·spi·nal r.
clasp·ing r.
co·chle·o-or·bic·u·lar r.
co·chle·o·pal·pe·bral r.
co·chle·o·pu·pil·lary r.
co·chle·o·sta·pe·di·al r.
con·di·tioned r.
con·junc·ti·val r.
con·sen·su·al light r.
con·tra·lat·er·al r.
con·vul·sive r.
co·or·di·nat·ed r.
cor·ne·al r.
cor·ti·co·pu·pil·lary r.
cos·tal arch r.
cos·to·pec·to·ral r.
cough r.
cra·ni·o·car·di·ac r.
crem·as·ter·ic r.
crossed r.
crossed ad·duc·tor r.
crossed ex·ten·sion r.
crossed knee r.
crossed r. of pel·vis
crossed spi·no-ad·duc·tor r.
cry r.
cu·boi·do·dig·i·tal r.
cu·ta·ne·ous r.
cu·ta·ne·ous pu·pil r.
cu·ta·ne·ous-pu·pil·lary r.
dar·win·i·an r.
deep r.
deep ab·dom·i·nal r.'s
de·fense r.
de·glu·ti·tion r.
Dejerine's r.
de·layed r.
de·pres·sor r.
dif·fused r.
dig·i·tal r.
div·ing r.
dor·sal r.
dor·sam of foot r.
dor·sum pe·dis r.
el·bow r.
en·ter·o·gas·tric r.
ep·i·gas·tric r.
erec·tor-spi·nal r.
esoph·a·go·sal·i·vary r.
ex·ter·nal ob·lique r.
eye r.
eye-clo·sure r.
fa·cial r.
fau·cial r.

fem·o·ral r.
fem·o·ro·ab·dom·i·nal r.
fin·ger-thumb r.
flex·or r.
forced grasp·ing r.
front-tap r.
fun·dus r.
gag r.
Galant's r.
gal·van·ic skin r.
gas·tro·co·lic r.
gas·tro·il·e·ac r.
Gei·gel's r.
Gifford's r.
glu·te·al r.
Gordon r.
grasp r.
grasp·ing r.
great-toe r.
Guillain-Barré r.
gus·ta·to·ry-su·do·rif·ic r.
H r.
Haab's r.
heart r.
he·pa·to·jug·u·lar r.
Hering-Breuer r.
Hoffmann's r.
hy·po·chon·dri·al r.
hy·po·gas·tric r.
in·nate r.
in·ter·scap·u·lar r.
in·trin·sic r.
in·vert·ed r.
in·vert·ed ra·di·al r.
in·ves·ti·ga·to·ry r.
ip·si·lat·er·al r.
Jacobson's r.
jaw r.
jaw-work·ing r.
Joffroy's r.
Kisch's r.
knee r.
knee-jerk r.
lab·y·rin·thine r.'s
lab·y·rin·thine right·ing r.'s
lac·ri·mal r.
lac·ri·mo-gus·ta·to·ry r.
la·ryn·ge·al r.
la·ryn·go·spas·tic r.
la·tent r.
laugh·ter r.
lid r.
Liddell-Sherrington r.
light r.
lip r.
lor·do·sis r.
Lovén r.

re·flex *(continued)*

low·er ab·dom·i·nal per·i·os·te·al r.
mag·net r.
man·dib·u·lar r.
mass r.
mas·se·ter r.
Mayer's r.
McCarthy's r.'s
me·di·o·pu·bic r.
Mendel-Bechterew r.
Mendel's in·step r.
met·a·car·po·hy·po·the·nar r.
met·a·car·po·the·nar r.
met·a·tar·sal r.
mic·tu·ri·tion r.
milk-e·jec·tion r.
Mondonesi's r.
Moro r.
mus·cu·lar r.
my·en·ter·ic r.
my·o·tat·ic r.
na·sal r.
na·so·men·tal r.
near r.
neck r.'s
no·ci·cep·tive r.
no·ci·fen·sor r.
nose-bridge-lid r.
nose-eye r.
oc·u·lo·car·di·ac r.
oc·u·lo·ce·phal·ic r.
oc·u·lo·ceph·a·lo·gy·ric r.
olec·ra·non r.
Oppenheim's r.
op·ti·cal right·ing r.'s
op·ti·co·fa·cial r.
or·bi·cu·la·ris oc·u·li r.
or·bi·cu·la·ris pu·pil·lary r.
or·i·ent·ing r.
pal·a·tal r.
pal·a·tine r.
pal·mar r.
palm-chin r.
pal·mo·men·tal r.
par·a·chute r.
par·a·dox·i·cal r.
par·a·dox·i·cal ex·ten·sor r.
par·a·dox·i·cal flex·or r.
par·a·dox·i·cal pa·tel·lar r.
par·a·dox·i·cal pu·pil·lary r.
par·a·dox·i·cal tri·ceps r.
pa·tel·lar r.
pa·tel·lar ten·don r.
pa·tel·lo-ad·duc·tor r.
Pavlov's r.
pec·to·ral r.

Perez r.
per·i·car·di·al r.
per·i·os·te·al r.
pha·ryn·ge·al r.
pha·sic r.
Phillipson's r.
pi·lo·mo·tor r.
plan·tar r.
plan·tar mus·cle r.
pne·o·car·di·ac r.
pne·o·pne·ic r.
pos·tur·al r.
pres·so·re·cep·tor r.
pro·na·tor r.
pro·pri·o·cep·tive r.'s
pro·pri·o·cep·tive-oc·u·lo·ceph·al·ic r.
pro·tec·tive la·ryn·ge·al r.
psy·cho·car·di·ac r.
psy·cho·gal·van·ic r.
psy·cho·gal·van·ic skin r.
pul·mo·no·cor·o·nary r.
pu·pil·lary r.
pu·pil·lary-skin r.
quad·ri·ceps r.
qua·dri·pe·dal ex·ten·sor r.
ra·di·al r.
ra·di·o·bi·cip·i·tal r.
ra·di·o·per·i·os·te·al r.
rec·tal r.
rec·to·car·di·ac r.
rec·to·la·ryn·ge·al r.
red r.
Remak's r.
re·nal r.
right·ing r.'s
Roger's r.
root·ing r.
Rossolimo's r.
scap·u·lar r.
scap·u·lo·hu·mer·al r.
scap·u·lo·per·i·os·te·al r.
Schäffer's r.
scratch r. in dogs
sem·i·mem·bra·no·sus r.
sem·i·ten·di·no·sus r.
shot-silk r.
si·nus r.
skin r.'s
skin-mus·cle r.'s
skin-pu·pil·lary r.
snap·ping r.
snout r.
sole r.
sole tap r.
spi·nal r.
spi·no-ad·duc·tor r.
Starling's r.

star·tle r.
stat·ic r.
stat·o·ki·net·ic r.
stat·o·ton·ic r.'s
step·ping r.
ster·no·brach·i·al r.
stretch r.
Strümpell's r.
sty·lo·ra·di·al r.
suck·ling r.
su·per·fi·cial r.
su·pi·na·tion r.
su·pi·na·tor r.
su·pi·na·tor lon·gus r.
sup·port·ing r.'s
su·pra·or·bit·al r.
su·pra·pa·tel·lar r.
su·pra·um·bil·i·cal r.
swal·low·ing r.
syn·chro·nous r.
ta·pe·tal light r.
tar·so·pha·lan·ge·al r.
ten·do Achil·lis r.
ten·don r.
thumb r.
toe r.
ton·ic r.
trace con·di·tioned r.
trained r.
tri·ceps r.
tri·ceps su·rae r.
tri·ge·mi·no·fa·cial r.
tro·chan·ter r.
Trömner's r.
ul·nar r.
un·con·di·tion·ed r.
up·per ab·dom·i·nal per·i·
  os·te·al r.
uri·nary r.
utric·u·lar r.'s
va·go·va·gal r.
va·so·pres·sor r.
ve·no·res·pi·ra·to·ry r.
ver·te·bra pro·mi·nens r.
ves·i·cal r.
ves·tib·u·lo·spi·nal r.
vis·cer·al trac·tion r.
vis·cer·o·gen·ic r.
vis·cer·o·mo·tor r.
vis·cer·o·pan·nic·u·lar r.
vis·cer·o·sen·sory r.
vis·cer·o·tro·phic r.
vi·su·al or·bi·cu·la·ris r.
vom·it·ing r.
Weingrow's r.
Westphal's pu·pil·lary r.
white pu·pil·lary r.
wink r.

with·draw·al r.
wrist clo·nus r.
re·flex
an·gi·na
arc
asth·ma
con·trol
cough
dys·pep·sia
ep·i·lep·sy
head·ache
in·con·ti·nence
in·hi·bi·tion
ir·i·do·ple·gia
lig·a·ment
move·ment
otal·gia
sen·sa·tion
symp·tom
ther·a·py
re·flex neu·ro·gen·ic
blad·der
re·flex·o·gen·ic
pres·so·sen·si·tiv·i·ty
zone
re·flex·og·e·nous
re·flex·o·graph
re·flex·ol·o·gy
re·flex·om·e·ter
re·flex·o·phil
re·flex·o·phile
re·flex·o·ther·a·py
re·flux
ab·dom·i·no·jug·u·lar r.
esoph·a·ge·al r.
gas·tro·e·soph·a·ge·al r.
he·pa·to·jug·u·lar r.
ure·ter·o·re·nal r.
ves·i·co·u·re·ter·al r.
re·flux
esoph·a·gi·tis
oti·tis me·dia
re·fract
re·fract·ed
light
re·fract·ing
an·gle of a prism
re·frac·tion
dou·ble r.
dy·nam·ic r.
stat·ic r.
re·frac·tion·ist
re·frac·tion·om·e·ter
re·frac·tive
am·bly·o·pia
in·dex
ker·a·tot·o·my

re·frac·tive ac·com·mo·da·tive
  es·o·tro·pia
re·frac·tiv·i·ty
re·frac·tom·e·ter
re·frac·tom·e·try
re·frac·to·ry
  ane·mia
  cast
  flask
  in·vest·ment
  pe·ri·od
  pe·ri·od of elec·tron·ic
    pace·mak·er
  state
re·frac·ture
re·fran·gi·ble
re·fresh
re·frig·er·ant
re·frig·er·a·tion
  an·es·the·sia
re·frin·gence
re·frin·gent
Refsum's
  dis·ease
  syn·drome
re·fu·sion
re·gain·er
Regaud's
  fix·a·tive
re·gen·er·ate
re·gen·er·a·tion
  ab·er·rant r.
re·gen·er·a·tive
  pol·yp
reg·i·men
re·gio
  r. in·fra·cla·vic·u·la·ris
re·gion
  ab·dom·i·nal r.'s
  anal r.
  an·kle r.
  an·te·ri·or car·pal r.
  an·te·ri·or cu·bi·tal r.
  an·te·ri·or r. of fore·arm
  an·te·ri·or r. of neck
  ax·il·lary r.
  r.'s of back
  r.'s of body
  buc·cal r.
  cal·ca·ne·al r.
  r.'s of chest
  r. of chest
  chro·mo·som·al r.
  con·stant r.
  del·toid r.
  ep·i·gas·tric r.
  r.'s of face
  fem·o·ral r.

fron·tal r. of head
glu·te·al r.
r.'s of head
hinge r.
hy·po·chon·dri·ac r.
il·i·ac r.
r.'s of in·fe·ri·or limb
in·fra·mam·ma·ry r.
in·fra·or·bit·al r.
in·fra·scap·u·lar r.
in·gui·nal r.
K r.
lat·er·al r.
lat·er·al r. of neck
lum·bar r.
mam·ma·ry r.
men·tal r.
na·sal r.
r.'s of neck
oc·cip·i·tal r. of head
ol·fac·to·ry r. of tu·ni·ca
  mu·co·sa of nose
oral r.
or·bi·tal r.
pa·ri·e·tal r.
pec·to·ral r.'s
pec·to·ral r.
per·i·ne·al r.
pop·lit·e·al r.
pos·te·ri·or car·pal r.
pos·te·ri·or cu·bi·tal r.
pos·te·ri·or r. of fore·arm
pos·te·ri·or r. of neck
pre·op·tic r.
pre·ster·nal r.
pre·sump·tive r.
pre·tec·tal r.
pu·bic r.
res·pi·ra·to·ry r. of tu·ni·ca
  mu·co·sa of nose
sa·cral r.
scap·u·lar r.
ster·no·clei·do·mas·toid r.
r.'s of su·pe·ri·or limb
su·ral r.
tem·po·ral r. of head
um·bil·i·cal r.
uro·gen·i·tal r.
var·i·a·ble r.
ver·te·bral r.
Wernicke's r.
zy·go·mat·ic r.
re·gion·al
  anat·o·my
  an·es·the·sia
  en·ter·i·tis
  en·ter·o·co·li·tis
  hy·po·ther·mia

il·e·i·tis
per·fu·sion
re·gion·al gran·u·lom·a·tous
lym·phad·e·ni·tis
re·gi·o·nes
re·gi·o·nis
reg·is·tered
nurse
reg·is·tra·tion
max·il·lo·man·dib·u·lar r.
tis·sue r.
reg·nan·cy
re·gress·ing atyp·i·cal
his·ti·o·cy·to·sis
re·gres·sion
pho·ne·mic r.
re·gres·sive
stain·ing
re·gres·sive-re·con·struc·tive
ap·proach
reg·u·lar
astig·ma·tism
reg·u·lar in·su·lin
in·jec·tion
reg·u·la·tion
reg·u·la·tor
gene
reg·u·la·to·ry
al·bu·min·ur·ia
se·quence
re·gur·gi·tant
frac·tion
mur·mur
re·gur·gi·tate
re·gur·gi·ta·tion
aor·tic r.
mi·tral r.
re·gur·gi·ta·tion
jaun·dice
re·ha·bil·i·ta·tion
mouth r.
re·hears·al
Rehfuss
meth·od
Rehfuss stom·ach
tube
re·hy·dra·tion
Reichel-Pólya stom·ach
re·sec·tion
Reichert-Meissl
num·ber
Reichert's
car·ti·lage
Reichert's co·chle·ar
re·cess
Reid's base
line

Reifenstein's
syn·drome
Reil's
an·sa
band
rib·bon
tri·an·gle
re·im·plan·ta·tion
re·in·fec·tion
tu·ber·cu·lo·sis
re·in·forced
an·chor·age
re·in·force·ment
pri·mary r.
sec·on·dary r.
re·in·forc·er
Reinke
crys·tal·loids
re·in·ner·va·tion
re·in·oc·u·la·tion
Reinsch's
test
re·in·te·gra·tion
re·in·ver·sion
Reisseisen's
mus·cles
Reissner's
fi·ber
mem·brane
Reiter
test
Reiter's
dis·ease
syn·drome
re·jec·tion
ac·cel·er·at·ed r.
acute cel·lu·lar r.
chron·ic r.
chron·ic al·lo·graft r.
hy·per·a·cute r.
pa·ren·tal r.
pri·mary r.
re·ju·ve·nes·cence
re·lapse
re·laps·ing
fe·ver
ma·lar·ia
per·i·chon·dri·tis
pol·y·chon·dri·tis
re·la·tion
ac·quired cen·tric r.
ac·quired ec·cen·tric r.
buc·co·lin·gual r.
cen·tric r.
cen·tric jaw r.
dy·nam·ic r.'s
ec·cen·tric r.
in·ter·max·il·lary r.

re·la·tion *(continued)*
  max·il·lo·man·dib·u·lar r.
  me·di·an r.
  me·di·an re·trud·ed r.
  oc·clud·ing r.
  pro·tru·sive r.
  pro·tru·sive jaw r.
  rest r.
  rest jaw r.
  ridge r.
  stat·ic r.'s
  un·strained jaw r.
re·la·tion·al
  thresh·old
re·la·tion·ship
  blood r.
  hyp·not·ic r.
  ob·ject r.
  sa·do·mas·och·is·tic r.
rel·a·tive
  ac·com·mo·da·tion
  am·bly·o·pia
  de·hy·dra·tion
  hem·i·a·nop·sia
  hu·mid·i·ty
  im·mu·ni·ty
  in·com·pe·tence
  leu·ko·cy·to·sis
  pol·y·cy·the·mia
  sco·to·ma
  sen·si·tiv·i·ty
  spec·i·fic·i·ty
  ste·ril·i·ty
  vis·cos·i·ty
rel·a·tive re·frac·to·ry
  pe·ri·od
re·lax
re·lax·ant
  de·po·lar·iz·ing r.
  mus·cu·lar r.
  neu·ro·mus·cu·lar r.
  non·de·po·lar·iz·ing r.
  smooth mus·cle r.
re·lax·ant
  re·ver·sal
re·lax·a·tion
  fac·tor
  re·sponse
  su·ture
re·lax·a·tion
  car·di·o·e·soph·a·ge·al r.
  iso·met·ric r.
  iso·vol·u·met·ric r.
  iso·vol·u·mic r.
re·lax·in
re·learn·ing
re·lease
  phe·nom·e·non

re·leased
  sub·stance
re·leas·ing
  fac·tor
  hor·mone
re·li·a·bil·i·ty
  co·ef·fi·cient
re·li·a·bil·i·ty
  equiv·a·lent form r.
  in·ter·judge r.
  test-re·test r.
re·lief
  ar·ea
  cham·ber
re·lieve
re·line
REM
  sleep
  syn·drome
Remak's
  fi·bers
  gan·glia
  plex·us
  re·flex
  sign
Remak's nu·cle·ar
  di·vi·sion
re·me·di·a·ble
re·me·di·al
rem·e·dy
re·min·er·al·i·za·tion
rem·i·nis·cence
rem·i·nis·cent
  au·ra
  neu·ral·gia
re·mis·sion
  spon·ta·ne·ous r.
re·mit
re·mit·tence
re·mit·tent
  ma·lar·ia
re·mit·tent ma·lar·i·al
  fe·ver
re·mod·el·ing
re·mote
  mem·o·ry
re·mov·a·ble
  bridge
re·mov·a·ble par·tial
  den·ture
re·nal
  ad·e·no·car·ci·no·ma
  agen·e·sis
  am·y·loi·do·sis
  ar·tery
  bal·lotte·ment
  cal·cu·lus
  cap·su·lot·o·my

car·bun·cle
car·ci·no·sar·co·ma
cast
col·ic
col·lar
col·umns
cor·pus·cle
cor·tex
di·a·be·tes
ep·i·stax·is
fas·cia
gan·glia
gly·cos·ur·ia
he·ma·tu·ria
he·mo·phil·ia
hem·or·rhage
hy·per·ten·sion
hy·po·pla·sia
im·pres·sion
in·fan·ti·lism
in·suf·fi·cien·cy
lab·y·rinth
lobe
os·te·i·tis fi·bro·sa
os·te·o·dys·tro·phy
pa·pil·la
pel·vis
plex·us
pyr·a·mid
re·flex
ret·i·nop·a·thy
rick·ets
seg·ments
si·nus
sur·face
thresh·old
trans·plan·ta·tion
veins
re·nal cell
    car·ci·no·ma
re·nal cor·ti·cal
    ad·e·no·ma
    lob·ule
re·nal fi·bro·cys·tic
    os·te·o·sis
re·nal pap·il·lary
    ne·cro·sis
re·nal-splanch·nic
    steal
re·nal-splen·ic ve·nous
    shunt
re·nal tu·bu·lar
    ac·i·do·sis
ren·cu·lus
Rendu-Osler-Weber
    dis·ease
    syn·drome
ren·i·cap·sule

ren·i·car·di·ac
re·nic·u·li
re·nic·u·lus
re·ni·fleur
ren·i·form
    pel·vis
re·nin
re·nin-an·gi·o·ten·sin
    sys·tem
ren·i·por·tal
ren·nase
ren·net
ren·nin
ren·nin·o·gen
ren·no·gen
re·no·cu·ta·ne·ous
re·no·gas·tric
re·no·gen·ic
re·no·gram
re·nog·ra·phy
re·no·in·tes·ti·nal
re·no·meg·a·ly
re·nop·a·thy
re·no·pri·val
re·no·pul·mo·nary
re·no·tro·phic
re·no·tro·phin
re·no·tro·pic
re·no·tro·pin
re·no·vas·cu·lar
    hy·per·ten·sion
Renpenning's
    syn·drome
Renshaw
    cells
re·nun·cu·lus
Re·o·vir·i·dae
Re·o·vi·rus
re·o·vi·rus-like
    agent
re·pair
    chem·i·cal r.
re·pand
re·par·a·tive
    den·tin
re·par·a·tive gi·ant cell
    gran·u·lo·ma
re·peat ac·tion
    tab·let
re·pel·lent
rep·e·ti·tion
    rate
rep·e·ti·tion-com·pul·sion
    prin·ci·ple
re·pet·i·tive
    DNA
re·place·ment
    bone

re·place·ment *(continued)*
  fi·bro·sis
  ther·a·py
re·plant
re·plan·ta·tion
  in·ten·tion·al r.
re·ple·tion
rep·li·ca
rep·li·case
rep·li·cate
rep·li·ca·tion
rep·li·ca·tive
  form
rep·li·ca·tor
rep·li·con
rep·li·some
re·po·lar·i·za·tion
re·port·a·ble
  dis·ease
re·po·si·tion·ing
  gin·gi·val r.
  jaw r.
  mus·cle r.
re·pos·i·tor
re·pressed
re·press·i·ble
  en·zyme
re·pres·sion
  pri·mal r.
re·pres·sor
  ac·tive r.
  in·ac·tive r.
re·pres·sor
  gene
re·pro·duc·tion
  asex·u·al r.
  cy·to·gen·ic r.
  sex·u·al r.
  so·mat·ic r.
re·pro·duc·tive
  as·sim·i·la·tion
  cy·cle
  nu·cle·us
  sys·tem
Rep·til·ia
re·pul·lu·la·tion
re·pul·sion
re·quired arch
  length
res·a·zu·rin
res·cin·na·mine
re·sect
re·sect·a·ble
re·sec·tion
  gum r.
  Miles r.
  mus·cle r.
  Reichel-Pólya stom·ach r.

root r.
scle·ral r.
trans·u·re·thral r.
wedge r.
re·sec·to·scope
  sheath
re·ser·pine
re·serve
  al·ka·li r.
  breath·ing r.
  car·di·ac r.
re·serve
  air
  force
re·serve tooth
  germ
res·er·voir
  bag
  host
res·er·voir
  r. of in·fec·tion
  Ommaya r.
  Pecquet's r.
  r. of sper·ma·to·zoa
  vi·tel·line r.
re·set no·dus si·nu·a·tri·a·lis
res·i·dent
re·sid·ua
re·sid·u·al
  ab·scess
  af·fin·i·ty
  air
  body
  body of Regaud
  ca·pac·i·ty
  cleft
  in·hi·bi·tion
  in·hib·i·tor
  lu·men
  ridge
  schiz·o·phre·nia
  urine
  vol·ume
re·sid·u·al ova·ry
  syn·drome
res·i·due
  day r.
re·sid·u·um
re·sil·ience
res·in
  acryl·ic r.
  ac·ti·vat·ed r.
  an·i·on-ex·change r.
  au·to·pol·y·mer r.
  au·to·po·ly·mer·iz·ing r.
  car·ba·cryl·a·mine r.'s
  cat·i·on-ex·change r.
  cho·le·styr·a·mine r.

cold cure r.
cold-cur·ing r.
com·pos·ite r.
co·pol·y·mer r.
cross-linked r.
di·rect fill·ing r.
ep·ox·y r.
gum r.
heat-cur·ing r.
In·di·an pod·o·phyl·lum r.
ion-ex·change r.
ip·o·mea r.
jal·ap r.
mel·a·mine r.
meth·ac·ry·late r.
pod·o·phyl·lum r.
pol·y·a·mine-meth·yl·ene r.
pol·y·es·ter r.
quick cure r.
qui·nine car·ba·cryl·ic r.
self-cur·ing r.
res·in ac·ids
res·in·oid
res·in·ous
re·sis·tance
  air·way r.
  bac·te·ri·o·phage r.
  ex·pi·ra·to·ry r.
  im·pact r.
  in·duc·tive r.
  in·su·lin r.
  mu·tu·al r.
  pe·riph·e·ral r.
  syn·ap·tic r.
  sys·tem·ic vas·cu·lar r.
  to·tal pe·riph·e·ral r.
re·sis·tance
  fac·tors
  form
  plas·mids
  py·rom·e·ter
  ther·mom·e·ter
re·sis·tance-in·duc·ing
  fac·tor
re·sis·tance-trans·fer
  fac·tor
re·sis·tance-trans·fer·ring
  ep·i·somes
re·sis·tant ova·ry
  syn·drome
re·sis·tive
  move·ment
re·sis·tor
res·o·lu·tion
  acu·i·ty
re·solve
re·sol·vent

re·solv·ing
  pow·er
res·o·nance
  the·o·ry of hear·ing
res·o·nance
  am·phor·ic r.
  band·box r.
  bell·met·al r.
  cav·ern·ous r.
  cracked-pot r.
  elec·tron spin r.
  hy·da·tid r.
  nu·cle·ar mag·net·ic r.
  sko·da·ic r.
  tym·pa·nit·ic r.
  ve·sic·u·lar r.
  ve·sic·u·lo·tym·pa·ni·tic r.
  vo·cal r.
  wood·en r.
res·o·na·tor
re·sorb
res·or·cin
res·or·cin·ol
  r. mon·o·ac·e·tate
  r. phthal·ic an·hy·dride
res·or·cin·ol
  test
res·or·cin·ol·phtha·lein
  r. so·di·um
re·sorp·tion
  bone r.
  gin·gi·val r.
  hor·i·zon·tal r.
  in·ter·nal r.
  ridge r.
  root r.
re·sorp·tion
  la·cu·nae
res·pi·ra·ble
  aer·o·sols
res·pi·ra·tion
  rate
res·pi·ra·tion
  ab·dom·i·nal r.
  aer·o·bic r.
  am·phor·ic r.
  an·aer·o·bic r.
  ar·ti·fi·cial r.
  as·sist·ed r.
  Biot's r.
  bron·chi·al r.
  bron·cho·ve·sic·u·lar r.
  cav·ern·ous r.
  Cheyne-Stokes r.
  cog·wheel r.
  con·trolled r.
  cos·tal r.
  dif·fu·sion r.

res·pi·ra·tion *(continued)*
  elec·tro·phren·ic r.
  ex·ter·nal r.
  forced r.
  in·ter·nal r.
  in·ter·rupt·ed r.
  jerky r.
  Kussmaul r.
  Kussmaul-Kien r.
  mouth-to-mouth r.
  ni·trate r.
  par·a·dox·i·cal r.
  pu·er·ile r.
  sul·fate r.
  tho·rac·ic r.
  tis·sue r.
  tu·bu·lar r.
  ve·sic·u·lar r.
  ve·sic·u·lo·cav·ern·ous r.

res·pi·ra·tor
  cui·rass r.
  Drinker r.
  pres·sure-con·trolled r.
  tank r.
  vol·ume-con·trolled r.

res·pi·ra·tor
  brain

res·pi·ra·to·ry
  ac·i·do·sis
  air·way
  al·ka·lo·sis
  ap·pa·ra·tus
  ar·rhyth·mia
  bron·chi·oles
  burst
  ca·pac·i·ty
  cen·ter
  chain
  co·ef·fi·cient
  en·zyme
  ep·i·the·li·um
  fre·quen·cy
  hip·pus
  in·suf·fi·cien·cy
  lob·ule
  me·tab·o·lism
  met·al
  mu·co·sa
  mur·mur
  pause
  pig·ments
  pulse
  quo·tient
  re·gion of tu·ni·ca mu·co·sa of nose
  scle·ro·ma
  sound
  sys·tem
  tract

res·pi·ra·to·ry dead
  space
res·pi·ra·to·ry dis·tress
  syn·drome of the new·born
res·pi·ra·to·ry ex·change
  ra·ti·o
res·pi·ra·to·ry min·ute
  vol·ume
res·pi·ra·to·ry syn·cy·tial
  vi·rus
re·spire
res·pi·rom·e·ter
  Dräger r.
  Wright r.
re·spon·dent
  be·hav·ior
  con·di·tion·ing
re·sponse
  hi·er·ar·chy
re·sponse
  bi·pha·sic r.
  con·di·tioned r.
  curve r.
  Cushing r.
  de·ple·tion r.
  ear·ly-phase r.
  e·voked r.
  flight or fight r.
  gal·van·ic skin r.
  Henry-Gauer r.
  im·mune r.
  iso·mor·phic r.
  late-phase r.
  oc·u·lo·mo·tor r.
  or·i·ent·ing r.
  pri·mary im·mune r.
  psy·cho·gal·van·ic r.
  psy·cho·gal·van·ic skin r.
  re·cruit·ing r.
  re·lax·a·tion r.
  sec·on·dary im·mune r.
  son·o·mo·tor r.
  tar·get r.
  tri·ple r.
  un·con·di·tion·ed r.
re·sponse-pro·duced
  cues
rest
  ar·ea
  bite
  body
  ni·tro·gen
  pain
  po·si·tion
  re·la·tion
  seat

rest
  ad·re·nal r.
  cin·gu·lum r.
  in·ci·sal r.
  lin·gual r.
  Malassez' ep·i·the·li·al r.'s
  Marchand's r.
  mes·o·neph·ric r.
  oc·clu·sal r.
  pre·ci·sion r.
  Walthard's cell r.
  wolff·i·an r.
re·ste·no·sis
res·ti·form
  body
  em·i·nence
rest·ing
  cell
  sa·li·va
  stage
rest·ing tid·al
  vol·ume
rest·ing wan·der·ing
  cell
res·ti·tu·tion
rest jaw
  re·la·tion
rest·less
  legs
rest·less legs
  syn·drome
res·to·ra·tion
  ac·id-etched r.
  com·bi·na·tion r.
  com·pound r.
  di·rect acryl·ic r.
  di·rect com·pos·ite res·in r.
  di·rect res·in r.
  over·hang·ing r.
  per·ma·nent r.
  root ca·nal r.
  sil·i·cate r.'s
  tem·po·rary r.
re·stor·a·tive
  den·tis·try
re·stor·a·tive den·tal
  ma·te·ri·als
re·stored
  cy·cle
re·strained
  beam
re·straint
re·stric·tion
  en·do·nu·cle·ase
  en·zyme
  site
re·stric·tion length
  pol·y·mor·phism

re·stric·tion-site
  pol·y·mor·phism
re·stric·tive
  car·di·o·my·op·a·thy
re·struc·tured
  cell
rest ver·ti·cal
  di·men·sion
re·sus·ci·tate
re·sus·ci·ta·tion
  car·di·o·pul·mo·nary r.
  mouth-to-mouth r.
re·sus·ci·ta·tor
re·tained
  men·stru·a·tion
  pla·cen·ta
  tes·tis
re·tain·er
  con·tin·u·ous bar r.
  di·rect r.
  ex·tra·cor·o·nal r.
  Hawley r.
  in·di·rect r.
  in·tra·cor·o·nal r.
  ma·trix r.
  space r.
re·tard·ate
re·tar·da·tion
  men·tal r.
  psy·cho·mo·tor r.
re·tard·ed
  den·ti·tion
re·tard·er
retch
retch·ing
re·te
  r. ca·na·lis hy·po·glos·si
  r. car·pi pos·te·ri·us
  r. cu·ta·ne·um co·rii
  r. fo·ra·mi·nis ova·lis
  r. hal·leri
  Haller's r.
  mal·pi·ghi·an r.
  r. ova·rii
  r. sub·pa·pil·la·re
re·te
  cords
  cyst of ova·ry
  pegs
  ridg·es
re·ten·tion
  ar·ea
  arm
  cyst
  form
  groove
  jaun·dice
  point

re·ten·tion *(continued)*
  pol·yp
  su·ture
  vom·it·ing
re·ten·tion
  den·ture r.
  di·rect r.
  in·di·rect r.
  par·tial den·ture r.
re·ten·tive
  arm
re·ten·tive cir·cum·fer·en·tial clasp
  arm
re·ten·tive ful·crum
  line
re·tia
re·ti·al
re·tic·u·la
re·tic·u·lar
  car·ti·lage
  cell
  de·gen·er·a·tion
  dys·tro·phy of cor·nea
  fi·bers
  for·ma·tion
  lam·i·na
  lay·er of co·ri·um
  mem·brane
  nu·clei of the brain·stem
  nu·cle·us of thal·a·mus
  sub·stance
  tis·sue
re·tic·u·lar ac·ti·vat·ing
  sys·tem
re·tic·u·lar er·y·them·a·tous
  mu·ci·no·sis
re·tic·u·la·ris
  cell
re·tic·u·lated
  bone
  cor·pus·cle
re·tic·u·lat·ing
  col·li·qua·tion
re·tic·u·la·tion
re·tic·u·lin
re·tic·u·li·tis
re·tic·u·lo·cyte
re·tic·u·lo·cy·to·pe·nia
re·tic·u·lo·cy·to·sis
re·tic·u·lo·en·do·the·li·al
  cell
  sys·tem
re·tic·u·lo·en·do·the·li·o·ma
re·tic·u·lo·en·do·the·li·o·sis
  avi·an r.
  leu·ke·mic r.
re·tic·u·lo·en·do·the·li·um

re·tic·u·lo·his·ti·o·cyt·ic
  gran·u·lo·ma
re·tic·u·lo·his·ti·o·cy·to·ma
re·tic·u·lo·his·ti·o·cy·to·sis
  mul·ti·cen·tric r.
re·tic·u·loid
  ac·tin·ic r.
re·tic·u·lo·pe·nia
re·tic·u·lo·sis
  be·nign in·oc·u·la·tion r.
  his·ti·o·cyt·ic med·ul·lary r.
  leu·ke·mic r.
  lip·o·me·lan·ic r.
  my·e·loid r.
  pag·et·oid r.
  pol·y·mor·phic r.
re·tic·u·lo·spi·nal
  tract
re·tic·u·lot·o·my
re·tic·u·lum
  agran·u·lar en·do·plas·mic r.
  Ebner's r.
  en·do·plas·mic r.
  Golgi in·ter·nal r.
  gran·u·lar en·do·plas·mic r.
  Kölliker's r.
  rough-sur·faced en·do·plas·mic r.
  sar·co·plas·mic r.
  smooth-sur·faced en·do·plas·mic r.
  stel·late r.
  tra·bec·u·lar r.
re·tic·u·lum cell
  sar·co·ma
ret·i·form
  car·ti·lage
  tis·sue
ret·i·na
  co·arc·tate r.
  de·tached r.
  fleck r.
  flecked r.
  fleck r. of Kandori
  leop·ard r.
  shot-silk r.
  ti·groid r.
ret·i·nac·u·la
ret·i·nac·u·li
ret·i·nac·u·lum
  r. cap·su·lae ar·ti·cu·la·ris cox·ae
  cau·dal r.
  ex·ten·sor r.
  ret·i·nac·u·la of ex·ten·sor mus·cles
  flex·or r.

r. of flex·or mus·cles
in·fe·ri·or r. of ex·ten·sor
  mus·cles
lat·er·al r. of pa·tel·la
me·di·al r. of pa·tel·la
Morgagni's r.
ret·i·nac·u·la of nail
r. pa·tel·lae me·di·a·le
ret·i·nac·u·la of per·o·ne·al
  mus·cles
r. of skin
su·pe·ri·or r. of ex·ten·sor
  mus·cles
r. ten·di·num
ret·i·nal
r. de·hy·dro·gen·ase
r. isom·er·ase
r. re·duc·tase
ret·i·nal
ad·ap·ta·tion
as·the·no·pia
cam·era
cones
de·tach·ment
dis·par·i·ty
dys·pla·sia
em·bo·lism
fold
im·age
trans-**ret·i·nal**
ret·i·nal an·la·ge
tu·mor
ret·i·nal·de·hyde
r. de·hy·dro·gen·ase
r. isom·er·ase
r. re·duc·tase
ret·i·nene
ret·i·ni·tis
al·bu·min·ur·ic r.
ap·o·plec·tic r.
az·o·tem·ic r.
cen·tral an·gi·o·spas·tic r.
cir·ci·nate r.
di·a·bet·ic r.
r. ex·u·da·ti·va
ex·ud·a·tive r.
gra·vid·ic r.
leu·ke·mic r.
met·a·stat·ic r.
r. pig·men·to·sa
r. pro·li·fe·rans
punc·tate r.
pu·ru·lent r.
re·cur·rent cen·tral r.
r. sclo·pe·ta·ria
sec·on·dary r.
sep·tic r.

se·rous r.
sim·ple r.
syph·i·lit·ic r.
r. syph·i·li·ti·ca
ret·i·no·blas·to·ma
ret·i·no·cer·e·bral
an·gi·o·ma·to·sis
ret·i·no·cho·roid
ret·i·no·cho·roid·i·tis
bird shot r.
r. jux·ta·pa·pil·la·ris
ret·i·no·di·al·y·sis
ret·i·no·ic ac·id
ret·i·noid
ret·i·noids
ret·i·nol
r. de·hy·dro·gen·ase
ret·i·no·pap·il·li·tis
r. of pre·ma·ture in·fants
ret·i·nop·a·thy
an·gi·o·path·ic r.
ar·te·ri·o·scle·rot·ic r.
cen·tral an·gi·o·spas·tic r.
cen·tral se·rous r.
cir·ci·nate r.
com·pres·sion r.
di·a·bet·ic r.
dys·or·ic r.
dys·pro·tein·e·mic r.
ec·lamp·tic r.
elec·tric r.
ex·ter·nal ex·ud·a·tive r.
gra·vid·ic r.
hy·per·ten·sive r.
hy·po·ten·sive r.
Leber's id·i·o·path·ic stel·
  late r.
leu·ke·mic r.
li·pe·mic r.
mac·u·lar r.
pho·to r.
pig·men·tary r.
r. of pre·ma·tu·ri·ty
pro·lif·er·a·tive r.
punc·ta·ta al·bes·cens r.
re·nal r.
ru·bel·la r.
sick·le cell r.
so·lar r.
stel·late r.
ta·pe·to·ret·i·nal r.
tox·e·mic r. of preg·nan·cy
tox·ic r.
trau·mat·ic r.
ve·nous-sta·sis r.
ret·i·no·pexy
ret·i·no·pi·e·sis

ret·i·nos·chi·sis
  ju·ve·nile r.
  se·nile r.
ret·i·no·scope
  lu·mi·nous r.
  re·flect·ing r.
ret·i·nos·co·py
  cyl·in·der r.
  fog·ging r.
ret·o·per·i·the·li·um
re·tort
Re·tor·tam·o·nas
ret·o·the·li·o·ma
re·tract
re·trac·tile
  tes·tis
re·trac·tion
  nys·tag·mus
  syn·drome
re·trac·tion
  gin·gi·val r.
  man·dib·u·lar r.
re·trac·tor
re·trad
re·tra·hens au·rem
re·tra·hens au·ric·u·lam
re·treat from re·al·i·ty
re·trench·ment
re·triev·al
ret·ro·ac·tive
  in·hi·bi·tion
ret·ro·au·ric·u·lar
ret·ro·au·ric·u·lar lymph
  nodes
ret·ro·buc·cal
ret·ro·bul·bar
  ab·scess
  an·es·the·sia
  neu·ri·tis
ret·ro·cal·ca·ne·o·bur·si·tis
ret·ro·ce·cal
  ab·scess
  re·cess
ret·ro·ce·cal lymph
  nodes
ret·ro·ced·ent
  gout
ret·ro·cer·vi·cal
ret·ro·ces·sion
ret·ro·clu·sion
ret·ro·co·chle·ar
  deaf·ness
ret·ro·co·lic
ret·ro·col·lic
  spasm
ret·ro·col·lis
ret·ro·con·duc·tion

ret·ro·cur·sive
  ab·sence
ret·ro·cus·pid
  pa·pil·la
ret·ro·de·vi·a·tion
ret·ro·dis·place·ment
ret·ro·du·o·de·nal
  ar·tery
  fos·sa
  re·cess
ret·ro·e·soph·a·ge·al
ret·ro·fil·ling
ret·ro·flect·ed
ret·ro·flec·tion
ret·ro·flex
  fas·cic·u·lus
ret·ro·flexed
ret·ro·flex·ion
  r. of iris
ret·ro·gas·se·ri·an
  neu·rec·to·my
  neu·rot·o·my
ret·ro·gnath·ic
ret·ro·gnath·ism
ret·ro·grade
  am·ne·sia
  aor·tog·ra·phy
  beat
  block
  chro·ma·tol·y·sis
  con·duc·tion
  de·gen·er·a·tion
  em·bo·lism
  her·nia
  in·tus·sus·cep·tion
  mem·o·ry
  men·stru·a·tion
  met·a·mor·pho·sis
  urog·ra·phy
ret·ro·grade P
  wave
ret·rog·ra·phy
ret·ro·gres·sion
ret·ro·hy·oid
  bur·sa
ret·ro·in·gui·nal
  space
ret·ro·i·rid·i·an
ret·ro·jec·tion
ret·ro·jec·tor
ret·ro·len·tal
  fi·bro·pla·sia
ret·ro·len·tic·u·lar
  limb of in·ter·nal cap·sule
ret·ro·lin·gual
ret·ro·mam·ma·ry
  mas·ti·tis

ret·ro·man·dib·u·lar
  fos·sa
  vein
ret·ro·mas·toid
ret·ro·mo·lar
  fos·sa
  pad
ret·ro·mor·pho·sis
ret·ro·my·lo·hy·oid
  space
ret·ro·na·sal
ret·ro-oc·u·lar
ret·ro·per·i·to·ne·al
  fi·bro·sis
  her·nia
  space
ret·ro·per·i·to·ne·um
ret·ro·per·i·to·ni·tis
  id·i·o·path·ic fi·brous r.
ret·ro·pha·ryn·ge·al
  ab·scess
  space
ret·ro·pha·ryn·ge·al lymph
  nodes
ret·ro·phar·ynx
ret·ro·pla·cen·tal
ret·ro·pla·sia
ret·ro·posed
ret·ro·po·si·tion
ret·ro·pos·on
ret·ro·pu·bic
  her·nia
  space
ret·ro·pul·sion
ret·ro·py·lor·ic
  nodes
ret·ro·spec·tion
ret·ro·spec·tive
  fal·si·fi·ca·tion
ret·ro·spon·dy·lo·lis·the·sis
ret·ro·ster·nal
  her·nia
ret·ro·ste·roid
ret·ro·tar·sal
  fold
ret·ro·u·ter·ine
ret·ro·ver·si·o·flex·ion
ret·ro·ver·sion
ret·ro·vert·ed
Ret·ro·vir·i·dae
ret·ro·vi·rus
re·tru·sion
re·tru·sive
  oc·clu·sion
Rett's
  syn·drome
re·turn
  ex·tra·sys·to·le

re·turn·ing
  cy·cle
Retzius'
  cav·i·ty
  fi·bers
  fo·ra·men
  gy·rus
  lig·a·ment
  space
  stri·ae
  veins
re·u·ni·ent
Reuss'
  for·mu·la
  test
Reuss' col·or
  ta·bles
re·vac·ci·na·tion
re·vas·cu·lar·i·za·tion
re·ver·ber·at·ing
  cir·cuit
Reverdin
  graft
Reverdin's
  meth·od
re·ver·sal
  adren·a·line r.
  ep·i·neph·rine r.
  nar·cot·ic r.
  pres·sure r.
  re·lax·ant r.
  sex r.
re·verse
  band·ing
  bev·el
  curve
  mu·ta·tion
  os·mo·sis
  tran·scrip·tase
re·versed
  an·a·phy·lax·is
  astig·ma·tism
  co·arc·ta·tion
  per·i·stal·sis
  shunt
re·versed par·a·dox·i·cal
  pulse
re·versed pas·sive
  an·a·phy·lax·is
re·versed Prausnitz-Küstner
  re·ac·tion
re·versed re·cip·ro·cal
  rhythm
re·verse Eck
  fis·tu·la
re·verse Kingsley
  splint

re·verse pas·sive
  he·mag·glu·ti·na·tion
re·vers·i·ble
  am·bly·o·pia
  cal·ci·no·sis
  col·loid
  de·cor·ti·ca·tion
  hy·dro·col·loid
  pulp·i·tis
  re·ac·tion
  shock
re·ver·sion
re·ver·tant
Revilliod's
  sign
rev·i·ves·cence
re·viv·i·fi·ca·tion
re·vul·sion
re·ward
re·warm·ing
Rexed
  lam·i·na
Reye's
  syn·drome
Rh
  an·ti·gens
rha·bar·ber·one
Rhab·di·tis
rhab·do·cyte
rhab·doid
rhab·do·my·o·blast
rhab·do·my·ol·y·sis
  acute re·cur·rent r.
  ex·er·tion·al r.
  fa·mil·i·al par·ox·ys·mal r.
  id·i·o·path·ic par·ox·ys·mal
    r.
rhab·do·my·o·ma
rhab·do·my·o·sar·co·ma
  em·bry·o·nal r.'s
rhab·do·pho·bia
rhab·do·sar·co·ma
rhab·do·sphinc·ter
Rhab·do·vir·i·dae
rhab·do·vi·rus
rhag·a·des
rha·gad·i·form
rha·gi·o·crine
  cell
ʟ-rham·nose
rham·no·side
rham·no·xan·thin
Rhamnus
rha·pha·nia
rha·phe
rha·thy·mia
Rh block·ing
  test

RH$_o$(D) im·mune
  glob·u·lin
rheg·ma
rheg·ma·tog·e·nous
rheg·ma·tog·e·nous ret·i·nal
  de·tach·ment
rhe·ic
Rheinberg
  mi·cro·scope
rhe·ni·um
rhe·o·base
rhe·o·ba·sic
rhe·o·car·di·og·ra·phy
rhe·o·chrys·i·din
rhe·o·en·ceph·a·lo·gram
rhe·o·en·ceph·a·log·ra·phy
rhe·o·gram
rhe·ol·o·gist
rhe·ol·o·gy
rhe·om·e·ter
rhe·om·e·try
rhe·o·pexy
rhe·o·stat
rhe·os·to·sis
rhe·o·tax·is
rhe·ot·ro·pism
rhes·to·cy·the·mia
rhe·sus
  dis·ease
rheum
rheu·ma·tal·gia
rheu·mat·ic
  ar·te·ri·tis
  car·di·tis
  cho·rea
  dis·ease
  en·do·car·di·tis
  fe·ver
  per·i·car·di·tis
  pneu·mo·nia
  tet·a·ny
  tor·ti·col·lis
  val·vu·li·tis
rheu·mat·ic heart
  dis·ease
rheu·ma·tid
rheu·ma·tism
  ar·tic·u·lar r.
  chron·ic r.
  gon·or·rhe·al r.
  in·flam·ma·to·ry r.
  lum·bar r.
  Macleod's r.
  mus·cu·lar r.
  no·dose r.
  sub·a·cute r.
  tu·ber·cu·lous r.
rheu·ma·tis·mal

rheu·ma·to·ce·lis
rheu·ma·toid
  ar·te·ri·tis
  ar·thri·tis
  dis·ease
  fac·tors
  nod·ules
  spon·dy·li·tis
rheu·ma·tol·o·gist
rheu·ma·tol·o·gy
rhex·is
rhi·go·sis
rhi·got·ic
rhi·nal
  fis·sure
  sul·cus
rhi·nal·gia
rhi·nar·ia
rhi·nar·i·um
rhin·e·de·ma
rhin·en·ce·phal·ic
rhin·en·ceph·a·lon
rhin·en·chy·sis
rhin·eu·ryn·ter
rhin·i·on
rhi·nism
rhi·ni·tis
  acute r.
  al·ler·gic r.
  atroph·ic r.
  atroph·ic r. of swine
  r. ca·se·o·sa
  ca·se·ous r.
  chron·ic r.
  croup·ous r.
  eo·sin·o·phil·ic non·al·ler·
   gic r.
  fi·brin·ous r.
  gan·gre·nous r.
  hy·per·tro·phic r.
  r. me·di·ca·men·to·sa
  mem·bra·nous r.
  ne·crot·ic r. of pigs
  r. ner·vo·sa
  pseu·do·mem·bra·nous r.
  pu·ru·lent r.
  r. pu·ru·len·ta
  scrof·u·lous r.
  r. sic·ca
  va·so·mo·tor r.
rhi·no·an·e·mom·e·ter
rhi·no·an·tri·tis
rhi·no·by·on
rhi·no·can·thec·to·my
rhi·no·cele
rhi·no·ce·pha·lia
rhi·no·ceph·a·ly
rhi·no·chei·lo·plas·ty

rhi·no·chi·lo·plas·ty
Rhi·no·clad·i·el·la
rhi·no·clei·sis
rhi·no·dac·ry·o·lith
rhi·no·dym·ia
rhi·no·dyn·ia
rhi·no·es·tro·sis
Rhi·no·es·trus pur·pu·re·us
rhi·nog·e·nous
rhi·no·ky·phec·to·my
rhi·no·ky·pho·sis
rhi·no·la·lia
  r. aper·ta
  r. clausa
rhi·no·lar·yn·gi·tis
rhi·no·lar·yn·gol·o·gy
rhi·no·lite
rhi·no·lith
rhi·no·li·thi·a·sis
rhi·no·log·ic
rhi·nol·o·gist
rhi·nol·o·gy
rhi·no·ma·nom·e·ter
rhi·no·ma·nom·e·try
rhi·no·mu·cor·my·co·sis
rhi·no·my·co·sis
rhi·no·ne·cro·sis
rhi·nop·a·thy
rhi·no·pha·ryn·ge·al
rhi·no·phar·yn·gi·tis
  r. mu·ti·lans
rhi·no·pha·ryn·go·lith
rhi·no·phar·ynx
rhi·no·pho·nia
rhi·no·phy·co·my·co·sis
rhi·no·phy·ma
rhi·no·plas·ty
  English r.
  In·di·an r.
  Ital·ian r.
  Joseph r.
rhi·no·pneu·mo·ni·tis
  equine r.
rhi·nor·rha·gia
rhi·nor·rhea
  cer·e·bro·spi·nal flu·id r.
  gus·ta·to·ry r.
rhi·no·sal·pin·gi·tis
rhi·no·scle·ro·ma
rhi·no·scope
rhi·no·scop·ic
rhi·nos·co·py
  an·te·ri·or r.
  me·di·an r.
  pos·te·ri·or r.
rhi·no·spo·rid·i·o·sis
Rhi·no·spo·rid·i·um see·beri
rhi·no·ste·no·sis

rhi·not·o·my
rhi·no·tra·che·i·tis
  fe·line vi·ral r.
  in·fec·tious bo·vine r.
Rhi·no·vi·rus
rhi·no·vi·rus
  bo·vine r.'s
  equine r.'s
Rhi·pi·ceph·a·lus
  R. ap·pen·di·cu·la·tus
  R. evert·si
  R. pul·chel·lus
  R. san·gui·ne·us
rhi·zoid
rhi·zome
rhi·zo·me·lia
rhi·zo·me·nin·go·my·e·li·tis
rhi·zo·plast
Rhi·zop·o·da
Rhi·zo·po·das·i·da
Rhi·zo·po·dea
rhi·zop·ter·in
Rhi·zo·pus
rhi·zot·o·my
  an·te·ri·or r.
  fac·et r.
  pos·te·ri·or r.
  tri·gem·i·nal r.
Rh null
  syn·drome
rho·da·mine B
rho·da·nate
rho·da·nese
rho·dan·ic ac·id
rho·da·nile blue
rho·de·ose
Rho·de·sian
  try·pan·o·so·mi·a·sis
Rho·de·sian ma·lig·nant
  thei·le·ri·o·sis
rho·din
rho·di·um
rho·do·gen·e·sis
rho·do·phy·lac·tic
rho·do·phy·lax·is
rho·dop·sin
meta-rho·dop·sin I
meta-rho·dop·sin II
meta-rho·dop·sin III
Rho·do·tor·u·la
rhomb·en·ce·phal·ic
  isth·mus
rhomb·en·ce·phal·ic gus·ta·to·ry
  nu·cle·us
rhomb·en·ceph·a·lon

rhom·bic
  grooves
  lip
rhom·bo·at·loi·de·us
rhom·bo·cele
rhom·boid
  fos·sa
  im·pres·sion
  lig·a·ment
rhom·boi·dal
  si·nus
rhom·boi·de·us
rhom·bo·mere
rhon·chal
  frem·i·tus
rhon·chi
rhon·chi·al
rhon·chus
  cav·ern·ous r.
rho·phe·o·cy·to·sis
rhop·tries
rhop·try
rho·ta·cism
rhu·barb
Rhus
rhus
  der·ma·ti·tis
Rhus tox·i·co·den·dron
  an·ti·gen
Rhus ve·ne·na·ta
  an·ti·gen
rhy·pa·ria
rhy·poph·a·gy
rhy·po·pho·bia
rhythm
  ag·o·nal r.
  al·pha r.
  atri·o·ven·tric·u·lar no·dal r.
  A-V no·dal r.
  Berger r.
  be·ta r.
  bi·gem·i·nal r.
  can·ter·ing r.
  cir·ca·di·an r.
  cir·cus r.
  cor·o·nary no·dal r.
  cor·o·nary si·nus r.
  cou·pled r.
  del·ta r.
  di·ur·nal r.
  ec·top·ic r.
  es·cape r.
  fast r.
  gal·lop r.
  id·i·o·nod·al r.
  id·i·o·ven·tric·u·lar r.
  low·er no·dal r.

mid·no·dal r.
no·dal r.
pen·du·lum r.
quad·ri·gem·i·nal r.
quad·ru·ple r.
re·cip·ro·cal r.
re·cip·ro·cat·ing r.
re·versed re·cip·ro·cal r.
si·nus r.
the·ta r.
tic-tac r.
train·wheel r.
tri·gem·i·nal r.
tri·ple r.
ul·tra·di·an r.
up·per no·dal r.
ven·tric·u·lar r.
rhythm
meth·od
rhyth·meur
rhyth·mic
cho·rea
rhyt·i·dec·tomy
rhyt·i·do·plas·ty
rhyt·i·do·sis
rib
bi·cip·i·tal r.
bi·fid r.
cer·vi·cal r.
false r.'s
float·ing r.'s
lum·bar r.
slip·ping r.
true r.'s
ver·te·bral r.'s
ver·te·bro·chon·dral r.'s
ver·te·bro·ster·nal r.'s
rib
spread·er
ri·ba·vi·rin
Ribbert's
the·o·ry
rib·bon
arch
rib·bon
Reil's r.
rib·bon arch
ap·pli·ance
Ribes'
gan·gli·on
ri·bi·tol
ri·bi·tyl
ri·bo·fla·vin
r. ki·nase
meth·yl·ol r.
ri·bo·fla·vin
de·fi·cien·cy
unit

ri·bo·fla·vine
ri·bo·fu·ra·nose
ri·bo·fu·ran·o·syl·thy·mine
ri·bo·nu·cle·ase
al·ka·line
al·pha
Esch·e·rich·ia co·li   I
mi·cro·bi·al   II
pan·cre·at·ic
plant
yeast
ri·bo·nu·cle·ase (Ba·cil·lus sub·ti·lis)
ri·bo·nu·cle·ase (pan·cre·at·ic)
ri·bo·nu·cle·ic ac·id
het·er·o·ge·neous
in·for·ma·tion·al
mes·sen·ger
nu·cle·ar
pol·y·mer·ase
ri·bo·som·al
sol·u·ble
tem·plate
trans·fer
ri·bo·nu·cle·i·nase
ri·bo·nu·cle·o·pro·tein
ri·bo·nu·cle·o·side
ri·bo·nu·cle·o·tide
ri·bo·pyr·a·nose
ri·bose
ri·bo·side
ri·bo·som·al
RNA
ri·bo·some
ri·bo·some-la·mel·la
com·plex
ri·bo·su·ria
ri·bo·syl
ri·bo·syl·pur·ine
ri·bo·thy·mi·dine
ri·bo·thy·mi·dyl·ic ac·id
ri·bo·tide
ri·bo·vi·rus
ri·bu·lose
ri·bu·lose-bis·phos·phate car·box·yl·ase
Riccò's
law
rice
body
itch
rice·field
fe·ver
rice-Tween
agar
rice-wa·ter
stool

Richard's
  fring·es
Richards-Rundel
  syn·drome
Richter-Monro
  line
Richter's
  her·nia
  syn·drome
ri·cin
ric·i·nism
ri·cin·o·le·ate
ri·cin·o·le·ic ac·id
Ric·i·nus
rick·ets
  acute r.
  adult r.
  ce·li·ac r.
  hem·or·rhag·ic r.
  late r.
  re·nal r.
  scur·vy r.
  vi·ta·min D-re·sis·tant r.
Rick·ett·sia
  R. akari
  R. aus·tra·lis
  R. bur·ne·tii
  R. co·no·ri
  R. co·no·rii
  R. pro·wa·ze·kii
  R. psit·ta·ci
  R. rick·ett·sii
  R. ru·mi·nan·ti·um
  R. si·bi·ri·ca
  R. tsu·tsu·ga·mu·shi
  R. ty·phi
rick·ett·sia
  vac·cine, at·ten·u·at·ed
rick·ett·si·al
rick·ett·si·al·pox
rick·ett·si·o·sis
  ve·sic·u·lar r.
rick·ett·si·o·stat·ic
rick·e·ty
Rickles
  test
Rida
  vi·rus
Rideal-Walker
  co·ef·fi·cient
  meth·od
Ridell's
  op·er·a·tion
rid·er's
  bone
  bur·sa
  leg
  mus·cles

ridge
  ex·ten·sion
  re·la·tion
  re·sorp·tion
ridge
  al·ve·o·lar r.
  ap·i·cal ec·to·der·mal r.
  ba·sal r.
  bi·cip·i·tal r.'s
  buc·co·cer·vi·cal r.
  buc·co·gin·gi·val r.
  bul·bar r.
  bul·bo·ven·tric·u·lar r.
  den·tal r.
  ep·i·der·mal r.'s
  ep·i·per·i·car·di·al r.
  ex·ter·nal ob·lique r.
  gan·gli·on r.
  gen·i·tal r.
  glu·te·al r.
  go·nad·al r.
  in·ter·pap·il·lary r.'s
  key r.
  lat·er·al ep·i·con·dy·lar r.
  lat·er·al su·pra·con·dy·lar r.
  lin·guo·cer·vi·cal r.
  lin·guo·gin·gi·val r.
  Mall's r.'s
  mam·ma·ry r.
  mar·gi·nal r.
  me·di·al ep·i·con·dy·lar r.
  me·di·al su·pra·con·dy·lar
    r.
  mes·o·neph·ric r.
  milk r.
  my·lo·hy·oid r.
  na·sal r.
  ob·lique r.
  ob·lique r. of tra·pe·zi·um
  pal·a·tine r.
  Passavant's r.
  pec·to·ral r.
  prim·i·tive r.
  pro·na·tor r.
  pter·y·goid r. of sphe·noid
    bone
  pul·mo·nary r.'s
  re·sid·u·al r.
  re·te r.'s
  skin r.'s
  su·per·cil·i·ary r.
  sup·ple·men·tal r.
  su·pra·or·bit·al r.
  taste r.
  tem·po·ral r.
  trans·verse r.
  trans·verse pal·a·tine r.
  trap·e·zoid r.

tri·an·gu·lar r.
uro·gen·i·tal r.
wolff·i·an r.
rid·ing
em·bo·lism
Ridley's
cir·cle
si·nus
Riedel's
dis·ease
lobe
stru·ma
thy·roid·i·tis
Rieder
cells
Rieder cell
leu·ke·mia
Rieder's
lym·pho·cyte
Riegel's
pulse
Rieger's
anom·a·ly
syn·drome
Riehl's
mel·a·no·sis
ri·fam·pi·cin
rif·am·pin
rif·a·my·cin
rif·o·my·cin
Rift Val·ley
fe·ver
Rift Val·ley fe·ver
vi·rus
Riga-Fede
dis·ease
right
atri·um
au·ri·cle
crus of atri·o·ven·tric·u·lar
trunk
crus of di·a·phragm
duct of cau·date lobe
heart
lobe
lobe of liv·er
mar·gin of heart
part
plate of thy·roid car·ti·lage
ven·tri·cle
right atri·o·ven·tric·u·lar
valve
right au·ric·u·lar
ap·pend·age
right ax·is
de·vi·a·tion
right col·ic
ar·tery

flex·ure
vein
right col·ic lymph
nodes
right cor·o·nary
ar·tery
right-eyed
right fi·brous
tri·gone
right-foot·ed
right gas·tric
ar·tery
vein
right gas·tric lymph
nodes
right gas·tro·ep·i·plo·ic
ar·tery
vein
right gas·tro·ep·i·plo·ic lymph
nodes
right gas·tro·o·men·tal
vein
right gas·tro-o·men·tal
ar·tery
right gas·tro-o·men·tal lymph
nodes
right-hand·ed
right he·pa·tic
duct
veins
right in·fe·ri·or pul·mo·nary
vein
right·ing
re·flex·es
right lum·bar lymph
nodes
right lym·phat·ic
duct
right main
bron·chus
right ovar·i·an
vein
right ovar·i·an vein
syn·drome
right pul·mo·nary
ar·tery
right sag·it·tal
fis·sure
right su·pe·ri·or in·ter·cos·tal
vein
right su·pe·ri·or pul·mo·nary
vein
right su·pra·re·nal
vein
right tes·tic·u·lar
vein
right-to-left
shunt

right tri·an·gu·lar
  lig·a·ment
right ven·tric·u·lar
  fail·ure
  hy·po·pla·sia
rig·id
  pu·pil
ri·gid·i·ty
  an·a·tom·ic r.
  ca·dav·er·ic r.
  cat·a·ton·ic r.
  cer·e·bel·lar r.
  clasp-knife r.
  cog·wheel r.
  de·cer·e·brate r.
  lead-pipe r.
  myd·ri·at·ic r.
  oc·u·lar r.
  path·o·log·ic r.
  post·mor·tem r.
  scle·ral r.
rig·or
  ac·id r.
  cal·ci·um r.
  heat r.
  r. mor·tis
  my·o·car·di·al r. mor·tis
Riley-Day
  syn·drome
rim
  bite r.
  oc·clu·sal r.
  oc·clu·sion r.
  rec·ord r.
ri·ma
  r. res·pi·ra·tor·ia
  r. vo·ca·lis
  r. vul·vae
ri·mae
Rimini's
  test
ri·mose
rim·u·la
rin·der·pest
  vi·rus
Rindfleisch's
  cells
  folds
ring
  ab·scess
  chro·mo·some
  com·pound
  fin·ger
  lig·a·ment
  pes·sa·ry
  sco·to·ma
  sy·ringe

  test
  ul·cer of cor·nea
ring
  ab·dom·i·nal r.
  am·ni·on r.
  an·te·ri·or lim·it·ing r.
  Bandl's r.
  ben·zene r.
  Bickel's r.
  Cannon's r.
  car·di·ac lym·phat·ic r.
  cast·ing r.
  cho·roi·dal r.
  cil·i·ary r.
  com·mon ten·di·nous r.
  con·junc·ti·val r.
  con·stric·tion r.
  cru·ral r.
  deep in·gui·nal r.
  Donders' r.'s
  ex·ter·nal in·gui·nal r.
  fem·o·ral r.
  fi·bro·car·ti·lag·i·nous r.
  fi·brous r.
  Fleischer's r.
  Flieringa's r.
  glau·co·ma·tous r.
  Graefenberg r.
  Imlach's r.
  in·ter·nal in·gui·nal r.
  r. of iris
  Kayser-Fleischer r.
  Liesegang r.'s
  Lower's r.
  Löwe's r.
  lym·phat·ic r. of car·dia
  lym·phoid r.
  Maxwell's r.
  ne·o·na·tal r.
  path·o·log·ic re·trac·tion r.
  phys·i·o·log·ic re·trac·tion r.
  po·lar r.
  pre·pu·ti·al r.
  Schatzki's r.
  Schwalbe's r.
  scle·ral r.
  sig·net r.
  r. of Soemmering
  sub·cu·ta·ne·ous r.
  su·per·fi·cial in·gui·nal r.
  ton·sil·lar r.
  tra·che·al r.
  tym·pan·ic r.
  um·bil·i·cal r.
  vas·cu·lar r.
  Vieussens' r.
  Vossius' len·tic·u·lar r.

Waldeyer's throat r.
Zinn's r.
ring·bone
false r.
ringed
hair
Ringer's
in·jec·tion
so·lu·tion
ring-knife
ring-like cor·ne·al
dys·tro·phy
ring pre·cip·i·tin
test
ring-wall
le·sion
ring·worm
yaws
ring·worm
r. of beard
black-dot r.
r. of body
crust·ed r.
r. of foot
r. of gen·i·to·cru·ral re·gion
hon·ey·comb r.
hy·per·tro·phic r.
r. of nails
Or·i·en·tal r.
r. of scalp
scaly r.
To·ke·lau r.
Rinne's
test
Riolan's
anas·to·mo·sis
ar·cade
bones
bou·quet
mus·cle
ri·par·i·an
Ripault's
sign
ripe
cat·a·ract
rip·en·ing
rise
time
risk
fac·tor
risk
em·pir·ic r.
re·cur·rence r.
Risley's ro·ta·ry
prism
ri·so·ri·us
mus·cle
ris·to·ce·tin

ri·sus ca·ni·nus
ri·sus sar·do·ni·cus
Ritgen's
ma·neu·ver
ri·to·drine
Ritter-Rollet
phe·nom·e·non
Ritter's
dis·ease
law
Ritter's open·ing
tet·a·nus
rit·u·al
rit·u·al·is·tic
be·hav·ior
ri·val·ry
bin·oc·u·lar r.
r. of ret·i·na
sib·ling r.
Riv·ea co·rym·bo·sa
riv·er
blind·ness
Rivero-Carvallo
ef·fect
Rivers'
cock·tail
Rivière's
salt
Rivinus'
ca·nals
ducts
gland
in·ci·sure
mem·brane
notch
ri·vus la·cri·ma·lis
riz·i·form
RNA
vi·rus
RNA splic·ing
RNA tu·mor
vi·rus·es
Roach
clasp
Roaf's
syn·drome
roar·ing
Roberts
syn·drome
Robert's
pel·vis
Robertshaw
tube
Robertson
pu·pil
ro·bert·so·ni·an
trans·lo·ca·tion

Robin's
syn·drome
Robinson
cath·e·ter
in·dex
Robinson's
dis·ease
Robison
es·ter
Robison-Embden
es·ter
Robison es·ter
de·hy·dro·gen·ase
Robles'
dis·ease
ro·bot·ic
roc·cel·lin
Ro·cha·li·maea
Ro·chelle
salt
Rocher's
sign
rock·et
im·mu·no·e·lec·tro·pho·re·sis
rock oil
Rocky Moun·tain spot·ted
fe·ver
Rocky Moun·tain spot·ted fe·ver
vac·cine
rod
achro·ma·top·sia
cell of ret·i·na
disks
fi·ber
gran·ule
mon·o·chro·ma·sy
my·op·a·thy
vi·sion
rod
an·a·lyz·ing r.
Auer r.'s
ba·sal r.
Corti's r.'s
enam·el r.'s
ger·mi·nal r.
Maddox's r.
ro·dent
ul·cer
Ro·den·tia
ro·den·ti·cide
rod nu·cle·ar
cell
ro·don·al·gia
Roenne's na·sal
step

roent·gen
ray
unit
roent·gen
r.-equiv·a·lent-man
r.-equiv·a·lent-phys·i·cal
roent·ge·nism
roent·gen·i·za·tion
roent·gen·ky·mo·gram
roent·gen·ky·mo·graph
roent·gen·ky·mog·ra·phy
roent·gen·o·gram
ceph·a·lo·met·ric r.
lat·er·al ob·lique r.
lat·er·al ra·mus r.
lat·er·al skull r.
max·il·lary si·nus r.
ob·lique lat·er·al jaw r.
pan·o·ram·ic r.
per·i·ap·i·cal r.
scout r.
sub·men·tal ver·tex r.
Towne pro·jec·tion r.
trans·cra·ni·al r.
Waters' view r.
roent·gen·o·graph
roent·gen·og·ra·phy
mu·co·sal re·lief r.
sec·tion·al r.
se·ri·al r.
spot-film r.
roent·gen·ol·o·gist
roent·gen·ol·o·gy
roent·gen·om·e·ter
roent·gen·om·e·try
roent·gen·o·scope
roent·gen·os·co·py
roent·gen·o·ther·a·py
roeth·eln
Roger-Anderson pin fix·a·tion
ap·pli·ance
Rogers'
sphyg·mo·ma·nom·e·ter
Roger's
dis·ease
mur·mur
re·flex
Röhrer's
in·dex
Rohr's
stri·a
Rokitansky-Aschoff
si·nus·es
Rokitansky-Küster-Hauser
syn·drome
Rokitansky's
dis·ease

her·nia
pel·vis
ro·lan·dic
ep·i·lep·sy
Rolando's
an·gle
ar·ea
cells
col·umn
sub·stance
tu·ber·cle
Rolando's ge·lat·i·nous
sub·stance
role
con·flict
role
com·ple·men·ta·ry r.
gen·der r.
non·com·ple·men·ta·ry r.
sex r.
sick r.
role-play·ing
ro·li·tet·ra·cy·cline
roll
il·i·ac r.
scle·ral r.
roll
sul·fur
tube
roll·er
ban·dage
Roller's
nu·cle·us
Rolleston's
rule
Rollet's
stro·ma
roll-tube
cul·ture
Ro·man
fe·ver
Romaña's
sign
Romano-Ward
syn·drome
Romanowsky's blood
stain
Romberg
test
Romberg-Howship
symp·tom
rom·berg·ism
Romberg's
dis·ease
sign
symp·tom
syn·drome
troph·o·neu·ro·sis

Römer's
test
ron·geur
R-on-T
phe·nom·e·non
roof
nu·cle·us
plate
roof
r. of fourth ven·tri·cle
r. of mouth
r. of or·bit
r. of skull
r. of tym·pa·num
roof·plate
room
tem·per·a·ture
root
ab·scess
am·pu·ta·tion
apex
ca·nal of tooth
car·ies
de·his·cence
fil·a·ments
fo·ra·men
re·sec·tion
re·sorp·tion
sheath
tip
root
an·a·tom·i·cal r.
an·te·ri·or r.
clin·i·cal r.
co·chle·ar r. of ves·tib·u·
lo·co·chle·ar nerve
con·joined nerve r.
cra·ni·al r.'s
dor·sal r.
fa·cial r.
r. of fa·cial nerve
r. of foot
hair r.
in·fe·ri·or r.
in·fe·ri·or r. of cer·vi·cal
loop
in·fe·ri·or r. of ves·tib·u·
lo·co·chle·ar nerve
lat·er·al r. of me·di·an
nerve
lat·er·al r. of op·tic tract
long r. of cil·i·ary gan·gli·
on
r. of lung
me·di·al r. of me·di·an
nerve
me·di·al r. of op·tic tract
r. of mes·en·try

root *(continued)*
 mo·tor r. of cil·i·ary gan·
  gli·on
 mo·tor r. of tri·gem·i·nal
  nerve
 r. of nail
 na·so·cil·i·ary r.
 nerve r.
 r. of nose
 ol·fac·to·ry r.'s
 r.'s of ol·fac·to·ry tract,
  lat·er·al and me·di·al
 par·a·sym·pa·thet·ic r. of
  cil·i·ary gan·gli·on
 r. of pe·nis
 pos·te·ri·or r.
 sen·so·ry r. of cil·i·ary
  gan·gli·on
 sen·so·ry r. of tri·gem·i·nal
  nerve
 short r. of cil·i·ary gan·gli·
  on
 spi·nal r.'s
 su·pe·ri·or r.
 su·pe·ri·or r. of cer·vi·cal
  loop
 su·pe·ri·or r. of ves·tib·u·
  lo·co·chle·ar nerve
 sym·pa·thet·ic r. of cil·i·ary
  gan·gli·on
 r. of tongue
 r. of tooth
 r.'s of tri·gem·i·nal nerve
 tu·ber·ous r.
 ven·tral r.
 ves·tib·u·lar r. of ves·tib·u·
  lo·co·chle·ar nerve
root ca·nal
 file
 or·i·fice
 plug·ger
 res·to·ra·tion
 spread·er
 ther·a·py
 treat·ment
root car·ies
 in·dex
root end
 cyst
 gran·u·lo·ma
root·ing
 re·flex
root·lets
root plan·ing
ro·pal·o·cy·to·sis
rope
 burn
 flap

Ropes
 test
Rorschach
 test
Ro·sa
ro·sa·cea
 hy·per·tro·phic r.
ro·sa·cea-like
 tu·ber·cu·lid
ros·an·i·lin
 dyes
ro·sa·ry
 ra·chit·ic r.
Roscoe-Bunsen
 law
rose
 cold
 spots
rose
 r. oil
rose ben·gal
Rose-Bradford
 kid·ney
rose·mary oil
Rosenbach-Gmelin
 test
Rosenbach's
 dis·ease
 law
 sign
 test
Rosenmüller's
 fos·sa
 gland
 node
 re·cess
 valve
Rosenthal
 fi·ber
Rosenthaler-Turk
 re·a·gent
Rosenthal's
 ca·nal
 vein
ro·se·o·la
 ep·i·dem·ic r.
 id·i·o·path·ic r.
 r. in·fan·ti·lis
 r. in·fan·tum
 syph·i·lit·ic r.
ro·se·o·lous
Roser-Nélaton
 line
Rose's
 po·si·tion
Rose's ce·phal·ic
 tet·a·nus

ro·sette
  Wintersteiner r.'s
ro·sette-form·ing
  cells
Rose-Waaler
  test
ros·in
p-ro·so·lic ac·id
Ross-Jones
  test
Rossolimo's
  re·flex
  sign
Ross River
  fe·ver
  vi·rus
ros·tel·lum
  armed r.
  un·armed r.
ros·tra
ros·trad
ros·tral
  lam·i·na
  lay·er
  neu·ro·pore
ros·tra·lis
ros·tral trans·ten·to·ri·al
  her·ni·a·tion
ros·trate
  pel·vis
ros·tri·form
ros·trum
ros·trums
rot
  Bar·coo r.
  foot r.
ro·tam·e·ter
ro·ta·ry
  joint
  ver·ti·go
ro·ta·tion
  cen·ter
  flap
ro·ta·tion
  in·tes·ti·nal r.
  mo·lec·u·lar r.
  op·ti·cal r.
  spe·cif·ic r.
ro·ta·tion·al
  ax·is
  nys·tag·mus
ro·ta·tor
  cuff of shoul·der
  mus·cles
ro·ta·tor
  me·di·al r.
ro·ta·to·ry
  joint

nys·tag·mus
  spasm
  tic
ro·ta·vi·rus
Rotch's
  sign
rote
  learn·ing
röt·eln
ro·te·none
Roth-Bernhardt
  dis·ease
Roth·era's ni·tro·prus·side
  test
Roth·ia
Rothmund's
  syn·drome
Rothmund-Thomson
  syn·drome
Roth's
  dis·ease
  spots
  vas aber·rans
Rotor's
  syn·drome
ro·to·sco·li·o·sis
ro·to·tome
ro·tox·a·mine
Rouget
  cell
Rouget-Neumann
  sheath
Rouget's
  bulb
  mus·cle
rough
  col·o·ny
rough·age
rough-sur·faced en·do·plas·mic
  re·tic·u·lum
Roughton-Scholander
  ap·pa·ra·tus
  sy·ringe
Rougnon-Heberden
  dis·ease
rou·leaux
  for·ma·tion
round
  at·el·ec·ta·sis
  bur
  em·i·nence
  fo·ra·men
  lig·a·ment of el·bow joint
  lig·a·ment of fe·mur
  lig·a·ment of liv·er
  lig·a·ment of uter·us
  pel·vis
  win·dow

round cell
  sar·co·ma
round pro·na·tor
  mus·cle
round·worm
Rous
  sar·co·ma
  tu·mor
Rous-as·so·ci·at·ed
  vi·rus
Rous sar·co·ma
  vi·rus
Roussy-Lévy
  dis·ease
  syn·drome
Roux
  spat·u·la
Roux-en-Y
  anas·to·mo·sis
  op·er·a·tion
Roux's
  meth·od
  stain
Rovsing's
  sign
Rowntree and Geraghty
  test
RPR
  test
R-R
  in·ter·val
Rs
  vi·rus
RST
  seg·ment
rub
  fric·tion r.
  per·i·car·di·al r.
  per·i·car·di·al fric·tion r.
  pleu·rit·ic r.
Rubarth's dis·ease
  vi·rus
rub·ber
  dam
  pel·vis
  tis·sue
rub·ber-bulb
  sy·ringe
rub·ber dam
  clamp
rub·ber dam clamp
  for·ceps
rub·ber po·lice·man
rub·bing
  al·co·hol
ru·be·an·ic ac·id
ru·be·do
ru·be·fa·cient

ru·be·fac·tion
ru·bel·la
  cat·a·ract
  ret·i·nop·a·thy
  vi·rus
ru·bel·la HI
  test
ru·bel·la vi·rus
  vac·cine, live
ru·bel·lin
ru·be·o·la
  vi·rus
ru·be·o·sis
  r. ir·i·dis di·a·be·ti·ca
ru·bes·cent
ru·bid·i·um
Rubin
  test
ru·bine
ru·bin S
Rubinstein-Taybi
  syn·drome
Ru·bi·vi·rus
Rubner's
  laws of growth
  test
ru·bor
ru·bra·tox·in
ru·bre·dox·ins
ru·bri·blast
  per·ni·cious ane·mia type r.
ru·bri·cyte
ru·bro·bul·bar
  tract
ru·bro·re·tic·u·lar
  tract
ru·bro·spi·nal
  de·cus·sa·tion
  tract
ru·by
  spots
ruc·tus
ru·di·ment
ru·di·men·ta
ru·di·men·ta·ry
ru·di·men·tum
  r. hip·po·cam·pi
Rud's
  syn·drome
Ruffini's
  cor·pus·cles
ru·fous
  al·bi·nism
ru·ga
  r. gas·tri·ca
  r. pa·la·ti·na
ru·gae
ru·gine

ru·gi·tus
ru·gose
ru·gos·i·ty
ru·gous
rule
   Abegg's r.
   Amer·i·can Law In·sti·tute r.
   r. of bi·gem·i·ny
   Clark's weight r.
   Cowling's r.
   Durham r.
   Goriaew's r.
   Haase's r.
   His' r.
   iso·prene r.
   Jackson's r.
   Le Bel-van't Hoff r.
   Liebermeister's r.
   M'Naghten r.
   Nägele's r.
   New Hampshire r.
   Ogino-Knaus r.
   r. of out·let
   phase r.
   Prentice's r.
   Rolleston's r.
   Schütz r.
   Young's r.
rul·er
   iso·met·ric r.
rum
   nose
rum-blos·som
ru·men
ru·men·i·tis
ru·men·ot·o·my
ru·mi·na
ru·mi·nant
ru·mi·na·tion
ru·mi·na·tive
ru·mi·no·re·tic·u·lum
Rumpel-Leede
   sign
   test
run·a·round
Runeberg's
   for·mu·la
run·round
runt
   dis·ease
ru·pia
   r. es·cha·ro·ti·ca
ru·pi·al
   syph·i·lid
ru·pi·oid

rup·ture
rup·tured
   disk
ru·ral cu·ta·ne·ous
   leish·man·i·a·sis
Russell
   bod·ies
   ef·fect
   trac·tion
Russell's
   sign
   syn·drome
   vi·per
Russell's Per·i·o·don·tal In·dex
Russell's vi·per
   ven·om
Rus·sian
   fly
Rus·sian au·tumn
   en·ceph·a·li·tis
Rus·sian au·tumn en·ceph·a·li·tis
   vi·rus
Rus·sian spring-sum·mer
   en·ceph·a·li·tis (East·ern sub·type)
   en·ceph·a·li·tis (West·ern sub·type)
Rus·sian spring-sum·mer en·ceph·a·li·tis
   vi·rus
Rus·sian tick-borne
   en·ceph·a·li·tis
Rust's
   dis·ease
   phe·nom·e·non
rusts
rusty
   spu·tum
ru·the·ni·um
ru·the·ni·um red
ruth·er·ford
ru·ti·do·sis
ru·tin
ru·tin·ose
ru·to·side
Ruysch's
   mem·brane
   mus·cle
   tube
   veins
Rye
   clas·si·fi·ca·tion
rye smut
Ryle's
   tube

S

S

an·ti·gen
fac·tor
pep·tide
phase
po·ten·tial
pro·tein
unit of strep·to·my·cin
wave
sab·a·dil·la
sa·ber
shin
tib·ia
Sabin
vac·cine
Sabin-Feldman dye
test
sa·bot
heart
Sabouraud-Noiré
in·stru·ment
Sabouraud's
agar
pas·tils
sab·u·lous
sa·bur·ra
sa·bur·ral
am·au·ro·sis
sac
ab·dom·i·nal s.
air s.
al·lan·to·ic s.
al·ve·o·lar s.
am·ni·ot·ic s.
anal s.
an·eu·rys·mal s.
aor·tic s.
cho·ri·on·ic s.
con·junc·ti·val s.
cu·pu·lar blind s.
den·tal s.
en·do·lym·phat·ic s.
heart s.
her·nial s.
Hilton's s.
lac·ri·mal s.
less·er per·i·to·ne·al s.
lymph s.'s

na·sal s.'s
omen·tal s.
pre·pu·ti·al s.
pu·den·dal s.
tear s.
tooth s.
ves·tib·u·lar blind s.
vi·tel·line s.
yolk s.
sac·brood
sac·cad·ic
move·ment
sac·cate
sac·cha·rase
sac·cha·rate
sac·char·eph·i·dro·sis
sac·char·ic
sac·char·ic ac·id
sac·cha·rides
sac·cha·rif·er·ous
sac·char·i·fi·ca·tion
sac·char·i·fy
sac·cha·rim·e·ter
sac·cha·rin
sac·cha·rine
sac·cha·ro·gen am·y·lase
sac·cha·ro·lyt·ic
sac·cha·ro·met·a·bol·ic
sac·cha·ro·me·tab·o·lism
sac·cha·rom·e·ter
Sac·cha·ro·my·ces
Sac·cha·ro·my·ce·ta·ce·ae
Sac·cha·ro·my·ce·ta·les
sac·cha·ror·rhea
sac·cha·rose
sac·cha·ro·su·ria
sac·cha·rum
s. can·a·dense
s. lac·tis
sac·ci
sac·ci·form
re·cess
sac·cu·lar
an·eu·rysm
bron·chi·ec·ta·sis
gland
nerve
spot

sac·cu·lat·ed
  an·eu·rysm
  pleu·ri·sy
sac·cu·la·tion
sac·cule
  s. of lar·ynx
sac·cu·li
sac·cu·lo·co·chle·ar
sac·cu·lus
  sac·cu·li al·ve·o·la·res
  s. al·ve·o·la·ris
  s. com·mu·nis
  s. en·do·lym·pha·ti·cus
  s. la·cri·ma·lis
  s. pro·pri·us
  s. ves·tib·u·li
sac·cus
  s. re·u·ni·ens
  s. va·gi·na·lis
Sachs'
  ba·cil·lus
Sachs-Georgi
  test
sa·cra
sa·crad
sa·cral
  an·es·the·sia
  ca·nal
  crest
  flex·ure
  flex·ure of rec·tum
  fo·ra·men
  gan·glia
  hi·a·tus
  horn
  in·dex
  nerves
  part of spi·nal cord
  plex·us
  re·gion
  tri·an·gle
  tu·ber·os·i·ty
  veins
  ver·te·brae
sa·cral·gia
sa·cral·i·za·tion
sa·cral lymph
  nodes
sa·cral splanch·nic
  nerves
sa·cral ve·nous
  plex·us
sa·crec·to·my
sa·cred
  bone
sa·cro·an·te·ri·or
  po·si·tion

sa·cro·coc·cyg·e·al
  disk
  joint
  junc·tion
sa·cro·coc·cyg·e·us
sa·cro·du·ral
  lig·a·ment
sa·cro·dyn·ia
sa·cro·gen·i·tal
  folds
sa·cro·il·i·ac
  ar·tic·u·la·tion
  joint
sa·cro·il·i·i·tis
sa·cro·lis·the·sis
sa·cro·lum·ba·lis
sa·cro·lum·bar
sa·cro·pel·vic
  sur·face of il·i·um
sa·cro·pos·te·ri·or
  po·si·tion
sa·cro·sci·at·ic
  notch
sa·cro·spi·nal
sa·cro·spi·nous
  lig·a·ment
sa·crot·o·my
sa·cro·trans·verse
  po·si·tion
sa·cro·tu·ber·ous
  lig·a·ment
sa·cro·ver·te·bral
sa·crum
  as·sim·i·la·tion s.
sad·dle
  Turk·ish s.
sad·dle
  back
  em·bo·lism
  head
  joint
  nose
sad·dle block
  an·es·the·sia
sa·dism
sa·dist
sa·dis·tic
sa·do·mas·och·ism
sa·do·mas·och·is·tic
  re·la·tion·ship
Saemisch's
  op·er·a·tion
  sec·tion
  ul·cer
Saenger
  pu·pil
Saenger's
  mac·u·la

op·er·a·tion
sign
safe
pe·ri·od
safe·ty
lens
spec·ta·cles
saf·flow·er
saf·flow·er oil
saf·fron
mead·ow s.
saf·ra·nin O
saf·ra·no·phil
saf·ra·no·phile
saf·role
sage
sa·git·ta
sag·it·tal
ax·is
bor·der
crest
fon·ta·nel
groove
line
plane
sec·tion
sul·cus
su·ture
sa·git·ta·lis
sag·it·tal split man·dib·u·lar
os·te·ot·o·my
sa·go
spleen
Sai·gon
cin·na·mon
sail
sound
sail·or's
skin
Saint Anthony's
dance
Saint Ignatius'
itch
Saint John's
dance
Sainton's
sign
Saint's
tri·ad
Saint Vitus
dance
Sakaguchi
re·ac·tion
sa·ku·shu
fe·ver
sal
s. alem·broth
s. am·mo·ni·ac

s. di·u·re·ti·cum
s. so·da
s. vol·a·tile
sa·laam
at·tack
con·vul·sions
spasm
Salah's ster·nal punc·ture
nee·dle
sal·bu·ta·mol
sales
sal·i·cin
sal·i·cyl
s. al·co·hol
s. al·de·hyde
sal·i·cyl·am·ide
sal·i·cyl·an·i·lide
sa·lic·y·late
sa·lic·y·lat·ed
sal·i·cyl·az·o·sul·fa·pyr·i·dine
sal·i·cyl·ic ac·id
col·lo·di·on
sal·i·cyl·ic al·de·hyde
sal·i·cyl·ism
sal·i·cyl·ize
sal·i·cyl·sal·i·cyl·ic ac·id
sal·i·cyl·sul·fon·ic ac·id
sal·i·cyl·u·ric ac·id
sa·lient
pul·mo·nary s.
sal·i·fi·a·ble
sal·i·fy
sal·i·gen·in
sal·i·gen·ol
sa·lim·e·ter
sa·line
phys·i·o·log·i·cal s.
sa·line
ag·glu·ti·nin
pur·ga·tive
so·lu·tion
wa·ter
sa·li·nom·e·ter
Salis·bury com·mon cold
vi·rus·es
sa·li·va
ejec·tor
pump
sa·li·va
chor·da s.
gan·gli·on·ic s.
rest·ing s.
sym·pa·thet·ic s.
sal·i·vant
sal·i·vary
cal·cu·lus
col·ic
cor·pus·cle

sal·i·vary *(continued)*
  di·ges·tion
  duct
  fis·tu·la
  gland
  gland of ab·do·men
  vi·rus
sal·i·vary gland
  hor·mone
  vi·rus
sal·i·vary gland vi·rus
  dis·ease
sal·i·vate
sal·i·va·tion
sal·i·va·tor
sa·li·vo·li·thi·a·sis
Salk
  vac·cine
salm·on
  dis·ease
  patch
  poi·son·ing
Sal·mo·nel·la
  S. abor·ti·vo·e·quina
  S. abor·tus-o·vis
  S. chol·er·ae-suis
  S. en·ter·it·i·dis
  S. gal·li·na·rum
  S. hirsch·fel·dii
  S. pa·ra·ty·phi
  S. schott·mül·leri
  S. ty·phi
  S. ty·phi·mu·ri·um
  S. ty·pho·sa
Sal·mo·nel·la food
  poi·son·ing
sal·mo·nel·lo·sis
sal·ol
sal·pin·gec·to·my
  ab·dom·i·nal s.
sal·pin·gem·phrax·is
sal·pin·ges
sal·pin·gi·an
sal·pin·gi·o·ma
sal·pin·git·ic
sal·pin·gi·tis
  chron·ic in·ter·sti·tial s.
  for·eign body s.
  gon·or·rhe·al s.
  s. isth·mi·ca no·do·sa
  py·o·gen·ic s.
sal·pin·go·cele
sal·pin·go·cy·e·sis
sal·pin·gog·ra·phy
sal·pin·gol·y·sis
sal·pin·go-o·o·pho·rec·to·my
  ab·dom·i·nal s.
sal·pin·go-o·o·pho·ri·tis

sal·pin·go-o·oph·o·ro·cele
sal·pin·go-o·var·i·ec·to·my
sal·pin·go·pal·a·tine
  fold
sal·pin·go·per·i·to·ni·tis
sal·pin·go·pexy
sal·pin·go·pha·ryn·ge·al
  fold
  mus·cle
sal·pin·go·pha·ryn·ge·us
sal·pin·go·plas·ty
sal·pin·gor·rha·gia
sal·pin·gor·rha·phy
sal·pin·gos·co·py
sal·pin·go·sto·mat·o·my
sal·pin·gos·to·my
sal·pin·got·o·my
  ab·dom·i·nal s.
sal·pinx
salt
  ac·id s.
  ar·ti·fi·cial Carlsbad s.
  ar·ti·fi·cial Kis·sin·gen s.
  ar·ti·fi·cial Vichy s.
  ba·sic s.
  bile s.'s
  bone s.
  com·mon s.
  di·a·zo·ni·um s.'s
  dou·ble s.
  ef·fer·ves·cent s.'s
  Ep·som s.'s
  Glauber's s.
  hex·a·zo·ni·um s.'s
  Rivière's s.
  Ro·chelle s.
  Seignette's s.
  smell·ing s.'s
  ta·ble s.
  tet·ra·zo·ni·um s.'s
  s. of wis·dom
salt
  ac·tion
  de·ple·tion
  dye
  ede·ma
  fe·ver
  load·ing
  poi·son·ing
  sen·si·tiv·i·ty
  so·lu·tion
  wast·ing
sal·ta·tion
sal·ta·to·ry
  cho·rea
  con·duc·tion
  ev·o·lu·tion
  spasm

salt de·ple·tion
syn·drome
salt·ed
plas·ma
se·rum
Salter-Harris
clas·si·fi·ca·tion of ep·i·
phys·i·al frac·tures
Salter's in·cre·men·tal
lines
salt·ing out
salt-los·ing
ne·phri·tis
salt·pe·ter
Chil·e·an s.
salt sub·sti·tute
salt wa·ter
boils
soap
sa·lu·bri·ous
sal·u·re·sis
sal·u·ret·ic
sal·u·ta·ri·um
sal·u·tary
sal·vage
che·mo·ther·a·py
Sal·var·san
salve
sal·via
Salzmann's nod·u·lar cor·ne·al
de·gen·er·a·tion
sa·mar·i·um
sam·bu·cus
sam·ple
end-tid·al s.
Haldane-Priestley s.
Rahn-Otis s.
ran·dom s.
Sanarelli
phe·nom·e·non
Sanarelli-Shwartzman
phe·nom·e·non
san·a·tive
san·a·to·ri·um
san·a·to·ry
Sanchez Sa·lo·rio
syn·drome
sand
bath
bod·ies
tu·mor
sand
brain s.
hy·da·tid s.
in·tes·ti·nal s.
uri·nary s.
san·dal
foot

san·dal strap
der·ma·ti·tis
san·dal·wood oil
sand-crack
sand·fly
fe·ver
sand·fly fe·ver
vi·rus·es
Sand·hoff's
dis·ease
Sandison-Clark
cham·ber
sand·pa·per
disks
gall·blad·der
Sandström's
bod·ies
sand·worm
dis·ease
sane
Sanfilippo's
syn·drome
Sanger's
re·a·gent
san·gui·fa·ci·ent
san·guif·er·ous
san·gui·fi·ca·tion
san·guin·a·rine
san·guine
san·guin·e·ous
cyst
san·guin·o·lent
san·gui·no·pu·ru·lent
san·guis
San·gui·su·ga
san·guiv·or·ous
sa·ni·es
sa·ni·o·pu·ru·lent
sa·ni·o·se·rous
sa·ni·ous
pus
san·i·tar·i·an
san·i·tar·i·um
san·i·tary
san·i·ta·tion
san·i·ti·za·tion
san·i·ty
San Joaquin
fe·ver
San Mi·guel sea li·on
vi·rus
Sansom's
sign
Sanson's
im·ag·es
san·tal oil
Santini's boom·ing
sound

san·to·nin
Santorini's
  ca·nal
  car·ti·lage
  con·cha
  duct
  fis·sures
  in·ci·sures
  lab·y·rinth
  mus·cle
  tu·ber·cle
  vein
Santorini's ma·jor
  ca·run·cle
Santorini's mi·nor
  ca·run·cle
São Pau·lo
  fe·ver
sap
  nu·cle·ar s.
sa·phe·na
saph·e·nec·to·my
sa·phe·nous
  nerve
  open·ing
  veins
sap·o·gen·in
sap·o·na·ceous
sap·o·na·tus
sa·pon·i·fi·ca·tion
  num·ber
sa·pon·i·fy
sap·o·nins
Sappey's
  fi·bers
  plex·us
  veins
sap·phism
sa·pre·mia
sap·robe
sa·pro·bic
sap·ro·don·tia
sap·ro·gen
sap·ro·gen·ic
sa·prog·e·nous
sa·proph·i·lous
sap·ro·phyte
  fac·ul·ta·tive s.
sap·ro·phyt·ic
sap·ro·zo·ic
sap·ro·zo·o·no·sis
sar·al·a·sin ac·e·tate
Sar·ci·na
  S. max·i·ma
  S. ven·tric·u·li
sar·cine
sar·co·blast
sar·co·cele

Sar·co·cys·tis
  S. fu·si·for·mis
  S. hom·i·nis
  S. lin·de·man·ni
  S. mie·sche·ri·a·na
  S. su·i·ho·mi·nis
  S. te·nel·la
sar·co·cys·to·sis
sar·code
Sar·co·di·na
sar·co·gen·ic
  cell
sar·cog·lia
sar·coid
  Boeck's s.
  Spiegler-Fendt s.
sar·coid·al
  gran·u·lo·ma
sar·coid·o·sis
  hy·per·cal·ce·mic s.
sar·co·lem·ma
sar·co·lem·mal
sar·co·lem·mic
sar·co·lem·mous
sar·col·o·gy
sar·co·ly·sine
sar·co·ma
  al·ve·o·lar soft part s.
  am·e·lo·blas·tic s.
  an·gi·o·lith·ic s.
  avi·an s.
  bot·ry·oid s.
  en·do·me·tri·al stro·mal s.
  Ewing's s.
  fas·cic·u·lar s.
  gi·ant cell s.
  gran·u·lo·cyt·ic s.
  im·mu·no·blas·tic s.
  Jensen's s.
  jux·ta·cor·ti·cal os·te·o·gen·
    ic s.
  Kaposi's s.
  leu·ko·cyt·ic s.
  lym·phat·ic s.
  med·ul·lary s.
  mul·ti·ple id·i·o·path·ic
    hem·or·rhag·ic s.
  my·e·lo·gen·ic s.
  my·e·loid s.
  os·te·o·gen·ic s.
  per·i·os·te·al s.
  re·tic·u·lum cell s.
  round cell s.
  Rous s.
  spin·dle cell s.
  syn·o·vi·al s.
  tel·an·gi·ec·tat·ic os·te·o·
    gen·ic s.

Sar·co·mas·ti·goph·o·ra
sar·co·ma·toid
  car·ci·no·ma
sar·co·ma·to·sis
sar·com·a·tous
sar·co·mere
sar·co·neme
sar·co·plasm
sar·co·plas·mic
  re·tic·u·lum
sar·co·plast
sar·co·poi·et·ic
Sar·cop·syl·la pen·e·trans
Sar·cop·syl·li·dae
Sar·cop·tes sca·biei
sar·cop·tic
  ac·a·ri·a·sis
  mange
sar·cop·tid
sar·co·sine
  s. de·hy·dro·gen·ase
sar·co·si·ne·mia
sar·co·sis
sar·co·some
sar·cos·to·sis
sar·cot·ic
sar·co·trip·sy
sar·co·tu·bules
sar·cous
sar·don·ic grin
sa·rin
sar·mas·sa·tion
sar·sa·pa·ril·la
sar·to·ri·us
  bur·sas
sas·sa·fras
sat·el·lite
  chro·mo·some s.
  nu·cle·o·lar s.
  per·i·neu·ro·nal s.
sat·el·lite
  ab·scess
  cells
  cell of skel·e·tal mus·cle
  DNA
  me·tas·ta·sis
sat·el·lite-rich
  het·er·o·chro·ma·tin
sat·el·lit·o·sis
sa·ti·a·tion
sa·ti·e·ty
  cen·ter
Sattler's
  veil
Sattler's elas·tic
  lay·er
sat·u·rate

sat·u·rat·ed
  col·or
  fat
  fat·ty ac·id
  hy·dro·car·bon
  so·lu·tion
sat·u·ra·tion
  anal·y·sis
  in·dex
sat·u·ra·tion
  sec·on·dary s.
sat·ur·nine
  col·ic
  en·ceph·a·lop·a·thy
  gout
  trem·or
sat·urn·ism
sat·y·ri·a·sis
sat·y·rism
sau·cer·i·za·tion
sau·cer-shaped
  cat·a·ract
Sauerbruch's
  cab·i·net
Saundby's
  test
sau·ri·a·sis
sau·ri·der·ma
sau·ri·o·sis
sau·ro·der·ma
sau·sage
  fin·gers
Savage
  syn·drome
Savage's per·i·ne·al
  body
saw
  Gigli's s.
  Stryker s.
sax·i·tox·in
Sayre's
  jack·et
Sayre's sus·pen·sion
  ap·pa·ra·tus
  trac·tion
S-BP
  line
scab
scab·bard
  tra·chea
scab·i·ci·dal
scab·i·cide
sca·bies
  Nor·we·gian s.
sca·bi·et·i·cide
sca·bi·ous
sca·brit·i·es
  s. un·gui·um

scab·wort
sca·la
  Löwenberg's s.
  s. me·dia
sca·lae
scald
scald·ed skin
  syn·drome
scald·ing
scale
  ab·so·lute s.
  adap·tive be·hav·ior s.'s
  Ångström s.
  Baumé s.
  Bay·ley s.'s of In·fant
   De·vel·op·ment
  Benois s.
  Binet s.
  Binet-Simon s.
  Cel·si·us s.
  cen·ti·grade s.
  Charrière s.
  Co·lum·bia Men·tal
   Ma·tu·ri·ty S.
  co·ma s.
  Fahr·en·heit s.
  French s.
  Gaffky s.
  gray s.
  hard·ness s.
  ho·mi·grade s.
  in·ter·val s.
  Kar·nof·sky s.
  Kelvin s.
  Lei·ter In·ter·na·tion·al
   Per·form·ance S.
  mas·cu·lin·i·ty-fem·i·nin·i·ty
   s.
  Mohs s.
  pH s.
  Rankine s.
  ra·ti·o s.
  Réaumur s.
  Shipley-Hartford s.
  Sörensen s.
  Stanford-Binet in·tel·li·gence
   s.
  Wechsler-Bellevue s.
  Wechsler in·tel·li·gence s.'s
sca·lene
  tu·ber·cle of Lisfranc
sca·le·nec·to·my
sca·le·not·o·my
sca·le·nus
sca·le·nus an·te·ri·or
  syn·drome

scal·er
  hoe s.
  son·ic s.
scal·ing
scall
  hon·ey·comb s.
  milk s.
scal·lop·ing
scalp
  con·tu·sion
  in·fec·tion
  lac·er·a·tion
  mus·cle
scal·pel
  plas·ma s.
scal·pri·form
  in·ci·sors
scal·prum
scaly
  leg
  ring·worm
  tet·ter
scam·mo·ny
scamp·ing
  speech
scan
  Meckel s.
  ven·ti·la·tion-per·fu·sion s.
scan·di·um
scan·ner
scan·ning
  speech
scan·ning elec·tron
  mi·cro·scope
scan·so·ri·us
Scanzoni's
  ma·neu·ver
Scanzoni's sec·ond
  os
sca·pha
scaph·o·ce·phal·ic
scaph·o·ceph·a·lism
scaph·o·ceph·a·lous
scaph·o·ceph·a·ly
scaph·o·hy·dro·ceph·a·lus
scaph·o·hy·dro·ceph·a·ly
scaph·oid
  ab·do·men
  bone
  fos·sa
  scap·u·la
  tu·ber·os·i·ty
sca·pi
scap·u·la
  s. ala·ta
  s. el·e·va·ta
  scaph·oid s.

scaph·oid type of s.
winged s.
scap·u·lae
scap·u·lal·gia
scap·u·lar
line
notch
re·flex
re·gion
scap·u·lary
scap·u·lec·to·my
scap·u·lo·cla·vic·u·lar
scap·u·lo·cos·tal
syn·drome
scap·u·lo·dyn·ia
scap·u·lo·hu·mer·al
at·ro·phy
re·flex
scap·u·lo·per·i·os·te·al
re·flex
scap·u·lo·pexy
sca·pus
s. pe·nis
s. pi·li
scar
cig·a·rette-pa·per s.'s
hy·per·tro·phic s.
pap·y·ra·ceous s.'s
ra·di·al s.
shil·ling s.'s
scar
can·cer
car·ci·no·ma
Scardino ver·ti·cal flap
py·e·lo·plas·ty
scarf
ban·dage
scar·i·fi·ca·tion
test
scar·i·fi·ca·tor
scar·i·fy
scar·la·ti·na
s. an·gi·no·sa
an·gi·nose s.
s. hem·or·rha·gi·ca
s. la·tens
la·tent s.
s. ma·lig·na
s. rheu·ma·ti·ca
s. sim·plex
scar·la·ti·nal
ne·phri·tis
scar·la·ti·nel·la
scar·la·ti·ni·form
er·y·the·ma
scar·la·ti·noid
scar·let
fe·ver

scar·let fe·ver
an·ti·tox·in
scar·let fe·ver eryth·ro·gen·ic
tox·in
scar·let red sul·fo·nate
Scarpa's
fas·cia
flu·id
fo·ram·i·na
gan·gli·on
ha·ben·u·la
hi·a·tus
li·quor
mem·brane
meth·od
sheath
staph·y·lo·ma
tri·an·gle
sca·te·mia
scat·o·log·ic
sca·tol·o·gy
sca·to·ma
sca·toph·a·gy
sca·tos·co·py
scat·ter
scat·tered
ra·di·a·tion
scat·u·la
scav·eng·er
cell
Sced·os·por·i·um ap·i·o·sper·mum
sce·lal·gia
scel·o·tyr·be
scent
glands
Schacher's
gan·gli·on
Schaef·fer-Ful·ton
stain
Schaer's
re·a·gent
Schäfer's
meth·od
Schaffer's
test
Schäffer's
re·flex
Schamberg's
der·ma·ti·tis
dis·ease
Schanz
syn·drome
Schapiro's
sign
Schardinger
en·zyme
re·ac·tion

schar·lach red
Schat·zki's
 ring
Schaudinn's
 fix·a·tive
Schaumann
 bod·ies
Schaumann's
 lym·pho·gran·u·lo·ma
 syn·drome
Schaum·berg's
 dis·ease
Schauta vag·i·nal
 op·er·a·tion
Schede's
 clot
 meth·od
sched·ule
 con·tin·u·ous re·in·force·
  ment s.
 fixed-in·ter·val re·in·force·
  ment s.
 fixed-ra·tio re·in·force·ment
  s.
 in·ter·mit·tent re·in·force·
  ment s.
 s.'s of re·in·force·ment
 var·i·a·ble-in·ter·val re·in·
  force·ment s.
sched·uled
 drug
Scheele's
 green
Scheibe's
 deaf·ness
Scheibler's
 re·a·gent
Scheie's
 syn·drome
Scheiner's
 ex·per·i·ment
Schellong
 test
Schellong-Strisower
 phe·nom·e·non
sche·ma
 body s.
sche·ma·ta
sche·mat·ic
 eye
sche·mat·o·graph
scheme
 oc·clu·sal s.
Schenck's
 dis·ease
Scheuermann's
 dis·ease

Schick
 meth·od
 test
Schick test
 tox·in
Schiff
 base
Schiff's
 re·a·gent
Schiff-Sherrington
 phe·nom·e·non
Schilder's
 dis·ease
Schiller's
 test
Schilling
 test
Schilling's
 blood count
 in·dex
Schilling's band
 cell
Schilling type of mon·o·cyt·ic
 leu·ke·mia
schin·dy·le·sis
schin·dy·let·ic
 joint
Schiötz
 to·nom·e·ter
Schirmer
 test
Schirmer's
 syn·drome
schis·to·ce·lia
schis·to·cor·mia
schis·to·cys·tis
schis·to·cyte
schis·to·cy·to·sis
schis·to·glos·sia
schis·tor·rha·chis
Schis·to·so·ma
 S. bo·vis
 S. hae·ma·to·bi·um
 S. in·di·cum
 S. in·ter·ca·la·tum
 S. ja·po·ni·cum
 S. man·so·ni
 S. mat·the·ei
 S. me·kongi
 S. spin·da·le
schis·to·some
 der·ma·ti·tis
 gran·u·lo·ma
schis·to·so·mia
schis·to·so·mi·a·sis
 Asi·at·ic s.
 blad·der s.
 ec·top·ic s.

s. hae·ma·to·bi·um
in·tes·ti·nal s.
Jap·a·nese s.
s. ja·pon·i·ca
s. man·so·ni
Manson's s.
s. me·kongi
Or·i·en·tal s.
uri·nary s.
schis·to·som·u·la
schis·to·som·u·lum
schis·to·ster·nia
schis·to·tho·rax
schiz·am·ni·on
schiz·ax·on
schiz·en·ce·phal·ic
mi·cro·ceph·a·ly
schiz·en·ceph·aly
schiz·o-af·fec·tive
psy·cho·sis
schiz·o·cyte
schiz·o·cy·to·sis
schiz·o·gen·e·sis
schi·zog·o·ny
schiz·o·gy·ria
schiz·oid
per·son·al·i·ty
schiz·oid·ism
schiz·o·my·cete
Schiz·o·my·ce·tes
schiz·o·my·cet·ic
schiz·o·my·co·sis
schiz·ont
schi·zon·ti·cide
schiz·o·nych·ia
schiz·o·pha·sia
schiz·o·phre·nia
am·bu·la·to·ry s.
cat·a·ton·ic s.
dis·or·ga·nized s.
he·be·phren·ic s.
la·tent s.
par·a·noid s.
pro·cess s.
pseu·do·neu·rot·ic s.
re·ac·tive s.
re·sid·u·al s.
sim·ple s.
schiz·o·phren·ic
schiz·o·phren·i·form
dis·or·der
schiz·o·the·mia
schiz·o·to·nia
schiz·o·trich·ia
Schiz·o·tryp·a·num cru·zi
schiz·o·typ·i·cal
per·son·al·i·ty
schiz·o·zo·ite

Schlatter-Osgood
dis·ease
Schlatter's
dis·ease
Schlemm's
ca·nal
Schlesinger's
sign
Schmidel's
anas·to·mo·ses
Schmid-Fraccaro
syn·drome
Schmidt-Lanterman
clefts
in·ci·sures
Schmidt's
syn·drome
Schmidt-Thannhauser
meth·od
Schmorl's
ba·cil·lus
nod·ule
Schmorl's fer·ric-fer·ri·cy·a·nide
re·duc·tion
stain
Schmorl's pic·ro·thi·o·nin
stain
schnei·de·ri·an
mem·brane
schnei·de·ri·an first rank
symp·toms
Schneider's
car·mine
Schneider's first rank
symp·toms
Schnei·der·sitz
Scholander
ap·pa·ra·tus
Scholz'
dis·ease
Schönbein's
test
Schönlein-Henoch
syn·drome
Schönlein's
dis·ease
pur·pu·ra
Schott
treat·ment
Schottmüller's
ba·cil·lus
dis·ease
Schreger's
lines
Schridde's can·cer
hairs
Schroeder's
op·er·a·tion

Schuchardt's
op·er·a·tion
Schüffner's
dots
gran·ules
Schüller's
dis·ease
ducts
phe·nom·e·non
syn·drome
Schultz
re·ac·tion
stain
Schultz-Charlton
phe·nom·e·non
re·ac·tion
Schultz-Dale
re·ac·tion
Schultze's
cells
fold
mech·a·nism
mem·brane
phan·tom
pla·cen·ta
sign
Schütz
rule
Schütz'
bun·dle
law
Schwabach
test
Schwachman
syn·drome
Schwalbe's
cor·pus·cle
nu·cle·us
ring
spac·es
Schwann
cells
schwan·no·ma
acous·tic s.
schwan·no·sis
Schwann's white
sub·stance
Schwartz
syn·drome
trac·tot·o·my
Schwarz's
test
Schweninger-Buzzi
an·e·to·der·ma
sci·age
sci·at·ic
fo·ra·men
her·nia

nerve
neu·ral·gia
neu·ri·tis
plex·us
sco·li·o·sis
spine
sci·at·i·ca
scil·la
scil·la·ren
s. A
s. B
scim·i·tar
sign
scin·ti·cis·tern·og·ra·phy
scin·ti·gram
scin·ti·graph·ic
scin·tig·ra·phy
scin·til·la·scope
scin·til·lat·ing
sco·to·ma
scin·til·la·tion
count·er
scin·til·la·tor
scin·til·lom·e·ter
scin·ti·pho·to·graph
scin·ti·pho·tog·ra·phy
scin·ti·scan
scin·ti·scan·ner
sci·on
sci·os·o·phy
scir·rhen·can·this
scir·rhos·i·ty
scir·rhous
car·ci·no·ma
scir·rhus
scis·sion
scis·si·par·i·ty
scis·sor
gait
scis·sors
de Wecker's s.
Smellie's s.
scis·sors-shad·ow
scis·su·ra
s. pi·lo·rum
scis·su·rae
scis·sure
scle·ra
blue s.
scler·ad·e·ni·tis
scler·ae
scle·ral
ec·ta·sia
re·sec·tion
ri·gid·i·ty
ring
roll
spur

staph·y·lo·ma
veins
scle·ral buck·ling
op·er·a·tion
scle·ras
scle·ra·tog·e·nous
scle·rec·ta·sia
par·tial s.
to·tal s.
scle·rec·to·ir·i·dec·to·my
scle·rec·to·ir·i·do·di·al·y·sis
scle·rec·to·my
scle·re·de·ma
s. adul·to·rum
scle·re·ma
s. adi·po·sum
s. ne·o·na·to·rum
scle·ren·ce·pha·lia
scle·ren·ceph·a·ly
scle·ri·a·sis
scle·ri·rit·o·my
scle·ri·tis
an·nu·lar s.
an·te·ri·or s.
brawny s.
deep s.
ge·lat·i·nous s.
ma·lig·nant s.
nec·ro·tiz·ing s.
nod·u·lar s.
pos·te·ri·or s.
scle·ro·at·ro·phy
scle·ro·blas·te·ma
scle·ro·cho·roi·dal
scle·ro·cho·roid·i·tis
s. an·te·ri·or
s. pos·te·ri·or
scle·ro·con·junc·ti·val
scle·ro·cor·nea
scle·ro·cor·ne·al
junc·tion
scle·ro·cys·tic
dis·ease of the ova·ry
scle·ro·dac·tyl·ia
scle·ro·dac·ty·ly
scle·ro·der·ma
lo·cal·ized s.
scle·ro·der·ma·ti·tis
scle·ro·der·ma·tous
scle·ro·gen·ic
scle·rog·e·nous
scle·roid
scle·ro·i·ri·tis
scle·ro·ker·a·ti·tis
scle·ro·ker·a·to·i·ri·tis
scle·ro·ma
res·pi·ra·to·ry s.
scle·ro·ma·la·cia

scle·ro·mere
scle·rom·e·ter
scle·ro·myx·e·de·ma
scle·ro·nych·ia
scle·ro-o·o·pho·ri·tis
scle·roph·thal·mia
scle·ro·plas·ty
scle·ro·pro·tein
scle·ro·sal
scle·ro·sant
scle·rose
scle·ro·ses
scle·ros·ing
ad·e·no·sis
agent
he·man·gi·o·ma
in·flam·ma·tion
ker·a·ti·tis
mas·toid·i·tis
os·te·i·tis
ther·a·py
scle·ro·sis
Alzheimer's s.
amy·o·tro·phic lat·er·al s.
ar·te·ri·al s.
ar·te·ri·o·cap·il·lary s.
ar·te·ri·o·lar s.
bone s.
Canavan's s.
cen·tral are·o·lar cho·roi·dal s.
com·bined s.
s. co·rii
s. cu·ta·nea
dif·fuse in·fan·tile fa·mil·i·al s.
dis·sem·i·nat·ed s.
en·do·car·di·al s.
fo·cal s.
glo·mer·u·lar s.
hip·po·cam·pal s.
id·i·o·path·ic hy·per·cal·ce·mic s. of in·fants
in·su·lar s.
lam·i·nar cor·ti·cal s.
lat·er·al spi·nal s.
lo·bar s.
man·tle s.
men·stru·al s.
Mönckeberg's s.
mul·ti·ple s.
nod·u·lar s.
nu·cle·ar s.
o·vu·la·tion·al s.
phys·i·o·log·ic s.
pos·te·ri·or s.
pos·te·ri·or spi·nal s.
pro·gress·ive sys·tem·ic s.

scle·ro·sis *(continued)*
  tu·ber·ous s.
  uni·cel·lu·lar s.
  vas·cu·lar s.
  s. of white mat·ter
scle·ro·ste·no·sis
Scle·ros·to·ma
scle·ros·to·my
scle·ro·ther·a·py
scle·ro·thrix
scle·ro·tia
scle·rot·ic
  bod·ies
  coat
  den·tin
  gas·tri·tis
  kid·ney
  stom·ach
  teeth
scle·rot·i·ca
scle·rot·ic ce·ment·al
  mass
scle·rot·i·co·cho·roid·i·tis
scle·ro·ti·um
scle·ro·tome
scle·rot·o·my
  an·te·ri·or s.
  pos·te·ri·or s.
scle·ro·trich·ia
scle·ro·ty·lo·sis
scle·rous
scol·e·ces
sco·le·ci·a·sis
sco·le·ci·form
sco·le·coid
sco·le·col·o·gy
sco·lex
scol·i·ces
sco·li·o·ky·pho·sis
sco·li·om·e·ter
sco·li·o·sis
  cox·it·ic s.
  em·py·e·mic s.
  hab·it s.
  my·o·path·ic s.
  oc·u·lar s.
  oph·thal·mic s.
  os·te·o·path·ic s.
  par·a·lyt·ic s.
  ra·chit·ic s.
  sci·at·ic s.
  stat·ic s.
sco·li·ot·ic
  pel·vis
sco·li·o·tone
Scol·o·pen·dra
scom·broid
  poi·son·ing

s-cone
scoop
sco·pine
sco·pol·a·mine
  s. hy·dro·bro·mide
  s. meth·yl·bro·mide
sco·po·lia
  s. ja·pon·i·ca
sco·po·line
sco·pom·e·ter
sco·po·mor·phi·nism
sco·po·phil·ia
sco·po·pho·bia
Scop·u·lar·i·op·sis
scor·bu·tic
scor·bu·ti·gen·ic
scor·bu·tus
scor·di·ne·ma
score
  Ap·gar s.
  Du·bo·witz s.
  Glea·son's s.
  raw s.
  re·cov·ery s.
  stan·dard s.
scor·pi·on
Scor·pi·on·i·da
scot·o·chro·mo·gens
scot·o·graph
sco·to·ma
  ab·so·lute s.
  an·nu·lar s.
  ar·cu·ate s.
  Bjerrum's s.
  ce·co·cen·tral s.
  cen·tral s.
  col·or s.
  flit·ter·ing s.
  glau·co·ma·tous nerve-fi·ber
    bun·dle s.
  hem·i·a·nop·ic s.
  in·su·lar s.
  men·tal s.
  neg·a·tive s.
  par·a·cen·tral s.
  per·i·cen·tral s.
  pe·riph·e·ral s.
  phys·i·o·log·ic s.
  pos·i·tive s.
  quad·ran·tic s.
  rel·a·tive s.
  ring s.
  scin·til·lat·ing s.
  Sei·del's s.
  sick·le s.
  zo·nu·lar s.
sco·to·ma·ta
sco·tom·a·tous

sco·tom·e·ter
sco·tom·e·try
scot·o·phil·ia
scot·o·pho·bia
sco·to·pia
sco·top·ic
  ad·ap·ta·tion
  eye
  pe·rim·e·try
  vi·sion
sco·top·sin
sco·tos·co·py
Scott
  op·er·a·tion
Scott-Wilson
  re·a·gent
scout
  roent·gen·o·gram
scrape
scrap·ie
scratch
  re·flex in dogs
  test
scratch·es
screen
  Bjerrum s.
  flu·o·res·cent s.
  Hess s.
  tan·gent s.
  ves·tib·u·lar s.
screen
  de·fense
  mem·o·ry
screen·ing
  au·di·om·e·try
  test
screen·ing
  car·ri·er s.
  cy·to·log·ic s.
  fa·mil·i·al s.
  mul·ti·pha·sic s.
  ne·o·na·tal s.
  pre·na·tal s.
screw
  af·ter·load·ing s.
screw
  ar·ter·ies
  el·e·va·tor
  joint
screw·driv·er
  teeth
screw-worm
  pri·mary s.
  sec·on·dary s.
scribe
Scribner
  shunt

scriv·en·er's
  pal·sy
scro·bic·u·late
scro·bic·u·lus cor·dis
scrof·u·la
scrof·u·lo·der·ma
  s. gum·mo·sa
  pap·u·lar s.
  tu·ber·cu·lous s.
  ul·cer·a·tive s.
  ver·ru·cous s.
scrof·u·lo·tu·ber·cu·lo·sis
scrof·u·lous
  ker·a·ti·tis
  oph·thal·mia
  rhi·ni·tis
scroll
  bones
  ear
scro·ta
scro·tal
  ar·ter·ies
  her·nia
  ra·phe
  sep·tum
  swell·ing
  tongue
  veins
scro·tec·to·my
scro·ti·form
scro·ti·tis
scro·to·cele
scro·to·plas·ty
scro·tum
  lymph s.
  wa·ter·ing-can s.
scro·tums
scrub
  nurse
  ty·phus
scru·ple
Scul·te·tus'
  ban·dage
  po·si·tion
scum
scurf
scur·vy
  Al·pine s.
  in·fan·tile s.
  land s.
  sea s.
scur·vy
  rick·ets
scu·ta
scu·tate
scute
  tym·pan·ic s.
scu·ti·form

Scu·tig·e·ra
scu·tu·la
scu·tu·lar
scu·tu·lum
scu·tum
scyb·a·la
scyb·a·lous
scyb·a·lum
scy·phi·form
scy·phoid
sea
   scur·vy
sea-blue
   his·ti·o·cyte
sea-blue his·ti·o·cyte
   dis·ease
sea gull
   mur·mur
seal
   bor·der s.
   pal·a·tal s.
   pe·riph·e·ral s.
   pos·te·ri·or pal·a·tal s.
   post·pal·a·tal s.
   vel·o·pha·ryn·ge·al s.
seal·ant
   fis·sure s.
sealed jar
   tech·nique
seal-fin
   de·for·mi·ty
seam·stress's
   cramp
search·er
Seashore
   test
sea·sick·ness
sea·son
   mat·ing s.
seat
   ba·sal s.
   rest s.
seat·worm
sea ur·chin
   gran·u·lo·ma
se·ba·ceous
   ad·e·no·ma
   cyst
   ep·i·the·li·o·ma
   fol·li·cles
   glands
   horn
   tu·ber·cle
se·ba·ceus
seb·i·a·gog·ic
se·bif·er·ous

Sebileau's
   hol·low
   mus·cle
se·bip·a·rous
seb·o·lith
seb·or·rhea
   s. adi·po·sa
   s. ca·pi·tis
   s. ce·rea
   con·crete s.
   s. cor·po·ris
   ec·ze·ma·toid s.
   s. of face
   s. fa·ci·ei
   s. fur·fu·ra·cea
   s. nig·ra
   s. ole·o·sa
   s. sic·ca
   s. squa·mo·sa ne·o·na·to·rum
seb·or·rhe·ic
   bleph·a·ri·tis
   der·ma·ti·tis
   der·ma·to·sis
   ec·ze·ma
   ker·a·to·sis
   ver·ru·ca
   wart
Se·bright ban·tam
   syn·drome
se·bum
   s. cu·ta·ne·um
   s. pal·pe·bra·le
   s. pre·pu·ti·a·le
Se·cer·nen·tas·i·da
Se·cer·nen·tia
Seckel
   dwarf·ism
   syn·drome
se·clu·sion of pu·pil
sec·o·bar·bi·tal
sec·ond
   fin·ger
   in·ci·sor
   law of ther·mo·dy·nam·ics
   mes·sen·ger
   mo·lar
   sight
   tooth
sec·on·dar·ies
sec·on·dary
   ad·he·sion
   aer·o·don·tal·gia
   agam·ma·glob·u·lin·e·mia
   al·co·hol
   al·do·ste·ron·ism
   amen·or·rhea
   am·pu·ta·tion

am·y·loi·do·sis
an·es·thet·ic
an·oph·thal·mia
at·el·ec·ta·sis
ax·is
buff·er
bu·tyl al·co·hol
cal·ci·um phos·phate
car·ci·no·ma
car·di·o·my·op·a·thy
car·ies
car·ti·lage
cat·a·ract
ce·men·tum
cen·ter of os·si·fi·ca·tion
cho·a·na
coc·cid·i·oi·do·my·co·sis
con·stric·tion
de·gen·er·a·tion
de·men·tia
den·tin
den·ti·tion
de·vi·a·tion
dex·tro·car·dia
di·ges·tion
dis·ease
drives
dys·men·or·rhea
elab·o·ra·tion
en·ceph·a·li·tis
fail·ure
fis·sure of the cer·e·bel·lum
fol·li·cle
gain
glau·co·ma
gout
he·mo·chro·ma·to·sis
hem·or·rhage
host
hy·dro·ceph·a·lus
hy·per·par·a·thy·roid·ism
hy·per·thy·roid·ism
hy·po·gam·ma·glob·u·lin·e·
  mia
hy·po·go·nad·ism
hy·po·thy·roid·ism
im·mu·no·de·fi·cien·cy
in·fec·tion
ly·so·somes
mes·o·derm
met·he·mo·glo·bi·ne·mia
nar·cis·sism
nod·ule
non·dis·junc·tion
oo·cyte
pal·ate
pel·lag·ra
point of os·si·fi·ca·tion

pro·cess
pro·te·ose
py·o·der·ma
rays
re·in·force·ment
ret·i·ni·tis
sat·u·ra·tion
screw-worm
sper·ma·to·cyte
su·ture
syph·i·lid
syph·i·lis
throm·bus
tu·ber·cu·lo·sis
un·ion
vil·lus
vit·re·ous
sec·on·dary ab·dom·i·nal
  preg·nan·cy
sec·on·dary adre·no·cor·ti·cal
  in·suf·fi·cien·cy
sec·on·dary am·ide
sec·on·dary amine
sec·on·dary an·ti·body
  de·fi·cien·cy
sec·on·dary egg
  mem·brane
sec·on·dary gen·er·al·ized
  ep·i·lep·sy
sec·on·dary im·mune
  re·sponse
sec·on·dary in·ter·a·tri·al
  fo·ra·men
sec·on·dary med·i·cal
  care
sec·on·dary mu·ci·no·sis
sec·on·dary my·e·loid
  met·a·pla·sia
sec·on·dary pul·mo·nary
  lob·ule
sec·on·dary re·frac·to·ry
  ane·mia
sec·on·dary re·nal
  cal·cu·lus
sec·on·dary re·nal tu·bu·lar
  ac·i·do·sis
sec·on·dary sen·so·ry
  cor·tex
  nu·clei
sec·on·dary sex
  char·ac·ters
sec·on·dary spi·ral
  plate
sec·on·dary tym·pan·ic
  mem·brane
sec·on·dary uter·ine
  in·er·tia

sec·on·dary vi·su·al
  ar·ea
  cor·tex
sec·on·dary X
  zone
sec·ond cra·ni·al
  nerve
sec·ond cu·ne·i·form
  bone
sec·ond de·gree
  burn
  pro·lapse
sec·ond de·gree A-V
  block
sec·ond gas
  ef·fect
sec·ond heart
  sound
sec·ond-look
  op·er·a·tion
sec·ond-or·der
  con·di·tion·ing
sec·ond par·al·lel pel·vic
  plane
sec·ond sig·nal·ing
  sys·tem
sec·ond stage
sec·ond tem·po·ral
  con·vo·lu·tion
sec·ond tib·i·al
  mus·cle
se·cre·ta
se·cre·ta·gogue
Se·cré·tan's
  syn·drome
se·crete
se·cre·tin
  test
se·cre·tion
  cy·to·crine s.
  neu·ro·hu·mor·al s.
se·cre·to·gogue
se·cre·to·mo·tor
se·cre·to·mo·tory
se·cre·tor
  fac·tor
se·cre·to·ry
  can·a·lic·u·lus
  car·ci·no·ma
  cyst
  duct
  gran·ule
  nerve
  oti·tis me·dia
sec·tile
sec·tio
sec·tion
  ab·dom·i·nal s.

at·tached cra·ni·al s.
ce·sar·e·an s.
clas·si·cal ce·sar·e·an s.
cor·o·nal s.
de·tached cra·ni·al s.
fro·zen s.
Latzko's ce·sar·e·an s.
low cer·vi·cal ce·sar·e·an s.
mi·cro·scop·ic s.
per·i·ne·al s.
pi·tu·i·tary stalk s.
Saemisch's s.
sag·it·tal s.
se·ri·al s.
thin s.
ul·tra·thin s.
sec·tion·al
  im·pres·sion
  roent·gen·og·ra·phy
sec·ti·o·nes
sec·tor
  ir·i·dec·to·my
sec·tor·an·o·pia
sec·to·ri·al
se·cun·di·grav·i·da
se·cun·di·na
se·cun·di·nae
se·cun·dines
se·cun·dip·a·ra
se·date
se·da·tion
sed·a·tive
se·dig·i·tate
sed·i·ment
sed·i·men·ta·ry
  cat·a·ract
sed·i·men·tate
sed·i·men·ta·tion
  con·stant
  rate
sed·i·men·ta·tor
sed·i·men·tom·e·ter
sed·i·men·tum
  s. la·te·ri·ti·um
se·do·hep·tu·lose
seed
  corn
Seeligmüller's
  sign
see·saw
  mur·mur
  nys·tag·mus
Seessel's
  pock·et
  pouch
seg·ment
  an·te·ri·or s.
  an·te·ri·or ba·sal s.

an·te·ri·or in·fe·ri·or s.
an·te·ri·or oc·u·lar s.
an·te·ri·or su·pe·ri·or s.
ap·i·cal s.
ap·i·co·pos·te·ri·or s.
ar·te·ri·al s.'s of kid·ney
bron·cho·pul·mo·nary s.
car·di·ac s.
he·pa·tic s.'s
he·pa·tic ve·nous s.'s
in·fe·ri·or s.
in·fe·ri·or lin·gu·lar s.
in·ter·an·nu·lar s.
in·ter·max·il·lary s.
in·ter·nod·al s.
Lanterman's s.'s
lat·er·al s.
lat·er·al ba·sal s.
s.'s of liv·er
low·er uter·ine s.
me·di·al s.
me·di·al ba·sal s.
mes·o·blas·tic s.
neu·ral s.
pos·te·ri·or s.
pos·te·ri·or ba·sal s.
P-R s.
Ranvier's s.
re·nal s.'s
RST s.
s.'s of spi·nal cord
s.'s of spleen
ST s.
sub·ap·i·cal s.
sub·su·pe·ri·or s.
su·pe·ri·or s.
su·pe·ri·or lin·gu·lar s.
sym·pa·thet·ic s.
up·per uter·ine s.
ve·nous s.'s of the kid·ney
ve·nous s.'s of liv·er
seg·men·ta
seg·men·tal
an·es·the·sia
ar·tery
bron·chus
frac·ture
glo·mer·u·lo·ne·phri·tis
neu·ri·tis
neu·rop·a·thy
plate
sphinc·ter
zone
seg·men·tal al·ve·o·lar
os·te·ot·o·my
seg·men·ta·tion
cav·i·ty
nu·cle·us

seg·men·tec·to·my
seg·ment·ed
cell
leu·ko·cyte
neu·tro·phil
seg·ment·er
Seg·men·ti·na
seg·ment·ing
body
seg·men·tum
s. an·te·ri·us
s. ap·i·ca·le
seg·men·ta hep·a·tis
s. in·ter·no·da·le
s. la·te·ra·le
seg·men·ta li·e·nis
s. me·di·a·le
s. pos·te·ri·us
s. sub·a·pi·ca·le
s. sub·su·pe·ri·us
seg·re·ga·tion
anal·y·sis
ra·ti·o
seg·re·ga·tor
Seidel's
sco·to·ma
sign
Seignette's
salt
Seiler's
car·ti·lage
seis·mo·ther·a·py
Seitelberger's
dis·ease
sei·zure
ab·sence s.
ano·sog·no·sic s.
com·plex par·tial s.
gen·er·al·ized ton·ic-clo·nic
s.
par·tial s.
psy·chic s.
psy·cho·mo·tor s.
se·junc·tion
se·la·pho·bia
Seldinger
tech·nique
se·lec·tion
co·ef·fi·cient
pres·sure
se·lec·tion
ar·ti·fi·cial s.
med·i·cal s.
nat·u·ral s.
sex·u·al s.
se·lec·tive
an·gi·og·ra·phy
grind·ing

se·lec·tive *(continued)*
  hy·po·al·dos·ter·on·ism
  in·at·ten·tion
  in·hi·bi·tion
  me·di·um
  mem·o·ry
  stain
se·le·ne un·gui·um
se·le·ni·um
  s. sul·fide
se·le·ni·um
  poi·son·ing
se·le·no·cys·teine
se·len·o·dont
se·le·no·me·thi·o·nine
Se·le·no·mo·nas
self
  sub·lim·i·nal s.
self
  con·cept
self-ac·cu·sa·tion
self-a·naly·sis
self-a·ware·ness
self-cen·tered·ness
self-com·mit·ment
self-con·trol
self-cur·ing
  res·in
self-dif·fer·en·ti·a·tion
self-dis·cov·e·ry
self-fer·til·i·za·tion
self-in·fec·tion
self-knowl·edge
self-lim·it·ed
self-love
self-poi·son·ing
self-reg·is·ter·ing
  ther·mom·e·ter
self-re·tain·ing
  cath·e·ter
self-stim·u·la·tion
Selivanoff's
  test
sel·la
  emp·ty s.
sel·lar
Sellick's
  ma·neu·ver
Selters
  wa·ter
Selter's
  dis·ease
Selt·zer
  wa·ter
se·man·tic
  apha·sia
se·man·tics
se·mei·og·ra·phy

se·mei·o·log·ic
se·mei·ol·o·gy
se·mei·o·path·ic
se·mei·ot·ic
se·mei·ot·ics
sem·el·in·ci·dent
se·men
se·mens
se·me·nu·ria
sem·i·al·de·hyde
sem·i·ca·nal
sem·i·ca·na·les
sem·i·ca·na·lis
sem·i·car·ti·lag·i·nous
sem·i·cir·cu·lar
  ca·nals
  ducts
  line
sem·i-closed
  an·es·the·sia
  cir·cle
sem·i·co·ma
sem·i·com·a·tose
sem·i·con·duc·tor
sem·i·con·scious
sem·i·cris·ta
  s. in·ci·si·va
sem·i·de·cus·sa·tion
sem·i·di·rect
  leads
sem·i·flex·ion
sem·i·hor·i·zon·tal
  heart
sem·i·len·te
  in·su·lin
sem·i·lu·nar
  bone
  car·ti·lage
  fas·cia
  fas·cic·u·lus
  fi·bro·car·ti·lage
  fold
  fold of co·lon
  gan·gli·on
  hi·a·tus
  line
  notch
  nu·cle·us of Flechsig
  valve
sem·i·lu·nar con·junc·ti·val
  fold
sem·i·lu·na·re
sem·i·lux·a·tion
sem·i·mem·bra·no·sus
  mus·cle
  re·flex
sem·i·mem·bra·nous
sem·i·na

sem·i·nal
  cap·sule
  col·lic·u·lus
  duct
  flu·id
  gland
  gran·ule
  hil·lock
  lake
  ves·i·cle
sem·i·na·tion
sem·i·nif·er·ous
  ep·i·the·li·um
  tu·bule
sem·i·nif·er·ous tu·bule
  dys·gen·e·sis
sem·i·no·ma
  sper·ma·cyt·ic s.
se·mi·no·ma·tous
sem·i·nor·mal
sem·i·nose
sem·i·nu·ria
se·mi·og·ra·phy
se·mi·o·log·ic
se·mi·ol·o·gy
sem·i·o·path·ic
sem·i-o·pen
  an·es·the·sia
sem·i·or·bic·u·lar
se·mi·ot·ic
se·mi·ot·ics
sem·i·o·val
  cen·ter
sem·i·pen·ni·form
sem·i·per·me·a·ble
  mem·brane
sem·i·pla·cen·ta
sem·i·po·lar
  bond
sem·i·pro·na·tion
sem·i·prone
  po·si·tion
sem·i·qui·none
sem·i·spi·nal
  mus·cle
  mus·cle of head
  mus·cle of neck
  mus·cle of tho·rax
Sem·i·sul·co·spi·na
sem·i·sul·cus
sem·i·sul·fur
  mus·tard
sem·i·su·pi·na·tion
sem·i·su·pine
sem·i·syn·thet·ic
sem·i·sys·tem·at·ic name

sem·i·ten·di·no·sus
  mus·cle
  re·flex
sem·i·ten·di·nous
  mus·cle
sem·i·ter·tian
sem·i·triv·i·al name
sem·i·va·lent
sem·i·ver·ti·cal
  heart
Semon-Hering
  the·o·ry
Semon's
  law
Semple
  vac·cine
Sendai
  vi·rus
Senear-Usher
  dis·ease
  syn·drome
Sen·e·ca
  snake·root
Se·ne·cio
se·ne·ci·o·ic ac·id
se·ne·ci·o·sis
sen·e·ga
sen·e·gal
  gum
se·nes·cence
  den·tal s.
se·nes·cent
Sengstaken-Blakemore
  tube
se·nile
  am·y·loi·do·sis
  ar·te·ri·o·scle·ro·sis
  at·ro·pho·der·ma
  at·ro·phy
  cat·a·ract
  cho·rea
  de·gen·er·a·tion
  de·lir·i·um
  de·men·tia
  de·te·ri·o·ra·tion
  dwarf·ism
  ec·ta·sia
  em·phy·se·ma
  fi·bro·ma
  gan·grene
  ha·lo
  he·man·gi·o·ma
  in·vo·lu·tion
  ker·a·to·der·ma
  ker·a·to·ma
  ker·a·to·sis
  len·ti·go
  mel·a·no·der·ma

se·nile *(continued)*
  mem·o·ry
  neph·ro·scle·ro·sis
  os·te·o·ma·la·cia
  par·a·ple·gia
  plaque
  pru·ri·tus
  psy·cho·sis
  ret·i·nos·chi·sis
  trem·or
  vag·i·ni·tis
  wart
se·nile den·tal
  car·ies
se·nile gut·tate
  cho·roi·dop·a·thy
se·nile hip
  dis·ease
se·nile len·tic·u·lar
  my·o·pia
se·nile se·ba·ceous
  hy·per·pla·sia
se·nil·i·ty
sen·ior
  syn·o·nym
se·ni·um
sen·na
  s. pod
Sen·net·su
  fe·ver
sen·no·side A
sen·no·side B
sen·sate
sen·sa·tion
  cinc·ture s.
  de·layed s.
  gen·er·al s.
  gir·dle s.
  ob·jec·tive s.
  pri·mary s.
  re·ferred s.
  re·flex s.
  spe·cial s.
  sub·jec·tive s.
  trans·ferred s.
sen·sa·tion
  time
sense of
  iden·ti·ty
sense
  or·gans
sense
  col·or s.
  s. of equi·lib·ri·um
  joint s.
  kin·es·thet·ic s.
  light s.
  mus·cu·lar s.

ob·sta·cle s.
po·si·tion s.
pos·ture s.
pres·sure s.
sev·enth s.
sixth s.
space s.
spe·cial s.
stat·ic s.
tac·tile s.
tem·per·a·ture s.
ther·mal s.
ther·mic s.
time s.
vis·cer·al s.
sen·si·bil·i·ty
  ar·tic·u·lar s.
  bone s.
  cor·ti·cal s.
  deep s.
  dis·so·ci·a·tion s.
  elec·tro·mus·cu·lar s.
  ep·i·crit·ic s.
  mes·o·blas·tic s.
  pall·es·thet·ic s.
  pro·pri·o·cep·tive s.
  pro·to·path·ic s.
  splanch·nes·the·tic s.
  vi·bra·to·ry s.
sen·si·ble
  heat
  pers·pi·ra·tion
  tem·per·a·ture
sen·sif·er·ous
sen·sig·e·nous
sen·sim·e·ter
sen·si·tive
sen·si·tiv·i·ty
  ac·quired s.
  an·ti·bi·ot·ic s.
  con·trast s.
  di·ag·nos·tic s.
  id·i·o·syn·crat·ic s.
  in·duced s.
  pace·mak·er s.
  pho·to·al·ler·gic s.
  pho·to·tox·ic s.
  pri·ma·quine s.
  rel·a·tive s.
  salt s.
  spec·tral s.
sen·si·tiv·i·ty train·ing
  group
sen·si·ti·za·tion
  au·to·e·ryth·ro·cyte s.
  cov·ert s.
  pho·to·dy·nam·ic s.
sen·si·tize

sen·si·tized
  an·ti·gen
  cell
  cul·ture
sen·si·tiz·er
sen·si·tiz·ing
  dose
  in·jec·tion
  sub·stance
sen·so·mo·bile
sen·so·mo·bil·i·ty
sen·so·mo·tor
sen·sor
sen·so·ria
sen·so·ri·al
  ar·e·as
sen·so·ri·glan·du·lar
sen·so·ri·mo·tor
  ar·ea
  the·o·ry
sen·so·ri·mus·cu·lar
sen·so·ri·neu·ral
  deaf·ness
sen·so·ri·um
sen·so·ri·ums
sen·so·ri·vas·cu·lar
sen·so·ri·vas·o·mo·tor
sen·so·ry
  am·bly·o·pia
  amu·sia
  apha·sia
  ar·e·as
  cor·tex
  cross·way
  de·cus·sa·tion of me·dul·la
    ob·lon·ga·ta
  dep·ri·va·tion
  ep·i·lep·sy
  gan·gli·on
  im·age
  in·at·ten·tion
  nerve
  neu·ro·nop·a·thy
  pa·ral·y·sis
  re·cep·tors
  root of cil·i·ary gan·gli·on
  root of tri·gem·i·nal nerve
  tract
  ur·gen·cy
sen·so·ry alex·ia
sen·so·ry pre·cip·i·tat·ed
  ep·i·lep·sy
sen·so·ry speech
  cen·ter
sen·su·al
sen·su·al·ism
sen·su·al·i·ty
sen·tient

sen·ti·ment
sen·ti·nel
  an·i·mal
  gland
  pile
  tag
sen·ti·nel spi·nous pro·cess
  frac·ture
sen·ti·sec·tion
sep·a·rat·ing
  me·di·um
  wire
sep·a·ra·tion
  anx·i·e·ty
sep·a·ra·tion
  jaw s.
  s. of ret·i·na
  s. of teeth
sep·a·ra·tor
sep·ses
sep·sis
  in·tes·ti·nal s.
  s. len·ta
  pu·er·per·al s.
sep·ta
sep·tal
  ar·ea
  ar·tery
  bone
  car·ti·lage
  cell
  cusp
  gin·gi·va
sep·tan
sep·tate
  hy·men
  my·ce·li·um
  uter·us
sep·tec·to·my
sep·te·mia
sep·ti
sep·tic
  abor·tion
  en·do·car·di·tis
  fe·ver
  in·farct
  in·tox·i·ca·tion
  phle·bi·tis
  pneu·mo·nia
  ret·i·ni·tis
  shock
sep·ti·ce·mia
  acute ful·mi·nat·ing
    me·nin·go·coc·cal s.
  an·thrax s.
  cryp·to·gen·ic s.
  hem·or·rhag·ic s.
  s. plu·ri·for·mis

sep·ti·ce·mia *(continued)*
pu·er·per·al s.
ty·phoid s.
sep·ti·ce·mic
ab·scess
plague
sep·ti·co·py·e·mia
sep·ti·co·py·e·mic
sep·tic sore
throat
sep·ti·me·tri·tis
sep·ti·va·lent
sep·to·der·mo·plas·ty
sep·to·mar·gi·nal
fas·cic·u·lus
tra·bec·u·la
tract
sep·to·na·sal
sep·to-op·tic
dys·pla·sia
sep·to·plas·ty
sep·to·rhi·no·plas·ty
sep·tos·to·my
sep·tot·o·my
sep·tu·la
sep·tu·lum
sep·tum
s. ac·ces·so·ri·um
al·ve·o·lar s.
aor·to·pul·mo·nary s.
atri·o·ven·tric·u·lar s.
s. of au·di·to·ry tube
Bigelow's s.
bony na·sal s.
bul·bar s.
s. bul·bi ure·thrae
car·ti·lag·i·nous s.
s. cli·to·ri·dis
Cloquet's s.
comb·like s.
cru·ral s.
dis·tal s.
s. en·do·ve·no·sum
en·do·ve·nous s.
fem·o·ral s.
s. of fron·tal si·nus·es
gin·gi·val s.
s. of glans
hang·ing s.
in·ter·al·ve·o·lar s.
in·ter·a·tri·al s.
in·ter·den·tal s.
s. in·ter·me·di·um
in·ter·mus·cu·lar s.
in·ter·pul·mo·nary s.
in·ter·ra·dic·u·lar sep·ta
in·ter·ven·tric·u·lar s.
s. lu·ci·dum

s. me·di·a·sti·na·le
s. mem·bra·na·ce·um ven·
tri·cu·lo·rum
mem·bra·nous s.
s. mo·bile na·si
s. mus·cu·la·re ven·tri·cu·
lo·rum
s. of mus·cu·lo·tu·bal
ca·nal
na·sal s.
pec·tin·i·form s.
s. pec·ti·ni·for·me
pla·cen·tal sep·ta
pre·com·mis·sur·al s.
s. pri·mum
prox·i·mal s.
prox·i·mal spi·ral s.
rec·to·vag·i·nal s.
rec·to·ves·i·cal s.
scro·tal s.
s. se·cun·dum
si·nus s.
s. of sphe·noi·dal si·nus·es
spi·ral s.
spi·ral bul·bar s.
s. spu·ri·um
s. of tongue
trans·par·ent s.
trans·verse s.
s. tu·bae
uro·gen·i·tal s.
uro·rec·tal s.
ven·tric·u·lar s.
se·que·la
se·que·lae
se·quence
cod·ing s.
in·ser·tion s.
in·ter·ven·ing s.
pal·in·drom·ic s.
reg·u·la·to·ry s.
ter·mi·na·tion s.
se·quence
hy·poth·e·sis
se·quence lad·der
se·quen·tial
se·quen·tial mul·ti·chan·nel
au·to·an·a·lyz·er
se·quen·tial oral
con·tra·cep·tive
se·ques·ter
se·ques·tra
se·ques·tral
se·ques·tra·tion
bron·cho·pul·mo·nary s.
se·ques·tra·tion
cyst
der·moid

se·ques·trec·to·my
se·ques·trot·o·my
se·ques·trum
 pri·mary s.
se·quoi·o·sis
se·ra
ser·al·bu·min
ser·en·dip·i·ty
Sergent's white
 line
se·ri·al
 ex·trac·tion
 roent·gen·og·ra·phy
 sec·tion
se·ries
 ar·o·mat·ic s.
 eryth·ro·cyt·ic s.
 fat·ty s.
 gran·u·lo·cyt·ic s.
 Hofmeister s.
 ho·mol·o·gous s.
 lym·pho·cyt·ic s.
 lym·phoid s.
 ly·o·tro·pic s.
 my·e·loid s.
 throm·bo·cyt·ic s.
ser·ine
 s. de·am·i·nase
 s. de·hy·drase
 s. di·az·o·ac·e·tate
 s. sulf·hy·drase
ser·ine
 car·box·y·pep·ti·dase
L-ser·ine de·hy·dra·tase
se·ri·o·graph
se·ri·og·ra·phy
se·ri·os·co·py
ser·i·scis·sion
se·ro·co·li·tis
se·ro·con·ver·sion
se·ro·cys·tic
se·ro·di·ag·no·sis
se·ro·en·ter·i·tis
se·ro·ep·i·de·mi·ol·o·gy
se·ro·fast
se·ro·fi·brin·ous
 in·flam·ma·tion
 pleu·ri·sy
se·ro·fi·brous
se·ro·log·ic
se·rol·o·gy
se·ro·ma
se·ro·mem·bra·nous
se·ro·mu·coid
 ac·id s.
se·ro·mu·cous
 cells
 gland

se·ro·neg·a·tive
se·ro·pos·i·tive
se·ro·pu·ru·lent
se·ro·pus
se·ro·sa
se·ro·sae
se·ro·sa·mu·cin
se·ro·san·guin·e·ous
se·ro·se·rous
se·ro·si·tis
 mul·ti·ple s.
se·ros·i·ty
se·ro·syn·o·vi·al
se·ro·syn·o·vi·tis
se·ro·tax·is
se·ro·ther·a·py
se·ro·tho·rax
ser·o·ti·na
se·ro·to·ner·gic
se·ro·to·nin
se·ro·type
se·rous
 ap·o·plexy
 at·ro·phy
 cell
 coat
 cyst
 dem·i·lunes
 di·ar·rhea
 gland
 hem·or·rhage
 in·flam·ma·tion
 iri·tis
 lig·a·ment
 mem·brane
 men·in·gi·tis
 oti·tis
 pleu·ri·sy
 ret·i·ni·tis
 syn·o·vi·tis
 tu·nic
se·ro·vac·ci·na·tion
se·ro·var
se·ro·zyme
ser·pent
 ul·cer of cor·nea
ser·pen·tar·ia
ser·pen·tine
 an·eu·rysm
ser·pig·i·nous
 cho·roi·dop·a·thy
 ker·a·ti·tis
 ul·cer
ser·pi·go
ser·rate
 su·ture
ser·rat·ed

Ser·ra·tia
  S. mar·ces·cens
ser·ra·tion
serre·fine
ser·re·no·eud
Serres'
  an·gle
  glands
ser·ru·late
ser·ru·lat·ed
Sertoli cell
  tu·mor
Sertoli-cell-on·ly
  syn·drome
Sertoli's
  cells
  col·umns
se·rum
  ac·cel·er·a·tor
  ac·ci·dent
  agar
  ag·glu·ti·nin
  al·bu·min
  dis·ease
  erup·tion
  hep·a·ti·tis
  ne·phri·tis
  rash
  re·ac·tion
  shock
  sick·ness
  ther·a·py
se·rum
  an·ti·com·ple·men·ta·ry s.
  an·ti·ep·i·the·li·al s.
  an·ti·lym·pho·cyte s.
  an·ti·ra·bies s.
  an·ti·re·tic·u·lar cy·to·
    tox·ic s.
  an·ti·tox·ic s.
  bac·te·ri·o·lyt·ic s.
  blood s.
  con·va·les·cent s.
  Coombs' s.
  dried hu·man s.
  for·eign s.
  hu·man s.
  hu·man mea·sles im·mune
    s.
  hu·man per·tus·sis im·mune
    s.
  hu·man scar·let fe·ver
    im·mune s.
  im·mune s.
  s. lac·tis
  liq·uid hu·man s.
  mea·sles con·va·les·cent s.
  mus·cle s.

non·im·mune s.
nor·mal s.
nor·mal horse s.
nor·mal hu·man s.
pol·y·va·lent s.
pooled s.
pooled blood s.
salt·ed s.
spe·cif·ic s.
thy·ro·tox·ic s.
truth s.
se·rum ac·cel·er·a·tor
  glob·u·lin
se·rum·al
  cal·cu·lus
se·rum-fast
se·rum glu·tam·ic-ox·a·lo·ace·
  tic trans·am·i·nase
se·rum glu·tam·ic-py·ru·vic
  trans·am·i·nase
se·rum hep·a·ti·tis
  vi·rus
se·rum pro·throm·bin con·ver·
  sion
  ac·cel·er·a·tor
se·rums
ser·va·tion
Servetus'
  cir·cu·la·tion
ser·vo·mech·a·nism
ser·yl
ses·a·me
  s. oil
ses·a·moid
  bone
  car·ti·lage of lar·ynx
  car·ti·lag·es of nose
ses·a·moid·i·tis
ses·qui·hy·drates
ses·sile
  hy·da·tid
  pol·yp
set
  learn·ing s.
  pos·tur·al s.
se·ta
se·ta·ceous
set·ae
Se·tar·ia
  S. cer·vi
  S. equi·na
se·ta·ri·a·sis
set·back
se·tif·er·ous
se·tig·er·ous
se·ton
  op·er·a·tion
  wound

set·ting
  ex·pan·sion
set-up
sev·en-day
  fe·ver
sev·enth
  sense
sev·enth cra·ni·al
  nerve
se·vere com·bined
  im·mu·no·de·fi·cien·cy
Severinghaus
  elec·trode
se·vo·flu·rane
se·vum
sew·er
  gas
sew·ing
  spasm
sex
  cell
  chro·ma·tin
  chro·mo·somes
  cords
  de·ter·mi·na·tion
  fac·tor
  hor·mones
  link·age
  ob·ject
  ra·ti·o
  re·ver·sal
  role
  skin
sex chro·mo·some
  im·bal·ance
sex·dig·i·tate
sex·duc·tion
sex-in·flu·enced
  in·her·i·tance
sex·i·va·lent
sex-lim·it·ed
  in·her·i·tance
sex-linked
  char·ac·ter
  gene
  in·her·i·tance
  lo·cus
sex·ol·o·gy
sex·tan
sex·u·al
  con·trary s.
sex·u·al
  de·vi·a·tion
  di·mor·phism
  dwarf·ism
  dys·func·tion
  gen·er·a·tion
  gland

in·fan·ti·lism
in·stinct
in·ter·course
life
neur·as·the·nia
per·ver·sion
po·ten·cy
re·pro·duc·tion
se·lec·tion
sex·u·al·i·ty
  in·fan·tile s.
sex·u·al·i·za·tion
sex·u·al·ly trans·mit·ted
  dis·ease
sex·u·al pref·er·ence
Sézary
  cell
  eryth·ro·der·ma
  syn·drome
shad·ow
  cells
  cor·pus·cle
  nu·cle·us
  test
shad·ow
  Gumprecht's s.'s
  Ponfick's s.
shad·ow-cast·ing
Shaffer-Hartman
  meth·od
shaft
  s. of fe·mur
  hair s.
  s. of hu·mer·us
  s. of ra·di·us
  s. of tib·ia
shag·gy
  cho·ri·on
  per·i·car·di·um
sha·green
  patch
  skin
shake
  cul·ture
  test
shak·ing
  pal·sy
shal·low
  breath·ing
sham
  feed·ing
  rage
sham-move·ment
  ver·ti·go
shank
  bone
shap·ing
shark liv·er oil

sharp
spoon
Sharpey's
fi·bers
shave
bi·op·sy
Shaver's
dis·ease
shav·ing
cramp
shawl
mus·cle
shear
rate
stress
thin·ning
shear·ing
edge
shears
Liston's s.
sheath
ca·rot·id s.
cau·dal s.
com·mon flex·or s.
cru·ral s.
den·ti·nal s.
du·ral s.
enam·el rod s.
ex·ter·nal root s.
s. of eye·ball
fem·o·ral s.
fen·es·trat·ed s.
fi·brous s.'s
Henle's s.
Hertwig's s.
Huxley's s.
in·fun·dib·u·li·form s.
in·ter·nal root s.
in·ter·tu·ber·cu·lar s.
s. of Key and Retzius
Mauthner's s.
med·ul·lary s.
mi·cro·fi·lar·i·al s.
mi·to·chon·dri·al s.
mu·cous s. of ten·don
my·e·lin s.
Neumann's s.
no·to·chor·dal s.
re·sec·to·scope s.
root s.
Rouget-Neumann s.
Scarpa's s.
s. of Schwann
s. of Schweigger-Seidel
s. of sty·loid pro·cess
s. of su·pe·ri·or ob·lique
mus·cle
syn·o·vi·al s.

syn·o·vi·al s.'s of dig·its of
foot
syn·o·vi·al s.'s of dig·its of
hand
tail s.
s.'s of ves·sels
Waldeyer's s.
sheath
lig·a·ments
pro·cess of sphe·noid bone
sheathed
ar·tery
Sheehan's
syn·drome
sheep
bots
sheep-pox
vi·rus
shelf
pro·ce·dure
shelf
Blumer's s.
den·tal s.
pal·a·tal s.
rec·tal s.
vo·cal s.
shell
cy·to·tro·pho·blas·tic s.
dif·fu·sion s.
shell
nail
shock
shel·lac
base
Shenton's
line
Shepherd's
frac·ture
Sherman
unit
Sherman-Munsell
unit
Sherrington
phe·nom·e·non
Sherrington's
law
sher·ry
wine
shield
em·bry·on·ic s.
nip·ple s.
oral s.'s
shift
an·ti·gen·ic s.
ax·is s.
chlo·ride s.
Doppler s.
s. to the left

lu·te·o·pla·cen·tal s.
Purkinje s.
s. to the right
thresh·old s.

shift·ing
dull·ness
pace·mak·er

Shiga
ba·cil·lus

Shiga-Kruse
ba·cil·lus

Shi·gel·la
S. boy·dii
S. dys·en·te·ri·ae
S. flex·neri
S. pa·ra·dy·sen·te·ri·ae
S. son·nei

shig·el·lo·sis
shi·kim·ate de·hy·dro·gen·ase
shi·kim·ic ac·id
shil·ling
scars

shi·ma·mu·shi
dis·ease

shin
bone
splints

shin
sa·ber s.
sore s.'s
toast·ed s.'s

shin·gles
shin-splints
ship
Fabricius' s.

ship
fe·ver

Shipley-Hartford
scale

ship·ping
fe·ver

ship·ping fe·ver
vi·rus

Shirodkar
op·er·a·tion

shirt-stud
ab·scess

shiv·er
shiv·er·ing
shoat
shock
an·a·phy·lac·tic s.
an·a·phy·lac·toid s.
an·es·thet·ic s.
break s.
car·di·o·gen·ic s.
chron·ic s.
counter-s.

cul·tur·al s.
de·clamp·ing s.
de·ferred s.
de·layed s.
de·lir·i·ous s.
di·a·stol·ic s.
elec·tric s.
en·do·tox·in s.
er·e·this·tic s.
hem·or·rhag·ic s.
his·ta·mine s.
hy·po·vo·le·mic s.
in·su·lin s.
ir·re·vers·i·ble s.
ni·troid s.
ol·i·ge·mic s.
os·mot·ic s.
pri·mary s.
pro·tein s.
re·vers·i·ble s.
sep·tic s.
se·rum s.
shell s.
spi·nal s.
sys·tol·ic s.
tox·ic s.
va·so·gen·ic s.
wet s.

shock
an·ti·gen
in·dex
lung
ther·a·py
treat·ment

shock·ing
dose

shoe
boil

shoe dye
der·ma·ti·tis

Shone's
anom·a·ly

shook jong
Shope
fi·bro·ma

Shope fi·bro·ma
vi·rus

short
bone
chain
crus of in·cus
gy·ri of the in·su·la
head
pro·cess of mal·le·us
root of cil·i·ary gan·gli·on
sight
vin·cu·lum

short ab·duc·tor
  mus·cle of thumb
short ad·duc·tor
  mus·cle
short cen·tral
  ar·tery
short cil·i·ary
  nerve
short·en·ing
  re·ac·tion
short ex·ten·sor
  mus·cle of great toe
  mus·cle of thumb
  mus·cle of toes
short fib·u·lar
  mus·cle
short flex·or
  mus·cle of great toe
  mus·cle of lit·tle fin·ger
  mus·cle of lit·tle toe
  mus·cle of thumb
  mus·cle of toes
short gas·tric
  ar·ter·ies
  veins
short in·cu·ba·tion
  hep·a·ti·tis
short lu·te·al
  phase
short pal·mar
  mus·cle
short per·o·ne·al
  mus·cle
short pos·te·ri·or cil·i·ary
  ar·tery
short ra·di·al ex·ten·sor
  mus·cle of wrist
short sa·phe·nous
  nerve
  vein
short·sight·ed·ness
short-term
  mem·o·ry
short-term ex·po·sure
  lim·it
short wave
  di·a·ther·my
shote
shot-feel
shot·gun
  pre·scrip·tion
shot-silk
  phe·nom·e·non
  re·flex
  ret·i·na
shot·ted
  su·ture

shoul·der
  bur·si·tis
  gir·dle
  joint
  pre·sen·ta·tion
shoul·der
  fro·zen s.
shoul·der blade
shoul·der-gir·dle
  syn·drome
shoul·der-hand
  syn·drome
show
Shrapnell's
  mem·brane
shud·der
  ca·rot·id s.
Shulman's
  syn·drome
shunt
  ar·te·ri·o·ve·nous s.
  Denver s.
  di·al·y·sis s.
  Dickens s.
  dis·tal sple·no·re·nal s.
  H s.
  hex·ose mon·o·phos·phate s.
  je·ju·no·il·e·al s.
  left-to-right s.
  LeVeen s.
  mes·o·ca·val s.
  per·i·to·ne·o·ve·nous s.
  por·ta·ca·val s.
  por·ta·sys·tem·ic s.
  Rapoport-Luebering s.
  re·nal-splen·ic ve·nous s.
  re·versed s.
  right-to-left s.
  Scribner s.
  sple·no·re·nal s.
  Torkildsen s.
  Warburg-Lipmann-Dickens s.
  Warren s.
  Waterston s.
shut-in
  per·son·al·i·ty
Shwartzman
  phe·nom·e·non
  re·ac·tion
Shy-Drager
  syn·drome
SI
  units
si·a·gon·an·tri·tis
si·al·a·den
si·al·ad·e·ni·tis
si·al·ad·en·on·cus
si·al·ad·e·no·sis

si·al·ad·e·no·tro·pic
si·al·a·gogue
si·al·a·po·ria
si·al·ec·ta·sis
si·al·e·me·sia
si·al·em·e·sis
si·al·ic
si·al·ic ac·ids
si·al·i·dase
si·al·i·do·sis
si·a·line
si·a·lism
si·a·lis·mus
si·a·lo·ad·e·nec·to·my
si·a·lo·ad·e·ni·tis
si·a·lo·ad·e·not·o·my
si·a·lo·aer·oph·a·gy
si·a·lo·an·gi·ec·ta·sis
si·a·lo·an·gi·i·tis
si·a·lo·cele
si·a·lo·do·chi·tis
si·a·lo·do·cho·plas·ty
si·a·log·e·nous
si·a·lo·gogue
si·a·lo·gram
si·a·log·ra·phy
si·a·lo·lith
si·a·lo·li·thi·a·sis
si·a·lo·li·thot·o·my
si·al·o·met·a·pla·sia
   nec·ro·tiz·ing s.
si·a·lom·e·try
si·a·lor·rhea
si·a·los·che·sis
si·a·lo·se·mei·ol·o·gy
si·a·lo·se·mi·ol·o·gy
si·a·lo·sis
si·a·lo·ste·no·sis
si·a·lo·syr·inx
Si·a·mese
   twins
sib·i·lant
   rale
sib·i·lant rhon·chus
sib·i·lus
sib·ling
   ri·val·ry
sib·ship
Sibson's
   ap·o·neu·ro·sis
   fas·cia
   groove
   mus·cle
Sibson's aor·tic
   ves·ti·bule
sic·ca
   com·plex
   syn·drome

sic·cant
sic·ca·tive
sic·cha·sia
sic·co·la·bile
sic·co·sta·bile
sic·co·sta·ble
sick
   head·ache
   role
sick·le
   cell
   flap
   form
   sco·to·ma
sick·le cell
   ane·mia
   cri·sis
   dac·ty·li·tis
   dis·ease
   he·mo·glo·bin
   ret·i·nop·a·thy
   test
   trait
sick·le cell C
   dis·ease
sick·le cell-thal·as·se·mia
   dis·ease
sick·le·mia
sick·ling
sick·ness
   acute Af·ri·can sleep·ing s.
   Af·ri·can horse s.
   Af·ri·can sleep·ing s.
   air s.
   al·ti·tude s.
   black s.
   bush s.
   car s.
   chron·ic Af·ri·can sleep·ing
     s.
   chron·ic moun·tain s.
   de·com·pres·sion s.
   East Af·ri·can sleep·ing s.
   fall·ing s.
   green s.
   In·di·an s.
   Ja·mai·can vom·it·ing s.
   lamb·ing s.
   laugh·ing s.
   milk s.
   Mon·day morn·ing s.
   morn·ing s.
   mo·tion s.
   moun·tain s.
   ra·di·a·tion s.
   se·rum s.
   sleep·ing s.
   spot·ted s.

sick·ness *(continued)*
   sweat·ing s.
   West Af·ri·can sleep·ing s.
sick si·nus
   syn·drome
side
   chain
side
   bal·anc·ing s.
   work·ing s.
side·bones
side-chain
   the·o·ry
side ef·fect
sid·er·a·tic
   cat·a·ract
sid·er·a·tion
sid·er·o·a·chres·tic
   ane·mia
sid·er·o·blast
sid·er·o·blas·tic
   ane·mia
sid·er·o·cyte
sid·er·o·der·ma
sid·er·o·fi·bro·sis
sid·er·og·en·ous
sid·er·o·pe·nia
sid·er·o·pe·nic
   dys·pha·gia
sid·er·o·phage
sid·er·o·phil
sid·er·o·phile
sid·er·oph·i·lin
sid·er·oph·i·lous
sid·er·o·phone
sid·er·o·phore
sid·er·o·scope
sid·er·o·sil·i·co·sis
sid·er·o·sis
sid·er·ot·ic
   nod·ules
Siegert's
   sign
Siegle's
   oto·scope
sie·mens
Siemerling-Creutzfeldt
   dis·ease
sieve
   bone
   graft
   plate
sieve
   mo·lec·u·lar s.
sie·vert
Siggaard-Andersen
   nom·o·gram
sigh

sight
   day s.
   far s.
   long s.
   near s.
   night s.
   sec·ond s.
   short s.
sig·ma
   ef·fect
   pep·tide
sig·ma·tism
sig·moid
   ar·ter·ies
   co·lon
   flex·ure
   fos·sa
   groove
   notch
   si·nus
   sul·cus
   veins
sig·moi·dec·to·my
sig·moid·i·tis
sig·moid lymph
   nodes
sig·moi·do·pexy
sig·moi·do·proc·tos·to·my
sig·moi·do·rec·tos·to·my
sig·moi·do·scope
sig·moi·dos·co·py
sig·moi·dos·to·my
sig·moi·dot·o·my
sig·moi·do·ves·i·cal
   fis·tu·la
sig·mo·scope
sign
   Aaron's s.
   Abadie's s. of ex·oph·thal·mic goi·ter
   Abadie's s. of ta·bes dor·sa·lis
   Abrahams' s.
   ac·ces·so·ry s.
   Allis' s.
   Amoss' s.
   Anghelescu's s.
   an·te·ced·ent s.
   Ar·royo's s.
   as·si·dent s.
   Auenbrugger's s.
   Aufrecht's s.
   Babinski's s.
   Baccelli's s.
   Ballance's s.
   Ballet's s.
   Bamberger's s.
   ban·dage s.

Bárány's s.
Bard's s.
Barré's s.
Bassler's s.
Bastedo's s.
Battle's s.
Bechterew's s.
Beevor's s.
Bezold's s.
Biederman's s.
Bielschowsky's s.
Biermer's s.
Biernacki's s.
Bird's s.
Bjerrum's s.
Blumberg's s.
Bonhoeffer's s.
Boston's s.
Bozzolo's s.
Branham's s.
Braxton Hicks' s.
Broadbent's s.
Brockenbrough s.
Brudzinski's s.
Bryant's s.
burn·ing drops s.
Calkins' s.
Cantelli's s.
Carnett's s.
Carvallo's s.
Castellani-Low s.
Chaddock s.
Chadwick's s.
Chaussier's s.
Chvostek's s.
Claybrook's s.
Cleemann's s.
clenched fist s.
Codman's s.
Comby's s.
com·mem·o·ra·tive s.
Comolli's s.
con·tra·lat·er·al s.
con·ven·tion·al s.'s
Coopernail's s.
Courvoisier's s.
Crichton-Browne's s.
Cruveilhier-Baumgarten s.
Cullen's s.
Dalrymple's s.
Dance's s.
Danforth's s.
Darier's s.
Dawbarn's s.
Dejerine's s.
Delbet's s.
D'És·pine's s.
dim·ple s.

doll's eye s.
Dorendorf's s.
draw·er s.
Drummond's s.
Duchenne's s.
Dupuytren's s.
ear s.
Ebstein's s.
s. of ede·ma of low·er eye·lid
Enroth's s.
Erb's s.
Erb-Westphal s.
Erichsen's s.
Escherich's s.
Ewart's s.
Ewing's s.
ex·ter·nal mal·le·o·lar s.
eye·lash s.
Faget's s.
fan s.
Fischer's s.
flag s.
Forchheimer's s.
Fothergill's s.
Friedreich's s.
Froment's s.
Gaenslen's s.
Gauss' s.
Gerhardt's s.
Gifford's s.
Glasgow's s.
Goggia's s.
Goldstein's toe s.
Goldthwait's s.
Goodell's s.
Goppert's s.
Gordon's s.
Gorlin's s.
Graefe's s.
Grasset's s.
Grey Turner's s.
Griffith's s.
Grisolle's s.
Grocco's s.
groove s.
Gunn's s.
Guyon's s.
ha·lo s.
ha·lo s. of hy·drops
Hamman's s.
Hegar's s.
Heim-Kreysig s.
Helbings' s.
Hi·gou·me·nak·ia s.
Hill's s.
Hoffmann's s.
Hoglund's s.

sign *(continued)*

Homans' s.
Hoover's s.'s
Hueter's s.
icon·ic s.'s
in·dex·i·cal s.'s
Jackson's s.
Jellinek's s.
Joffroy's s.
Keen's s.
Kehr's s.
Kernig's s.
Kestenbaum's s.
Knies' s.
Kocher's s.
Kreysig's s.
Kussmaul's s.
Lancisi's s.
Landolfi's s.
Lasègue's s.
Laugier's s.
Legendre's s.
Leichtenstern's s.
Leri's s.
Leser-Trélat s.
Lhermitte's s.
Lichtheim's s.
lo·cal s.
Loewi's s.
Lorenz' s.
Lovibond's pro·file s.
Ludloff's s.
Macewen's s.
Magendie-Hertwig s.
Magnan's s.
Magnus' s.
Mannkopf's s.
Marañón's s.
Marcus Gunn's s.
Masini's s.
Means' s.
Metenier's s.
Mirchamp's s.
Möbius' s.
Müller's s.
Munson's s.
Musset's s.
neck s.
Néri's s.
Nikolsky's s.
ob·jec·tive s.
s. of the or·bi·cu·la·ris
Osler's s.
Pastia's s.
Payr's s.
Perez' s.
Pfuhl's s.
phys·i·cal s.

Piltz s.
Pins' s.
Pitres' s.
pla·cen·tal s.
Pool-Schlesinger s.
Potain's s.
pro·dro·mic s.
pseu·do-Grae·fe s.
pud·dle s.
pyr·a·mid s.
Quant's s.
Quénu-Muret s.
Quincke's s.
Ransohoff's s.
Remak's s.
Revilliod's s.
Ripault's s.
Rocher's s.
Romaña's s.
Romberg's s.
Rosenbach's s.
Rossolimo's s.
Rotch's s.
Rovsing's s.
Rumpel-Leede s.
Russell's s.
Saenger's s.
Sainton's s.
Sansom's s.
Schapiro's s.
Schlesinger's s.
Schultze's s.
scim·i·tar s.
Seeligmüller's s.
Sei·del's s.
Siegert's s.
Signorelli's s.
Simon's s.
Skoda's s.
spi·nal s.
spine s.
Steinberg thumb s.
Stellwag's s.
Stewart-Holmes s.
Stierlin's s.
Straus' s.
sub·jec·tive s.
Sumner's s.
ten Horn's s.
Thomson's s.
Tinel's s.
Toma's s.
Topolanski's s.
Tournay s.
Trélat's s.
Trendelenburg's s.
Tresilian's s.
Trousseau's s.

Uhthoff s.
Vierra's s.
Vipond's s.
vi·tal s.'s
von Graefe's s.
Weber's s.
Weiss' s.
Wernicke's s.
Westphal-Erb s.
Westphal's s.
Wilder's s.
Winterbottom's s.
wrist s.
sign
blind·ness
sig·nal
node
sig·na·ture
sig·net ring
cells
sig·net ring cell
car·ci·no·ma
sig·nif·i·cant
Signorelli's
sign
si·lane
si·lent
al·lele
ar·ea
elec·trode
gall·stones
gap
is·che·mia
mu·tant
mu·ta·tion
pe·ri·od
si·lent my·o·car·di·al
in·farc·tion
sil·i·ca
s. gel
sil·i·cate
ce·ment
res·to·ra·tions
sil·i·ca·to·sis
si·li·ceous
si·lic·ic
si·lic·ic ac·id
si·lic·ic an·hy·dride
si·li·cious
sil·i·co·flu·o·ride
sil·i·con
gran·u·lo·ma
sil·i·con di·ox·ide
col·loi·dal s. d.
sil·i·cone
sil·i·co·pro·te·i·no·sis
sil·i·co·sid·er·o·sis
sil·i·co·sis

sil·i·co·tu·ber·cu·lo·sis
si·lic·u·lose
cat·a·ract
si·li·qua oli·vae
sil·i·quose
cat·a·ract
silk
floss s.
sur·gi·cal s.
vir·gin s.
si·lo·fil·ler's
dis·ease
sil·ver
cell
cone
point
poi·son·ing
stain
sil·ver
s. chlo·ride
col·loi·dal s. io·dide
s. flu·o·ride
fused s. ni·trate
s. io·date
s. lac·tate
mild s. pro·tein
s. ni·trate
s. ox·ide
s. pic·rate
strong s. pro·tein
s. sul·fa·di·a·zine
tough·ened s. ni·trate
sil·ver-am·mo·ni·a·cal sil·ver
stain
sil·ver-fork
de·for·mi·ty
frac·ture
sil·ver im·preg·na·tion
sil·ver·ized
cat·gut
Silverman-Lilly
pneu·mo·tach·o·graph
sil·ver pro·tein
stain
Silver-Russell
dwarf·ism
syn·drome
Silverskiöld's
syn·drome
sil·ver-tin
al·loy
Sim·bu
vi·rus
si·meth·i·cone
sim·i·an
crease
fis·sure

sim·i·an *(continued)*
  ma·lar·ia
  vi·rus
sim·i·an vac·u·o·lat·ing
  vi·rus
si·mi·lia si·mi·li·bus cur·an·tur
si·mil·i·mum
si·mil·li·mum
Simmonds'
  dis·ease
Simmons' cit·rate
  me·di·um
Simonart's
  bands
  lig·a·ments
  threads
Si·mo·nea fol·lic·u·lo·rum
Simons'
  dis·ease
Simon's
  po·si·tion
  sign
sim·ple
  ab·sence
  ac·ne
  an·chor·age
  beam
  col·or
  con·junc·ti·vi·tis
  di·plo·pia
  dis·lo·ca·tion
  ep·i·the·li·um
  fis·sion
  frac·ture
  glau·co·ma
  goi·ter
  het·er·o·chro·mia
  hy·per·tro·phy
  joint
  lip·ids
  lob·ule
  lym·phan·gi·ec·ta·sis
  mas·tec·to·my
  mi·cro·scope
  my·o·pia
  ne·cro·sis
  obe·si·ty
  pro·tein
  ret·i·ni·tis
  schiz·o·phre·nia
  ul·cer
  ure·thri·tis
sim·ple hy·per·o·pic
  astig·ma·tism
sim·ple mem·bra·nous
  limb of sem·i·cir·cu·lar
   duct

sim·ple my·o·pic
  astig·ma·tism
sim·ple pul·mo·nary
  eo·sin·o·phil·ia
sim·ple skull
  frac·ture
sim·ple squa·mous
  ep·i·the·li·um
Sim·pli·fied Oral Hy·giene
In·dex
Simpson
  light
Simpson's
  for·ceps
Simpson uter·ine
  sound
Sims'
  po·si·tion
Sims uter·ine
  sound
sim·u·lat·ed
  hy·per·tro·phy
sim·u·la·tion
  com·put·er s.
sim·u·la·tor
Sim·u·lium
  S. dam·no·sum
  S. ne·a·vei
  S. och·ra·ce·um
  S. or·na·tum
  S. rug·glesi
si·mul·tan·ag·no·sia
si·mul·ta·ne·ous
  con·trast
  per·cep·tion
sin·ca·lide
sin·cip·i·ta
sin·cip·i·tal
  pre·sen·ta·tion
sin·ci·put
sin·ci·puts
Sind·bis
  fe·ver
  vi·rus
sin·ew
sing·er's
  nodes
  nod·ules
sin·gle
  as·cer·tain·ment
  bond
  im·mu·no·dif·fu·sion
  mi·cro·scope
sin·gle (gel) dif·fu·sion pre·cip·i·tin
  test in one di·men·sion
  test in two di·men·sions

sin·gle pho·ton emis·sion com·
  put·ed
    to·mog·ra·phy
sin·gle-strand·ed nu·cle·ate
  en·do·nu·cle·ase
sin·glet
  ox·y·gen
  state
sin·gul·ta·tion
sin·gul·tous
sin·gul·tus
sin·i·grase
sin·i·gri·nase
sin·is·ter
sin·is·trad
sin·is·tral
sin·is·tral·i·ty
sin·is·tro·car·dia
sin·is·tro·ce·re·bral
sin·is·troc·u·lar
sin·is·tro·gy·ra·tion
sin·is·tro·man·u·al
sin·is·tro·ped·al
sin·is·tro·ro·ta·tion
sin·is·trorse
sin·is·tro·tor·sion
sin·is·trous
si·no·a·tri·al
  block
  node
si·no·a·tri·al con·duc·tion
  time
si·no·a·tri·al re·cov·ery
  time
si·no·au·ric·u·lar
  block
si·nog·ra·phy
si·no·pul·mo·nary
si·no·vag·i·nal
sin·ter
si·nu·a·tri·al
  cham·ber
si·nus
  ar·rest
  ar·rhyth·mia
  bar·o·trau·ma
  block
  bra·dy·car·dia
  his·ti·o·cy·to·sis with mas·
    sive lym·phad·e·nop·a·thy
  nerve of Hering
  node
  pause
  phle·bi·tis
  re·flex
  rhythm
  sep·tum
  stand·still

tach·y·car·dia
tu·ber·cle
si·nus
  s. alae par·vae
  anal si·nus·es
  s. an·a·les
  an·te·ri·or si·nus·es
  aor·tic s.
  Arlt's s.
  bar·ber's pi·lo·ni·dal s.
  bas·i·lar s.
  Breschet's s.
  ca·rot·id s.
  cav·ern·ous s.
  ce·re·bral si·nus·es
  cer·vi·cal s.
  cir·cu·lar s.
  s. cir·cu·la·ris
  coc·cyg·eal s.
  cor·o·nary s.
  cos·to·me·di·as·ti·nal s.
  cra·ni·al si·nus·es
  der·mal s.
  du·ral si·nus·es
  si·nus·es of du·ra mat·er
  Englisch's s.
  eth·moi·dal si·nus·es
  fron·tal s.
  Guérin's s.
  Huguier's s.
  in·fe·ri·or lon·gi·tu·di·nal
    s.
  in·fe·ri·or pe·tro·sal s.
  in·fe·ri·or sag·it·tal s.
  in·ter·cav·ern·ous si·nus·es
  jug·u·lar s.
  s. ju·gu·la·ris
  lac·tif·er·ous s.
  la·ryn·ge·al s.
  s. la·ryn·ge·us
  lat·er·al s.
  lon·gi·tu·di·nal s.
  Luschka's s.
  lymph s.
  lym·phat·ic s.
  Maier's s.
  mar·gi·nal s. of pla·cen·ta
  mas·toid si·nus·es
  max·il·lary s.
  Meyer's s.
  mid·dle si·nus·es
  Morgagni's s.
  s. of nail
  ob·lique s. of per·i·car·di·
    um
  oc·cip·i·tal s.
  Palfyn's s.
  par·a·na·sal si·nus·es

si·nus *(continued)*
  par·a·si·noi·dal si·nus·es
  Petit's s.
  pe·tro·sal s.
  phren·i·co·cos·tal s.
  pi·lo·ni·dal s.
  pir·i·form s.
  pleu·ral si·nus·es
  s. po·cu·la·ris
  pre·cer·vi·cal s.
  pros·tat·ic s.
  rec·tal si·nus·es
  re·nal s.
  s. re·u·ni·ens
  rhom·boi·dal s.
  s. rhom·boi·da·lis
  Ridley's s.
  Rokitansky-Aschoff si·nus·es
  sig·moid s.
  sphe·noi·dal s.
  sphe·no·pa·ri·e·tal s.
  splen·ic s.
  straight s.
  su·pe·ri·or lon·gi·tu·di·nal s.
  su·pe·ri·or pe·tro·sal s.
  su·pe·ri·or sag·it·tal s.
  tar·sal s.
  ten·to·ri·al s.
  ter·mi·nal s.
  s. ter·mi·na·lis
  s. ton·sil·la·ris
  Tourtual's s.
  trans·verse s.
  trans·verse s. of per·i·car·di·um
  tym·pan·ic s.
  s. un·guis
  uro·gen·i·tal s.
  s. uro·ge·ni·ta·lis
  uter·ine s.
  uter·o·pla·cen·tal s.
  Valsalva's s.
  ve·nous si·nus·es
  ve·nous s. of scle·ra
  s. ver·te·bra·les lon·gi·tu·di·na·les

si·nus·es
si·nus·i·tis
  s. ab·scen·dens
  fron·tal s.
  in·fec·tious s. of tur·keys
si·nus·oid
  uter·ine s.
si·nus·oi·dal
  cap·il·lary
si·nus·ot·o·my

si·nu·ver·te·bral
  nerve
si·phon
si·phon·age
Si·pho·na ir·ri·tans
Si·pho·nap·tera
Sipple's
  syn·drome
Sippy
  di·et
si·ren·i·form
si·re·no·me·lia
si·ri·a·sis
sir·up
SISI
  test
sis·mo·ther·a·py
sis·o·mi·cin sul·fate
sis·ter
sis·ter chro·ma·tid
  ex·change
Sister Joseph's
  nod·ule
Sis·trunk
  op·er·a·tion
site
  ac·tive s.
  al·lo·ste·ric s.
  cleav·age s.
  frag·ile s.
  priv·i·leged s.
  re·cep·tor s.
  re·stric·tion s.
  switch·ing s.
si·to·stane
si·to·tax·is
si·to·tox·in
si·to·tox·ism
si·tot·ro·pism
in si·tu
sit·u·a·tion
  psy·cho·an·a·lyt·ic s.
sit·u·a·tion
  anx·i·e·ty
sit·u·a·tion·al
  psy·cho·sis
  test
si·tus
  s. in·ver·sus
  s. in·ver·sus vis·ce·rum
  s. per·ver·sus
  s. so·li·tus
  s. trans·ver·sus
sitz
  bath
sixth
  dis·ease

sense
ven·tri·cle
sixth cra·ni·al
nerve
sixth ve·ne·re·al
dis·ease
sixth-year
mo·lar
siz·er
Sjögren-Larsson
syn·drome
Sjögren's
dis·ease
syn·drome
Sjöqvist
trac·tot·o·my
skat·ole
skat·ox·yl
skein
cho·roid s.
test s.'s
skein
cell
skel·e·tal
ex·ten·sion
mus·cle
sys·tem
trac·tion
skel·e·tal mus·cle
fi·bers
tis·sue
skel·e·tol·o·gy
skel·e·ton
ap·pen·dic·u·lar s.
ar·tic·u·lat·ed s.
ax·i·al s.
car·di·ac s.
s. of free in·fe·ri·or limb
s. of free su·pe·ri·or limb
gill arch s.
jaw s.
vis·cer·al s.
skel·e·ton
hand
ske·nei·tis
skene·o·scope
Skene's
glands
tu·bules
ske·ni·tis
skew
de·vi·a·tion
form
ski·as·co·py
ski·a·sco·tom·e·try
Skillern's
frac·ture

skim
milk
skimmed
milk
skin
bot·flies
dose
flap
graft
grooves
heart
re·ac·tion
re·flex·es
ridg·es
stones
tag
test
trac·tion
skin
al·li·ga·tor s.
bronzed s.
de·cid·u·ous s.
di·a·mond s.
elas·tic s.
farm·er's s.
fish s.
gla·brous s.
glossy s.
loose s.
nail s.
parch·ment s.
pie·bald s.
pig s.
por·cu·pine s.
sail·or's s.
sex s.
sha·green s.
s. of teeth
toad s.
yel·low s.
skin·bound
dis·ease
skin-mus·cle
re·flex·es
Skinner
box
skin·ner·i·an
con·di·tion·ing
skin-punc·ture
test
skin-pu·pil·lary
re·flex
skin writ·ing
skip
ar·e·as
skipped
gen·er·a·tion

Sklowsky
symp·tom
sko·da·ic
res·o·nance
Skoda's
rale
sign
tym·pa·ny
skull
frac·ture
skull
clo·ver·leaf s.
map·like s.
stee·ple s.
tow·ers s.
skull·cap
sky blue
slab-off
lens
slaked
lime
slant
cul·ture
slaty
ane·mia
sleep
ap·nea
dis·so·ci·a·tion
drunk·en·ness
ep·i·lep·sy
pa·ral·y·sis
spin·dle
sleep
cre·scen·do s.
elec·tric s.
elec·tro·ther·a·peu·tic s.
hyp·not·ic s.
light s.
par·a·dox·i·cal s.
par·ox·ys·mal s.
rap·id eye move·ment s.
REM s.
twi·light s.
win·ter s.
sleep-in·duced
ap·nea
sleep·i·ness
sleep·ing
sick·ness
sleep·less·ness
sleep·talk·ing
sleep·walk·er
sleep·walk·ing
sleeve
graft
slen·der
fas·cic·u·lus

lob·ule
pro·cess of mal·le·us
slew
rate
slide
mi·cro·me·ter
slid·ing
flap
her·nia
hook
slid·ing esoph·a·ge·al hi·a·tal
her·nia
slid·ing fil·a·ment
hy·poth·e·sis
slid·ing hi·a·tal
her·nia
slid·ing ob·lique
os·te·ot·o·my
slime
fun·gus
sling
psy·chrom·e·ter
slipped
her·nia
ten·don
slipped ten·don
dis·ease
slip·ping
pa·tel·la
rib
slip·ping rib
car·ti·lage
slit
pores
slit
Cheatle s.
fil·tra·tion s.'s
pu·den·dal s.
vul·var s.
slit·lamp
slit ven·tri·cle
syn·drome
slope
cul·ture
slope
low·er ridge s.
slot·ted
at·tach·ment
slough
slough·ing
phag·e·de·na
ul·cer
slow
com·bus·tion
fe·ver
vi·rus
slow chan·nel-block·ing
agent

slow-re·act·ing
fac·tor of an·a·phy·lax·is
sub·stance
sub·stance of an·a·phy·lax·
is
slow vi·rus
dis·ease
SLR
fac·tor
Sluder's
neu·ral·gia
sludge
ac·ti·vat·ed s.
sludged
blood
slug·gish
lay·er
sluice
sluice·way
slur·ring
speech
slur·ry
slyke
Sm
an·ti·gen
small
ar·ter·ies
cal·o·rie
ca·nal of chor·da tym·pa·ni
in·tes·tine
pan·cre·as
pel·vis
tro·chan·ter
vein
small car·di·ac
vein
small cell
car·ci·no·ma
small cleaved
cell
small deep pe·tro·sal
nerve
small·er
mus·cle of he·lix
small·er pec·to·ral
mus·cle
small·er pos·te·ri·or rec·tus
mus·cle of head
small·er pso·as
mus·cle
small·est car·di·ac
veins
small·est sca·lene
mus·cle
small·est splanch·nic
nerve
small in·cre·ment sen·si·tiv·i·ty
in·dex

small in·cre·ment sen·si·tiv·i·ty
in·dex
test
small in·ter·arch
dis·tance
small lym·pho·cyt·ic
lym·pho·ma
small·pox
vac·cine
vi·rus
small·pox
con·flu·ent s.
dis·crete s.
ful·mi·nat·ing s.
hem·or·rhag·ic s.
ma·lig·nant s.
mod·i·fied s.
var·i·cel·loid s.
West In·di·an s.
small pu·den·dal
lip
small sa·phe·nous
vein
small sci·at·ic
nerve
smear
cul·ture
smear
al·i·men·ta·ry tract s.
bron·cho·scop·ic s.
buc·cal s.
cer·vi·cal s.
co·lon·ic s.
cul-de-sac s.
cy·to·log·ic s.
du·o·de·nal s.
ec·to·cer·vi·cal s.
en·do·cer·vi·cal s.
en·do·me·tri·al s.
esoph·a·ge·al s.
fast s.
fe·male gen·i·tal tract
cy·to·log·ic s.
FGT cy·to·log·ic s.
gas·tric s.
lat·er·al vag·i·nal wall s.
low·er res·pi·ra·to·ry tract
s.
oral s.
pan·cer·vi·cal s.
Pap s.
Papanicolaou s.
spu·tum s.
uri·nary s.
vag·i·nal s.
VCE s.

smeg·ma
s. cli·to·ri·dis
s. pre·pu·tii
smeg·ma·lith
smell
blind·ness
smell-brain
Smellie's
scis·sors
smell·ing
salts
Smith-Boyce
op·er·a·tion
Smith-Indian
op·er·a·tion
Smith-Lemli-Opitz
syn·drome
Smith-Petersen
nail
Smith-Riley
syn·drome
Smith-Robinson
op·er·a·tion
Smith's
frac·ture
op·er·a·tion
smog
smok·er's
patch·es
tongue
smok·er's res·pi·ra·to·ry
syn·drome
smooth
broach
cho·ri·on
col·o·ny
di·et
lep·ro·sy
mus·cle
smooth mus·cle
re·lax·ant
tis·sue
smooth mus·cu·lar
sphinc·ter
smooth sur·face
car·ies
smooth-sur·faced en·do·plas·mic
re·tic·u·lum
smudge
cells
smut
S-N
line
S-N-A
an·gle
snail
fe·ver
snake

snake·root
Can·a·da s.
Eu·ro·pe·an s.
Sen·e·ca s.
Tex·as s.
Vir·gin·ia s.
snap
clos·ing s.
open·ing s.
snap
fin·ger
snap·ping
hip
re·flex
snare
cold s.
gal·va·no·caus·tic s.
hot s.
S-N-B
an·gle
Sneddon's
syn·drome
Sneddon-Wilkinson
dis·ease
sneeze
sneez·ing
gas
Snellen's
test types
Snell's
law
snore
snout
re·flex
snow
blind·ness
con·junc·ti·vi·tis
snow·ball
opac·i·ty
snow·shoe hare
vi·rus
snub-nose
dwarf·ism
snuff
snuff-box
snuf·fles
rab·bit s.
Snyder's
test
soap
an·i·mal s.
Cas·tile s.
curd s.
do·mes·tic s.
green s.
hard s.
in·sol·u·ble s.
ma·rine s.

me·dic·i·nal soft s.
salt wa·ter s.
soft s.
sol·u·ble s.
su·per·fat·ted s.
tal·low s.
soap·stone
soap·suds
en·e·ma
Soave
op·er·a·tion
so·cal·o·in
so·cial
ad·ap·ta·tion
con·trol
dis·eas·es
in·stinct
in·tel·li·gence
mal·ad·just·ment
psy·chi·a·try
ther·a·py
so·cial·i·za·tion
so·cial·ized
med·i·cine
so·cial net·work
ther·a·py
so·cia pa·ro·ti·dis
so·ci·o·cen·tric
so·ci·o·cen·trism
so·ci·o·cosm
so·ci·o·gen·e·sis
so·ci·o·gram
so·ci·o·med·i·cal
so·ci·o·met·ric
dis·tance
so·ci·om·e·try
so·ci·o·path
so·ci·op·a·thy
sock·et
dry s.
eye s.
tooth s.
sock·et
joint
so·da
bak·ing s.
caus·tic s.
s. lime
wash·ing s.
so·dic
so·di·um
s. ac·e·tate
s. ac·id car·bon·ate
s. ac·id cit·rate
s. ac·id phos·phate
s. al·gi·nate
s. *p*-ami·no·hip·pu·rate

s. *p*-ami·no·phen·yl·ar·so·nate
s. ami·no·sa·lic·y·late
s. an·ti·mo·nyl·glu·co·nate
s. an·ti·mo·nyl tar·trate
s. ar·san·i·late
s. ascor·bate
s. au·ro·thi·o·ma·late
s. au·ro·thi·o·sul·fate
s. ben·zo·ate
s. bi·car·bon·ate
s. bi·phos·phate
s. bi·sul·fite
s. bo·rate
s. bro·mide
s. cac·o·dyl·ate
s. cal·ci·um ed·e·tate
s. car·bon·ate
s. car·box·y·meth·yl cel·lu·lose
s. chlo·ride
s. cit·rate
s. cit·rate, ac·id
s. cro·mo·gly·cate
s. de·hy·dro·cho·late
s. di·a·tri·zo·ate
di·ba·sic s. phos·phate
s. di·hy·dro·gen phos·phate
s. di·meth·yl·ar·se·nate
s. do·de·cyl sul·fate
ef·fer·ves·cent s. phos·phate
s. eth·yl·sul·fate
ex·sic·cat·ed s. sul·fite
s. flu·o·ride
s. flu·o·sil·i·cate
s. fo·late
s. fu·si·date
s. glyc·er·o·phos·phate
s. hex·a·flu·o·ro·sil·i·cate
s. hy·dro·gen car·bon·ate
s. hy·dro·gen sul·fite
s. hy·drox·ide
s. hy·po·phos·phite
s. hy·po·sul·fite
s. ich·thy·ol·sul·fo·nate
s. in·dig·o·tin·di·sul·fo·nate
s. io·dide
s. lac·tate
s. lau·ryl sul·fate
s. le·vo·thy·rox·ine
s. li·o·thy·ro·nine
s. met·a·bi·sul·fite
s. meth·i·cil·lin
s. meth·yl·ar·so·nate
s. ni·trate
s. ni·trite
s. ni·tro·fer·ri·cy·a·nide
s. ni·tro·prus·side

so·di·um *(continued)*
s. nu·cle·ate
s. nu·cle·i·nate
s. or·tho·phos·phate
s. per·bo·rate
s. per·ox·ide
s. per·tech·ne·tate
s. phe·nol·sul·fo·nate
s. phos·phate
s. pol·y·an·hy·dro·man·nu·
ron·ic ac·id sul·fate
s. pol·y·sty·rene sul·fo·nate
s. po·tas·si·um tar·trate
pri·mary s. phos·phate
s. pro·pi·o·nate
s. psyl·li·ate
s. pter·o·yl·glu·ta·mate
s. py·ro·bo·rate
s. py·ro·sul·fite
s. rho·da·nate
s. ric·i·nate
s. ri·cin·o·le·ate
s. sa·lic·y·late
s. sil·i·co·flu·o·ride
s. ste·a·rate
s. suc·ci·nate
s. sul·fate
s. sul·fite
s. sul·fo·car·bo·late
s. sul·fo·cy·a·nate
s. sul·fo·ric·i·nate
s. sul·fo·ric·in·ol·e·ate
s. sul·fo·vi·nate
s. tar·trate
s. tau·ro·cho·late
s. tet·ra·bo·rate
s. tet·ra·dec·yl sul·fate
s. thi·o·cy·a·nate
s. thi·o·sul·fate
s. tung·sto·bo·rate

so·di·um
meth·yl·pred·nis·o·lone suc·
ci·nate
pump

so·di·um group

so·di·um-po·tas·si·um
pump

**so·di·um-re·spon·sive pe·ri·od·
ic**
pa·ral·y·sis

so·do·ku

sod·om·ist

sod·om·ite

sod·o·my

Soemmering's
gan·gli·on
lig·a·ment

mus·cle
spot

soft
cat·a·ract
chan·cre
corn
di·et
pal·ate
pap·il·lo·ma
parts
pulse
rays
soap
sore
sul·fur
tu·ber·cle
ul·cer
wart
wa·ter

Sohval-Soffer
syn·drome

so·ja

so·ko·sho

So·la·na·ce·ae

so·la·na·ceous

sol·a·no·chro·mene

so·lap·sone

so·lar
blind·ness
chei·li·tis
der·ma·ti·tis
elas·to·sis
en·er·gy
fe·ver
gan·glia
ker·a·to·sis
plex·us
ret·i·nop·a·thy
ur·ti·car·ia

sol·a·sul·fone

sol·a·tion

sol·der

sol·dier's
heart
patch·es

sole
nu·clei
plate
re·flex

so·le·al
line

So·le·nog·ly·pha

so·le·noid

So·le·no·po·tes cap·il·la·tus

so·le·nop·sin A

sole-plate
end·ing

sole tap
re·flex
so·le·us
mus·cle
sol·id
ede·ma
sol·id
sol·id phase
im·mu·no·as·say
sol·i·dus
sol·i·ped
sol·ip·sism
sol·i·tary
bun·dle
fol·li·cles
fo·ra·men
glands
nod·ules of in·tes·tine
tract
sol·i·tary bone
cyst
sol·i·tary os·te·o·car·ti·lag·i·nous
ex·os·to·sis
sol·u·bil·i·ty
test
sol·u·ble
an·ti·gen
fer·ric phos·phate
glass
lig·a·ture
RNA
soap
starch
tar·tar
sol·u·ble gun
cot·ton
sol·u·ble spe·cif·ic
sub·stance
so·lum
sol·ute
so·lu·tio
so·lu·tion
ace·tic s.
Benedict's s.
Burow's s.
chem·i·cal s.
col·loi·dal s.
s. of con·ti·gu·i·ty
s. of con·ti·nu·i·ty
Dakin's s.
dis·clos·ing s.
Earle's s.
ethe·re·al s.
Fehling's s.
Fonio's s.
Gallego's dif·fer·en·ti·at·ing
s.

Gey's s.
Hanks' s.
Hartmann's s.
Hartman's s.
Hayem's s.
Krebs-Ringer s.
lac·tat·ed Ringer's s.
Lange's s.
Locke-Ringer s.
Locke's s.'s
Lu·gol's io·dine s.
mo·lec·u·lar dis·persed s.
nor·mal s.
oph·thal·mic s.'s
Ringer's s.
sa·line s.
salt s.
sat·u·rat·ed s.
stan·dard s.
stan·dard·ized s.
su·per·sat·u·rat·ed s.
test s.
Tyrode's s.
vol·u·met·ric s.
Weigert's io·dine s.
so·lu·tion
pres·sure
sol·vate
sol·va·tion
sol·vent
drag
ether
in·ha·la·tion
sol·vent
am·phi·pro·tic s.
fat s.'s
non·po·lar s.'s
po·lar s.'s
uni·ver·sal s.
sol·vol·y·sis
so·ma
so·man
so·mas·the·nia
so·ma·tag·no·sia
so·ma·tal·gia
so·ma·tas·the·nia
so·ma·tes·the·sia
so·mat·es·the·tic
so·mat·ic
ag·glu·ti·nin
an·ti·gen
ar·ter·ies
cells
cross·ing-o·ver
death
de·lu·sion
lay·er
mes·o·derm

so·mat·ic *(continued)*
  mi·to·sis
  mu·ta·tion
  nerve
  nu·cle·us
  re·pro·duc·tion
  swal·low
  te·ni·a·sis
so·mat·ic cell
  ge·net·ics
  hy·brid·i·za·tion
so·mat·ic mo·tor
  neu·ron
  neu·rons
  nu·clei
so·mat·ic mu·ta·tion
  the·o·ry of can·cer
so·mat·i·co·splanch·nic
so·mat·i·co·vis·cer·al
so·mat·ic sen·so·ry
  cor·tex
so·ma·tist
so·ma·ti·za·tion
  dis·or·der
so·ma·to·chrome
so·mat·o·form
  dis·or·ders
so·ma·to·gen·ic
so·ma·to·lib·er·in
so·ma·tol·o·gy
so·ma·to·mam·mo·tro·pin
  hu·man cho·ri·on·ic s.
so·ma·to·me·din
so·ma·to·meg·a·ly
so·ma·tom·e·try
so·ma·top·a·gus
so·ma·to·path·ic
so·ma·top·a·thy
so·ma·to·phre·nia
so·ma·to·plasm
so·ma·to·pleu·ral
so·ma·to·pleure
so·ma·to·pros·thet·ics
so·ma·to·psy·chic
so·ma·to·psy·cho·sis
so·ma·tos·co·py
so·ma·to·sen·so·ry
  cor·tex
so·ma·to·sex·u·al
so·ma·to·stat·in
so·ma·to·stat·i·no·ma
so·ma·to·ther·a·py
so·ma·to·top·ag·no·sis
so·ma·to·top·ic
so·ma·tot·o·py
so·ma·to·troph
so·ma·to·tro·phic

so·ma·to·tro·pic
  hor·mone
so·ma·to·tro·pin
so·ma·to·tro·pin re·lease-
  in·hib·it·ing
  fac·tor
so·ma·to·tro·pin-re·leas·ing
  fac·tor
so·ma·to·type
so·ma·to·ty·pol·o·gy
so·ma·trem
som·es·the·sia
som·es·thet·ic
  ar·ea
  sys·tem
so·mite
  cav·i·ty
so·mite
  oc·cip·i·tal s.
so·mit·ic
  mes·o·derm
som·nam·bu·lance
som·nam·bu·lic
  ep·i·lep·sy
som·nam·bu·lism
som·nam·bu·list
som·nam·bu·lis·tic
  trance
som·ni·fa·cient
som·nif·er·ous
som·nif·ic
som·nif·u·gous
som·nil·o·quence
som·nil·o·quism
som·nil·o·quist
som·nil·o·quy
som·nip·a·thist
som·nip·a·thy
som·no·cin·e·mat·o·graph
som·no·cin·e·ma·tog·ra·phy
som·no·lence
som·no·len·cy
som·no·lent
som·no·len·tia
som·no·les·cent
som·no·lism
So·mog·yi
  ef·fect
  meth·od
  phe·nom·e·non
  unit
son·co·gene
Sondermann's
  ca·nal
sone
son·ic
  scal·er
  waves

son·i·cate
son·i·ca·tion
son·i·fi·ca·tion
son·i·fi·er
son·i·fy
Sonne
   ba·cil·lus
   dys·en·tery
son·o·chem·is·try
son·o·gram
son·o·graph
so·nog·ra·pher
so·nog·ra·phy
son·o·lu·cent
son·o·mo·tor
   re·sponse
so·no·rous
   rale
so·no·rous rhon·chus
soot
   wart
so·phis·ti·cate
soph·o·re·tin
so·por
so·po·rif·er·ous
so·po·rif·ic
sop·o·rose
so·po·rous
sor·be·fa·cient
sor·bic ac·id
sor·bin
sor·bin·ose
sor·bi·tan
sor·bite
sor·bi·tol
sor·bi·tose
ʟ-sor·bose
sor·des
sore
   bay s.
   bed s.
   can·ker s.'s
   cold s.
   de·sert s.
   fun·gat·ing s.
   hard s.
   Or·i·en·tal s.
   pres·sure s.
   soft s.
   sum·mer s.'s
   trop·i·cal s.
   veldt s.
   ve·ne·re·al s.
   wa·ter s.
sore
   mouth
   shins
   throat

sore·head
sore·mouth
   vi·rus
sore·muz·zle
Sörensen
   scale
Soret
   band
Soret's
   phe·nom·e·non
so·ro·che
   chron·ic s.
sorp·tion
Sorsby's
   syn·drome
Sorsby's mac·u·lar
   de·gen·er·a·tion
so·ta·lol hy·dro·chlo·ride
So·tos
   syn·drome
souf·fle
   car·di·ac s.
   fe·tal s.
   fu·nic s.
   fu·nic·u·lar s.
   mam·ma·ry s.
   pla·cen·tal s.
   um·bil·i·cal s.
   uter·ine s.
soul
   pain
sound
   af·ter-s.
   am·phor·ic voice s.
   an·vil s.
   atri·al s.
   aus·cul·ta·to·ry s.
   bell s.
   Béniqué's s.
   bow·el s.'s
   Campbell s.
   can·non s.
   car·di·ac s.
   cav·ern·ous voice s.
   co·co·nut s.
   cracked-pot s.
   Davis in·ter·lock·ing s.
   dou·ble-shock s.
   ed·dy s.'s
   ejec·tion s.
   first heart s.
   fourth heart s.
   fric·tion s.
   gal·lop s.
   heart s.
   hip·po·crat·ic suc·cus·sion
      s.
   Jewett s.

sound *(continued)*
  Korotkoff s.'s
  Le Fort s.
  McCrea s.
  Mercier's s.
  mus·cle s.
  per·cus·sion s.
  per·i·car·di·al fric·tion s.
  pis·tol-shot fem·o·ral s.
  post·tus·sis suc·tion s.
  res·pi·ra·to·ry s.
  sail s.
  Santini's boom·ing s.
  sec·ond heart s.
  Simpson uter·ine s.
  Sims uter·ine s.
  tam·bour s.
  third heart s.
  tic-tac s.'s
  Van Buren s.
  wa·ter-whis·tle s.
  Winternitz' s.
  xiph·i·ster·nal crunch·ing s.
sound pres·sure
  lev·el
South Af·ri·can tick-bite
  fe·ver
South Af·ri·can type
  por·phyr·ia
South Amer·i·can
  blas·to·my·co·sis
  try·pan·o·so·mi·a·sis
South·ern blot
  anal·y·sis
Southey's
  tubes
soy·a
soy·bean
  s. oil
space
  al·ve·o·lar dead s.
  an·a·tom·i·cal dead s.
  an·te·cu·bi·tal s.
  ap·i·cal s.
  ax·il·lary s.
  Berger's s.
  Bogros' s.
  Böttcher's s.
  Bowman's s.
  Burns' s.
  cap·su·lar s.
  car·ti·lage s.
  Chassaignac's s.
  Cloquet's s.
  Colles' s.
  cor·ne·al s.
  Cotunnius' s.
  dead s.

  deep per·i·ne·al s.
  den·ture s.
  Disse's s.
  s. of Donders
  ep·i·du·ral s.
  ep·i·scle·ral s.
  ep·i·tym·pan·ic s.
  fil·tra·tion s.
  Fontana's s.'s
  free·way s.
  gin·gi·val s.
  ha·ver·si·an s.'s
  Henke's s.
  His' per·i·vas·cu·lar s.
  in·fra·glot·tic s.
  in·ter·al·ve·o·lar s.
  in·ter·cos·tal s.
  in·ter·fas·cial s.
  in·ter·glob·u·lar s.
  in·ter·glob·u·lar s. of Owen
  in·ter·oc·clu·sal rest s.
  in·ter·pleu·ral s.
  in·ter·prox·i·mal s.
  in·ter·ra·dic·u·lar s.
  in·ter·sep·to·val·vu·lar s.
  in·ter·sheath s.'s of op·tic
    nerve
  in·ter·vil·lous s.'s
  in·tra·ret·i·nal s.
  s.'s of ir·i·do·cor·ne·al an·
    gle
  Kiernan's s.
  Kretschmann's s.
  Kuhnt's s.'s
  lat·er·al pha·ryn·ge·al s.
  lee·way s.
  lymph s.
  Magendie's s.'s
  Malacarne's s.
  Meckel's s.
  me·di·as·ti·nal s.
  med·ul·lary s.
  Mohrenheim's s.
  Nuel's s.
  pal·mar s.
  par·a·pha·ryn·ge·al s.
  Parona's s.
  per·fo·rat·ed s.
  per·i·cho·roid s.
  per·i·lym·phat·ic s.
  per·i·ne·al s.'s
  per·i·nu·cle·ar s.
  per·i·pha·ryn·ge·al s.
  per·i·por·tal s. of Mall
  per·i·si·nu·soi·dal s.
  per·i·vi·tel·line s.
  per·son·al s.
  pha·ryn·ge·al s.

pha·ryn·go·max·il·lary s.
phys·i·o·log·ic dead s.
plan·tar s.
pleu·ral s.
pneu·mat·ic s.
Poiseuille's s.
pop·lit·e·al s.
post·pha·ryn·ge·al s.
Proust's s.
Prussak's s.
pter·y·go·man·dib·u·lar s.
res·pi·ra·to·ry dead s.
ret·ro·in·gui·nal s.
ret·ro·my·lo·hy·oid s.
ret·ro·per·i·to·ne·al s.
ret·ro·pha·ryn·ge·al s.
ret·ro·pu·bic s.
Retzius' s.
Schwalbe's s.'s
sub·a·rach·noid s.
sub·cho·ri·al s.
sub·du·ral s.
sub·gin·gi·val s.
su·pra·he·pat·ic s.'s
su·pra·ster·nal s.
Tarin's s.
Tenon's s.
the·nar s.
Traube's s.
Trautmann's tri·an·gu·lar s.
Virchow-Robin s.
Waldeyer's s.
Westberg's s.
zo·nu·lar s.'s

space
main·tain·er
med·i·cine
my·o·pia
nerve
re·tain·er
sense

spaced
teeth

spade
fin·gers
hand

spall

Spallanzani's
law

spall·a·tion
pro·duct

span
mem·o·ry s.

Span·ish
fly
in·flu·en·za

span·nungs-P

spar·ga·no·ma

spar·ga·no·sis
oc·u·lar s.

spar·ga·num

spar·ing
ac·tion

spar·te·ine

spasm
s. of ac·com·mo·da·tion
af·fect s.'s
ano·rec·tal s.
Bell's s.
ca·dav·er·ic s.
ca·nine s.
car·po·ped·al s.
clo·nic s.
cyn·ic s.
danc·ing s.
ep·i·dem·ic tran·sient di·a·phrag·mat·ic s.
fa·cial s.
func·tion·al s.
hab·it s.
his·tri·on·ic s.
in·fan·tile s.
in·ten·tion s.
mas·ti·ca·to·ry s.
mim·ic s.
mo·bile s.
mus·cle s.
nic·ti·tat·ing s.
nod·ding s.
oc·cu·pa·tion·al s.
phon·ic s.
pro·fes·sion·al s.
pro·gress·ive tor·sion s.
ret·ro·col·lic s.
ro·ta·to·ry s.
sa·laam s.
sal·ta·to·ry s.
sew·ing s.
syn·clon·ic s.
tai·lor's s.
ton·ic s.
ton·o·clon·ic s.
tooth s.'s
tor·sion s.
va·so·mo·tor s.
wink·ing s.

spas·mod·ic
ap·o·plexy
asth·ma
di·ath·e·sis
dys·men·or·rhea
lar·yn·gi·tis
my·dri·a·sis
stric·ture
tic
tor·ti·col·lis

spas·mo·gen
spas·mo·gen·ic
spas·mol·o·gy
spas·mo·lyg·mus
spas·mol·y·sis
spas·mo·lyt·ic
spas·mo·phil·ia
spas·mo·phil·ic
  di·ath·e·sis
spas·mus
  s. ag·i·tans
  s. ca·ni·nus
  s. co·or·di·na·tus
  s. glot·ti·dis
  s. nic·ti·tans
  s. nu·tans
spas·tic
  aba·si·a
  ane·mia
  apho·nia
  di·ple·gia
  ec·tro·pi·on
  en·tro·pi·on
  gait
  hem·i·ple·gia
  il·e·us
  mi·o·sis
  my·dri·a·sis
  par·a·ple·gia
  speech
  syn·drome in cat·tle
spas·tic flat
  foot
spas·tic·i·ty
  clasp-knife s.
  s. of con·ju·gate gaze
spas·tic spi·nal
  pa·ral·y·sis
spa·tia
spa·tial
  acu·i·ty
  for·mu·la
  lo·cal·i·za·tion
  vec·tor
  vec·tor·car·di·og·ra·phy
spa·tial con·ti·gu·i·ty
spa·ti·um
  s. in·ter·fas·ci·a·le
  s. in·ter·va·gi·na·le bul·bi
    oc·u·li
  s. ret·ro·in·gui·na·le
spat·u·la
  Roux s.
spat·u·la
  nee·dle
spat·u·late
spat·u·lat·ed
spat·u·la·tion

spav·in
  blood s.
  bog s.
  bone s.
spav·ined
spay
spear·mint
  s. oil
spe·cial
  anat·o·my
  hos·pi·tal
  sen·sa·tion
  sense
spe·cial·ist
spe·cial·i·za·tion
spe·cial·ize
spe·cial·ized
  trans·duc·tion
spe·cial so·mat·ic af·fer·ent
  col·umn
spe·cial·ty
spe·cial vis·cer·al
  col·umn
spe·cial vis·cer·al ef·fer·ent
  nu·clei
spe·cial vis·cer·al mo·tor
  nu·clei
spe·ci·a·tion
spe·cies
  type s.
spe·cies
spe·cies
  tol·er·ance
spe·cies-spe·cif·ic
  an·ti·gen
spe·cif·ic
  ab·sor·bance
  ac·tion
  ac·tiv·i·ty
  an·er·gy
  an·ti·gens
  an·ti·se·rum
  bac·te·ri·cide
  cause
  cho·lin·es·ter·ase
  com·pli·ance
  dis·ease
  ep·i·thet
  ex·tinc·tion
  grav·i·ty
  heat
  he·mo·ly·sin
  im·mu·ni·ty
  op·so·nin
  par·a·site
  re·ac·tion
  ro·ta·tion
  se·rum

trans·duc·tion
ure·thri·tis
spe·cif·ic ab·sorp·tion
  co·ef·fi·cient
spe·cif·ic ac·tive
  im·mu·ni·ty
spe·cif·ic cap·su·lar
  sub·stance
spe·cif·ic dy·nam·ic
  ac·tion
spe·cif·ic im·mune
  glob·u·lin (hu·man)
spe·cif·ic in·di·ca·tion
spec·i·fic·i·ty
  di·ag·nos·tic s.
  rel·a·tive s.
spe·cif·ic pas·sive
  im·mu·ni·ty
spe·cif·ic sol·u·ble
  pol·y·sac·char·ide
  sug·ar
spe·cil·la
spe·cil·lum
spec·i·men
  cy·to·log·ic s.
spec·ta·cle
  eyes
  plane
spec·ta·cles
  Bartels' s.
  bi·fo·cal s.
  cler·i·cal s.
  div·ers' s.
  di·vid·ed s.
  Franklin s.
  half-glass s.
  hem·i·a·nop·ic s.
  Masselon's s.
  or·tho·scop·ic s.
  pan·to·scop·ic s.
  pho·to·chro·mic s.
  pro·tec·tive s.
  pul·pit s.
  safe·ty s.
  sten·o·pa·ic s.
  sten·o·pe·ic s.
  tel·e·scop·ic s.
spec·ti·no·my·cin hy·dro·chlo·ride
spec·tra
spec·tral
  pho·no·car·di·o·graph
  sen·si·tiv·i·ty
spec·trin
spec·tro·chem·is·try
spec·tro·col·or·im·e·ter
spec·tro·flu·o·rom·e·ter
spec·tro·gram

spec·tro·graph
  mass s.
spec·trog·ra·phy
spec·trom·e·ter
spec·trom·e·try
  clin·i·cal s.
spec·tro·pho·bia
spec·tro·pho·to·flu·o·rim·e·try
spec·tro·pho·tom·e·ter
spec·tro·pho·tom·e·try
  atom·ic ab·sorp·tion s.
  flame emis·sion s.
spec·tro·po·lar·im·e·ter
spec·tro·scope
  di·rect vi·sion s.
spec·tro·scop·ic
spec·tros·co·py
  clin·i·cal s.
  in·fra·red s.
spec·trum
  ab·sorp·tion s.
  an·ti·mi·cro·bi·al s.
  broad s.
  chro·mat·ic s.
  col·or s.
  con·tin·u·ous s.
  ex·ci·ta·tion s.
  flu·o·res·cence s.
  for·ti·fi·ca·tion s.
  in·fra·red s.
  in·vis·i·ble s.
  Raman s.
  ther·mal s.
  tox·in s.
  vis·i·ble s.
  wide s.
spec·trums
spec·u·la
spec·u·lar
  glare
  im·age
spec·u·lum
  for·ceps
spec·u·lum
  bi·valve s.
  Cooke's s.
  duck·bill s.
  eye s.
  Kelly's rec·tal s.
  Pedersen's s.
  stop-s.
speech
  cer·e·bel·lar s.
  clipped s.
  echo s.
  esoph·a·ge·al s.
  ex·plo·sive s.
  he·li·um s.

speech *(continued)*
  mir·ror s.
  scamp·ing s.
  scan·ning s.
  slur·ring s.
  spas·tic s.
  stac·ca·to s.
  sub·vo·cal s.
  syl·lab·ic s.
speech
  au·di·o·gram
  au·di·om·e·ter
  au·di·om·e·try
  bulb
  cen·ters
  pa·thol·o·gy
spe·len·ceph·a·ly
spe·le·os·to·my
Spens'
  syn·drome
sperm
  as·ter
  cell
  crys·tal
  nu·cle·us
sper·ma·ce·ti
sper·ma·cyt·ic
  sem·i·no·ma
sperm·ag·glu·ti·na·tion
sperm-as·ter
sper·mat·ic
  cord
  duct
  fil·a·ment
  fis·tu·la
  plex·us
  vein
sper·ma·tid
sper·ma·tin
sper·ma·to·blast
sper·ma·to·cele
sper·ma·to·ci·dal
sper·ma·to·cide
sper·ma·to·cyst
sper·ma·to·cy·tal
sper·ma·to·cyte
  pri·mary s.
  sec·on·dary s.
sper·ma·to·cy·to·gen·e·sis
sper·ma·to·gen·e·sis
sper·ma·to·ge·net·ic
sper·ma·to·gen·ic
sper·ma·tog·e·nous
sper·ma·tog·e·ny
sper·ma·to·gone
sper·ma·to·go·ni·um
sper·ma·toid
sper·ma·tol·o·gy

sper·ma·tol·y·sin
sper·ma·tol·y·sis
sper·ma·to·lyt·ic
sper·ma·to·pho·bia
sper·ma·to·phore
sper·ma·to·poi·et·ic
sper·ma·tor·rhea
sper·ma·tox·in
sper·ma·to·zoa
sper·ma·to·zo·al
sper·ma·to·zo·an
sper·ma·to·zo·on
sper·ma·tu·ria
sper·mia
sper·mi·ci·dal
sper·mi·cide
sper·mi·dine
sper·mi·duct
sperm·in
  crys·tal
sperm·ine
sper·mi·o·gen·e·sis
sper·mi·um
sper·mo·lith
sper·mol·y·sis
sphac·e·late
sphac·e·la·tion
sphac·el·ism
sphac·e·lo·der·ma
sphac·e·lous
sphac·e·lus
Sphae·roph·o·rus
sphag·num
  moss
sphen·eth·moid
sphe·ni·on
sphe·no·bas·i·lar
sphe·noc·cip·i·tal
sphe·no·ceph·a·ly
sphe·no·eth·moid
sphe·no·eth·moi·dal
  re·cess
  su·ture
  syn·chon·dro·sis
sphe·no·fron·tal
  su·ture
sphe·noid
  an·gle
  bone
  crest
  pro·cess
  pro·cess of sep·tal car·ti·
  lage
sphe·noi·dal
  an·gle
  bor·der
  con·chae
  fis·sure

fon·ta·nel
her·ni·a·tion
part
si·nus
spine
sphe·noi·da·le
sphe·noi·dal si·nus
ap·er·ture
sphe·noi·dal tur·bi·nat·ed
bones
sphe·noid·i·tis
sphe·noi·dos·to·my
sphe·noi·dot·o·my
sphe·no·ma·lar
sphe·no·man·dib·u·lar
lig·a·ment
sphe·no·max·il·lary
fis·sure
fos·sa
su·ture
sphe·no-oc·cip·i·tal
joint
su·ture
sphe·no-or·bit·al
su·ture
sphe·no·pal·a·tine
ar·tery
fo·ra·men
gan·gli·on
neu·ral·gia
notch
sphe·no·pa·ri·e·tal
si·nus
su·ture
sphe·no·pe·tro·sal
fis·sure
syn·chon·dro·sis
sphe·no·pet·rous
syn·chon·dro·sis
sphe·nor·bit·al
sphe·no·sal·pin·go·staph·y·li·nus
sphe·no·squa·mo·sal
sphe·no·squa·mous
su·ture
sphe·no·tem·po·ral
sphe·not·ic
cen·ter
fo·ra·men
sphe·no·tur·bi·nal
sphe·no·vo·mer·ine
su·ture
sphe·no·zy·go·mat·ic
su·ture
sphere
at·trac·tion s.
Morgagni's s.'s
sphe·res·the·sia

spher·i·cal
ab·er·ra·tion
amal·gam
lens
nu·cle·us
re·cess
spher·i·cal form of
oc·clu·sion
sphe·ro·cyl·in·der
sphe·ro·cy·lin·dri·cal
lens
sphe·ro·cyte
sphe·ro·cyt·ic
ane·mia
jaun·dice
sphe·ro·cy·to·sis
he·red·i·tary s.
sphe·roid
ar·tic·u·la·tion
col·o·ny
joint
sphe·roi·dal
sphe·rom·e·ter
sphe·ro·pha·ki·a
sphe·ro·pha·ki·a-brach·y·mor·phia
syn·drome
Sphe·roph·o·rus
sphe·ro·plast
sphe·ro·prism
sphe·ro·sper·mia
spher·ule
sphinc·ter
anal s.
an·a·tom·i·cal s.
an·gu·lar s.
s. an·gu·la·ris
s. ani
s. ani ter·ti·us
an·nu·lar s.
an·tral s.
s. an·tri
s. of an·trum
ar·ti·fi·cial s.
ba·sal s.
bi·can·a·lic·u·lar s.
Boyden's s.
can·a·lic·u·lar s.
cho·le·doch·al s.
col·ic s.
s. of com·mon bile duct
s. con·stric·tor car·di·ae
du·o·de·nal s.
du·o·de·no·je·ju·nal s.
ex·trin·sic s.
first du·o·de·nal s.
func·tion·al s.
s. of gas·tric an·trum

sphinc·ter *(continued)*
  Glisson's s.
  s. of he·pa·tic flex·ure of
    co·lon
  Hyrtl's s.
  il·e·al s.
  il·e·o·ce·co·co·lic s.
  il·i·o·pel·vic s.
  s. in·ter·me·di·us
  in·trin·sic s.
  mac·ro·scop·ic s.
  mar·gi·nal s.
  me·di·o·col·ic s.
  mi·cro·scop·ic s.
  mid·gas·tric trans·verse s.
  mid·sig·moid s.
  my·o·vas·cu·lar s.
  my·o·ve·nous s.
  Nélaton's s.
  O'Beirne's s.
  s. oc·u·li
  Oddi's s.
  s. oris
  os·ti·al s.
  pan·cre·at·ic s.
  path·o·log·ic s.
  pel·vi·rec·tal s.
  phys·i·o·log·i·cal s.
  post·py·lor·ic s.
  pre·pap·il·lary s.
  pre·py·lor·ic s.
  s. pu·pil·lae
  py·lor·ic s.
  ra·di·o·log·i·cal s.
  rec·to·sig·moid s.
  seg·men·tal s.
  smooth mus·cu·lar s.
  stri·at·ed mus·cu·lar s.
  s. of third por·tion of du·
    o·de·num
  uni·can·a·lic·u·lar s.
  s. ure·thrae
  s. va·gi·nae
  Varolius' s.
  s. ve·si·cae
  s. ve·si·cae fel·le·ae
sphinc·ter
  mus·cle
  mus·cle of com·mon bile
    duct
  mus·cle of pan·cre·at·ic
    duct
  mus·cle of pu·pil
  mus·cle of py·lo·rus
  mus·cle of ure·thra
  mus·cle of uri·nary blad·der
sphinc·ter·al
sphinc·ter·al·gia

sphinc·ter·ec·to·my
sphinc·te·ri·al
sphinc·ter·ic
sphinc·ter·is·mus
sphinc·ter·i·tis
sphinc·ter·oid
  tract of il·e·um
sphinc·ter·ol·y·sis
sphinc·ter·o·plas·ty
sphinc·ter·o·scope
sphinc·ter·os·co·py
sphinc·ter·o·tome
sphinc·ter·ot·o·my
  trans·du·o·de·nal s.
  ure·thral s.
sphin·ga·nine
sphing·ol
sphin·go·lip·id
sphin·go·lip·i·do·sis
  adult type
  ce·re·bral s.
  ear·ly ju·ve·nile type
  in·fan·tile type
  late ju·ve·nile type
sphin·go·lip·o·dys·tro·phy
sphin·go·my·e·lin
  lip·i·do·sis
sphin·go·my·e·li·nase
sphin·go·my·e·lin phos·pho·di·
  es·ter·ase
sphin·go·my·e·lins
sphin·go·sine
sphyg·mic
  in·ter·val
sphyg·mo·car·di·o·graph
sphyg·mo·car·di·o·scope
sphyg·mo·chron·o·graph
sphyg·mo·gram
sphyg·mo·graph
sphyg·mo·graph·ic
sphyg·mog·ra·phy
sphyg·moid
sphyg·mo·ma·nom·e·ter
  Mosso's s.
  Rogers' s.
sphyg·mo·ma·nom·e·try
sphyg·mom·e·ter
sphyg·mo·met·ro·scope
sphyg·mo-os·cil·lom·e·ter
sphyg·mo·pal·pa·tion
sphyg·mo·phone
sphyg·mo·scope
  Bishop's s.
sphyg·mos·co·py
sphyg·mo·sys·to·le
sphyg·mo·ton·o·graph
sphyg·mo·to·nom·e·ter
sphyg·mo·vis·co·sim·e·try

sphy·rec·to·my
sphy·ro·to·my
spi·ca
  ban·dage
spi·cae
spic·u·la
spic·u·lar
spic·ule
spic·u·lum
spi·der
  ar·te·ri·al s.
  vas·cu·lar s.
spi·der
  an·gi·o·ma
  can·cer
  cell
  fin·ger
  mole
  ne·vus
  pel·vis
  tel·an·gi·ec·ta·sia
spi·der-burst
Spiegelberg's
  cri·te·ria
Spiegler-Fendt
  pseu·do·lym·pho·ma
  sar·coid
Spielmeyer's acute
  swell·ing
Spielmeyer-Sjögren
  dis·ease
Spielmeyer-Stock
  dis·ease
Spielmeyer-Vogt
  dis·ease
spi·ge·li·an
  her·nia
Spigelius'
  line
  lobe
spike
  po·ten·tial
spike and wave
  com·plex
spill
  cel·lu·lar s.
spill·way
spi·lo·ma
spi·lo·plax·ia
spi·lus
spi·na
  s. an·gu·la·ris
  s. bi·fi·da
  s. bi·fi·da
  s. bi·fi·da aper·ta
  s. bi·fi·da cys·ti·ca
  s. bi·fi·da man·i·fes·ta
  s. bi·fi·da oc·cul·ta

  s. dor·sa·lis
  s. fron·ta·lis
  s. me·a·tus
  s. pe·dis
  s. pe·ro·ne·a·lis
  s. pu·bis
  s. su·pra·me·a·tum
  s. ven·to·sa
spin·a·cene
spin·ach
  stools
spi·nae
spi·nal
  an·al·ge·sia
  an·es·the·sia
  an·es·thet·ic
  an·gi·og·ra·phy
  ap·o·plexy
  ar·te·ri·og·ra·phy
  atax·ia
  at·ro·phy
  block
  ca·nal
  col·umn
  con·cus·sion
  cord
  cur·va·ture
  de·com·pres·sion
  fu·sion
  gan·gli·on
  head·ache
  in·duc·tion
  mar·row
  mus·cle
  mus·cle of head
  mus·cle of neck
  mus·cle of tho·rax
  nerves
  nu·cle·us of ac·ces·so·ry
    nerve
  nu·cle·us of the tri·gem·i·
    nus
  pa·ral·y·sis
  part of ac·ces·so·ry nerve
  point
  punc·ture
  py·ram·i·dot·o·my
  quo·tient
  re·flex
  roots
  shock
  sign
  stroke
  tap
  tract
  trac·tot·o·my
  tract of tri·gem·i·nal nerve
  veins

spi·nal ac·ces·so·ry
  nerve
spi·na·lis
spi·nant
spi·nate
spin·dle
  aor·tic s.
  cen·tral s.
  cleav·age s.
  His' s.
  Krukenberg's s.
  Kühne's s.
  mi·tot·ic s.
  mus·cle s.
  neu·ro·mus·cu·lar s.
  neu·ro·ten·di·nous s.
  nu·cle·ar s.
  sleep s.
spin·dle
  cat·a·ract
  cell
  fi·ber
spin·dle cell
  car·ci·no·ma
  li·po·ma
  ne·vus
  sar·co·ma
spin·dle-celled
  lay·er
spin·dle-shaped
  mus·cle
spine
  cell
  fu·sion
  sign
spine
  alar s.
  an·gu·lar s.
  an·te·ri·or in·fe·ri·or il·i·ac
    s.
  an·te·ri·or na·sal s.
  an·te·ri·or su·pe·ri·or il·i·
    ac s.
  cleft s.
  den·drit·ic s.'s
  dor·sal s.
  great·er tym·pan·ic s.
  s. of he·lix
  he·mal s.
  Henle's s.
  il·i·ac s.
  is·chi·ad·ic s.
  less·er tym·pan·ic s.
  me·a·tal s.
  men·tal s.
  na·sal s. of fron·tal bone
  neu·ral s.
  pal·a·tine s.'s

pe·nis s.'s
pok·er s.
pos·te·ri·or in·fe·ri·or il·i·
  ac s.
pos·te·ri·or na·sal s.
pos·te·ri·or pal·a·tine s.
pos·te·ri·or su·pe·ri·or il·i·
  ac s.
pu·bic s.
s. of scap·u·la
sci·at·ic s.
sphe·noi·dal s.
Spix's s.
su·pra·me·a·tal s.
tho·rac·ic s.
troch·le·ar s.
Spinelli
  op·er·a·tion
spi·nif·u·gal
spi·nip·e·tal
spinn·bar·keit
spin·ning disk
  neb·u·liz·er
spi·no-ad·duc·tor
  re·flex
spi·no·bul·bar
spi·no·cer·e·bel·lar
  tracts
spi·no·cer·e·bel·lum
spi·no·col·lic·u·lar
spi·no·cos·ta·lis
spi·no·gal·va·ni·za·tion
spi·no·gle·noid
  lig·a·ment
spi·no·mus·cu·lar
spi·no·neu·ral
spi·no-ol·i·vary
  tract
spi·nose
spi·no·tec·tal
  tract
spi·no·tha·lam·ic
  cor·dot·o·my
  tract
  trac·tot·o·my
spi·no·trans·ver·sar·i·us
spi·nous
  lay·er
  pro·cess
  pro·cess of tib·ia
spin·thar·i·con
spin·thar·i·scope
spip·e·rone
spi·ra·cle
spi·rad·e·ni·tis
spi·rad·e·no·ma
  ec·crine s.

spi·ral
    Curschmann's s.'s
    s. of Tillaux
spi·ral
    ar·tery
    ban·dage
    ca·nal of co·chlea
    ca·nal of mo·di·o·lus
    crest
    fold of cys·tic duct
    frac·ture
    gan·gli·on of co·chlea
    groove
    hy·phae
    joint
    lig·a·ment of co·chlea
    line
    mem·brane
    or·gan
    plate
    prom·i·nence
    sep·tum
    su·ture
    tu·bule
    valve
    vein of mo·di·o·lus
spi·ral bul·bar
    sep·tum
spi·ral fo·ram·i·nous
    tract
spi·ral tip
    cath·e·ter
spir·a·my·cin
spi·rem
spi·reme
spi·ril·la
Spi·ril·la·ce·ae
spi·ril·lar
    dys·en·tery
spi·ril·li·ci·dal
spi·ril·lo·sis
Spi·ril·lum
    S. mi·nus
    S. vo·lu·tans
spi·ril·lum
    fe·ver
spir·it
    lamp
    ther·mom·e·ter
spir·it
    ar·dent s.'s
    in·dus·tri·al meth·yl·at·ed
      s.
    meth·yl·at·ed s.
    proof s.
    py·ro·lig·ne·ous s.
    pyr·ox·yl·ic s.
    rec·ti·fied s.

wine s.
wood s.
spir·i·tu·ous
    li·quor
spir·i·tus
spiro-
    in·dex
Spi·ro·cer·ca lu·pi
Spi·ro·chae·ta
    S. ober·mei·e·ri
    S. pli·ca·ti·lis
Spi·ro·chae·ta·ce·ae
Spi·ro·chae·ta·les
spi·ro·chet·al
spi·ro·chete
spi·ro·chet·e·mia
spi·ro·che·ti·cide
spi·ro·che·tol·y·sis
spi·ro·che·to·sis
    avi·an s.
    bron·cho·pul·mo·nary s.
spi·ro·che·tot·ic
spi·ro·gram
spi·ro·graph
spi·rom·e·ter
    chain-com·pen·sat·ed s.
    Krogh s.
    Tissot s.
    wedge s.
Spi·ro·me·tra
    S. man·so·ni
    S. man·so·noi·des
spi·rom·e·try
spi·ro·no·lac·tone
    test
spi·ro·scope
spi·ro·stan
spi·ru·roid
    lar·va mi·grans
Spi·ru·roi·dea
spis·si·tude
spit·ting
spit·tle
Spitz
    ne·vus
Spitzer's
    the·o·ry
Spitzka's
    nu·cle·us
Spitzka's mar·gi·nal
    tract
    zone
Spix's
    spine
splanch·nap·o·phys·e·al
splanch·nap·o·phys·i·al
splanch·na·poph·y·sis
splanch·nec·to·pia

splanch·nem·phrax·is
splanch·nes·the·sia
splanch·nes·the·tic
  sen·si·bil·i·ty
splanch·nic
  an·es·the·sia
  cav·i·ty
  gan·gli·on
  lay·er
  mes·o·derm
  nerve
  wall
splanch·nic af·fer·ent
  col·umn
splanch·ni·cec·to·my
splanch·nic ef·fer·ent
  col·umn
splanch·ni·cot·o·my
splanch·no·cele
splanch·no·cra·ni·um
splanch·no·di·as·ta·sis
splanch·nog·ra·phy
splanch·no·lith
splanch·no·lo·gia
splanch·nol·o·gy
splanch·no·meg·a·ly
splanch·no·mic·ria
splanch·nop·a·thy
splanch·no·pleu·ral
splanch·no·pleure
splanch·no·pleu·ric
splanch·nop·to·sia
splanch·nop·to·sis
splanch·no·scle·ro·sis
splanch·no·skel·e·tal
splanch·no·skel·e·ton
splanch·no·so·mat·ic
splanch·not·o·my
splanch·no·tribe
splay
splay·foot
spleen
  ac·ces·so·ry s.
  dif·fuse waxy s.
  float·ing s.
  lar·da·ceous s.
  mov·a·ble s.
  sa·go s.
  sug·ar-coat·ed s.
  waxy s.
spleen
  de·ox·y·ri·bo·nu·cle·ase
  en·do·nu·cle·ase
  phos·pho·di·es·ter·as·es
splen
sple·nal·gia
sple·nauxe

Splendore-Hoeppli
  phe·nom·e·non
sple·nec·to·my
sple·nec·to·pia
sple·nec·to·py
sple·nel·co·sis
sple·nem·phrax·is
sple·ne·o·lus
sple·net·ic
sple·nia
sple·ni·al
  gy·rus
splen·ic
  ane·mia
  ap·o·plexy
  ar·tery
  cells
  cords
  cor·pus·cles
  flex·ure
  in·dex
  leu·ke·mia
  plex·us
  pulp
  re·cess
  si·nus
  vein
  ve·nog·ra·phy
splen·ic flex·ure
  syn·drome
splen·ic lymph
  fol·li·cles
  nodes
  nod·ules
splen·ic por·tal
  ve·nog·ra·phy
sple·ni·cu·lus
splen·i·form
splen·i·ser·rate
sple·ni·tis
sple·ni·um
sple·ni·us
  mus·cle of head
  mus·cle of neck
sple·no·cele
sple·no·clei·sis
sple·no·co·lic
sple·no·dyn·ia
sple·nog·ra·phy
sple·no·he·pa·to·me·ga·lia
sple·no·he·pa·to·meg·a·ly
sple·noid
sple·no·lym·phat·ic
sple·no·ma
sple·no·ma·la·cia
sple·no·med·ul·lary
sple·no·me·ga·lia

sple·no·meg·a·ly
  con·ges·tive s.
  Egyp·tian s.
  he·mo·lyt·ic s.
  hy·per·re·ac·tive ma·lar·i·
    ous s.
  trop·i·cal s.
sple·no·my·e·log·e·nous
sple·no·my·e·lo·ma·la·cia
sple·non·cus
sple·no·neph·ric
sple·no·pan·cre·at·ic
sple·nop·a·thy
sple·no·pex·ia
sple·no·pexy
sple·no·phren·ic
sple·no·por·to·gram
sple·no·por·tog·ra·phy
sple·nop·to·sia
sple·nop·to·sis
sple·no·re·nal
  lig·a·ment
  shunt
sple·nor·rha·gia
sple·nor·rha·phy
sple·not·o·my
sple·no·tox·in
splen·ule
splen·u·li
splen·u·lus
sple·nun·cu·li
sple·nun·cu·lus
splic·ing
splint
  ac·id etch ce·ment·ed s.
  ac·tive s.
  air s.
  air·plane s.
  an·chor s.
  Anderson s.
  back·board s.
  Bal·kan s.'s
  cap s.
  co·ap·ta·tion s.
  con·tact s.
  Cramer wire s.
  Denis Browne s.
  dy·nam·ic s.
  Essig s.
  Frejka pil·low s.
  func·tion·al s.
  Gunning s.
  Hodgen s.
  in·flat·a·ble s.
  in·ter·den·tal s.
  Kingsley s.
  la·bi·al s.
  lad·der s.

lin·gual s.
Liston's s.
plas·ter s.
re·verse Kingsley s.
shin s.'s
Stader s.
sur·gi·cal s.
Taylor's s.
Thomas s.
Tobruk s.
wire s.
splint
  bone
splint·ed
  abut·ment
splin·ter
  hem·or·rhage
splin·tered
  frac·ture
splint·ing
splints
split
  brain
  fat
  gene
  hand
  pap·ules
  pel·vis
  tol·er·ance
split cast
  meth·od
  mount·ing
split re·nal func·tion
  test
split-skin
  graft
split-thick·ness
  flap
  graft
split·ting
  en·zymes
split·ting
spo·dog·e·nous
spod·o·gram
spo·dog·ra·phy
spo·doph·o·rous
spoke-shave
spon·da·ic
spon·dee
Spond·we·ni
  vi·rus
spon·dy·lal·gia
spon·dy·lar·thri·tis
spon·dy·lar·throc·a·ce
spon·dy·lit·ic
spon·dy·li·tis
  an·ky·los·ing s.
  s. de·for·mans

spon·dy·li·tis *(continued)*
  Kümmell's s.
  rheu·ma·toid s.
  tu·ber·cu·lous s.
spon·dy·loc·a·ce
spon·dy·lo·ep·i·phys·i·al
  dys·pla·sia
spon·dy·lo·lis·the·sis
spon·dy·lo·lis·thet·ic
  pel·vis
spon·dy·lol·y·sis
spon·dy·lo·ma·la·cia
spon·dy·lop·a·thy
spon·dy·lop·to·sis
spon·dy·lo·py·o·sis
spon·dy·los·chi·sis
spon·dy·lo·sis
  cer·vi·cal s.
  hy·per·os·tot·ic s.
spon·dy·lo·syn·de·sis
spon·dy·lo·tho·rac·ic
spon·dy·lot·o·my
spon·dyl·ous
sponge
  ab·sorb·a·ble gel·a·tin s.
  Bernays' s.
  bron·cho·scop·ic s.
  com·pressed s.
  con·tra·cep·tive s.
sponge
  bi·op·sy
  tent
spon·gia
spon·gi·form
  en·ceph·a·lop·a·thy
  pus·tule of Kogoj
spon·gi·o·blast
spon·gi·o·blas·to·ma
spon·gi·o·cyte
spon·gi·oid
spon·gi·ose
  part of the male ure·thra
spon·gi·o·sis
spon·gi·o·si·tis
spongy
  body of pe·nis
  bone
  de·gen·er·a·tion
  iri·tis
  spot
  sub·stance
  ure·thra
spon·ta·ne·ous
  abor·tion
  ag·glu·ti·na·tion
  am·pu·ta·tion
  com·bus·tion

  cor·rec·tion of pla·cen·ta
  pre·via
  ev·o·lu·tion
  frac·ture
  gan·grene of new·born
  mu·ta·tion
  phag·o·cy·to·sis
  pneu·mo·thor·ax
  re·cov·ery
  re·mis·sion
  ver·sion
spon·ta·ne·ous ce·phal·ic
  de·liv·ery
spon·ta·ne·ous in·ter·mit·tent
  man·da·to·ry
  ven·ti·la·tion
spoon
  nail
spoon
  cat·a·ract s.
  Daviel's s.
  sharp s.
  Volkmann's s.
spo·rad·ic
spo·rad·ic bo·vine
  leu·ko·sis
spo·ra·din
spo·ran·gia
spo·ran·gi·o·phore
spo·ran·gi·um
spore
  black s.
spo·ri·ci·dal
spo·ri·cide
spo·rid·ia
spo·rid·i·um
spo·ro·ag·glu·ti·na·tion
spo·ro·blast
spo·ro·cyst
Spo·ro·cys·tin·ea
spo·ro·do·chi·um
spo·ro·gen·e·sis
spo·rog·e·nous
spo·rog·e·ny
spo·rog·o·ny
spo·ront
spo·ro·phore
spo·ro·plasm
spo·ro·the·ca
Spo·ro·thrix
spo·ro·tri·cho·sis
spo·ro·tri·cho·sit·ic
  chan·cre
Spo·ro·tri·chum
spo·ro·zo·an
Spo·ro·zo·as·i·da
Spor·o·zo·ea
spo·ro·zo·ite

spo·ro·zo·oid
spo·ro·zo·on
sport
sports
   med·i·cine
spor·u·lar
spor·u·la·tion
spor·ule
spot
   acous·tic s.'s
   Bitot's s.'s
   blind s.
   blood s.'s
   blue s.
   Brushfield's s.'s
   ca·fé au lait s.'s
   cher·ry-red s.
   cor·ne·al s.
   cot·ton-wool s.'s
   De Morgan's s.'s
   Elschnig's s.'s
   Filatov's s.'s
   flame s.'s
   Fordyce's s.'s
   Fuchs' black s.
   Gaule's s.'s
   ger·mi·nal s.
   Graefe's s.'s
   hot s.
   hyp·no·gen·ic s.
   Koplik's s.'s
   liv·er s.
   Mariotte's blind s.
   Maxwell's s.
   milk s.'s
   mon·go·li·an s.
   mul·ber·ry s.'s
   rose s.'s
   Roth's s.'s
   ru·by s.'s
   sac·cu·lar s.
   Soemmering's s.
   spongy s.
   Tardieu's s.'s
   Tay's cher·ry-red s.
   tem·per·a·ture s.
   ten·di·nous s.
   Trousseau's s.
   utric·u·lar s.
   white s.
   yel·low s.
spot
   test for in·fec·tious mon·o·
     nu·cle·o·sis
spot-film
   roent·gen·og·ra·phy

spot·ted
   fe·ver
   sick·ness
sprain
   frac·ture
spray
spread·er
   gut·ta-per·cha s.
   rib s.
   root ca·nal s.
spread·ing
   de·pres·sion
   fac·tor
Sprengel's
   de·for·mi·ty
spring
   con·junc·ti·vi·tis
   fin·ger
   lan·cet
   lig·a·ment
   oph·thal·mia
spring·ing
   my·dri·a·sis
Sprinz-Nelson
   syn·drome
sprout
   syn·cy·tial s.
sprue
   non·trop·i·cal s.
   trop·i·cal s.
sprue-form·er
spud
Spu·ma·vir·i·nae
Spu·ma·vi·rus
spur
   Fuchs' s.
   Grunert's s.
   Michel's s.
   Morand's s.
   scle·ral s.
   vas·cu·lar s.
spu·ri·ous
   an·ky·lo·sis
   cast
   me·nin·go·cele
   preg·nan·cy
   tor·ti·col·lis
spu·ta
spu·tum
   s. aer·o·ge·no·sum
   glob·u·lar s.
   green s.
   num·mu·lar s.
   prune-juice s.
   rusty s.
spu·tum
   smear
squa·lene

squa·ma
  tem·po·ral s.
  s. tem·po·ra·lis
squa·mae
squa·mate
squa·ma·ti·za·tion
squame
squa·mo·cel·lu·lar
squa·mo·co·lum·nar
  junc·tion
squa·mo·fron·tal
squa·mo·mas·toid
  su·ture
squa·mo-oc·cip·i·tal
squa·mo·pa·ri·e·tal
  su·ture
squa·mo·pe·tro·sal
squa·mo·sa
squa·mo·sae
squa·mo·sal
squa·mo·sphe·noid
squa·mo·tem·po·ral
squa·mo·tym·pan·ic
  fis·sure
squa·mous
  cell
  mar·gin
  met·a·pla·sia
  met·a·pla·sia of am·ni·on
  pearl
  su·ture
squa·mous al·ve·o·lar
  cells
squa·mous cell
  car·ci·no·ma
squa·mous odon·to·gen·ic
  tu·mor
squa·mo·zy·go·mat·ic
square wave
  stim·u·li
squar·rose
squar·rous
squill
squint
  con·ver·gent s.
  di·ver·gent s.
  ex·ter·nal s.
  in·ter·nal s.
squint
  hook
squint·ing
  eye
squir·rel
  por·phyr·ia
squir·rel plague
  con·junc·ti·vi·tis
S ro·ma·num

ST
  junc·tion
  seg·ment
stab
  cell
  cul·ture
  drain
  neu·tro·phil
  wound
sta·bi·late
sta·bile
stab·i·lim·e·ter
sta·bil·i·ty
  den·ture s.
  di·men·sion·al s.
  en·dem·ic s.
  en·zo·ot·ic s.
  sus·pen·sion s.
sta·bi·li·za·tion
sta·bi·lized
  base·plate
sta·bi·liz·er
  en·do·don·tic s.
sta·bi·liz·ing cir·cum·fer·en·tial clasp
  arm
sta·bi·liz·ing ful·crum
  line
sta·ble
  col·loid
  equi·lib·ri·um
  fac·tor
  frac·ture
  iso·tope
stac·ca·to
  speech
stach·ybot·ry·o·tox·i·co·sis
stach·y·drine
stach·y·ose
stac·tom·e·ter
Stader
  splint
Staderini's
  nu·cle·us
sta·dia
sta·di·om·e·ter
sta·di·um
staff
  con·sult·ing s.
staff
  cell
Staf·ne bone
  cyst
stage
  al·gid s.
  Arneth s.'s
  cap s.
  cold s.

de·fer·ves·cent s.
end s.
ex·o·e·ryth·ro·cyt·ic s.
im·per·fect s.
in·cu·ba·tive s.
in·tu·i·tive s.
s. of in·va·sion
s.'s of la·bor
la·tent s.
per·fect s.
pre·con·cep·tu·al s.
pro·dro·mal s.
rest·ing s.
Tanner s.
try·pan·o·some s.
tu·mor s.
veg·e·ta·tive s.

stag·es of la·bor
stag·ger
stag·gers
blind s.
brack·en s.
stag·horn
cal·cu·lus
stag·ing
Jewett and Strong s.
TMN s.
stag·nant
an·ox·ia
hy·pox·ia
stag·na·tion
mas·ti·tis
Stahl's
ear
line
stain
Abbott's s. for spores
ac·e·to-or·ce·in s.
ac·id s.
Ag-AS s.
Albert's s.
Altmann's an·i·lin-ac·id
fuch·sin s.
au·ra·mine O flu·o·res·cent
s.
ba·sic s.
ba·sic fuch·sin-meth·yl·ene
blue s.
Bauer's chro·mic ac·id leu·
co·fuch·sin s.
Becker's s. for spi·ro·chetes
Benn·hold's Con·go red s.
Berg's s.
Best's car·mine s.
Bielschowsky's s.
Biondi-Heidenhain s.
Birch-Hirschfeld s.

Bodian's cop·per-PRO·TAR·GOL
s.
Borrel's blue s.
Bowie's s.
Brown-Brenn s.
Cajal's as·tro·cyte s.
car·bol-thi·o·nin s.
C-band·ing s.
cen·tro·mere band·ing s.
chro·mate s. for lead
chrome al·um he·ma·tox·y·
lin-phlox·ine s.
Ciaccio's s.
con·trast s.
Da Fano's s.
Dane's s.
DAPI s.
di·a·zo s. for ar·gen·taf·fin
gran·ules
Dieterle's s.
dif·fer·en·tial s.
dou·ble s.
Ehrlich's ac·id he·ma·tox·y·
lin s.
Ehrlich's an·i·line crys·tal
vi·o·let s.
Ehrlich's tri·ac·id s.
Ehrlich's tri·ple s.
Einarson's gal·lo·cy·a·nin-
chrome al·um s.
Eranko's flu·o·res·cence s.
Feulgen s.
Field's rap·id s.
Fink-Heim·er s.
Flemming's tri·ple s.
flu·o·res·cence plus Giemsa
s.
flu·o·res·cent s.
Fon·ta·na-Mas·son sil·ver s.
Fontana's s.
Foot's re·tic·u·lin im·preg·
na·tion s.
Fouchet's s.
Fraser-Lendrum s. for fi·
brin
Friedländer's s. for cap·sules
G-band·ing s.
Giemsa s.
Giemsa chro·mo·some
band·ing s.
Glenner-Lillie s. for pi·tu·i·
tary
GMS s.
Golgi's s.
Gomori-Jones pe·ri·od·ic
ac·id-me·the·na·mine-sil·ver
s.

stain *(continued)*

Gomori's al·de·hyde fuch·sin s.

Gomori's chrome al·um he·ma·tox·y·lin-phlox·ine s.

Gomori's meth·en·a·mine-sil·ver s.'s

Gomori's non·spe·cif·ic ac·id phos·pha·tase s.

Gomori's non·spe·cif·ic al·ka·line phos·pha·tase s.

Gomori's one-step tri·chrome s.

Gomori's sil·ver im·preg·na·tion s.

Goodpasture's s.

Gordon and Sweet s.

Gram's s.

green s.

Gridley's s.

Gridley's s. for fun·gi

Grocott-Gomori meth·en·a·mine-sil·ver s.

Hale's col·loi·dal iron s.

Heidenhain's azan s.

Heidenhain's iron he·ma·tox·y·lin s.

he·ma·tox·y·lin and eo·sin s.

he·ma·tox·y·lin-mal·a·chite green-ba·sic fuch·sin s.

he·ma·tox·y·lin-phlox·ine B s.

Hirsch-Peiffer s.

Hiss' s.

Holmes' s.

Hortega's neu·rog·lia s.

Hucker-Conn s.

im·mu·no·flu·o·res·cent s.

In·dia ink cap·sule s.

in·tra·vi·tal s.

io·dine s.

Jenner's s.

Kasten's flu·o·res·cent Feulgen s.

Kasten's flu·o·res·cent PAS s.

Kin·youn s.

Kittrich's s.

Kleihauer's s.

Klinger-Ludwig ac·id-thi·o·nin s. for sex chro·ma·tin

Klüver-Barrera Luxol fast blue s.

Kossa s.

Kronecker's s.

Laquer's s. for al·co·hol·ic hy·a·lin

Lawless' s.

lead hy·drox·ide s.

Leishman's s.

Lendrum's phlox·ine-tar·tra·zine s.

Lepehne-Pickworth s.

Levaditi s.

Lillie's al·lo·chrome con·nec·tive tis·sue s.

Lillie's az·ure-e·o·sin s.

Lillie's fer·rous iron s.

Lillie's sul·fu·ric ac·id Nile blue s.

Lison-Dunn s.

Loeffler's s.

Loeffler's caus·tic s.

Luna-Ishak s.

Macchiavello's s.

MacNeal's tet·ra·chrome blood s.

ma·lar·i·al pig·ment s.

Maldonado-San Jose s.

Mallory's s. for ac·ti·no·my·ces

Mallory's an·i·line blue s.

Mallory's col·la·gen s.

Mallory's s. for he·mo·fuch·sin

Mallory's io·dine s.

Mallory's phlox·ine s.

Mallory's phos·pho·tung·stic ac·id he·ma·tox·y·lin s.

Mallory's tri·chrome s.

Mallory's tri·ple s.

Mann's meth·yl blue-e·o·sin s.

Marchi's s.

Masson-Fontana am·mo·ni·a·cal sil·ver s.

Masson's ar·gen·taf·fin s.

Masson's tri·chrome s.

Maximow's s. for bone mar·row

Mayer's he·mal·um s.

Mayer's mu·ci·car·mine s.

Mayer's mu·ci·he·ma·te·in s.

May-Grünwald s.

met·a·chro·mat·ic s.

meth·yl green-py·ro·nin s.

Mowry's col·loi·dal iron s.

MSB tri·chrome s.

mul·ti·ple s.

Nakanishi's s.

Nau·ta's s.

neg·a·tive s.

Neisser's s.

neu·tral s.

Nicolle's s. for cap·sules
nin·hy·drin-Schiff s. for
 pro·teins
Nissl's s.
Noble's s.
nu·cle·ar s.
Orth's s.
ox·y·ta·lan fi·ber s.
Padykula-Herman s. for my·
 o·sin ATPase
Paget-Eccleston s.
pan·op·tic s.
Papanicolaou s.
Pappenheim's s.
par·a·car·mine s.
PAS s.
pe·ri·od·ic ac·id-Schiff s.
Perls' Prus·sian blue s.
per·ox·i·dase s.
phos·pho·tung·stic ac·id s.
pic·ro·car·mine s.
pic·ro-Mallory tri·chrome s.
pic·ro·ni·gro·sin s.
plas·ma s.
plas·mat·ic s.
plas·mic s.
plas·tic sec·tion s.
port-wine s.
pos·i·tive s.
Prus·sian blue s.
PTA s.
Puchtler-Sweat s. for base·
 ment mem·branes
Puchtler-Sweat s. for he·mo·
 glo·bin and he·mo·sid·er·
 in
Q-band·ing s.
quin·a·crine chro·mo·some
 band·ing s.
Rambourg's chro·mic ac·id-
 phos·pho·tung·stic ac·id s.
Rambourg's pe·ri·od·ic
 ac·id-chro·mic meth·en·
 a·mine-sil·ver s.
R-band·ing s.
Ro·ma·now·sky's blood s.
Roux's s.
Schaef·fer-Ful·ton s.
Schmorl's fer·ric-fer·ri·cy·a·
 nide re·duc·tion s.
Schmorl's pic·ro·thi·o·nin s.
Schultz s.
se·lec·tive s.
sil·ver s.
sil·ver-am·mo·ni·a·cal sil·
 ver s.
sil·ver pro·tein s.

Stirling's mod·i·fi·ca·tion of
 Gram's s.
su·pra·vi·tal s.
Taenzer's s.
Takayama's s.
tel·o·mer·ic R-band·ing s.
thi·o·fla·vine T s.
Tiz·zo·ni's s.
Toison's s.
tri·chrome s.
tryp·sin G-band·ing s.
Unna-Pappenheim s.
Unna's s.
Unna-Taenzer s.
ura·nyl ac·e·tate s.
urate crys·tals s.
van Ermengen's s.
van Gieson's s.
Verhoeff's elas·tic tis·sue s.
vi·tal s.
von Kossa s.
Wach·stein-Meis·sel s. for
 cal·ci·um-mag·ne·si·um-
 ATPase
Warthin-Starry sil·ver s.
Weigert-Gram s.
Weigert's s. for ac·ti·no·
 my·ces
Weigert's s. for elas·tin
Weigert's s. for fi·brin
Weigert's iron he·ma·tox·y·
 lin s.
Weigert's s. for my·e·lin
Weigert's s. for neu·rog·lia
Wilder's s. for re·tic·u·lum
Williams' s.
Wright's s.
Ziehl-Neelsen s.
Ziehl's s.
stain·ing
 pro·gress·ive s.
 re·gres·sive s.
stains-all
stair·case
 phe·nom·e·non
stal·ag·mom·e·ter
stalk
 al·lan·to·ic s.
 body s.
 con·nect·ing s.
 in·fun·dib·u·lar s.
 op·tic s.
 pin·e·al s.
 pi·tu·i·tary s.
 yolk s.
stalked
 hy·da·tid
stal·tic

Stamey
  test
stam·mer
stam·mer·ing
  s. of the blad·der
Stam·no·so·ma
stan·dard
  at·mo·sphere
  bi·car·bon·ate
  cell
  de·vi·a·tion
  lead
  pres·sure
  score
  so·lu·tion
  tem·per·a·ture
  vol·ume
stan·dard er·ror of the
  mean
stan·dard er·ror of
  dif·fer·ence
stan·dard·i·za·tion
  s. of a test
stan·dard·ized
  so·lu·tion
stan·dard se·ro·log·ic
  tests for syph·i·lis
stan·dard urea
  clear·ance
stand·by pulse
  gen·er·a·tor
stand·ing
  test
stand·ing plas·ma
  test
stand·still
  atri·al s.
  au·ric·u·lar s.
  car·di·ac s.
  si·nus s.
  ven·tric·u·lar s.
Stanford-Binet in·tel·li·gence
  scale
Stanley's cer·vi·cal
  lig·a·ments
Stanley Way
  pro·ce·dure
stan·nic
stan·nic chlo·ride
stan·nic ox·ide
Stannius
  lig·a·ture
stan·nous
stan·nous flu·o·ride
stan·num
stan·o·lone
stan·o·zo·lol
sta·pe·dec·to·my

sta·pe·des
sta·pe·di·al
  ar·tery
  fold
  mem·brane
sta·pe·dii
sta·pe·di·o·te·not·o·my
sta·pe·di·o·ves·tib·u·lar
sta·pe·di·us
  mus·cle
sta·pes
  mo·bi·li·za·tion
sta·pes mo·bi·li·za·tion
  op·er·a·tion
staph·y·lag·ra
staph·y·lec·to·my
staph·yl·e·de·ma
staph·y·line
sta·phyl·i·on
staph·y·lo·coc·cal
  en·ter·o·tox·in
  pneu·mo·nia
staph·y·lo·coc·cal scald·ed skin
  syn·drome
staph·y·lo·coc·ce·mia
staph·y·lo·coc·ci
staph·y·lo·coc·cia
staph·y·lo·coc·cic
staph·y·lo·coc·col·y·sin
staph·y·lo·coc·col·y·sis
staph·y·lo·coc·co·ses
staph·y·lo·coc·co·sis
Sta·phy·lo·coc·cus
  S. au·re·us
  S. ep·i·derm·i·dis
  S. hy·i·cus
  S. py·og·e·nes al·bus
  S. py·og·e·nes au·re·us
staph·y·lo·coc·cus
  an·ti·tox·in
  vac·cine
Sta·phy·lo·coc·cus food
  poi·son·ing
staph·y·lo·der·ma
staph·y·lo·der·ma·ti·tis
staph·y·lo·di·al·y·sis
staph·y·lo·he·mia
staph·y·lo·he·mo·ly·sin
staph·y·lo·ki·nase
staph·y·lol·y·sin
staph·y·lo·ma
  an·nu·lar s.
  an·te·ri·or s.
  cil·i·ary s.
  cor·ne·al s.
  equa·to·ri·al s.
  in·ter·ca·lary s.
  pos·te·ri·or s.

Scarpa's s.
scle·ral s.
uve·al s.
staph·y·lom·a·tous
staph·y·lon·cus
staph·y·lo-op·son·ic
in·dex
staph·y·lo·phar·yn·gor·rha·phy
staph·y·lo·plas·ty
staph·y·lo·ple·gia
staph·y·lop·to·sis
staph·y·lor·rha·phy
staph·y·los·chi·sis
staph·y·lo·tome
staph·y·lot·o·my
staph·y·lo·tox·in
sta·pling
gas·tric s.
star
daugh·ter s.
lens s.'s
moth·er s.
po·lar s.
ve·nous s.
Verheyen's s.'s
Winslow's s.'s
starch
an·i·mal s.
liv·er s.
moss s.
sol·u·ble s.
starch
equiv·a·lent
glyc·er·ite
gum
sug·ar
starch-eat·ing
starch-i·o·dine
test
stare
post·ba·sic s.
Stargardt's
dis·ease
Starling's
curve
hy·poth·e·sis
law
re·flex
start·ing
fric·tion
star·tle
ep·i·lep·sy
re·ac·tion
re·flex
star·va·tion
di·a·be·tes
starve
sta·ses

stas·i·mor·phia
sta·sis
pap·il·lary s.
pres·sure s.
sta·sis
cir·rho·sis
der·ma·ti·tis
ec·ze·ma
ul·cer
Stas-Otto
meth·od
stat·am·pere
stat·cou·lomb
state
ab·sent s.
ac·ti·vat·ed s.
anx·i·e·ty s.
apal·lic s.
car·ri·er s.
cen·tral ex·cit·a·to·ry s.
con·vul·sive s.
dreamy s.
eu·nuch·oid s.
ex·cit·ed s.
ground s.
hyp·not·ic s.
hy·po·met·a·bol·ic s.
im·per·fect s.
lo·cal ex·cit·a·to·ry s.
mul·ti·ple ego s.'s
per·fect s.
re·frac·to·ry s.
sin·glet s.
steady s.
trip·let s.
twi·light s.
state
hos·pi·tal
state-de·pen·dent
learn·ing
stat·far·ad
stat·hen·ry
stath·mo·ki·ne·sis
stat·ic
ar·throp·a·thy
atax·ia
com·pli·ance
con·vul·sion
fric·tion
gan·grene
hys·ter·e·sis
in·fan·ti·lism
pe·rim·e·try
re·flex
re·frac·tion
re·la·tions
sco·li·o·sis
sense

stat·ic *(continued)*
  sys·tem
  trem·or
stat·ic bone
  cyst
sta·tim
sta·tion
  test
sta·tion·ary
  an·chor·age
  cat·a·ract
  phase
sta·tis·ti·cal
  ge·net·ics
sta·tis·tics
  de·scrip·tive s.
  in·fer·en·tial s.
  vi·tal s.
stat·o·a·cou·stic
stat·o·co·nia
stat·o·co·ni·al
  mem·brane
stat·o·co·ni·um
stat·o·ki·net·ic
  re·flex
stat·o·ki·net·ics
stat·o·liths
sta·tom·e·ter
stat·o·sphere
stat·o·ton·ic
  re·flex·es
stat·ure
sta·tus
  s. an·gi·no·sus
  s. ar·thri·ti·cus
  s. asth·mat·i·cus
  s. cho·le·ra·i·cus
  s. cho·re·i·cus
  s. con·vul·si·vus
  s. cri·bro·sus
  s. cri·ti·cus
  s. dys·my·e·li·ni·sa·tus
  s. dys·ra·phi·cus
  s. ep·i·lep·ti·cus
  s. hem·i·cra·ni·cus
  s. hyp·no·ti·cus
  s. la·cu·na·ris
  s. lym·pha·ti·cus
  s. mar·mo·ra·tus
  s. ner·vo·sus
  s. prae·sens
  s. rap·tus
  s. spon·gi·o·sus
  s. ster·nu·ens
  s. thy·mi·co·lym·pha·ti·cus
  s. thy·mi·cus
  s. ty·pho·sus
  s. ver·ti·gi·no·sus

stat·u·vo·lence
sta·tu·vo·lent
stat·volt
Staub-Traugott
  ef·fect
stau·ri·on
stau·ro·ple·gia
steady
  state
steal
  phe·nom·e·non
steal
  il·i·ac s.
  re·nal-splanch·nic s.
  sub·cla·vi·an s.
steam-fit·ter's
  asth·ma
ste·ap·sin
ste·a·ral
ste·a·ral·de·hyde
ste·a·rate
ste·ar·ic ac·id
ste·a·rin
Stearns al·co·hol·ic
  amen·tia
ste·ar·rhea
ste·a·ryl al·co·hol
ste·a·tite
ste·a·ti·tis
ste·a·to·cys·to·ma
  s. mul·ti·plex
ste·a·to·gen·e·sis
ste·a·tol·y·sis
ste·a·to·ly·tic
ste·a·to·ne·cro·sis
ste·a·to·py·ga
ste·a·to·py·gia
ste·a·to·py·gous
ste·a·tor·rhea
  bil·i·ary s.
  in·tes·ti·nal s.
  pan·cre·at·ic s.
ste·a·to·sis
  s. cor·dis
  he·pa·tic s.
ste·a·to·zo·on
Steele-Richardson-Olszewski
  dis·ease
  syn·drome
Steell's
  mur·mur
Steenbock
  unit
stee·ple
  skull
ste·ge
steg·no·sis
steg·not·ic

Steidele's
com·plex
Steinberg thumb
sign
Steinert's
dis·ease
Stein-Leventhal
syn·drome
Steinmann
pin
Stein's
test
stel·la
s. len·tis hy·a·loi·dea
s. len·tis iri·di·ca
stel·lae
stel·late
ab·scess
block
cat·a·ract
cells of ce·re·bral cor·tex
cells of liv·er
frac·ture
gan·gli·on
hair
lig·a·ment
re·tic·u·lum
ret·i·nop·a·thy
veins
ven·ules
stel·late skull
frac·ture
stel·lec·to·my
stel·lu·la
stel·lu·lae
stel·lu·lae vas·cu·lo·sae
stel·lu·lae ver·hey·en·ii
stel·lu·lae win·slow·ii
Stellwag's
sign
stem
bron·chus
cell
stem
brain s.
in·fun·dib·u·lar s.
stem cell
leu·ke·mia
Stender
dish
Stenger
test
ste·ni·on
sten·o·breg·mat·ic
sten·o·car·dia
sten·o·ce·pha·lia
sten·o·ce·phal·ic
sten·o·ceph·a·lous

sten·o·ceph·a·ly
sten·o·cho·ria
sten·o·com·pres·sor
sten·o·cro·ta·phia
sten·o·crot·a·phy
sten·o·pa·ic
disk
spec·ta·cles
sten·o·pe·ic
disk
ir·i·dec·to·my
spec·ta·cles
Steno's
duct
ste·no·sal
mur·mur
ste·nosed
ste·no·ses
ste·no·sis
aor·tic s.
but·ton·hole s.
cal·cif·ic nod·u·lar aor·tic
s.
con·gen·i·tal py·lor·ic s.
cor·o·nary os·ti·al s.
Dittrich's s.
dou·ble aor·tic s.
fish-mouth mi·tral s.
hy·per·tro·phic py·lor·ic s.
id·i·o·path·ic hy·per·tro·
phic sub·a·or·tic s.
in·fun·dib·u·lar s.
la·ryn·ge·al s.
mi·tral s.
mus·cu·lar sub·a·or·tic s.
pul·mo·nary s.
py·lor·ic s.
sub·a·or·tic s.
sub·val·var s.
su·pra·val·var s.
tri·cus·pid s.
sten·o·ste·no·sis
sten·o·sto·mia
sten·o·ther·mal
sten·o·tho·rax
ste·not·ic
sten·ox·e·nous
sten·ox·ous
par·a·site
Stensen's
duct
ex·per·i·ment
fo·ra·men
plex·us
veins
Stent
graft
stent

Stenvers
  pro·jec·tion
  view
step
  Krönig's s.'s
  Roenne's na·sal s.
ste·pha·ni·al
ste·pha·ni·on
Ste·pha·no·fi·la·ria sti·le·si
Steph·a·nu·rus den·ta·tus
step·page
  gait
step·ping
  re·flex
ste·ra·di·an
ster·ane
ster·co·bi·lin
l-ster·co·bi·lin·o·gen
ster·co·lith
ster·co·ra·ceous
  vom·it·ing
ster·co·ral
  ab·scess
  ap·pen·di·ci·tis
  fis·tu·la
  ul·cer
ster·co·rin
ster·co·ro·ma
ster·co·rous
ster·cu·lia
  gum
ster·cus
stere
ster·e·o·ag·no·sis
ster·e·o·an·es·the·sia
ster·e·o·ar·throl·y·sis
ster·e·o·cam·pim·e·ter
ster·e·o·chem·i·cal
  for·mu·la
  isom·er·ism
ster·e·o·chem·is·try
ster·e·o·cil·ia
ster·e·o·cil·i·um
ster·e·o·cin·e·flu·o·rog·ra·phy
ster·e·o·col·po·gram
ster·e·o·col·po·scope
ster·e·o·e·lec·tro·en·ceph·a·log·
  ra·phy
ster·e·o·en·ceph·a·lom·e·try
ster·e·o·en·ceph·a·lot·o·my
ster·e·og·no·sis
ster·e·og·nos·tic
ster·e·o·gram
ster·e·o·graph
ster·e·o·i·so·mer
ster·e·o·i·so·mer·ic
ster·e·o·i·som·er·ism
ster·e·ol·o·gy

ster·e·om·e·ter
ster·e·om·e·try
ster·e·o-or·thop·ter
ster·e·op·a·thy
ster·e·o·phan·to·scope
ster·e·o·pho·rom·e·ter
ster·e·o·phor·o·scope
ster·e·o·pho·to·mi·cro·graph
ster·e·op·sis
ster·e·o·ra·di·og·ra·phy
ster·e·o·roent·gen·og·ra·phy
ster·e·o·scope
ster·e·o·scop·ic
  acu·i·ty
  mi·cro·scope
  par·al·lax
  pel·vim·e·try
  vi·sion
ster·e·os·co·py
ster·e·o·se·lec·tive
ster·e·o·spe·cif·ic
ster·e·o·tac·tic
  cor·dot·o·my
  in·stru·ment
  sur·gery
ster·e·o·tax·ic
  in·stru·ment
  lo·cal·i·za·tion
  sur·gery
ster·e·o·tax·is
ster·e·o·taxy
ster·e·o·tro·pic
ster·e·ot·ro·pism
ster·e·o·typy
  oral s.
ste·ric
ste·ric hin·drance
ster·id
ste·rig·ma
ste·rig·ma·ta
ster·ile
  ab·scess
  cyst
ster·ile in·sect
  tech·nique
ste·ril·i·ty
  ab·so·lute s.
  ad·o·les·cent s.
  asper·mat·o·gen·ic s.
  dys·sper·mat·o·gen·ic s.
  fe·male s.
  male s.
  nor·mo·sper·ma·to·gen·ic s.
  one-child s.
  rel·a·tive s.
ster·il·i·za·tion
  dis·con·tin·u·ous s.

frac·tion·al s.
in·ter·mit·tent s.
ster·il·ize
ster·il·iz·er
glass bead s.
hot salt s.
ster·na
ster·nad
ster·nal
an·gle
ar·ter·ies
bar
car·ti·lage
ex·trem·i·ty of clav·i·cle
joints
line
mem·brane
mus·cle
notch
part of di·a·phragm
plane
punc·ture
syn·chon·dro·ses
ster·nal ar·tic·u·lar
sur·face of clav·i·cle
ster·nal·gia
ster·na·lis
Sternberg
cells
Sternberg-Reed
cells
ster·ne·bra
ster·ne·brae
ster·nen
ster·ni
ster·no·brach·i·al
re·flex
ster·no·chon·dro·scap·u·lar
mus·cle
ster·no·chon·dro·sca·pu·la·ris
ster·no·cla·vic·u·lar
an·gle
disk
joint
lig·a·ment
mus·cle
ster·no·cla·vic·u·lar ar·tic·u·lar
disk
ster·no·cla·vi·cu·la·ris
ster·no·clei·dal
ster·no·clei·do·mas·toid
mus·cle
re·gion
vein
ster·no·clei·do·mas·toi·de·us
ster·no·cos·tal
ar·tic·u·la·tions
joints

part
sur·face of heart
tri·an·gle
ster·no·dyn·ia
ster·no·fas·ci·a·lis
ster·no·glos·sal
ster·no·hy·oid
mus·cle
ster·no·hy·oi·de·us
ster·noid
ster·no·mas·toid
ar·tery
mus·cle
ster·no·pa·gia
ster·no·per·i·car·di·al
lig·a·ment
ster·nos·chi·sis
ster·no·thy·roid
mus·cle
ster·no·thy·roi·de·us
ster·not·o·my
ster·no·tra·che·al
ster·no·try·pe·sis
ster·no·ver·te·bral
Stern's
pos·ture
ster·num
ster·nu·ta·tion
ster·nu·ta·tor
ster·nu·ta·to·ry
ab·sence
ste·roid
ac·ne
di·a·be·tes
fe·ver
hor·mones
nu·cle·us
ul·cer
ste·roid
s. hy·drox·y·las·es
s. mon·o·ox·y·ge·na·ses
ste·roi·dal
ste·roid met·a·bol·ic clear·ance
rate
ste·roi·do·gen·e·sis
ste·roid pro·duc·tion
rate
ste·roids
ste·roid se·cre·to·ry
rate
ste·roid with·draw·al
syn·drome
ste·rol
ster·tor
hen-cluck s.
ster·to·rous
ste·thal·gia
steth·ar·te·ri·tis

steth·en·do·scope
steth·o·cyr·to·graph
steth·o·cyr·tom·e·ter
steth·o·go·ni·om·e·ter
steth·o·graph
steth·o·kyr·to·graph
steth·o·my·i·tis
steth·o·my·o·si·tis
steth·o·pa·ral·y·sis
steth·o·scope
  bin·au·ral s.
  Bowles type s.
  dif·fer·en·tial s.
steth·o·scop·ic
  pho·no·car·di·o·graph
ste·thos·co·py
steth·o·spasm
Stevens-Johnson
  syn·drome
Stewart-Holmes
  sign
Stewart-Morel
  syn·drome
Stewart's
  test
Stewart-Treves
  syn·drome
sthe·nia
sthen·ic
sthe·nom·e·ter
sthe·nom·e·try
stib·a·mine glu·co·side
stib·e·nyl
stib·i·al·ism
stib·i·a·ted
stib·i·a·tion
stib·i·um
stib·o·cap·tate
stib·o·glu·co·nate so·di·um
sti·bo·ni·um
stib·o·phen
stich·o·chrome
  cell
Sticker's
  dis·ease
Stickler
  syn·drome
Stieda's
  pro·cess
Stierlin's
  sign
sties
stiff
  neck
  toe
stiff lamb
  dis·ease

stiff-man
  syn·drome
sti·fle
  bone
  joint
stig·ma
  fol·lic·u·lar s.
  mal·pi·ghi·an stig·mas
  s. ven·tric·u·li
stig·mas
stig·mas·tane
stig·ma·ta
stig·ma·ta may·dis
stig·mat·ic
stig·ma·tism
stig·ma·ti·za·tion
stig·ma·tom·e·ter
stil·bam·i·dine
stil·baz·i·um io·dide
stil·bene
stil·bes·trol
Stiles-Crawford
  ef·fect
sti·let
sti·lette
still
  lay·er
still·birth
  rate
still·born
  in·fant
Still-Chauffard
  syn·drome
Stilling col·or
  ta·bles
Stilling's
  ca·nal
  col·umn
  nu·cle·us
  ra·phe
Stilling's ge·lat·i·nous
  sub·stance
Still's
  dis·ease
  mur·mur
sti·lus
stim·u·lant
  dif·fus·i·ble s.
  gen·er·al s.
  lo·cal s.
stim·u·la·tion
  dor·sal col·umn s.
  Ganzfeld s.
  per·cu·ta·ne·ous s.
  pho·tic s.
stim·u·la·tor
  long-act·ing thy·roid s.
stim·u·li

stim·u·lus
ad·e·quate s.
con·di·tioned s.
dis·crim·i·nant s.
het·er·ol·o·gous s.
ho·mol·o·gous s.
in·ad·e·quate s.
lim·i·nal s.
max·i·mal s.
square wave stim·u·li
sub·lim·i·nal s.
sub·thresh·old s.
su·pra·max·i·mal s.
thresh·old s.
train-of-four s.
un·con·di·tion·ed s.
stim·u·lus
con·trol
gen·er·al·i·za·tion
sub·sti·tu·tion
thresh·old
stim·u·lus sen·si·tive
my·oc·lo·nus
stim·u·lus word
sting
stink weed
stip·pled
epiph·y·sis
tongue
stip·pling
ge·o·graph·ic s. of nails
Ziemann's s.
Stirling's mod·i·fi·ca·tion of
Gram's
stain
stir·rup
stitch
ab·scess
St. Louis en·ceph·a·li·tis
vi·rus
Sto·bo
an·ti·gen
stock
cul·ture
strain
vac·cine
Stocker's
line
Stock·holm
syn·drome
stock·ing
an·es·the·sia
Stoerk's
blen·nor·rhea
Stoffel's
op·er·a·tion
stoi·chi·ol·o·gy
stoi·chi·o·met·ric

stoi·chi·om·e·try
stoke
stok·er's
cramps
Stokes
am·pu·ta·tion
Stokes'
law
Stokes-Adams
dis·ease
syn·drome
sto·lon
sto·ma
Fuchs' sto·mas
loop s.
stom·ach
bi·loc·u·lar s.
cas·cade s.
drain-trap s.
hour·glass s.
leath·er-bot·tle s.
min·i·a·ture s.
Pavlov s.
pow·dered s.
scle·rot·ic s.
tho·rac·ic s.
tri·fid s.
wal·let s.
wa·ter-trap s.
stom·ach
ache
cough
drops
pump
reef·ing
tooth
tube
stom·ach·al
stom·a·chal·gia
sto·mach·ic
stom·a·cho·dyn·ia
sto·mal
ul·cer
sto·mas
sto·ma·ta
sto·ma·tal
sto·ma·tal·gia
sto·mat·ic
sto·ma·ti·tis
an·gu·lar s.
aph·tho·bul·lous s.
aph·thous s.
bo·vine pap·u·lar s.
gan·gre·nous s.
gon·o·coc·cal s.
lead s.
s. me·di·ca·men·to·sa
mer·cu·ri·al s.

sto·ma·ti·tis *(continued)*
  s. pa·pu·lo·sa
  pri·mary her·pet·ic s.
  re·cur·rent aph·thous s.
  re·cur·rent her·pet·ic s.
  re·cur·rent ul·cer·a·tive s.
  ul·cer·a·tive s.
  s. ve·ne·na·ta
  ve·sic·u·lar s.
sto·ma·to·ca·thar·sis
sto·ma·to·cyte
sto·ma·to·cy·to·sis
sto·ma·to·de·um
sto·ma·to·dyn·ia
sto·ma·to·dys·o·dia
sto·ma·to·gnath·ic
  sys·tem
sto·ma·to·log·ic
sto·ma·tol·o·gist
sto·ma·tol·o·gy
sto·ma·to·ma·la·cia
sto·mat·o·my
sto·ma·to·my·co·sis
sto·ma·to·ne·cro·sis
sto·ma·to·no·ma
sto·ma·top·a·thy
sto·ma·to·plas·tic
sto·ma·to·plas·ty
sto·ma·tor·rha·gia
sto·ma·to·scope
sto·ma·to·sis
sto·ma·tot·o·my
sto·mi·on
sto·mo·ceph·a·lus
sto·mo·de·al
sto·mo·de·um
Sto·mox·ys cal·ci·trans
stone
  ar·ti·fi·cial s.
  pulp s.
  skin s.'s
  tear s.
  vein s.
stone
  bas·ket
  heart
stone-ma·sons'
  dis·ease
Stookey-Scarff
  op·er·a·tion
stool
  but·ter s.'s
  rice-wa·ter s.
  spin·ach s.'s
  Trélat's s.'s
stop-nee·dle
stop-spec·u·lum
stops

stor·age
  dis·ease
  os·cil·lo·scope
sto·rax
sto·ri·form
  neu·ro·fi·bro·ma
storm
  thy·roid s.
Stout's
  wir·ing
stra·bis·mal
stra·bis·mic
  am·bly·o·pia
  nys·tag·mus
stra·bis·mom·e·ter
stra·bis·mus
  A-s.
  ac·com·mo·da·tive s.
  al·ter·nate day s.
  al·ter·nat·ing s.
  con·com·i·tant s.
  con·ver·gent s.
  cy·clic s.
  s. de·or·sum ver·gens
  di·ver·gent s.
  ex·ter·nal s.
  in·com·i·tant s.
  in·ter·nal s.
  ki·net·ic s.
  man·i·fest s.
  me·chan·i·cal s.
  mo·noc·u·lar s.
  par·a·lyt·ic s.
  s. sur·sum ver·gens
  ver·ti·cal s.
  X-s.
stra·bom·e·ter
strab·o·tome
stra·bot·o·my
strad·dling
  em·bo·lism
straight
  gy·rus
  jack·et
  part
  si·nus
  tu·bule
  ven·ules of kid·ney
straight back
  syn·drome
strain
  frac·ture
  gauge
strain
  aux·o·tro·phic s.'s
  car·ri·er s.
  cell s.
  con·gen·ic s.

HFR s.
Hfr s.
hy·po·thet·i·cal mean s.
iso·gen·ic s.
ly·so·gen·ic s.
ne·o·type s.
pro·to·tro·phic s.'s
pseu·do·ly·so·gen·ic s.
re·com·bi·nant s.
stock s.
type s.
wild-type s.

strait
strait·jack·et
stra·mo·ni·um
strand
com·ple·men·ta·ry s.
mi·nus s.
plus s.
vi·ral s.
stran·gal·es·the·sia
stran·gle
stran·gles
stran·gu·lat·ed
her·nia
stran·gu·la·tion
stran·gu·ry
strap
cell
mus·cles
Strassburg's
test
Strassman's
phe·nom·e·non
stra·ta
stra·ti
strat·i·fi·ca·tion
strat·i·fied
ep·i·the·li·um
throm·bus
strat·i·fied cil·i·at·ed co·lum·
nar
ep·i·the·li·um
strat·i·fied squa·mous
ep·i·the·li·um
strat·i·form
fi·bro·car·ti·lage
stra·tig·ra·phy
stra·to·graph·ic
anal·y·sis
stra·tum
s. acu·le·a·tum
s. al·bum pro·fun·dum
s. ba·sa·le
s. ba·sa·le ep·i·derm·i·dis
s. ce·re·bra·le ret·i·nae
s. ci·ne·re·um col·lic·u·li
su·pe·ri·o·ris

s. cir·cu·la·re mem·bra·nae
tym·pa·ni
s. com·pac·tum
s. cor·ne·um ep·i·derm·i·
dis
s. cor·ne·um un·guis
s. cu·ta·ne·um mem·bra·nae
tym·pa·ni
s. cy·lin·dri·cum
s. dis·junc·tum
s. func·tio·na·le
s. gan·gli·o·na·re ner·vi op·
ti·ci
s. gan·gli·o·na·re ret·i·nae
s. gan·gli·o·sum ce·re·bel·li
s. ger·mi·na·ti·vum
s. ger·mi·na·ti·vum un·guis
s. gran·u·lo·sum fol·lic·u·li
ova·ri·ci ve·si·cu·lo·si
s. gran·u·lo·sum ova·rii
s. gris·e·um me·di·um
s. gris·e·um pro·fun·dum
s. gris·e·um su·per·fi·ci·a·le
s. in·ter·ol·i·va·re lem·nis·
ci
s. lem·nis·ci
s. lu·ci·dum
mal·pi·ghi·an s.
s. mo·le·cu·la·re
s. mo·le·cu·la·re ret·i·nae
s. neu·ro·ep·i·the·li·a·le
ret·i·nae
s. nu·cle·a·re ex·ter·num et
in·ter·num ret·i·nae
s. nu·cle·a·re ex·ter·num
ret·i·nae
s. nu·cle·a·re in·ter·num
ret·i·nae
s. op·ti·cum
s. pa·pil·la·re co·rii
s. pig·men·ti bul·bi
s. pig·men·ti cor·po·ris cil·
i·ar·is
s. pig·men·ti ir·i·dis
s. pig·men·ti ret·i·nae
s. plex·i·for·me ex·ter·num
et in·ter·num ret·i·nae
s. ra·di·a·tum mem·bra·nae
tym·pa·ni
s. re·ti·cu·la·re co·rii
s. re·ti·cu·la·re cu·tis
s. spi·no·sum ep·i·derm·i·
dis
s. spon·gi·o·sum
s. sub·cu·ta·ne·um
Straus
re·ac·tion

Straus'
  sign
straw
  itch
straw-bed
  itch
straw·ber·ry
  birth·mark
  gall·blad·der
  mark
  ne·vus
  tongue
straw·ber·ry-cream
  blood
streak
  cul·ture
  hy·per·os·to·sis
streak
  an·gi·oid s.'s
  go·nad·al s.
  Knapp's s.'s
  men·in·git·ic s.
  Moore's light·ning s.'s
  prim·i·tive s.
streaked
  go·nad
stream
  hair s.'s
stream·ing
  move·ment
streb·lo·dac·ty·ly
street
  vi·rus
Streeter's
  bands
Streeter's ho·ri·zon
strem·ma
strength
  as·so·ci·a·tive s.
  bit·ing s.
  com·pres·sive s.
  fa·tigue s.
  ion·ic s.
  ten·sile s.
  ul·ti·mate s.
  yield s.
strength-du·ra·tion
  curve
streph·o·sym·bo·lia
stre·pi·tus
strep·ti·ce·mia
Strep·to·ba·cil·lus
  S. mo·nil·i·for·mis
strep·to·bi·o·sa·mine
strep·to·bi·ose
strep·to·cer·ci·a·sis

strep·to·coc·cal
  fi·bri·nol·y·sin
  pneu·mo·nia
strep·to·coc·ce·mia
strep·to·coc·ci
strep·to·coc·cic
strep·to·coc·co·sis
Strep·to·coc·cus
  S. ac·i·do·min·i·mus
  S. ag·a·lac·ti·ae
  S. an·gi·no·sus
  S. bo·vis
  S. du·rans
  S. dys·ga·lac·ti·ae
  S. equi
  S. equi·nus
  S. equi·si·mi·lis
  S. fae·ca·lis
  S. lac·tis
  S. mi·tis
  S. mu·tans
  S. pneu·mo·ni·ae
  S. py·og·e·nes
  S. sa·li·va·ri·us
  S. san·guis
  S. ube·ris
  S. vir·i·dans
  S. zo·o·e·pi·de·mi·cus
strep·to·coc·cus
  he·mo·lyt·ic strep·to·coc·ci
strep·to·coc·cus eryth·ro·gen·ic
  tox·in
Strep·to·coc·cus lac·tis R
  fac·tor
Strep·to·coc·cus M
  an·ti·gen
strep·to·der·ma
strep·to·der·ma·ti·tis
strep·to·dor·nase
strep·to·fu·ra·nose
strep·to·ki·nase
strep·to·ki·nase-strep·to·dor·nase
strep·to·ly·sin
  s. O
Strep·to·my·ces
  S. al·bus
  S. gib·so·nii
  S. so·ma·li·en·sis
Strep·to·my·ce·ta·ce·ae
strep·to·my·cete
strep·to·my·cin
  units
strep·to·my·cin A
strep·to·my·co·sis
strep·to·ni·vi·cin
strep·tose
strep·to·sep·ti·ce·mia

strep·to·thri·cho·sis
Strep·to·thrix
strep·to·tri·chi·a·sis
strep·to·tri·cho·sis
strep·to·zo·cin
stress
   life s.
   shear s.
   ten·sile s.
   yield s.
stress
   frac·ture
   im·mu·ni·ty
   in·oc·u·la·tion
   re·ac·tion
   ul·cers
stress-bear·ing
   ar·ea
stress break·er
stress ris·er
stress shield·ing
stress-strain
   curve
stretch
   re·cep·tors
   re·flex
stretch·er
stri·a
   acous·tic stri·ae
   stri·ae atro·phi·cae
   au·di·to·ry stri·ae
   brown stri·ae
   stri·ae ci·li·a·res
   stri·ae cu·tis dis·ten·sae
   s. for·ni·cis
   Gennari's s.
   stri·ae grav·i·dar·um
   Knapp's stri·ae
   stri·ae lan·ci·si
   Langhans' s.
   lat·er·al lon·gi·tu·di·nal s.
   me·di·al lon·gi·tu·di·nal s.
   med·ul·lary stri·ae of the
     fourth ven·tri·cle
   med·ul·lary s. of the thal·
     a·mus
   s. na·si trans·ver·sa
   Nitabuch's s.
   ol·fac·to·ry stri·ae
   stri·ae pa·ral·le·lae
   stri·ae ret·i·nae
   Retzius' stri·ae
   Rohr's s.
   s. spi·no·sa
   s. tec·ta
   ter·mi·nal s.
   s. ven·tric·u·li ter·tii

Wickham's stri·ae
stri·ae of Zahn
stri·ae
stri·a·tal
stri·ate
   ar·ea
   at·ro·phy of skin
   body
   cor·tex
   ker·a·top·a·thy
   veins
stri·at·ed
   bor·der
   duct
   mem·brane
   mus·cle
stri·at·ed mus·cu·lar
   sphinc·ter
stri·a·tion
   ba·sal s.'s
   tab·by cat s.
   ti·groid s.
stri·a·to·ni·gral
stri·a·tum
stric·ture
   anas·to·mot·ic s.
   an·nu·lar s.
   bri·dle s.
   con·trac·tile s.
   func·tion·al s.
   Hunner's s.
   or·gan·ic s.
   per·ma·nent s.
   re·cur·rent s.
   spas·mod·ic s.
   tem·po·rary s.
   ure·thral s.
stric·tur·o·tome
stric·tur·ot·o·my
stri·dent
stri·dor
   con·gen·i·tal s.
   s. den·ti·um
   ex·pi·ra·to·ry s.
   in·spi·ra·to·ry s.
   la·ryn·ge·al s.
   s. ser·ra·ti·cus
strid·u·lous
string
   au·di·to·ry s.'s
string
   test
stringed in·stru·ment
   the·o·ry
strip
   abra·sive s.
   amal·gam s.

strip *(continued)*
cel·lu·loid s.
light·ning s.
stripe
s. of Gennari
Hensen's s.
mal·le·ar s.
Mees' s.'s
vas·cu·lar s.
stripped
at·om
strip·per
strip·per's
asth·ma
stro·bi·la
stro·bi·lae
strob·i·lo·cer·cus
strob·i·loid
stro·bo·scope
stro·bo·scop·ic
disk
mi·cro·scope
Stroganoff's
meth·od
stroke
out·put
vol·ume
stroke
heart s.
heat s.
spi·nal s.
sun s.
stroke work
in·dex
strok·ing
stro·ma
s. of iris
lym·phat·ic s.
s. of ova·ry
Rollet's s.
s. of thy·roid gland
s. of vit·re·ous
stro·ma
plex·us
stro·mal
hy·per·the·co·sis
stro·ma·ta
stro·ma·tin
stro·ma·tol·y·sis
stro·ma·to·sis
strom·ic
stro·muhr
Ludwig's s.
thermo-s.
strong sil·ver
pro·tein
Strong vo·ca·tion·al in·ter·est
test

stron·gyle
Stron·gyl·i·dae
Stron·gy·loi·dea
Stron·gy·loi·des
stron·gy·loi·di·a·sis
stron·gy·loi·do·sis
stron·gy·lo·sis
Stron·gy·lus
S. as·ini
S. eden·ta·tus
S. equi·nus
S. ra·di·a·tus
S. ven·tri·co·sus
S. vul·ga·ris
stron·ti·um
stro·phan·thin
Stro·phan·thus
stroph·o·ceph·a·ly
stroph·o·so·mia
stroph·u·lus
s. can·di·dus
s. in·ter·tinc·tus
s. pru·ri·gi·no·sus
Stroud's pec·ti·nat·ed
ar·ea
struck
struc·tur·al
for·mu·la
gene
in·ter·face
isom·er·ism
struc·tur·al·ism
struc·ture
brush heap s.
crys·tal s.
den·ture-sup·port·ing s.'s
fine s.
gel s.
men·tal s.
tu·bo·re·tic·u·lar s.
stru·ma
s. aber·ra·ta
s. col·loi·des
Hashimoto's s.
lig·ne·ous s.
s. lym·pho·ma·to·sa
s. ma·lig·na
s. me·di·ca·men·to·sa
s. ova·rii
Riedel's s.
stru·mae
stru·mec·to·my
me·di·an s.
stru·mi·form
stru·mi·tis
stru·mous
Strümpell-Marie
dis·ease

Strümpell's
dis·ease
phe·nom·e·non
re·flex
Strümpell-Westphal
dis·ease
stru·vite
cal·cu·lus
strych·nine
strych·nin·ism
Strych·nos
Stryker
frame
saw
Stryker-Halbeisen
syn·drome
Stuart
fac·tor
Stuart-Prower
fac·tor
stuck
fin·ger
Stu·dent's *t*
test
study
blind s.
case-con·trol s.
co·hort s.
cross-sec·tion·al s.
di·a·chron·ic s.
dou·ble blind s.
lon·gi·tu·di·nal s.
mul·ti·var·i·ate s.'s
syn·chron·ic s.
stump
can·cer
hal·lu·ci·na·tion
neu·ral·gia
stun
stupe
stu·pe·fa·cient
stu·pe·fac·tive
stu·por
be·nign s.
cat·a·ton·ic s.
de·pres·sive s.
ma·lig·nant s.
stu·por·ous
cat·a·to·nia
Sturge-Kalischer-Weber
syn·drome
Sturge's
dis·ease
Sturge-Weber
dis·ease
syn·drome
Sturmdorf's
op·er·a·tion

Sturm's
co·noid
in·ter·val
stut·ter
stut·ter·ing
uri·nary s.
stut·ter·ing
uri·na·tion
Stuttgart
dis·ease
sty
mei·bo·mi·an s.
zeis·i·an s.
stye
styes
style
sty·let
en·do·tra·che·al s.
sty·lette
sty·li·form
sty·lo·au·ric·u·lar
mus·cle
sty·lo·au·ri·cu·la·ris
sty·lo·glos·sus
mus·cle
sty·lo·hy·al
sty·lo·hy·oid
lig·a·ment
mus·cle
sty·loid
cor·nu
pro·cess of fib·u·la
pro·cess of ra·di·us
pro·cess of tem·po·ral bone
pro·cess of third met·a·car·pal bone
pro·cess of ul·na
prom·i·nence
sty·loi·di·tis
sty·lo·la·ryn·ge·us
sty·lo·man·dib·u·lar
lig·a·ment
sty·lo·mas·toid
ar·tery
fo·ra·men
vein
sty·lo·max·il·lary
lig·a·ment
sty·lo·pha·ryn·ge·al
mus·cle
sty·lo·pha·ryn·ge·us
sty·lo·po·di·um
sty·lo·ra·di·al
re·flex
sty·lo·staph·y·line
sty·los·te·o·phyte
Sty·lo·vir·i·dae

sty·lus
  trac·ing
stype
"s"-type
  cho·lin·es·ter·ase
styp·tic
  col·lo·di·on
  col·loid
  cot·ton
styr·a·mate
sty·rax
sty·rene
sty·rol
sty·rone
sub·ab·dom·i·nal
sub·ab·dom·i·no·per·i·to·ne·al
sub·ac·e·tate
sub·a·cro·mi·al
  bur·sa
  bur·si·tis
sub·a·cute
  ab·scess
  glo·mer·u·lo·ne·phri·tis
  hep·a·ti·tis
  in·flam·ma·tion
  ne·phri·tis
  rheu·ma·tism
sub·a·cute bac·te·ri·al
  en·do·car·di·tis
sub·a·cute com·bined
  de·gen·er·a·tion of the spi·
  nal cord
sub·a·cute gran·u·lom·a·tous
  thy·roid·i·tis
sub·a·cute in·clu·sion body
  en·ceph·a·li·tis
sub·a·cute mi·gra·to·ry
  pan·nic·u·li·tis
sub·a·cute nec·ro·tiz·ing
  my·e·li·tis
sub·a·cute scle·ros·ing
  leu·ko·en·ceph·a·li·tis
  pan·en·ceph·a·li·tis
sub·a·cute spon·gi·form
  en·ceph·a·lop·a·thy
sub·ad·ven·ti·tial
  fi·bro·sis
sub·al·i·men·ta·tion
sub·a·nal
sub·an·co·ne·us
  mus·cle
sub·a·or·tic
  ste·no·sis
sub·a·or·tic lymph
  nodes
sub·ap·i·cal
  seg·ment
sub·ap·o·neu·rot·ic

sub·a·rach·noid
  an·es·the·sia
  cav·i·ty
  hem·or·rhage
  space
sub·ar·ach·noi·dal
  cis·terns
sub·ar·cu·ate
  fos·sa
sub·a·re·o·lar
sub·a·re·o·lar duct
  pap·il·lo·ma·to·sis
sub·as·trag·a·lar
  am·pu·ta·tion
sub·a·tom·ic
sub·au·ral
sub·au·ric·u·lar
sub·ax·i·al
sub·ax·il·lary
sub·bas·al
sub·brach·y·ce·phal·ic
sub·cal·ca·rine
sub·cal·lo·sal
  ar·ea
  fas·cic·u·lus
  gy·rus
sub·cap·i·tal
  frac·ture
sub·cap·su·lar
  cat·a·ract
sub·car·bon·ate
sub·car·di·nal
sub·car·ti·lag·i·nous
sub·ce·cal
  fos·sa
sub·cel·lu·lar
sub·cep·tion
sub·chlo·ride
sub·chon·dral
sub·cho·ri·al
  lake
  space
sub·cho·ri·on·ic
sub·cho·roi·dal
sub·class
sub·cla·vi·an
  ar·tery
  duct
  groove
  loop
  mus·cle
  nerve
  plex·us
  steal
  sul·cus
  tri·an·gle
  trunk
  vein

sub·cla·vi·an steal
  syn·drome
sub·cla·vic·u·lar
sub·cla·vi·us
sub·clin·i·cal
  ab·sence
  di·a·be·tes
sub·col·lat·er·al
sub·com·mis·sur·al
  or·gan
sub·con·junc·ti·val
sub·con·junc·ti·vi·tis
sub·con·scious
  mem·o·ry
  mind
sub·con·scious·ness
sub·cor·a·coid
sub·cor·ne·al pus·tu·lar
  der·ma·ti·tis
  der·ma·to·sis
sub·cor·tex
sub·cor·ti·cal
sub·cor·ti·cal ar·te·ri·o·scle·
  rot·ic
  en·ceph·a·lop·a·thy
sub·cos·tal
  ar·tery
  groove
  line
  mus·cle
  nerve
  plane
sub·cos·tal·gia
sub·cos·to·ster·nal
sub·cra·ni·al
sub·crep·i·tant
  rale
sub·crep·i·ta·tion
sub·crest·al
  pock·et
sub·cru·ral
  mus·cle
sub·cru·ra·lis
sub·cru·re·us
sub·cul·ture
sub·cu·ra·tive
sub·cu·ta·ne·ous
  bur·sa of tib·i·al tu·ber·os·
   i·ty
  em·phy·se·ma
  flap
  im·plan·ta·tion
  mas·tec·to·my
  my·i·a·sis
  op·er·a·tion
  part
  ring
  te·not·o·my

  tis·sue
  trans·fu·sion
  veins of ab·do·men
sub·cu·ta·ne·ous cal·ca·ne·al
  bur·sa
sub·cu·ta·ne·ous fat
  ne·cro·sis of new·born
sub·cu·ta·ne·ous in·fra·pa·tel·
  lar
  bur·sa
sub·cu·tic·u·lar
  su·ture
sub·cu·tis
sub·de·lir·i·um
sub·del·toid
  bur·sa
  bur·si·tis
sub·den·tal
sub·der·mic
sub·di·a·phrag·mat·ic
  ab·scess
  py·o·pneu·mo·tho·rax
sub·di·gas·tric
  node
sub·dor·sal
sub·duce
sub·duct
sub·du·ral
  cav·i·ty
  he·ma·to·ma
  he·ma·tor·rha·chis
  hem·or·rhage
  hy·gro·ma
  space
sub·en·do·car·di·al
  lay·er
sub·en·do·car·di·al my·o·car·
  di·al
  in·farc·tion
sub·en·do·the·li·al
  lay·er
sub·en·do·the·li·um
sub·en·dy·mal
sub·ep·en·dy·mal
sub·ep·en·dy·mo·ma
sub·ep·i·der·mal
  ab·scess
sub·ep·i·der·mic
sub·ep·i·der·mic bul·la
sub·ep·i·the·li·al
sub·ep·i·the·li·um
su·ber·o·sis
sub·fal·cial
  her·ni·a·tion
sub·fam·i·ly
sub·fas·cial
sub·fas·cial pre·pa·tel·lar
  bur·sa

sub·fer·til·i·ty
sub·fis·sure
sub·fo·li·um
sub·ga·le·al
  em·phy·se·ma
  hem·or·rhage
sub·gal·late
sub·gem·mal
sub·ge·nus
sub·ger·mi·nal
  cav·i·ty
sub·gin·gi·val
  cal·cu·lus
  cu·ret·tage
  space
sub·gle·noid
sub·glos·sal
sub·glos·si·tis
sub·glot·tic
sub·gran·u·lar
sub·grun·da·tion
sub·he·pat·ic
  re·cess
sub·hy·a·loid
sub·hy·oid
  bur·sa
sub·hy·oid·e·an
sub·ic·ter·ic
su·bic·u·la
su·bic·u·lar
su·bic·u·lum
sub·il·i·ac
sub·il·i·um
sub·in·fec·tion
sub·in·flam·ma·to·ry
sub·in·gui·nal
  fos·sa
  tri·an·gle
sub·in·teg·u·men·tal
sub·in·ti·mal
sub·in·trant
sub·in·vo·lu·tion
sub·i·o·dide
sub·ja·cent
sub·ject
sub·jec·tive
  frem·i·tus
  psy·chol·o·gy
  sen·sa·tion
  sign
  symp·tom
  syn·o·nyms
  vi·sion
sub·jec·tive ver·ti·go
sub·ju·gal
sub·king·dom
sub·la·tion

sub·len·tic·u·lar
  limb of in·ter·nal cap·sule
sub·le·thal
sub·leu·ke·mia
sub·leu·ke·mic
  leu·ke·mia
  my·e·lo·sis
sub·li·mate
  cor·ro·sive s.
sub·li·ma·tion
sub·lime
sub·limed
  sul·fur
sub·lim·i·nal
  self
  stim·u·lus
  thirst
sub·li·mis
sub·lin·gual
  ar·tery
  cres·cent
  cyst
  fold
  fos·sa
  gan·gli·on
  gland
  nerve
  pit
  tab·let
  vein
sub·lin·gui·tis
sub·lob·u·lar
sub·lum·bar
sub·lu·mi·nal
sub·lux·a·tion
sub·lym·phe·mia
sub·mam·ma·ry
  mas·ti·tis
sub·man·dib·u·lar
  duct
  fos·sa
  gan·gli·on
  gland
  tri·an·gle
sub·man·dib·u·lar lymph
  nodes
sub·mar·gin·al
sub·max·il·la
sub·max·il·lar·i·tis
sub·max·il·lary
  duct
  fos·sa
  gan·gli·on
  gland
  tri·an·gle
sub·max·il·li·tis
sub·me·di·al
sub·me·di·an

sub·mem·bra·nous
sub·men·tal
  ar·tery
  tri·an·gle
  vein
sub·men·tal lymph
  nodes
sub·men·tal ver·tex
  roent·gen·o·gram
sub·merged
  ton·sil
sub·met·a·cen·tric
  chro·mo·some
sub·mi·cron·ic
sub·mi·cro·scop·ic
sub·mor·phous
sub·mu·co·sa
sub·mu·co·sal
  im·plant
  plex·us
sub·mu·cous
sub·nar·co·tic
sub·na·sal
  point
sub·na·si·on
sub·neu·ral
  ap·pa·ra·tus
sub·ni·trate
sub·nor·mal
sub·nor·mal·i·ty
sub·nu·cle·us
sub·oc·cip·i·tal
  de·com·pres·sion
  mus·cles
  nerve
  neu·ral·gia
  neu·ri·tis
  tri·an·gle
sub·oc·cip·i·tal ve·nous
  plex·us
sub·oc·cip·i·to·breg·mat·ic
  di·am·e·ter
sub·oc·clud·ing
  lig·a·ture
sub·oc·clu·sal
  sur·face
sub·op·ti·mal
sub·or·bit·al
sub·or·der
sub·ox·i·da·tion
sub·ox·ide
sub·pap·il·lary
  lay·er
  net·work
sub·pap·u·lar
sub·pa·ri·e·tal
  sul·cus
sub·pa·tel·lar

sub·pec·to·ral
sub·pel·lic·u·lar
  fi·bril
  mi·cro·tu·bule
sub·pel·vi·per·i·to·ne·al
sub·per·i·car·di·al
sub·pe·ri·od·ic
  per·i·o·dic·i·ty
sub·per·i·os·te·al
  ab·scess
  am·pu·ta·tion
  frac·ture
  im·plant
sub·per·i·to·ne·al
  ap·pen·di·ci·tis
  fas·cia
sub·per·i·to·ne·o·ab·dom·i·nal
sub·per·i·to·ne·o·pel·vic
sub·pe·tro·sal
sub·pha·ryn·ge·al
sub·phren·ic
  ab·scess
  py·o·pneu·mo·tho·rax
  re·cess·es
sub·phy·lum
sub·pi·al
sub·pla·cen·tal
sub·plas·ma·lem·mal dense
  zone
sub·pleu·ral
sub·plex·al
sub·pop·lit·e·al
  re·cess
sub·pre·pu·tial
sub·pu·bic
  an·gle
sub·pul·mo·nary
sub·py·lor·ic
  node
sub·py·ram·i·dal
sub·quad·ri·cip·i·tal
  mus·cle
sub·ret·i·nal
sub·salt
sub·sar·to·ri·al
  ca·nal
sub·scap·u·lar
  ar·tery
  bur·sa
  fos·sa
  mus·cle
  nerve
sub·scap·u·la·ris
sub·scap·u·lar lymph
  nodes
sub·scle·ral
sub·scle·rot·ic
sub·scrip·tion

sub·sep·tate
  uter·us
sub·se·ro·sal
sub·se·rous
  plex·us
sub·sib·i·lant
sub·si·dence
sub·sid·i·ary atri·al
  pace·mak·er
sub·spi·na·le
sub·spi·nous
sub·stage
sub·stance
  al·pha s.
  an·te·ri·or per·fo·rat·ed s.
  bac·te·ri·o·tro·pic s.
  ba·so·phil s.
  be·ta s.
  blood group s.
  blood group-spe·cif·ic s.'s A
    and B
  cen·tral gray s.
  chro·mid·i·al s.
  chro·mo·phil s.
  com·pact s.
  con·trolled s.
  cor·ti·cal s.
  ex·oph·thal·mos-pro·duc·ing
    s.
  fi·lar s.
  ge·lat·i·nous s.
  glan·du·lar s. of pros·tate
  gray s.
  ground s.
  H s.
  in·nom·i·nate s.
  in·ter·spon·gi·o·plas·tic s.
  s. of lens of eye
  med·ul·lary s.
  mus·cu·lar s. of pros·tate
  neu·ro·se·cre·to·ry s.
  Nissl s.
  s. P
  pos·te·ri·or per·fo·rat·ed s.
  pres·sor s.
  prop·er s.
  re·leased s.
  re·tic·u·lar s.
  Rolando's s.
  Rolando's ge·lat·i·nous s.
  Schwann's white s.
  sen·si·tiz·ing s.
  slow-re·act·ing s.
  slow-re·act·ing s. of an·a·
    phy·lax·is
  sol·u·ble spe·cif·ic s.
  spe·cif·ic cap·su·lar s.
  spongy s.

  Stilling's ge·lat·i·nous s.
  thresh·old s.
  ti·groid s.
  white s.
  zy·mo·plas·tic s.
sub·stance
  abuse
sub·stance abuse
  dis·or·ders
sub·stan·tia
  s. ad·a·man·ti·na
  s. ba·so·phil·ia
  s. ci·ne·rea
  s. com·pac·ta os·si·um
  s. ebur·nea
  s. fun·da·men·ta·lis
  s. gel·at·i·no·sa cen·tra·lis
  s. glan·du·la·ris pros·ta·tae
  s. in·no·mi·na·ta
  s. me·dul·la·ris
  s. met·a·chro·mat·i·co·gran·
    u·lar·is
  s. os·sea den·tis
  s. pro·pria mem·bra·nae
    tym·pa·ni
  s. re·tic·u·la·ris
  s. re·tic·u·lo·fi·la·men·to·sa
  s. vi·trea
sub·stan·ti·ae
sub·ster·nal
  an·gle
  goi·ter
sub·ster·no·mas·toid
sub·sti·tute
  blood s.
  plas·ma s.
  vol·ume s.
sub·sti·tu·tion
  stim·u·lus s.
  symp·tom s.
sub·sti·tu·tion
  pro·duct
  ther·a·py
  trans·fu·sion
sub·sti·tu·tive
  ther·a·py
sub·strate
sub·stra·tum
sub·struc·ture
  im·plant den·ture s.
sub·sul·fate
sub·sul·tus
  s. clo·nus
  s. ten·di·num
sub·su·pe·ri·or
  seg·ment
sub·sur·face
  cis·ter·na

sub·ta·lar
  joint
sub·tar·sal
sub·teg·u·men·tal
sub·tem·po·ral
  de·com·pres·sion
sub·ten·di·nous
  bur·sa of gas·troc·ne·mi·us
sub·ten·di·nous il·i·ac
  bur·sa
sub·ten·di·nous pre·pa·tel·lar
  bur·sa
sub·ten·to·ri·al
sub·ter·mi·nal
sub·te·tan·ic
sub·tha·lam·ic
  nu·cle·us
sub·thal·a·mus
sub·thresh·old
  stim·u·lus
sub·thy·roid·e·us
sub·til·i·sin
sub·ti·lo·pep·ti·dase
sub·to·tal
  hys·ter·ec·to·my
sub·trac·tion
sub·tra·pe·zi·al
sub·tribe
sub·tro·chan·ter·ic
sub·troch·le·ar
sub·tu·ber·al
sub·tym·pan·ic
sub·um·bil·i·cal
sub·un·gual
  ab·scess
  mel·a·no·ma
sub·un·gui·al
sub·u·nit
  vac·cine
sub·u·re·thral
sub·vag·i·nal
sub·val·var
  ste·no·sis
sub·val·vu·lar
sub·ver·te·bral
sub·vir·ile
sub·vit·ri·nal
sub·vo·cal
  speech
sub·vo·lu·tion
sub·wak·ing
sub·zon·al
sub·zy·go·mat·ic
suc·ca·gogue
suc·ce·da·ne·ous
  den·ti·tion
  tooth
suc·ce·da·ne·um

suc·cen·tu·ri·ate
  pla·cen·ta
suc·ces·sive
  con·trast
suc·ci
suc·ci·nate
  s. de·hy·dro·gen·ase
suc·ci·nate-CoA li·gase
suc·cin·ic ac·id
  cy·cle
suc·cin·ic thi·o·ki·nase
suc·ci·nyl·cho·line
suc·ci·nyl-CoA
suc·ci·nyl-CoA syn·the·tase
suc·ci·nyl·co·en·zyme
suc·ci·nyl·di·cho·line
O-suc·ci·nyl·ho·mo·ser·ine
  (thi·ol)-ly·ase
suc·ci·nyl·sul·fa·thi·a·zole
suc·ci·sul·fone im·i·no·di·eth·
  a·nol
suc·cor·rhea
suc·cu·bus
suc·cus
suc·cuss
suc·cus·sion
  hip·po·crat·ic s.
suck
suck·ing
  cush·ion
  louse
  pad
  wound
suck·le
suck·ling
  re·flex
Sucquet-Hoyer
  anas·to·mo·ses
  ca·nals
Sucquet's
  anas·to·mo·ses
  ca·nals
su·cral·fate
su·crase
su·crate
su·crose
  s. oc·ta·ac·e·tate
su·crose he·mol·y·sis
  test
su·cro·se·mia
su·cro·su·ria
suc·tion
  post·tus·sive s.
  Wangensteen s.
suc·tion
  cup
  drain·age

suc·tion *(continued)*
  oph·thal·mo·dy·na·mom·e·
    ter
  plate
suc·to·ri·al
  pad
su·da·men
su·dam·i·na
su·dam·i·nal
Su·dan black B
Su·dan brown
Su·dan III
Su·dan IV
su·dan·o·phil·ia
su·dan·o·phil·ic
su·dan·o·pho·bic
  zone
Su·dan red III
Su·dan yel·low
su·da·tion
sud·den in·fant death
  syn·drome
Su·deck's
  at·ro·phy
  syn·drome
Su·deck's crit·i·cal
  point
su·do·mo·tor
  fi·bers
su·dor
  s. san·gui·ne·us
  s. uri·no·sus
su·dor·al
su·do·re·sis
su·do·rif·er·ous
  duct
  glands
su·do·rif·ic
su·dor·i·ker·a·to·sis
su·do·rip·a·rous
  ab·scess
su·do·rom·e·ter
su·dor·rhea
su·et
  pre·pared s.
su·fen·ta·nil cit·rate
suf·fo·cate
suf·fo·cat·ing
  gas
suf·fo·ca·tion
suf·fo·ca·tive
  goi·ter
suf·fu·sion
sug·ar
  ami·no s.'s
  beech·wood s.
  beet s.
  blood s.

brain s.
cane s.
corn s.
de·oxy s.
fruit s.
gel·a·tin s.
grape s.
in·vert s.
s. of lead
malt s.
man·na s.
ma·ple s.
milk s.
oil s.
pec·tin s.
re·duc·ing s.
spe·cif·ic sol·u·ble s.
starch s.
wood s.
sug·ar
  al·co·hol
  cat·a·ract
  tu·mor
sug·ar ac·ids
sug·ar-coat·ed
  spleen
sug·ar-ic·ing
  liv·er
sug·ars
  Fischer pro·jec·tion for·mu·
    las of s.
  Haworth con·for·ma·tion·al
    for·mu·las of cy·clic s.
  Haworth per·spec·tive for·
    mu·las of cy·clic s.
sug·gest·i·bil·i·ty
sug·gest·i·ble
sug·ges·tion
  post·hyp·not·ic s.
sug·ges·tive
  psy·cho·ther·a·py
  ther·a·peu·tics
sug·gil·la·tion
  post·mor·tem s.
Sugiura
  pro·ce·dure
su·i·cide
  ges·ture
sui·cid·ol·o·gy
su·int
suit
sul·ben·tine
sul·cal
  ar·tery
sul·cate
sul·cat·ed
sul·ci
sul·ci·form

sul·co·mar·gin·al
  tract
sul·cu·lar
  ep·i·the·li·um
  flu·id
sul·cu·li
sul·cu·lus
sul·cus
  al·ve·o·lo·buc·cal s.
  al·ve·o·lo·la·bi·al s.
  al·ve·o·lo·lin·gual s.
  am·pul·la·ry s.
  s. an·gu·la·ris
  an·te·ri·or par·ol·fac·to·ry
    s.
  an·ter·o·lat·er·al s.
  aor·tic s.
  s. aor·ti·cus
  atri·o·ven·tric·u·lar s.
  s. au·ric·u·lae an·te·ri·or
  bas·i·lar s.
  cal·ca·ne·al s.
  cal·ca·rine s.
  cal·lo·sal s.
  s. cal·lo·so·mar·gi·na·lis
  ca·rot·id s.
  cen·tral s.
  cer·e·bel·lar sul·ci
  ce·re·bral sul·ci
  chi·as·mat·ic s.
  s. of cin·gu·lum
  cir·cu·lar s. of Reil
  col·lat·er·al s.
  cor·o·nary s.
  s. of cor·pus col·la·sum
  ex·ter·nal spi·ral s.
  fim·bri·o·den·tate s.
  s. fim·bri·o·den·ta·tus
  s. fron·ta·lis me·di·us
  s. fron·to·mar·gi·na·lis
  gin·gi·val s.
  gin·gi·vo·buc·cal s.
  gin·gi·vo·la·bi·al s.
  gin·gi·vo·lin·gual s.
  s. for great·er pal·a·tine
    nerve
  hy·po·tha·lam·ic s.
  in·fe·ri·or fron·tal s.
  in·fe·ri·or pe·tro·sal s.
  in·fe·ri·or tem·po·ral s.
  s. in·fra·pal·pe·bra·lis
  s. in·ter·me·di·us an·te·ri·
    or
  in·ter·nal spi·ral s.
  in·ter·pa·ri·e·tal s.
  in·ter·tu·ber·cu·lar s.
  s. in·ter·ven·tri·cu·la·ris
    cor·dis

  s. in·tra·grac·i·lis
  in·tra·pa·ri·e·tal s.
  in·tra·pa·ri·e·tal s. of
    Turner
  la·bi·al s.
  lat·er·al ce·re·bral s.
  lat·er·al oc·cip·i·tal s.
  lim·it·ing s. of Reil
  lim·it·ing s. of rhom·boid
    fos·sa
  lip s.
  lon·gi·tu·di·nal s. of heart
  lu·nate s.
  mal·le·o·lar s.
  s. ma·tri·cis un·guis
  me·di·an s. of fourth ven·
    tri·cle
  me·di·an fron·tal s.
  s. men·to·la·bi·a·lis
  mid·dle fron·tal s.
  mid·dle tem·po·ral s.
  s. for mid·dle tem·po·ral
    ar·tery
  Monro's s.
  s. na·so·la·bi·a·lis
  s. ner·vi o·cu·lo·mo·to·rii
  nym·pho·ca·run·cu·lar s.
  s. nym·pho·ca·run·cu·laris
  nym·pho·hy·men·al s.
  s. of oc·cip·i·tal ar·tery
  ol·fac·to·ry s. of nose
  s. oc·ci·pi·ta·lis la·te·ra·lis
  s. oc·ci·pi·ta·lis su·pe·ri·or
  oc·cip·i·to·tem·po·ral s.
  ol·fac·to·ry s.
  ol·fac·to·ry s. of nose
  or·bi·tal sul·ci
  par·a·glen·oid s.
  s. pa·ra·gle·noi·da·lis
  pa·ri·e·to-oc·cip·i·tal s.
  s. pa·rol·fac·to·ri·us an·te·
    ri·or
  s. pa·rol·fac·to·ri·us pos·te·
    ri·or
  per·i·con·chal s.
  s. pop·li·te·us
  post·cen·tral s.
  pos·te·ri·or me·di·an s. of
    me·dul·la ob·lon·ga·ta
  pos·te·ri·or me·di·an s. of
    spi·nal cord
  pos·te·ri·or par·ol·fac·
    to·ry s.
  pos·ter·o·lat·er·al s.
  pre·au·ric·u·lar s.
  pre·cen·tral s.
  pre·chi·as·mat·ic s.
  s. of pter·y·goid ham·u·lus
  s. pte·ry·go·pa·la·ti·nus

sul·cus *(continued)*
  pul·mo·nary s.
  rhi·nal s.
  sag·it·tal s.
  s. of scle·ra
  sig·moid s.
  s. spi·no·sus
  sub·cla·vi·an s.
  s. sub·cla·vi·a·nus
  s. sub·cla·vi·us
  sub·pa·ri·e·tal s.
  su·pe·ri·or fron·tal s.
  su·pe·ri·or lon·gi·tu·
    di·nal s.
  su·pe·ri·or oc·cip·i·tal s.
  su·pe·ri·or pe·tro·sal s.
  su·pe·ri·or tem·po·ral s.
  su·pra-ac·e·tab·u·lar s.
  ta·lar s.
  s. tem·po·ra·lis me·di·us
  ter·mi·nal s.
  ton·sil·lo·lin·gual s.
  trans·verse oc·cip·i·tal s.
  s. for trans·verse si·nus
  trans·verse tem·po·ral sul·ci
  Turner's s.
  s. for ve·na ca·va
  s. ve·nae ca·vae cra·ni·a·lis
  s. ven·tra·lis
  s. for ver·te·bral ar·tery
  s. ver·ti·ca·lis
  vo·mer·al s.
sul·fa
sul·fa·benz·am·ide
sul·fa·cet·a·mide
sulf·ac·id
sul·fac·tam
sul·fa·cy·tine
sul·fa·di·a·zine
sul·fa·di·me·thox·ine
sul·fa·dim·i·dine
sul·fa·dox·ine
sul·fa·eth·i·dole
sul·fa·fur·a·zole
sul·fa·gua·ni·dine
sul·fa·lene
sul·fa·mer·a·zine
sul·fa·me·ter
sul·fa·meth·a·zine
sul·fa·meth·i·zole
sul·fa·meth·ox·a·zole
sul·fa·me·thox·y·di·a·zine
sul·fa·me·thox·y·py·rid·a·zine
sul·fa·mox·ole
p-**sul·fa·myl·ac·e·tan·il·ide**
sul·fa·nil·a·mide
N-**sul·fan·i·lyl·a·cet·a·mide**
N-**sul·fan·i·lyl·benz·a·mide**

sul·fan·i·lyl·gua·ni·dine
sul·fa·ni·tran
sul·fa·per·in
sul·fa·phen·a·zole
sul·fa·pyr·a·zine
sul·fa·pyr·i·dine
sul·fa·sal·a·zine
sul·fa·tase
sul·fate
  ac·id s.
  ac·tive s.
sul·fate
  res·pi·ra·tion
  wa·ter
sul·fa·thi·a·zole
sul·fa·ti·dates
sul·fa·tide
  lip·i·do·sis
sul·fa·tides
sul·fa·ti·do·sis
sul·fa·tion
  fac·tor
sulf·he·mo·glo·bin
sulf·he·mo·glo·bi·ne·mia
sulf·hy·drate
sulf·hy·dryl
sul·fide
sul·fin·di·got·ic ac·id
sul·fin·py·ra·zone
sul·fi·so·mi·dine
sul·fi·sox·a·zole
  s. di·ol·a·mine
sul·fite
  s. de·hy·dro·gen·ase
  s. ox·i·dase
  s. re·duc·tase
sulf·met·he·mo·glo·bin
sul·fo·ac·id
sul·fo·bro·mo·phtha·lein
  so·di·um
sul·fo·cy·a·nate
sul·fo·cy·an·ic ac·id
sul·fo·gel
sul·fo·hy·drate
sul·fol·y·sis
sul·fo·mu·cin
sul·fo·myx·in so·di·um
sul·fon·a·mides
sul·fo·nate
sul·fone
sul·fon·ic ac·id
sul·fo·ni·um
  ion
sul·fo·nyl·u·re·as
sul·fo·pro·tein
sul·fo·rho·da·mine B
sul·for·me·thox·ine
sul·fo·sal·i·cyl·ic ac·id

sul·fo·sal·i·cyl·ic ac·id tur·bid·
i·ty
   test
sul·fo·sol
sul·fo·trans·fer·ase
sulf·ox·ide
sulf·ox·one so·di·um
sul·fur
   s. di·ox·ide
   s. io·dide
   liv·er of s.
   pre·cip·i·tat·ed s.
   roll s.
   soft s.
   sub·limed s.
   s. tri·ox·ide
   veg·e·ta·ble s.
   washed s.
   wet·ta·ble s.
sul·fur
   mus·tard
   wa·ter
sul·fu·rat·ed
   lime
   pot·ash
sul·fu·ret
sul·fu·ret·ed
   hy·dro·gen
sul·fur group
sul·fu·ric ac·id
   fum·ing s. a.
   Nordhausen s. a.
sul·fu·ric ether
sul·fu·ric ox·ide
sul·fu·rous
sul·fu·rous ac·id
sul·fu·rous ox·ide
sul·fur·yl
sul·fy·drate
sul·in·dac
sul·i·so·ben·zone
Sulkowitch's
   re·a·gent
sul·pir·ide
sul·thi·ame
Sulzberger-Garbe
   dis·ease
   syn·drome
sum·ma·tion
   beat
   gal·lop
sum·ma·tion
   s. of stim·u·li
sum·mer
   asth·ma
   di·ar·rhea
   itch
   pru·ri·go

   rash
   sores
Sumner's
   sign
sump
   drain
   syn·drome
sun
   stroke
sun·burn
sun·flow·er seed oil
sun pro·tec·tion
   fac·tor
sun·screen
sun·stroke
su·per·ab·duc·tion
su·per·a·cid·i·ty
su·per·a·cro·mi·al
su·per·ac·tiv·i·ty
su·per·a·cute
su·per·al·i·men·ta·tion
su·per·a·nal
su·per·cil·ia
su·per·cil·i·ary
   arch
   ridge
su·per·cil·i·um
su·per·di·crot·ic
su·per·dis·ten·tion
su·per·duct
su·per·e·go
su·per·ex·ci·ta·tion
su·per·ex·ten·sion
su·per·fat·ted
   soap
su·per·fe·ta·tion
su·per·fi·cial
   an·gi·o·ma
   burn
   cleav·age
   ec·to·derm
   fas·cia
   fas·cia of per·i·ne·um
   head
   im·plan·ta·tion
   lay·er
   part
   re·flex
   ton·sil·li·tis
   vein
su·per·fi·cial an·te·ri·or cer·vi·
cal lymph
   nodes
su·per·fi·cial brach·i·al
   ar·tery
su·per·fi·cial car·di·ac
   plex·us

su·per·fi·cial ce·re·bral
  veins
su·per·fi·cial cer·vi·cal
  ar·tery
  nerve
su·per·fi·cial cir·cum·flex
  il·i·ac
  ar·tery
  vein
su·per·fi·cial dor·sal
  veins of clit·o·ris
  veins of pe·nis
su·per·fi·cial dor·sal sa·cro·
  coc·cyg·e·al
  lig·a·ment
su·per·fi·cial ep·i·gas·tric
  ar·tery
  vein
su·per·fi·cial fib·u·lar
  nerve
su·per·fi·cial flex·or
  mus·cle of fin·gers
su·per·fi·cial in·gui·nal
  pouch
  ring
su·per·fi·cial in·gui·nal lymph
  nodes
su·per·fi·ci·a·lis
  s. vo·lae
su·per·fi·cial lat·er·al cer·vi·cal
  lymph
  nodes
su·per·fi·cial lin·e·ar
  ker·a·ti·tis
su·per·fi·cial lin·gual
  mus·cle
su·per·fi·cial lym·phat·ic
  ves·sel
su·per·fi·cial mid·dle ce·re·bral
  vein
su·per·fi·cial or·i·gin
su·per·fi·cial pal·mar
  arch
  ar·tery
su·per·fi·cial pal·mar ve·nous
  arch
su·per·fi·cial pa·rot·id lymph
  nodes
su·per·fi·cial per·o·ne·al
  nerve
su·per·fi·cial pos·te·ri·or sa·
  cro·coc·cyg·e·al
  lig·a·ment
su·per·fi·cial punc·tate
  ker·a·ti·tis
su·per·fi·cial pus·tu·lar
  per·i·fol·lic·u·li·tis

su·per·fi·cial spread·ing
  mel·a·no·ma
su·per·fi·cial tem·po·ral
  ar·tery
  plex·us
  veins
su·per·fi·cial trans·verse
  mus·cle of per·i·ne·um
su·per·fi·cial trans·verse met·a·
  car·pal
  lig·a·ment
su·per·fi·cial trans·verse met·a·
  tar·sal
  lig·a·ment
su·per·fi·cial vo·lar
  ar·tery
su·per·fi·cies
su·per·flex·ion
su·per·fuse
su·per·fu·sion
su·per·gen·u·al
su·per·im·posed
  ec·lamp·sia
  pre·e·clamp·sia
su·per·im·preg·na·tion
su·per·in·duce
su·per·in·fec·tion
su·per·in·vo·lu·tion
su·pe·ri·or
  an·gle of scap·u·la
  bor·der of pet·rous part of
    tem·po·ral bone
  bur·sa of bi·ceps fe·mo·ris
  col·lic·u·lus
  con·cha
  ex·trem·i·ty
  fas·cia of pel·vic di·a·
    phragm
  fas·cia of uro·gen·i·tal
    di·a·phragm
  flex·ure of du·o·de·num
  gan·gli·on of glos·so·pha·
    ryn·ge·al nerve
  gan·gli·on of the va·gus
    nerve
  horn
  horn of sa·phe·nous open·
    ing
  horn of thy·roid car·ti·lage
  lar·yn·got·o·my
  lig·a·ment of ep·i·did·y·mis
  lig·a·ment of in·cus
  lig·a·ment of mal·le·us
  limb
  lobe of lung
  mar·gin
  ol·ive
  par·a·ple·gia

part
part of ves·tib·u·lo·
co·chle·ar nerve
pole
po·li·o·en·ceph·a·li·tis
re·cess of less·er per·i·to·
ne·al sac
re·cess of tym·pan·ic mem·
brane
ret·i·nac·u·lum of ex·ten·
sor mus·cles
root
root of cer·vi·cal loop
root of ves·tib·u·lo·co·chle·
ar nerve
seg·ment
sur·face of cer·e·bel·lar
hem·i·sphere
sur·face of ta·lus
trunk
veins of cer·e·bel·lar hem·
i·sphere
vein of ver·mis
ve·na ca·va
wall of or·bit
su·pe·ri·or al·ve·o·lar
nerves
su·pe·ri·or anas·to·mot·ic
vein
su·pe·ri·or ar·tic·u·lar
pit of at·las
pro·cess of sa·crum
sur·face of tib·ia
su·pe·ri·or au·ric·u·lar
mus·cle
su·pe·ri·or ba·sal
vein
su·pe·ri·or ca·rot·id
tri·an·gle
su·pe·ri·or cer·e·bel·lar
ar·tery
pe·dun·cle
su·pe·ri·or cer·e·bel·lar ar·tery
syn·drome
su·pe·ri·or ce·re·bral
veins
su·pe·ri·or cer·vi·cal
gan·gli·on
su·pe·ri·or cer·vi·cal car·di·ac
nerve
su·pe·ri·or cho·roid
vein
su·pe·ri·or clu·ne·al
nerves
su·pe·ri·or con·stric·tor
mus·cle of phar·ynx
su·pe·ri·or cor·o·nary
ar·tery

su·pe·ri·or cos·tal
pit
su·pe·ri·or cos·to·trans·verse
lig·a·ment
su·pe·ri·or den·tal
arch
nerves
plex·us
su·pe·ri·or du·o·de·nal
fold
fos·sa
re·cess
su·pe·ri·or ep·i·gas·tric
ar·tery
veins
su·pe·ri·or fa·cial
in·dex
su·pe·ri·or fron·tal
con·vo·lu·tion
gy·rus
sul·cus
su·pe·ri·or gas·tric lymph
nodes
su·pe·ri·or ge·mel·lus
mus·cle
su·pe·ri·or glu·te·al
ar·tery
nerve
veins
su·pe·ri·or hem·or·rhag·ic
po·li·o·en·ceph·a·li·tis
su·pe·ri·or hem·or·rhoi·dal
ar·tery
plex·us
vein
su·pe·ri·or hy·po·gas·tric
plex·us
su·pe·ri·or hy·po·phy·si·al
ar·tery
su·pe·ri·or il·e·o·ce·cal
re·cess
su·pe·ri·or in·ter·nal pa·ri·e·
tal
ar·tery
su·pe·ri·or·i·ty
com·plex
su·pe·ri·or la·bi·al
ar·tery
vein
su·pe·ri·or la·ryn·ge·al
ar·tery
nerve
vein
su·pe·ri·or lim·bic
ker·a·to·con·junc·ti·vi·tis
su·pe·ri·or lin·gu·lar
seg·ment

su·pe·ri·or lon·gi·tu·di·nal
fas·cic·u·lus
si·nus
sul·cus

su·pe·ri·or mac·u·lar
ar·te·ri·ole
ven·ule

su·pe·ri·or max·il·lary
nerve

su·pe·ri·or med·ul·lary
ve·lum

su·pe·ri·or mes·en·ter·ic
ar·tery
gan·gli·on
plex·us
vein

su·pe·ri·or mes·en·ter·ic
ar·tery
syn·drome

su·pe·ri·or mes·en·ter·ic lymph
nodes

su·pe·ri·or na·sal
ar·te·ri·ole of ret·i·na
ven·ule of ret·i·na

su·pe·ri·or nu·chal
line

su·pe·ri·or ob·lique
mus·cle
mus·cle of head

su·pe·ri·or oc·cip·i·tal
gy·rus
sul·cus

su·pe·ri·or ol·i·vary
nu·cle·us

su·pe·ri·or omen·tal
re·cess

su·pe·ri·or oph·thal·mic
vein

su·pe·ri·or or·bi·tal
fis·sure

su·pe·ri·or pan·cre·at·i·co·du·
o·de·nal
ar·tery

su·pe·ri·or pa·ri·e·tal
gy·rus
lob·ule

su·pe·ri·or pe·tro·sal
si·nus
sul·cus

su·pe·ri·or phren·ic
ar·tery
veins

su·pe·ri·or phren·ic lymph
nodes

su·pe·ri·or pos·te·ri·or ser·ra·
tus
mus·cle

su·pe·ri·or pu·bic
lig·a·ment

su·pe·ri·or pul·mo·nary sul·cus
tu·mor

su·pe·ri·or quad·ri·gem·i·nal
bra·chi·um

su·pe·ri·or ra·di·o·ul·nar
joint

su·pe·ri·or rec·tal
ar·tery
plex·us
vein

su·pe·ri·or rec·tal lymph
nodes

su·pe·ri·or rec·tus
mus·cle

su·pe·ri·or sag·it·tal
si·nus

su·pe·ri·or sal·i·vary
nu·cle·us

su·pe·ri·or sem·i·lu·nar
lob·ule

su·pe·ri·or strait

su·pe·ri·or su·pra·re·nal
ar·tery

su·pe·ri·or tar·sal
mus·cle

su·pe·ri·or tem·po·ral
ar·te·ri·ole of ret·i·na
con·vo·lu·tion
fis·sure
gy·rus
line
sul·cus
ven·ule of ret·i·na

su·pe·ri·or thal·a·mo·stri·ate
vein

su·pe·ri·or tho·rac·ic
ap·er·ture
ar·tery

su·pe·ri·or thy·roid
ar·tery
notch
plex·us
tu·ber·cle
vein

su·pe·ri·or tib·i·al
ar·tic·u·la·tion

su·pe·ri·or tib·i·o·fib·u·lar
joint

su·pe·ri·or tra·che·o·bron·chi·
al lymph
nodes

su·pe·ri·or trans·verse scap·u·
lar
lig·a·ment

su·pe·ri·or tur·bi·nat·ed
bone

su·pe·ri·or tym·pan·ic
  ar·tery
su·pe·ri·or ul·nar col·lat·er·al
  ar·tery
su·pe·ri·or ve·na ca·val
  syn·drome
su·pe·ri·or ves·i·cal
  ar·tery
su·pe·ri·or ves·tib·u·lar
  ar·ea
  nu·cle·us
su·per·lac·ta·tion
su·per·lig·a·men
su·per·me·di·al
su·per·mo·til·i·ty
su·per·na·tant
  flu·id
su·per·nor·mal re·cov·ery
  phase
su·per·nu·mer·ary
  kid·ney
  mam·ma
  or·gans
  pla·cen·ta
su·per·nu·tri·tion
su·per·o·lat·er·al
  sur·face of cer·e·brum
su·per·o·me·di·al
  mar·gin
su·per·ov·u·la·tion
su·per·ox·ide
  s. dis·mu·tase
su·per·par·a·site
su·per·par·a·sit·ism
su·per·pe·tro·sal
su·per·pig·men·ta·tion
su·per·sat·u·rate
su·per·sat·u·rat·ed
  so·lu·tion
su·per·scrip·tion
su·per·son·ic
  rays
  waves
su·per·son·ic vi·bra·tion
  tech·nique
su·per·struc·ture
  im·plant den·ture s.
su·per·ten·sion
su·per·trac·tion
  co·nus
su·per·volt·age
su·pi·nate
su·pi·na·tion
  s. of the foot
  s. of the fore·arm
su·pi·na·tion
  re·flex

su·pi·na·tor
  crest
  jerk
  mus·cle
  re·flex
su·pi·na·tor lon·gus
  re·flex
su·pine
  po·si·tion
su·pine hy·po·ten·sive
  syn·drome
sup·pe·da·nia
sup·pe·da·ni·um
sup·ple·men·tal
  air
  groove
  lobe
  ridge
sup·ple·men·tary
  men·stru·a·tion
sup·ple·men·tary mo·tor
  cor·tex
sup·port
  me·di·um
sup·port·er
sup·port·ing
  ar·ea
  cell
  re·ac·tions
  re·flex·es
sup·port·ive
  psy·cho·ther·a·py
sup·pos·i·to·ry
sup·pressed
  men·stru·a·tion
sup·pres·sion
sup·pres·sor
  cell
  gene
  mu·ta·tion
sup·pres·sor-sen·si·tive
  mu·tant
sup·pu·rant
sup·pu·rate
sup·pu·ra·tion
sup·pu·ra·tive
  ap·pen·di·ci·tis
  ar·thri·tis
  cer·e·bri·tis
  cho·roid·i·tis
  en·ceph·a·li·tis
  gin·gi·vi·tis
  hep·a·ti·tis
  hy·a·li·tis
  in·flam·ma·tion
  mas·ti·tis
  ne·cro·sis
  ne·phri·tis

sup·pu·ra·tive *(continued)*
  per·i·o·don·ti·tis
  pleu·ri·sy
  pneu·mo·nia
  pulp·i·tis
  syn·o·vi·tis
su·pra-ac·e·tab·u·lar
  groove
  sul·cus
su·pra-a·cro·mi·al
su·pra-a·nal
su·pra-ar·y·te·noid
  car·ti·lage
su·pra-au·ric·u·lar
  point
su·pra-ax·il·lary
su·pra·buc·cal
su·pra·bulge
su·pra·cal·lo·sal
  gy·rus
su·pra·car·di·nal
su·pra·cer·e·bel·lar
su·pra·ce·re·bral
su·pra·cer·vi·cal
  hys·ter·ec·to·my
su·pra·cho·roid
  lay·er
su·pra·cho·roi·dea
su·pra·cil·i·ary
su·pra·cla·vic·u·lar
  mus·cle
  part of brach·i·al plex·us
su·pra·cla·vic·u·lar·is
su·pra·cla·vic·u·lar lymph
  nodes
su·pra·cli·noid
  an·eu·rysm
su·pra·con·dy·lar
  frac·ture
  pro·cess
su·pra·con·dy·loid
su·pra·cos·tal
su·pra·cot·y·loid
su·pra·crest·al
  line
  plane
su·pra·cris·tal
su·pra·di·a·phrag·mat·ic
su·pra·duc·tion
su·pra·du·o·de·nal
  ar·tery
su·pra·ep·i·con·dy·lar
  pro·cess
su·pra·gin·gi·val
  cal·cu·lus
su·pra·gle·noid
  tu·ber·cle
su·pra·glot·tic

su·pra·he·pat·ic
  spac·es
su·pra·his·i·an
  block
su·pra·hy·oid
  gland
  mus·cles
su·pra·in·gui·nal
su·pra·in·ter·pa·ri·e·tal
  bone
su·pra·in·tes·ti·nal
su·pra·lim·i·nal
su·pra·lum·bar
su·pra·mal·le·o·lar
su·pra·mam·ma·ry
su·pra·man·dib·u·lar
su·pra·mar·gin·al
  con·vo·lu·tion
  gy·rus
su·pra·mas·toid
  crest
  fos·sa
su·pra·max·il·la
su·pra·max·il·lary
su·pra·max·i·mal
  stim·u·lus
su·pra·me·a·tal
  pit
  spine
  tri·an·gle
su·pra·men·tal
su·pra·men·ta·le
su·pra·na·sal
  point
su·pra·neu·ral
su·pra·nor·mal
  con·duc·tion
  ex·cit·a·bil·i·ty
su·pra·nu·cle·ar
  le·sion
  pa·ral·y·sis
su·pra·oc·clu·sion
su·pra·op·tic
  com·mis·sures
  nu·cle·us
su·pra·op·ti·co·hy·po·phy·si·al
  tract
su·pra·or·bit·al
  arch
  ar·tery
  fo·ra·men
  mar·gin
  nerve
  neu·ral·gia
  notch
  point
  re·flex

ridge
vein
su·pra·or·bi·to·me·a·tal
plane
su·pra·pa·tel·lar
bur·sa
re·flex
su·pra·pel·vic
su·pra·per·i·os·te·al
im·plant
su·pra·phys·i·o·log·ic
su·pra·phys·i·o·log·i·cal
su·pra·pin·e·al
re·cess
su·pra·pleu·ral
mem·brane
su·pra·pu·bic
cys·tot·o·my
li·thot·o·my
su·pra·py·lor·ic
node
su·pra·re·nal
body
cap·sule
cor·tex
gland
im·pres·sion
plex·us
veins
su·pra·re·nal·ec·to·my
su·pra·scap·u·lar
ar·tery
lig·a·ment
nerve
notch
vein
su·pra·scle·ral
su·pra·sel·lar
cyst
su·pra·spi·nal
su·pra·spi·na·lis
su·pra·spi·na·tus
syn·drome
su·pra·spi·nous
fos·sa
lig·a·ment
mus·cle
su·pra·sta·pe·di·al
su·pra·ster·nal
bone
notch
plane
space
su·pra·syl·vi·an
su·pra·sym·phys·ary
su·pra·tem·po·ral
su·pra·ten·to·ri·al
su·pra·tho·rac·ic

su·pra·ton·sil·lar
fos·sa
re·cess
su·pra·trag·ic
tu·ber·cle
su·pra·troch·le·ar
ar·tery
nerve
veins
su·pra·tur·bi·nal
su·pra·tym·pan·ic
su·pra·um·bil·i·cal
re·flex
su·pra·vag·i·nal
su·pra·val·var
ste·no·sis
su·pra·val·var aor·tic ste·no·sis
syn·drome
su·pra·val·var aor·tic ste·no·
sis-in·fan·tile hy·per·cal·ce·
mia
syn·drome
su·pra·val·vu·lar
su·pra·ven·tric·u·lar
crest
ex·tra·sys·to·le
su·pra·ver·gence
su·pra·ver·sion
su·pra·ves·i·cal
fos·sa
su·pra·vi·tal
stain
su·preme
con·cha
su·preme in·ter·cos·tal
ar·tery
su·preme tur·bi·nat·ed
bone
su·pro·fen
su·ra
su·ral
ar·tery
nerve
re·gion
sur·al·i·men·ta·tion
sur·a·min so·di·um
sur·do·car·di·ac
syn·drome
sur·face
an·al·ge·sia
anat·o·my
ca·tal·y·sis
ep·i·the·li·um
ten·sion
ther·mom·e·ter
sur·face
acro·mi·al ar·tic·u·lar s. of
clav·i·cle

sur·face *(continued)*

an·te·ri·or s.

an·te·ri·or ar·tic·u·lar s. of dens

an·te·ri·or cal·ca·ne·al ar·tic·u·lar s.

an·te·ri·or s. of eye·lids

an·te·ri·or s. of leg

an·te·ri·or s. of max·il·la

an·te·ri·or s. of pet·rous part

an·ter·o·lat·er·al s. of hu·mer·us

an·ter·o·me·di·al s. of hu·mer·us

ar·tic·u·lar s. of acro·mi·on

ar·tic·u·lar s. of ar·y·te·noid car·ti·lage

ar·tic·u·lar s. of head of fib·u·la

ar·tic·u·lar s. of head of rib

ar·tic·u·lar s. of pa·tel·la

ar·tic·u·lar s. of tem·po·ral bone

ar·tic·u·lar s. of tu·ber·cle of rib

ar·y·te·noi·dal ar·tic·u·lar s. of cri·coid

au·ric·u·lar s. of il·i·um

au·ric·u·lar s. of sa·crum

ax·i·al s.

bal·anc·ing oc·clu·sal s.

ba·sal s.

buc·cal s.

cal·ca·ne·al ar·tic·u·lar s. of ta·lus

car·pal ar·tic·u·lar s. of ra·di·us

ce·re·bral s.

col·ic s. of spleen

con·tact s. of tooth

cos·tal s.

cos·tal s. of lung

cos·tal s. of scap·u·la

cu·boi·dal ar·tic·u·lar s. of cal·ca·ne·us

den·ture ba·sal s.

den·ture foun·da·tion s.

den·ture im·pres·sion s.

den·ture oc·clu·sal s.

den·ture pol·ished s.

di·a·phrag·mat·ic s.

dis·tal s. of tooth

dor·sal s. of dig·it

dor·sal s. of sa·crum

dor·sal s. of scap·u·la

ex·ter·nal s. of fron·tal bone

ex·ter·nal s. of pa·ri·e·tal bone

fa·cial s. of tooth

fib·u·lar ar·tic·u·lar s. of tib·ia

gas·tric s. of spleen

gle·noid s.

glu·te·al s. of il·i·um

grind·ing s.

in·ci·sal s.

in·fe·ri·or ar·tic·u·lar s. of tib·ia

in·fe·ri·or s. of cer·e·bel·lar hem·i·sphere

in·fe·ri·or s. of pan·cre·as

in·fe·ri·or s. of pet·rous part of tem·po·ral bone

in·fe·ri·or s. of tongue

in·fe·ro·lat·er·al s. of pros·tate

in·fra·tem·po·ral s. of max·il·la

in·ter·lo·bar s.'s of lung

in·ter·nal s.

in·ter·nal s. of fron·tal bone

in·ter·nal s. of pa·ri·e·tal bone

in·tes·ti·nal s. of uter·us

la·bi·al s.

lat·er·al s.

lat·er·al s. of leg

lat·er·al mal·le·o·lar s. of ta·lus

lat·er·al s. of ova·ry

lin·gual s.

lu·nate s. of ac·e·tab·u·lum

mal·le·o·lar ar·tic·u·lar s. of fib·u·la

mal·le·o·lar ar·tic·u·lar s. of tib·ia

mas·ti·cat·ing s.

mas·ti·ca·to·ry s.

max·il·lary s.

me·di·al s.

me·di·al s. of ar·y·te·noid car·ti·lage

me·di·al s. of ce·re·bral hem·i·sphere

me·di·al s. of fib·u·la

me·di·al s. of lung

me·di·al mal·le·o·lar s. of ta·lus

me·di·al s. of ova·ry

me·di·al s. of tes·tis

me·di·al s. of tib·ia

me·di·al s. of ul·na
me·si·al s. of tooth
mid·dle cal·ca·ne·al ar·tic·
 u·lar s.
na·sal s. of max·il·la
na·sal s. of pal·a·tine bone
na·vic·u·lar ar·tic·u·lar s.
 of ta·lus
oc·clu·sal s.
or·bi·tal s.
pal·a·tine s.
pa·tel·lar s. of fe·mur
pel·vic s. of sa·crum
pop·lit·e·al s. of fe·mur
pos·te·ri·or s.
pos·te·ri·or ar·tic·u·lar s.
 of dens
pos·te·ri·or cal·ca·ne·al ar·
 tic·u·lar s.
pos·te·ri·or s. of eye·lids
pos·te·ri·or s. of pet·rous
 part
pul·mo·nary s. of heart
re·nal s.
sa·cro·pel·vic s. of il·i·um
ster·nal ar·tic·u·lar s. of
 clav·i·cle
ster·no·cos·tal s. of heart
sub·oc·clu·sal s.
su·pe·ri·or ar·tic·u·lar s. of
 tib·ia
su·pe·ri·or s. of cer·e·bel·
 lar hem·i·sphere
su·pe·ri·or s. of ta·lus
su·per·o·lat·er·al s. of cer·
 e·brum
sym·phys·i·al s. of pu·bis
ta·lar ar·tic·u·lar s. of cal·
 ca·ne·us
tem·po·ral s.
thy·roi·dal ar·tic·u·lar s. of
 cri·coid
ure·thral s. of pe·nis
ven·tral s. of dig·it
ves·i·cal s. of uter·us
ves·tib·u·lar s. of tooth
vis·cer·al s. of liv·er
vis·cer·al s. of the spleen
work·ing oc·clu·sal s.'s
sur·face-ac·tive
sur·face mu·cous
 cells of stom·ach
sur·face ten·sion
 the·o·ry of nar·co·sis
sur·face tha·lam·ic
 veins
sur·fac·tant

sur·geon
 den·tal s.
 oral s.
sur·geon-gen·er·al
sur·gery
 am·bu·la·to·ry s.
 asep·tic s.
 closed s.
 cos·met·ic s.
 cra·ni·o·fa·cial s.
 es·thet·ic s.
 fea·tur·al s.
 ma·jor s.
 mi·nor s.
 open heart s.
 oral s.
 or·thog·nath·ic s.
 or·tho·pae·dic s.
 or·tho·pe·dic s.
 plas·tic s.
 re·con·struc·tive s.
 ster·e·o·tac·tic s.
 ster·e·o·tax·ic s.
 trans·sex·u·al s.
sur·gi·cal
 ab·do·men
 anat·o·my
 an·es·the·sia
 ap·pli·ance
 di·a·ther·my
 em·phy·se·ma
 erup·tion
 er·y·sip·e·las
 li·ga·tion
 mag·got
 mi·cro·scope
 neck of hu·mer·us
 or·tho·don·tics
 pa·thol·o·gy
 pros·the·sis
 silk
 splint
 tem·plate
surg·ing
 far·a·dism
sur·ra
sur·re·nal
sur·ro·gate
 moth·er s.
sur·ro·gate
 moth·er
sur·sa·nure
sur·sum·duc·tion
sur·sum·ver·gence
sur·sum·ver·sion
sur·veil·lance
 im·mune s.
 im·mu·no·log·i·cal s.

sur·vey
line
sur·vey·ing
sur·vey·or
sur·viv·al
time
sus·pend·ed
an·i·ma·tion
heart
sus·pen·sion
col·loid
lar·yn·gos·co·py
sta·bil·i·ty
sus·pen·sion
amor·phous in·su·lin zinc s.
Coffey s.
crys·tal·line in·su·lin zinc s.
ex·tend·ed in·su·lin zinc s.
in·su·lin zinc s.
mag·ne·sia and alu·mi·na
oral s.
prompt in·su·lin zinc s.
sus·pen·soid
sus·pen·so·ry
ban·dage
lig·a·ment of ax·il·la
lig·a·ment of clit·o·ris
lig·a·ment of esoph·a·gus
lig·a·ment of eye·ball
lig·a·ment of go·nad
lig·a·ment of lens
lig·a·ment of ova·ry
lig·a·ment of pe·nis
lig·a·ments of breast
lig·a·ments of Cooper
lig·a·ment of tes·tis
lig·a·ment of thy·roid gland
mus·cle of du·o·de·num
sus·tained ac·tion
tab·let
sus·tained re·lease
tab·let
sus·ten·tac·u·la
sus·ten·tac·u·lar
cell
fi·bers of ret·i·na
sus·ten·tac·u·lum
s. li·e·nis
su·sur·rus
s. au·ri·um
Sutter blood group
Sutton's
dis·ease
ne·vus
ul·cer
su·tu·ra
s. in·fra·or·bi·ta·lis
s. in·ter·pa·ri·e·ta·lis

s. na·so·fron·ta·lis
s. no·tha
s. sphe·no·or·bi·ta·lis
s. zy·go·ma·ti·co·fron·ta·lis
s. zy·go·ma·ti·co·tem·po·ra·
lis
su·tu·rae
su·tur·al
bones
cat·a·ract
lig·a·ment
su·ture
joint
lig·a·ture
su·ture
ab·sorb·a·ble sur·gi·cal s.
Albert's s.
ap·po·si·tion s.
ap·prox·i·ma·tion s.
atrau·mat·ic s.
blan·ket s.
bri·dle s.
Bunnell's s.
bur·ied s.
but·ton s.
cat·gut s.
co·ap·ta·tion s.
cob·bler's s.
Connell's s.
con·tin·u·ous s.
cor·o·nal s.
cra·ni·al s.'s
Cushing's s.
Czerny-Lembert s.
Czerny's s.
de·layed s.
den·tate s.
dou·bly armed s.
Dupuytren's s.
end-on mat·tress s.
eth·moi·do·lac·ri·mal s.
eth·moi·do·max·il·lary s.
Fa·den s.
false s.
far-and-near s.
fron·tal s.
fron·to·eth·moi·dal s.
fron·to·lac·ri·mal s.
fron·to·max·il·lary s.
fron·to·na·sal s.
fron·to·zy·go·mat·ic s.
Frost s.
Gély's s.
glov·er's s.
Gould's s.
Gussenbauer's s.
Halsted's s.
har·mon·ic s.

im·plant·ed s.
in·ci·sive s.
in·fra·or·bit·al s.
in·ter·max·il·lary s.
in·ter·na·sal s.
in·ter·pa·ri·e·tal s.
in·ter·rupt·ed s.
Jobert de Lamballe's s.
lac·ri·mo·con·chal s.
lac·ri·mo·max·il·lary s.
lamb·doid s.
Lembert s.
lens s.'s
mat·tress s.
me·di·an pal·a·tine s.
me·top·ic s.
na·so·max·il·lary s.
nerve s.
neu·ro·cen·tral s.
non·ab·sorb·a·ble sur·gi·cal s.
oc·cip·i·to·mas·toid s.
pal·a·to·eth·moi·dal s.
pal·a·to·max·il·lary s.
Pancoast's s.
Paré's s.
pa·ri·e·to·mas·toid s.
Parker-Kerr s.
pet·ro·squa·mous s.
plane s.
pre·max·il·lary s.
purse-string s.
quilt·ed s.
re·lax·a·tion s.
re·ten·tion s.
sag·it·tal s.
sec·on·dary s.
ser·rate s.
shot·ted s.
sphe·no·eth·moi·dal s.
sphe·no·fron·tal s.
sphe·no·max·il·lary s.
sphe·no-oc·cip·i·tal s.
sphe·no-or·bit·al s.
sphe·no·pa·ri·e·tal s.
sphe·no·squa·mous s.
sphe·no·vo·mer·ine s.
sphe·no·zy·go·mat·ic s.
spi·ral s.
squa·mo·mas·toid s.
squa·mo·pa·ri·e·tal s.
squa·mous s.
sub·cu·tic·u·lar s.
tem·po·ro·zy·go·mat·ic s.
ten·don s.
ten·sion s.
trans·fix·ion s.
trans·verse pal·a·tine s.

tym·pa·no·mas·toid s.
un·in·ter·rupt·ed s.
wedge-and-groove s.
zy·go·mat·i·co·max·il·lary s.
su·tur·ec·to·my
Suzanne's
   gland
Svedberg
   unit
Svedberg of flo·ta·tion
Sw^a
   an·ti·gen
swab
swage
swal·low
   so·mat·ic s.
   vis·cer·al s.
swal·low·ing
   re·flex
   thresh·old
swamp
   fe·ver
   itch
swamp fe·ver
   vi·rus
Swan-Ganz
   cath·e·ter
Swann
   an·ti·gens
swan-neck
   de·for·mi·ty
swarm·ing
sway-back
sweat
   col·liq·ua·tive s.
   night s.'s
   red s.
sweat
   duct
   glands
   pore
   test
sweat duct
   ad·e·no·ma
sweat gland
   car·ci·no·ma
sweat·ing
   sick·ness
   test
Swediauer's
   dis·ease
Swed·ish
   gym·nas·tics
   move·ments
sweep
sweet
   balm
   pre·cip·i·tate

sweet clo·ver
dis·ease
poi·son·ing
Sweet's
dis·ease
swelled
head
swell·head
swell·ing
al·bu·min·ous s.
ar·y·te·noid s.
brain s.
Cal·a·bar s.
cloudy s.
fu·gi·tive s.
gen·i·tal s.'s
hun·ger s.
la·bi·al s.
la·bi·o·scro·tal s.'s
lat·er·al lin·gual s.'s
le·va·tor s.
Neufeld cap·su·lar s.
scro·tal s.
Spielmeyer's acute s.
Swift's
dis·ease
swim
blad·der
swim·mer's
itch
swim·ming
test
swim·ming pool
con·junc·ti·vi·tis
gran·u·lo·ma
swine
dys·en·tery
er·y·sip·e·las
fe·ver
ic·ter·o·a·ne·mia
in·flu·en·za
pest
por·phyr·ia
swine ede·ma
dis·ease
swine en·ceph·a·li·tis
vi·rus
swine fe·ver
vi·rus
swine·herd's
dis·ease
swine in·flu·en·za
vi·rus·es
swine·pox
vi·rus
swine ve·sic·u·lar
dis·ease

Swiss cheese
en·do·me·tri·um
Swiss mouse leu·ke·mia
vi·rus
Swiss type
agam·ma·glob·u·lin·e·mia
switch·ing
site
sword·fish
test
Swy·er-James
syn·drome
sy·co·ma
sy·co·si·form
sy·co·sis
s. fram·be·si·for·mis
lu·poid s.
s. nu·chae ne·cro·ti·sans
Sydenham's
cho·rea
dis·ease
Syd·ney
crease
line
syl·lab·ic
speech
syl·la·ble-stum·bling
syl·vat·ic
plague
Sylvest's
dis·ease
syl·vi·an
an·gle
aq·ue·duct
fis·sure
line
point
valve
ven·tri·cle
sym·bal·lo·phone
sym·bi·on
sym·bi·ont
sym·bi·o·sis
dy·ad·ic s.
tri·ad·ic s.
sym·bi·ote
sym·bi·ot·ic
sym·bi·ot·ic fer·men·ta·tion
phe·nom·e·non
sym·bleph·a·ron
an·te·ri·or s.
pos·te·ri·or s.
sym·bleph·a·rop·te·ryg·i·um
sym·bol
sym·bo·lia
sym·bol·ism
sym·bol·i·za·tion
sym·brach·y·dac·ty·ly

Syme's
  am·pu·ta·tion
  op·er·a·tion
Syming·ton's ano·coc·cyg·e·al
  body
sym·me·lia
Symmers'
  fi·bro·sis
Symmers' clay pipe·stem
  fi·bro·sis
sym·met·ric
  ad·e·no·lip·o·ma·to·sis
  as·phyx·ia
sym·met·ri·cal
  gan·grene
sym·met·ric dis·tal
  neu·rop·a·thy
sym·me·try
  in·verse s.
sym·pa·thec·to·my
  chem·i·cal s.
  per·i·ar·te·ri·al s.
  pre·sa·cral s.
sym·pa·the·tec·to·my
sym·pa·thet·ic
  agent
  amine
  block·ade
  gan·glia
  het·er·o·chro·mia
  hor·mone
  hy·per·to·nia
  im·bal·ance
  ir·i·do·ple·gia
  iri·tis
  nerve
  oph·thal·mia
  part
  plex·us·es
  root of cil·i·ary gan·gli·on
  sa·li·va
  seg·ment
  symp·tom
  trunk
  uve·i·tis
sym·pa·thet·ic form·a·tive
  cell
sym·pa·thet·ic ner·vous
  sys·tem
sym·pa·thet·ic re·flex
  dys·tro·phy
sym·pa·thet·o·blast
sym·pa·thet·o·blas·to·ma
sym·pa·thic
sym·path·i·cec·to·my
sym·path·i·co·blast
sym·path·i·co·blas·to·ma
sym·path·i·co·go·ni·o·ma

sym·path·i·co·lyt·ic
sym·path·i·co·mi·met·ic
sym·path·i·co·neu·ri·tis
sym·path·i·co·cop·a·thy
sym·path·i·co·to·nia
sym·path·i·co·ton·ic
sym·path·i·co·trip·sy
sym·path·i·co·tro·pic
  cells
sym·pa·thin
sym·pa·thism
sym·pa·thist
sym·pa·thiz·er
sym·pa·thiz·ing
  eye
sym·pa·tho·ad·re·nal
sym·pa·tho·blast
sym·pa·tho·blas·to·ma
sym·pa·tho·chro·maf·fin
  cell
sym·pa·tho·go·nia
sym·pa·tho·go·ni·o·ma
sym·pa·tho·lyt·ic
sym·pa·tho·mi·met·ic
  amine
sym·pa·tho·par·a·lyt·ic
sym·pa·thy
sym·per·i·to·ne·al
sym·pex·is
sym·pha·lan·gism
sym·pha·lan·gy
sym·phy·o·ge·net·ic
sym·phys·e·al
sym·phys·e·o·tome
sym·phys·e·ot·o·my
sym·phy·ses
sym·phys·i·al
  sur·face of pu·bis
sym·phys·ic
  ter·a·to·sis
sym·phys·i·on
sym·phys·i·o·tome
sym·phys·i·ot·o·my
sym·phy·sis
  car·di·ac s.
  in·ter·ver·te·bral s.
  s. man·dib·u·lae
  ma·nu·bri·o·ster·nal s.
  men·tal s.
  s. men·ta·lis
  s. men·ti
  pu·bic s.
  s. sa·cro·coc·cy·gea
sym·plas·mat·ic
sym·plast
sym·po·dia
sym·port
sym·port·er

symp·tom
ab·sti·nence s.'s
ac·ces·so·ry s.
ac·ci·den·tal s.
as·si·dent s.
Baumès s.
Bezold's s.
Bolognini's s.
car·di·nal s.
con·com·i·tant s.
con·sti·tu·tion·al s.
de·fi·cien·cy s.
Demarquay's s.
Duroziez' s.
Epstein's s.
equiv·o·cal s.
first rank s.'s
Fischer's s.
Frenkel's s.
Gordon's s.
Griesinger's s.
Haenel's s.
in·car·cer·a·tion s.
in·duced s.
Kerandel's s.
Kussmaul's s.
lo·cal s.
lo·cal·iz·ing s.
Macewen's s.
ob·jec·tive s.
Oehler's s.
path·og·no·mon·ic s.
Pratt's s.
rain·bow s.
re·flex s.
Romberg-Howship s.
Romberg's s.
schnei·de·ri·an first rank
s.'s
Schneider's first rank s.'s
Sklowsky s.
sub·jec·tive s.
sym·pa·thet·ic s.
Trendelenburg's s.
Trunecek's s.
Wartenberg's s.
with·draw·al s.'s
symp·tom
com·plex
for·ma·tion
group
sub·sti·tu·tion
symp·to·mat·ic
ep·i·lep·sy
er·y·the·ma
fe·ver
head·ache
im·po·tence

neu·ral·gia
par·a·my·o·to·nia
por·phyr·ia
pru·ri·tus
re·ac·tion
tor·ti·col·lis
ul·cer
var·i·co·cele
symp·to·mat·ic in·di·ca·tion
symp·to·mat·ic my·e·loid
met·a·pla·sia
symp·tom·a·tol·o·gy
symp·to·mat·o·lyt·ic
symp·to·mo·lyt·ic
symp·to·sis
sym·pus
s. apus
s. di·pus
s. mon·o·pus
Syms
trac·tor
syn·a·del·phus
syn·al·gia
syn·al·gic
syn·a·nas·to·mo·sis
syn·an·che
syn·an·dro·gen·ic
sy·nan·them
syn·an·the·ma
sy·naph·o·cep·tors
syn·apse
ax·o·ax·on·ic s.
ax·o·den·drit·ic s.
ax·o·so·mat·ic s.
elec·tro·ton·ic s.
per·i·cor·pus·cu·lar s.
syn·aps·es
syn·ap·sis
syn·ap·tic
bou·tons
cleft
con·duc·tion
end·ings
phase
re·sis·tance
ter·mi·nals
trough
ves·i·cles
syn·ap·ti·ne·mal
com·plex
syn·ap·tol·o·gy
syn·ap·to·some
syn·ar·thro·dia
syn·ar·thro·di·al
joint
syn·ar·thro·phy·sis
syn·ar·thro·ses
syn·ar·thro·sis

syn·can·thus
syn·car·y·on
syn·ceph·a·lus
   s. asym·me·tros
syn·ceph·a·ly
syn·chei·lia
syn·chei·ria
syn·chi·lia
syn·chi·ria
syn·chon·dro·di·al
   joint
syn·chon·dro·se·ot·o·my
syn·chon·dro·ses
syn·chon·dro·sis
   s. ar·y·cor·ni·cu·la·ta
   cra·ni·al syn·chon·dro·ses
   s. epiph·y·se·os
   syn·chon·dro·ses in·ter·ster·
     ne·bra·les
   neu·ro·cen·tral s.
   sphe·no·eth·moi·dal s.
   sphe·no·pe·tro·sal s.
   sphe·no·pet·rous s.
   ster·nal syn·chon·dro·ses
syn·chon·dro·to·my
syn·cho·ri·al
syn·chro·nia
syn·chron·ic
   study
syn·chro·nism
syn·chro·nized in·ter·mit·tent
   man·da·to·ry
   ven·ti·la·tion
syn·chro·nous
   re·flex
syn·chro·ny
   bi·lat·er·al s.
syn·chro·tron
syn·chy·sis
   s. scin·til·lans
syn·ci·ne·sis
syn·cli·nal
syn·clit·ic
syn·cli·tism
syn·clon·ic
   spasm
syn·clo·nus
syn·co·pal
syn·co·pe
   ca·rot·id si·nus s.
   hys·ter·i·cal s.
   la·ryn·ge·al s.
   lo·cal s.
   mic·tu·ri·tion s.
   pos·tur·al s.
   va·so·va·gal s.
syn·cop·ic
syn·cre·tio

syn·cy·a·nin
syn·cy·tia
syn·cy·tial
   bud
   knot
   sprout
   troph·o·blast
syn·cy·ti·o·tro·pho·blast
syn·cy·ti·um
syn·dac·tyl
syn·dac·tyle
syn·dac·tyl·ia
syn·dac·ty·lism
syn·dac·ty·lous
syn·dac·ty·ly
syn·der·ma·tot·ic
   cat·a·ract
syn·de·sis
syn·des·mec·to·my
syn·des·mec·to·pia
syn·des·mi·tis
   s. me·ta·tar·sea
syn·des·mo·cho·ri·al
   pla·cen·ta
syn·des·mo·di·al
   joint
syn·des·mog·ra·phy
syn·des·mo·lo·gia
syn·des·mol·o·gy
syn·des·mo·pexy
syn·des·mo·phyte
syn·des·mo·plas·ty
syn·des·mor·rha·phy
syn·des·mo·ses
syn·des·mo·sis
   ra·di·o·ul·nar s.
   tib·i·o·fib·u·lar s.
syn·des·mot·ic
   joint
syn·des·mot·o·my
syn·drome
   Aarskog-Scott s.
   ab·dom·i·nal mus·cle de·fi·
     cien·cy s.
   Achard s.
   Achard-Thiers s.
   Ach·en·bach s.
   ac·quired im·mu·no·de·fi·
     cien·cy s.
   ac·ro·fa·cial s.
   ac·ro·par·es·the·sia s.
   acute ra·di·a·tion s.
   Adams-Stokes s.
   ad·ap·ta·tion s. of Sel·ye
   ad·her·ence s.
   Adie s.
   ad·i·po·so·gen·i·tal s.
   ad·re·nal cor·ti·cal s.

syn·drome *(continued)*

ad·re·nal vir·i·liz·ing s.
adre·no·gen·i·tal s.
adult res·pi·ra·to·ry dis·tress s.
af·fer·ent loop s.
aglos·sia-adac·tyl·ia s.
Ahu·ma·da-Del Castillo s.
Aicardi's s.
Albright's s.
al·co·hol am·nes·tic s.
Aldrich s.
Alezzandrini's s.
Alice in Won·der·land s.
Allen-Masters s.
Alport's s.
Alström's s.
amen·or·rhea-ga·lac·tor·rhea s.
am·nes·tic s.
am·ni·ot·ic flu·id s.
Am·ster·dam s.
Angelucci's s.
an·gi·o-os·te·o·hy·per·tro·phy s.
an·ky·lo·glos·sia su·pe·ri·or s.
ano·rec·tal s.
an·te·ri·or cham·ber cleav·age s.
an·te·ri·or tib·i·al com·part·ment s.
an·ti·body de·fi·cien·cy s.
Anton's s.
anx·i·e·ty s.
aor·tic arch s.
apal·lic s.
Apert-Crouzon s.
Apert's s.
s. of ap·prox·i·mate rel·e·vant an·swers
Argonz-Del Castillo s.
Arndt-Gottron s.
Arnold-Chia·ri s.
Ascher's s.
Asherman's s.
au·ric·u·lo·tem·po·ral nerve s.
au·to·e·ryth·ro·cyte sen·si·ti·za·tion s.
Avellis' s.
A-V stra·bis·mus s.
Axenfeld's s.
Ayerza's s.
Balint's s.
Bamberger-Marie s.
Banti's s.
Bardet-Biedl s.

bare lym·pho·cyte s.
Barlow s.
Barrett s.
Bart's s.
Bartter's s.
ba·sal cell ne·vus s.
Basan's s.
Basex's s.
Bassen-Kornzweig s.
bat·tered child s.
Bauer's s.
Beckwith-Wiedemann s.
Behçet's s.
Behr's s.
Benedikt's s.
Be·ra·di·nel·li's s.
Bernard-Horner s.
Bernard-Sergent s.
Bernard-Soulier s.
Bernhardt-Roth s.
Bernheim's s.
Besnier-Boeck-Schaumann s.
Beu·ren s.
Biemond s.
Bjornstad's s.
B-K mole s.
Blatin's s.
blind loop s.
Bloch-Sulzberger s.
Bloom's s.
Boerhaave's s.
Bonnevie-Ullrich s.
Bonnier's s.
Böök s.
Börjeson-Forssman-Lehmann s.
bow·el by·pass s.
Briquet's s.
Brissaud-Marie s.
Brock's s.
Brown's s.
Brown-Séquard's s.
Brugsch's s.
Budd-Chiari s.
Budd's s.
Bürger-Grütz s.
Burnett's s.
Buschke-Ollendorf s.
Caffey's s.
Caffey-Silverman s.
Cap·gras' s.
Caplan's s.
car·ci·noid s.
ca·rot·id si·nus s.
car·pal tun·nel s.
Carpenter's s.
cat·a·ract-ol·i·go·phre·nia s.
cat-cry s.

cat's-eye s.
cau·da equi·na s.
cav·ern·ous si·nus s.
Ceelen-Gellerstadt s.
cel·lu·lar im·mu·ni·ty
  de·fi·cien·cy s.
cen·tral cord s.
cer·e·bel·lar s.
cer·e·bel·lo·med·ul·lary
  mal·for·ma·tion s.
cer·e·bel·lo·pon·tine an·gle
  s.
cer·e·bro·hep·a·to·re·nal s.
cer·vi·cal com·pres·sion s.
cer·vi·cal disc s.
cer·vi·cal fu·sion s.
cer·vi·cal rib s.
cer·vi·cal ten·sion s.
cer·vi·co-oc·u·lo-a·cous·tic
  s.
Cestan-Chenais s.
chan·cri·form s.
Chan·dler s.
Charcot's s.
Charcot-Weiss-Baker s.
Charlin's s.
Chauffard's s.
Chédiak-Steinbrinck-Higashi
  s.
Cheney s.
cher·ry-red spot my·oc·lo·
  nus s.
Chiari-Budd s.
Chiari-Frommel s.
Chiari II s.
Chiari's s.
chi·as·ma s.
Chilaiditi's s.
CHILD s.
"Chi·nese res·tau·rant" s.
Chotzen s.
Christian's s.
Christ-Siemens s.
chro·mo·som·al s.
chro·mo·som·al break·age
  s.'s
chro·mo·som·al in·sta·bil·i·
  ty s.'s
chron·ic hy·per·ven·ti·la·
  tion s.
Churg-Strauss s.
Clarke-Hadfield s.
Claude's s.
cli·mac·ter·ic s.
clo·ver·leaf skull s.
Cobb s.
Cockayne's s.
Coffin-Lowry s.

Coffin-Siris s.
Cogan-Reese s.
Cogan's s.
Collet-Sicard s.
com·part·men·tal s.
com·pres·sion s.
Conn's s.
Cornelia de Lange s.
cor·pus lu·te·um de·fi·cien·
  cy s.
Costen's s.
cos·to·chon·dral s.
cos·to·cla·vic·u·lar s.
Cotard's s.
Crandall's s.
CREST s.
cri-du-chat s.
Crigler-Najjar s.
croc·o·dile tears s.
Cronkhite-Canada s.
Crouzon's s.
CRST s.
crush s.
Cruveilhier-Baumgarten s.
cryp·toph·thal·mus s.
Cushing's s.
Cushing's s. med·i·ca·men·
  to·sus
cu·ta·ne·o·mu·cou·veal s.
DaCosta's s.
Dandy-Walker s.
dead fe·tus s.
de Clerambault s.
Degos s.
Dejerine-Roussy s.
de Lange s.
Del Castillo s.
de Morsier's s.
den·gue shock s.
De Sanctis-Cacchione s.
De Toni-Fanconi s.
s. of de·vi·ous·ly rel·e·vant
  an·swers
di·al·y·sis dis·e·qui·lib·ri·
  um s.
di·al·y·sis en·ceph·a·lop·a·
  thy s.
Di·a·mond-Black·fan s.
di·en·ce·phal·ic s. of
  in·fan·cy
DiGeorge s.
Di Guglielmo's s.
dis·con·nec·tion s.
disk s.
Doose s.
Dorfman-Chanarin s.
Down's s.
Dressler's s.

syn·drome *(continued)*

dry eye s.
Duane's s.
Dubin-Johnson s.
Dubreuil-Chambardel s.
Duchenne's s.
dump·ing s.
Dyggve-Melchior-Clausen s.
dys·mne·sic s.
dys·plas·tic ne·vus s.
Eagle s.
Eaton-Lambert s.
ec·top·ic ACTH s.
Edwards' s.
ef·fort s.
egg-white s.
Ehlers-Danlos s.
Eisenlohr's s.
Eisenmenger s.
Ekbom s.
Ellis-van Creveld s.
EMG s.
en·ceph·a·lo·tri·gem·i·nal
  vas·cu·lar s.
en·do·crine pol·y·glan·du·lar
  s.
eryth·ro·dys·es·the·sia s.
Evans' s.
ex·tra·py·ram·i·dal s.
Faber's s.
Fanconi's s.
Farber's s.
Felty's s.
fe·tal al·co·hol s.
fe·tal as·pi·ra·tion s.
fe·tal face s.
fe·tal hy·dan·to·in s.
fe·tal tri·meth·a·di·one s.
fe·tal war·fa·rin s.
fi·brin·o·gen-fi·brin con·ver·
  sion s.
Fiessinger-Leroy-Reiter s.
Figueira's s.
first arch s.
Fisher's s.
Fitz-Hugh and Curtis s.
flash·ing pain s.
flecked ret·i·na s.
flop·py valve s.
Flynn-Aird s.
fo·cal der·mal hy·po·pla·sia
  s.
Foix's s.
fold·ed-lung s.
Forbes-Albright s.
Forney's s.
Foster Kennedy's s.
Foville's s.

frag·ile X s.
Fraley s.
Franceschetti-Jadassohn s.
Franceschetti's s.
Fraser's s.
Freeman-Sheldon s.
Frenkel's an·te·ri·or oc·u·
  lar trau·mat·ic s.
Frey's s.
Friderichsen-Waterhouse s.
Fröhlich's s.
Froin's s.
Fuchs' s.
func·tion·al pre·pu·ber·tal
  cas·tra·tion s.
G s.
Gaisböck's s.
Ganser's s.
Gardner-Diamond s.
Gardner's s.
gas·tro·car·di·ac s.
gas·tro·je·ju·nal loop ob·
  struc·tion s.
Gélineau's s.
gen·er·al-ad·ap·ta·tion s.
Gerstmann s.
Gerstmann-Sträussler s.
Gianotti-Crosti s.
Gilbert's s.
Gilles de la Tourette's s.
Glanzmann-Riniker s.
glo·man·gi·o·ma·tous os·se·
  ous mal·for·ma·tion s.
glu·ca·gon·o·ma s.
Goldberg-Maxwell s.
Goldenhar's s.
Goltz s.
Goodpasture's s.
Gop·a·lan's s.
Gorlin-Chaudhry-Moss s.
Gorlin's s.
Gor·man's s.
Gougerot-Carteaud s.
Gowers' s.
grac·i·lis s.
Gradenigo's s.
Graham Little s.
gray s.
gray ba·by s.
Greig's s.
Grönblad-Strandberg s.
Gruber's s.
Gubler's s.
Guillain-Barré s.
Gunn's s.
gus·ta·to·ry sweat·ing s.
Haber's s.
Hallermann-Streiff s.

Hallervorden s.
Hallervorden-Spatz s.
Hallgren's s.
Hamman-Rich s.
Hamman's s.
hand-and-foot s.
Hanhart's s.
hap·py pup·pet s.
Harada's s.
Hartnup s.
Hayem-Widal s.
head-bob·bing doll s.
heart-hand s.
Hegglin's s.
Helweg-Larssen s.
he·man·gi·o·ma-throm·bo·
cy·to·pe·nia s.
he·mo·lyt·ic ure·mic s.
Henoch-Schönlein s.
hep·a·to·ne·pho·ric s.
he·pa·to·re·nal s.
Her·litz s.
Herrmann's s.
Hinman s.
Hirschowitz s.
hol·i·day s.
hol·i·day heart s.
Holmes-Adie s.
Holt-Oram s.
Horner's s.
Houssay s.
Hunter's s.
Hunt's s.
Hurler's s.
Hutchinson-Gilford s.
Hutchison s.
hy·dral·a·zine s.
hy·per·ab·duc·tion s.
hy·per·e·o·sin·o·phil·ic s.
hy·per·im·mu·no·glob·u·lin
E s.
hy·per·ki·net·ic s.
hy·per·sen·si·tive xi·phoid
s.
hy·per·tro·phied fren·u·la s.
hy·per·ven·ti·la·tion s.
hy·per·vis·cos·i·ty s.
hy·po·met·a·bol·ic s.
hy·po·par·a·thy·roid·ism s.
hy·po·phy·si·al s.
hy·po·phys·i·o-sphe·noi·dal
s.
hy·po·plas·tic left heart s.
im·mo·tile cil·ia s.
im·mu·no·de·fi·cien·cy s.
im·mu·no·log·i·cal de·fi·
cien·cy s.

s. of in·ap·pro·pri·ate se·
cre·tion of an·ti·di·u·ret·ic
hor·mone
in·dif·fer·ence to pain s.
in·ter·nal cap·sule s.
in·versed jaw-wink·ing s.
ir·i·do·cor·ne·al en·do·the·
li·al s.
iris-ne·vus s.
Ir·vine-Gass s.
Ive·mark's s.
Jacod's s.
Ja·das·sohn-Le·wan·dow·ski
s.
Jahnke's s.
jaw-wink·ing s.
Jeghers-Peutz s.
Jervell and Lange-Nielsen s.
Jeune's s.
Job s.
Jou·bert's s.
jug·u·lar fo·ra·men s.
Kallmann's s.
Kanner's s.
Kartagener's s.
Kasabach-Merritt s.
Katayama s.
Kearns-Sayre s.
Kennedy's s.
Kimmelstiel-Wilson s.
Kleine-Levin s.
Klinefelter's s.
Klippel-Feil s.
Klippel-Trenaunay-Weber s.
Klumpke-Dejerine s.
Klüver-Bucy s.
Kniest s.
Koenig's s.
Koerber-Salus-Elschnig s.
Korsakoff's s.
Krabbe's s.
Krause's s.
Kus·ko·kwim s.
Laband's s.
Labbé's neu·ro·cir·cu·la·to·
ry s.
LAMB s.
Lambert-Eaton s.
Landau-Kleffner s.
Landry s.
Landry-Guillain-Barré s.
Larsen's s.
Lasègue's s.
lat·er·al med·ul·lary s.
Launois-Bensaude s.
Launois-Cléret s.
Laurence-Biedl s.
Laurence-Moon s.

syn·drome *(continued)*

Laurence-Moon-Bardet-Biedl s.
Lawford's s.
Lawrence-Seip s.
Le·jeune s.
Le·nègre's s.
Lennox s.
Lennox-Gastaut s.
Leriche's s.
Leri-Weill s.
Lermoyez' s.
Lesch-Nyhan s.
Lev's s.
Libman-Sacks s.
Li-Frau·me·ni can·cer s.
Lignac-Fanconi s.
Lobstein's s.
locked-in s.
loc·u·la·tion s.
Löffler's s.
Lorain-Lévi s.
Louis-Bar s.
Lowe's s.
Lowe-Terrey-MacLachlan s.
Lown-Ganong-Levine s.
low salt s.
low so·di·um s.
Lutembacher's s.
Ly·ell's s.
Macleod's s.
Mad Hat·ter s.
Maffucci's s.
Magendie-Hertwig s.
mal·ab·sorp·tion s.
male Turner's s.
ma·lig·nant car·ci·noid s.
Mallory-Weiss s.
man·dib·u·lo·fa·cial dys·o·to·sis s.
man·dib·u·lo-oc·u·lo·fa·cial s.
Marañón's s.
Marchesani s.
Marchiafava-Micheli s.
Marcus Gunn s.
Marfan's s.
Marie-Robinson s.
Marinesco-Garland s.
Marinesco-Sjögren s.
Maroteaux-Lamy s.
Marshall s.
Martorell's s.
mas·sive bow·el re·sec·tion s.
Mauriac's s.
Mayer-Rokitansky-Küster-Hauser s.

May-White s.
McCune-Albright s.
Mead·ows' s.
Meckel s.
Meckel-Gruber s.
me·co·ni·um block·age s.
meg·a·cys·tic s.
Meigs' s.
Melkersson-Rosenthal s.
Melnick-Needles s.
Mendelson's s.
Ménétrièr's s.
Ménière's s.
Menkes' s.
men·o·pau·sal s.
met·a·stat·ic car·ci·noid s.
Meyenburg-Altherr-Uehlinger s.
Meyer-Betz s.
Meyer-Schwickerath and Weyers s.
mid·dle lobe s.
Mikulicz' s.
milk-al·ka·li s.
Milkman's s.
Millard-Gubler s.
Milles' s.
min·i·mal-change neph·rot·ic s.
Mir·riz·zi's s.
Möbius' s.
Monakow's s.
Morgagni-Adams-Stokes s.
Morgagni's s.
morn·ing glo·ry s.
Morquio's s.
Morris s.
Morton's s.
Mounier-Kuhn s.
Mucha-Habermann s.
Muckle-Wells s.
mu·co·cu·ta·ne·ous lymph node s.
Muir-Torre s.
mul·ti·ple ham·ar·to·ma s.
mul·ti·ple len·tig·i·nes s.
mul·ti·ple mu·co·sal neu·ro·ma s.
Munchausen s.
Münchhausen s.
my·e·lo·pro·lif·er·a·tive s.'s
my·o·fa·cial pain-dys·func·tion s.
my·o·fas·ci·al s.
Naegeli s.
Naffziger s.
nail-pa·tel·la s.
NAME s.

Nelson s.
ne·phrit·ic s.
neph·rot·ic s.
Netherton's s.
neu·ral crest s.
neu·ro·cu·ta·ne·ous s.
neu·ro·lep·tic ma·lig·nant s.
Nezelof s.
Nieden's s.
non·sense s.
Noonan's s.
Nothnagel's s.
nys·tag·mus block·age s.
OAV s.
oc·u·lar-mu·cous mem·brane s.
oc·u·lo·buc·co·gen·i·tal s.
oc·u·lo·cer·e·bro·re·nal s.
oc·u·lo·cu·ta·ne·ous s.
oc·u·lo·den·to·dig·i·tal s.
oc·u·lo·pha·ryn·ge·al s.
oc·u·lo·ver·te·bral s.
oc·u·lo·ves·tib·u·lo-au·di·to·ry s.
ODD s.
OFD s.
Omenn's s.
OMM s.
Oppenheim's s.
or·bi·tal s.
or·gan·ic brain s.
or·gan·ic men·tal s.
or·o·fa·ci·o·dig·i·tal s.
os·te·o·my·e·lo·fi·brot·ic s.
Othel·lo s.
oto·man·dib·u·lar s.
oto·pal·a·to·dig·i·tal s.
pach·y·der·mo·per·i·os·to·sis s.
Pag·et-von Schröt·ter s.
pain·ful-bruis·ing s.
pa·le·o·stri·a·tal s.
pal·li·dal s.
Pancoast s.
pap·il·lary mus·cle s.
Papillon-Léage and Psaume s.
Papillon-Lefèvre s.
par·a·ne·o·plas·tic s.
Parinaud's s.
Parinaud's oc·u·lo·glan·du·lar s.
Patau's s.
Paterson-Kelly s.
Pellizzi's s.
Pendred's s.
Pepper s.
per·i·col·ic mem·brane s.

pet·ro·sphe·noid·al s.
Peutz-Jeghers s.
Peutz's s.
Pfaundler-Hurler s.
Pfeiffer s.
pha·ryn·ge·al pouch s.
PHC s.
Picchini's s.
Pick's s.
Pick·wick·i·an s.
Pierre Robin s.
Pins' s.
pla·cen·tal dys·func·tion s.
Plummer-Vinson s.
PNP s.
POEMS s.
pol·y·cys·tic ova·ry s.
pol·y·en·do·crine de·fi·cien·cy s.
pol·y·glan·du·lar de·fi·cien·cy s.
pol·y·sple·nia s.
pop·lit·e·al en·trap·ment s.
post·a·dre·nal·ec·to·my s.
post·car·di·ot·o·my s.
post·cho·le·cys·tec·to·my s.
post·com·mis·sur·ot·o·my s.
post·con·cus·sion s.
pos·te·ri·or in·fe·ri·or cer·e·bel·lar ar·tery s.
post·gas·trec·to·my s.
post·ma·tur·i·ty s.
post·my·o·car·di·al in·farc·tion s.
post·par·tum pi·tu·i·tary ne·cro·sis s.
post·per·i·car·di·ot·o·my s.
post·phle·bit·ic s.
post·ru·bel·la s.
post·trau·mat·ic s.
post·trau·mat·ic neck s.
post·trau·mat·ic stress s.
Potter's s.
Prader-Willi s.
pre·cor·di·al catch s.
pre·ex·ci·ta·tion s.
pre·in·farc·tion s.
pre·ma·ture se·nil·i·ty s.
pre·men·stru·al s.
pre·men·stru·al sal·i·vary s.
pre·men·stru·al ten·sion s.
pre·mo·tor s.
prune bel·ly s.
pseu·do·tha·lid·o·mide s.
pseu·do-Tur·ner's s.
psy·cho·gen·ic noc·tur·nal pol·y·dip·sia s.
pte·ryg·i·um s.

syn·drome *(continued)*

pul·mo·nary dys·ma·tu·ri·ty s.

punch·drunk s.

Putnam-Dana s.

ra·di·al apla·sia-throm·bo·cy·to·pe·nia s.

ra·dic·u·lar s.

Raeder's par·a·tri·gem·i·nal s.

Ramsay Hunt's s.

Raynaud's s.

Refetoff s.

Refsum's s.

Reifenstein's s.

Reiter's s.

REM s.

Rendu-Osler-Weber s.

Renpenning's s.

re·sid·u·al ova·ry s.

re·sis·tant ova·ry s.

res·pi·ra·to·ry dis·tress s. of the new·born

rest·less legs s.

re·trac·tion s.

Rett's s.

Reye's s.

Rh null s.

Richards-Rundel s.

Richter's s.

Rieger's s.

right ovar·i·an vein s.

Riley-Day s.

Roaf's s.

Rob·erts s.

Robin's s.

Rokitansky-Küster-Hauser s.

Romano-Ward s.

Romberg's s.

Rothmund's s.

Rothmund-Thomson s.

Ro·tor's s.

Roussy-Lévy s.

Rubinstein-Taybi s.

Rud's s.

Russell's s.

salt de·ple·tion s.

Sanchez Sa·lo·rio s.

Sanfilippo's s.

Savage s.

scald·ed skin s.

sca·le·nus an·te·ri·or s.

scap·u·lo·cos·tal s.

Schanz s.

Schaumann's s.

Scheie's s.

Schirmer's s.

Schmid-Fraccaro s.

Schmidt's s.

Schönlein-Henoch s.

Schüller's s.

Schwach·man s.

Schwartz s.

Se·bright ban·tam s.

Seckel s.

Secrétan's s.

Senear-Usher s.

Ser·to·li-cell-on·ly s.

Sézary s.

Sheehan's s.

shoul·der-gir·dle s.

shoul·der-hand s.

Shulman's s.

Shy-Drager s.

sic·ca s.

sick si·nus s.

Silver-Russell s.

Silverskiöld's s.

Sipple's s.

Sjögren-Larsson s.

Sjögren's s.

slit ven·tri·cle s.

Smith-Lemli-Opitz s.

Smith-Ri·ley s.

smok·er's res·pi·ra·to·ry s.

Sneddon's s.

Sohval-Soffer s.

Sorsby's s.

So·tos s.

spas·tic s. in cat·tle

Spens' s.

sphe·ro·pha·ki·a-brach·y·mor·phia s.

splen·ic flex·ure s.

Sprinz-Nelson s.

staph·y·lo·coc·cal scald·ed skin s.

Steele-Richardson-Olszewski s.

Stein-Leventhal s.

ste·roid with·draw·al s.

Stevens-Johnson s.

Stewart-Morel s.

Stewart-Treves s.

Stickler s.

stiff-man s.

Still-Chauffard s.

Stock·holm s.

Stokes-Adams s.

straight back s.

Stryker-Halbeisen s.

Sturge-Kalischer-Weber s.

Sturge-Weber s.

sub·cla·vi·an steal s.

sud·den in·fant death s.

Su·deck's s.

Sulzberger-Garbe s.
sump s.
su·pe·ri·or cer·e·bel·lar
  ar·tery s.
su·pe·ri·or mes·en·ter·ic
  ar·tery s.
su·pe·ri·or ve·na ca·val s.
su·pine hy·po·ten·sive s.
su·pra·spi·na·tus s.
su·pra·val·var aor·tic ste·
  no·sis s.
su·pra·val·var aor·tic ste·
  no·sis-in·fan·tile hy·per·
  cal·ce·mia s.
sur·do·car·di·ac s.
Swy·er-James s.
tach·y·car·dia-brad·y·car·dia
  s.
Takayasu's s.
Tapia's s.
TAR s.
tar·sal tun·nel s.
Taussig-Bing s.
teg·men·tal s.
tem·po·ro·man·dib·u·lar s.
tem·po·ro·man·dib·u·lar
  joint pain-dys·func·tion s.
ten·don sheath s.
Terry's s.
tes·tic·u·lar fem·i·ni·za·tion
  s.
teth·ered cord s.
tha·lam·ic s.
third and fourth pha·ryn·
  ge·al pouch s.
tho·rac·ic out·let s.
Thorn's s.
throm·bo·cy·to·pe·nia-
  ab·sent ra·di·us s.
throm·bo·path·ic s.
thy·ro·hy·po·phy·si·al s.
Tietze's s.
To·lo·sa-Hunt s.
tooth-and-nail s.
TORCH s.
Tornwaldt's s.
Torre's s.
Torsten Sjögren's s.
Tourette's s.
tox·ic shock s.
trans·plant lung s.
Treacher Collins' s.
tri·ad s.
trich·o·rhi·no·pha·lan·ge·al
  s.
tri·ple X s.
tri·so·my C s.
tri·so·my D s.

tri·so·my E s.
tro·chan·ter·ic s.
trop·i·cal sple·no·meg·a·ly
  s.
Trousseau's s.
tu·mor ly·sis s.
Turcot s.
Turner's s.
Uehlinger's s.
Ulysses s.
Usher's s.
uve·o·cu·ta·ne·ous s.
uve·o-en·ceph·a·lit·ic s.
uve·o·men·in·gi·tis s.
VACTERL s.
Van Buch·em's s.
van der Hoeve's s.
van·ish·ing lung s.
vas·cu·lo·car·di·ac s. of
  hy·per·se·ro·to·ne·mia
va·so·va·gal s.
Verner-Morrison s.
Vernet's s.
ver·ti·cal re·trac·tion s.
vi·bra·tion s.
vi·rus-as·so·ci·at·ed
  he·mo·phag·o·cyt·ic s.
vit·re·o·ret·i·nal
  cho·roi·dop·a·thy s.
vit·re·o·ret·i·nal trac·tion s.
Vogt s.
Vogt-Koyanagi s.
Voh·wink·el s.
von Hippel-Lindau s.
von Willebrand's s.
vul·ner·a·ble child s.
Waardenburg s.
Wagner's s.
Waldenström's s.
Wallenberg's s.
Waterhouse-Friderichsen s.
WDHA s.
Weber-Cockayne s.
Weber's s.
Weill-Marchesani s.
Wells' s.
Wermer's s.
Werner's s.
Wernicke-Korsakoff s.
Wernicke's s.
West's s.
Weyers-Thier s.
whis·tling face s.
white-out s.
Widal's s.
Wildervanck s.
Williams s.
Wilson-Mikity s.

syn·drome *(continued)*
  Wilson's s.
  Wiskott-Aldrich s.
  Wissler's s.
  Wolff-Parkinson-White s.
  Wyburn-Mason s.
  XO s.
  XXY s.
  XYY s.
  Zellweger s.
  Zieve's s.
  Zollinger-Ellison s.
syn·drom·ic
syn·ech·ia
  an·nu·lar s.
  an·te·ri·or s.
  s. pe·ri·car·dii
  pe·riph·e·ral an·te·ri·or s.
  pos·te·ri·or s.
  to·tal s.
syn·ech·i·ae
syn·ech·i·ot·o·my
syn·ech·o·tome
syn·ec·ten·ter·ot·o·my
syn·en·ceph·a·lo·cele
syn·er·e·sis
syn·er·get·ic
syn·er·gia
syn·er·gic
  con·trol
syn·er·gism
syn·er·gist
syn·er·gis·tic
  mus·cles
syn·er·gy
syn·es·the·sia
  s. al·gi·ca
  au·di·to·ry s.
syn·es·the·si·al·gia
Syn·gam·i·dae
Syn·ga·mus
  S. tra·chea
syn·ga·my
syn·ge·ne·ic
  graft
syn·ge·ne·si·o·plas·ty
syn·ge·ne·si·o·trans·plan·ta·tion
syn·gen·e·sis
syn·ge·net·ic
syn·gen·ic
syn·gna·thia
syn·graft
syn·i·dro·sis
syn·i·ze·sis
syn·kar·y·on
syn·ki·ne·sis
syn·ki·net·ic
syn·ne·ma·tin B

syn·o·nych·ia
syn·o·nym
  ob·jec·tive s.'s
  sen·ior s.
  sub·jec·tive s.'s
syn·oph·rys
syn·oph·thal·mia
syn·oph·thal·mus
syn·op·to·phore
syn·or·chi·dism
syn·or·chism
syn·os·che·os
syn·os·te·ol·o·gy
syn·os·te·o·sis
syn·os·to·sis
  tri·bas·i·lar s.
syn·os·tot·ic
sy·no·tia
syn·o·vec·to·my
syn·o·via
syn·o·vi·al
  bur·sa
  cell
  chon·dro·ma·to·sis
  crypt
  cyst
  flu·id
  fold
  fre·na
  fren·u·la
  fringe
  glands
  her·nia
  joint
  lig·a·ment
  mem·brane
  mes·en·chyme
  os·te·o·chon·dro·ma·to·sis
  sar·co·ma
  sheath
  sheaths of dig·its of foot
  sheaths of dig·its of hand
  tufts
  vil·li
syn·o·vi·al troch·le·ar
  bur·sa
syn·o·vi·o·ma
  ma·lig·nant s.
syn·o·vip·a·rous
syn·o·vi·tis
  bur·sal s.
  chron·ic hem·or·rhag·ic vil·lous s.
  dry s.
  fi·lar·i·al s.
  pig·ment·ed vil·lo·nod·u·lar s.
  pu·ru·lent s.

se·rous s.
s. sic·ca
sup·pu·ra·tive s.
ten·di·nous s.
vag·i·nal s.
syn·o·vi·um
syn·pol·y·dac·ty·ly
syn·tac·ti·cal
apha·sia
syn·tac·tics
syn·tal·i·ty
syn·tec·tic
syn·ten·ic
syn·te·ny
syn·tex·is
syn·thase
syn·ther·mal
syn·the·ses
syn·the·sis
s. of con·ti·nu·i·ty
en·zy·mat·ic s.
pro·tein s.
syn·the·sis
pe·ri·od
syn·the·size
syn·the·tase
syn·thet·ic
chem·is·try
dyes
syn·tho·rax
syn·ton·ic
per·son·al·i·ty
syn·tro·phism
syn·tro·pho·blast
syn·tro·pic
syn·tro·py
in·verse s.
Sy·pha·cia
syph·i·le·mia
syph·i·lid
ac·ne·form s.
acu·mi·nate pap·u·lar s.
an·nu·lar s.
bul·lous s.
cor·ym·bose s.
ec·thym·a·tous s.
er·y·them·a·tous s.
flat pap·u·lar s.
fol·lic·u·lar s.
fram·be·si·form s.
gum·ma·tous s.
im·pe·tig·i·nous s.
len·tic·u·lar s.
mac·u·lar s.
mil·i·a·ry pap·u·lar s.
nod·u·lar s.
num·mu·lar s.
pal·mar s.

pap·u·lar s.
pap·u·lo·squa·mous s.
pem·phi·goid s.
pig·men·tary s.
plan·tar s.
pus·tu·lar s.
ru·pi·al s.
sec·on·dary s.
ter·ti·ary s.
var·i·ol·i·form s.
syph·i·lim·e·try
syph·i·li·on·thus
syph·i·lis
con·gen·i·tal s.
s. d'em·blée
equine s.
s. he·re·di·ta·ria
s. he·re·di·ta·ria tar·da
he·red·i·tary s.
me·nin·go·vas·cu·lar s.
pri·mary s.
qua·ter·na·ry s.
sec·on·dary s.
ter·ti·ary s.
syph·i·lit·ic
ab·scess
an·eu·rysm
aor·ti·tis
fe·ver
leu·ko·der·ma
me·nin·go·en·ceph·a·li·tis
ne·phri·tis
os·te·o·chon·dri·tis
ret·i·ni·tis
ro·se·o·la
teeth
ul·cer
syph·i·lo·derm
syph·i·lo·der·ma
syph·i·loid
syph·i·lol·o·gist
syph·i·lol·o·gy
syph·i·lo·ma
s. of Fournier
syph·i·lom·a·tous
Syr·i·ac
ul·cer
Syr·i·an
ul·cer
sy·rig·mus
syr·ing·ad·e·no·ma
syr·ing·ad·e·no·sus
sy·ringe
air s.
chip s.
con·trol s.
Davidson s.
den·tal s.

sy·ringe *(continued)*
  foun·tain s.
  hy·po·der·mic s.
  Luer s.
  Luer-Lok s.
  Neisser's s.
  Pitkin s.
  probe s.
  ring s.
  Roughton-Scholander s.
  rub·ber-bulb s.
sy·rin·ge·al
sy·rin·gec·to·my
sy·ring·es
sy·rin·gi·tis
sy·rin·go·ad·e·no·ma
sy·rin·go·bul·bia
sy·rin·go·car·ci·no·ma
sy·rin·go·cele
sy·rin·go·cys·tad·e·no·ma
  s. pa·pil·li·fe·rum
sy·rin·go·cys·to·ma
sy·rin·go·en·ceph·a·lo·my·e·lia
sy·rin·goid
sy·rin·go·ma
  chon·droid s.
sy·rin·go·me·nin·go·cele
sy·rin·go·my·e·lia
sy·rin·go·my·el·ic
  dis·so·ci·a·tion
  hem·or·rhage
sy·rin·go·my·e·lo·cele
sy·rin·go·my·e·lus
sy·rin·go·pon·tia
sy·rin·go·tome
sy·rin·got·o·my
syr·inx
sy·ro·sing·o·pine
syr·up
syr·u·pus
syr·upy
sys·sar·co·sic
sys·sar·co·sis
sys·sar·cot·ic
sys·tal·tic
sys·tem
  ab·so·lute s. of units
  ab·sor·bent s.
  al·i·men·ta·ry s.
  arch-loop-whorl s.
  as·so·ci·a·tion s.
  au·to·nom·ic ner·vous s.
  blood group s.'s
  blood-vas·cu·lar s.
  bul·bo·sa·cral s.
  car·di·o·vas·cu·lar s.
  cau·dal neu·ro·se·cre·to·ry s.

cen·ti·me·ter-gram-sec·ond s.
cen·tral ner·vous s.
cer·e·bro·spi·nal s.
chro·maf·fin s.
cir·cu·la·to·ry s.
col·loid s.
con·duct·ing s. of heart
cra·ni·o·sa·cral s.
cy·to·chrome s.
der·mal s.
der·moid s.
di·ges·tive s.
ec·o·log·i·cal s.
elec·tron-trans·port s.
en·do·crine s.
es·the·si·od·ic s.
ex·ter·o·fec·tive s.
ex·tra·py·ram·i·dal mo·tor s.
feed·back s.
foot-pound-second s.
Galton's s. of clas·si·fi·ca·tion of fin·ger·prints
gam·ma mo·tor s.
gen·i·tal s.
gen·i·to·u·ri·nary s.
glan·du·lar s.
ha·ver·si·an s.
he·ma·to·poi·et·ic s.
het·er·o·ge·neous s.
hex·ax·i·al ref·er·ence s.
His-Tawara s.
ho·mo·ge·neous s.
hy·po·thal·a·mo·hy·po·phy·si·al por·tal s.
hy·pox·ia warn·ing s.
im·mune s.
in·di·ca·tor s.
in·teg·u·men·ta·ry s.
in·ter·me·di·ary s.
In·ter·na·tion·al S. of Units
in·ter·o·fec·tive s.
in·vol·un·tary ner·vous s.
kal·li·kre·in s.
ki·net·ic s.
lat·er·al line s.
lim·bic s.
lin·nae·an s. of no·men·cla·ture
lym·phat·ic s.
s. of mac·ro·phag·es
mas·ti·ca·to·ry s.
met·a·mer·ic ner·vous s.
me·ter-kil·o·gram-sec·ond s.
met·ric s.
mon·o·nu·cle·ar phag·o·cyte s.
mus·cu·lar s.

ner·vous s.
neu·ro·mus·cu·lar s.
non·spe·cif·ic s.
oc·clu·sal s.
oc·u·lo·mo·tor s.
O-R s.
ox·i·da·tion-re·duc·tion s.
par·a·sym·pa·thet·ic ner·
  vous s.
ped·al s.
pe·ri·od·ic s.
pe·riph·e·ral ner·vous s.
Pinel's s.
por·tal s.
pres·so·re·cep·tor s.
pro·jec·tion s.
pro·per·din s.
Purkinje s.
re·dox s.
re·nin-an·gi·o·ten·sin s.
re·pro·duc·tive s.
res·pi·ra·to·ry s.
re·tic·u·lar ac·ti·vat·ing s.
re·tic·u·lo·en·do·the·li·al s.
sec·ond sig·nal·ing s.
skel·e·tal s.
som·es·thet·ic s.
stat·ic s.
sto·ma·to·gnath·ic s.
sym·pa·thet·ic ner·vous s.
T s.
tho·ra·co·lum·bar s.
tri·ax·i·al ref·er·ence s.
uri·nary s.
uro·gen·i·tal s.
uro·poi·e·tic s.
vas·cu·lar s.
veg·e·ta·tive ner·vous s.
ver·te·bral-bas·i·lar s.
ver·te·bral ve·nous s.
vis·cer·al ner·vous s.
sys·te·ma
sys·tem·at·ic
anat·o·my
bac·te·ri·ol·o·gy
de·sen·si·tiz·a·tion
ver·ti·go
sys·tem·at·ic name
sys·tem·a·ti·za·tion
sys·tem·a·tized
de·lu·sion
ne·vus

Sys·tème In·ter·na·tion·al
  d'Un·i·tés
sys·tem·ic
an·a·phy·lax·is
anat·o·my
chon·dro·ma·la·cia
cir·cu·la·tion
death
heart
hy·a·li·no·sis
lu·pus er·y·the·ma·to·sus
my·e·li·tis
poi·son·ing
sys·tem·ic au·to·im·mune
dis·eas·es
sys·tem·ic feb·rile
dis·eas·es
sys·tem·ic vas·cu·lar
re·sis·tance
sys·te·moid
sys·to·le
abort·ed s.
s. al·ter·nans
atri·al s.
au·ric·u·lar s.
elec·tro·me·chan·i·cal s.
ex·tra-s.
late s.
pre·ma·ture s.
ven·tric·u·lar s.
sys·tol·ic
click
gal·lop
gra·di·ent
honk
mur·mur
pres·sure
shock
thrill
whoop
sys·tol·ic time
in·ter·vals
sys·to·lom·e·ter
sys·trem·ma
sy·zyg·i·al
sy·zyg·i·ol·o·gy
sy·zyg·i·um
syz·y·gy

T
ag·glu·tin·o·gen
an·ti·gens
cell
en·zyme
group
lym·pho·cyte
my·e·lot·o·my
sys·tem
tube
tu·bule
wave

T₃
tox·i·co·sis

T-
ban·dage
bind·er

t
test

T.A.B.
vac·cine

tab·a·nid
Ta·ban·i·dae
Ta·ba·nus
ta·bar·dil·lo
ta·ba·tière an·a·to·mique
tab·by cat
stri·a·tion
ta·bel·la
ta·bel·lae
ta·bes
t. di·a·be·ti·ca
t. dor·sa·lis
t. er·go·ti·ca
t. mes·en·te·ri·ca
pe·riph·e·ral t.
t. spas·mo·di·ca
t. spi·na·lis
ta·bes·cence
ta·bes·cent
ta·bet·ic
ar·throp·a·thy
cri·sis
cui·rass
dis·so·ci·a·tion
ta·bet·i·form
tab·ic
tab·id
tab·la·ture

ta·ble
Aub-DuBois t.
ex·am·in·ing t.
Gaffky t.
in·ner t. of skull
life t.
oc·clu·sal t.
op·er·at·ing t.
out·er t. of skull
Reuss' col·or t.'s
Stilling col·or t.'s
tilt t.
vit·re·ous t.
ta·ble
salt
ta·ble·spoon
tab·let
trit·u·rate
tab·let
buc·cal t.
com·pressed t.
dis·pens·ing t.
en·ter·ic coat·ed t.
hy·po·der·mic t.
pro·longed ac·tion t.
re·peat ac·tion t.
sub·lin·gual t.
sus·tained ac·tion t.
sus·tained re·lease t.
t. trit·u·rate
ta·boo
ta·bo·pa·re·sis
ta·bu
tab·u·lar
tab·ule
ta·bun
Tac·a·ribe
com·plex of vi·rus·es
vi·rus
tache
t. blanche
t. bleu·âtre
t. cé·ré·bra·le
t. lai·teuse
t. mé·nin·gé·a·le
t. noire
t. spi·na·le
ta·chet·ic
ta·chis·tes·the·sia

ta·chis·to·scope
tach·o·gram
tach·o·graph
ta·chog·ra·phy
ta·chom·e·ter
tach·y·ar·rhyth·mia
tach·y·aux·e·sis
tach·y·car·dia
  atri·al t.
  atri·al cha·ot·ic t.
  atri·o·ven·tric·u·lar no·dal
    t.
  au·ric·u·lar t.
  A-V no·dal t.
  bi·di·rec·tion·al ven·tric·u·
    lar t.
  dou·ble t.
  ec·top·ic t.
  t. en salves
  es·sen·tial t.
  t. ex·oph·thal·mi·ca
  fe·tal t.
  no·dal t.
  par·ox·ys·mal t.
  si·nus t.
  ven·tric·u·lar t.
tach·y·car·dia
  win·dow
tach·y·car·dia-brad·y·car·dia
  syn·drome
tach·y·car·di·ac
tach·y·crot·ic
tach·y·ki·nin
tach·y·la·lia
tach·y·lo·gia
tach·y·pac·ing
tach·y·pha·gia
tach·y·pha·sia
tach·y·phe·mia
tach·y·phra·sia
tach·y·phy·lax·is
tach·yp·nea
tach·y·rhyth·mia
ta·chys·ter·ol
tach·y·sys·to·le
tach·y·zo·ite
tac·rine
tac·tile
  ag·no·sia
  an·es·the·sia
  cell
  cor·pus·cle
  disk
  el·e·va·tions
  frem·i·tus
  hair
  hy·per·es·the·sia
  im·age

  me·nis·cus
  pa·pil·la
  sense
tac·tion
tac·tom·e·ter
tac·tor
tac·tu·al
Tae·nia
  T. af·ri·ca·na
  T. ar·ma·ta
  T. cras·si·col·lis
  T. dem·e·rar·i·en·sis
  T. den·ta·ta
  T. equi·na
  T. hom·i·nis
  T. hy·da·ti·ge·na
  T. mad·a·gas·ca·ri·en·sis
  T. min·i·ma
  T. ovis
  T. phi·lip·pi·na
  T. pi·si·for·mis
  T. quad·ri·lo·ba·ta
  T. sa·gi·na·ta
  T. so·li·um
  T. tae·ni·ae·for·mis
tae·nia
Tae·ni·a·rhyn·chus
tae·ni·a·sis
tae·ni·id
Tae·ni·i·dae
tae·ni·oid
Tae·ni·o·rhyn·chus
Taenzer's
  stain
tag
  anal skin t.
  sen·ti·nel t.
  skin t.
tag·a·tose
tagged
  at·om
tag·li·a·co·ti·an
  op·er·a·tion
Ta·hy·na
  vi·rus
tail
  bone
  bud
  fold
  sheath
  ver·te·brae
tail
  t. of cau·date nu·cle·us
  t. of den·tate gy·rus
  t. of ep·i·did·y·mis
  t. of he·lix
  t. of pan·cre·as
tail·gut

tai·lor's
　cramp
　mus·cle
　spasm
Tait's
　law
Takahara's
　dis·ease
Takayama's
　stain
Takayasu's
　dis·ease
　syn·drome
take
ta·lal·gia
ta·lar
　sul·cus
ta·lar ar·tic·u·lar
　sur·face of cal·ca·ne·us
tal·bu·tal
talc
　op·er·a·tion
tal·co·sis
tal·cum
ta·li
tal·i·on
tal·i·on dread
tal·i·ped·ic
tal·i·pes
　t. ar·cu·a·tus
　t. cal·ca·ne·o·val·gus
　t. cal·ca·ne·o·var·us
　t. cal·ca·ne·us
　t. cav·us
　t. equi·no·val·gus
　t. equi·no·var·us
　t. equi·nus
　t. plan·tar·is
　t. pla·nus
　t. spas·mo·di·cus
　t. trans·ver·so·pla·nus
　t. val·gus
　t. var·us
tal·i·pom·a·nus
tal·low
　pre·pared mut·ton t.
tal·low
　soap
Talma's
　dis·ease
ta·lo·cal·ca·ne·al
　joint
　lig·a·ment
ta·lo·cal·ca·ne·an
ta·lo·cal·ca·ne·o·na·vic·u·lar
　joint
ta·lo·cru·ral
　ar·tic·u·la·tion

ta·lo·fib·u·lar
tal·on
ta·lo·na·vic·u·lar
　lig·a·ment
ta·lo·scaph·oid
tal·ose
ta·lo·tib·i·al
ta·lus
tam·a·rind
tam·bour
　sound
tamed
　io·dine
Tamm-Horsfall
　mu·co·pro·tein
　pro·tein
ta·mox·i·fen cit·rate
tam·pon
　Corner's t.
tam·pon·ade
　car·di·ac t.
tam·pon·age
tam·pon·ing
tam·pon·ment
ta·nace·tol
tan·a·ce·tone
tan·gent
　screen
tan·gen·tial
　wound
tan·gen·ti·al·i·ty
Tan·gier
　dis·ease
tank
　res·pi·ra·tor
tan·nase
tan·nate
tanned red
　cells
Tanner
　stage
Tanner growth
　chart
tan·ner's
　ul·cer
tan·nic
tan·nic ac·id
　glyc·er·ite
tan·nin
tan·nyl·ac·e·tate
tan·ta·lum
tan·trum
tan·y·cyte
tan·y·pho·nia
tap
　heel t.
　mi·tral t.
　spi·nal t.

tape
   ad·he·sive t.
ta·pered
   bou·gie
ta·pe·ta
ta·pe·tal light
   re·flex
ta·pe·to·cho·roi·dal
ta·pe·to·ret·i·nal
   de·gen·er·a·tion
   ret·i·nop·a·thy
ta·pe·to·ret·in·op·a·thy
ta·pe·tum
   t. al·ve·o·li
   t. ni·grum
   t. oc·u·li
tape·worm
taph·o·phil·ia
taph·o·pho·bia
Tapia's
   syn·drome
tap·i·no·ce·phal·ic
tap·i·no·ceph·a·ly
tap·i·o·ca
ta·pir
   mouth
ta·pir·oid
ta·pote·ment
tap·ping
TAR
   syn·drome
tar
   ac·ne
   cam·phor
   ker·a·to·sis
tar·an·tism
ta·ran·tu·la
   Amer·i·can t.
   black t.
   Eu·ro·pe·an t.
   Pe·ru·vi·an t.
ta·rax·a·cum
Tardieu's
   ec·chy·mos·es
   pe·te·chi·ae
   spots
tar·dive
   cy·a·no·sis
tar·dive oral
   dys·ki·ne·sia
tar·dy
   ep·i·lep·sy
tar·get
   be·hav·ior
   cell
   gland
   or·gan

pa·tient
   re·sponse
tar·get cell
   ane·mia
Tarin's
   space
   te·nia
   valve
ta·rir·ic ac·id
Tarlov's
   cyst
Tarnier's
   for·ceps
tar·ra·gon oil
tar·ry
   cyst
tars·ad·e·ni·tis
tar·sal
   arch
   bones
   ca·nal
   car·ti·lage
   cyst
   fold
   glands
   joints
   lig·a·ments
   plates
   si·nus
tar·sa·le
tars·al·gia
tar·sa·lia
tar·sa·lis
tar·sal tun·nel
   syn·drome
tars·ec·to·my
tar·sec·to·pia
tar·sec·to·py
tar·sen
tar·si
tar·si·tis
tar·so·chi·lo·plas·ty
tar·so·cla·sia
tar·soc·la·sis
tar·so·ma·la·cia
tar·so·meg·a·ly
tar·so·met·a·tar·sal
   joints
   lig·a·ments
tar·so·met·a·tar·sus
tar·so-or·bit·al
tar·so·pha·lan·ge·al
   re·flex
tar·so·phy·ma
tar·sor·rha·phy
tar·so·tar·sal
tar·so·tib·i·al
   am·pu·ta·tion

tar·sot·o·my
tar·sus
tart
  cell
tar·tar
  cream of t.
  t. emet·ic
  sol·u·ble t.
tar·tar·ic ac·id
tar·trate
  ac·id t.
  nor·mal t.
tar·trat·ed
  an·ti·mo·ny
tar·tra·zine
task-o·ri·ent·ed
  group
taste
  blind·ness
  bud
  bulb
  cells
  cor·pus·cle
  de·fi·cien·cy
  hairs
  pore
  ridge
taste
  af·ter-t.
  col·or t.
  frank·lin·ic t.
  vol·ta·ic t.
TATA
  box
tat·too
  amal·gam t.
tau·rine
tau·ro·cho·late
tau·ro·cho·lic ac·id
tau·ro·don·tism
Taussig-Bing
  dis·ease
  syn·drome
tau·to·me·ni·al
tau·to·mer·ic
  fi·bers
tau·tom·er·ism
Tawara's
  node
taxa
tax·is
  bi·po·lar t.
  neg·a·tive t.
  pos·i·tive t.
tax·on
tax·o·nom·ic
tax·on·o·my
  nu·mer·i·cal t.

Taylor's
  ap·pa·ra·tus
  dis·ease
  splint
Taylor's back
  brace
Tay's
  dis·ease
Tay-Sachs
  dis·ease
Tay's cher·ry-red
  spot
tea
  Hot·ten·tot t.
  Jes·u·it t.
  Mex·i·can t.
  Par·a·guay t.
teach·ers'
  nodes
teach·ing
  hos·pi·tal
TEAE-cel·lu·lose
Teale's
  am·pu·ta·tion
tear
  film
  gas
  sac
  stone
tear
  ar·ti·fi·cial t.'s
  croc·o·dile t.'s
tear
  buck·et-han·dle t.
  Mallory-Weiss t.
tear·drop
  heart
tear·ing
tease
tea·spoon
teat
teb·u·tate
tech·ne·ti·um
tech·nic
tech·ni·cal
tech·ni·cian
tech·nique
  air·bra·sive t.
  atri·al-well t.
  Barcroft-Warburg t.
  Begg light wire dif·fer·en·
    tial force t.
  di·rect t.
  Fi·coll-Hy·paque t.
  flick·er fu·sion fre·quen·cy
    t.
  flu·o·res·cent an·ti·body t.
  flush t.

tech·nique *(continued)*
  Hampton t.
  Hartel t.
  im·mu·no·per·ox·i·dase t.
  in·di·rect t.
  Judkins t.
  long cone t.
  McGoon's t.
  Merendino's t.
  Mohs' fresh tis·sue che·mo·
    sur·gery t.
  PAP t.
  re·breath·ing t.
  Re·buck skin win·dow t.
  sealed jar t.
  Sel·din·ger t.
  ster·ile in·sect t.
  su·per·son·ic vi·bra·tion t.
  washed field t.
tech·no·cau·sis
tech·nol·o·gist
tech·nol·o·gy
tec·lo·thi·a·zide
tec·ta
tec·tal
tec·ti·form
tec·to·bul·bar
  tract
tec·to·ce·phal·ic
tec·to·ceph·a·ly
tec·tol·o·gy
tec·ton·ic
  ker·a·to·plas·ty
tec·to·pon·tine
  tract
tec·to·ri·al
  mem·brane
  mem·brane of co·chle·ar
    duct
tec·to·ri·um
tec·to·spi·nal
  de·cus·sa·tion
  tract
tec·tum
teel oil
teeth
teeth·ing
tef·lu·rane
teg·men
  t. cru·ris
  t. mas·toi·de·um
teg·men·ta
teg·men·tal
  de·cus·sa·tions
  fields of Forel
  syn·drome
  wall of mid·dle ear
teg·men·tot·o·my

teg·men·tum
  mes·en·ce·phal·ic t.
  mid·brain t.
  t. of pons
  t. of rhomb·en·ceph·a·lon
teg·mi·na
teg·mi·nis
teg·u·ment
teg·u·men·tal
teg·u·men·ta·ry
Teichmann's
  crys·tals
tei·cho·ic ac·ids
tei·chop·sia
te·la
  t. cho·roi·dea
  t. cho·roi·dea in·fe·ri·or
  t. cho·roi·dea su·pe·ri·or
  cho·roid t. of fourth ven·
    tri·cle
  cho·roid t. of third ven·tri·
    cle
  t. con·junc·ti·va
  t. elas·ti·ca
  t. sub·mu·co·sa pha·ryn·gis
  t. vas·cu·lo·sa
Te·la·dor·sa·gia dav·ti·ani
te·lae
tel·al·gia
tel·an·gi·ec·ta·ses
tel·an·gi·ec·ta·sia
  ceph·a·lo·oc·u·lo·cu·ta·ne·
    ous t.
  es·sen·tial t.
  he·red·i·tary hem·or·rhag·ic
    t.
  t. lym·pha·ti·ca
  t. ma·cu·la·ris erup·ti·va
    per·stans
  spi·der t.
  t. ver·ru·co·sa
tel·an·gi·ec·ta·sis
tel·an·gi·ec·tat·ic
  an·gi·o·ma
  an·gi·o·ma·to·sis
  can·cer
  fi·bro·ma
  gli·o·ma
  li·po·ma
  wart
tel·an·gi·ec·tat·ic os·te·o·gen·ic
  sar·co·ma
tel·an·gi·ec·to·des
tel·an·gi·o·ma
tel·an·gi·on
tel·an·gi·o·sis
tel·e·can·thus
tel·e·car·di·o·gram

tel·e·car·di·o·phone
tel·e·co·balt
tel·e·di·ag·no·sis
tel·e·di·a·stol·ic
tel·e·lec·tro·car·di·o·gram
te·lem·e·ter
te·lem·e·try
   car·di·ac t.
tel·en·ce·phal·ic
   flex·ure
   ves·i·cle
tel·en·ceph·al·i·za·tion
tel·en·ceph·a·lon
te·le·ol·o·gy
tel·e·o·mi·to·sis
tel·e·o·nom·ic
tel·e·on·o·my
tel·e·op·sia
tel·e·or·gan·ic
tel·e·ost
tel·e·path·ine
te·lep·a·thy
tel·e·phone
   the·o·ry
tel·e·ra·di·og·ra·phy
tel·e·ra·di·um
   ther·a·py
tel·e·re·cep·tor
tel·er·gy
tel·e·roent·gen·o·gram
tel·e·roent·gen·og·ra·phy
tel·e·roent·gen·ther·a·py
tel·e·scop·ic
   den·ture
   spec·ta·cles
tel·e·sis
tel·e·sys·tol·ic
tel·e·tac·tor
tel·e·ther·a·py
tel·e·vi·sion
   mi·cro·scope
TeLinde
   op·er·a·tion
tel·lu·ric
tel·lu·rism
tel·lu·ri·um
tel·o·cen·tric
   chro·mo·some
tel·o·den·dron
tel·o·gen
   ef·flu·vi·um
te·log·lia
tel·og·no·sis
tel·o·ki·ne·sia
tel·o·lec·i·thal
   egg
   ovum
tel·o·mere

tel·o·mer·ic R-band·ing
   stain
tel·o·pep·tide
tel·o·phase
Te·lo·spo·rea
Te·lo·spo·rid·ia
tel·o·tism
te·maz·e·pam
tem·per
tem·per·a·ment
tem·per·ance
tem·per·ate
   bac·te·ri·o·phage
tem·per·a·ture
   co·ef·fi·cient
   sense
   spot
tem·per·a·ture
   ab·so·lute t.
   crit·i·cal t.
   de·na·tur·a·tion t. of DNA
   ef·fec·tive t.
   equiv·a·lent t.
   eu·tec·tic t.
   fu·sion t.
   max·i·mum t.
   mean t.
   melt·ing t.
   melt·ing t. of DNA
   t. mid·point
   min·i·mum t.
   op·ti·mum t.
   room t.
   sen·si·ble t.
   stan·dard t.
tem·per·a·ture-com·pen·sat·ed
   va·por·iz·er
tem·per·a·ture-sen·si·tive
   mu·tant
tem·plate
   RNA
tem·plate
   sur·gi·cal t.
tem·ple
tem·po·la·bile
tem·po·ra
tem·po·ral
   ap·o·neu·ro·sis
   apoph·y·sis
   ar·te·ri·tis
   bone
   ca·nal
   cor·tex
   dis·per·sion
   fas·cia
   fos·sa
   horn
   line

tem·po·ral *(continued)*
  lobe
  mus·cle
  plane
  pole
  pro·cess
  re·gion of head
  ridge
  squa·ma
  sur·face
  veins
  ven·ules of ret·i·na
tem·po·ral con·ti·gu·i·ty
tem·po·ra·lis
tem·po·ral lobe
  ep·i·lep·sy
tem·po·rary
  base
  cal·lus
  car·ti·lage
  den·ture
  par·a·site
  res·to·ra·tion
  stric·ture
  tooth
tem·po·ris
tem·po·ro·au·ric·u·lar
tem·po·ro·fron·tal
  tract
tem·po·ro·hy·oid
tem·po·ro·ma·lar
tem·po·ro·man·dib·u·lar
  ar·thro·sis
  ar·tic·u·la·tion
  joint
  lig·a·ment
  nerve
  syn·drome
tem·po·ro·man·dib·u·lar ar·tic·u·lar
  disk
tem·po·ro·man·dib·u·lar joint
  dys·func·tion
tem·po·ro·man·dib·u·lar joint
  pain-dys·func·tion
  syn·drome
tem·po·ro·max·il·lary
  vein
tem·po·ro-oc·cip·i·tal
tem·po·ro·pa·ri·e·tal
  mus·cle
tem·po·ro·pon·tine
  tract
tem·po·ro·sphe·noid
tem·po·ro·zy·go·mat·ic
  su·ture
tem·po·sta·bile
tem·po·sta·ble

temps utile
tem·pus
te·na·cious
te·nac·i·ty
  cel·lu·lar t.
te·nac·u·la
  t. ten·di·num
te·nac·u·lum
  for·ceps
te·nal·gia
  t. crep·i·tans
ten·der
  lines
  points
  zones
ten·der·ness
  pen·cil t.
  re·bound t.
ten·di·nes
ten·di·nis
ten·di·ni·tis
ten·di·no·plas·ty
ten·di·no·su·ture
ten·di·nous
  arch
  arch of le·va·tor ani
    mus·cle
  arch of pel·vic fas·cia
  arch of so·le·us mus·cle
  cords
  in·scrip·tion
  in·ter·sec·tion
  open·ing
  spot
  syn·o·vi·tis
ten·do
  t. cal·ca·ne·us com·mu·nis
  t. oc·u·li
  t. pal·pe·bra·rum
ten·do Achil·lis
  re·flex
ten·dol·y·sis
ten·do·mu·cin
ten·do·mu·coid
ten·don
  Achil·les t.
  bowed t.
  cal·ca·ne·an t.
  cen·tral t. of di·a·phragm
  cen·tral t. of per·i·ne·um
  con·joined t.
  con·joint t.
  con·tract·ed t.
  cor·o·nary t.
  cri·co·e·soph·a·ge·al t.
  Gerlach's an·nu·lar t.
  ham·string t.
  heel t.

slipped t.
Todaro's t.
tre·foil t.
Zinn's t.
ten·don
ad·vance·ment
bun·dle
cells
graft
re·ces·sion
re·flex
su·ture
trans·plan·ta·tion
ten·don·i·tis
ten·don sheath
syn·drome
ten·doph·o·ny
ten·do·plas·ty
ten·do·syn·o·vi·tis
ten·dot·o·my
ten·do·vag·i·nal
ten·do·vag·i·ni·tis
ra·di·al sty·loid t.
te·nec·to·my
te·nes·mic
te·nes·mus
ten Horn's
sign
te·nia
te·ni·ae acus·ti·cae
col·ic te·ni·ae
t. fim·bri·ae
t. of the for·nix
t. of fourth ven·tri·cle
t. hip·po·cam·pi
med·ul·lary te·ni·ae
t. sem·i·cir·cu·la·ris
Tarin's t.
t. tec·ta
t. ter·mi·na·lis
tha·lam·ic t.
te·ni·ae of Valsalva
t. ven·tric·u·li ter·tii
te·ni·a·cide
te·ni·ae
te·ni·a·fuge
ten·i·al
te·ni·a·sis
so·mat·ic t.
ten·i·cide
ten·i·form
te·nif·u·gal
ten·i·fuge
te·ni·oid
te·ni·o·la
t. cor·po·ris cal·losi
ten·nis
el·bow

leg
thumb
te·no·de·sis
ten·o·dyn·ia
ten·o·fi·bril
ten·ol·y·sis
ten·o·my·o·plas·ty
ten·o·my·ot·o·my
ten·o·nec·to·my
ten·o·ni·tis
ten·o·nom·e·ter
Tenon's
cap·sule
space
ten·on·ti·tis
te·non·to·dyn·ia
te·non·tog·ra·phy
te·non·to·lem·mi·tis
te·non·tol·o·gy
te·non·to·my·o·plas·ty
te·non·to·my·ot·o·my
te·non·to·plas·tic
te·non·to·plas·ty
te·non·to·the·ci·tis
te·noph·o·ny
ten·o·phyte
ten·o·plas·tic
ten·o·plas·ty
ten·o·re·cep·tor
te·nor·rha·phy
ten·o·si·tis
ten·os·to·sis
ten·o·sus·pen·sion
ten·o·su·ture
ten·o·syn·o·vec·to·my
ten·o·syn·o·vi·tis
t. crep·i·tans
lo·cal·ized nod·u·lar t.
vil·lo·nod·u·lar pig·ment·ed
t.
vil·lous t.
te·not·o·my
curb t.
grad·u·at·ed t.
sub·cu·ta·ne·ous t.
ten·o·vag·i·ni·tis
tense
part of the tym·pan·ic
mem·brane
pulse
ten·sile
strength
stress
ten·si·om·e·ter
ten·sion
ar·te·ri·al t.
in·ter·fa·cial sur·face t.
oc·u·lar t.

ten·sion *(continued)*
  pre·men·stru·al t.
  sur·face t.
  tis·sue t.
ten·sion
  cav·i·ty
  curve
  head·ache
  pneu·mo·thor·ax
  su·ture
ten·sor
  mus·cle of fas·cia la·ta
  mus·cle of soft pal·ate
  mus·cle of tym·pan·ic
   mem·brane
ten·so·res
ten·sor tar·si
  mus·cle
tent
  ox·y·gen t.
  sponge t.
ten·ta·cle
tenth cra·ni·al
  nerve
ten·to·ria
ten·to·ri·al
  an·gle
  nerve
  si·nus
ten·to·ri·um
  t. of hy·poph·y·sis
teph·ro·ma·la·cia
teph·ry·lom·e·ter
tep·ro·tide
ter·as
ter·a·ta
ter·at·ic
ter·a·tism
ter·a·to·blas·to·ma
ter·a·to·car·ci·no·ma
te·rat·o·gen
ter·a·to·gen·e·sis
ter·a·to·ge·net·ic
ter·a·to·gen·ic
ter·a·to·ge·nic·i·ty
ter·a·tog·e·ny
ter·a·toid
  tu·mor
ter·a·to·log·ic
ter·a·tol·o·gy
ter·a·to·ma
  t. or·bi·tae
  tri·phyl·lo·ma·tous t.
ter·a·tom·a·tous
  cyst
ter·a·to·pho·bia
ter·a·to·sis
  atre·sic t.

ce·as·mic t.
ec·to·gen·ic t.
ec·top·ic t.
hy·per·gen·ic t.
sym·phys·ic t.
ter·a·to·sper·mia
te·ra·zo·sin hy·dro·chlo·ride
ter·bi·um
ter·bu·ta·line sul·fate
ter·e·bene
ter·e·bin·thi·nate
ter·e·bin·thine
ter·e·bin·thin·ism
ter·e·brant
ter·e·brat·ing
ter·e·bra·tion
te·res
te·res ma·jor
  mus·cle
te·res mi·nor
  mus·cle
ter·e·tes
ter·e·tis
ter·fen·a·dine
ter·gal
ter·gum
term
  in·fant
ter·mi·nad
ter·mi·nal
  ax·on t.'s
  syn·ap·tic t.'s
ter·mi·nal
  ar·tery
  bar
  bou·tons
  bron·chi·ole
  cis·ter·nae
  crest
  de·le·tion
  en·do·car·di·tis
  fi·lum
  gan·gli·on
  hair
  he·ma·tu·ria
  il·e·i·tis
  il·e·us
  in·fec·tion
  leu·ko·cy·to·sis
  line
  nerves
  notch of au·ri·cle
  nu·clei
  part
  plate
  pneu·mo·nia
  si·nus
  stri·a

sul·cus
thread
vein
ven·tri·cle
web
ter·mi·nal ad·di·tion
en·zyme
ter·mi·nal de·ox·y·nu·cle·o·ti·
dyl trans·fer·ase
ter·mi·nal hinge
po·si·tion
ter·mi·nal jaw re·la·tion
rec·ord
ter·mi·nal nerve
cor·pus·cles
ter·mi·na·tio
ter·mi·na·tion
co·don
se·quence
ter·mi·na·ti·o·nes
ter·mi·ni
ter·mi·no-ter·mi·nal
anas·to·mo·sis
ter·mi·nus
C-t.
ter·mone
ter·na·ry
com·plex
ter·ox·ide
ter·pene
p-**ter·phen·yl**
ter·pin
t. hy·drate
ter·pin·e·ol
ter·pi·nol
ter·race
ter·ra ja·pon·i·ca
Terrien's mar·gi·nal
de·gen·er·a·tion
Terrier's
valve
ter·ri·to·ri·al
ma·trix
ter·ri·to·ri·al·i·ty
Terry's
nails
syn·drome
Terson's
glands
ter·tian
fe·ver
ma·lar·ia
par·a·site
ter·tian
dou·ble t.
ter·ti·a·rism
ter·ti·a·ris·mus

ter·ti·ary
al·co·hol
am·pu·ta·tion
am·yl al·co·hol
bu·tyl al·co·hol
cal·ci·um phos·phate
cor·tex
den·tin
syph·i·lid
syph·i·lis
vil·lus
vit·re·ous
ter·ti·ary am·ide
ter·ti·ary amine
ter·ti·ary egg
mem·brane
ter·ti·ary med·i·cal
care
Teschen
dis·ease
Teschen dis·ease
vi·rus
Tesla
cur·rent
tesla
tes·sel·lat·ed
fun·dus
test
cross
meal
ob·ject
pro·file
skeins
so·lu·tion
tube
type
test
ABLB t.
abor·tus-Bang-ring t.
ac·e·tone t.
achieve·ment t.
acid·i·fied se·rum t.
ac·id per·fu·sion t.
ac·id phos·pha·tase t. for
se·men
ac·id re·flux t.
ACTH stim·u·la·tion t.
ac·tive ro·sette t.
ad·he·sion t.
Adler's t.
ad·re·nal ascor·bic ac·id
de·ple·tion t.
Adson's t.
Al·bar·ran's t.
al·ka·li de·na·tur·a·tion t.
Allen t.
Allen-Doisy t.
Allen's t.

test *(continued)*

Al·mén's t. for blood
al·ter·nate bin·au·ral loud·ness bal·ance t.
al·ter·nate cov·er t.
Ames t.
Amsler t.
Anderson-Collip t.
an·ox·e·mia t.
an·ti·bi·ot·ic sen·si·tiv·i·ty t.
an·ti·glob·u·lin t.
an·ti·hu·man glob·u·lin t.
ap·ti·tude t.
Aschheim-Zondek t.
ascor·bate-cy·a·nide t.
as·so·ci·a·tion t.
Ast·wood's t.
at·ro·pine t.
aug·ment·ed his·ta·mine t.
aus·sa·ge t.
au·to·he·mol·y·sis t.
A.-Z. t.
Bachman-Pettit t.
Bagolini t.
BALB t.
Bárány's ca·lor·ic t.
BEI t.
belt t.
Bender ge·stalt t.
Benedict's t. for glu·cose
ben·tir·o·mide t.
ben·ton·ite floc·cu·la·tion t.
ben·zi·dine t.
Bern·stein t.
Berson t.
Betke-Kleihauer t.
Bettendorff's t.
Bi·al's t.
bile ac·id tol·er·ance t.
bin·au·ral al·ter·nate loud·ness bal·ance t.
Binet t.
Binz' t.
bi·u·ret t.
blind t.
block de·sign t.
breath anal·y·sis t.
breath-hold·ing t.
brom·phe·nol t.
brom·sul·pha·lein t.
BSP t.
bu·ta·nol-ex·tract·a·ble io·dine t.
Cal·i·for·nia psy·cho·log·i·cal in·ven·to·ry t.
Calmette t.
ca·lor·ic t.

CAMP t.
cap·il·lary fra·gil·i·ty t.
cap·il·lary re·sis·tance t.
ca·pon-comb-growth t.
car·bo·hy·drate uti·li·za·tion t.
Casoni in·tra·der·mal t.
Casoni skin t.
cat·a·tor·u·lin t.
Chick-Martin t.
chi square t.
Clauberg t.
clo·mi·phene t.
coc·cid·i·oi·din t.
coin t.
cold bend t.
col·or·i·met·ric car·ies sus·cep·ti·bil·i·ty t.
comb-growth t.
com·ple·ment-fix·a·tion t.
Coombs' t.
Corner-Allen t.
cov·er t.
cov·er-un·cov·er t.
Crampton t.
t.'s of crim·i·nal re·spon·si·bil·i·ty
cu·ta·ne·ous t.
cu·ta·ne·ous tu·ber·cu·lin t.
cu·ti·re·ac·tion t.
cy·an·ide-ni·tro·prus·side t.
cy·to·tro·pic an·ti·body t.
DA preg·nan·cy t.
Day's t.
Dehio's t.
de·hy·dro·cho·late t.
dex·a·meth·a·sone sup·pres·sion t.
Dick t.
dif·fer·en·tial re·nal func·tion t.
dif·fer·en·tial ure·ter·al cath·e·ter·i·za·tion t.
di·ni·tro·phen·yl·hy·dra·zine t.
di·rect Coombs' t.
di·rect flu·o·res·cent an·ti·body t.
dis·con·tin·u·a·tion t.
Doerfler-Stewart t.
dou·ble (gel) dif·fu·sion pre·cip·i·tin t. in one di·men·sion
dou·ble (gel) dif·fu·sion pre·cip·i·tin t. in two di·men·sions
Dragendorff's t.
draw·er t.

D-S t.
Ducrey t.
Dugas' t.
dye ex·clu·sion t.
Ebbinghaus t.
Ellsworth-Howard t.
Emmens' S/L t.
E-ro·sette t.
eryth·ro·cyte ad·her·ence t.
eryth·ro·cyte fra·gil·i·ty t.
ether t.
ex·er·cise t.
FANA t.
Farnsworth-Munsell col·or t.
fern t.
fer·ric chlo·ride t.
Fevold t.
Finckh t.
fin·ger-nose t.
fin·ger-to-fin·ger t.
fish t.
Fishberg con·cen·tra·tion t.
fis·tu·la t.
FIT t.
Fleitmann's t.
floc·cu·la·tion t.
flu·o·res·ce·in in·stil·la·tion t.
flu·o·res·ce·in string t.
flu·o·res·cent an·ti·nu·cle·ar an·ti·body t.
flu·o·res·cent trep·o·ne·mal an·ti·body-ab·sorp·tion t.
foam sta·bil·i·ty t.
Folin-Looney t.
Folin's t.
Fosdick-Hansen-Epple t.
Foshay t.
fra·gil·i·ty t.
Frei t.
Fridenberg's stig·o·met·ric card t.
FTA-ABS t.
fu·sion-in·ferred thresh·old t.
Gad·dum and Schild t.
ga·lac·tose tol·er·ance t.
gel dif·fu·sion pre·cip·i·tin t.'s
gel dif·fu·sion pre·cip·i·tin t.'s in one di·men·sion
gel dif·fu·sion pre·cip·i·tin t.'s in two di·men·sions
Gellé t.
Geraghty's t.
Gerhardt's t. for ac·e·to·a·ce·tic ac·id

Gerhardt's t. for uro·bi·lin in the urine
germ tube t.
glu·cose ox·i·dase pa·per strip t.
glu·cose tol·er·ance t.
Gmelin's t.
Gofman t.
Goldscheider's t.
gold sol t.
Göthlin's t.
group t.
guai·ac t.
Günzberg's t.
Guthrie t.
Gutzeit's t.
Habel t.
Hallion's t.
Ham's t.
Hardy-Rand-Ritter t.
Harrington-Flocks t.
Harris t.
Harris and Ray t.
head-drop·ping t.
heat co·ag·u·la·tion t.
heat in·sta·bil·i·ty t.
heel-tap t.
Heinz body t.
he·mad·sorp·tion vi·rus t.
he·moc·cult t.
Hering's t.
Hess' t.
Hinton t.
His·ta·log t.
his·ta·mine t.
his·to·plas·min-la·tex t.
Hollander t.
Holmgren's t.
ho·mo·va·nil·lic ac·id t.
Hooker-Forbes t.
Howard t.
Huhner t.
HVA t.
hy·per·e·mia t.
hy·per·ven·ti·la·tion t.
hy·pox·e·mia t.
im·mune ad·he·sion t.
im·mu·no·log·ic preg·nan·cy t.
in·di·rect t.
in·di·rect Coombs' t.
in·di·rect flu·o·res·cent an·ti·body t.
in·di·rect he·mag·glu·ti·na·tion t.
in·su·lin hy·po·gly·ce·mia t.
in·tel·li·gence t.
Ishihara t.

test *(continued)*

iso·pro·pa·nol pre·cip·i·ta·tion t.
Ito-Reenstierna t.
Jacquemin's t.
Jaffe's t.
Janet's t.
Jolles' t.
Katayama's t.
ke·to·gen·ic cor·ti·coids t.
Knoop hard·ness t.
Kober t.
Kolmer t.
Korotkoff's t.
Kurzrok-Ratner t.
Kveim t.
Kveim-Stilzbach t.
Landsteiner-Donath t.
Lange's t.
la·tex ag·glu·ti·na·tion t.
la·tex fix·a·tion t.
LE cell t.
Legal's t.
lep·ro·min t.
leu·ko·cyte ad·her·ence as·say t.
leu·ko·cyte bac·te·ri·cid·al as·say t.
Liebermann-Burchard t.
li·mu·lus ly·sate t.
line t.
Lombard voice-re·flex t.
Lücke's t.
lu·pus band t.
lu·pus er·y·the·ma·to·sus cell t.
Machado-Guerreiro t.
mac·ro·phage mi·gra·tion in·hi·bi·tion t.
Man·toux t.
Mas·ter's t.
Mas·ter's two-step ex·er·cise t.
Mauthner's t.
max·i·mal His·ta·log t.
Mazzotti t.
McMurray t.
McPhail t.
Meinicke t.
Meltzer-Lyon t.
met·a·bi·sul·fite t.
me·tro·tro·phic t.
MHA-TP t.
mi·cro·he·mag·glu·ti·na·tion-Trep·o·ne·ma pal·li·dum t.
mi·cro·pre·cip·i·ta·tion t.
mi·gra·tion in·hi·bi·tion t.

milk-ring t.
Millon-Nasse t.
Min·ne·so·ta mul·ti·pha·sic per·son·al·i·ty in·ven·to·ry t.
mixed ag·glu·ti·na·tion t.
mixed lym·pho·cyte cul·ture t.
MLC t.
Molisch's t.
Moloney t.
Morner's t.
Moszkowicz' t.
Motulsky dye re·duc·tion t.
mu·cin clot t.
mul·ti·ple punc·ture tu·ber·cu·lin t.
mumps sen·si·tiv·i·ty t.
Nagel's t.
neu·tral·i·za·tion t.
ni·a·cin t.
Nickerson-Kveim t.
Nicklès' t.
ni·tro·blue tet·ra·zo·li·um t.
ni·tro·prus·side t.
nys·tag·mus t.
Obermayer's t.
oral lac·tose tol·er·ance t.
or·cin·ol t.
Ouchterlony t.
ovar·i·an ascor·bic ac·id de·ple·tion t.
Pachon's t.
Palmer ac·id t. for pep·tic ul·cer
pal·min t.
pal·mi·tin t.
pan·cre·o·zy·min-se·cre·tin t.
Pandy's t.
Pap t.
Papanicolaou smear t.
par·al·lax t.
patch t.
Patrick's t.
Paul's t.
PBI t.
pen·ta·gas·trin t.
per·form·ance t.
Perls' t.
per·son·al·i·ty t.
Perthes' t.
phe·nol·sul·fon·phthal·e·in t.
phen·tol·a·mine t.
pho·to-patch t.
pho·to·stress t.
phren·ic pres·sure t.

phthal·ein t.
Pirquet's t.
piv·ot shift t.
plas·ma·crit t.
plate·let ag·gre·ga·tion t.
pol·y·u·ria t.
Porges-Meier t.
Porter-Silber chro·mo·gens t.
P and P t.
pre·cip·i·ta·tion t.
pre·cip·i·tin t.
prism ver·gence t.
pro·jec·tive t.
pro·tec·tion t.
pro·tein-bound io·dine t.
pro·throm·bin t.
pro·throm·bin and pro·con·ver·tin t.
pro·voc·a·tive t.
pro·voc·a·tive Wassermann t.
psy·cho·log·i·cal t.'s
psy·cho·mo·tor t.'s
pulp t.
Queckenstedt-Stookey t.
quel·lung t.
Quick's t.
qui·nine car·ba·cryl·ic res·in t.
Quinlan's t.
ra·di·o·ac·tive io·dide up·take t.
ra·di·o·al·ler·go·sor·bent t.
RAI t.
rap·id plas·ma re·a·gin t.
Rapoport t.
Rayleigh t.
red t.
red cell ad·her·ence t.
Reinsch's t.
Reiter t.
res·or·cin·ol t.
Reuss' t.
Rh block·ing t.
Rickles t.
Rimini's t.
ring t.
ring pre·cip·i·tin t.
Rinne's t.
Romberg t.
Römer's t.
Ropes t.
Rorschach t.
Rosenbach-Gmelin t.
Rosenbach's t.
Rose-Waal·er t.
Ross-Jones t.
Roth·era's ni·tro·prus·side t.

Rowntree and Geraghty t.
RPR t.
ru·bel·la HI t.
Rubin t.
Rubner's t.
Rumpel-Leede t.
Sabin-Feldman dye t.
Sachs-Georgi t.
Saundby's t.
scar·i·fi·ca·tion t.
Schaffer's t.
Schellong t.
Schick t.
Schiller's t.
Schilling t.
Schirmer t.
Schönbein's t.
Schwabach t.
Schwarz's t.
scratch t.
screen·ing t.
Seashore t.
se·cre·tin t.
Selivanoff's t.
shad·ow t.
shake t.
sick·le cell t.
sin·gle (gel) dif·fu·sion pre·cip·i·tin t. in one di·men·sion
sin·gle (gel) dif·fu·sion pre·cip·i·tin t. in two di·men·sions
SISI t.
sit·u·a·tion·al t.
skin t.
skin-punc·ture t.
small in·cre·ment sen·si·tiv·i·ty in·dex t.
Snyder's t.
sol·u·bil·i·ty t.
spi·ro·no·lac·tone t.
split re·nal func·tion t.
spot t. for in·fec·tious mon·o·nu·cle·o·sis
Stamey t.
stan·dard se·ro·log·ic t.'s for syph·i·lis
stand·ing t.
stand·ing plas·ma t.
starch-i·o·dine t.
sta·tion t.
Stein's t.
Stenger t.
Stewart's t.
Strassburg's t.
string t.

test *(continued)*

Strong vo·ca·tion·al in·ter·
est t.
STS for syph·i·lis
Stu·dent's *t* t.
su·crose he·mol·y·sis t.
sul·fo·sal·i·cyl·ic ac·id tur·
bid·i·ty t.
sweat t.
sweat·ing t.
swim·ming t.
sword·fish t.
t t.
the·mat·ic ap·per·cep·tion t.
ther·mo·sta·ble op·so·nin t.
Thompson's t.
Thormählen's t.
Thorn t.
three-glass t.
thy·roid-stim·u·lat·ing hor·
mone stim·u·la·tion t.
thy·roid sup·pres·sion t.
thy·rot·ro·pin-re·leas·ing
hor·mone stim·u·la·tion t.
tine t.
ti·trat·a·ble acid·i·ty t.
tol·bu·ta·mide t.
tone de·cay t.
Töpfer's t.
to·tal cat·e·chol·a·mine t.
tour·ni·quet t.
TPH t.
TPHA t.
TPI t.
Trendelenburg's t.
Trep·o·ne·ma pal·li·dum
he·mag·glu·ti·na·tion t.
Trep·o·ne·ma pal·li·dum
im·mo·bi·li·za·tion t.
TRH stim·u·la·tion t.
tri·i·o·do·thy·ro·nine up·
take t.
TSH stim·u·lat·ing t.
tu·ber·cu·lin t.
Tuffier's t.
two-glass t.
two-step ex·er·cise t.
Tzanck t.
urea clear·ance t.
ure·ase t.
uri·nary con·cen·tra·tion t.
vag·i·nal cor·ni·fi·ca·tion t.
vag·i·nal mu·ci·fi·ca·tion t.
Val·en·tine's t.
Valsalva t.
van Deen's t.
van den Bergh's t.
van der Vel·den's t.

va·nil·lyl·man·del·ic ac·id t.
VDRL t.
vi·tal·i·ty t.
vi·ta·min C t.
VMA t.
Volhard's t.
Vollmer t.
Wada t.
Waldenström's t.
Wang's t.
wash·out t.
Wassén t.
Wassermann t.
Watson-Schwartz t.
Weber's t. for hear·ing
Webster's t.
Weil-Felix t.
Werner's t.
Wheeler-Johnson t.
Wormley's t.
Wurster's t.
Xi·phoph·o·rus t.
xy·lose t.
Yvon's t.
Zimmermann t.
Zondek-Aschheim t.
Zsigmondy's t.

tes·ta
Tes·ta·ce·a·lo·bo·sia
tes·tal·gia
tes·tane
tes·tec·to·my
tes·tes
test han·dle
in·stru·ment
tes·ti·cle
tes·tic·u·lar
ar·tery
cord
duct
dys·gen·e·sis
fem·i·ni·za·tion
plex·us
veins
tes·tic·u·lar fem·i·ni·za·tion
syn·drome
tes·tic·u·lar tu·bu·lar
ad·e·no·ma
tes·tic·u·lus
tes·tis
cryp·tor·chid t.
ec·top·ic t.
in·vert·ed t.
ir·ri·ta·ble t.
mov·a·ble t.
ob·struct·ed t.
t. re·dux
re·tained t.

re·trac·tile t.
un·de·scend·ed t.

tes·tis
cords

tes·ti·tis

test let·ter

tes·toid
hy·per·the·co·sis

tes·to·lac·tone

tes·top·a·thy

tes·tos·ter·one
t. cyp·i·o·nate
t. enan·thate
t. phen·yl·pro·pi·o·nate
t. pro·pi·o·nate

test-re·test
re·li·a·bil·i·ty

test sym·bols

test-tube
ba·by

test types
Jaeger's t. t.
point sys·tem t. t.
Snellen's t. t.

te·ta·nia
t. ep·i·dem·i·ca
t. gas·tri·ca
t. grav·i·dar·um
t. ne·o·na·to·ri·um
t. par·a·thy·re·o·pri·va
t. rheu·ma·ti·ca

te·tan·ic
con·trac·tion
con·vul·sion

te·tan·i·form

tet·a·nig·e·nous

tet·a·nil·la

tet·a·nism

tet·a·ni·za·tion

tet·a·nize

tet·a·node

tet·a·noid
cho·rea
par·a·ple·gia

tet·a·no·ly·sin

tet·a·nom·e·ter

tet·a·no·mo·tor

tet·a·no·spas·min

tet·a·no·toxin

tet·a·nus
acous·tic t.
anod·al clo·sure t.
anod·al du·ra·tion t.
anod·al open·ing t.
t. an·ti·cus
apy·ret·ic t.
be·nign t.
cath·o·dal clo·sure t.

cath·o·dal du·ra·tion t.
cath·o·dal open·ing t.
ce·phal·ic t.
ce·re·bral t.
com·plete t.
t. com·ple·tus
t. dor·sa·lis
drug t.
ex·ten·sor t.
flex·or t.
gen·er·al·ized t.
head t.
hy·dro·pho·bic t.
im·i·ta·tive t.
in·com·plete t.
in·ter·mit·tent t.
lo·cal t.
t. ne·o·na·to·rum
t. pos·ti·cus
post·par·tum t.
pu·er·per·al t.
Ritter's open·ing t.
Rose's ce·phal·ic t.
tox·ic t.
trau·mat·ic t.
uter·ine t.

tet·a·nus
an·ti·tox·in
im·mu·no·glob·u·lin
tox·in
vac·cine

tet·a·nus an·ti·tox·in
unit

tet·a·nus and gas gan·grene
an·ti·tox·ins

tet·a·nus im·mune
glob·u·lin

tet·a·nus-per·frin·gens
an·ti·tox·in

tet·a·ny
cat·a·ract

tet·a·ny
t. of al·ka·lo·sis
du·ra·tion t.
ep·i·dem·ic t.
gas·tric t.
grass t.
hy·per·ven·ti·la·tion t.
hy·po·par·a·thy·roid t.
in·fan·tile t.
la·tent t.
man·i·fest t.
ne·o·na·tal t.
par·a·thy·roid t.
par·a·thy·ro·pri·val t.
phos·phate t.
post·op·er·a·tive t.

tet·a·ny *(continued)*
  rheu·mat·ic t.
  trans·port t.
te·tar·ta·no·pia
te·tar·ta·nop·sia
Tete
  vi·rus·es
teth·ered cord
  syn·drome
tet·ra-a·me·lia
tet·ra·ba·sic
tet·ra·ben·a·zine
tet·ra·bo·ric ac·id
tet·ra·bra·chi·us
tet·ra·bro·mo·phe·nol·phthal·ein
  so·di·um
tet·ra·caine hy·dro·chlo·ride
tet·ra·chi·rus
tet·ra·chlor·eth·y·lene
tet·ra·chlo·ride
tet·ra·chlor·me·thi·a·zide
tet·ra·chlo·ro·eth·ane
tet·ra·chlo·ro·eth·yl·ene
tet·ra·chlo·ro·meth·ane
tet·ra·coc·ci
tet·ra·coc·cus
tet·ra·co·sac·tide
tet·ra·co·sac·tin
tet·ra·co·sa·no·ic ac·id
tet·ra·crot·ic
tet·ra·cus·pid
tet·ra·cy·clic
  an·ti·de·pres·sant
tet·ra·cy·clic ste·roid
  nu·cle·us
tet·ra·cy·cline
tet·rad
  Fallot's t.
  nar·co·lep·tic t.
tet·ra·dac·tyl
tet·ra·dec·a·no·ic ac·id
te·trad·ic
tet·ra·eth·yl
  poi·son·ing
tet·ra·eth·yl·am·mo·ni·um
  chlo·ride
tet·ra·eth·yl·lead
tet·ra·eth·yl·mon·o·thi·o·no·py·
  ro·phos·phate
tet·ra·eth·yl py·ro·phos·phate
tet·ra·eth·yl·thi·u·ram di·sul·
  fide
tet·ra·gly·cine hy·dro·per·i·o·
  dide
tet·ra·gon
  t. lum·ba·le
tet·ra·go·num
tet·ra·go·nus

tet·ra·hy·dric
tet·ra·hy·dro·can·nab·i·nol
tet·ra·hy·dro·fo·late de·hy·dro·
  gen·ase
tet·ra·hy·droz·o·line hy·dro·
  chlo·ride
Tet·ra·hy·me·na pyr·i·for·mis
tet·ra·i·o·do·phe·nol·phthal·ein
  so·di·um
te·tral·o·gy
  Eisenmenger's t.
  Fallot's t.
tet·ra·mas·tia
tet·ra·mas·ti·gote
tet·ra·mas·tous
te·tram·e·lus
Tet·ra·meres
tet·ra·mer·ic
te·tram·er·ous
tet·ra·meth·yl
  ac·ri·dine
tet·ra·meth·yl·am·mo·ni·um
  io·dide
tet·ra·meth·yl·di·ar·sine
tet·ra·meth·yl·pu·tres·cine
tet·ra·ni·trol
tet·ra·nu·cle·o·tide
tet·ra·pa·re·sis
tet·ra·pep·tide
tet·ra·pe·ro·me·lia
tet·ra·pho·co·me·lia
tet·ra·ple·gia
tet·ra·ple·gic
tet·ra·ploid
tet·ra·pus
tet·ra·pyr·role
tet·ra·sac·cha·ride
te·tras·ce·lus
tet·ra·so·mic
tet·ras·ter
tet·ra·sti·chi·a·sis
tet·ra·ter·penes
tet·ra·tom·ic
Tet·ra·trich·o·mo·nas
  T. ovis
tet·ra·va·lent
tet·ra·zole
tet·ra·zo·li·um
  ni·tro·blue t.
tet·ra·zo·ni·um
  salts
tet·ro·do·tox·in
tet·rose
te·tro·tus
te·trox·ide
tet·ter
  bran·ny t.
  crust·ed t.

dry t.
hon·ey·comb t.
hu·mid t.
milk t.
moist t.
scaly t.
wet t.
Teutleben's
lig·a·ment
Tex·as
fe·ver
snake·root
text
blind·ness
tex·ti·form
tex·tur·al
tex·ture
tex·tus
TGE
vi·rus
Thal
pro·ce·dure
thal·a·mec·to·my
thal·a·men·ce·phal·ic
thal·a·men·ceph·a·lon
thal·a·mi
tha·lam·ic
syn·drome
te·nia
tha·lam·ic gus·ta·to·ry
nu·cle·us
thal·a·mo·cor·ti·cal
thal·a·mo·stri·ate
veins
thal·a·mot·o·my
thal·a·mus
thal·as·sa·ne·mia
thal·as·se·mia
F t.
Le·pore t.
t. ma·jor
t. mi·nor
tha·las·so·pho·bia
tha·las·so·po·sia
tha·las·so·ther·a·py
tha·lid·o·mide
thal·lic
thal·li·um
poi·son·ing
Thal·lo·phy·ta
thal·lo·phyte
thal·lo·spore
thal·lo·tox·i·co·sis
thal·lus
tha·mu·ria
than·a·to·bi·o·log·ic
than·a·to·gno·mon·ic
than·a·tog·ra·phy

than·a·toid
than·a·tol·o·gy
than·a·to·ma·nia
than·a·to·phid·ia
than·a·to·pho·bia
than·a·to·phor·ic
dwarf·ism
than·a·top·sy
than·a·tos
Thane's
meth·od
thau·mat·ro·py
Thayer-Martin
me·di·um
thea
the·a·ism
the·a·ter
the·ba·ic
the·ba·ine
the·be·si·an
fo·ram·i·na
valve
veins
the·ca
cells of stom·ach
the·ca
t. cor·dis
t. ex·ter·na
t. fol·lic·u·li
t. in·ter·na
t. ten·di·nis
t. ver·te·bra·lis
the·ca cell
tu·mor
the·cae
the·ca in·ter·na
cone
the·cal
ab·scess
whit·low
the·ca lu·te·in
cell
the·ci·tis
thec·o·dont
the·co·ma
the·co·ma·to·sis
the·co·steg·no·sia
the·co·steg·no·sis
Theden's
meth·od
Thei·ler·ia
T. an·nu·la·ta
T. bo·vis
T. fe·lis
T. hir·ci
T. law·ren·cei
T. mu·tans
T. or·i·en·ta·lis

Thei·ler·ia *(continued)*
  T. par·va
  T. par·va bo·vis
  T. par·va law·ren·cei
  T. par·va par·va
  T. ser·genti
  T. tau·ro·tra·gi
thei·le·ri·a·sis
Thei·le·ri·i·dae
thei·le·ri·o·sis
  be·nign bo·vine t.
  ma·lig·nant ovine and cap·
    rine t.
  Med·i·ter·ra·ne·an t.
  Rho·de·sian ma·lig·nant t.
  trop·i·cal t.
Theiler's
  dis·ease
  vi·rus
Theiler's orig·i·nal
  vi·rus
Theile's
  ca·nal
  glands
  mus·cle
the·in
the·in·ism
the·ism
the·lar·che
The·la·zia
  T. cal·i·for·ni·en·sis
  T. cal·li·pae·da
thel·a·zi·a·sis
the·le
the·le·plas·ty
the·lia
the·li·um
the·lon·cus
the·lor·rha·gia
the·mat·ic
  par·a·lo·gia
  par·a·pha·sia
the·mat·ic ap·per·cep·tion
  test
the·nad
the·nal
the·nal·dine
the·nar
  em·i·nence
  prom·i·nence
  space
the·nen
then·yl
then·yl·di·a·mine hy·dro·
  chlo·ride
Theobald Smith's
  phe·nom·e·non

the·o·bro·ma
  t. oil
the·o·bro·mine
the·o·ma·nia
the·o·pho·bia
the·o·phyl·line
  t. ami·no·i·so·bu·ta·nol
  t. cal·ci·um sa·lic·y·late
  t. eth·a·nol·a·mine
  t. eth·yl·ene·di·a·mine
  t. iso·pro·pa·nol·a·mine
  t. so·di·um ac·e·tate
  t. so·di·um gly·cin·ate
the·o·rem
  Bayes t.
  Bernoulli's t.
  Gibbs' t.
the·o·ry
  ad·sorp·tion t. of nar·co·sis
  Altmann's t.
  Arrhenius-Madsen t.
  atom·ic t.
  Baeyer's t.
  bal·ance t.
  bal·ance t. of sex
  be·ta-ox·i·da·tion-con·den·
    sa·tion t.
  Bohr's t.
  Bordeau t.
  Bordeu t.
  Bowman's t.
  Brønsted t.
  Burn and Rand t.
  Cannon-Bard t.
  Cannon's t.
  ce·lom·ic met·a·pla·sia t. of
    en·do·me·tri·o·sis
  clo·a·cal t.
  clo·nal se·lec·tion t.
  cog·ni·tive dis·so·nance t.
  Cohnheim's t.
  col·loid t. of nar·co·sis
    de Bordeau t.
  de·cay t.
  De Vries' t.
  Dieulafoy's t.
  di·pole t.
  du·plic·i·ty t. of vi·sion
  Ehrlich's t.
  Ehrlich's side-chain t.
  t. of elec·tro·lyt·ic dis·so·
    ci·a·tion
  emer·gen·cy t.
  em·i·gra·tion t.
  en·zyme in·hi·bi·tion t. of
    nar·co·sis
  Flourens' t.
  Frerich's t.

Freud's t.
gam·e·toid t.
gas·trea t.
gate-con·trol t.
germ t.
germ lay·er t.
ge·stalt t.
Haeckel's gas·trea t.
Helmholtz t. of ac·com·mo·da·tion
Helmholtz t. of col·or vi·sion
Helmholtz-Gibbs t.
Helmholtz t. of hear·ing
he·ma·tog·e·nous t. of en·do·me·tri·o·sis
Hering's t. of col·or vi·sion
hy·drate mi·cro·crys·tal t. of an·es·the·sia
im·plan·ta·tion t. of the pro·duc·tion of en·do·me·tri·o·sis
in·case·ment t.
in·for·ma·tion t.
James-Lange t.
kern-plas·ma re·la·tion t.
Knoop's t.
Ladd-Franklin t.
learn·ing t.
li·bi·do t.
Liebig's t.
lip·oid t. of nar·co·sis
lym·phat·ic dis·sem·i·na·tion t. of en·do·me·tri·o·sis
mass ac·tion t.
t. of med·i·cine
mem·brane ex·pan·sion t.
Metchnikoff's t.
Meyer-Overton t. of nar·co·sis
mi·gra·tion t.
Miller's chem·i·co·par·a·sit·ic t.
mne·mic t.
mo·lec·u·lar dis·so·ci·a·tion t.
mon·o·phy·let·ic t.
my·o·e·las·tic t.
my·o·gen·ic t.
Nernst's t.
neu·ro·chro·nax·ic t.
neu·ro·gen·ic t.
Ollier's t.
ome·ga-ox·i·da·tion t.
over·pro·duc·tion t.
ox·y·gen dep·ri·va·tion t. of nar·co·sis

Pauling's t.
per·me·a·bil·i·ty t. of nar·co·sis
place t.
Planck's t.
pol·y·phy·let·ic t.
quan·tum t.
re·ca·pi·tu·la·tion t.
reed in·stru·ment t.
re·en·try t.
res·o·nance t. of hear·ing
Ribbert's t.
Semon-Hering t.
sen·so·ri·mo·tor t.
side-chain t.
so·mat·ic mu·ta·tion t. of can·cer
Spitzer's t.
stringed in·stru·ment t.
sur·face ten·sion t. of nar·co·sis
tel·e·phone t.
ther·mo·dy·nam·ic t. of nar·co·sis
two-sym·pa·thin t.
van't Hoff's t.
Warburg's t.
Weismann's t.
Wollaston's t.
Young-Helmholtz t. of col·or vi·sion
the·o·ther·a·py
thèque
ther·a·peu·sis
ther·a·peu·tic
  abor·tion
  an·es·the·sia
  an·gi·og·ra·phy
  com·mu·ni·ty
  cri·sis
  elec·trode
  fe·ver
  group
  in·com·pat·i·bil·i·ty
  in·dex
  ir·i·dec·to·my
  ma·lar·ia
  ni·hil·ism
  op·ti·mism
  pes·si·mism
  pneu·mo·thor·ax
  ra·ti·o
ther·a·peu·tics
  ray t.
  sug·ges·tive t.
ther·a·peu·tist
the·ra·pia
  t. mag·na ste·ri·li·sans

the·ra·pia *(continued)*
   t. ste·ri·li·sans co·ver·gens
   t. ste·ri·li·sans di·ver·gens
   t. ste·ri·li·sans frac·tio·na·ta
ther·a·pist
ther·a·py
   al·ka·li t.
   an·a·lyt·ic t.
   an·ti·co·ag·u·lant t.
   au·to·se·rum t.
   aver·sion t.
   be·hav·ior t.
   cli·ent-cen·tered t.
   cog·ni·tive t.
   col·lapse t.
   con·joint t.
   cy·to·re·duc·tive t.
   de·pot t.
   di·a·ther·mic t.
   elec·tro·con·vul·sive t.
   elec·tro·shock t.
   elec·tro·ther·a·peu·tic sleep
    t.
   ex·tend·ed fam·i·ly t.
   fam·i·ly t.
   fe·ver t.
   for·eign pro·tein t.
   func·tion·al or·tho·don·tic
    t.
   ger·i·at·ric t.
   ge·stalt t.
   het·er·o·vac·cine t.
   hy·per·bar·ic ox·y·gen t.
   im·plo·sive t.
   in·di·vid·u·al t.
   in·ha·la·tion t.
   in·su·lin co·ma t.
   in·tra·le·sion·al t.
   main·te·nance drug t.
   mar·riage t.
   mi·cro·wave t.
   mil·ieu t.
   my·o·func·tion·al t.
   non·spe·cif·ic t.
   oc·cu·pa·tion·al t.
   or·tho·don·tic t.
   or·tho·mo·lec·u·lar t.
   ox·y·gen t.
   par·en·ter·al t.
   pho·to·ra·di·a·tion t.
   phys·i·cal t.
   plas·ma t.
   play t.
   pro·lif·er·a·tion t.
   pro·tein shock t.
   psy·che·del·ic t.
   psy·cho·an·a·lyt·ic t.
   pulse t.

   qua·dran·gu·lar t.
   ra·di·a·tion t.
   ra·di·um beam t.
   ra·tion·al t.
   re·flex t.
   re·place·ment t.
   root ca·nal t.
   scle·ros·ing t.
   se·rum t.
   shock t.
   so·cial t.
   so·cial net·work t.
   sub·sti·tu·tion t.
   sub·sti·tu·tive t.
   tel·e·ra·di·um t.
   thy·roid t.
   to·tal push t.
   ul·tra·son·ic t.
   x-ray t.
ther·en·ceph·a·lous
the·ri·a·ca
the·ri·at·rics
the·ri·o·gen·o·log·ic
the·ri·o·gen·o·log·i·cal
the·ri·o·gen·ol·o·gy
the·ri·o·mor·phism
therm
ther·ma·co·gen·e·sis
ther·mal
   an·es·the·sia
   burn
   ca·pac·i·ty
   sense
   spec·trum
ther·mal·ge·sia
ther·mal·gia
therm·an·al·ge·sia
therm·an·es·the·sia
ther·ma·tol·o·gy
ther·me·lom·e·ter
therm·es·the·sia
therm·es·the·si·om·e·ter
ther·mic
   an·es·the·sia
   fe·ver
   sense
therm·is·tor
thermo-
   stro·muhr
ther·mo·al·ge·sia
ther·mo·an·al·ge·sia
ther·mo·an·es·the·sia
ther·mo·cau·ter·ec·to·my
ther·mo·cau·tery
ther·mo·chem·is·try
ther·mo·chro·ic
ther·moch·ro·ism
ther·mo·chrose

ther·mo·chro·sis
ther·moch·ro·sy
ther·mo·co·ag·u·la·tion
ther·mo·cou·ple
ther·mo·cur·rent
ther·mo·dif·fu·sion
ther·mo·di·lu·tion
ther·mo·du·ric
ther·mo·dy·nam·ic
  po·ten·tial
  the·o·ry of nar·co·sis
ther·mo·dy·nam·ics
ther·mo·e·lec·tric
  pile
ther·mo·e·lec·tric·i·ty
ther·mo·es·the·sia
ther·mo·es·the·si·om·e·ter
ther·mo·ex·ci·to·ry
ther·mo·gen·e·sis
ther·mo·ge·net·ic
ther·mo·gen·ic
  ac·tion
ther·mo·gen·ics
ther·mog·e·nous
ther·mo·gram
ther·mo·graph
ther·mog·ra·phy
  in·fra·red t.
  liq·uid crys·tal t.
ther·mo·hy·per·al·ge·sia
ther·mo·hy·per·es·the·sia
ther·mo·hyp·es·the·sia
ther·mo·hy·po·es·the·sia
ther·mo·in·hib·i·to·ry
ther·mo·in·te·gra·tor
ther·mo·junc·tion
ther·mo·ker·a·to·plas·ty
ther·mo·la·bile
  op·so·nin
ther·mo·lamp
ther·mol·o·gy
ther·mo·lu·mi·nes·cence
  do·sim·e·try
ther·mol·y·sis
ther·mo·lyt·ic
ther·mo·mas·sage
ther·mom·e·ter
  air t.
  clin·i·cal t.
  dif·fer·en·tial t.
  gas t.
  re·sis·tance t.
  self-reg·is·ter·ing t.
  spir·it t.
  sur·face t.
  wet and dry bulb t.
ther·mo·met·ric
ther·mom·e·try

ther·mo·neu·ro·sis
ther·mo·nu·cle·ar
ther·mo·pen·e·tra·tion
ther·mo·phil
ther·mo·phile
ther·mo·phil·ic
ther·mo·pho·bia
ther·mo·phore
ther·mo·phy·lic
ther·mo·pile
ther·mo·plac·en·tog·ra·phy
Ther·mo·plas·ma
  T. ac·i·do·phi·lum
ther·mo·plas·ma
ther·mo·plas·ma·ta
ther·mo·plas·tic
ther·mo·ple·gia
ther·mo·pre·cip·i·tin
  re·ac·tion
ther·mo·re·cep·tor
ther·mo·reg·u·la·tion
ther·mo·reg·u·la·tor
ther·mo·scope
ther·mo·set
ther·mo·sta·bile
ther·mo·sta·ble
  op·so·nin
ther·mo·sta·ble op·so·nin
  test
ther·mo·stat
ther·mo·ste·re·sis
ther·mo·stro·muhr
ther·mo·sys·tal·tic
ther·mo·sys·tal·tism
ther·mo·tac·tic
ther·mo·tax·ic
ther·mo·tax·is
  neg·a·tive t.
  pos·i·tive t.
ther·mo·ther·a·py
ther·mot·ic
ther·mot·ics
ther·mo·to·nom·e·ter
ther·mot·ro·pism
the·roid
the·rol·o·gy
the·sau·ris·mo·sis
the·sau·ris·mot·ic
the·sau·ro·sis
the·ta
  rhythm
  wave
the·tins
thi·a·ben·da·zole
thi·a·bu·ta·zide
thi·a·cet·a·zone
thi·al·bar·bi·tal
thi·am·bu·to·sine

thi·a·min
    t. hy·dro·chlo·ride
    t. mon·o·ni·trate
    t. pyr·i·din·y·lase
    t. py·ro·phos·phate
thi·am·i·nase
    t. I
    t. II
thi·a·min chlo·ride
    unit
thi·a·mine
thi·a·min hy·dro·chlo·ride
    unit
thi·am·phen·i·col
thi·am·y·lal so·di·um
thi·a·phor·as·es
Thi·a·ra
thi·a·zide
    di·a·be·tes
thi·a·zides
thi·a·zin
    dyes
thi·a·zol·sul·fone
thick·ness
    Bres·low's t.
thi·e·mia
thi·e·nyl
thi·e·nyl·al·a·nine
Thiersch
    graft
Thiersch's
    can·a·lic·u·li
    meth·od
thi·eth·yl·per·a·zine ma·le·ate
thigh
    driv·er's t.
    Heilbronner's t.
thigh
    bone
    joint
thig·mes·the·sia
thig·mo·tax·is
thig·mot·ro·pism
thi·mer·o·sal
thin
    sec·tion
think·ing
    ab·stract t.
    ar·cha·ic-par·a·log·i·cal t.
    con·crete t.
    cre·a·tive t.
    mag·i·cal t.
    pre·log·i·cal t.
think·ing through
thin-lay·er
    chro·ma·tog·ra·phy
    elec·tro·pho·re·sis
    im·mu·no·as·say

thin·ning
    shear t.
thi·o·ac·id
thi·o·al·co·hol
thi·o·am·ide
thi·o·ate
thi·o·bar·bi·tu·rates
thi·o·car·bam·ide
thi·o·car·lide
thi·o·chrome
    meth·od
thi·o·clas·tic
    cleav·age
thi·oc·tic ac·id
thi·o·cy·a·nate
thi·o·cy·an·ic ac·id
thi·o·cy·an·o·gen
    num·ber
    val·ue
thi·o·di·phen·yl·a·mine
thi·o·eth·a·nol·a·mine ace·tyl·
    trans·fer·ase
thi·o·e·ther
thi·o·fla·vine S
thi·o·fla·vine T
    stain
thi·o·fla·vin T
thi·o·fu·ran
thi·o·glu·co·si·dase
thi·o·glyc·er·ol
thi·o·gly·co·late
thi·o·gly·col·ic ac·id
thi·o·gly·col·late
thi·o·gua·nine
thi·o·ki·nase
thi·ol
thi·o·lase
thi·ole
thi·ol·his·ti·dyl·be·ta·ine
thi·ol·trans·a·cet·y·lase A
thi·ol·y·sis
thi·o·mer·sal
thi·o·mer·sa·late
thi·o·meth·yl·a·den·o·sine
thi·o·ne·ine
thi·on·ic
thi·o·nine
thi·o·pan·ic ac·id
thi·o·pen·tal so·di·um
thi·o·phene
thi·o·phe·ni·col
thi·o·phor·as·es
thi·o·pro·pa·zate hy·dro·chlo·
    ride
thi·o·pro·per·a·zine
thi·o·rid·a·zine hy·dro·chlo·ride
thi·o·sem·i·car·ba·zide
thi·o·sem·i·car·ba·zone

thi·o·sul·fate
    t. cy·a·nide trans·sul·fu·rase
    t. sul·fur·trans·fer·ase
    t. thi·o·trans·fer·ase
thi·o·sul·fur·ic ac·id
thi·o·te·pa
thi·o·thix·ene
thi·o·trans·a·cet·y·lase B
thi·o·u·rea
thi·o·xan·thene
thi·ox·o·lone
thi·phen·a·mil hy·dro·chlo·ride
third
    cor·pus·cle
    dis·ease
    eye·lid
    fin·ger
    mo·lar
    ova·ry
    ton·sil
    tro·chan·ter
    ven·tri·cle
    ven·tric·u·los·to·my
third cra·ni·al
    nerve
third cu·ne·i·form
    bone
third de·gree
    burn
    pro·lapse
third and fourth pha·ryn·ge·al
  pouch
    syn·drome
third heart
    sound
third oc·cip·i·tal
    nerve
third par·al·lel pel·vic
    plane
third per·o·ne·al
    mus·cle
third s
third tem·po·ral
    con·vo·lu·tion
thirst
    fe·ver
thirst
    false t.
    in·sen·si·ble t.
    mor·bid t.
    sub·lim·i·nal t.
    true t.
Thiry's
    fis·tu·la
Thiry-Vella
    fis·tu·la
thix·o·la·bile

thix·o·tro·pic
    flu·id
thix·ot·ro·py
Thomas
    splint
Thoma's
    am·pul·la
    fix·a·tive
    laws
Thoma's count·ing
    cham·ber
Thompson's
    test
Thomsen's
    dis·ease
Thomson's
    sign
thon·zo·ni·um bro·mide
thon·zyl·a·mine hy·dro·
  chlo·ride
tho·ra·cal
tho·ra·cal·gia
tho·ra·cec·to·my
tho·ra·cen·te·sis
tho·ra·ces
tho·rac·ic
    ax·is
    cage
    cav·i·ty
    choke
    com·pli·ance
    duct
    fis·tu·la
    gan·glia
    gir·dle
    glands
    goi·ter
    in·dex
    limb
    nerves
    nu·cle·us
    part
    part of aor·ta
    part of esoph·a·gus
    part of spi·nal cord
    part of tho·rac·ic duct
    res·pi·ra·tion
    spine
    stom·ach
    veins
    ver·te·brae
    wall
tho·rac·ic aor·tic
    plex·us
tho·rac·ic car·di·ac
    nerves
tho·rac·ic in·ter·spi·nal
    mus·cle

tho·rac·ic in·ter·trans·verse
  mus·cles
tho·rac·ic lon·gis·si·mus
  mus·cle
tho·rac·i·co·ab·dom·i·nal
tho·rac·i·co·a·cro·mi·al
tho·rac·i·co·hu·mer·al
tho·rac·ic out·let
  syn·drome
tho·rac·ic-pel·vic-pha·lan·ge·al
  dys·tro·phy
tho·rac·ic ro·ta·tor
  mus·cles
tho·ra·cis
tho·ra·co·ab·dom·i·nal
tho·ra·co·a·cro·mi·al
  ar·tery
  vein
tho·ra·co·ce·los·chi·sis
tho·ra·co·cen·te·sis
tho·ra·co·cyl·lo·sis
tho·ra·co·cyr·to·sis
tho·ra·co·del·phus
tho·ra·co·dor·sal
  ar·tery
  nerve
tho·ra·co·dyn·ia
tho·ra·co·ep·i·gas·tric
  vein
tho·ra·co·gas·tros·chi·sis
tho·ra·co·graph
tho·ra·co·lap·a·rot·o·my
tho·ra·co·lum·bar
  ap·o·neu·ro·sis
  sys·tem
tho·ra·co·lum·bar ve·nous
  line
tho·ra·col·y·sis
tho·ra·com·e·lus
tho·ra·com·e·ter
tho·ra·co·my·o·dyn·ia
tho·ra·cop·a·gus
tho·ra·co·par·a·ceph·a·lus
tho·ra·cop·a·thy
tho·ra·co·plas·ty
  con·ven·tion·al t.
tho·ra·co·pneu·mo·plas·ty
tho·ra·cos·chi·sis
tho·ra·co·scope
tho·ra·cos·co·py
tho·ra·co·ste·no·sis
tho·ra·cos·to·my
tho·ra·cot·o·my
tho·ra·del·phus
tho·rax
  Peyrot's t.
tho·ri·um
  em·a·na·tion

Thormählen's
  test
Thorn
  test
thorn
  den·drit·ic t.'s
  pe·nis t.'s
thorn ap·ple
  crys·tals
Thorn's
  syn·drome
Thornwaldt's
  dis·ease
thor·ough·bred
thor·ough-pin
thought broad·cast·ing
thought in·ser·tion
thought pro·cess
  dis·or·der
thought with·draw·al
thread
  Simonart's t.'s
  ter·mi·nal t.
thread·worm
thready
  pulse
threat·en·ed
  abor·tion
three-cor·nered
  bone
three-day
  fe·ver
  mea·sles
three-di·men·sion·al
  rec·ord
three-glass
  test
thre·on·ic ac·id
thre·o·nine
  t. de·am·i·nase
  t. de·hy·dra·tase
thre·ose
thresh·er's
  lung
thresh·old
  body
  dif·fer·en·tial
  per·cus·sion
  shift
  stim·u·lus
  sub·stance
thresh·old
  ab·so·lute t.
  ach·ro·mat·ic t.
  au·di·to·ry t.
  bright·ness dif·fer·ence t.
  t. of con·scious·ness
  con·vul·sant t.

dif·fer·en·tial t.
dis·place·ment t.
dou·ble-point t.
er·y·the·ma t.
fi·bril·la·tion t.
gal·van·ic t.
light dif·fer·en·tial t.
min·i·mum light t.
t. of nose
pain t.
re·la·tion·al t.
re·nal t.
stim·u·lus t.
swal·low·ing t.
vi·su·al t.
t. of vi·su·al sen·sa·tion
thresh·old lim·it
val·ue
thrill
di·a·stol·ic t.
hy·da·tid t.
pre·sys·tol·ic t.
sys·tol·ic t.
thrix
t. an·nu·la·ta
throat
pu·trid t.
sep·tic sore t.
sore t.
throb
throm·base
throm·bas·the·nia
Glanzmann's t.
he·red·i·tary hem·or·rhag·ic
t.
throm·bec·to·my
throm·bi
throm·bin
time
throm·bin
hu·man t.
throm·bin·o·gen
throm·bi·no·gen·e·sis
throm·bin·ti·mec·to·my
throm·bo·an·gi·i·tis
t. ob·li·te·r·ans
throm·bo·ar·te·ri·tis
throm·bo·as·the·nia
throm·bo·blast
throm·boc·la·sis
throm·bo·clas·tic
throm·bo·cyst
throm·bo·cys·tis
throm·bo·cy·tas·the·nia
throm·bo·cyte
throm·bo·cy·the·mia
throm·bo·cyt·ic
se·ries

throm·bo·cy·tin
throm·bo·cy·top·a·thy
throm·bo·cy·to·pe·nia
au·to·im·mune t.
es·sen·tial t.
im·mune t.
iso·im·mune t.
throm·bo·cy·to·pe·nia-ab·sent
ra·di·us
syn·drome
throm·bo·cy·to·pe·nic
pur·pu·ra
throm·bo·cy·to·poi·e·sis
throm·bo·cy·to·sis
throm·bo·e·las·to·gram
throm·bo·e·las·to·graph
throm·bo·em·bo·lec·to·my
throm·bo·em·bo·lism
throm·bo·end·ar·ter·ec·to·my
throm·bo·en·do·car·di·tis
throm·bo·gen
throm·bo·gene
throm·bo·gen·ic
throm·boid
throm·bo·kat·i·ly·sin
throm·bo·ki·nase
throm·bol·ic
throm·bo·lus
throm·bo·lym·phan·gi·tis
throm·bol·y·sis
throm·bo·lyt·ic
throm·bon
throm·bo·ne·cro·sis
throm·bo·path·ic
syn·drome
throm·bop·a·thy
con·sti·tu·tion·al t.
throm·bo·pe·nia
throm·bo·phil·ia
throm·bo·phle·bi·tis
t. mi·grans
t. sal·tans
throm·bo·plas·tic plas·ma
com·po·nent
throm·bo·plas·tid
throm·bo·plas·tin
throm·bo·plas·tin·o·gen
throm·bo·plas·tin·o·ge·nase
throm·bo·plas·tin·o·ge·ne·mia
throm·bo·poi·e·sis
throm·bosed
throm·bose par ef·fort
throm·bo·ses
throm·bo·sin
throm·bo·sis
atroph·ic t.
ce·re·bral t.
com·pres·sion t.

throm·bo·sis *(continued)*
  cor·o·nary t.
  creep·ing t.
  di·la·tion t.
  ef·fort t.
  jump·ing t.
  ma·ran·tic t.
  ma·ras·mic t.
  mu·ral t.
  pla·cen·tal t.
  plate t.
  plate·let t.
  post·trau·mat·ic ar·te·ri·al
    t.
  post·trau·mat·ic ve·nous t.
throm·bo·sta·sis
throm·bo·sthe·nin
throm·bot·ic
  ap·o·plexy
  gan·grene
  hy·dro·ceph·a·lus
  in·farct
  mi·cro·an·gi·op·a·thy
  phleg·ma·sia
throm·bot·ic throm·bo·cy·to·
  pe·nic
  pur·pu·ra
throm·bo·to·nin
throm·box·ane
throm·box·anes
throm·bo·zyme
throm·bus
  ag·glu·ti·na·tive t.
  ag·o·nal t.
  an·te·mor·tem t.
  ball t.
  ball-valve t.
  bile t.
  fi·brin t.
  glob·u·lar t.
  hy·a·line t.
  in·fec·tive t.
  lam·i·nat·ed t.
  ma·ran·tic t.
  ma·ras·mic t.
  mixed t.
  mu·ral t.
  ob·struc·tive t.
  pale t.
  pa·ri·e·tal t.
  post·mor·tem t.
  prop·a·gat·ed t.
  red t.
  sec·on·dary t.
  strat·i·fied t.
  val·vu·lar t.
  white t.

through
  drain·age
through-and-through **my·o·car·**
  di·al
  in·farc·tion
throw·back
thrush
  fun·gus
thu·ja
  t. oil
thu·jol
thu·jone
thu·li·um
thumb
  game·keep·er's t.
  hitch·hik·er t.'s
  ten·nis t.
thumb
  for·ceps
  lan·cet
  re·flex
thumb·print·ing
thumps
thun·der
  hu·mor
thus
thu·ya
thu·yol
thu·yone
Thygeson's
  dis·ease
thy·la·ci·tis
thyme
  t. oil
  oil of t.
thyme
  cam·phor
thy·mec·to·my
thy·mel·co·sis
thy·mi
thy·mic
  ab·scess·es
  agen·e·sis
  alym·pho·pla·sia
  cor·pus·cle
  hy·po·pla·sia
  veins
thy·mic ac·id
thy·mic lym·pho·poi·et·ic
  fac·tor
thy·mi·co·lym·phat·ic
thy·mi·dine
  t. phos·pho·ryl·ase
  trit·i·at·ed t.
thy·mi·dyl·ate syn·thase
thy·mi·dyl·ic ac·id
thy·min

thy·mine
    t. de·ox·y·ri·bo·nu·cle·o·side
    t. de·ox·y·ri·bo·nu·cle·o·tide
    t. nu·cle·o·tide

thy·mine
    di·mer

thym·i·on

thym·i·o·sis

thy·mi·tis

thy·mo·cyte

thy·mo·gen·ic

thy·mo·ki·net·ic

thy·mol
    t. blue
    t. io·dide

thy·mo·ma

thy·mo·nu·cle·ase

thy·mo·poi·et·in

thy·mo·pri·val

thy·mo·priv·ic

thy·mo·pri·vous

thy·mo·sin

thy·mox·a·mine

thy·mus
    gland

thy·mus-de·pen·dent
    zone

thy·mus·es

thy·ro·a·ce·tic ac·id

thy·ro·ad·e·ni·tis

thy·ro·a·pla·sia

thy·ro·ar·y·te·noid
    mus·cle

thy·ro·cal·ci·to·nin

thy·ro·car·di·ac
    dis·ease

thy·ro·cele

thy·ro·cer·vi·cal
    trunk

thy·ro·chon·drot·o·my

thy·ro·col·loid

thy·ro·cri·co·to·my

thy·ro·ep·i·glot·tic
    lig·a·ment
    mus·cle

thy·ro·e·pi·glot·tid·e·an
    lig·a·ment
    mus·cle

thy·ro·e·soph·a·ge·us

thy·ro·fis·sure

thy·ro·gen·ic

thy·rog·e·nous

thy·ro·glob·u·lin

thy·ro·glos·sal
    di·ver·tic·u·lum
    duct

thy·ro·glos·sal duct
    cyst

thy·ro·hy·al

thy·ro·hy·oid
    mem·brane
    mus·cle

thy·ro·hy·po·phy·si·al
    syn·drome

thy·roid
    ax·is
    body
    bru·it
    car·ti·lage
    col·loid
    cri·sis
    di·ver·tic·u·lum
    em·i·nence
    fo·ra·men
    gland
    storm
    ther·a·py
    tox·i·co·sis
    veins

thy·roid
    ac·ces·so·ry t.

thy·roi·dal ar·tic·u·lar
    sur·face of cri·coid

thy·roi·dea
    t. ac·ces·so·ria
    t. ima

thy·roid·ec·to·my
    "chem·i·cal t.

thy·roid·ism

thy·roid·i·tis
    au·to·im·mune t.
    chron·ic atroph·ic t.
    de Quervain's t.
    fo·cal lym·pho·cyt·ic t.
    gi·ant cell t.
    Hashimoto's t.
    lig·ne·ous t.
    par·a·sit·ic t.
    Riedel's t.
    sub·a·cute gran·u·lom·a·tous t.

thy·roid lymph
    nodes

thy·roi·dol·o·gy

thy·roid·o·to·my

thy·roid-stim·u·lat·ing
    hor·mone

thy·roid-stim·u·lat·ing hor·mone-re·leas·ing
    fac·tor

thy·roid-stim·u·lat·ing hor·mone stim·u·la·tion
    test

thy·roid sup·pres·sion
  test
thy·ro·la·ryn·ge·al
thy·ro·lib·er·in
thy·ro·lin·gual
  cyst
  duct
thy·ro·lyt·ic
thy·ro·meg·a·ly
thy·ro·nine
thy·ro·pal·a·tine
thy·ro·par·a·thy·roid·ec·to·my
thy·rop·a·thy
thy·ro·pha·ryn·ge·al
  part
thy·ro·pri·val
thy·ro·priv·ia
thy·ro·priv·ic
thy·ro·pri·vous
thy·ro·pro·tein
thy·rop·to·sis
thy·rot·o·my
thy·ro·tox·ic
  co·ma
  cri·sis
  en·ceph·a·lop·a·thy
  my·op·a·thy
  se·rum
thy·ro·tox·ic com·ple·ment-
  fix·a·tion
  fac·tor
thy·ro·tox·i·co·sis
  ap·a·thet·ic t.
  t. me·di·ca·men·to·sa
thy·ro·tox·in
thy·ro·troph
thy·ro·tro·phic
thy·rot·ro·phin
thy·ro·tro·pic
  hor·mone
thy·rot·ro·pin
thy·rot·ro·pin-pro·duc·ing
  ad·e·no·ma
thy·rot·ro·pin-re·leas·ing
  fac·tor
  hor·mone
thy·rot·ro·pin-re·leas·ing hor·
  mone stim·u·la·tion
  test
thy·rox·in
thy·rox·ine
  ra·di·o·ac·tive t.
  t. so·di·um
thy·rox·ine-bind·ing
  glob·u·lin
  pre·al·bu·min
  pro·tein

Thys·a·no·so·ma ac·ti·noi·des
tib·ia
  sa·ber t.
  t. val·ga
  t. va·ra
tib·i·ad
tib·i·ae
tib·i·al
  bor·der
  crest
  nerve
  phe·nom·e·non
  tu·ber·os·i·ty
tib·i·al col·lat·er·al
  lig·a·ment
tib·i·al com·mu·ni·cat·ing
  nerve
tib·i·a·le pos·ti·cum
tib·i·al·gia
tib·i·al in·ter·ten·di·nous
  bur·sa
tib·i·a·lis
tib·i·o·cal·ca·ne·al
  part
tib·i·o·cal·ca·ne·an
tib·i·o·fas·ci·a·lis
tib·i·o·fem·o·ral
  in·dex
tib·i·o·fib·u·lar
  ar·tic·u·la·tion
  joint, in·fe·ri·or
  joint, su·pe·ri·or
  lig·a·ment
  syn·des·mo·sis
tib·i·o·na·vic·u·lar
  lig·a·ment
  part
tib·i·o·per·o·ne·al
tib·i·o·scaph·oid
tib·i·o·tar·sal
tic
  con·vul·sive t.
  t. de pen·sée
  t. dou·lou·reux
  fa·cial t.
  glos·so·pha·ryn·ge·al t.
  hab·it t.
  lo·cal t.
  mim·ic t.
  psy·chic t.
  ro·ta·to·ry t.
  spas·mod·ic t.
ti·car·cil·lin di·so·di·um
tick
  fe·ver
  pa·ral·y·sis
  ty·phus

tick-borne
en·ceph·a·li·tis (Cen·tral
Eu·ro·pe·an sub·type)
en·ceph·a·li·tis (East·ern
sub·type)
tick-borne en·ceph·a·li·tis
vi·rus
tick·ling
ti·cryn·a·fen
tic-tac
rhythm
sounds
tid·al
air
drain·age
vol·ume
wave
tide
ac·id t.
al·ka·line t.
fat t.
Tiedemann's
gland
nerve
tie-o·ver
dress·ing
Tier·fell·nae·vus
Tietze's
syn·drome
ti·ger
heart
tight
junc·tion
tig·late
tig·li·an
tig·lic ac·id
ti·gre·ti·er
ti·groid
bod·ies
fun·dus
ret·i·na
stri·a·tion
sub·stance
ti·grol·y·sis
tilt
ta·ble
tim·bre
time
ac·ti·vat·ed par·tial
throm·bo·plas·tin t.
A-H con·duc·tion t.
as·so·ci·a·tion t.
bi·o·log·ic t.
bleed·ing t.
cal·ci·um t.
cir·cu·la·tion t.
clot re·trac·tion t.
clot·ting t.

co·ag·u·la·tion t.
eu·glob·u·lin clot ly·sis t.
fad·ing t.
forced ex·pi·ra·to·ry t.
half-t.
H-R con·duc·tion t.
H-V con·duc·tion t.
in·er·tia t.
in·tra-a·tri·al con·duc·tion
t.
left ven·tric·u·lar ejec·tion
t.
P-A con·duc·tion t.
par·tial throm·bo·plas·tin t.
P-H con·duc·tion t.
pro·throm·bin t.
re·ac·tion t.
rec·og·ni·tion t.
rise t.
sen·sa·tion t.
si·no·a·tri·al con·duc·tion t.
si·no·a·tri·al re·cov·ery t.
sur·viv·al t.
throm·bin t.
tis·sue throm·bo·plas·tin
in·hi·bi·tion t.
uti·li·za·tion t.
time
con·stant
mark·er
sense
time com·pen·sa·tion
gain
time-var·ied gain
con·trol
ti·mo·lol ma·le·ate
tim·o·thy hay
ba·cil·lus
tin
t. ox·ide
tinct
tinc·ta·ble
tinc·tion
tinc·to·ri·al
tinc·tu·ra
tinc·tu·rae
tinc·tu·ra·tion
tinc·ture
al·co·hol·ic t.
am·mo·ni·at·ed t.
ethe·re·al t.
glyc·er·in·at·ed t.
hy·dro·al·co·hol·ic t.
tine
test
tin·ea
t. am·i·an·ta·cea
t. ax·il·la·ris

tin·ea *(continued)*
  t. bar·bae
  t. ca·pi·tis
  t. ci·li·o·rum
  t. cir·ci·na·ta
  t. cor·po·ris
  t. cru·ris
  t. fa·vo·sa
  t. fur·fu·ra·cea
  t. gla·bro·sa
  t. im·bri·ca·ta
  t. in·gui·na·lis
  t. ke·ri·on
  t. ma·nus
  t. nig·ra
  t. pe·dis
  t. sy·co·sis
  t. tar·si
  t. ton·dens
  t. ton·su·rans
  t. tro·pi·ca·lis
  t. un·gui·um
  t. ve·ra
  t. ver·si·col·or
Tinel's
  sign
tin·foil
tin·gi·bil·i·ty
tin·gi·ble
tin·gle
tin·gling
ti·nid·a·zole
tin·ni·tus
  t. au·ri·um
  t. ce·re·bri
  click·ing t.
  Leu·det's t.
tint
tint·ed den·ture
  base
ti·o·con·a·zole
tip
  t. of au·ri·cle
  t. of el·bow
  t. of nose
  t. of pos·te·ri·or horn
  root t.
  t. of tongue
  Woolner's t.
tip·ping
ti·pren·o·lol hy·dro·chlo·ride
tir·ing
Tiselius
  ap·pa·ra·tus
Tiselius elec·tro·pho·re·sis
  cell
Tissot
  spi·rom·e·ter

tis·sue
  ba·so·phil
  cul·ture
  dis·place·a·bil·i·ty
  dis·place·ment
  flu·id
  lymph
  mold·ing
  reg·is·tra·tion
  res·pi·ra·tion
  ten·sion
tis·sue
  ad·e·noid t.
  ad·i·pose t.
  are·o·lar t.
  bone t.
  can·cel·lous t.
  car·di·ac mus·cle t.
  car·ti·lag·i·nous t.
  cav·ern·ous t.
  chon·droid t.
  chro·maf·fin t.
  con·nec·tive t.
  dar·to·ic t.
  elas·tic t.
  ep·i·the·li·al t.
  erec·tile t.
  fat·ty t.
  fi·bro·hy·a·line t.
  fi·brous t.
  Gam·gee t.
  ge·lat·i·nous t.
  gin·gi·val t.'s
  gran·u·la·tion t.
  Haller's vas·cu·lar t.
  hard t.
  he·mo·poi·et·ic t.
  in·dif·fer·ent t.
  in·ter·sti·tial t.
  in·vest·ing t.'s
  is·let t.
  lym·phat·ic t.
  lym·phoid t.
  me·sen·chy·mal t.
  mes·o·neph·ric t.
  met·a·neph·ro·gen·ic t.
  mu·cous con·nec·tive t.
  mul·ti·loc·u·lar ad·i·pose t.
  mus·cu·lar t.
  my·e·loid t.
  na·si·on soft t.
  neph·ro·gen·ic t.
  ner·vous t.
  no·dal t.
  os·se·ous t.
  os·te·o·gen·ic t.
  os·te·oid t.
  per·i·ap·i·cal t.

re·tic·u·lar t.
ret·i·form t.
rub·ber t.
skel·e·tal mus·cle t.
smooth mus·cle t.
sub·cu·ta·ne·ous t.
tis·sue-bear·ing
ar·ea
tis·sue cul·ture in·fec·tious
dose
tis·sue plas·min·o·gen
ac·ti·va·tor
tis·sue-spe·cif·ic
an·ti·gen
tis·sue throm·bo·plas·tin in·hi·
bi·tion
time
tis·sue-trim·ming
tis·su·lar
ti·ta·ni·um
t. di·ox·ide
ti·ter
tit·il·la·tion
ti·trant
ti·trat·a·ble acid·i·ty
test
ti·trate
ti·tra·tion
col·or·i·met·ric t.
for·mol t.
po·ten·ti·o·met·ric t.
tit·u·ba·tion
Tiz·zo·ni's
stain
Tj
an·ti·gen
TM-mode
TMN
stag·ing
T-my·co·plas·ma
TO
vi·rus
toad
skin
to-and-fro
an·es·the·sia
mur·mur
toast·ed
shins
to·bac·co
heart
to·bac·co
wild t.
Tobia
fe·ver
to·bra·my·cin
To·bruk
splint

to·cai·nide hy·dro·chlo·ride
to·cam·phyl
toc·o·dy·na·graph
toc·o·dy·na·mom·e·ter
toc·o·graph
to·cog·ra·phy
to·col
to·col·o·gy
to·co·lyt·ic
to·com·e·ter
to·coph·er·ol
mixed t.'s con·cen·trate
to·coph·er·ol·qui·none
to·coph·er·yl·qui·none
toc·o·pho·bia
to·co·qui·none
to·co·tri·en·ol
to·co·tri·en·ol·qui·none
Todaro's
ten·don
Todd's
pa·ral·y·sis
Todd's post·ep·i·lep·tic
pa·ral·y·sis
Tod's
mus·cle
toe
clo·nus
itch
phe·nom·e·non
re·flex
toe
great t.
ham·mer t.
Hong Kong t.
pain·ful t.
stiff t.
webbed t.'s
toe-crack
toe-drop
toe·nail
in·grow·ing t.
to·fen·a·cin hy·dro·chlo·ride
To·ga·vir·i·dae
to·ga·vi·rus
toi·let
train·ing
Toison's
stain
To·ke·lau
ring·worm
to·laz·a·mide
to·laz·o·line hy·dro·chlo·ride
tol·bu·ta·mide
test
tol·cy·cla·mide

Toldt's
    fas·cia
    mem·brane
tol·er·ance
    dose
tol·er·ance
    acous·tic t.
    cross t.
    frus·tra·tion t.
    im·mu·no·log·i·cal t.
    in·di·vid·u·al t.
    pain t.
    spe·cies t.
    split t.
    vi·bra·tion t.
tol·er·ant
tol·er·o·gen·ic
tol·hex·a·mide
tol·met·in
tol·naf·tate
to·lo·ni·um chlo·ride
To·lo·sa-Hunt
    syn·drome
tol·pro·pa·mine
To·lu
    bal·sam
tol·u·ene
to·lu·ic ac·id
to·lu·i·dine
    al·ka·line t. blue O
    t. blue O
tol·u·ol
tol·u·o·yl
tol·u·yl·ene red
tol·yl
Toma's
    sign
to·men·tum
to·men·tum ce·re·bri
Tomes'
    fi·bers
    pro·cess·es
Tomes' gran·u·lar
    lay·er
Tommaselli's
    dis·ease
to·mo·gram
to·mo·graph
to·mog·ra·phy
    com·put·ed t.
    com·put·er·ized ax·i·al t.
    hy·po·cy·cloi·dal t.
    pos·i·tron emis·sion t.
    sin·gle pho·ton emis·sion
      com·put·ed t.
to·mo·lev·el
to·mo·ma·nia
ton·a·pha·sia

tone
    af·fec·tive t.
    emo·tion·al t.
    feel·ing t.
    fun·da·men·tal t.
    Traube's dou·ble t.
tone
    col·or
tone de·cay
    test
ton·er
tongue
    baked t.
    bald t.
    beet-t.
    bi·fid t.
    black t.
    t. of cer·e·bel·lum
    cleft t.
    coat·ed t.
    dot·ted t.
    fis·sured t.
    furred t.
    ge·o·graph·ic t.
    grooved t.
    hairy t.
    hob·nail t.
    ma·gen·ta t.
    man·dib·u·lar t.
    rasp·ber·ry t.
    scro·tal t.
    smok·er's t.
    stip·pled t.
    straw·ber·ry t.
    wood·en t. of cat·tle
tongue
    bone
    de·pres·sor
    flap
    phe·nom·e·non
tongue crib
tongue-swal·low·ing
tongue thrust
tongue-tie
ton·ic
    bit·ter t.
ton·ic
    con·trac·tion
    con·trol
    con·vul·sion
    ep·i·lep·sy
    pu·pil
    re·flex
    spasm
to·nic·i·ty
ton·i·co·clon·ic
to·nin
ton·ing

ton·i·tro·pho·bia
ton·o·clon·ic
  spasm
ton·o·fi·bril
ton·o·fil·a·ment
ton·o·graph
to·nog·ra·phy
to·nom·e·ter
  ap·pla·na·tion t.
  Gärtner's t.
  Goldmann's ap·pla·na·tion
    t.
  Mackay-Marg t.
  Mueller elec·tron·ic t.
  pneu·mat·ic t.
  Schiötz t.
to·nom·e·try
ton·o·phant
ton·o·plast
to·nos·cil·lo·graph
to·no·top·ic
to·no·tro·pic
ton·sil
  cer·e·bel·lar t.
  eu·sta·chi·an t.
  fau·cial t.
  Gerlach's t.
  la·ryn·ge·al t.'s
  lin·gual t.
  Luschka's t.
  pal·a·tine t.
  pha·ryn·ge·al t.
  sub·merged t.
  third t.
  tub·al t.
ton·sil·la
  t. in·tes·ti·na·lis
ton·sil·lae
ton·sil·lar
  cal·cu·lus
  crypt
  fos·sa
  fos·su·lae
  her·ni·a·tion
  ring
ton·sil·lary
ton·sil·lec·to·my
ton·sil·lith
ton·sil·li·tis
  la·cu·nar t.
  par·en·chym·a·tous t.
  su·per·fi·cial t.
  Vincent's t.
ton·sil·lo·lin·gual
  sul·cus
ton·sil·lo·lith
ton·sil·lop·a·thy
ton·sil·lo·tome

ton·sil·lot·o·my
to·nus
  base·line t.
tooth
  acryl·ic res·in t.
  an·a·tom·ic teeth
  an·ky·losed t.
  an·te·ri·or teeth
  au·di·to·ry teeth
  ba·by t.
  back teeth
  bi·cus·pid t.
  buck t.
  ca·nine t.
  car·nas·si·al t.
  cheek t.
  Corti's au·di·to·ry teeth
  cross-bite teeth
  cus·pid t.
  cus·pi·date t.
  cusp·less t.
  cut·ting teeth
  dead t.
  de·cid·u·ous t.
  de·vi·tal·ized t.
  ex·trud·ed teeth
  eye t.
  flu·o·ri·dat·ed teeth
  fused teeth
  gem·i·nat·ed teeth
  ghost t.
  green t.
  Horner's teeth
  Huschke's au·di·to·ry teeth
  Hutchinson's teeth
  im·pact·ed t.
  in·ci·sor t.
  met·al in·sert teeth
  mi·grat·ing teeth
  milk t.
  mo·lar t.
  mot·tled t.
  mul·ti·cus·pid t.
  na·tal t.
  ne·o·na·tal t.
  non-an·a·tom·ic teeth
  non·vit·al t.
  nor·mal·ly posed t.
  notched teeth
  oral teeth
  pegged t.
  per·ma·nent t.
  per·pet·u·al·ly grow·ing t.
  per·sis·tent·ly grow·ing t.
  plas·tic teeth
  pos·te·ri·or teeth
  pre·mo·lar t.
  pri·mary t.

tooth *(continued)*
  pro·trud·ing teeth
  pulp·less t.
  scle·rot·ic teeth
  screw·driv·er teeth
  sec·ond t.
  spaced teeth
  stom·ach t.
  suc·ce·da·ne·ous t.
  syph·i·lit·ic teeth
  tem·po·rary t.
  tri·an·gu·lar·i·ty of the
    teeth
  tri·cus·pid t.
  tube teeth
  Turner's t.
  un·e·rup·ted t.
  vi·tal t.
  wis·dom t.
  wolf t.
  ze·ro de·gree teeth
tooth
  abra·sion
  avul·sion
  bud
  ce·ment
  cough
  form
  germ
  li·ga·tion
  plane
  pol·yp
  pulp
  sac
  sock·et
  spasms
  trans·plan·ta·tion
tooth·ache
tooth-and-nail
  syn·drome
tooth ar·range·ment
tooth-borne
  base
toothed
  ver·te·bra
top·ag·no·sis
to·pal·gia
to·pec·to·my
top·er's
  nose
top·es·the·sia
Töpfer's
  test
to·pha·ceous
  gout
to·phi
to·phus
  gouty t.

top·i·ca
top·i·cal
  an·es·the·sia
Topinard's
  line
Topinard's fa·cial
  an·gle
to·pis·tic
top·o·an·es·the·sia
top·og·no·sia
top·og·no·sis
top·o·gom·e·ter
top·o·graph·ic
  anat·o·my
to·pog·ra·phy
Topolanski's
  sign
to·pol·o·gy
top·o·nar·co·sis
top·o·nym
to·pon·y·my
top·o·path·o·gen·e·sis
top·o·pho·bia
top·o·phy·lax·is
top·o·scope
top·o·therm·es·the·si·om·e·ter
TORCH
  syn·drome
tor·cu·lar he·roph·i·li
Torek
  op·er·a·tion
to·ri
to·ric
  lens
Torkildsen
  shunt
tor·na·do
  ep·i·lep·sy
Tornwaldt's
  ab·scess
  cyst
  dis·ease
  syn·drome
to·roi·dal
  valve
to·rose
to·rous
tor·pent
tor·pid
tor·pid·i·ty
tor·por
  t. ret·i·nae
torque
torr
tor·re·fac·tion
tor·re·fy
Torre's
  syn·drome

tor·sade de pointes
tor·si·om·e·ter
tor·sion
    t. of tes·tis
    t. of a tooth
tor·sion
    dys·to·nia
    frac·ture
    neu·ro·sis
    spasm
tor·sion·al
    de·for·mi·ty
tor·sion·om·e·ter
tor·sive
    oc·clu·sion
tor·si·ver·sion
tor·so
tor·so·clu·sion
Torsten Sjögren's
    syn·drome
tor·ti·col·lar
tor·ti·col·lis
    con·gen·i·tal t.
    der·mat·o·gen·ic t.
    dys·ton·ic t.
    fixed t.
    in·ter·mit·tent t.
    lab·y·rin·thine t.
    oc·u·lar t.
    psy·cho·gen·ic t.
    rheu·mat·ic t.
    spas·mod·ic t.
    t. spas·ti·ca
    spu·ri·ous t.
    symp·to·mat·ic t.
tor·ti·pel·vis
tor·tu·ous
tor·u·li
tor·u·lo·ma
Tor·u·lop·sis
tor·u·lop·so·sis
tor·u·lus
to·rus
    t. fron·ta·lis
    man·dib·u·lar t.
    t. man·di·bu·la·ris
    t. ma·nus
    t. oc·ci·pi·ta·lis
    pal·a·tine t.
    t. pal·a·ti·nus
    t. ure·te·ri·cus
    t. uter·i·nus
to·rus
    frac·ture
tos·yl
tos·yl·ate
to·tal
    acid·i·ty

apha·sia
cat·a·ract
cys·tec·to·my
elas·tic·i·ty of mus·cle
en·er·gy
he·ma·tu·ria
hy·per·o·pia
ker·a·to·plas·ty
mas·tec·to·my
ne·cro·sis
pla·cen·ta pre·via
scle·rec·ta·sia
syn·ech·ia
trans·fu·sion
to·tal body
    hy·po·ther·mia
to·tal cat·e·chol·a·mine
    test
to·tal end-di·a·stol·ic
    di·am·e·ter
to·tal end-sys·tol·ic
    di·am·e·ter
to·tal fa·cial
    in·dex
to·tal joint
    ar·thro·plas·ty
to·tal lung
    ca·pac·i·ty
to·tal par·en·ter·al
    nu·trit·ion
to·tal pel·vic
    ex·en·ter·a·tion
to·tal pe·riph·e·ral
    re·sis·tance
to·tal push
    ther·a·py
to·tal re·frac·to·ry
    pe·ri·od
to·tal spi·nal
    an·es·the·sia
to·tem
to·tem·ism
to·tem·is·tic
to·tip·o·tence
to·tip·o·ten·cy
to·tip·o·tent
    cell
to·ti·po·ten·tial
    pro·to·plasm
touch
    cell
    cor·pus·cle
tough·ened
    sil·ver ni·trate
Tourette's
    dis·ease
    syn·drome

Tournay
  sign
Tournay's
  phe·nom·e·non
tour·ni·quet
  po·di·tis
  test
tour·ni·quet
  Dupuytren's t.
  Esmarch t.
Tourtual's
  mem·brane
  si·nus
Touton gi·ant
  cell
To·vell
  tube
tow·ers
  skull
Towne
  pro·jec·tion
  view
Towne pro·jec·tion
  roent·gen·o·gram
tox·a·ne·mia
tox·a·phene
Tox·as·ca·ris le·o·ni·na
tox·e·mia
tox·e·mic
  jaun·dice
  ret·i·nop·a·thy of preg·
   nan·cy
tox·ic
  am·au·ro·sis
  am·bly·o·pia
  ane·mia
  cat·a·ract
  cir·rho·sis
  cy·a·no·sis
  de·lir·i·um
  de·men·tia
  equiv·a·lent
  goi·ter
  he·mo·glo·bi·nu·ria
  hy·dro·ceph·a·lus
  meg·a·co·lon
  ne·phro·sis
  neu·ri·tis
  psy·cho·sis
  ret·i·nop·a·thy
  shock
  tet·a·nus
  unit
tox·i·cant
tox·i·ce·mia
tox·ic ep·i·der·mal
  ne·crol·y·sis

tox·ic·i·ty
  ox·y·gen t.
Tox·i·co·den·dron
tox·i·co·der·ma
tox·i·co·der·ma·ti·tis
tox·i·co·der·ma·to·sis
tox·i·co·gen·ic
  con·junc·ti·vi·tis
tox·i·coid
tox·i·co·log·ic
tox·i·col·o·gist
tox·i·col·o·gy
tox·i·co·path·ic
tox·i·co·pho·bia
tox·i·co·sis
  en·do·gen·ic t.
  ex·o·gen·ic t.
  T_3 t.
  thy·roid t.
  tri·i·o·do·thy·ro·nine t.
tox·ic shock
  syn·drome
tox·if·er·ines
tox·if·er·ous
tox·i·gen·ic
tox·i·ge·nic·i·ty
tox·il·ic ac·id
tox·in
  an·i·mal t.
  an·thrax t.
  Ba·cil·lus an·thra·cis t.
  bac·te·ri·al t.
  bot·u·li·nus t.
  chol·era t.
  di·ag·nos·tic diph·the·ria t.
  Dick test t.
  di·no·flag·el·late t.
  diph·the·ria t.
  eryth·ro·gen·ic t.
  ex·tra·cel·lu·lar t.
  in·tra·cel·lu·lar t.
  nor·mal t.
  plant t.
  scar·let fe·ver eryth·ro·
   gen·ic t.
  Schick test t.
  strep·to·coc·cus eryth·ro·
   gen·ic t.
  tet·a·nus t.
tox·in
  spec·trum
  unit
tox·in·ic
tox·i·no·gen·ic
tox·i·no·ge·nic·i·ty
tox·i·nol·o·gy
tox·i·no·sis
tox·i·path·ic

tox·ip·a·thy
tox·i·pho·bia
tox·is·ter·ol
Tox·o·ca·ra
  T. ca·nis
  T. mys·tax
tox·o·ca·ri·a·sis
tox·oid
tox·on
tox·one
tox·o·neme
tox·o·no·sis
tox·o·phil
tox·o·phile
tox·o·phore
tox·oph·o·rous
Tox·o·plas·ma gon·dii
Tox·o·plas·mat·i·dae
tox·o·plas·mo·sis
  ac·quired t. in adults
  con·gen·i·tal t.
tox·o·py·rim·i·dine
Toynbee's
  cor·pus·cles
  ex·per·i·ment
  mus·cle
  tube
TPH
  test
TPHA
  test
TPI
  test
Tr^a
  an·ti·gen
tra·bec·u·la
  an·te·ri·or cham·ber t.
  tra·bec·u·lae cra·nii
  sep·to·mar·gi·nal t.
  t. tes·tis
tra·bec·u·lae
tra·bec·u·lar
  bone
  car·ci·no·ma
  mesh·work
  net·work
  re·tic·u·lum
  zone
tra·bec·u·late
tra·bec·u·la·tion
tra·bec·u·lec·to·my
tra·bec·u·lo·plas·ty
  la·ser t.
tra·bec·u·lot·o·my
trace
  mem·o·ry t.

trace
  con·di·tion·ing
  el·e·ments.
trace con·di·tioned
  re·flex
trac·er
tra·chea
  scab·bard t.
tra·che·ae
tra·che·al
  car·ti·lag·es
  fen·es·tra·tion
  fis·tu·la
  glands
  pain
  ring
  tri·an·gle
  tube
  tug
  ul·cer·a·tion
  veins
tra·che·al·gia
tra·che·a·lis
tra·che·al lymph
  nodes
tra·che·i·tis
trach·e·lag·ra
trach·e·la·lis
trach·e·lec·to·my
trach·e·le·ma·to·ma
trach·e·li·an
trach·e·lism
trach·e·lis·mus
trach·e·li·tis
trach·e·lo·breg·mat·ic
  di·am·e·ter
trach·e·lo·cele
trach·e·lo·cla·vic·u·lar
  mus·cle
trach·e·lo·cyr·to·sis
trach·e·lo·cys·ti·tis
trach·e·lo·dyn·ia
trach·e·lo·ky·pho·sis
trach·e·lol·o·gy
trach·e·lo·mas·toid
trach·e·lo·my·i·tis
trach·e·lo-oc·cip·i·ta·lis
trach·e·lo·pa·nus
trach·e·lo·pex·ia
trach·e·lo·pexy
trach·e·lo·phy·ma
trach·e·lo·plas·ty
trach·e·lor·rha·phy
trach·e·los
trach·e·los·chi·sis
trach·e·lot·o·my
tra·che·o·aer·o·cele

tra·che·o·bil·i·ary
  fis·tu·la
tra·che·o·bron·chi·al
  dys·ki·ne·sia
  groove
tra·che·o·bron·chi·tis
tra·che·o·bron·cho·meg·a·ly
tra·che·o·bron·chos·co·py
tra·che·o·cele
tra·che·o·e·soph·a·ge·al
  fis·tu·la
tra·che·o·la·ryn·ge·al
tra·che·o·ma·la·cia
tra·che·o·meg·a·ly
tra·che·o·path·ia
  t. os·te·o·plas·ti·ca
tra·che·op·a·thy
tra·che·o·pha·ryn·ge·al
tra·che·o·pho·ne·sis
tra·che·oph·o·ny
tra·che·o·plas·ty
tra·che·o·py·o·sis
tra·che·or·rha·gia
tra·che·os·chi·sis
tra·che·o·scope
tra·che·o·scop·ic
tra·che·os·co·py
tra·che·o·ste·no·sis
tra·che·os·to·ma
tra·che·os·to·my
tra·che·o·tome
tra·che·ot·o·my
  hook
  tube
tra·chi·tis
tra·cho·ma
  fol·lic·u·lar t.
  gran·u·lar t.
tra·cho·ma
  bod·ies
  glands
  vi·rus
tra·chom·a·tous
  con·junc·ti·vi·tis
  ker·a·ti·tis
  pan·nus
tra·chy·chro·mat·ic
tra·chy·pho·nia
trac·ing
  ar·row point t.
  ceph·a·lo·met·ric t.
  Goth·ic arch t.
  nee·dle point t.
  sty·lus t.
tract
  al·i·men·ta·ry t.
  an·te·ri·or cor·ti·co·spi·nal
    t.

an·te·ri·or py·ram·i·dal t.
an·te·ri·or spi·no·cer·e·bel·
  lar t.
an·te·ri·or spi·no·tha·lam·ic
  t.
Arnold's t.
as·so·ci·a·tion t.
au·di·to·ry t.
Burdach's t.
cen·tral teg·men·tal t.
cer·e·bel·lo·ru·bral t.
cer·e·bel·lo·tha·lam·ic t.
Collier's t.
com·ma t. of Schultze
cor·ti·co·bul·bar t.
cor·ti·co·pon·tine t.
cor·ti·co·spi·nal t.
crossed py·ram·i·dal t.
cu·ne·o·cer·e·bel·lar t.
dead t.'s
de·it·er·o·spi·nal t.
den·ta·to·tha·lam·ic t.
de·scend·ing t. of tri·gem·i·
  nal nerve
di·ges·tive t.
di·rect py·ram·i·dal t.
dor·sal spi·no·cer·e·bel·lar
  t.
dor·so·lat·er·al t.
fas·tig·i·o·bul·bar t.
Flechsig's t.
fron·to·pon·tine t.
fron·to·tem·po·ral t.
gas·tro·in·tes·ti·nal t.
ge·nic·u·lo·cal·ca·rine t.
gen·i·tal t.
t. of Goll
Gowers' t.
ha·ben·u·lo·in·ter·pe·dun·
  cu·lar t.
Hoche's t.
hy·po·thal·a·mo·hy·po·phy·
  si·al t.
James t.'s
lat·er·al cor·ti·co·spi·nal t.
lat·er·al py·ram·i·dal t.
lat·er·al spi·no·tha·lam·ic t.
Lissauer's t.
Loewenthal's t.
mam·il·lo·tha·lam·ic t.
Marchi's t.
mes·en·ce·phal·ic t. of tri·
  gem·i·nal nerve
Monakow's t.
t. of Münzer and Wiener
nerve t.
oc·cip·i·to·col·lic·u·lar t.
oc·cip·i·to·pon·tine t.

oc·cip·i·to·tec·tal t.
ol·fac·to·ry t.
ol·i·vo·cer·e·bel·lar t.
ol·i·vo·spi·nal t.
op·tic t.
pa·ri·e·to·pon·tine t.
pos·te·ri·or spi·no·cer·e·bel·
lar t.
pre·py·ram·i·dal t.
py·ram·i·dal t.
res·pi·ra·to·ry t.
re·tic·u·lo·spi·nal t.
ru·bro·bul·bar t.
ru·bro·re·tic·u·lar t.
ru·bro·spi·nal t.
t. of Schütz
sen·so·ry t.
sep·to·mar·gi·nal t.
sol·i·tary t.
sphinc·ter·oid t. of il·e·um
spi·nal t.
spi·nal t. of tri·gem·i·nal
nerve
spi·no·cer·e·bel·lar t.'s
spi·no-ol·i·vary t.
spi·no·tec·tal t.
spi·no·tha·lam·ic t.
spi·ral fo·ram·i·nous t.
Spitzka's mar·gi·nal t.
sul·co·mar·gin·al t.
su·pra·op·ti·co·hy·po·phy·
si·al t.
tec·to·bul·bar t.
tec·to·pon·tine t.
tec·to·spi·nal t.
tem·po·ro·fron·tal t.
tem·po·ro·pon·tine t.
tu·ber·o·in·fun·dib·u·lar t.
Türck's t.
uri·nary t.
uve·al t.
ven·tral spi·no·cer·e·bel·lar
t.
ven·tral spi·no·tha·lam·ic t.
ves·tib·u·lo·spi·nal t.
Waldeyer's t.
trac·tel·la
trac·tel·lum
trac·tion
ax·is t.
Bryant's t.
Buck's t.
ex·ter·nal t.
ha·lo t.
in·ter·max·il·lary t.
in·ter·nal t.
iso·met·ric t.
iso·ton·ic t.

max·il·lo·man·dib·u·lar t.
Russell t.
Sayre's sus·pen·sion t.
skel·e·tal t.
skin t.
trac·tion
al·o·pe·cia
an·eu·rysm
at·ro·phy
di·ver·tic·u·lum
epiph·y·sis
trac·tor
Lowsley t.
Syms t.
Young pros·tat·ic t.
trac·tot·o·my
an·ter·o·lat·er·al t.
in·tra·med·ul·lary t.
py·ram·i·dal t.
Schwartz t.
Sjöqvist t.
spi·nal t.
spi·no·tha·lam·ic t.
tri·gem·i·nal t.
Walker t.
trac·tus
trac·tus
t. cen·tra·lis teg·men·ti
t. cor·ti·co·bul·ba·ris
t. de·scen·dens ner·vi tri·
gem·i·ni
t. fas·tig·i·o·bul·ba·ris
t. ha·ben·u·lo·pe·dun·cu·la·
ris
t. spi·no·tha·la·mi·cus
t. spi·ra·lis fo·ra·mi·nu·lo·
sus
t. tec·to·bul·ba·ris
t. tec·to·pon·ti·nus
t. tu·ber·o·in·fun·di·bu·la·
ris
trag·a·canth
trag·a·can·tha
tra·gal
tra·gi
tra·gi·cus
trag·i·on
trag·o·mas·chal·ia
trag·o·pho·nia
tra·goph·o·ny
tra·gus
train
trained
re·flex
train·ing
anal·y·sis
group

train·ing
    as·ser·tive t.
    aver·sive t.
    toi·let t.
train-of-four
    stim·u·lus
train·wheel
    rhythm
trait
    Bom·bay t.
    cat·e·gor·i·cal t.
    chro·mo·som·al t.
    co·dom·i·nant t.
    dom·i·nant t.
    in·ter·me·di·ate t.
    lim·i·nal t.
    mark·er t.
    non·pen·e·trant t.
    qual·i·ta·tive t.
    re·ces·sive t.
    sick·le cell t.
tra·jec·tor
tra·maz·o·line hy·dro·chlo·ride
trance
    death t.
    in·duced t.
    som·nam·bu·lis·tic t.
trance
    co·ma
tran·ex·am·ic ac·id
tran·quil·iz·er
    ma·jor t.
    mi·nor t.
trans
    phase
trans·a·cet·y·lase
trans·a·cet·y·la·tion
trans·ac·tion
trans·ac·tion·al
    anal·y·sis
    psy·cho·ther·a·py
trans·ac·yl·as·es
trans·al·dol·ase
trans·al·do·la·tion
trans·am·i·di·nas·es
trans·am·i·di·na·tion
trans·am·i·nas·es
trans·am·i·na·tion
trans·an·i·ma·tion
trans·au·di·ent
trans·ca·lent
trans·cap·si·da·tion
trans·car·bam·o·y·las·es
trans·car·box·yl·as·es
trans·cel·lu·lar
    flu·ids
tran·scen·den·tal
    anat·o·my

trans·cer·vi·cal
    frac·ture
trans·co·bal·a·mins
trans·con·dy·lar
    frac·ture
trans·cor·ti·cal
    apha·sia
    aprax·ia
trans·cor·tin
trans·cra·ni·al
    roent·gen·o·gram
tran·scrip·tase
    re·verse t.
tran·scrip·tion
trans·cu·ta·ne·ous
trans·cy·to·sis
trans·der·mic
trans·duce
trans·duc·er
    cell
trans·duc·ing
trans·duc·tant
trans·duc·tion
    abor·tive t.
    com·plete t.
    gen·er·al t.
    high fre·quen·cy t.
    low fre·quen·cy t.
    spe·cial·ized t.
    spe·cif·ic t.
trans·du·o·de·nal
    sphinc·ter·ot·o·my
tran·sec·tion
trans·eth·moi·dal
trans·fec·tion
trans·fer
    cop·ing
    fac·tor
    genes
    RNA
trans·fer
    em·bryo t.
trans·fer·as·es
trans·fer·ence
    ex·tra·sen·so·ry thought t.
    neg·a·tive t.
    pas·sive t.
    pos·i·tive t.
trans·fer·ence
    neu·ro·sis
trans·fer·ence love
trans·ferred
    oph·thal·mia
    sen·sa·tion
trans·fer·rin
trans·fer·ring
    en·zymes
trans·fer-RNA

trans·fix
trans·fix·ion
  su·ture
trans·form·ant
trans·for·ma·tion
  cell t.
  Haldane t.
  Lobry de Bruyn-van
    Ekenstein t.
  lo·git t.
  lym·pho·cyte t.
  nod·u·lar t. of the liv·er
trans·formed
  lym·pho·cyte
trans·form·ing
  agent
  fac·tor
  gene
trans·fuse
trans·fu·sion
  ar·te·ri·al t.
  di·rect t.
  drip t.
  ex·change t.
  ex·san·gui·na·tion t.
  im·me·di·ate t.
  in·di·rect t.
  me·di·ate t.
  per·i·to·ne·al t.
  re·cip·ro·cal t.
  sub·cu·ta·ne·ous t.
  sub·sti·tu·tion t.
  to·tal t.
  twin-twin t.
trans·fu·sion
  hep·a·ti·tis
  ne·phri·tis
trans·glu·co·syl·ase
trans·gly·co·syl·ase
trans·hi·a·tal
  e·soph·a·gec·to·my
tran·sient
  agam·ma·glob·u·lin·e·mia
  al·bu·min·ur·ia
  hy·po·gam·ma·glob·u·lin·e·
    mia of in·fan·cy
  my·o·pia
tran·sient acan·tho·lyt·ic
  der·ma·to·sis
tran·sient is·che·mic
  at·tack
trans·il·i·ac
tran·sil·i·ent
trans·il·lu·mi·na·tion
trans·in·su·lar
trans·is·chi·ac
trans·isth·mi·an

tran·si·tion
  cer·vi·co·tho·rac·ic t.
  iso·mer·ic t.
tran·si·tion
  mu·ta·tion
  rays
tran·si·tion·al
  cell
  con·vo·lu·tion
  den·ture
  ep·i·the·li·um
  gy·rus
  leu·ko·cyte
  zone
tran·si·tion·al cell
  car·ci·no·ma
  pap·il·lo·ma
trans·ke·tol·ase
trans·ke·to·la·tion
trans·la·tion
trans·la·to·ry
  move·ment
trans·lo·ca·tion
  car·ri·er
  chro·mo·some
  mon·go·lism
trans·lo·ca·tion
  bal·anced t.
  re·cip·ro·cal t.
  ro·bert·so·ni·an t.
  un·bal·anced t.
trans·lu·cent
trans·lum·bar
  aor·tog·ra·phy
trans·mem·brane
  po·ten·tial
trans·meth·yl·ase
trans·meth·yl·a·tion
  fac·tor
trans·mi·gra·tion
  di·rect o·vu·lar t.
  ex·ter·nal o·vu·lar t.
  in·di·rect o·vu·lar t.
  in·ter·nal o·vu·lar t.
  o·vu·lar t.
trans·mis·si·ble
  en·ceph·a·lop·a·thy of mink
  en·ter·i·tis
  gas·tro·en·ter·i·tis of swine
  plas·mid
trans·mis·si·ble gas·tro·en·ter·
i·tis
  vi·rus of swine
trans·mis·si·ble tur·key en·ter·
i·tis
  vi·rus
trans·mis·si·ble ve·ne·re·al
  tu·mor

trans·mis·sion
du·plex t.
hor·i·zon·tal t.
iat·ro·gen·ic t.
neu·ro·hu·mor·al t.
trans·o·var·i·al t.
trans·sta·di·al t.
ver·ti·cal t.
trans·mit·ted
light
trans·mu·ral
pres·sure
trans·mu·ral my·o·car·di·al
in·farc·tion
trans·mu·ta·tion
trans·neu·ro·nal
at·ro·phy
trans·nex·us
chan·nel
trans·oc·u·lar
tran·so·nance
trans·or·bit·al
leu·kot·o·my
lo·bot·o·my
trans·os·se·ous
ve·nog·ra·phy
trans·o·var·i·al
trans·mis·sion
trans·par·ent
den·tin
sep·tum
ul·cer of the cor·nea
trans·pa·ri·e·tal
trans·pep·ti·dase
trans·pep·ti·da·tion
trans·per·i·to·ne·al
trans·phos·pha·tas·es
trans·phos·pho·ryl·as·es
trans·phos·pho·ryl·a·tion
tran·spir·a·ble
tran·spi·ra·tion
pul·mo·nary t.
tran·spire
trans·pla·cen·tal
trans·plant
Gallie's t.
trans·plan·tar
trans·plan·ta·tion
bone mar·row t.
t. of cor·nea
cor·ne·al t.
heart t.
pan·cre·at·i·co·du·o·de·nal
t.
re·nal t.
ten·don t.
tooth t.

trans·plan·ta·tion
ge·net·ics
trans·plant lung
syn·drome
trans·pleu·ral
trans·po·ri·on·ic
ax·is
trans·port
host
max·i·mum
me·di·um
num·ber
tet·a·ny
trans·port
ac·tive t.
ax·o·plas·mic t.
hy·dro·gen t.
ve·sic·u·lar t.
trans·pos·a·ble
el·e·ment
trans·pos·ase
trans·pose
trans·po·si·tion
t. of ar·te·ri·al stems
t. of the great ves·sels
trans·po·son
trans·pul·mo·nary
pres·sure
trans·py·lor·ic
plane
trans·sec·tion
trans·seg·men·tal
trans·sep·tal
fi·bers
or·chi·o·pexy
trans·sex·u·al
sur·gery
trans·sex·u·al·ism
trans·sphe·noi·dal
trans·sta·di·al
trans·mis·sion
trans·sul·fu·rase
trans·syn·ap·tic
chro·ma·tol·y·sis
de·gen·er·a·tion
trans·ten·to·ri·al
her·ni·a·tion
trans·tha·lam·ic
trans·ther·mia
trans·tho·rac·ic
e·soph·a·gec·to·my
pres·sure
trans·tho·ra·cot·o·my
tran·sub·stan·ti·a·tion
tran·su·date
tran·su·da·tion
tran·sude
tran·sul·fu·rase

trans·u·re·ter·o·u·re·ter·al
anas·to·mo·sis
trans·u·re·ter·o·u·re·ter·os·to·
my
trans·u·re·thral
re·sec·tion
trans·vag·i·nal
trans·vec·tor
trans·ver·sa·lis
trans·verse
am·pu·ta·tion
arch of foot
ar·tery of neck
co·lon
crest
di·am·e·ter
disk
duc·tules of ep·o·oph·o·ron
fas·cic·u·li
fi·bers of pons
fis·sure of cer·e·bel·lum
fis·sure of cer·e·brum
fis·sure of the lung
folds of rec·tum
fo·ra·men
for·nix
frac·ture
head
her·maph·ro·dit·ism
lie
lig·a·ment of ac·e·tab·u·
lum
lig·a·ment of at·las
lig·a·ment of el·bow
lig·a·ment of knee
lig·a·ment of leg
lig·a·ment of pel·vis
lig·a·ment of per·i·ne·um
line
mus·cle of ab·do·men
mus·cle of au·ri·cle
mus·cle of chin
mus·cle of nape
mus·cle of tho·rax
mus·cle of tongue
my·e·li·tis
nerve of neck
part
plane
pre·sen·ta·tion
pro·cess
ridge
sep·tum
si·nus
si·nus of per·i·car·di·um
vein of face
vein of scap·u·la
veins of neck

trans·verse ar·y·te·noid
mus·cle
trans·verse car·pal
lig·a·ment
trans·verse cer·vi·cal
ar·tery
trans·verse cru·ral
lig·a·ment
trans·ver·sec·to·my
trans·verse fa·cial
ar·tery
frac·ture
trans·verse hor·i·zon·tal
ax·is
trans·verse hu·mer·al
lig·a·ment
trans·verse met·a·car·pal
lig·a·ment
trans·verse met·a·tar·sal
lig·a·ment
trans·verse na·sal
groove
trans·verse oc·cip·i·tal
sul·cus
trans·verse oval
pel·vis
trans·verse pal·a·tine
ridge
su·ture
trans·verse pan·cre·at·ic
ar·tery
trans·verse rhomb·en·ce·phal·ic
flex·ure
trans·verse scap·u·lar
ar·tery
trans·verse tar·sal
ar·tic·u·la·tion
joint
trans·verse tem·po·ral
con·vo·lu·tions
gy·ri
sul·ci
trans·verse tib·i·o·fib·u·lar
lig·a·ment
trans·verse ves·i·cal
fold
trans·ver·sion
mu·ta·tion
trans·ver·so·cos·tal
trans·ver·so·spi·nal
mus·cle
trans·ver·so·u·re·thra·lis
trans·ver·so·ver·ti·cal
in·dex
trans·ver·sus
trans·ves·tism
trans·ves·tite
trans·ves·ti·tism

Trantas'
  dots
tran·yl·cyp·ro·mine sul·fate
tra·pe·zia
tra·pe·zi·al
tra·pe·zi·form
tra·pe·zi·o·met·a·car·pal
tra·pe·zi·um
  bone
tra·pe·zi·ums
tra·pe·zi·us
  mus·cle
trap·e·zoid
  body
  bone
  lig·a·ment
  line
  ridge
trap·i·dil
Trapp-Häser
  for·mu·la
Trapp's
  for·mu·la
Traube-Hering
  curves
  waves
Traube's
  bru·it
  cor·pus·cle
  dysp·nea
  plugs
  space
Traube's dou·ble
  tone
trau·ma
  birth t.
  t. from oc·clu·sion
  oc·clu·sal t.
  psy·chic t.
trau·mas
trau·mas·the·nia
trau·ma·ta
trau·mat·ic
  al·o·pe·cia
  amen·or·rhea
  am·pu·ta·tion
  ane·mia
  an·es·the·sia
  an·eu·rysm
  as·phyx·ia
  cat·a·ract
  der·ma·ti·tis
  en·ceph·a·lop·a·thy
  fe·ver
  gas·tri·tis
  her·pes
  me·nin·go·cele
  my·i·a·sis

  neur·as·the·nia
  neu·ri·tis
  neu·ro·ma
  neu·ro·sis
  oc·clu·sion
  or·chi·tis
  pneu·mo·nia
  psy·cho·sis
  ret·i·nop·a·thy
  tet·a·nus
trau·mat·ic cer·vi·cal
  dis·cop·a·thy
trau·mat·ic pro·gress·ive
  en·ceph·a·lop·a·thy
trau·ma·tism
trau·ma·tize
trau·ma·to·gen·ic
  oc·clu·sion
trau·ma·tol·o·gy
trau·ma·to·ne·sis
trau·ma·top·a·thy
trau·ma·top·nea
trau·ma·top·ne·ic
  wound
trau·ma·to·py·ra
trau·ma·to·sep·sis
trau·ma·to·ther·a·py
Trautmann's tri·an·gu·lar
  space
trav·el·er's
  di·ar·rhea
tra·verse
tray
  acryl·ic res·in t.
  an·neal·ing t.
  im·pres·sion t.
traz·o·done hy·dro·chlo·ride
Treacher Collins'
  syn·drome
trea·cle
treat
treat·ment
  Carrel's t.
  Dakin-Carrel t.
  Goeckerman t.
  heat t.
  in·su·lin co·ma t.
  iso·se·rum t.
  Kenny's t.
  light t.
  med·i·cal t.
  Mitchell's t.
  mor·al t.
  Nau·heim t.
  pal·li·a·tive t.
  pre·ven·tive t.
  pro·phy·lac·tic t.
  root ca·nal t.

Schott t.
shock t.
Tweed edge·wise t.
Weir Mitchell t.
treat·ment
den·ture
tre·foil
der·ma·ti·tis
ten·don
tre·ha·la
tre·ha·lose
Treitz'
arch
her·nia
lig·a·ment
mus·cle
Treitz's
fas·cia
fos·sa
Trélat's
sign
stools
tre·ma
Trem·a·to·da
trem·a·tode
trem·a·toid
trem·bles
trem·bling
pal·sy
trem·el·loid
trem·el·lose
trem·o·gram
trem·o·graph
trem·o·la·bile
trem·o·pho·bia
trem·or
ac·tion t.
al·ter·nat·ing t.
ar·sen·i·cal t.
t. ar·tu·um
be·nign es·sen·tial t.
coarse t.
con·tin·u·ous t.
ep·i·dem·ic t.
fi·bril·lary t.
fine t.
flap·ping t.
head t.'s
her·e·do·fa·mil·i·al t.
in·ten·tion t.
ki·net·ic t.
mer·cu·ri·al t.
me·tal·lic t.
t. opi·o·pha·go·rum
pas·sive t.
per·sis·tent t.
pos·tur·al t.
t. po·ta·to·rum

pro·gress·ive cer·e·bel·lar t.
sat·ur·nine t.
se·nile t.
stat·ic t.
t. ten·di·num
vo·li·tion·al t.
trem·or·gram
trem·o·sta·ble
trem·u·lor
trem·u·lous
iris
trench
fe·ver
foot
hand
lung
mouth
ne·phri·tis
Trendelenburg's
op·er·a·tion
po·si·tion
sign
symp·tom
test
trend of thought
tre·pan
trep·a·na·tion
t. of cor·nea
cor·ne·al t.
treph·i·na·tion
tre·phine
bi·op·sy
treph·o·cyte
trep·i·dant
trep·i·da·tio cor·dis
trep·i·da·tion
Trep·o·ne·ma
T. cal·li·gy·rum
T. ca·ra·te·um
T. cu·nic·u·li
T. gen·i·tal·is
T. hy·o·dys·en·te·ri·ae
T. mi·cro·den·ti·um
T. mu·co·sum
T. pal·li·dum
T. per·ten·ue
trep·o·ne·ma-im·mo·bi·liz·ing
an·ti·body
trep·o·ne·mal
an·ti·body
Trep·o·ne·ma pal·li·dum he·mag·glu·ti·na·tion
test
Trep·o·ne·ma pal·li·dum im·mo·bi·li·za·tion
re·ac·tion
test
trep·o·ne·ma·to·sis

trep·o·neme
trep·o·ne·mi·a·sis
trep·o·ne·mi·ci·dal
trep·pe
Tresilian's
  sign
tre·sis
tret·i·noin
Treves'
  fold
TRH stim·u·la·tion
  test
tri·a·ce·tic ac·id
tri·ac·e·tin
tri·a·ce·tyl·glyc·er·ol
tri·a·ce·tyl·o·le·an·do·my·cin
tri·ac·yl·glyc·er·ol
  t. li·pase
tri·ad
  acute com·pres·sion t.
  Beck's t.
  Bezold's t.
  Charcot's t.
  Fallot's t.
  he·pa·tic t.
  Hull's t.
  Hutchinson's t.
  Kartagener's t.
  Saint's t.
tri·ad
  syn·drome
tri·ad·ic
  sym·bi·o·sis
tri·age
tri·al
  base
  case
  den·ture
  frame
  lens·es
tri·al and er·ror
tri·am·cin·o·lone
  t. ac·e·to·nide
  t. di·ac·e·tate
tri-a·me·lia
tri·am·ter·ene
tri·an·gle
  anal t.
  an·te·ri·or t.
  Assézat's t.
  au·ric·u·lar t.
  t. of aus·cul·ta·tion
  ax·il·lary t.
  Béclard's t.
  Bonwill t.
  Bryant's t.
  Burow's t.
  Calot's t.

car·di·o·he·pat·ic t.
ca·rot·id t.'s
ce·phal·ic t.
cer·vi·cal t.
Codman's t.
cru·ral t.
del·toi·de·o·pec·to·ral t.
di·gas·tric t.
Einthoven's t.
Elaut's t.
t. of el·bow
fa·cial t.
Farabeuf's t.
fem·o·ral t.
t. of fil·let
fron·tal t.
Garland's t.
Gombault's t.
Grocco's t.
Grynfeltt's t.
Hesselbach's t.
il·i·o·fem·o·ral t.
in·fe·ri·or ca·rot·id t.
in·fe·ri·or oc·cip·i·tal t.
in·fra·cla·vic·u·lar t.
in·gui·nal t.
Koch's t.
Labbé's t.
Langenbeck's t.
Lesser's t.
Lesshaft's t.
Lieutaud's t.
lum·bar t.
lum·bo·cos·to·ab·dom·i·nal
  t.
Macewen's t.
Malgaigne's t.
Marcille's t.
mus·cu·lar t.
oc·cip·i·tal t.
omo·cla·vic·u·lar t.
omo·tra·che·al t.
pal·a·tal t.
par·a·ver·te·bral t.
Petit's lum·bar t.
Philippe's t.
Pirogoff's t.
pos·te·ri·or t. of neck
pu·bo·u·re·thral t.
Reil's t.
sa·cral t.
t. of safe·ty
Scarpa's t.
ster·no·cos·tal t.
sub·cla·vi·an t.
sub·in·gui·nal t.
sub·man·dib·u·lar t.
sub·max·il·lary t.

sub·men·tal t.
sub·oc·cip·i·tal t.
su·pe·ri·or ca·rot·id t.
su·pra·me·a·tal t.
tra·che·al t.
Tweed t.
um·bil·i·co·mam·mil·la·ry t.
uro·gen·i·tal t.
ves·i·cal t.
Ward's t.
Weber's t.
Wilde's t.
tri·an·gu·lar
  ban·dage
  bone
  car·ti·lage
  crest
  disk of wrist
  fas·cia
  fold
  fos·sa
  la·mel·la
  lig·a·ment
  lig·a·ments of liv·er
  mus·cle
  pit of ar·y·te·noid car·ti·
   lage
  re·cess
  ridge
  uter·us
tri·an·gu·la·ris
tri·an·gu·lar·i·ty of the
  teeth
tri·an·gu·lum
Tri·at·o·ma
Tri·a·tom·i·nae
tri·ax·i·al ref·er·ence
  sys·tem
tri·a·zo·lam
tri·az·o·lo·gua·nine
tri·a·zol·o·pyr·i·dine
  an·ti·de·pres·sant
trib·ade
trib·a·dism
trib·a·dy
tri·ba·sic
  cal·ci·um phos·phate
  mag·ne·si·um phos·phate
tri·bas·i·lar
  syn·os·to·sis
tribe
tri·bol·o·gy
tri·bo·lu·mi·nes·cence
tri·bra·chia
tri·bra·chi·us
tri·bro·mo·eth·a·nol
tri·brom·sa·lan
tri·bu·ty·rase

tri·bu·tyr·in
tri·bu·tyr·in·ase
tri·bu·tyr·yl·glyc·er·ol
TRIC
  agents
tri·cal·ci·um phos·phate
tri·car·box·yl·ic ac·id
  cy·cle
tri·ceph·a·lus
tri·ceps
  bur·sa
  mus·cle of arm
  mus·cle of calf
  re·flex
tri·ceps su·rae
  re·flex
trich·al·gia
trich·an·gi·on
trich·a·tro·phia
trich·aux·is
tri·chi·a·sis
trich·i·lem·mal
  cyst
trich·i·lem·mo·ma
Tri·chi·na
tri·chi·na
tri·chi·nae
Trich·i·nel·la
  T. spi·ra·lis
trich·i·nel·li·a·sis
Trich·i·nel·li·cae
Trich·i·nel·loi·dea
trich·i·nel·lo·sis
trich·i·ni·a·sis
trich·i·nif·er·ous
trich·i·ni·za·tion
tri·chi·no·scope
trich·i·no·sis
tri·chi·nous
trich·i·on
trich·ite
tri·chi·tis
tri·chlo·ral
tri·chlor·fon
tri·chlo·ride
tri·chlor·me·thi·a·zide
tri·chlor·meth·ine
tri·chlo·ro·a·ce·tic ac·id
tri·chlo·ro·eth·ane
tri·chlo·ro·eth·a·nol
tri·chlo·ro·eth·ene
tri·chlo·ro·eth·yl al·co·hol
tri·chlo·ro·eth·yl·ene
tri·chlo·ro·flu·o·ro·meth·ane
tri·chlo·ro·meth·ane
tri·chlo·ro·mon·o·flu·o·ro·meth·
  ane
tri·chlo·ro·phe·nol

trich·o·be·zoar
Trich·o·ceph·a·lus
trich·o·cla·sia
tri·choc·la·sis
trich·o·cryp·to·sis
trich·o·cyst
Trich·o·dec·tes
Trich·o·der·ma
trich·o·dis·co·ma
trich·o·dyn·ia
trich·o·ep·i·the·li·o·ma
  ac·quired t.
  des·mo·plas·tic t.
  he·red·i·tary mul·ti·ple t.
  t. pa·pil·lo·sum mul·ti·plex
trich·o·es·the·sia
trich·o·fol·lic·u·lo·ma
trich·o·gen
tri·chog·e·nous
trich·o·glos·sia
trich·o·hy·a·lin
trich·oid
trich·o·lem·mo·ma
trich·o·lith
trich·o·lo·gia
tri·chol·o·gy
tri·cho·ma
tri·cho·ma·tose
tri·cho·ma·to·sis
tri·chom·a·tous
trich·o·meg·a·ly
trich·o·mo·na·cide
trich·o·mon·ad
Trich·o·mo·nad·i·dae
Trich·o·mon·as
  T. buc·ca·lis
  T. foe·tus
  T. gal·li·nae
  T. gal·li·na·rum
  T. hom·i·nis
  T. ovis
  T. su·is
  T. te·nax
  T. va·gi·na·lis
trich·o·mo·ni·a·sis
  avi·an t.
  bo·vine t.
  t. vag·i·ni·tis
trich·o·my·ce·to·sis
trich·o·my·co·sis
  t. ax·il·la·ris
  t. chro·ma·ti·ca
  t. no·do·sa
  t. no·du·la·ris
  t. pal·mel·li·na
  t. pus·tu·lo·sa
trich·o·no·car·di·o·sis
  t. ax·il·la·ris

trich·o·no·do·sis
trich·o·no·sis
tri·cho·no·sus
  t. ver·si·col·or
trich·o·path·ic
trich·o·path·o·pho·bia
tri·chop·a·thy
tri·choph·a·gy
trich·o·pho·bia
trich·o·phyt·ic
trich·o·phy·tid
tri·choph·y·tin
trich·o·phy·to·be·zoar
Trich·o·phy·ton
  T. con·cen·tri·cum
  T. equi·num
  T. meg·ni·nii
  T. men·tag·ro·phytes
  T. ru·brum
  T. schoen·lei·nii
  T. si·mii
  T. ton·su·rans
  T. ver·ru·co·sum
  T. vi·o·la·ce·um
trich·o·phyt·o·sis
  t. bar·bae
  t. ca·pi·tis
  t. cor·po·ris
  t. cru·ris
  t. un·gui·um
Trich·o·pleu·ris
trich·o·po·li·o·sis
Tri·chop·tera
trich·o·pti·lo·sis
trich·o·rhi·no·pha·lan·ge·al
syn·drome
trich·or·rhex·is
  t. in·va·gi·na·ta
  t. no·do·sa
tri·chos·chi·sis
tri·chos·co·py
tri·cho·sis
  t. ca·run·cu·lae
  t. sen·si·ti·va
  t. se·to·sa
trich·o·so·ma·tous
Tri·cho·spo·ron
trich·o·spo·ro·sis
trich·o·sta·sis spi·nu·lo·sa
trich·o·stron·gyle
Trich·o·stron·gyl·i·dae
trich·o·stron·gy·lo·sis
Trich·o·stron·gy·lus
  T. ax·ei
  T. cap·ri·co·la
  T. co·lu·bri·for·mis
  T. lon·gi·spi·cu·la·ris

T. ten·u·is
T. vit·ri·nus
Trich·o·the·ci·um
trich·o·thi·o·dys·tro·phy
trich·o·til·lo·ma·nia
tri·chot·o·my
trich·o·tox·in
tri·chot·ro·phy
tri·chro·ic
tri·chro·ism
tri·chro·mat
tri·chro·mat·ic
tri·chro·ma·tism
anom·a·lous t.
tri·chro·ma·top·sia
tri·chrome
stain
tri·chro·mic
trich·ter·brust
trich·u·ri·a·sis
Trich·u·ris
T. trich·i·u·ra
tri·cip·i·tal
tri·clo·bi·so·ni·um chlo·ride
tri·clo·fen·ol pi·per·a·zine
tri·corn
tri·cor·nute
tri·cre·sol
tri·crot·ic
tri·cro·tism
tri·cro·tous
Tric·u·la
tri·cus·pid
ar·ea
atre·sia
in·com·pe·tence
in·suf·fi·cien·cy
mur·mur
or·i·fice
ste·no·sis
tooth
valve
tri·cus·pi·dal
tri·cus·pi·date
tri·cy·cla·mol chlo·ride
tri·cyc·lic
an·ti·de·pres·sant
tri·dac·ty·lous
tri·dent
hand
tri·den·tate
tri·der·mic
tri·der·mo·ma
tri·dig·i·tate
tri·di·hex·eth·yl chlo·ride
trid·y·mite
trid·y·mus
tri·el·con

tri·en·tine hy·dro·chlo·ride
tri·eth·a·nol·a·mine
tri·eth·yl·ene gly·col
tri·eth·yl·ene mel·a·mine
tri·eth·yl·ene phos·phor·a·mide
tri·eth·yl·ene·tet·ra·mine di·hy·dro·chlo·ride
tri·eth·yl·ene·thi·o·phos·phor·a·mide
tri·fa·cial
nerve
neu·ral·gia
tri·fid
stom·ach
tri·flu·o·per·a·zine hy·dro·chlo·ride
tri·flu·per·i·dol hy·dro·chlo·ride
tri·flu·pro·ma·zine hy·dro·chlo·ride
tri·flur·i·dine
tri·fo·cal
lens
tri·fo·li·o·sis
tri·fur·ca·tion
tri·gas·tric
tri·gem·i·nal
cav·i·ty
cough
crest
de·com·pres·sion
gan·gli·on
im·pres·sion
lem·nis·cus
nerve
neu·ral·gia
pulse
rhi·zot·o·my
rhythm
trac·tot·o·my
tri·ge·mi·no·fa·cial
re·flex
tri·gem·i·nus
tri·gem·i·ny
trig·e·nol·line
trig·ger
ar·ea
fin·ger
point
zone
trig·gered
ac·tiv·i·ty
tri·glyc·er·ide
tri·go·na
trig·o·nal
tri·gone
t. of au·di·to·ry nerve
t. of blad·der
col·lat·er·al t.

tri·gone *(continued)*
  del·toi·de·o·pec·to·ral t.
  fi·brous t.'s of heart
  t. of fil·let
  t. of ha·ben·u·la
  t. of hy·po·glos·sal nerve
  in·gui·nal t.
  t. of lat·er·al ven·tri·cle
  left fi·brous t.
  Lieutaud's t.
  Müller's t.
  ol·fac·to·ry t.
  right fi·brous t.
  t. of va·gus nerve
  ver·te·bro·cos·tal t.
trig·o·nel·line
tri·go·nid
tri·go·ni·tis
trig·o·no·ce·phal·ic
trig·o·no·ceph·a·ly
tri·go·num
  t. acus·ti·ci
  t. ce·re·bra·le
  t. cer·vi·ca·le
  t. cer·vi·ca·le an·te·ri·us
  t. cer·vi·ca·le pos·te·ri·us
  t. col·li
  t. del·toi·de·o·pec·to·ra·le
  tri·go·na fi·bro·sa cor·dis
  t. hy·po·glos·si
  t. lem·nis·ci
  t. lum·bo·cos·ta·le
  t. pa·la·ti
  t. ster·no·cos·ta·le
  t. ven·tric·u·li
tri·hy·brid
tri·hy·dric
  al·co·hol
tri·hy·drox·y·es·trin
tri·in·i·od·y·mus
tri·i·o·dide
tri·i·o·do·meth·ane
tri·i·o·do·thy·ro·nine
  tox·i·co·sis
tri·i·o·do·thy·ro·nine up·take
  test
tri·ke·to·hy·drin·dene
  re·ac·tion
tri·ke·to·hy·drin·dene hy·drate
tri·ke·to·pu·rine
tri·labe
tri·lam·i·nar
  blas·to·derm
tri·lat·er·al
tri·lo·bate
tri·lobed
tri·loc·u·lar

tril·o·gy
  t. of Fallot
tri·lo·stane
tri·mal·le·o·lar
  frac·ture
tri·mas·ti·gote
tri·mep·ra·zine tar·trate
tri·mes·ter
tri·met·a·phan cam·sy·late
tri·me·taz·i·dine
tri·meth·a·di·one
tri·meth·a·phan cam·sy·late
tri·meth·i·di·um meth·o·sul·fate
tri·meth·o·benz·a·mide hy·dro·
  chlo·ride
tri·meth·o·prim
tri·meth·yl·a·mine
tri·meth·yl·am·i·nur·ia
tri·meth·yl·car·bin·ol
tri·meth·yl·ene
tri·meth·yl·eth·yl·ene
tri·meth·yl·gly·co·coll an·hy·
  dride
tri·meth·y·lo·mel·a·mine
tri·met·o·zine
tri·me·trex·ate
tri·mip·ra·mine
tri·mor·phic
tri·mor·phism
tri·mor·phous
tri·ni·tro·cel·lu·lose
tri·ni·tro·glyc·er·in
tri·ni·tro·tol·u·ene
tri·ni·tro·tol·u·ol
tri·nu·cle·o·tide
tri·o·ki·nase
tri·o·le·in
tri·oph·thal·mos
tri·or·chism
tri·ose
tri·ose·ki·nase
tri·ose·phos·phate isom·er·ase
tri·o·tus
tri·ox·ide
tri·ox·sa·len
tri·ox·y·meth·yl·ene
tri·pal·mi·tin
tri·par·a·nol
tri·pel·en·na·mine hy·dro·chlo·
  ride
tri·pha·lan·gia
trip·ham·mer
  pulse
tri·phen·yl·meth·ane
  dyes
tri·phos·pha·tase
tri·phos·pho·pyr·i·dine nu·cle·
  o·tide

tri·phyl·lo·ma·tous
   ter·a·to·ma
Tripier's
   am·pu·ta·tion
tri·plant
   im·plant
tri·ple
   ar·throd·e·sis
   bond
   phos·phate
   quar·tan
   re·sponse
   rhythm
   vi·sion
tri·ple·gia
tri·ple symp·tom
   com·plex
trip·let
   ox·y·gen
   state
trip·let
   non·sense t.
tri·ple X
   syn·drome
trip·lo·blas·tic
trip·loid
trip·loi·dy
trip·lo·pia
tri·pod
   Haller's t.
   vi·tal t.
tri·po·dia
tri·prol·i·dine hy·dro·chlo·ride
tri·pro·so·pus
trip·sis
tri·que·tral
   bone
tri·que·trous
   car·ti·lage
tri·que·trum
tri·ra·di·al
tri·ra·di·ate
tri·ra·di·us
tri·sac·cha·ride
tris(hy·drox·y·meth·yl)meth·yl·
   a·mine
tris·kai·dek·a·pho·bia
tris·mic
tris·moid
tris·mus
   t. cap·i·stra·tus
   t. do·lo·rif·i·cus
   t. nas·cen·ti·um
   t. ne·o·na·to·rum
   t. sar·do·ni·cus
tri·so·mic
tri·so·my

tri·so·my C
   syn·drome
tri·so·my D
   syn·drome
tri·so·my E
   syn·drome
tri·splanch·nic
tri·ste·a·rin
tri·stich·ia
tri·sul·cate
tri·symp·tome
tri·ta·nom·a·ly
trit·an·o·pia
tri·ter·penes
trit·i·at·ed
   thy·mi·dine
tri·ti·ce·o·glos·sus
tri·ti·ceous
tri·tic·e·um
trit·i·um
tri·to·cal·ine
tri·ton
   tu·mor
trit·o·qual·ine
Tri·trich·o·mon·as
tri·tu·ber·cu·lar
trit·u·ra·ble
trit·u·rate
   tab·let t.
trit·u·ra·tion
tri·tyl
tri·va·lence
tri·va·len·cy
tri·va·lent
tri·valve
triv·i·al name
tri·zon·al
tro·car
tro·chan·ter
   great·er t.
   less·er t.
   small t.
   third t.
tro·chan·ter
   re·flex
tro·chan·ter·i·an
tro·chan·ter·ic
   bur·sa
   bur·si·tis
   crest
   fos·sa
   syn·drome
tro·chan·ter·plas·ty
tro·chan·tin
tro·chan·tin·i·an
tro·che
tro·chis·ci
tro·chis·cus

troch·lea
    t. fe·mo·ris
    t. of hu·mer·us
troch·le·ae
troch·le·ar
    fos·sa
    nerve
    notch
    nu·cle·us
    pit
    pro·cess
    spine
troch·le·ar·i·form
troch·le·ar·is
troch·le·ar syn·o·vi·al
    bur·sa
troch·le·i·form
troch·o·car·dia
tro·choid
    ar·tic·u·la·tion
    joint
tro·chor·i·zo·car·dia
Trog·lo·tre·ma sal·min·co·la
Troisier's
    gan·gli·on
    node
tro·la·mine
tro·land
Trolard's
    vein
tro·le·an·do·my·cin
trol·ni·trate phos·phate
Tröltsch's
    cor·pus·cles
    fold
    pock·ets
    re·cess·es
Trom·bic·u·la
    T. ak·a·mu·shi
    T. al·fred·du·gesi
    T. de·li·en·sis
trom·bic·u·li·a·sis
trom·bic·u·lid
Trom·bic·u·li·dae
Trom·bi·di·i·dae
tro·meth·a·mine
Trömner's
    re·flex
tro·na
tro·pa·ic ac·id
tro·pane
tro·pate
tro·pe·ic ac·id
tro·pe·ine
tro·pen·tane
tro·pe·o·lins
troph·ec·to·derm
troph·e·de·ma

tro·phe·sic
troph·e·sy
tro·phic
    change
    gan·grene
    hor·mones
    nu·cle·us
    ul·cer
tro·phic·i·ty
tro·phism
troph·o·blast
    plas·mo·di·al t.
    syn·cy·tial t.
troph·o·blas·tic
    la·cu·na
    oper·cu·lum
troph·o·blas·to·ma
troph·o·chro·ma·tin
troph·o·chro·mid·ia
troph·o·cyte
troph·o·derm
troph·o·der·ma·to·neu·ro·sis
troph·o·dy·nam·ics
troph·o·neu·ro·sis
    fa·cial t.
    lin·gual t.
    mus·cu·lar t.
    Romberg's t.
troph·o·neu·rot·ic
    at·ro·phy
    lep·ro·sy
troph·o·nu·cle·us
troph·o·plasm
troph·o·plast
troph·o·spon·gia
troph·o·tax·is
troph·o·tro·pic
    zone of Hess
tro·phot·ro·pism
troph·o·zo·ite
tro·pia
tro·pic
    hor·mones
tro·pic ac·id
trop·i·cal
    ab·scess
    ac·ne
    ane·mia
    boil
    bu·bo
    di·ar·rhea
    ec·ze·ma
    eo·sin·o·phil·ia
    hy·phe·mia
    li·chen
    mask
    mea·sles
    med·i·cine

my·o·si·tis
py·o·my·o·si·tis
sore
sple·no·meg·a·ly
sprue
thei·le·ri·o·sis
ty·phus
ul·cer
trop·i·cal ca·nine
pan·cy·to·pe·nia
trop·i·cal sple·no·meg·a·ly
syn·drome
tro·pic·a·mide
tro·pine
t. man·del·ate
t. tro·pate
tro·pism
vi·ral t.
tro·po·col·la·gen
tro·pom·e·ter
tro·po·my·o·sin
tro·po·nin
trough
gin·gi·val t.
Langmuir t.
syn·ap·tic t.
Trousseau-Lallemand
bod·ies
Trousseau's
point
sign
spot
syn·drome
trox·e·ru·tin
trox·i·done
true
an·eu·rysm
an·ky·lo·sis
ap·nea
ce·men·to·ma
cho·lin·es·ter·ase
con·ju·gate
di·ver·tic·u·lum
dwarf·ism
glot·tis
her·maph·ro·dit·ism
hy·per·tro·phy
knot
knot of um·bil·i·cal cord
pel·vis
ribs
thirst
ver·te·bra
true uter·ine
in·er·tia
true vo·cal
cord
trun·cal

trun·cate
as·cer·tain·ment
trun·ci
trun·cus
t. ar·te·ri·o·sus
t. ar·te·ri·o·sus com·mu·nis
per·sis·tent t. ar·te·ri·o·sus
Trunecek's
symp·tom
trunk
atri·o·ven·tric·u·lar t.
t.'s of brach·i·al plex·us
bra·chi·o·ce·phal·ic t.
bron·cho·me·di·as·ti·nal t.
ce·li·ac t.
t. of cor·pus cal·lo·sum
cos·to·cer·vi·cal t.
in·fe·ri·or t.
in·tes·ti·nal t.'s
jug·u·lar t.
lum·bar t.'s
lum·bo·sa·cral t.
mid·dle t.
nerve t.
pul·mo·nary t.
sub·cla·vi·an t.
su·pe·ri·or t.
sym·pa·thet·ic t.
thy·ro·cer·vi·cal t.
va·gal t.
tru·sion
truss
truth
se·rum
try-in
try·pan blue
try·pan·i·ci·dal
try·pan·i·cide
tryp·a·nid
try·pan·o·ci·dal
try·pan·o·cide
Try·pan·o·plas·ma
Try·pan·o·so·ma
T. avi·um
T. brucei
T. brucei brucei
T. brucei gam·bi·ense
T. brucei rho·des·i·ense
T. con·go·lense
T. cru·zi
T. di·mor·phon
T. equi·num
T. equi·per·dum
T. es·com·e·lis
T. ev·an·si
T. gam·bi·ense
T. hip·pi·cum
T. hom·i·nis

Try·pan·o·so·ma *(continued)*
   T. ig·no·tum
   T. lew·isi
   T. mel·o·pha·gi·um
   T. ran·geli
   T. rho·des·i·ense
   T. sim·i·ae
   T. su·is
   T. thei·leri
   T. tri·at·o·mae
   T. ugan·den·se
   T. vi·vax
try·pan·o·so·mat·id
Try·pan·o·so·mat·i·dae
try·pan·o·some
   fe·ver
   stage
try·pan·o·so·mi·a·sis
   acute t.
   Af·ri·can t.
   chron·ic t.
   Cruz t.
   East Af·ri·can t.
   Gam·bi·an t.
   Rho·de·sian t.
   South Amer·i·can t.
   West Af·ri·can t.
try·pan·o·so·mic
try·pan·o·so·mi·cide
try·pan·o·so·mid
try·pan red
tryp·ar·sa·mide
tryp·o·mas·ti·gote
tryp·sin
   crys·tal·lized t.
tryp·sin
   in·hib·i·tor
tryp·sin G-band·ing
   stain
tryp·sin·o·gen
tryp·so·gen
trypt·a·mine
trypt·a·mine-stro·phan·thi·din
tryp·tic
tryp·tone
tryp·to·ne·mia
tryp·to·phan
   t. de·car·box·yl·ase
   t. des·mo·lase
   t. ox·y·gen·ase
   t. pyr·ro·lase
   t. syn·thase
   t. syn·the·tase
tryp·to·pha·nase
tryp·to·pha·nu·ria
   t. with dwarf·ism
tset·se

TSH stim·u·lat·ing
   test
tsu·tsu·ga·mu·shi
   dis·ease
   fe·ver
tu·a·mi·no·hep·tane
tu·ba
   t. acus·ti·ca
   t. eu·sta·chi·a·na
   t. eu·sta·chii
   t. fal·lo·pi·a·na
   t. fal·lo·pii
tu·bae
tub·age
tub·al
   abor·tion
   car·ti·lage
   col·ic
   dys·men·or·rhea
   ex·trem·i·ty
   in·fan·ti·lism
   in·suf·fla·tion
   li·ga·tion
   preg·nan·cy
   ton·sil
tub·al air
   cells
tu·ba·tor·sion
tub·ba
tub·bae
Tubbs'
   di·la·tor
tube
   cast
   teeth
tube
   Abbott's t.
   air t.
   au·di·to·ry t.
   Babcock t.
   Bouchut's t.
   Bourdon t.
   bron·chi·al t.'s
   Cantor t.
   car·di·ac t.
   Carlen's t.
   cath·ode ray t.
   Ce·les·tin t.
   Coolidge t.
   di·ges·tive t.
   drain·age t.
   Durham's t.
   em·py·e·ma t.
   en·do·bron·chi·al t.
   en·do·tra·che·al t.
   eu·sta·chi·an t.
   fal·lo·pi·an t.
   feed·ing t.

Ferrein's t.
Geiger-Müller t.
germ t.
Haldane t.
in·tra·tra·che·al t.
Levin t.
Martin's t.
med·ul·lary t.
Miescher's t.'s
Miller-Abbott t.
Moss t.
na·so·gas·tric t.
na·so·tra·che·al t.
neu·ral t.
O'Dwyer's t.
or·o·tra·che·al t.
oto·pha·ryn·ge·al t.
pha·ryn·go·tym·pan·ic t.
pho·to·mul·ti·pli·er t.
Pitot t.
pus t.
Rehfuss stom·ach t.
Robertshaw t.
roll t.
Ruysch's t.
Ryle's t.
Sengstaken-Blakemore t.
Southey's t.'s
stom·ach t.
T t.
test t.
Tovell t.
Toynbee's t.
tra·che·al t.
tra·che·ot·o·my t.
tym·pan·os·to·my t.
uter·ine t.
vac·u·um t.
Venturi t.
Wangensteen t.
x-ray t.
tu·bec·to·my
tubed
flap
tubed ped·i·cle
flap
tu·ber
t. an·te·ri·us
ash·en t.
cal·ca·ne·al t.
t. cal·cis
t. co·chle·ae
t. cor·po·ris cal·losi
t. dor·sa·le
eu·sta·chi·an t.
fron·tal t.
gray t.
t. of is·chi·um

omen·tal t.
pa·ri·e·tal t.
t. ra·dii
t. val·vu·lae
t. zy·go·ma·ti·cum
tu·bera
tu·be·ral
nu·clei
tu·ber·cle
ba·cil·lus
tu·ber·cle
ac·ces·so·ry t.
acous·tic t.
ad·duc·tor t.
amyg·da·loid t.
an·a·tom·i·cal t.
an·te·ri·or t. of at·las
an·te·ri·or t. of cer·vi·cal ver·te·brae
t. of an·te·ri·or sca·lene mus·cle
an·te·ri·or t. of thal·a·mus
ar·tic·u·lar t.
ash·en t.
au·ric·u·lar t.
cal·ca·ne·al t.
Carabelli t.
ca·rot·id t.
ca·se·ous t.
Chassaignac's t.
co·noid t.
cor·nic·u·late t.
crown t.
t. of cu·ne·ate nu·cle·us
cu·ne·i·form t.
dar·win·i·an t.
den·tal t.
dis·sec·tion t.
dor·sal t.
ep·i·glot·tic t.
fi·brous t.
ge·ni·al t.
gen·i·tal t.
Gerdy's t.
Ghon's t.
grac·ile t.
gray t.
great·er t. of hu·mer·us
hard t.
hy·a·line t.
il·i·ac t.
t. of il·i·ac crest
in·fe·ri·or thy·roid t.
in·fra·gle·noid t.
in·ter·con·dy·lar t.
in·ter·ve·nous t.
jug·u·lar t.
la·bi·al t.

tu·ber·cle *(continued)*
  lat·er·al t. of pos·te·ri·or
   pro·cess of ta·lus
  less·er t. of hu·mer·us
  Lisfranc's t.
  Lister's t.
  Low·er's t.
  mam·il·lary t.
  mam·il·lary t. of hy·po·
   thal·a·mus
  mar·gi·nal t.
  me·di·al t. of pos·te·ri·or
   pro·cess of ta·lus
  men·tal t.
  Montgomery's t.'s
  Morgagni's t.
  Müller's t.
  nu·chal t.
  t. of nu·cle·us grac·i·lis
  ob·tu·ra·tor t.
  ol·fac·to·ry t.
  or·bi·tal t.
  phal·lic t.
  pha·ryn·ge·al t.
  pos·te·ri·or t. of at·las
  pos·te·ri·or t. of cer·vi·cal
   ver·te·brae
  post·mor·tem t.
  Princeteau's t.
  pro·sec·tor's t.
  pter·y·goid t.
  pu·bic t.
  t. of rib
  Rolando's t.
  t. of sad·dle
  Santorini's t.
  sca·lene t. of Lisfranc
  t. of scaph·oid bone
  se·ba·ceous t.
  si·nus t.
  soft t.
  su·pe·ri·or thy·roid t.
  su·pra·gle·noid t.
  su·pra·trag·ic t.
  t. of tooth
  t. of tra·pe·zi·um
  t. of up·per lip
  wedge-shaped t.
  Whitnall's t.
  Wrisberg's t.
tu·ber·cu·la
tu·ber·cu·lar
tu·ber·cu·late
tu·ber·cu·lat·ed
tu·ber·cu·la·tion
tu·ber·cu·lid
  nod·u·lar t.
  pap·u·lar t.

pap·u·lo·ne·crot·ic t.
  ro·sa·cea-like t.
tu·ber·cu·lin
  Koch's old t.
  Koch's orig·i·nal t.
  pu·ri·fied pro·tein de·riv·a·
   tive of t.
tu·ber·cu·lin
  test
tu·ber·cu·li·tis
tu·ber·cu·li·za·tion
tu·ber·cu·lo·cele
tu·ber·cu·lo·che·mo·ther·a·peu·
tic
tu·ber·cu·lo·ci·dal
tu·ber·cu·lo·der·ma
tu·ber·cu·lo·fi·broid
tu·ber·cu·loid
  lep·ro·sy
tu·ber·cu·lo·ma
tu·ber·cu·lo-op·son·ic
  in·dex
tu·ber·cu·lo·pro·tein
tu·ber·cu·lo·sis
  acute t.
  acute mil·i·a·ry t.
  adult t.
  an·thra·cot·ic t.
  ar·rest·ed t.
  at·ten·u·at·ed t.
  ba·sal t.
  ce·re·bral t.
  child·hood type t.
  cu·ta·ne·ous t.
  t. cu·tis
  t. cu·tis fol·lic·u·la·ris dis·
   sem·i·na·ta
  t. cu·tis lu·po·sa
  t. cu·tis or·i·fi·ci·a·lis
  t. cu·tis ver·ru·co·sa
  der·mal t.
  dis·sem·i·nat·ed t.
  en·ter·ic t.
  gen·er·al t.
  healed t.
  in·ac·tive t.
  mil·i·a·ry t.
  open t.
  t. pap·u·lo·ne·crot·i·ca
  post·pri·mary t.
  pri·mary t.
  pul·mo·nary t.
  re·in·fec·tion t.
  sec·on·dary t.
  t. ul·ce·ro·sa
tu·ber·cu·lo·sis
  vac·cine
tu·ber·cu·lo·stat

tu·ber·cu·lo·stat·ic
tu·ber·cu·lous
  ab·scess
  bron·cho·pneu·mo·nia
  en·ter·i·tis
  lym·phad·e·ni·tis
  men·in·gi·tis
  ne·phri·tis
  per·i·to·ni·tis
  rheu·ma·tism
  scrof·u·lo·der·ma
  spon·dy·li·tis
  wart
tu·ber·cu·lum
  t. an·te·ri·us ver·te·bra·rum
    cer·vi·ca·li·um
  t. ar·thri·ti·cum
  t. ci·ne·re·um
  t. co·ro·nae
  tu·ber·cu·la do·lo·ro·sa
  t. hy·po·glos·si
  t. im·par
  t. mal·lei
  t. ol·fac·to·ri·um
  t. pos·te·ri·us ver·te·bra·
    rum cer·vi·ca·li·um
  t. se·ba·ce·um
  t. sep·ti na·ri·um
  t. su·pe·ri·us
  t. syph·i·li·ti·cum
tu·ber·if·er·ous
tu·ber·o·in·fun·dib·u·lar
  tract
tu·ber·ose
tu·ber·os·i·tas
  t. co·ra·coi·dea
  t. cos·ta·lis
  t. un·gui·cu·la·ris
tu·ber·os·i·ty
  bi·cip·i·tal t.
  cal·ca·ne·al t.
  cor·a·coid t.
  cos·tal t.
  t. of cu·boid bone
  del·toid t.
  t. of fifth met·a·tar·sal
  t. of first met·a·tar·sal
  glu·te·al t.
  great·er t. of hu·mer·us
  il·i·ac t.
  in·fra·gle·noid t.
  is·chi·al t.
  lat·er·al fem·o·ral t.
  less·er t. of hu·mer·us
  mas·se·ter·ic t.
  max·il·lary t.
  me·di·al fem·o·ral t.
  t. of na·vic·u·lar bone

  pter·y·goid t.
  t. of ra·di·us
  sa·cral t.
  scaph·oid t.
  tib·i·al t.
  t. of ul·na
  un·gual t.
tu·ber·os·i·ty
  re·duc·tion
tu·ber·ous
  root
  scle·ro·sis
tu·bi
Tü·bing·er
  pe·rim·e·ter
tu·bo·ab·dom·i·nal
  preg·nan·cy
tu·bo·cu·ra·rine chlo·ride
tu·bo·lig·a·men·tous
tu·bo·o·var·i·an
  ab·scess
  preg·nan·cy
  var·i·co·cele
tu·bo·o·var·i·ec·to·my
tu·bo·o·va·ri·tis
tu·bo·per·i·to·ne·al
tu·bo·plas·ty
tu·bo·re·tic·u·lar
  struc·ture
tu·bo·tor·sion
tu·bo·tym·pa·nal
tu·bo·tym·pan·ic
  ca·nal
  re·cess
tu·bo·u·ter·ine
  preg·nan·cy
tu·bo·vag·i·nal
tu·bu·lar
  ad·e·no·ma
  an·eu·rysm
  car·ci·no·ma
  cyst
  for·ceps
  gland
  max·i·mum
  res·pi·ra·tion
  vi·sion
tu·bu·lar ex·cre·to·ry
  mass
tu·bu·la·ture
tu·bule
  Albarran y Dominguez' t.'s
  col·lect·ing t.
  con·nect·ing t.
  con·vo·lut·ed t. of kid·ney
  con·vo·lut·ed sem·i·nif·er·
    ous t.
  den·tal t.'s

tu·bule *(continued)*
  den·ti·nal t.'s
  dis·charg·ing t.
  Henle's t.'s
  Kobelt's t.'s
  mal·pi·ghi·an t.'s
  mes·o·neph·ric t.
  met·a·neph·ric t.
  par·a·gen·i·tal t.'s
  pro·neph·ric t.
  sem·i·nif·er·ous t.
  Skene's t.'s
  spi·ral t.
  straight t.
  T t.
  uri·nif·er·ous t.
  wolff·i·an t.'s
tu·bu·li
tu·bu·li·form
tu·bu·lin
tu·bu·li·za·tion
tu·bu·lo·ac·i·nar
  gland
tu·bu·lo·al·ve·o·lar
  gland
tu·bu·lo·cyst
tu·bu·lo·der·moid
tu·bu·lo·in·ter·sti·tial
  ne·phri·tis
tu·bu·lo·rac·e·mose
tu·bu·lor·rhex·is
tu·bu·lose
tu·bu·lous
tu·bu·lus
  tu·bu·li bil·i·fe·ri
  t. con·tor·tus
  tu·bu·li den·ta·les
  tu·bu·li ep·o·oph·o·ri
  tu·bu·li ga·lac·to·pho·ri
  tu·bu·li lac·ti·fe·ri
  tu·bu·li pa·ro·o·pho·ri
  t. rec·tus
tu·bus
  t. di·ges·to·ri·us
  t. me·dul·la·ris
  t. ver·te·bra·lis
Tucker-McLean
  for·ceps
Tuffier's
  test
tuff·stone
  body
tuft
  enam·el t.
  mal·pi·ghi·an t.
  syn·o·vi·al t.'s

tufted
  cell
  pha·lanx
tug
  tra·che·al t.
tug·ging
tu·la·re·mia
tu·la·re·mic
  chan·cre
  con·junc·ti·vi·tis
  pneu·mo·nia
tulle gras
Tulpius'
  valve
Tulp's
  valve
tum·bu·der·mal
  my·i·a·sis
tu·me·fa·cient
tu·me·fac·tion
tu·me·fy
tu·men·tia
tu·mes·cence
tu·mes·cent
tu·mid
tu·mor
  ac·i·nar cell t.
  acute splen·ic t.
  ad·e·noid t.
  ad·e·no·ma·toid t.
  ad·e·no·ma·toid odon·to·gen·ic t.
  ad·i·pose t.
  am·e·lo·blas·tic ad·e·no·ma·toid t.
  am·y·loid t.
  an·gi·o·ma·toid t.
  aor·tic body t.
  Bednar t.
  be·nign t.
  blood t.
  Brenner t.
  Brooke's t.
  brown t.
  Buschke-Löwenstein t.
  cal·ci·fy·ing ep·i·the·li·al odon·to·gen·ic t.
  car·ci·noid t.
  ca·rot·id body t.
  cel·lu·lar t.
  cer·e·bel·lo·pon·tine an·gle t.
  che·mo·re·cep·tor t.
  chro·maf·fin t.
  Codman's t.
  col·li·sion t.
  con·nec·tive t.
  der·mal duct t.

der·moid t.
des·moid t.
eighth nerve t.
em·bry·o·nal t.
em·bry·o·nal t. of cil·i·ary
  body
em·bry·on·ic t.
en·do·der·mal si·nus t.
en·do·me·tri·oid t.
Erdheim t.
Ewing's t.
fe·cal t.
fi·broid t.
gi·ant cell t. of bone
gi·ant cell t. of ten·don
  sheath
glo·mus t.
glo·mus ju·gu·la·re t.
Godwin t.
gran·u·lar cell t.
gran·u·lo·sa cell t.
Grawitz' t.
Gubler's t.
haar·scheibe t.
het·er·ol·o·gous t.
hi·lar cell t. of ova·ry
his·toid t.
ho·mol·o·gous t.
Hürthle cell t.
hy·lic t.
in·no·cent t.
in·ter·sti·tial cell t. of
  tes·tis
Koenen's t.
Krukenberg's t.
Landschutz t.
Lindau's t.
ma·lig·nant t.
mel·a·not·ic neu·ro·ec·to·
  der·mal t.
Merkel cell t.
mes·o·neph·roid t.
mixed t.
mixed mes·o·der·mal t.
mixed t. of sal·i·vary gland
mixed t. of skin
mu·co·ep·i·der·moid t.
Nelson t.
oil t.
on·co·cyt·ic he·pa·to·cel·lu·
  lar t.
or·gan·oid t.
Pancoast t.
pap·il·lary t.
par·af·fin t.
pearl t.
phan·tom t.
phyl·lodes t.

pi·lar t. of scalp
Pindborg t.
pon·tine an·gle t.
po·ta·to t. of neck
Pott's puffy t.
preg·nan·cy t.
ra·nine t.
Rathke's pouch t.
Recklinghausen's t.
ret·i·nal an·la·ge t.
Rous t.
sand t.
Sertoli cell t.
squa·mous odon·to·gen·ic t.
sug·ar t.
su·pe·ri·or pul·mo·nary sul·
  cus t.
ter·a·toid t.
the·ca cell t.
trans·mis·si·ble ve·ne·re·al
  t.
tri·ton t.
tur·ban t.
vil·lous t.
Warthin's t.
Wilms' t.
Ya·ba t.
yolk sac t.
Zollinger-Ellison t.
tu·mor
  an·ti·gens
  em·bo·lism
  mark·er
  stage
  vi·rus
tu·mor·af·fin
tu·mor·al
  cal·ci·no·sis
tu·mor an·gi·o·gen·ic
  fac·tor
tu·mor bur·den
tu·mor·i·ci·dal
tu·mor·i·gen·e·sis
  for·eign body t.
tu·mor·i·gen·ic
tu·mor·lets
tu·mor ly·sis
  syn·drome
tu·mor ne·cro·sis
  fac·tor
tu·mor·ous
tu·mor-spe·cif·ic trans·plan·ta·
  tion
  an·ti·gens
tu·mul·tus cor·dis
Tun·ga pen·e·trans
tun·gi·a·sis
Tung·i·dae

tung·sten
t. car·bide
tu·nic
Bichat's t.
Brücke's t.
fi·brous t. of cor·pus spon·gi·o·sum
fi·brous t. of eye
mu·co·sal t.'s
mu·cous t.'s
mus·cu·lar t.'s
ner·vous t. of eye·ball
se·rous t.
tu·ni·ca
t. ab·do·mi·na·lis
t. al·bu·gin·ea oc·u·li
t. car·nea
t. elas·ti·ca
t. ex·ter·na oc·u·li
t. ex·ter·na the·cae fol·lic·u·li
t. ex·ti·ma
t. fi·bro·sa re·nis
Haller's t. vas·cu·lo·sa
t. in·ter·na the·cae fol·lic·u·li
t. ner·vea
t. pro·pria
t. pro·pria co·rii
t. pro·pria li·e·nis
t. re·flexa
t. scle·rot·i·ca
t. sub·mu·co·sa
t. va·gi·na·lis com·mu·nis
t. vas·cu·lo·sa
t. vas·cu·lo·sa len·tis
t. vas·cu·lo·sa oc·u·li
t. vas·cu·lo·sa tes·tis
t. vi·trea
tu·ni·cae
tun·ing
fork
tun·nel
cells
dis·ease
vi·sion
tun·nel
car·pal t.
Corti's t.
Tuo·hy
nee·dle
tu·ran·ose
tur·ban
tu·mor
Tur·ba·trix
tur·bid
tur·bi·dim·e·ter
tur·bi·di·met·ric

tur·bi·dim·e·try
tur·bid·i·ty
tur·bi·nal
var·ix
tur·bi·nate
tur·bi·nat·ed
body
bones
crest
tur·bi·nec·to·my
tur·bi·no·tome
tur·bi·not·o·my
Türck's
bun·dle
col·umn
de·gen·er·a·tion
tract
Turcot
syn·drome
tur·ges·cence
tur·ges·cent
tur·gid
tur·gom·e·ter
tur·gor
t. vi·ta·lis
tu·ris·ta
Türk
cell
tur·key me·nin·go·en·ceph·a·li·tis
vi·rus
tur·key red
Turk·ish
sad·dle
Türk's
leu·ko·cyte
Turlock
vi·rus
tur·mer·ic
turn
Turner's
sul·cus
syn·drome
tooth
turn·o·ver
flap
tur·pen·tine
en·e·ma
poi·son·ing
tur·pen·tine
Can·a·da t.
Chi·an t.
larch t.
Ven·ice t.
white t.
tur·pen·tine oil
rec·ti·fied t. o.
tur·pen·tine spir·it

turps
tur·ri·ceph·a·ly
tu·run·da
tu·run·dae
tush
tusk
tus·sal
tus·sic·u·lar
tus·sic·u·la·tion
tus·sis
tus·sive
  ab·sence
  frem·i·tus
tu·ta·men
  tu·ta·mi·na ce·re·bri
  tu·ta·mi·na oc·u·li
tu·ta·mi·na
Tuttle's
  proc·to·scope
Tweed
  tri·an·gle
Tweed edge·wise
  treat·ment
tweez·ers
twelfth cra·ni·al
  nerve
twelfth-year
  mo·lar
twen·ty-nail
  dys·tro·phy
twig
twi·light
  sleep
  state
  vi·sion
twin
  cone
  crys·tal
  he·lix
  pla·cen·ta
  preg·nan·cy
twin
  al·lan·toid·o·an·gi·op·a·gous
    t.'s
  con·joined t.'s
  con·joined asym·met·ri·cal
    t.'s
  con·joined equal t.'s
  con·joined sym·met·ri·cal
    t.'s
  con·joined un·e·qual t.'s
  di·cho·ri·al t.'s
  di·ov·u·lar t.'s
  di·zy·got·ic t.'s
  en·zy·got·ic t.'s
  fra·ter·nal t.'s
  het·er·ol·o·gous t.'s
  iden·ti·cal t.'s

in·com·plete con·joined t.'s
mon·o·am·ni·ot·ic t.'s
mon·o·cho·ri·al t.'s
mon·o·vu·lar t.'s
mon·o·zy·got·ic t.'s
om·pha·lo·an·gi·op·a·gous
  t.'s
par·a·sit·ic t.
pla·cen·tal par·a·sit·ic t.
pol·y·zy·got·ic t.'s
Si·a·mese t.'s
uni·ov·u·lar t.'s
twinge
twin·ning
twin-twin
  trans·fu·sion
twist
  form
twist·ed
  hairs
twitch
two-bel·lied
  mus·cle
two-car·bon
  frag·ment
two-di·men·sion·al
  chro·ma·tog·ra·phy
  ech·o·car·di·og·ra·phy
  im·mu·no·e·lec·tro·pho·re·
    sis
two-glass
  test
Twort
  phe·nom·e·non
Twort-d'Herelle
  phe·nom·e·non
two-step ex·er·cise
  test
two-sym·pa·thin
  the·o·ry
two-way
  cath·e·ter
ty·ba·mate
ty·le
ty·lec·to·my
tyl·ia
tyl·i·on
ty·lo·ma
  t. con·junc·ti·vae
ty·lo·ses
ty·lo·sis
  t. cil·i·ar·is
  t. lin·guae
  t. pal·mar·is et plan·tar·is
ty·lot·ic
ty·lox·a·pol
ty·maz·o·line
tym·pa·na

tym·pa·nal
tym·pa·nec·to·my
tym·pan·ia
tym·pan·ic
  an·trum
  at·tic
  body
  bone
  ca·nal
  cav·i·ty
  cells
  crest
  gan·gli·on
  gland
  groove
  in·ci·sure
  in·tu·mes·cence
  lip
  mem·brane
  nerve
  notch
  open·ing of au·di·to·ry tube
  open·ing of ca·nal for chor·
   da tym·pa·ni
  open·ing of eu·sta·chi·an
   tube
  part of tem·po·ral bone
  plate
  plex·us
  prom·on·to·ry
  ring
  scute
  si·nus
  veins
  wall of co·chle·ar duct
tym·pan·i·chord
tym·pan·i·chor·dal
tym·pa·nic·i·ty
tym·pa·nism
tym·pa·ni·tes
  uter·ine t.
tym·pa·nit·ic
  res·o·nance
tym·pa·ni·tis
tym·pa·no·cen·te·sis
tym·pa·no·eu·sta·chian
tym·pa·no·hy·al
  bone
tym·pa·no·mal·le·al
tym·pa·no·man·dib·u·lar
tym·pa·no·mas·toid
  fis·sure
  su·ture
tym·pa·no·mas·toid·i·tis
tym·pa·no·me·a·to·mas·toid·ec·
  to·my
tym·pa·no·pho·nia
tym·pa·noph·o·ny

tym·pa·no·plas·ty
tym·pa·no·squa·mo·sal
tym·pa·no·squa·mous
  fis·sure
tym·pa·no·sta·pe·di·al
  junc·tion
tym·pan·os·to·my
  tube
tym·pa·no·tem·po·ral
tym·pa·not·o·my
tym·pa·nous
tym·pa·num
tym·pa·nums
tym·pa·ny
  Skoda's t.
Tyndall
  phe·nom·e·non
tyn·dal·li·za·tion
type
  ba·sic per·son·al·i·ty t.
  blood t.
  no·men·cla·tur·al t.
  test t.
  wild t.
type
  cul·ture
  spe·cies
  strain
type A
  be·hav·ior
  per·son·al·i·ty
type B
  be·hav·ior
  per·son·al·i·ty
type I
  ac·ro·ceph·a·lo·syn·dac·ty·ly
  col·la·gen
  di·a·be·tes
  dip
  mu·co·pol·y·sac·cha·ri·do·
   sis
type I fa·mil·i·al
  hy·per·lip·o·pro·tein·e·mia
type II
  ac·ro·ceph·a·lo·syn·dac·ty·ly
  cells
  col·la·gen
  di·a·be·tes
  dip
  mu·co·pol·y·sac·cha·ri·do·
   sis
type II fa·mil·i·al
  hy·per·lip·o·pro·tein·e·mia
type III
  ac·ro·ceph·a·lo·syn·dac·ty·ly
  col·la·gen
  mu·co·pol·y·sac·cha·ri·do·
   sis

type III fa·mil·i·al
hy·per·lip·o·pro·tein·e·mia
type IS
mu·co·pol·y·sac·cha·ri·do·sis
type IV
col·la·gen
mu·co·pol·y·sac·cha·ri·do·sis
type IV fa·mil·i·al
hy·per·lip·o·pro·tein·e·mia
type V
ac·ro·ceph·a·lo·syn·dac·ty·ly
mu·co·pol·y·sac·cha·ri·do·sis
type V fa·mil·i·al
hy·per·lip·o·pro·tein·e·mia
type VI
mu·co·pol·y·sac·cha·ri·do·sis
type VII
mu·co·pol·y·sac·cha·ri·do·sis
ty·phin·ia
typh·lec·ta·sis
typh·lec·to·my
typh·len·ter·i·tis
typh·li·tis
typh·lo·dic·li·di·tis
typh·lo·em·py·e·ma
typh·lo·en·ter·i·tis
typh·lo·li·thi·a·sis
typh·lol·o·gy
typh·lo·meg·a·ly
typh·lon
typh·lo·pex·ia
typh·lo·pexy
typh·lor·rha·phy
typh·lo·sis
typh·los·to·my
typh·lot·o·my
typh·lo·u·re·ter·os·to·my
ty·phoid
ab·dom·i·nal t.
am·bu·la·to·ry t.
apy·ret·ic t.
bil·ious t. of Griesinger
fowl t.
la·tent t.
prov·o·ca·tion t.
walk·ing t.
ty·phoid
ba·cil·lus
bac·te·ri·o·phage
chol·era
fe·ver
pleu·ri·sy
pneu·mo·nia

sep·ti·ce·mia
vac·cine
ty·phoi·dal
ty·phoid-par·a·ty·phoid A and B
vac·cine
ty·phol·y·sin
ty·pho·ma·nia
ty·pho·sep·sis
ty·phous
ty·phus
en·dem·ic t.
ep·i·dem·ic t.
flea-borne t.
louse-borne t.
mite t.
t. mi·ti·or
mu·rine t.
North Queens·land tick t.
re·cru·des·cent t.
scrub t.
tick t.
trop·i·cal t.
ty·phus
vac·cine
typ·i·cal
ab·sence
achro·ma·top·sia
ac·ro·ceph·a·lo·syn·dac·ty·ly
pseu·do·cho·lin·es·ter·ase
typ·ing
bac·te·ri·o·phage t.
blood t.
typ·ist's
cramp
ty·ra·mi·nase
ty·ra·mine
t. ox·i·dase
tyr·an·nism
ty·rem·e·sis
ty·ro·ci·din
ty·ro·ci·dine
Ty·rode's
so·lu·tion
ty·rog·e·nous
Ty·rog·ly·phus lon·gi·or
ty·roid
ty·ro·ke·to·nu·ria
ty·ro·ma
ty·ro·pa·no·ate so·di·um
Ty·roph·a·gus pu·tres·cen·ti·ae
ty·ro·sin·ase
ty·ro·sine
t. io·di·nase
t. phe·nol·ly·ase
ty·ro·si·ne·mia
ty·ro·si·no·sis
ty·ro·si·nu·ria

ty·ro·sis
ty·ro·sy·lu·ria
ty·ro·thri·cin
ty·ro·tox·ism
Tyrrell's
  fas·cia

Tyson's
  glands
Tyz·ze·ria
Tzanck
  cells
  test

U
  wave
ubi·hy·dro·qui·none
ubi·qui·nol
ubi·qui·none
ubiq·ui·tin
ud·der
UDPga·lac·tose
UDPglu·cose
UDPglu·cur·o·nate.–bil·i·ru·bin
  glu·cu·ron·o·syl trans·fer·ase
Uehlinger's
  syn·drome
Uffelmann's
  re·a·gent
Uhl
  anom·a·ly
Uhthoff
  sign
ukam·bin
ul·cer
  acute de·cu·bi·tus u.
  Aden u.
  am·pu·tat·ing u.
  anas·to·mot·ic u.
  aton·ic u.
  Bu·ru·li u.
  chi·cle·ro's u.
  chrome u.
  chron·ic u.
  cocks·comb u.
  cold u.
  con·sti·tu·tion·al u.
  cor·ro·sive u.
  creep·ing u.
  Curling's u.
  de·cu·bi·tus u.
  den·drit·ic cor·ne·al u.
  den·tal u.
  diph·the·rit·ic u.
  dis·ten·tion u.
  elu·sive u.
  fas·cic·u·lar u.
  Fenwick-Hunner u.
  Ga·boon u.
  gas·tric u.
  grav·i·ta·tion·al u.
  groin u.
  gum·ma·tous u.

hard u.
healed u.
her·pet·ic u.
Hunner's u.
hy·po·py·on u.
in·do·lent u.
in·flamed u.
Ku·ru·ne·ga·la u.'s
Lipschütz' u.
lu·poid u.
Mann-Williamson u.
mar·gi·nal ring u. of
  cor·nea
Marjolin's u.
Meleney's u.
Mooren's u.
Or·i·en·tal u.
pen·e·trat·ing u.
pep·tic u.
per·am·bu·lat·ing u.
per·fo·rat·ed u.
per·fo·rat·ing u. of foot
phag·e·den·ic u.
phleg·mon·ous u.
pneu·mo·coc·cus u.
pu·den·dal u.
re·cur·rent aph·thous u.'s
ring u. of cor·nea
ro·dent u.
Saemisch's u.
ser·pent u. of cor·nea
ser·pig·i·nous u.
sim·ple u.
slough·ing u.
soft u.
sta·sis u.
ster·co·ral u.
ste·roid u.
sto·mal u.
stress u.'s
Sutton's u.
symp·to·mat·ic u.
syph·i·lit·ic u.
Syr·i·ac u.
Syr·i·an u.
tan·ner's u.
trans·par·ent u. of the
  cor·nea
tro·phic u.

ul·cer *(continued)*
  trop·i·cal u.
  un·der·min·ing u.
  var·i·cose u.
  ve·ne·re·al u.
  warty u.
  Zam·be·si u.
ul·ce·ra
ul·cer·ate
ul·cer·at·ed
ul·cer·at·ing
  gran·u·lo·ma of pu·den·da
ul·cer·a·tion
  lip and leg u.
  tra·che·al u.
ul·cer·a·tive
  co·li·tis
  der·ma·to·sis
  phar·yn·gi·tis
  scrof·u·lo·der·ma
  sto·ma·ti·tis
ul·cer·o·gen·ic
ul·cer·o·glan·du·lar
ul·cer·o·mem·bra·nous
  gin·gi·vi·tis
  phar·yn·gi·tis
ul·cer·ous
ul·cus
  u. am·bu·lans
  u. hy·po·sta·ti·cum
  u. ser·pens cor·ne·ae
  u. ter·e·brans
  u. ve·ne·re·um
  u. vul·vae acu·tum
ulec·to·my
ule·gy·ri·a
uler·y·the·ma
  u. oph·ry·og·e·nes
  u. sy·co·si·for·me
ulet·ic
ulet·omy
Ullmann's
  line
ul·na
ul·nad
ul·nae
ul·nar
  ar·tery
  bur·sa
  em·i·nence of wrist
  head
  mar·gin
  nerve
  notch
  re·flex
  veins

ul·nar col·lat·er·al
  lig·a·ment
  lig·a·ment of wrist
ul·nar ex·ten·sor
  mus·cle of wrist
ul·nar flex·or
  mus·cle of wrist
ul·na·ris
ul·nen
ul·no·car·pal
ul·no·ra·di·al
ulo·der·ma·ti·tis
uloid
ulot·o·my
ulot·ri·chous
ul·ti·mate
  prin·ci·ple
  strength
ul·ti·mo·bran·chi·al
  body
  pouch
ul·ti·mum mo·ri·ens
ultra-
  mi·cro·scope
ul·tra·brach·y·ce·phal·ic
ul·tra·cen·tri·fuge
ul·tra·cy·to·stome
ul·tra·di·an
  rhythm
ul·tra·dol·i·cho·ce·phal·ic
ul·tra·fil·ter
ul·tra·fil·tra·tion
  co·ef·fi·cient
  he·mo·di·a·lyz·er
ul·tra·len·te
  in·su·lin
ul·tra·li·ga·tion
ul·tra·mi·cro·scope
ul·tra·mi·cro·scop·ic
ul·tra·mi·cro·tome
ul·tra·mi·crot·o·my
ul·tra·son·ic
  ceph·a·lom·e·try
  clean·ing
  lith·o·tre·sis
  mi·cro·scope
  neb·u·liz·er
  rays
  ther·a·py
  waves
ul·tra·son·ic egg
  re·cov·ery
ul·tra·son·ics
ul·tra·son·o·gram
ul·tra·son·o·graph
ul·tra·so·nog·ra·pher

ul·tra·so·nog·ra·phy
  Doppler u.
  gray-scale u.
ul·tra·son·o·sur·gery
ul·tra·sound
  di·ag·nos·tic u.
  real-time u.
ul·tra·sound
  car·di·og·ra·phy
ul·tra·struc·tur·al
  anat·o·my
ul·tra·struc·ture
ul·tra·therm
ul·tra·thin
  sec·tion
ul·tra·vi·o·let
  ker·a·to·con·junc·ti·vi·tis
  lamp
  mi·cro·scope
  rays
ul·tra·vi·o·let
  ex·tra·vi·tal u.
  in·tra·vi·tal u.
  vi·tal u.
ul·tra·vi·rus
ul·tro·mo·tiv·i·ty
ul·tro·paque
  meth·od
ulu·la·tion
Ulysses
  syn·drome
um·bil·i·cal
  ar·tery
  cord
  cyst
  fis·sure
  fis·tu·la
  fos·sa
  fun·gus
  her·nia
  notch
  part
  re·gion
  ring
  souf·fle
  vein
  ves·i·cle
um·bil·i·cal pre·ves·i·cal
  fas·cia
um·bil·i·cate
um·bil·i·cat·ed
  cat·a·ract
um·bil·i·ca·tion
um·bil·i·ci
um·bil·i·co·mam·mil·la·ry
  tri·an·gle
um·bil·i·co·ves·i·cal
  fas·cia

um·bil·i·cus
um·bo
um·bo·nes
um·bo·nis
Um·bre
  vi·rus
un·armed
  ros·tel·lum
un·a·void·a·ble
  hem·or·rhage
un·bal·anced
  trans·lo·ca·tion
un·cal
  her·ni·a·tion
un·ci
un·cia
un·ci·form
  bone
  fas·cic·u·lus
  pan·cre·as
un·ci·for·me
Un·ci·nar·ia
un·ci·na·ri·a·sis
un·ci·nate
  at·tack
  bun·dle of Russell
  ep·i·lep·sy
  fas·cic·u·lus
  fas·cic·u·lus of Russell
  fit
  gy·rus
  pan·cre·as
  pro·cess of eth·moid bone
  pro·cess of pan·cre·as
un·ci·na·tum
un·ci·pres·sure
un·com·pen·sat·ed
  ac·i·do·sis
  al·ka·lo·sis
un·com·ple·ment·ed
un·con·di·tion·ed
  re·flex
  re·sponse
  stim·u·lus
un·con·ju·gat·ed
  bil·i·ru·bin
un·con·scious
  ho·mo·sex·u·al·i·ty
un·con·scious
  col·lec·tive u.
un·con·scious·ness
un·co-os·si·fied
un·cou·plers
un·cou·pling
  fac·tors
un·co·ver·te·bral
  joints
unc·tion

unc·tu·ous
unc·ture
un·cus
  u. gy·ri pa·ra·hip·po·cam·
  pa·lis
un·cus
  band of Giacomini
un·dec·e·no·ic ac·id
un·de·co·yl·i·um chlo·ride
un·de·co·yl·i·um chlo·ride-
  io·dine
un·dec·y·len·ate
un·dec·y·len·ic ac·id
un·der·a·chieve·ment
un·der·a·chiev·er
un·der·bite
un·der·cut
  gauge
un·der·drive pac·ing
un·der·horn
un·der·min·ing
  ul·cer
un·der·nu·tri·tion
un·der·shoot
un·der·ven·ti·la·tion
Underwood's
  dis·ease
un·de·scend·ed
  tes·tis
un·de·ter·mined
  ni·tro·gen
un·dif·fer·en·ti·at·ed
  cell
un·dif·fer·en·ti·at·ed cell
  ad·e·no·ma
un·dif·fer·en·ti·at·ed type
  fe·vers
un·dine
un·din·ism
un·di·ver·sion
un·do·ing
un·du·lant
  fe·ver
un·du·late
un·du·lat·ing
  mem·brane
  pulse
un·du·la·to·ry
  mem·brane
un·du·li·po·dia
un·du·li·po·di·um
un·e·qual
  cleav·age
  cross·ing-o·ver
un·e·qual ret·i·nal
  im·age
un·e·rup·ted
  tooth

un·e·ven
  cross·ing-o·ver
un·formed vi·su·al
  hal·lu·ci·na·tion
un·gual
  pha·lanx
  tu·ber·os·i·ty
un·guent
un·gues
Un·guic·u·la·ta
un·guic·u·late
un·guic·u·lus
un·gui·nal
un·guis
  u. adun·cus
  u. avis
  Haller's u.
  u. in·car·na·tus
Un·gu·la·ta
un·gu·late
un·gu·li·grade
u·ni·ar·tic·u·lar
uni·ax·i·al
  joint
uni·bas·al
Un·i·blue A
uni·cam·er·al
  cyst
uni·cam·er·al bone
  cyst
uni·cam·er·ate
uni·can·a·lic·u·lar
  sphinc·ter
uni·cel·lu·lar
  gland
  scle·ro·sis
u·ni·cen·tral
uni·corn
  uter·us
uni·cor·nous
uni·cus·pid
uni·cus·pi·date
uni·di·rec·tion·al
  block
  flux
uni·fa·mil·i·al
uni·fla·gel·late
uni·fo·rate
uni·form
uni·ger·mi·nal
uni·glan·du·lar
uni·lam·i·nar
uni·lam·i·nate
uni·lat·e·ral
  an·es·the·sia
  hem·i·a·nop·sia
  her·maph·ro·dit·ism
uni·lo·bar

uni·lo·cal
uni·loc·u·lar
  cyst
  fat
  joint
uni·loc·u·lar hy·da·tid
  cyst
uni·mo·lec·u·lar
  re·ac·tion
un·in·hib·i·ted neu·ro·gen·ic
  blad·der
un·in·ter·rupt·ed
  su·ture
uni·nu·cle·ar
uni·nu·cle·ate
uni·oc·u·lar
  hem·i·a·nop·sia
un·ion
  au·tog·e·nous u.
  faulty u.
  fi·brous u.
  pri·mary u.
  sec·on·dary u.
  vi·cious u.
uni·o·val
uni·ov·u·lar
  twins
uni·pen·nate
  mus·cle
uni·po·lar
  cell
  elec·tro·car·di·o·gram
  leads
  neu·ron
uni·port
uni·port·er
uni·sep·tate
unit
  ab·so·lute u.
  alex·in u.
  Allen-Doisy u.
  al·pha u.'s
  am·bo·cep·tor u.
  an·dro·gen u.
  Angström u.
  an·ti·gen u.
  an·ti·tox·in u.
  an·ti·ve·nene u.
  atom·ic mass u.
  base u.'s
  Be·thes·da u.
  bi·o·log·i·cal stan·dard u.
  bird u.
  Bodansky u.
  Brit·ish ther·mal u.
  cat u.
  cen·ti·me·ter-gram-sec·ond
    u.

CGS u.
cgs u.
chlo·ro·phyll u.
cho·ri·on·ic go·nad·o·tro·
  pin u.
Clauberg u.
com·ple·ment u.
Corner-Allen u.
cor·o·nary care u.
cor·pus lu·te·um hor·mone
  u.
crit·i·cal care u.
CT u.
Dam u.
dig·i·tal·is u.
diph·the·ria an·ti·tox·in u.
dog u.
elec·tro·mag·net·ic u.
elec·tro·stat·ic u.
u. of en·er·gy
equine go·nad·o·tro·pin u.
es·tra·di·ol ben·zo·ate u.
es·trone u.
Fishman-Lerner u.
Florey u.
foot-pound-second u.
u. of force
FPS u.
fps u.
grav·i·ta·tion·al u.'s
G u. of strep·to·my·cin
Hampson u.
u. of heat
he·mo·ly·sin u.
he·mo·lyt·ic u.
hep·a·rin u.
Holzknecht u.
Hounsfield u.
Howell u.
in·su·lin u.
in·ten·sive care u.
u. of in·ter·me·din
in·ter·na·tion·al u.
In·ter·na·tion·al Sys·tem of
  u.'s
Jenner-Kay u.
Karmen u.
Kienböck's u.
King u.
King-Armstrong u.
u. of length
u. of light
L u. of strep·to·my·cin
u. of lu·mi·nous flux
u. of lu·mi·nous in·ten·
  si·ty
lung u.

unit *(continued)*
  u. of lu·te·i·niz·ing ac·tiv·i·ty
  Mache u.
  u. of mag·net·ic field in·ten·si·ty
  u. of mass
  me·ter-kil·o·gram-sec·ond u.
  MKS u.
  mks u.
  mo·tor u.
  mouse u.
  u. of oc·u·lar con·ver·gence
  Ox·ford u.
  u. of ox·y·to·cin
  pan·to·then·ic ac·id u.
  u. of pen·i·cil·lin
  phos·pha·tase u.
  phys·i·o·log·ic u.
  prac·ti·cal u.'s
  u. of pro·ges·ta·tion·al ac·tiv·i·ty
  pro·ges·ter·one u.
  pro·lac·tin u.
  u. of ra·di·o·ac·tiv·i·ty
  ri·bo·fla·vin u.
  roent·gen u.
  Sherman u.
  Sherman-Munsell u.
  SI u.'s
  So·mog·yi u.
  S u. of strep·to·my·cin
  Steenbock u.
  strep·to·my·cin u.'s
  Svedberg u.
  tet·a·nus an·ti·tox·in u.
  thi·a·min chlo·ride u.
  thi·a·min hy·dro·chlo·ride u.
  u. of thy·ro·tro·phic ac·tiv·i·ty
  tox·ic u.
  tox·in u.
  ura·ni·um u.
  USP u.
  u. of va·so·pres·sin
  vi·ta·min A u.
  vi·ta·min C u.
  vi·ta·min D u.
  vi·ta·min E u.
  vi·ta·min K u.
  vol·ume u.
  u. of wave·length
  u. of weight
  u. of work
unit of
  con·ver·gence

unit
  char·ac·ter
  fi·brils
  mem·brane
unit·ing
  ca·nal
  car·ti·lage
  duct
uni·va·lence
uni·va·len·cy
uni·va·lent
  an·ti·body
uni·ver·sal
  ap·pli·ance
  do·nor
  in·fan·ti·lism
  sol·vent
un·med·ul·lat·ed
un·mod·i·fied zinc ox·ide-eu·ge·nol
  ce·ment
un·my·e·li·nat·ed
  fi·bers
Unna-Pappenheim
  stain
Unna's
  dis·ease
  mark
  stain
Unna-Taenzer
  stain
un·of·fi·cial
un·paired
  al·lo·some
  chro·mo·some
un·phys·i·o·log·ic
un·re·solved
  pneu·mo·nia
un·san·i·tary
un·sat·u·rat·ed
  al·co·hols
  fat
  fat·ty ac·id
un·sex
un·sound·ness
un·sta·ble
  an·gi·na
  col·loid
  equi·lib·ri·um
  frac·ture
  he·mo·glo·bins
un·strained jaw
  re·la·tion
un·stri·at·ed
  mus·cle
un·striped
  mus·cle

un·sys·tem·a·tized
   de·lu·sion
un·thrifty
un·u·nit·ed
   frac·ture
Unverricht's
   dis·ease
up·beat
   nys·tag·mus
up·per
   air·way
   ex·trem·i·ty
   ex·trem·i·ty of fib·u·la
   eye·lid
   jaw
   lip
   lobe of lung
up·per ab·dom·i·nal per·i·os·
   te·al
   re·flex
up·per jaw
   bone
up·per lat·er·al cu·ta·ne·ous
   nerve of arm
up·per mo·tor
   neu·ron
up·per mo·tor neu·ron
   le·sion
up·per no·dal
   ex·tra·sys·to·le
   rhythm
up·per uter·ine
   seg·ment
up-reg·u·la·tion
up·si·loid
up·take
ur-
   de·fens·es
ura·chal
   cyst
   fis·tu·la
   fold
   lig·a·ment
ura·chus
ura·cil
   u. de·hy·dro·gen·ase
   u. mus·tard
   u. ox·i·dase
ura·cil
   mus·tard
Ur·a·go·ga
ura·gogue
ur·a·mus·tine
ura·nin
ura·ni·nite
ura·nis·co·chasm
ura·nis·co·ni·tis
ura·nis·co·plas·ty

ura·nis·cor·rha·phy
ura·nis·cus
ura·ni·um
   ne·phri·tis
   unit
ura·no·plas·ty
ura·nor·rha·phy
ura·nos·chi·sis
ura·no·staph·y·lo·plas·ty
ura·no·staph·y·lor·rha·phy
ura·no·staph·y·los·chi·sis
ura·no·ve·los·chi·sis
ura·nyl
ura·nyl ac·e·tate
   stain
ura·ri
ura·ro·ma
urar·thri·tis
urate
   u. ox·i·dase
urate crys·tals
   stain
ura·te·mia
ur·ate·ri·bo·nu·cle·o·tide phos·
   pho·ryl·ase
urat·ic
ura·tol·y·sis
ura·to·ly·tic
ura·to·ma
ura·to·sis
ura·tu·ria
Urbach-Wiethe
   dis·ease
ur·ban cu·ta·ne·ous
   leish·man·i·a·sis
Urban's
   op·er·a·tion
ur·ce·i·form
ur·ce·o·late
urea
   u. per·ox·ide
   u. stib·a·mine
urea
   clear·ance
   cy·cle
   frost
   ni·tro·gen
urea clear·ance
   test
ure·a·gen·e·sis
ure·al
Ure·a·plas·ma
ure·a·poi·e·sis
ure·ase
   test
urec·chy·sis
ure·de·ma
ure·do

ure·ic
ure·ide
ure·i·do·suc·cin·ic ac·id
urel·co·sis
ure·mia
  hy·per·cal·ce·mic u.
ure·mic
  breath
  co·li·tis
  frost
  lung
  per·i·car·di·tis
  pneu·mo·nia
  pneu·mo·ni·tis
  pol·y·neu·rop·a·thy
ure·mi·gen·ic
ure·o·tel·ic
ur·er·y·thrin
ure·si·es·the·sia
ure·sis
ure·ter
  cur·li·cue u.
ure·ter·al
  me·a·tus
  open·ing
ure·ter·al·gia
ure·ter·cys·to·scope
ure·ter·ec·ta·sia
ure·ter·ec·to·my
ure·ter·ic
  bud
  dys·men·or·rhea
  fold
  plex·us
ure·ter·i·tis
ure·ter·o·cele
ure·ter·o·ce·lor·ra·phy
ure·ter·o·cer·vi·cal
ure·ter·o·co·lic
ure·ter·o·co·los·to·my
ure·ter·o·cu·ta·ne·ous
  fis·tu·la
ure·ter·o·cyst·a·nas·to·mo·sis
ure·ter·o·cys·to·scope
ure·ter·o·cys·tos·to·my
ure·ter·o·en·ter·ic
ure·ter·o·en·ter·os·to·my
ure·ter·og·ra·phy
ure·ter·o·hy·dro·ne·phro·sis
ure·ter·o-il·e·al
  anas·to·mo·sis
ure·ter·o·il·e·o·ne·o·cys·tos·to·my
ure·ter·o·il·e·os·to·my
ure·ter·o·lith
ure·ter·o·li·thi·a·sis
ure·ter·o·li·thot·o·my
ure·ter·ol·y·sis

ure·ter·o·ne·o·cys·tos·to·my
ure·ter·o·ne·o·py·e·los·to·my
ure·ter·o·ne·phrec·to·my
ure·ter·op·a·thy
ure·ter·o·pel·vic
  ob·struc·tion
ure·ter·o·plas·ty
ure·ter·o·proc·tos·to·my
ure·ter·o·py·e·li·tis
ure·ter·o·py·e·log·ra·phy
ure·ter·o·py·e·lo·ne·os·to·my
ure·ter·o·py·e·lo·ne·phri·tis
ure·ter·o·py·e·lo·ne·phros·to·my
ure·ter·o·py·e·lo·plasty
ure·ter·o·py·e·los·to·my
ure·ter·o·py·o·sis
ure·ter·o·rec·tos·to·my
ure·ter·o·re·nal
  re·flux
ure·ter·or·rha·gia
ure·ter·or·rha·phy
ure·ter·o·sig·moid
  anas·to·mo·sis
ure·ter·o·sig·moi·dos·to·my
ure·ter·o·steg·no·sis
ure·ter·o·sten·o·ma
ure·ter·o·sten·o·sis
ure·ter·os·to·ma
ure·ter·os·to·my
ure·ter·ot·o·my
ure·ter·o·tri·go·no·en·ter·os·to·my
ure·ter·o·tub·al
  anas·to·mo·sis
ure·ter·o·u·re·ter·al
  anas·to·mo·sis
ure·ter·o·u·re·ter·os·to·my
ure·ter·o·u·ter·ine
ure·ter·o·vag·i·nal
  fis·tu·la
ure·ter·o·ves·i·cal
  ob·struc·tion
ure·ter·o·ves·i·cos·to·my
ure·than
ure·thane
ure·thra
  fe·male u.
  male u.
  mem·bra·nous u.
  u. mu·li·e·bris
  pe·nile u.
  pros·tat·ic u.
  spongy u.
  u. vi·ri·lis
ure·thral
  ar·tery
  ca·run·cle
  crest

di·la·tion
di·ver·tic·u·lum
fe·ver
glands
groove
he·ma·tu·ria
la·cu·na
open·ings
pa·pil·la
plate
sphinc·ter·ot·o·my
stric·ture
sur·face of pe·nis
valves
ure·thral·gia
ure·thral pres·sure
  pro·file
ureth·ram·e·ter
ure·thra·scope
ure·thra·tre·sia
ure·threc·to·my
ure·threm·or·rha·gia
ure·threm·phrax·is
ure·threu·ryn·ter
ure·thrism
ure·thris·mus
ure·thri·tis
  an·te·ri·or u.
  fol·lic·u·lar u.
  gon·o·coc·cal u.
  gran·u·lar u.
  non·gon·o·coc·cal u.
  non·spe·cif·ic u.
  u. pet·ri·fi·cans
  pos·te·ri·or u.
  sim·ple u.
  spe·cif·ic u.
  u. ve·ne·rea
ure·thro·bal·a·no·plas·ty
ure·thro·bul·bar
ure·thro·cele
ure·thro·cys·ti·tis
ure·thro·cys·to·me·trog·ra·phy
ure·thro·cys·tom·e·try
ure·thro·cys·to·pexy
ure·thro·dyn·ia
ure·thro·graph
ure·throm·e·ter
ure·thro·pe·nile
ure·thro·per·i·ne·al
ureth·ro·per·i·ne·o·scro·tal
ure·thro·pexy
ure·thro·phrax·is
ure·thro·phy·ma
ure·thro·plasty
ure·thro·pros·ta·tic
ure·thro·rec·tal
ure·thror·rha·gia

ure·thror·rha·phy
ure·thror·rhea
ure·thro·scope
ure·thro·scop·ic
ure·thros·co·py
ure·thro·spasm
ure·thro·stax·is
ure·thro·ste·no·sis
ure·thros·to·my
  per·i·ne·al u.
ure·thro·tome
ure·throt·o·my
  ex·ter·nal u.
  in·ter·nal u.
  per·i·ne·al u.
ure·thro·vag·i·nal
  fis·tu·la
ure·thro·ves·i·cal
ure·thro·ves·i·co·pexy
urge
  in·con·ti·nence
ur·gen·cy
  in·con·ti·nence
ur·gen·cy
  mo·tor u.
  sen·so·ry u.
ur·gi·nea
ur·hi·dro·sis
uri·an
uric
uric ac·id
  u. a. ox·i·dase
uric ac·id
  in·farct
uri·case
uri·col·y·sis
uri·co·lyt·ic
  in·dex
uri·co·su·ria
uri·co·su·ric
uri·co·tel·ic
uri·dine
  u. di·phos·phate
  u. phos·phate
  u. phos·pho·ryl·ase
  u. tri·phos·phate
uri·dine·di·phos·pho·ga·lac·tose
uri·dine·di·phos·pho·glu·cose
uri·dine·di·phos·pho·glu·cu·ron·
  ic ac·id
uri·dro·sis
  u. cry·stal·li·na
uri·dyl·ic ac·id
uri·dyl·trans·fer·ase
uri·es·the·sia
uri·nal
uri·nal·y·sis

uri·nary
  ap·pa·ra·tus
  blad·der
  cal·cu·lus
  casts
  cyst
  fe·ver
  fis·tu·la
  ni·tro·gen
  or·gans
  re·flex
  sand
  schis·to·so·mi·a·sis
  smear
  stut·ter·ing
  sys·tem
  tract
uri·nary con·cen·tra·tion
  test
uri·nary ex·er·tion·al
  in·con·ti·nence
uri·nary stress
  in·con·ti·nence
uri·nate
uri·na·tion
  stut·ter·ing u.
urine
  am·mo·ni·a·cal u.
  black u.
  chy·lous u.
  cloudy u.
  crude u.
  feb·rile u.
  fe·ver·ish u.
  gouty u.
  hon·ey u.
  ma·ple syr·up u.
  milky u.
  neb·u·lous u.
  re·sid·u·al u.
uri·ne·mia
uri·nif·er·ous
  tu·bule
uri·nif·ic
uri·nip·a·rous
uri·no·gen·i·tal
uri·nog·e·nous
uri·no·ma
uri·nom·e·ter
uri·nom·e·try
uri·nos·co·py
uri·no·sex·u·al
uri·nous
uri·po·sia
uri·tis
uro·am·mo·ni·ac
uro·an·the·lone
uro·bi·lin

uro·bi·li·ne·mia
uro·bi·lin·o·gen
uro·bi·lin·u·ria
uro·can·ase
ur·o·can·ate
  u. hy·dra·tase
uro·can·ic ac·id
uro·can·i·case
uro·cele
uroch·er·as
uro·che·sia
uro·chrome
uro·chro·mo·gen
uro·cris·ia
uro·cri·sis
uro·cy·a·nin
uro·cy·an·o·gen
uro·cy·a·no·sis
uro·cyst
uro·cys·tic
uro·cys·tis
ur·o·cys·ti·tis
uro·dy·na·mics
uro·dyn·ia
uro·dys·func·tion
uro·e·de·ma
uro·en·ter·one
uro·er·y·thrin
uro·fla·vin
ur·o·fol·li·tro·pin
uro·fus·co·hem·a·tin
uro·gas·trone
uro·gen·i·tal
  ap·pa·ra·tus
  ca·nal
  cleft
  di·a·phragm
  fis·tu·la
  mem·brane
  mes·en·tery
  re·gion
  ridge
  sep·tum
  si·nus
  sys·tem
  tri·an·gle
urog·e·nous
uro·glau·cin
ur·o·go·nad·o·tro·pin
uro·gram
urog·ra·phy
  an·te·grade u.
  cys·to·scop·ic u.
  ex·cre·to·ry u.
  in·tra·ve·nous u.
  ret·ro·grade u.
uro·gra·vim·e·ter
uro·hem·a·tin

uro·hem·a·to·por·phy·rin
uro·hep·a·rin
uro·hy·per·ten·sin
uro·ki·nase
ur·o·lag·nia
uro·leu·cic ac·id
uro·leu·cin·ic ac·id
uro·lith
uro·li·thi·a·sis
uro·lith·ic
uro·li·thol·o·gy
uro·log·ic
uro·log·i·cal
urol·o·gist
urol·o·gy
uro·lu·te·in
uro·mel·a·nin
urom·e·ter
uron·cus
uro·ne·phro·sis
uron·ic ac·ids
uro·nos·co·py
urop·a·thy
uro·phan·ic
uro·phe·in
uro·pla·nia
uro·poi·e·sis
uro·poi·e·tic
  sys·tem
uro·por·phy·rin
ur·o·por·phy·rin·o·gen
uro·psam·mus
urop·ter·in
uro·pur·pur·in
uro·pyg·i·al
  gland
ur·o·ra·di·ol·o·gy
uro·rec·tal
  fold
  mem·brane
  sep·tum
uro·ro·se·in
uro·ru·bin
uro·ru·bro·hem·a·tin
uros·che·o·cele
uros·che·sis
uro·scop·ic
uros·co·py
uro·sem·i·ol·o·gy
uro·sep·sin
uro·sep·sis
uro·sep·tic
uro·spec·trin
ur·o·thi·on
ur·o·thor·ax
uro·u·re·ter
uro·xan·thin
urox·in

ur·ti·ca
ur·ti·cant
ur·ti·car·ia
  u. acu·ta
  acute u.
  u. bul·lo·sa
  cho·lin·er·gic u.
  chron·ic u.
  u. chron·i·ca
  cold u.
  u. con·fer·ta
  con·ge·la·tion u.
  u. en·de·mi·ca
  u. ep·i·dem·i·ca
  u. fac·ti·tia
  fac·ti·tious u.
  feb·rile u.
  u. fe·bri·lis
  gi·ant u.
  u. gi·gans
  u. gi·gan·tea
  heat u.
  u. hem·or·rha·gi·ca
  u. ma·cu·lo·sa
  u. me·di·ca·men·to·sa
  pap·u·lar u.
  u. pa·pu·lo·sa
  u. per·stans
  u. pig·men·to·sa
  so·lar u.
  u. sub·cu·ta·nea
  u. tu·be·ro·sa
  u. ve·si·cu·lo·sa
  vi·bra·to·ry u.
ur·ti·car·i·al
  fe·ver
ur·ti·car·i·ous
ur·ti·cate
ur·ti·ca·tion
uru·shi·ol
  u. ox·i·dase
Usher's
  syn·drome
USP
  unit
us·ti·lag·i·nism
Us·ti·la·go
  U. may·dis
  U. ze·ae
us·tu·la·tion
usur·pa·tion
uter·ec·to·my
uter·i
uter·ine
  ap·pend·ag·es
  ar·tery
  cal·cu·lus
  cav·i·ty

uter·ine *(continued)*
  col·ic
  con·trac·tion
  dys·men·or·rhea
  ex·trem·i·ty
  glands
  horn
  in·er·tia
  in·suf·fi·cien·cy
  milk
  part
  preg·nan·cy
  si·nus
  si·nus·oid
  souf·fle
  tet·a·nus
  tube
  tym·pa·ni·tes
  veins
uter·ine ve·nous
  plex·us
uter·is·mus
uter·i·tis
in utero
uter·o·ab·dom·i·nal
  preg·nan·cy
uter·o·cer·vi·cal
uter·o·cys·tos·to·my
uter·o·ep·i·cho·ri·al
  mem·brane
uter·o·fix·a·tion
uter·o·lith
uter·om·e·ter
uter·o-o·var·i·an
  var·i·co·cele
uter·o·pa·ri·e·tal
uter·o·pel·vic
uter·o·per·i·to·ne·al
  fis·tu·la
uter·o·pexy
uter·o·pla·cen·tal
  ap·o·plexy
  si·nus
uter·o·plas·ty
uter·o·sa·cral
  lig·a·ment
uter·o·sal·pin·gog·ra·phy
uter·o·scope
uter·os·co·py
uter·ot·o·my
uter·o·ton·ic
uter·o·tub·al
uter·o·tu·bog·ra·phy
uter·o·vag·i·nal
  ca·nal
  plex·us
uter·o·ven·tral
uter·o·ver·dine

uter·o·ves·i·cal
  fold
  pouch
uter·us
  u. acol·lis
  anom·a·lous u.
  ar·cu·ate u.
  u. ar·cu·a·tus
  u. bi·ca·me·ra·tus ve·tu·la·rum
  bi·cor·nate u.
  u. bi·cor·nate bi·col·lis
  u. bi·cor·nate uni·col·lis
  u. bi·cor·nis
  bi·fid u.
  u. bif·i·dus
  bi·fo·rate u.
  u. bi·fo·ris
  u. bi·lo·cu·la·ris
  bi·par·tite u.
  u. bi·par·ti·tus
  capped u.
  cor·di·form u.
  u. cor·di·for·mis
  Couvelaire u.
  u. di·del·phys
  dou·ble-mouthed u.
  du·plex u.
  u. du·plex
  grav·id u.
  heart-shaped u.
  in·cu·di·form u.
  u. in·cu·di·for·mis
  mas·cu·line u.
  u. mas·cu·li·nus
  one-horned u.
  u. par·vi·col·lis
  sep·tate u.
  u. sep·tus
  sub·sep·tate u.
  u. sub·sep·tus
  tri·an·gu·lar u.
  u. tri·an·gu·la·ris
  uni·corn u.
  u. uni·cor·nis
uti·li·za·tion
  time
utri·cle
  pros·tat·ic u.
utric·u·lar
  nerve
  re·flex·es
  spot
utric·u·li
utric·u·li·tis
utric·u·lo·am·pul·lar
  nerve

utric·u·lo·sac·cu·lar
  duct
utric·u·lus
utri·form
uvae·for·mis
uva ur·si
uvea
uve·al
  part
  staph·y·lo·ma
  tract
uve·it·ic
uve·i·ti·des
uve·i·tis
  an·te·ri·or u.
  Förster's u.
  Fuchs' u.
  het·er·o·chro·mic u.
  lens-in·duced u.
  phac·o·an·a·phy·lac·tic u.
  phac·o·gen·ic u.
  pos·te·ri·or u.
  sym·pa·thet·ic u.
uve·o·cu·ta·ne·ous
  syn·drome
uve·o-en·ceph·a·lit·ic
  syn·drome
uve·o·en·ceph·a·li·tis
uve·o·men·in·gi·tis
  syn·drome

uve·o·pa·rot·id
  fe·ver
uve·o·scle·ri·tis
uvi·form
uvi·o·fast
uvi·ol
  lamp
uvi·om·e·ter
uvi·o·re·sis·tant
uvi·o·sen·si·tive
uvu·la
  bi·fid u.
  u. ce·re·bel·li
  Lieutaud's u.
uvu·lap·to·sis
uvu·lar
uvu·la·ris
uvu·la·tome
uvu·lec·to·my
uvu·li
uvu·li·tis
uvu·lo·pal·a·to·pha·ryn·go·
  plas·ty
uvu·lo·pal·a·to·plas·ty
uvu·lop·to·sis
uvu·lo·tome
uvu·lot·o·my
Uz·bek·i·stan hem·or·rhag·ic
  fe·ver

V

V
an·ti·gen
lead
wave

V-
es·o·tro·pia
ex·o·tro·pia

V-A
con·duc·tion

vac·cen·ic ac·id

vac·ci·na

vac·ci·nal

vac·ci·nate

vac·ci·na·tion

vac·ci·na·tor

vac·cine
ad·ju·vant v.
aque·ous v.
au·tog·e·nous v.
ba·cil·lus Calmette-Guérin v.
BCG v.
Calmette-Guérin v.
chol·era v.
crys·tal vi·o·let v.
Da·kar v.
diph·the·ria, tet·a·nus tox·
oids, and per·tus·sis v.
duck em·bryo or·i·gin v.
Flury strain v.
foot-and-mouth dis·ease
vi·rus v.'s
Haffkine's v.
HEP v.
hep·a·ti·tis B v.
het·er·og·e·nous v.
high-egg-pas·sage v.
hog chol·era v.'s
hu·man dip·loid cell ra·bies
v.
in·ac·ti·vat·ed po·li·o·vi·rus
v.
in·flu·en·za vi·rus v.'s
LEP v.
live v.
live oral po·li·o·vi·rus v.
low-egg-pas·sage v.
mea·sles, mumps, and
ru·bel·la v.
mea·sles vi·rus v.

mul·ti·va·lent v.
mumps vi·rus v.
oil v.
oral po·li·o·vi·rus v.
Pasteur v.
per·tus·sis v.
plague v.
pneu·mo·coc·cal v.
po·li·o·my·e·li·tis v.'s
po·li·o·vi·rus v.'s
pol·y·va·lent v.
ra·bies v.
ra·bies v., Flury strain egg-
pas·sage
rick·ett·sia v., at·ten·
u·at·ed
Rocky Moun·tain spot·ted
fe·ver v.
ru·bel·la vi·rus v., live
Sabin v.
Salk v.
Semple v.
small·pox v.
staph·y·lo·coc·cus v.
stock v.
sub·u·nit v.
T.A.B. v.
tet·a·nus v.
tu·ber·cu·lo·sis v.
ty·phoid v.
ty·phoid-par·a·ty·phoid A
and B v.
ty·phus v.
whoop·ing-cough v.
yel·low fe·ver v.

vac·cine
bod·ies
lymph
vi·rus

vac·cin·ia
lymph
vi·rus

vac·cin·ia
v. gan·gre·no·sa
gen·er·al·ized v.
pro·gress·ive v.

vac·cin·i·al

vac·cin·i·form

vac·ci·nist

vac·cin·i·za·tion
vac·cin·o·gen
vac·ci·nog·e·nous
vac·ci·noid
  re·ac·tion
vac·ci·no·style
vac·ci·num
VACTERL
  syn·drome
in vac·uo
vac·u·o·lar
  de·gen·er·a·tion
  ne·phro·sis
vac·u·o·late
vac·u·o·lat·ed
vac·u·o·lat·ing
  vi·rus
vac·u·o·la·tion
vac·u·ole
  au·to·pha·gic v.
  con·trac·tile v.
  par·a·si·toph·or·ous v.
vac·u·o·li·za·tion
vac·u·ome
vac·u·tome
vac·u·um
  as·pi·ra·tor
  cast·ing
  des·ic·ca·tor
  ex·trac·tor
  flask
  head·ache
  in·vest·ing
  tube
va·dum
vag·a·bond's
  dis·ease
va·gal
  ap·nea
  at·tack
  part of ac·ces·so·ry nerve
  trunk
va·gec·to·my
va·gi
va·gi·na
  v. cel·lu·lo·sa
  v. mas·cu·li·na
  v. mu·co·sa ten·di·nis
  va·gi·nae ner·vi op·ti·ci
  v. oc·u·li
  v. sep·tate
  v. syn·o·vi·a·lis troch·le·ae
  va·gi·nae va·so·rum
va·gi·nae
vag·i·nal
  ar·tery
  atre·sia
  ce·li·ot·o·my

col·umns
dys·men·or·rhea
gland
hys·ter·ec·to·my
hys·ter·ot·o·my
lac·er·a·tion
li·thot·o·my
my·o·mec·to·my
nerves
open·ing
plug
pool
pro·cess
pro·cess of per·i·to·ne·um
pro·cess of tes·tis
smear
syn·o·vi·tis
vag·i·nal cor·ni·fi·ca·tion
  test
vag·i·na·li·tis
vag·i·nal mu·ci·fi·ca·tion
  test
vag·i·nal syn·o·vi·al
  mem·brane
vag·i·nal ve·nous
  plex·us
va·gi·na·pexy
vag·i·nate
vag·i·nec·to·my
vag·i·nism
vag·i·nis·mus
  pos·te·ri·or v.
vag·i·ni·ti·des
vag·i·ni·tis
  v. ad·he·si·va
  ad·he·sive v.
  ame·bic v.
  atroph·ic v.
  v. cys·ti·ca
  des·qua·ma·tive in·flam·ma·to·ry v.
  v. em·phy·se·ma·to·sa
  gran·u·lar v.
  pin·worm v.
  se·nile v.
  v. se·ni·lis
vag·i·no·ab·dom·i·nal
vag·i·no·cele
vag·i·no·dyn·ia
vag·i·no·fix·a·tion
vag·i·no·hys·ter·ec·to·my
vag·i·no·la·bi·al
vag·i·no·my·co·sis
vag·i·nop·a·thy
vag·i·no·per·i·ne·al
vag·i·no·per·i·ne·o·plas·ty
vag·i·no·per·i·ne·or·rha·phy
vag·i·no·per·i·ne·ot·o·my

vag·i·no·per·i·to·ne·al
vag·i·no·pexy
vag·i·no·plas·ty
vag·i·nos·co·py
vag·i·not·o·my
vag·i·no·ves·i·cal
vag·i·no·vul·var
Va·gin·u·lus ple·be·i·us
va·gi·tus uter·i·nus
va·go·ac·ces·so·ri·us
va·go·glos·so·pha·ryn·ge·al
va·gol·y·sis
va·go·lyt·ic
va·go·mi·met·ic
va·got·o·my
va·go·to·nia
va·go·ton·ic
va·go·tro·pic
va·go·va·gal
   re·flex
va·grant's
   dis·ease
va·gus
   ar·ea
   nerve
   pulse
va·lence
   elec·tron
va·lence
   neg·a·tive v.
   pos·i·tive v.
va·len·cy
va·lent
Val·en·tine's
   po·si·tion
   test
Valentin's
   cor·pus·cles
   gan·gli·on
   nerve
val·er·ate
va·le·ri·an
va·le·ri·a·nate
va·le·ric ac·id
va·leth·a·mate bro·mide
val·e·tu·di·nar·i·an
val·e·tu·di·nar·i·an·ism
val·goid
val·gus
val·id
val·i·da·tion
   con·sen·su·al v.
va·lid·i·ty
   con·cur·rent v.
   con·struct v.
   con·tent v.
   cri·te·ri·on-re·lat·ed v.

   face v.
   pre·dic·tive v.
va·line
val·la
val·late
   pa·pil·la
val·lec·u·la
   v. syl·vii
   v. un·guis
val·lec·u·lae
val·lec·u·lar
   dys·pha·gia
Valleix's
   points
val·ley
   fe·ver
val·lis
val·lum
val·meth·a·mide
val·noc·ta·mide
val·oid
val·pro·ic ac·id
Valsalva
   ma·neu·ver
   test
Valsalva's
   an·trum
   lig·a·ments
   mus·cle
   si·nus
val·ue
   ace·tyl v.
   buff·er v.
   buff·er v. of the blood
   ca·lor·ic v.
   glob·u·lar v.
   hom·ing v.
   io·dine v.
   mat·u·ra·tion v.
   nor·mal v.'s
   phe·no·typ·ic v.
   pre·dic·tive v.
   ref·er·ence v.'s
   thi·o·cy·an·o·gen v.
   thresh·old lim·it v.
val·va
   v. mi·tra·lis
   v. tri·cus·pi·da·lis
val·vae
val·val
val·var
val·vate
valve
   Amussat's v.
   anal v.'s
   an·te·ri·or ure·thral v.
   aor·tic v.
   atri·o·ven·tric·u·lar v.'s

valve *(continued)*
  ball v.
  Bauhin's v.
  Béraud's v.
  Bianchi's v.
  bi·cus·pid v.
  Bochdalek's v.
  Braune's v.
  ca·val v.
  con·gen·i·tal v.
  cor·o·nary v.
  v. of cor·o·nary si·nus
  eu·sta·chi·an v.
  Gerlach's v.
  Guérin's v.
  Hasner's v.
  Heister's v.
  Heyer-Pudenz v.
  Ho·bo·ken's v.'s
  Houston's v.'s
  Huschke's v.
  il·e·o·ce·cal v.
  il·e·o·co·lic v.
  v. of in·fe·ri·or ve·na
    ca·va
  Kerckring's v.'s
  Kohlrausch's v.'s
  Krause's v.
  left atri·o·ven·tric·u·lar v.
  Mercier's v.
  mi·tral v.
  Morgagni's v.'s
  na·sal v.
  non·re·breath·ing v.
  v. of oval fo·ra·men
  par·a·chute mi·tral v.
  por·cine v.
  pos·te·ri·or ure·thral v.'s
  pul·mo·nary v.
  v. of pul·mo·nary trunk
  py·lor·ic v.
  rec·tal v.'s
  re·duc·ing v.
  right atri·o·ven·tric·u·lar v.
  Rosenmüller's v.
  sem·i·lu·nar v.
  spi·ral v.
  syl·vi·an v.
  Tarin's v.
  Terrier's v.
  the·be·si·an v.
  to·roi·dal v.
  tri·cus·pid v.
  Tulpius' v.
  Tulp's v.
  ure·thral v.'s
  v. of Varolius
  ve·nous v.

  ves·i·co·u·re·ter·al v.
  Vieussens' v.
valve·less
val·vi·form
val·vo·plas·ty
val·vot·o·my
  rec·tal v.
val·vot·o·my
  knife
val·vu·la
  Amussat's v.
  v. bi·cus·pi·da·lis
  val·vu·lae con·ni·ven·tes
  Gerlach's v.
  v. pro·ces·sus ver·mi·for·
    mis
  v. py·lo·ri
  v. sem·i·lu·na·ris ta·ri·ni
  v. spi·ra·lis
  v. tri·cus·pi·da·lis
  v. ve·no·sa
  v. ves·tib·u·li
val·vu·lae
val·vu·lar
  en·do·car·di·tis
  in·com·pe·tence
  in·suf·fi·cien·cy
  pneu·mo·thor·ax
  throm·bus
val·vule
  Foltz' v.
  lym·phat·ic v.
val·vu·li·tis
  rheu·mat·ic v.
val·vu·lo·plas·ty
val·vu·lo·tome
val·vu·lot·o·my
val·yl
vam·pire
  bat
van·a·date
va·na·dic ac·id
va·na·di·um
va·na·di·um group
van Bogaert's
  dis·ease
Van Buchem's
  syn·drome
Van Buren
  sound
van Buren's
  dis·ease
van·co·my·cin
van·dal root
van Deen's
  test
van den Bergh's
  test

van der Hoeve's
 syn·drome
van der Kolk's
 law
van der Velden's
 test
van der Waals'
 forc·es
van Ermengen's
 stain
van Gieson's
 stain
van Helmont's
 mir·ror
van Horne's
 ca·nal
va·nil·la
va·nil·late
va·nil·lic ac·id
va·nil·lin
va·nil·lism
va·nil·lyl·man·del·ic ac·id
 test
van·ish·ing
 cream
 lung
van·ish·ing lung
 syn·drome
Van Slyke
 ap·pa·ra·tus
Van Slyke's
 for·mu·la
van't Hoff's
 law
 the·o·ry
va·por
 den·si·ty
 pres·sure
va·por
 an·es·thet·ic v.
va·por·i·za·tion
va·por·ize
va·por·iz·er
 Cop·per Ket·tle v.
 flow-over v.
 tem·per·a·ture-com·pen·
  sat·ed v.
 Ver·ni·trol v.
va·por·tho·rax
va·po·ther·a·py
Vaquez'
 dis·ease
var·i·a·bil·i·ty
 base·line v. of fe·tal heart
  rate
var·i·a·ble
 de·pen·dent v.

in·de·pen·dent v.
in·ter·ven·ing v.
var·i·a·ble
 cou·pling
 de·cel·er·a·tion
 re·gion
var·i·a·ble-in·ter·val re·in·
 force·ment
 sched·ule
var·i·ance
 ball v.
var·i·ant
 in·her·it·ed al·bu·min v.'s
 L-phase v.'s
var·i·ant
 an·gi·na pec·to·ris
 he·mo·glo·bin
var·i·ate
var·i·a·tion
 beat-to-beat v. of fe·tal
  heart rate
 con·tin·u·ous v.
 me·ris·tic v.
var·i·ca·tion
var·i·ce·al
var·i·cel·la
 v. gan·gre·no·sa
var·i·cel·la
 en·ceph·a·li·tis
var·i·cel·la·tion
var·i·cel·la-zos·ter
 vi·rus
var·i·cel·li·form
var·i·cel·loid
 small·pox
va·ri·ces
var·i·ci·form
var·i·co·bleph·a·ron
var·i·co·cele
 ovar·i·an v.
 symp·to·mat·ic v.
 tu·bo-o·var·i·an v.
 uter·o-o·var·i·an v.
var·i·co·ce·lec·to·my
var·i·cog·ra·phy
var·i·coid
var·i·cole
var·i·com·pha·lus
var·i·co·phle·bi·tis
var·i·cose
 an·eu·rysm
 ec·ze·ma
 ul·cer
 veins
var·i·cos·es
var·i·co·sis
var·i·cos·i·ty
var·i·cot·o·my

va·ric·u·la
var·i·cule
var·ie·gate
  por·phyr·ia
va·ri·o·la
  vi·rus
va·ri·o·la
  v. be·nig·na
  v. hem·or·rha·gi·ca
  v. ma·jor
  v. ma·lig·na
  v. mil·i·a·ris
  v. mi·nor
  v. pem·phi·go·sa
  v. sine erup·ti·o·ne
  v. vac·cine
  v. vac·cin·ia
  v. ve·ra
  v. ver·ru·co·sa
va·ri·o·lar
var·i·o·late
var·i·o·la·tion
var·i·ol·ic
var·i·ol·i·form
  syph·i·lid
var·i·o·li·za·tion
va·ri·o·loid
va·ri·o·lous
va·ri·o·lo·vac·cine
var·ix
  v. anas·to·mo·ti·cus
  an·eu·rys·mal v.
  cir·soid v.
  con·junc·ti·val v.
  esoph·a·ge·al va·ri·ces
  ge·lat·i·nous v.
  lymph v.
  tur·bi·nal v.
var·nish (den·tal)
Varolius'
  sphinc·ter
var·us
vas
  v. aber·rans
  v. aber·rans hep·a·tis
  va·sa aber·ran·tia hep·a·tis
  va·sa bre·via
  va·sa chy·li·fe·ra
  v. def·er·ens
  va·sa def·er·en·tia
  Ferrein's va·sa aber·ran·tia
  Haller's v. aber·rans
  va·sa pre·via
  va·sa rec·ta
  Roth's v. aber·rans
  va·sa vor·ti·co·sa
va·sa
va·sal

vas·cu·la
vas·cu·lar
  bud
  cat·a·ract
  cir·cle
  cir·cle of op·tic nerve
  cones
  de·men·tia
  den·tin
  fold of the ce·cum
  gland
  head·ache
  he·mo·phil·ia
  ker·a·ti·tis
  la·cu·na
  lay·er
  lay·er of cho·roid coat of
    eye
  lei·o·my·o·ma
  mur·mur
  nerve
  pa·pil·lae
  plex·us
  pol·yp
  ring
  scle·ro·sis
  spi·der
  spur
  stripe
  sys·tem
  zone
vas·cu·lar·i·ty
vas·cu·lar·i·za·tion
vas·cu·lar·ized
  graft
vas·cu·la·ture
vas·cu·li·tis
  cu·ta·ne·ous v.
  leu·ko·cy·to·clas·tic v.
  li·ve·do v.
  nod·u·lar v.
vas·cu·lo·car·di·ac
  syn·drome of hy·per·se·ro·
    to·ne·mia
vas·cu·lo·gen·e·sis
vas·cu·lo·mo·tor
vas·cu·lo·my·e·li·nop·a·thy
vas·cu·lop·a·thy
vas·cu·lum
va·sec·to·my
vas·i·fac·tion
vas·i·fac·tive
vas·i·form
va·sis
vas·i·tis
va·so·ac·tive
  amine

va·so·ac·tive in·tes·ti·nal
  pol·y·pep·tide
va·so·con·stric·tion
  ac·tive v.
  pas·sive v.
va·so·con·stric·tive
va·so·con·stric·tor
va·so·den·tin
va·so·de·pres·sion
va·so·de·pres·sor
va·so·di·la·ta·tion
va·so·di·la·tion
  ac·tive v.
  pas·sive v.
va·so·di·la·tive
va·so·di·la·tor
va·so·ep·i·did·y·mos·to·my
va·so·fac·tive
va·so·for·ma·tion
va·so·for·ma·tive
  cell
va·so·gan·gli·on
va·so·gen·ic
  shock
va·sog·ra·phy
va·so·hy·per·ton·ic
va·so·hy·po·ton·ic
va·so·in·hib·i·tor
va·so·in·hib·i·to·ry
va·so·la·bile
va·so·li·ga·tion
va·so·mo·tion
va·so·mo·tor
  ab·sence
  an·gi·na
  atax·ia
  ep·i·lep·sy
  im·bal·ance
  nerve
  pa·ral·y·sis
  rhi·ni·tis
  spasm
va·so·neu·rop·a·thy
va·so·neu·ro·sis
va·so-or·chi·dos·to·my
va·so·pa·ral·y·sis
va·so·pa·re·sis
va·so·pres·sin
  ar·gi·nine v.
va·so·pres·sin-re·sis·tant
  di·a·be·tes
va·so·pres·sor
  re·flex
va·so·punc·ture
va·so·re·flex
va·so·re·lax·a·tion
va·so·rum
va·so·sec·tion

va·so·sen·so·ry
va·so·spasm
va·so·spas·tic
va·so·stim·u·lant
va·sos·to·my
va·so·throm·bin
va·so·to·cin
  ar·gi·nine v.
va·sot·o·my
va·so·to·nia
va·so·ton·ic
va·so·tribe
va·so·trip·sy
va·so·tro·phic
va·so·tro·pic
va·so·va·gal
  at·tack
  ep·i·lep·sy
  syn·co·pe
  syn·drome
va·so·va·sos·to·my
va·so·ve·sic·u·lec·to·my
vas·tus
VATER
  com·plex
Vater-Pacini
  cor·pus·cles
Vater's
  am·pul·la
  cor·pus·cles
  fold
vault
V-bends
VCE
  smear
VDRL
  test
vec·tion
vec·tis
vec·tor
  bi·o·log·i·cal v.
  clon·ing v.
  ex·pres·sion v.
  in·stan·ta·ne·ous v.
  man·i·fest v.
  mean v.
  me·chan·i·cal v.
  spa·tial v.
vec·tor
  loop
vec·tor·car·di·o·gram
vec·tor·car·di·og·ra·phy
  spa·tial v.
vec·to·ri·al
ve·cu·ro·ni·um bro·mide
VEE
  vi·rus

veg·e·ta·ble
  al·ka·li
  base
  cal·o·mel
  char·coal
  gel·a·tin
  oph·thal·mia
  sul·fur
  wax
veg·e·tal
  pole
veg·e·tal·i·ty
veg·e·tar·i·an
veg·e·tar·i·an·ism
veg·e·ta·tion
veg·e·ta·tive
  bac·te·ri·o·phage
  en·do·car·di·tis
  life
  pole
  stage
veg·e·ta·tive ner·vous
  sys·tem
veg·e·to·an·i·mal
ve·hi·cle
veil
  aq·ue·duct v.
  Jackson's v.
  Sattler's v.
veil
  cell
veiled
  puff
veil·ing
  glare
Veil·lo·nel·la
  V. al·ca·les·cens subsp.
    al·ca·les·cens
  V. al·ca·les·cens subsp.
    cri·ce·ti
  V. al·ca·les·cens subsp.
    dis·par
  V. al·ca·les·cens subsp. *rat·ti*
  V. al·ca·le·sens
  V. par·vu·la
  V. par·vu·la subsp. *aty·pi·ca*
  V. par·vu·la subsp. *par·vu·la*
  V. par·vu·la subsp.
    ro·den·ti·um
Veil·lo·nel·la·ce·ae
vein
  ac·ces·so·ry ce·phal·ic v.
  ac·ces·so·ry hem·i·az·y·gos
    v.
  ac·ces·so·ry sa·phe·nous v.
  ac·ces·so·ry ver·te·bral v.
  ac·com·pa·ny·ing v.
  anas·to·mot·ic v.'s

an·gu·lar v.
anon·y·mous v.'s
an·te·ri·or au·ric·u·lar v.
an·te·ri·or car·di·ac v.'s
an·te·ri·or car·di·nal v.'s
an·te·ri·or car·di·nal v.'s
an·te·ri·or ce·re·bral v.
an·te·ri·or fa·cial v.
an·te·ri·or in·ter·cos·tal v.'s
an·te·ri·or jug·u·lar v.
an·te·ri·or la·bi·al v.'s
an·te·ri·or pon·to·mes·en·
  ce·phal·ic v.
an·te·ri·or scro·tal v.'s
an·te·ri·or v. of sep·tum
  pel·lu·ci·dum
an·te·ri·or tib·i·al v.'s
an·te·ri·or ver·te·bral v.
ap·pen·dic·u·lar v.
aque·ous v.
ar·ci·form v.'s of kid·ney
ar·cu·ate v.'s of kid·ney
ar·te·ri·al v.
as·cend·ing lum·bar v.
au·ric·u·lar v.'s
ax·il·lary v.
az·y·gos v.
ba·sal v.'s
ba·sal v. of Rosenthal
ba·sil·ic v.
ba·si·ver·te·bral v.
Baumgarten's v.'s
brach·i·al v.'s
bra·chi·o·ce·phal·ic v.'s
Breschet's v.
bron·chi·al v.'s
Browning's v.
v. of bulb of pe·nis
Burow's v.
cap·il·lary v.
car·di·ac v.'s
car·di·nal v.'s
v.'s of cau·date nu·cle·us
cen·tral v.'s of liv·er
cen·tral v. of ret·i·na
cen·tral v. of su·pra·re·nal
  gland
ce·phal·ic v.
cer·e·bel·lar v.'s
v.'s of cer·e·bel·lum
ce·re·bral v.'s
cer·vi·cal v.
cho·roid v.
cho·roid v.'s of eye
cil·i·ary v.'s
cir·cum·flex v.'s
v. of co·chle·ar aq·ue·duct

v. of co·chle·ar can·a·lic·u·lus
col·ic v.'s
com·mon ba·sal v.
com·mon car·di·nal v.'s
com·mon fa·cial v.
com·mon il·i·ac v.
com·pan·ion v.
com·pan·ion v.'s
con·dy·lar em·is·sary v.
con·junc·ti·val v.'s
cor·o·nary v.
v. of cor·pus stri·a·tum
cos·to·ax·il·lary v.
cu·ta·ne·ous v.
Cuvier's v.'s
cys·tic v.
deep ce·re·bral v.'s
deep cer·vi·cal v.
deep cir·cum·flex il·i·ac v.
deep v.'s of clit·o·ris
deep dor·sal v. of clit·o·ris
deep dor·sal v. of pe·nis
deep ep·i·gas·tric v.
deep fa·cial v.
deep fem·o·ral v.
deep lin·gual v.
deep mid·dle ce·re·bral v.
deep v. of pe·nis
deep tem·po·ral v.'s
dig·i·tal v.'s
di·plo·ic v.
dor·sal cal·lo·sal v.
dor·sal v.'s of clit·o·ris
dor·sal v. of cor·pus cal·lo·sum
dor·sal dig·i·tal v.'s of toes
dor·sal lin·gual v.
dor·sal met·a·car·pal v.'s
dor·sal met·a·tar·sal v.'s
dor·sal v.'s of pe·nis
dor·sal scap·u·lar v.
dor·si·spi·nal v.'s
em·is·sary v.
ep·i·gas·tric v.'s
ep·i·scle·ral v.'s
esoph·a·ge·al v.'s
eth·moi·dal v.'s
ex·ter·nal il·i·ac v.
ex·ter·nal jug·u·lar v.
ex·ter·nal na·sal v.'s
ex·ter·nal pu·den·dal v.'s
v.'s of eye·lids
fa·cial v.
fem·o·ral v.
fib·u·lar v.'s
fron·tal v.'s
v.'s of Galen

gas·tric v.'s
gas·tro·ep·i·plo·ic v.'s
glu·te·al v.'s
great car·di·ac v.
great ce·re·bral v.
great v. of Galen
great sa·phe·nous v.
hem·i·az·y·gos v.
hem·or·rhoi·dal v.'s
he·pa·tic v.'s
he·pa·tic por·tal v.
high·est in·ter·cos·tal v.
hy·po·gas·tric v.
il·e·al v.'s
il·e·o·co·lic v.
il·i·ac v.'s
il·i·o·lum·bar v.
in·fe·ri·or anas·to·mot·ic v.
in·fe·ri·or ba·sal v.
in·fe·ri·or car·di·ac v.
in·fe·ri·or v.'s of cer·e·bel·lar hem·i·sphere
in·fe·ri·or ce·re·bral v.'s
in·fe·ri·or cho·roid v.
in·fe·ri·or ep·i·gas·tric v.
v.'s of in·fe·ri·or eye·lid
in·fe·ri·or glu·te·al v.'s
in·fe·ri·or hem·or·rhoi·dal v.'s
in·fe·ri·or la·bi·al v.
in·fe·ri·or la·ryn·ge·al v.
in·fe·ri·or mes·en·ter·ic v.
in·fe·ri·or oph·thal·mic v.
in·fe·ri·or phren·ic v.
in·fe·ri·or rec·tal v.'s
in·fe·ri·or thal·a·mo·stri·ate v.'s
in·fe·ri·or thy·roid v.
in·fe·ri·or ven·tric·u·lar v.
in·fe·ri·or v. of ver·mis
in·fra·seg·men·tal v.'s
in·nom·i·nate v.'s
in·nom·i·nate car·di·ac v.'s
in·su·lar v.'s
in·ter·ca·pit·u·lar v.'s
in·ter·cos·tal v.'s
in·ter·lo·bar v.'s of kid·ney
in·ter·lob·u·lar v.'s of kid·ney
in·ter·lob·u·lar v.'s of liv·er
in·ter·me·di·ate an·te·brach·i·al v.
in·ter·me·di·ate ba·sil·ic v.
in·ter·me·di·ate ce·phal·ic v.
in·ter·me·di·ate cu·bi·tal v.
in·ter·me·di·ate v. of fore·arm

vein *(continued)*

in·ter·nal au·di·to·ry v.'s
in·ter·nal ce·re·bral v.'s
in·ter·nal il·i·ac v.
in·ter·nal jug·u·lar v.
in·ter·nal pu·den·dal v.
in·ter·nal tho·rac·ic v.
in·ter·seg·men·tal v.'s
in·ter·ver·te·bral v.
in·tra·seg·men·tal v.'s
je·ju·nal and il·e·al v.'s
jug·u·lar v.'s
key v.
v.'s of kid·ney
v.'s of knee
Krukenberg's v.'s
Labbé's v.
la·bi·al v.'s
lab·y·rin·thine v.'s
lac·ri·mal v.
large v.
large sa·phe·nous v.
la·ryn·ge·al v.'s
Latarget's v.
lat·er·al atri·al v.
lat·er·al cir·cum·flex fem·o·ral v.'s
lat·er·al di·rect v.'s
lat·er·al v. of lat·er·al ven·tri·cle
v. of lat·er·al re·cess of fourth ven·tri·cle
lat·er·al sa·cral v.'s
lat·er·al tho·rac·ic v.
left col·ic v.
left cor·o·nary v.
left gas·tric v.
left gas·tro·ep·i·plo·ic v.
left gas·tro·o·men·tal v.
left he·pa·tic v.'s
left in·fe·ri·or pul·mo·nary v.
left ovar·i·an v.
left su·pe·ri·or in·ter·cos·tal v.
left su·pe·ri·or pul·mo·nary v.
left su·pra·re·nal v.
left tes·tic·u·lar v.
left um·bil·i·cal v.
le·vo·a·trio-car·di·nal v.
lin·gual v.
long sa·phe·nous v.
long tho·rac·ic v.
lum·bar v.'s
Marshall's ob·lique v.
mas·se·ter·ic v.'s
mas·toid em·is·sary v.

max·il·lary v.
Mayo's v.
me·di·al atri·al v.
me·di·al cir·cum·flex fem·o·ral v.'s
me·di·al v. of lat·er·al ven·tri·cle
me·di·an an·te·brach·i·al v.
me·di·an ba·sil·ic v.
me·di·an ce·phal·ic v.
me·di·an cu·bi·tal v.
me·di·an v. of fore·arm
me·di·an v. of neck
me·di·an sa·cral v.
me·di·as·ti·nal v.'s
me·di·um v.
v.'s of me·dul·la ob·lon·ga·ta
me·nin·ge·al v.'s
mes·en·ce·phal·ic v.'s
mes·en·ter·ic v.'s
met·a·car·pal v.'s
mid·dle car·di·ac v.
mid·dle col·ic v.
mid·dle hem·or·rhoi·dal v.'s
mid·dle he·pa·tic v.'s
mid·dle me·nin·ge·al v.'s
mid·dle rec·tal v.'s
mid·dle tem·po·ral v.
mid·dle thy·roid v.
mus·cu·lo·phren·ic v.'s
na·so·fron·tal v.
ob·lique v. of left atri·um
ob·tu·ra·tor v.
oc·cip·i·tal v.
oc·cip·i·tal v.'s
oc·cip·i·tal em·is·sary v.
v. of ol·fac·to·ry gy·rus
oph·thal·mic v.'s
ovar·i·an v.'s
pal·a·tine v.
pal·mar dig·i·tal v.'s
pal·mar met·a·car·pal v.'s
pan·cre·at·ic v.'s
pan·cre·at·i·co·du·o·de·nal v.'s
par·a·um·bil·i·cal v.'s
pa·ri·e·tal v.'s
pa·ri·e·tal em·is·sary v.
pa·rot·id v.'s
pec·to·ral v.'s
pe·dun·cu·lar v.'s
per·fo·rat·ing v.'s
per·i·car·di·a·co·phren·ic v.'s
per·i·car·di·al v.'s
per·o·ne·al v.'s
pe·tro·sal v.

pha·ryn·ge·al v.'s
phren·ic v.'s
plan·tar dig·i·tal v.'s
plan·tar met·a·tar·sal v.'s
v.'s of pons
pon·tine v.'s
pop·lit·e·al v.
por·tal v.
pos·te·ri·or an·te·ri·or jug·
u·lar v.
pos·te·ri·or au·ric·u·lar v.
pos·te·ri·or car·di·nal v.'s
pos·te·ri·or fa·cial v.
v. of pos·te·ri·or horn
pos·te·ri·or in·ter·
cos·tal v.'s
pos·te·ri·or la·bi·al v.'s
pos·te·ri·or v. of left ven·
tri·cle
pos·te·ri·or mar·gi·nal v.
pos·te·ri·or pa·rot·id v.'s
pos·te·ri·or per·i·cal·lo·
sal v.
pos·te·ri·or scro·tal v.'s
pos·te·ri·or v. of sep·tum
pel·lu·ci·dum
pos·te·ri·or tib·i·al v.'s
pre·cen·tral cer·e·bel·lar v.
pre·fron·tal v.'s
pre·py·lor·ic v.
v. of pter·y·goid ca·nal
pu·den·dal v.'s
pul·mo·nary v.'s
py·lor·ic v.
ra·di·al v.'s
re·nal v.'s
ret·ro·man·dib·u·lar v.
Retzius' v.'s
right col·ic v.
right gas·tric v.
right gas·tro·ep·i·plo·ic v.
right gas·tro·o·men·tal v.
right he·pa·tic v.'s
right in·fe·ri·or pul·mo·
nary v.
right ovar·i·an v.
right su·pe·ri·or in·ter·cos·
tal v.
right su·pe·ri·or pul·mo·
nary v.
right su·pra·re·nal v.
right tes·tic·u·lar v.
Rosenthal's v.
Ruysch's v.'s
sa·cral v.'s
Santorini's v.
sa·phe·nous v.'s
Sappey's v.'s

scle·ral v.'s
scro·tal v.'s
v. of sep·tum pel·lu·ci·dum
short gas·tric v.'s
short sa·phe·nous v.
sig·moid v.'s
small v.
small car·di·ac v.
small·est car·di·ac v.'s
small sa·phe·nous v.
sper·mat·ic v.
spi·nal v.'s
spi·ral v. of mo·di·o·lus
splen·ic v.
stel·late v.'s
Stensen's v.'s
ster·no·clei·do·mas·toid v.
stri·ate v.'s
sty·lo·mas·toid v.
sub·cla·vi·an v.
sub·cu·ta·ne·ous v.'s of
ab·do·men
sub·lin·gual v.
sub·men·tal v.
su·per·fi·cial v.
su·per·fi·cial ce·re·bral v.'s
su·per·fi·cial cir·cum·flex
il·i·ac v.
su·per·fi·cial dor·sal v.'s of
clit·o·ris
su·per·fi·cial dor·sal v.'s of
pe·nis
su·per·fi·cial ep·i·gas·tric v.
su·per·fi·cial mid·dle ce·re·
bral v.
su·per·fi·cial tem·po·ral v.'s
su·pe·ri·or anas·to·mot·ic
v.
su·pe·ri·or ba·sal v.
su·pe·ri·or v.'s of cer·e·bel·
lar hem·i·sphere
su·pe·ri·or ce·re·bral v.'s
su·pe·ri·or cho·roid v.
su·pe·ri·or ep·i·gas·tric v.'s
v.'s of su·pe·ri·or eye·lid
su·pe·ri·or glu·te·al v.'s
su·pe·ri·or hem·or·rhoi·dal
v.
su·pe·ri·or la·bi·al v.
su·pe·ri·or la·ryn·ge·al v.
su·pe·ri·or mes·en·ter·ic v.
su·pe·ri·or oph·thal·mic v.
su·pe·ri·or phren·ic v.'s
su·pe·ri·or rec·tal v.
su·pe·ri·or thal·a·mo·stri·
ate v.
su·pe·ri·or thy·roid v.
su·pe·ri·or v. of ver·mis

vein *(continued)*
su·pra·or·bit·al v.
su·pra·re·nal v.'s
su·pra·scap·u·lar v.
su·pra·troch·le·ar v.'s
sur·face tha·lam·ic v.'s
tem·po·ral v.'s
v.'s of tem·po·ro·man·dib·u·lar joint
tem·po·ro·max·il·lary v.
ter·mi·nal v.
tes·tic·u·lar v.'s
thal·a·mo·stri·ate v.'s
the·be·si·an v.'s
tho·rac·ic v.'s
tho·ra·co·a·cro·mi·al v.
tho·ra·co·ep·i·gas·tric v.
thy·mic v.'s
thy·roid v.'s
tra·che·al v.'s
trans·verse v. of face
trans·verse v.'s of neck
trans·verse v. of scap·u·la
Trolard's v.
tym·pan·ic v.'s
ul·nar v.'s
um·bil·i·cal v.
v. of un·cus
uter·ine v.'s
var·i·cose v.'s
ver·te·bral v.
v.'s of ver·te·bral col·umn
Vesalius' v.
ves·i·cal v.'s
ves·tib·u·lar v.'s
v. of ves·tib·u·lar aq·ue·duct
v. of ves·tib·u·lar bulb
vid·i·an v.
Vieussens' v.'s
vi·tel·line v.'s
vor·tex v.'s
vor·ti·cose v.'s
vein
stone
veined
vein·let
Ve·jo·vis
Vel
an·ti·gen
ve·la
ve·la·men
v. vul·vae
vel·a·men·ta
vel·a·men·tous
in·ser·tion
vel·a·men·tum
ve·lam·i·na

ve·lar
veldt
sore
ve·li·form
Vella's
fis·tu·la
vel·li·cate
vel·li·ca·tion
vel·lus
v. oli·vae in·fe·ri·o·ris
vel·lus
hair
ve·loc·i·ty
co·ef·fi·cient
con·stants
ve·loc·i·ty
max·i·mum v.
nerve con·duc·tion v.
vel·o·gen·ic
ve·lo·no·ski·as·co·py
vel·o·pha·ryn·ge·al
clo·sure
in·suf·fi·cien·cy
seal
ve·lo·syn·the·sis
Velpeau's
ban·dage
ca·nal
fos·sa
her·nia
ve·lum
an·te·ri·or med·ul·lary v.
in·fe·ri·or med·ul·lary v.
v. in·ter·pos·i·tum
v. pen·du·lum pa·la·ti
pos·te·ri·or med·ul·lary v.
v. sem·i·lu·na·re
su·pe·ri·or med·ul·lary v.
v. ta·ri·ni
v. ter·mi·na·le
v. trans·ver·sum
v. tri·an·gu·la·re
vel·vet
ant
Ven
an·ti·gen
ve·na
v. ad·ve·hens
ve·nae ad·ve·hen·tes
v. ar·te·ri·o·sa
ve·nae ar·tic·u·la·res tem·po·ro·man·di·bu·la·res
v. az·y·gos ma·jor
v. az·y·gos mi·nor in·fe·ri·or
v. az·y·gos mi·nor su·pe·ri·or

Billroth's ve·nae ca·ver·no·sae
v. can·a·lic·u·li co·chle·ae
v. car·di·a·ca mag·na
ve·nae ce·re·bel·li in·fe·ri·o·res
ve·nae ce·re·bel·li su·pe·ri·o·res
v. cor·o·na·ria ven·tric·u·li
v. fa·ci·a·lis
v. fa·ci·a·lis an·te·ri·or
v. fa·ci·a·lis com·mu·nis
v. fa·ci·a·lis pos·te·ri·or
ve·nae fron·ta·les
ve·nae hem·or·rhoi·da·les in·fe·ri·o·res
ve·nae hem·or·rhoi·da·les me·di·ae
v. hem·or·rhoi·dal·is su·pe·ri·or
v. hy·po·gas·tri·ca
in·fe·ri·or v. ca·va
v. in·no·mi·na·ta
v. li·e·na·lis
v. mam·ma·ria in·ter·na
v. me·di·a·na an·te·bra·chii
v. me·di·a·na ba·sil·i·ca
v. me·di·a·na ce·pha·li·ca
v. me·di·a·na cu·bi·ti
v. por·ta·lis
v. pre·au·ri·cu·la·ris
ve·nae rec·tae
v. re·ve·hens
ve·nae re·ve·hen·tes
ve·nae ca·ver·no·sae of spleen
ve·nae stel·la·tae
ve·nae stri·a·tae
su·pe·ri·or v. ca·va
v. thy·roi·dea ima
v. trans·ver·sa scap·u·lae
v. vit·el·li·na
ve·na·ca·vog·ra·phy
ve·nae
ve·na·tion
ve·nec·ta·sia
ve·nec·to·my
ve·neer
ven·e·na·tion
ven·e·nif·er·ous
ven·e·no·sal·i·vary
ven·e·nos·i·ty
ven·e·nous
ve·ne·re·al
bu·bo
dis·ease
lym·pho·gran·u·lo·ma
sore

ul·cer
wart
ve·ne·re·ol·o·gy
ve·ne·re·o·pho·bia
ven·e·sec·tion
Ven·e·zu·e·lan equine en·ceph·a·lo·my·e·li·tis
Ven·e·zu·e·lan equine en·ceph·a·lo·my·e·li·tis vi·rus
Ven·ice tur·pen·tine
ven·in
ven·i·punc·ture
ve·no·cly·sis
ve·no·fi·bro·sis
ve·no·gram
ve·nog·ra·phy
splen·ic v.
splen·ic por·tal v.
trans·os·se·ous v.
ver·te·bral v.
ven·om
ko·koi v.
Russell's vi·per v.
ven·om he·mol·y·sis
ven·o·mo·sal·i·vary
ve·no·mo·tor
ve·no-oc·clu·sive dis·ease of the liv·er
ve·no·per·i·to·ne·os·to·my
ve·no·pres·sor
ve·no·res·pi·ra·to·ry re·flex
ve·no·scle·ro·sis
ve·nose
ve·no·si·nal
ve·nos·i·ty
ve·nos·ta·sis
ve·no·stat
ve·nos·to·my
ve·not·o·my
ve·nous
an·gle
ar·tery
blood
cap·il·lary
cir·cle of mam·ma·ry gland
con·ges·tion
em·bo·lism
gan·grene
grooves
heart
hum
hy·per·e·mia
in·suf·fi·cien·cy
lakes

ve·nous *(continued)*
  lig·a·ment
  mur·mur
  plex·us
  plex·us of blad·der
  plex·us of fo·ra·men ova·le
  plex·us of hy·po·glos·sal
    ca·nal
  pulse
  seg·ments of the kid·ney
  seg·ments of liv·er
  si·nus·es
  si·nus of scle·ra
  star
  valve
ve·nous oc·clu·sion
  pleth·ys·mog·ra·phy
ve·nous re·turn
ve·nous-sta·sis
  ret·i·nop·a·thy
ve·no·ve·nos·to·my
vent
ven·ter
  v. pro·pen·dens
ven·ti·late
ven·ti·la·tion
  al·ve·o·lar v.
  ar·ti·fi·cial v.
  as·sist-con·trol v.
  as·sist·ed v.
  con·tin·u·ous pos·i·tive
    pres·sure v.
  con·trolled v.
  con·trolled me·chan·i·cal v.
  in·ter·mit·tent man·da·to·ry
    v.
  in·ter·mit·tent pos·i·tive
    pres·sure v.
  man·u·al v.
  max·i·mum vol·un·tary v.
  me·chan·i·cal v.
  pul·mo·nary v.
  spon·ta·ne·ous in·ter·mit·
    tent man·da·to·ry v.
  syn·chro·nized in·ter·mit·
    tent man·da·to·ry v.
  wast·ed v.
ven·ti·la·tion
  me·ter
ven·ti·la·tion-per·fu·sion
  scan
ven·ti·la·tion/per·fu·sion
  ra·ti·o
ven·ti·la·to·ry
  com·pli·ance
vent·plant
ven·trad

ven·tral
  aor·tas
  col·umn of spi·nal cord
  glands
  her·nia
  horn
  mes·o·car·di·um
  nu·cle·us of thal·a·mus
  nu·cle·us of trap·e·zoid
    body
  pan·cre·as
  part of the pons
  plate
  plate of neu·ral tube
  root
  sur·face of dig·it
ven·tral an·te·ri·or
  nu·cle·us of thal·a·mus
ven·tral in·ter·me·di·ate
  nu·cle·us of thal·a·mus
ven·tra·lis
ven·tral lat·er·al
  nu·cle·us of thal·a·mus
ven·tral pos·te·ri·or
  nu·cle·us of thal·a·mus
ven·tral pos·te·ri·or in·ter·me·
  di·ate
  nu·cle·us of thal·a·mus
ven·tral pos·te·ri·or lat·er·al
  nu·cle·us of thal·a·mus
ven·tral pos·ter·o·lat·er·al
  nu·cle·us of thal·a·mus
ven·tral pos·ter·o·me·di·al
  nu·cle·us of thal·a·mus
ven·tral sa·cro·coc·cyg·e·al
  lig·a·ment
  mus·cle
ven·tral sa·cro·il·i·ac
  lig·a·ments
ven·tral spi·no·cer·e·bel·lar
  tract
ven·tral spi·no·tha·lam·ic
  tract
ven·tral splanch·nic
  ar·ter·ies
ven·tral teg·men·tal
  de·cus·sa·tion
ven·tral tha·lam·ic
  pe·dun·cle
ven·tral tier tha·lam·ic
  nu·clei
ven·tri·cle
  Arantius' v.
  ce·re·bral v.'s
  v. of ce·re·bral hem·i·
    sphere
  v. of di·en·ceph·a·lon
  Duncan's v.

fifth v.
fourth v.
v.'s of heart
la·ryn·ge·al v.
lat·er·al v.
left v.
Morgagni's v.
v. of rhomb·en·ceph·a·lon
right v.
sixth v.
syl·vi·an v.
ter·mi·nal v.
third v.
Verga's v.
Vieussens' v.
Wenzel's v.
ven·tri·cose
ven·tric·u·lar
ab·er·ra·tion
af·ter·load
an·eu·rysm
ar·ter·ies
band of lar·ynx
bi·gem·i·ny
bra·dy·car·dia
cap·ture
com·plex
con·duc·tion
di·ver·tic·u·lum
es·cape
ex·tra·sys·to·le
fi·bril·la·tion
flu·id
flut·ter
fold
gra·di·ent
lay·er
lig·a·ment
loop
pla·teau
pre·load
rhythm
sep·tum
stand·still
sys·to·le
tach·y·car·dia
ven·tric·u·lar fill·ing
pres·sure
ven·tric·u·lar fu·sion
beat
ven·tric·u·lar in·hib·it·ed pulse
gen·er·a·tor
ven·tric·u·lar·is
ven·tric·u·lar·i·za·tion
ven·tric·u·lar sep·tal
de·fect

ven·tric·u·lar syn·chro·nous pulse
gen·er·a·tor
ven·tric·u·lar trig·gered pulse
gen·er·a·tor
ven·tric·u·li
ven·tric·u·li·tis
ven·tric·u·lo·a·tri·al
con·duc·tion
ven·tric·u·lo·cis·ter·nos·to·my
ven·tric·u·log·ra·phy
ven·tric·u·lo·mas·toi·dos·to·my
ven·tric·u·lo·nec·tor
ven·tric·u·lo·pha·sic
ven·tric·u·lo·plas·ty
ven·tric·u·lo·punc·ture
ven·tric·u·lo·ra·di·al
dys·pla·sia
ven·tric·u·los·co·py
ven·tric·u·los·to·my
third v.
ven·tric·u·lo·sub·a·rach·noid
ven·tric·u·lot·o·my
ven·tric·u·lus
v. quin·tus
ven·tri·duct
ven·tri·duc·tion
ven·tro·ba·sal
nu·cle·us
ven·tro·cys·tor·rha·phy
ven·tro·dor·sad
ven·tro·in·gui·nal
ven·tro·lat·er·al
ven·tro·me·di·al
nu·cle·us of hy·po·thal·a·mus
ven·tro·me·di·an
ven·trop·to·sia
ven·trop·to·sis
ven·tros·co·py
ven·trot·o·my
Venturi
ef·fect
me·ter
tube
ven·u·la
ven·u·lae
ven·u·lar
ven·ule
high en·do·the·li·al post·cap·il·lary v.'s
in·fe·ri·or mac·u·lar v.
in·fe·ri·or na·sal v. of ret·i·na
in·fe·ri·or tem·po·ral v. of ret·i·na
me·di·al v. of ret·i·na
na·sal v.'s of ret·i·na

ven·ule *(continued)*
  per·i·cyt·ic v.'s
  post·cap·il·lary v.'s
  stel·late v.'s
  straight v.'s of kid·ney
  su·pe·ri·or mac·u·lar v.
  su·pe·ri·or na·sal v. of ret·i·na
  su·pe·ri·or tem·po·ral v. of ret·i·na
  tem·po·ral v.'s of ret·i·na
ven·u·lous
ve·rap·a·mil
ve·rat·ric ac·id
ver·a·trine
Ve·ra·trum
  V. al·bum
  V. vir·ide
ver·bal
  agraph·ia
ver·big·er·a·tion
ver·bo·ma·nia
ver·di·gris
ver·dine
ver·do·glo·bin
ver·do·he·mo·chrome
ver·do·he·mo·glo·bin
ver·do·per·ox·i·dase
Verga's
  ven·tri·cle
verge
  anal v.
ver·gence
  v. of lens
ver·ge·ture
Verheyen's
  stars
Verhoeff's elas·tic tis·sue
  stain
Ver·mes
ver·mes
ver·mi·an
  fos·sa
ver·mi·ci·dal
ver·mi·cide
ver·mic·u·lar
  col·ic
  move·ment
  pulse
ver·mic·u·la·tion
ver·mi·cule
ver·mic·u·lose
ver·mic·u·lous
ver·mi·cu·lus
ver·mi·form
  ap·pend·age
  ap·pen·dix
  pro·cess

ver·mif·u·gal
ver·mi·fuge
ver·mil·ion
  bor·der
  zone
ver·mil·ion·ec·to·my
ver·mil·ion tran·si·tion·al zone
ver·min
ver·mi·nal
ver·mi·na·tion
ver·min·ous
  ab·scess
  an·eu·rysm
  ap·pen·di·ci·tis
  bron·chi·tis
  il·e·us
ver·mis
ver·mix
ver·nal
  ca·tarrh
  con·junc·ti·vi·tis
  en·ceph·a·li·tis
  ker·a·to·con·junc·ti·vi·tis
Verner-Morrison
  syn·drome
Vernet's
  syn·drome
Verneuil's
  neu·ro·ma
Vernier
  acu·i·ty
Ver·ni·trol
  va·por·iz·er
ver·nix
  v. ca·se·o·sa
Ver·o·cay
  bod·ies
ver·ru·ca
  v. acu·mi·na·ta
  v. dig·i·ta·ta
  v. fi·li·for·mis
  v. gla·bra
  v. mol·lus·ci·for·mis
  v. nec·ro·ge·ni·ca
  v. pe·ru·ana
  v. pe·ru·vi·ana
  v. pla·na
  v. pla·na ju·ve·ni·lis
  v. pla·na se·ni·lis
  v. plan·tar·is
  seb·or·rhe·ic v.
  v. se·ni·lis
  v. sim·plex
  v. vul·ga·ris
ver·ru·cae
ver·ru·ci·form
ver·ru·cose

ver·ru·co·sis
  lym·pho·stat·ic v.
ver·ru·cous
  car·ci·no·ma
  en·do·car·di·tis
  he·man·gi·o·ma
  hy·per·pla·sia
  ne·vus
  scrof·u·lo·der·ma
  xan·tho·ma
ver·ru·ga
  v. pe·ru·ana
  v. pe·ru·vi·ana
ver·si·col·or
ver·sion
  bi·man·u·al v.
  bi·po·lar v.
  Braxton Hicks v.
  ce·phal·ic v.
  com·bined v.
  ex·ter·nal v.
  in·ter·nal v.
  pel·vic v.
  po·dal·ic v.
  pos·tur·al v.
  Potter's v.
  spon·ta·ne·ous v.
  Wright's v.
ver·te·bra
  bas·i·lar v.
  block ver·te·brae
  but·ter·fly v.
  cau·dal ver·te·brae
  cer·vi·cal ver·te·brae
  coc·cyg·eal ver·te·brae
  cod·fish ver·te·brae
  cra·ni·al v.
  v. den·ta·ta
  dor·sal ver·te·brae
  false ver·te·brae
  hour·glass ver·te·brae
  lum·bar ver·te·brae
  v. mag·na
  odon·toid v.
  v. pla·na
  sa·cral ver·te·brae
  ver·te·brae spu·ri·ae
  tail ver·te·brae
  tho·rac·ic ver·te·brae
  toothed v.
  true v.
  v. ve·ra
ver·te·brae
ver·te·bral
  arch
  ar·tery
  ca·nal
  col·umn

fo·ra·men
for·mu·la
fu·sion
gan·gli·on
groove
nerve
notch
part
part of di·a·phragm
plex·us
pol·y·ar·thri·tis
pulp
re·gion
ribs
vein
ve·nog·ra·phy
ver·te·bral-bas·i·lar
  sys·tem
ver·te·bral cer·vi·cal
  in·sta·bil·i·ty
ver·te·bral ve·nous
  plex·us
  sys·tem
ver·te·bra pro·mi·nens
  re·flex
ver·te·bra·ri·um
Ver·te·bra·ta
ver·te·brate
  no·to·chor·dal v.
ver·te·brat·ed
  cath·e·ter
  probe
ver·te·brec·to·my
ver·te·bro·ar·te·ri·al
  fo·ra·men
ver·te·bro·chon·dral
  ribs
ver·te·bro·cos·tal
  tri·gone
ver·te·bro·fem·o·ral
ver·te·bro·il·i·ac
ver·te·bro·pel·vic
  lig·a·ments
ver·te·bro·sa·cral
ver·te·bro·ster·nal
  ribs
ver·tex
  pre·sen·ta·tion
ver·tex
  v. cor·dis
  v. of cor·nea
ver·ti·cal
  ax·is
  di·men·sion
  elas·tic
  heart
  hy·men
  il·lu·mi·na·tion

ver·ti·cal *(continued)*
  in·dex
  mus·cle of tongue
  nys·tag·mus
  open·ing
  os·te·ot·o·my
  over·lap
  par·al·lax
  plate
  stra·bis·mus
  trans·mis·sion
  ver·ti·go
ver·ti·cal band·ed
  gas·tro·plas·ty
ver·ti·cal growth
  phase
ver·ti·ca·lis
ver·ti·cal re·trac·tion
  syn·drome
ver·ti·ces
ver·ti·cil
ver·ti·cil·late
Ver·ti·cil·li·um
ver·ti·co·men·tal
ver·ti·co·sub·men·tal
  view
ver·tig·i·nous
ver·ti·go
  v. ab au·re la·e·so
  au·di·to·ry v.
  au·ral v.
  Charcot's v.
  chron·ic v.
  en·dem·ic par·a·lyt·ic v.
  ep·i·dem·ic v.
  gal·van·ic v.
  gas·tric v.
  height v.
  hor·i·zon·tal v.
  lab·y·rin·thine v.
  la·ryn·ge·al v.
  lat·er·al v.
  me·chan·i·cal v.
  noc·tur·nal v.
  oc·u·lar v.
  or·gan·ic v.
  par·a·lyz·ing v.
  pos·tur·al v.
  ro·ta·ry v.
  sham-move·ment v.
  sys·tem·at·ic v.
  ver·ti·cal v.
  vol·ta·ic v.
ver·tom·e·ter
ver·u·mon·ta·ni·tis
ver·u·mon·ta·num
ve·sa·li·a·num

Vesalius'
  bone
  fo·ra·men
  vein
ve·si·ca
  v. pros·ta·ti·ca
ve·si·cae
ves·i·cal
  cal·cu·lus
  di·ver·tic·u·lum
  fis·tu·la
  gland
  he·ma·tu·ria
  li·thot·o·my
  plex·us
  re·flex
  sur·face of uter·us
  tri·an·gle
  veins
ves·i·cant
ves·i·cate
ves·i·cat·ing
  gas
ves·i·ca·tion
ves·i·ca·to·ry
ves·i·cle
  acous·tic v.
  ac·ro·so·mal v.
  air v.'s
  al·lan·to·ic v.
  am·ni·o·car·di·ac v.
  au·di·to·ry v.
  Baer's v.
  blas·to·der·mic v.
  ce·re·bral v.
  cer·vi·cal v.
  en·ce·phal·ic v.
  fore·brain v.
  ger·mi·nal v.
  hind·brain v.
  lens v.
  len·tic·u·lar v.
  mal·pi·ghi·an v.'s
  mid·brain v.
  oc·u·lar v.
  op·tic v.
  otic v.
  pin·o·cy·tot·ic v.
  pri·mary brain v.
  sem·i·nal v.
  syn·ap·tic v.'s
  tel·en·ce·phal·ic v.
  um·bil·i·cal v.
ves·i·cle
  her·nia
ves·i·co·ab·dom·i·nal
ves·i·co·bul·lous
ves·i·co·cele

ves·i·co·cer·vi·cal
ves·i·coc·ly·sis
ves·i·co·co·lic
  fis·tu·la
ves·i·co·cu·ta·ne·ous
  fis·tu·la
ves·i·co·fix·a·tion
ves·i·co·in·tes·ti·nal
  fis·tu·la
ves·i·co·li·thi·a·sis
ves·i·co·pros·ta·tic
ves·i·co·pu·bic
ves·i·co·pus·tu·lar
ves·i·co·pus·tule
ves·i·co·rec·tal
ves·i·co·rec·tos·to·my
ves·i·co·sig·moid
ves·i·co·sig·moi·dos·to·my
ves·i·co·spi·nal
ves·i·cos·to·my
ves·i·cot·o·my
ves·i·co·um·bi·li·cal
  lig·a·ment
ves·i·co·u·re·ter·al
  re·flux
  valve
ves·i·co·u·re·thral
  ca·nal
ves·i·co·u·ter·ine
  fis·tu·la
  lig·a·ment
  pouch
ves·i·co·u·ter·o·vag·i·nal
ves·i·co·vag·i·nal
  fis·tu·la
ves·i·co·vag·i·no·rec·tal
  fis·tu·la
ves·i·co·vis·cer·al
ve·sic·u·la
  v. fel·lis
  v. um·bi·li·ca·lis
ve·sic·u·lae
ve·sic·u·lar
  ap·pend·age
  ex·an·the·ma
  ker·a·ti·tis
  ker·a·top·a·thy
  mole
  mur·mur
  rale
  res·o·nance
  res·pi·ra·tion
  rick·ett·si·o·sis
  sto·ma·ti·tis
  trans·port
ve·sic·u·lar ex·an·the·ma of
  swine
  vi·rus

ve·sic·u·lar ovar·i·an
  fol·li·cle
ve·sic·u·lar sto·ma·ti·tis
  vi·rus
ve·sic·u·late
ve·sic·u·lat·ed
ve·sic·u·la·tion
ve·sic·u·lec·to·my
ve·sic·u·li·form
ve·sic·u·li·tis
ve·sic·u·lo·bron·chi·al
ve·sic·u·lo·cav·ern·ous
  res·pi·ra·tion
ve·sic·u·log·ra·phy
ve·sic·u·lo·pap·u·lar
ve·sic·u·lo·pros·ta·ti·tis
ve·sic·u·lo·pus·tu·lar
ve·si·cu·lose
ve·sic·u·lot·o·my
ve·sic·u·lo·tu·bu·lar
ve·sic·u·lo·tym·pan·ic
ve·sic·u·lo·tym·pa·ni·tic
  res·o·nance
ve·sic·u·lous
Ve·si·cu·lo·vi·rus
Vesling's
  line
ves·sel
  ab·sor·bent v.'s
  af·fer·ent v.
  blood v.
  cap·il·lary v.
  chyle v.
  col·lat·er·al v.
  deep lym·phat·ic v.
  ef·fer·ent v.
  lac·te·al v.
  lymph v.'s
  lym·phat·ic v.'s
  nu·tri·ent v.
  su·per·fi·cial lym·phat·ic v.
  v.'s of ves·sels
  vi·tel·line v.'s
ves·tib·u·la
ves·tib·u·lar
  anus
  ar·ea
  ca·nal
  crest
  fis·sure of co·chlea
  fold
  fos·sa
  gan·gli·on
  glands
  lab·y·rinth
  lig·a·ment
  lip
  mem·brane

ves·tib·u·lar *(continued)*
  nerve
  nu·clei
  nys·tag·mus
  or·gan
  part of ves·tib·u·lo·co·chle·
    ar nerve
  root of ves·tib·u·lo·co·chle·
    ar nerve
  screen
  sur·face of tooth
  veins
  wall of co·chle·ar duct
  win·dow
ves·tib·u·lar blind
  sac
ves·tib·u·lar hair
  cells
ves·ti·bu·la·ris
ves·tib·u·late
ves·ti·bule
  aor·tic v.
  buc·cal v.
  esoph·a·go·gas·tric v.
  gas·tro·e·soph·a·ge·al v.
  la·bi·al v.
  v. of lar·ynx
  v. of mouth
  v. of nose
  v. of omen·tal bur·sa
  Sibson's aor·tic v.
  v. of va·gi·na
ves·tib·u·lo·cer·e·bel·lar
  atax·ia
ves·tib·u·lo·cer·e·bel·lum
ves·tib·u·lo·co·chle·ar
  nerve
  or·gan
ves·tib·u·lo-e·quil·i·bra·to·ry
  con·trol
ves·tib·u·lo·plas·ty
ves·tib·u·lo·spi·nal
  re·flex
  tract
ves·tib·u·lot·o·my
ves·tib·u·lo·u·re·thral
ves·tib·u·lum
  v. aor·tae
  v. pu·den·di
ves·tige
  v. of vag·i·nal pro·cess
ves·tig·ia
ves·tig·i·al
  fold
  mus·cle
  or·gan
ves·tig·i·um
ve·su·vin

vet·er·i·nar·i·an
Vet·er·i·nar·i·an's Oath
vet·er·i·nary
  med·i·cine
Vi
  an·ti·body
  an·ti·gen
vi·a·bil·i·ty
vi·a·ble
vi·al
vi·bes·ate
vi·brat·ing
  line
vi·bra·tion
  syn·drome
  tol·er·ance
vi·bra·tive
vi·bra·tor
vi·bra·to·ry
  mas·sage
  sen·si·bil·i·ty
  ur·ti·car·ia
Vib·rio
  V. al·gi·no·lyt·i·cus
  V. chol·er·ae
  V. com·ma
  V. fe·tus
  V. flu·vi·a·lis
  V. fur·nis·sii
  V. metsch·ni·ko·vii
  V. mi·mi·cus
  V. par·a·hae·mo·lyt·i·cus
  V. spu·to·rum
  V. vul·ni·fi·cus
vib·rio
  El Tor v.
  Na·sik v.
vib·ri·on·ic
  abor·tion
vib·ri·on sep·tique
vib·ri·o·ses
vib·ri·o·sis
vi·bris·sa
vi·bris·sae
vi·bris·sal
vi·bro·car·di·o·gram
vi·bro·mas·seur
vi·bro·ther·a·peu·tics
vi·car·i·ous
  hy·per·tro·phy
  men·stru·a·tion
Vi·cat
  nee·dle
vi·cine
vi·cious
  cic·a·trix
  cir·cle
  un·ion

Vicq d'Azyr's
 bun·dle
 cen·trum sem·i·o·va·le
 fo·ra·men
Vic·to·ria blue
Vic·to·ria or·ange
Vidal's
 dis·ease
vi·dar·a·bine
vid·i·an
 ar·tery
 ca·nal
 nerve
 vein
Vierra's
 sign
Vieussens'
 an·nu·lus
 an·sa
 cen·trum
 fo·ram·i·na
 gan·gli·on
 isth·mus
 lim·bus
 loop
 ring
 valve
 veins
 ven·tri·cle
view
 ax·i·al v.
 base v.
 Caldwell v.
 Stenvers v.
 Towne v.
 ver·ti·co·sub·men·tal v.
vig·il
 co·ma v.
vig·il·am·bu·lism
vig·i·lance
vil·li
vil·lo·ma
vil·lo·nod·u·lar pig·ment·ed
 ten·o·syn·o·vi·tis
vil·lose
vil·lo·si·tis
vil·los·i·ty
vil·lous
 ad·e·no·ma
 car·ci·no·ma
 pap·il·lo·ma
 pla·cen·ta
 ten·o·syn·o·vi·tis
 tu·mor
vil·lus
 an·chor·ing v.
 arach·noid vil·li
 cho·ri·on·ic vil·li

 float·ing v.
 free v.
 in·tes·ti·nal vil·li
 vil·li pe·ri·car·di·a·ci
 per·i·car·di·al vil·li
 per·i·to·ne·al vil·li
 vil·li pe·ri·to·ne·a·les
 pleu·ral vil·li
 vil·li pleu·ra·les
 pri·mary v.
 sec·on·dary v.
 syn·o·vi·al vil·li
 ter·ti·ary v.
vil·lus·ec·to·my
vi·men·tin
vin·bar·bi·tal
vin·blas·tine sul·fate
vin·ca·leu·ko·blas·tine
Vin·ca ro·sea
Vincent's
 an·gi·na
 ba·cil·lus
 dis·ease
 in·fec·tion
 spi·ril·lum
 ton·sil·li·tis
Vincent's white
 my·ce·to·ma
vin·cris·tine sul·fate
vin·cu·la
vin·cu·lum
 v. lin·guae
 vin·cu·la lin·gu·lae ce·re·
  bel·li
 long v.
 v. pre·pu·tii
 short v.
 vin·cu·la of ten·dons
Vineberg
 pro·ce·dure
vin·e·gar
 py·ro·lig·ne·ous v.
 wood v.
vi·nic
vi·nous
 li·quor
vi·nyl
 v. car·bi·nol
 v. chlo·ride
vi·nyl·ben·zene
vi·nyl·ene
vi·nyl ether
vi·nyl·eth·yl ether
vi·nyl·i·dene
vi·o·la·ceous
vi·o·let
 vi·su·al v.

vi·o·lin·ist's
  cramp
vi·o·my·cin
vi·os·ter·ol
vi·per
  Russell's v.
Vi·per·i·dae
vi·po·ma
Vipond's
  sign
vip·ryn·i·um em·bo·nate
vir·a·gin·i·ty
vi·ral
  dys·en·tery
  en·ve·lope
  gas·tro·en·ter·i·tis
  he·mag·glu·ti·na·tion
  hep·a·ti·tis
  hep·a·ti·tis type A
  hep·a·ti·tis type B
  hep·a·ti·tis type D
  probe
  strand
  tro·pism
  wart
vi·ral hem·or·rhag·ic
  fe·ver
vi·ral hem·or·rhag·ic fe·ver
  vi·rus
Virchow-Hassall
  bod·ies
Virchow-Holder
  an·gle
Virchow-Robin
  space
Virchow's
  an·gle
  cells
  cor·pus·cles
  crys·tals
  dis·ease
  law
  node
  psam·mo·ma
vi·re·mia
vi·res
vir·ga
vir·gin
  gen·er·a·tion
  silk
vir·gin·al
  mem·brane
Vir·gin·ia
  snake·root
vir·gin·i·ty
vir·go·phre·nia
vir·i·ci·dal
vir·i·cide

vir·i·dans
  he·mol·y·sis
vir·ile
  mem·ber
vir·i·les·cence
vi·ril·ia
vir·i·lism
  ad·re·nal v.
vi·ril·i·ty
vir·i·li·za·tion
vir·i·liz·ing
vi·ri·on
vi·rip·o·tent
vi·roid
vi·rol·o·gist
vi·rol·o·gy
vi·ro·pex·is
vir·tu·al
  fo·cus
  im·age
vi·ru·ci·dal
vi·ru·cide
vi·ru·co·pria
vir·u·lence
vir·u·lent
  bac·te·ri·o·phage
  bu·bo
vir·u·lif·er·ous
vir·u·ria
vi·rus
  Abel·son mu·rine leu·ke·mia
    v.
  ad·e·no-as·so·ci·at·ed v.
  ad·e·noi·dal-pha·ryn·ge·al-
    con·junc·ti·val v.
  ad·e·no·sat·el·lite v.
  Af·ri·can horse sick·ness v.
  Af·ri·can swine fe·ver v.
  AIDS-re·lat·ed v.
  Ak·a·bane v.
  Aleu·tian dis·ease of mink
    v.
  am·pho·tro·pic v.
  an·i·mal vi·rus·es
  A-P-C v.
  at·ten·u·at·ed v.
  Aujeszky's dis·ease v.
  Aus·tra·li·an X dis·ease v.
  avi·an en·ceph·a·lo·my·e·li·
    tis v.
  avi·an eryth·ro·blas·to·sis v.
  avi·an in·fec·tious la·ryn·
    go·tra·che·i·tis v.
  avi·an in·flu·en·za v.
  avi·an leu·ko·sis-sar·co·ma
    v.
  avi·an lym·pho·ma·to·sis v.
  avi·an my·e·lo·blas·to·sis v.

avi·an neu·ro·lym·pho·ma·
to·sis v.
avi·an pneu·mo·en·ceph·a·
li·tis v.
avi·an sar·co·ma v.
avi·an vi·ral ar·thri·tis v.
B v.
bac·te·ri·al v.
BK v.
blue·comb v.
blue·tongue v.
Bor·na dis·ease v.
Bornholm dis·ease v.
bo·vine leu·ke·mia v.
bo·vine leu·ko·sis v.
bo·vine pap·u·lar sto·ma·ti·
tis v.
bo·vine vi·rus di·ar·rhea v.
Bun·yam·we·ra v.
Bwam·ba v.
CA v.
Cal·i·for·nia v.
ca·nar·y·pox v.
ca·nine dis·tem·per v.
Ca·pim vi·rus·es
Caraparu v.
cat dis·tem·per v.
cat·tle plague v.
Ca·tu v.
CELO v.
Cen·tral Eu·ro·pe·an tick-
borne en·ceph·a·li·tis v.
C group vi·rus·es
Chagres v.
chick·en em·bryo le·thal or·
phan v.
chick·en·pox v.
chi·kun·gun·ya v.
Coe v.
cold v.
Col·o·ra·do tick fe·ver v.
Co·lum·bia S. K. v.
com·mon cold v.
con·ta·gious ec·thy·ma
(pus·tu·lar der·ma·ti·tis) v.
of sheep
con·ta·gious pus·tu·lar sto·
ma·ti·tis v.
cow·pox v.
Cox·sack·ie v.
Cri·me·an-Con·go hem·or·
rhag·ic fe·ver v.
croup-as·so·ci·at·ed v.
cy·to·path·o·gen·ic v.
deer hem·or·rhag·ic fe·ver
v.
de·fec·tive v.
del·ta v.

den·gue v.
dis·tem·per v.
DNA v.
dog dis·tem·per v.
duck hep·a·ti·tis v.
duck in·flu·en·za v.
duck plague v.
east·ern equine en·ceph·a·
lo·my·e·li·tis v.
EB v.
E·bo·la v.
ECBO v.
ECHO v.
ECMO v.
ec·o·tro·pic v.
ECSO v.
ec·tro·me·lia v.
EEE v.
EMC v.
en·ceph·a·li·tis v.
en·ceph·a·lo·my·o·car·di·tis
v.
en·ter·ic vi·rus·es
en·ter·ic cy·to·path·o·gen·ic
bo·vine or·phan v.
en·ter·ic cy·to·path·o·gen·ic
hu·man or·phan v.
en·ter·ic cy·to·path·o·gen·ic
mon·key or·phan v.
en·ter·ic cy·to·path·o·gen·ic
swine or·phan v.
en·ter·ic or·phan vi·rus·es
en·zo·ot·ic en·ceph·a·lo·
my·e·li·tis v.
ephem·er·al fe·ver v.
ep·i·dem·ic gas·tro·en·ter·i·
tis v.
ep·i·dem·ic ker·a·to·con·
junc·ti·vi·tis v.
ep·i·dem·ic my·al·gia v.
ep·i·dem·ic par·o·ti·tis v.
ep·i·dem·ic pleu·ro·dyn·ia
v.
Epstein-Barr v.
equine abor·tion v.
equine ar·te·ri·tis v.
equine co·i·tal ex·an·the·ma
v.
equine in·fec·tious ane·mia
v.
equine in·flu·en·za vi·rus·es
equine rhi·no·pneu·mo·ni·tis
v.
FA v.
fe·line leu·ke·mia v.
fe·line pan·leu·ko·pe·nia v.
fe·line rhi·no·tra·che·i·tis v.

vi·rus *(continued)*
fi·bro·ma·to·sis v. of rab·
bits
fi·brous bac·te·ri·al
vi·rus·es
fil·a·men·tous bac·te·ri·al
vi·rus·es
fil·tra·ble v.
fixed v.
Flury strain ra·bies v.
FMD v.
foamy vi·rus·es
foot-and-mouth dis·ease v.
fowl eryth·ro·blas·to·sis v.
fowl lym·pho·ma·to·sis v.
fowl my·e·lo·blas·to·sis v.
fowl neu·ro·lym·pho·ma·to·
sis v.
fowl plague v.
fowl·pox v.
fox en·ceph·a·li·tis v.
Friend v.
Friend leu·ke·mia v.
GAL v.
gal·lus ad·e·no-like v.
gas·tro·en·ter·i·tis v. type
A
gas·tro·en·ter·i·tis v. type B
Ger·man mea·sles v.
goat·pox v.
Graffi's v.
green mon·key v.
Gross' v.
Gross' leu·ke·mia v.
Gu·a·ma v.
Gu·a·ro·a v.
hand-foot-and-mouth dis·ease
v.
Han·taan v.
hard pad v.
help·er v.
hep·a·ti·tis A v.
hep·a·ti·tis B v.
hep·a·ti·tis del·ta v.
her·pes v.
her·pes sim·plex v.
her·pes zos·ter v.
hog chol·era v.
horse·pox v.
hu·man im·mu·no·de·fi·
cien·cy v.
hu·man pap·il·lo·ma v.
hu·man T-cell lym·pho·
ma/leu·ke·mia v.
hu·man T-cell lym·pho·
trop·ic v.
Iba·ra·ki v.
IBR v.

v. III of rab·bits
Ilhé·us v.
in·clu·sion con·junc·ti·vi·tis
vi·rus·es
in·fan·tile gas·tro·en·ter·i·
tis v.
in·fec·tious ar·te·ri·tis v. of
hors·es
in·fec·tious bo·vine rhi·no·
tra·che·i·tis v.
in·fec·tious bron·chi·tis v.
in·fec·tious ca·nine hep·a·
ti·tis v.
in·fec·tious ec·tro·me·lia v.
in·fec·tious hep·a·ti·tis v.
in·fec·tious pap·il·lo·ma v.
in·fec·tious por·cine en·
ceph·a·lo·my·e·li·tis v.
in·flu·en·za vi·rus·es
in·sect vi·rus·es
James·town Can·yon v.
Jap·a·nese B en·ceph·a·li·
tis v.
JC v.
JH v.
Ju·nin v.
K v.
Ke·lev strain ra·bies v.
Kilham rat v.
Ki·sen·yi sheep dis·ease v.
Koongol vi·rus·es
Ky·as·a·nur For·est dis·ease
v.
La Crosse v.
lac·tate de·hy·dro·gen·ase v.
Lassa v.
la·tent rat v.
LCM v.
loup·ing-ill v.
Lucké's v.
lumpy skin dis·ease
vi·rus·es
Lun·yo v.
lymph·ad·e·nop·a·thy-
as·so·ci·at·ed v.
lym·pho·cyt·ic cho·ri·o·
men·in·gi·tis v.
lym·pho·gran·u·lo·ma
ve·ne·re·um v.
Ma·chu·po v.
mae·di v.
ma·lig·nant ca·tarrh·al
fe·ver v.
mam·ma·ry can·cer v. of
mice
mam·ma·ry tu·mor v. of
mice
Mar·burg v.

Marek's dis·ease v.
mar·mo·set v.
masked v.
Mayaro v.
mea·sles v.
me·di v.
Men·go v.
mink en·ter·i·tis v.
MM v.
Mo·ko·la v.
mol·lus·cum con·ta·gi·o·
   sum v.
Moloney's v.
mon·key B v.
mon·key·pox v.
mouse en·ceph·a·lo·my·e·li·
   tis v.
mouse hep·a·ti·tis v.
mouse leu·ke·mia vi·rus·es
mouse mam·ma·ry
   tu·mor v.
mouse pa·rot·id tu·mor v.
mouse po·li·o·my·e·li·tis v.
mouse·pox v.
mouse thy·mic v.
mu·co·sal dis·ease v.
mumps v.
mu·rine sar·co·ma v.
Murray Val·ley en·ceph·a·
   li·tis v.
Mu·ru·tu·cu v.
MVE v.
myx·o·ma·to·sis v.
Nai·ro·bi sheep dis·ease v.
na·ked v.
ND v.
Ne·bras·ka calf scours v.
Neeth·ling v.
neg·a·tive strand v.
Ne·gi·shi v.
ne·o·na·tal calf di·ar·
   rhea v.
neu·ro·tro·pic v.
New·cas·tle dis·ease v.
non·oc·clud·ed v.
oc·clud·ed v.
Omsk hem·or·rhag·ic
   fe·ver v.
on·co·gen·ic v.
O'ny·ong-ny·ong v.
orf v.
Ori·bo·ca v.
or·ni·tho·sis v.
or·phan vi·rus·es
Pa·che·co's par·rot
   dis·ease v.
pan·leu·ko·pe·nia v. of cats
pan·tro·pic v.

pap·pa·ta·ci fe·ver vi·rus·es
pap·u·lar sto·ma·ti·tis v. of
   cat·tle
par·a·in·flu·en·za vi·rus·es
par·a·vac·cin·ia v.
par·rot v.
Patois v.
pha·ryn·go·con·junc·ti·val
   fe·ver v.
phle·bot·o·mus fe·ver
   vi·rus·es
plant vi·rus·es
pneu·mo·nia v. of mice
po·li·o·my·e·li·tis v.
pol·y·o·ma v.
por·cine he·mag·glu·ti·nat·
   ing en·ceph·a·li·tis v.
Pow·as·san v.
pro·gress·ive pneu·mo·nia v.
pseu·do·cow·pox v.
pseu·do·lym·pho·cyt·ic cho·
   ri·o·men·in·gi·tis v.
pseu·do·ra·bies v.
psit·ta·co·sis v.
PVM v.
quail bron·chi·tis v.
Quar·an·fil v.
rab·bit fi·bro·ma v.
rab·bit myx·o·ma v.
rab·bit·pox v.
ra·bies v.
ra·bies v., Flury strain
ra·bies v., Ke·lev strain
Rauscher's v.
res·pi·ra·to·ry syn·cy·tial v.
Ri·da v.
Rift Val·ley fe·ver v.
rin·der·pest v.
RNA v.
RNA tu·mor vi·rus·es
Ross River v.
Rous-as·so·ci·at·ed v.
Rous sar·co·ma v.
Rs v.
Rubarth's dis·ease v.
ru·bel·la v.
ru·be·o·la v.
Rus·sian au·tumn en·ceph·
   a·li·tis v.
Rus·sian spring-sum·mer
   en·ceph·a·li·tis v.
Salis·bury com·mon cold
   vi·rus·es
sal·i·vary v.
sal·i·vary gland v.
sand·fly fe·ver vi·rus·es
San Mi·guel sea li·on v.
Sendai v.

vi·**rus** *(continued)*
se·rum hep·a·ti·tis v.
sheep-pox v.
ship·ping fe·ver v.
Shope fi·bro·ma v.
Sim·bu v.
sim·i·an v.
sim·i·an vac·u·o·lat·ing v.
Sind·bis v.
slow v.
small·pox v.
snow·shoe hare v.
sore·mouth v.
Spond·we·ni v.
St. Louis en·ceph·a·li·tis v.
street v.
swamp fe·ver v.
swine en·ceph·a·li·tis v.
swine fe·ver v.
swine in·flu·en·za vi·rus·es
swine·pox v.
Swiss mouse leu·ke·mia v.
Tac·a·ribe v.
Ta·hy·na v.
Teschen dis·ease v.
Tete vi·rus·es
TGE v.
Theiler's v.
Theiler's orig·i·nal v.
tick-borne en·ceph·a·li·tis v.
TO v.
tra·cho·ma v.
trans·mis·si·ble gas·tro·en·
ter·i·tis v. of swine
trans·mis·si·ble tur·key en·
ter·i·tis v.
tu·mor v.
tur·key me·nin·go·en·ceph·
a·li·tis v.
Turlock v.
Um·bre v.
vac·cine v.
vac·cin·ia v.
vac·u·o·lat·ing v.
var·i·cel·la-zos·ter v.
va·ri·o·la v.
VEE v.
Ven·e·zu·e·lan equine en·
ceph·a·lo·my·e·li·tis v.
ve·sic·u·lar ex·an·the·ma of
swine v.
ve·sic·u·lar sto·ma·ti·tis v.
vi·ral hem·or·rhag·ic fe·ver
v.
vis·cer·al dis·ease v.
vis·na v.
VS v.
WEE v.

Wesselsbron dis·ease v.
west·ern equine en·ceph·a·
lo·my·e·li·tis v.
West Nile v.
xen·o·tro·pic v.
Ya·ba mon·key v.
yel·low fe·ver v.
Zi·ka v.
vi·**rus**
block·ade
en·ceph·a·lo·my·e·li·tis
hep·a·ti·tis
hep·a·ti·tis of ducks
ker·a·to·con·junc·ti·vi·tis
pneu·mo·nia of pigs
vi·**rus A**
hep·a·ti·tis
vi·**rus-as·so·ci·at·ed he·mo·**
phag·o·cyt·ic
syn·drome
vi·**rus B**
hep·a·ti·tis
vi·**rus·es**
vi·**rus·oid**
vi·**rus shed·ding**
vi·**rus-trans·formed**
cell
vi·**rus X**
dis·ease
vis
v. con·ser·va·trix
v. a fron·te
v. a ter·go
v. vi·tae
v. vi·ta·lis
vis·cance
vis·cera
vis·cer·ad
vis·cer·al
an·es·the·sia
arch·es
brain
cav·i·ty
cleft
cra·ni·um
dis·or·der
ep·i·lep·sy
in·ver·sion
lar·va mi·grans
lay·er
leish·man·i·a·sis
lym·pho·ma·to·sis
mes·o·derm
nodes
plate
pleu·ra
pleu·ri·sy
sense

skel·e·ton
sur·face of liv·er
sur·face of the spleen
swal·low
vis·cer·al dis·ease
vi·rus
vis·cer·al·gia
vis·cer·al mo·tor
neu·ron
neu·rons
vis·cer·al ner·vous
sys·tem
vis·cer·al trac·tion
re·flex
vis·cer·i·mo·tor
vis·cer·o·cra·ni·um
car·ti·lag·i·nous v.
mem·bra·nous v.
vis·cer·o·gen·ic
re·flex
vis·cer·o·graph
vis·cer·o·in·hib·i·to·ry
vis·cer·o·meg·a·ly
vis·cer·o·mo·tor
re·flex
vis·cer·o·pan·nic·u·lar
re·flex
vis·cer·o·pa·ri·e·tal
vis·cer·o·per·i·to·ne·al
vis·cer·o·pleu·ral
vis·cer·op·to·sia
vis·cer·op·to·sis
vis·cer·o·sen·sory
re·flex
vis·cer·o·skel·e·tal
vis·cer·o·skel·e·ton
vis·cer·o·so·mat·ic
vis·cer·o·tome
vis·cer·ot·o·my
vis·cer·o·to·nia
vis·cer·o·tro·phic
re·flex
vis·cer·o·tro·pic
vis·cid
vis·cid·i·ty
vis·ci·do·sis
vis·co·e·las·tic·i·ty
vis·com·e·ter
vis·co·sim·e·ter
vis·co·sim·e·try
vis·cos·i·ty
ab·so·lute v.
anom·a·lous v.
ap·par·ent v.
dy·nam·ic v.
kin·e·mat·ic v.
new·to·ni·an v.
rel·a·tive v.

vis·cous
vis·cum
vis·cus
vis·i·bil·i·ty
acu·i·ty
vis·i·ble
spec·trum
vis·ile
vi·sion
ach·ro·mat·ic v.
bin·oc·u·lar v.
blue v.
cen·tral v.
chro·mat·ic v.
col·or v.
cone v.
di·rect v.
dou·ble v.
fa·cial v.
green v.
ha·lo v.
hap·lo·scop·ic v.
in·di·rect v.
mul·ti·ple v.
night v.
os·cil·lat·ing v.
pe·riph·e·ral v.
pho·top·ic v.
red v.
rod v.
sco·top·ic v.
ster·e·o·scop·ic v.
sub·jec·tive v.
tri·ple v.
tu·bu·lar v.
tun·nel v.
twi·light v.
yel·low v.
vis·it·ing
nurse
vis·na
vi·rus
vi·su·al
acu·i·ty
al·les·the·sia
an·gle
apha·sia
ar·ea
ax·is
black·out
cor·tex
cy·cle
ef·fi·cien·cy
ex·tinc·tion
field
im·age
in·at·ten·tion
pig·ments

vi·su·al *(continued)*
  pro·jec·tion
  pur·ple
  thresh·old
  vi·o·let
  yel·low
vi·su·al alex·ia
vi·su·al e·voked
  po·ten·tial
vi·su·al·ize
vi·su·al or·bi·cu·la·ris
  re·flex
vi·su·al re·cep·tor
  cells
vi·su·al-spa·tial
  ag·no·sia
vi·su·o·au·di·tory
vi·su·og·no·sis
vis·u·o·mo·tor
vi·su·o·psy·chic
vi·su·o·sen·so·ry
vis·u·o·spa·tial
vi·su·scope
vi·ta
  glass
vi·tal
  ca·pac·i·ty
  cen·ter
  force
  in·dex
  knot
  node
  pulp
  signs
  stain
  sta·tis·tics
  tooth
  tri·pod
  ul·tra·vi·o·let
vi·tal·ism
vi·tal·is·tic
vi·tal·i·ty
  test
vi·tal·ize
vi·ta·lom·e·ter
vi·tal red
vi·tals
vi·ta·mer
vi·ta·min
  v. A
  an·ti·ber·i·beri v.
  an·ti·hem·or·rhag·ic v.
  an·ti·neu·rit·ic v.
  an·ti·ra·chit·ic v.'s
  an·ti·scor·bu·tic v.
  an·ti·ste·ril·i·ty v.
  v. B
  v. B_T

  v. B_x
  v. B com·plex
  v. $B_c$con·ju·gase
  v. C
  v. D
  v. E
  v. F
  fat-sol·u·ble v.'s
  fer·til·i·ty v.
  v. H
  v. K
  mi·cro·bi·al v.
  v. P
  per·me·a·bil·i·ty v.
  v. U
vi·ta·min A
  unit
vi·ta·min C
  test
  unit
vi·ta·min D
  milk
  unit
vi·ta·min D-re·sis·tant
  rick·ets
vi·ta·min E
  unit
vi·ta·min K
  unit
vi·tel·lar·i·um
vi·tel·li·form
  de·gen·er·a·tion
vi·tel·lin
vi·tel·line
  ar·tery
  cord
  duct
  fis·tu·la
  mem·brane
  pole
  res·er·voir
  sac
  vein
  ves·sels
vi·tel·li·rup·tive
  de·gen·er·a·tion
vi·tel·lo·gen·e·sis
vi·tel·lo·in·tes·tin·al
  cyst
  duct
vi·tel·lo·lu·te·in
vitel·lo·ru·bin
vi·tel·lose
vi·tel·lus
  v. ovi
vi·ti·at·ed
  air
vi·ti·a·tion

vit·i·lig·i·nes
vit·i·lig·i·nous
vit·i·li·go
  v. ca·pi·tis
  Cazenave's v.
  Cel·sus' v.
  cir·cum·ne·vic v.
  v. ir·i·dis
vit·i·li·goi·dea
vit·rec·to·my
  an·te·ri·or v.
  pos·te·ri·or v.
vit·re·in
vit·re·i·tis
vit·re·o·den·tin
vit·re·o·ret·i·nal
vit·re·o·ret·i·nal cho·roi·dop·a·thy
  syn·drome
vit·re·o·ret·i·nal trac·tion
  syn·drome
vit·re·o·ret·i·nop·a·thy
  ex·ud·a·tive v.
vit·re·o-ta·pe·to·ret·i·nal
  dys·tro·phy
vit·re·ous
  body
  cam·era
  cell
  cham·ber of eye
  de·tach·ment
  her·nia
  hu·mor
  la·mel·la
  mem·brane
  ta·ble
vit·re·ous
  per·sis·tent an·te·ri·or hy·
    per·plas·tic pri·mary v.
  per·sis·tent pos·te·ri·or hy·
    per·plas·tic pri·mary v.
  pri·mary v.
  sec·on·dary v.
  ter·ti·ary v.
vit·re·um
vit·ri·fi·ca·tion
vit·ri·ol
in vit·ro
  fer·til·i·za·tion
vit·ro·sin
vi·var·ia
vi·var·i·um
vi·vax
  fe·ver
  ma·lar·ia
viv·i·di·al·y·sis
viv·i·dif·fu·sion
viv·i·fi·ca·tion

viv·i·par·i·ty
vi·vip·a·rous
viv·i·per·cep·tion
viv·i·sect
viv·i·sec·tion
viv·i·sec·tion·ist
viv·i·sec·tor
in vi·vo
  fer·til·i·za·tion
Vladimiroff-Mikulicz
  am·pu·ta·tion
VMA
  test
vo·cal
  amu·sia
  cord
  fold
  frem·i·tus
  lig·a·ment
  mus·cle
  pro·cess
  res·o·nance
  shelf
vo·cal cord
  nod·ules
Vogel's
  law
Voges-Proskauer
  re·ac·tion
Vogt
  syn·drome
Vogt-Koyanagi
  syn·drome
Vogt's
  an·gle
Vogt-Spielmeyer
  dis·ease
Vohwinkel
  syn·drome
voice
  am·phor·ic v.
  bron·chi·al v.
  cav·ern·ous v.
  ep·i·gas·tric v.
  eu·nuch·oid v.
  myx·e·de·ma v.
void
void·ing
  cys·to·gram
void·ing flow
  rate
void met·al com·pos·ite
Voigt's
  lines
vo·la
vo·lar
vo·lar car·pal
  lig·a·ment

vo·lar in·ter·os·se·ous
  ar·tery
  nerve
vo·la·ris
vol·a·tile
  an·es·thet·ic
  mus·tard oil
  oil
vol·a·tile fat·ty ac·id
  num·ber
vol·a·til·i·za·tion
vol·a·til·ize
vole
  ba·cil·lus
Volhard's
  test
vo·li·tion
vo·li·tion·al
  trem·or
Volkmann's
  ca·nals
  chei·li·tis
  con·trac·ture
  spoon
vol·ley
Vollmer
  test
Volpe-Manhold In·dex
vol·sel·la
volt
volt·age
volt·age-gat·ed
  chan·nel
vol·ta·ic
  taste
  ver·ti·go
vol·ta·ism
vol·tam·e·ter
volt·am·pere
volt·me·ter
Voltolini's
  dis·ease
vol·ume
  el·e·ment
  in·dex
  sub·sti·tute
  unit
vol·ume
  atom·ic v.
  clos·ing v.
  dis·tri·bu·tion v.
  end-di·a·stol·ic v.
  end-sys·tol·ic v.
  ex·pi·ra·to·ry re·serve v.
  forced ex·pi·ra·to·ry v.
  in·spi·ra·to·ry re·serve v.
  mean cell v.
  min·ute v.

packed cell v.
par·tial v.
re·sid·u·al v.
res·pi·ra·to·ry min·ute v.
rest·ing tid·al v.
stan·dard v.
stroke v.
tid·al v.
vol·ume-con·trolled
  res·pi·ra·tor
vol·ume-dis·place·ment
  ple·thys·mo·graph
vol·ume·nom·e·ter
vol·u·met·ric
  anal·y·sis
  flask
  so·lu·tion
vol·u·mom·e·ter
vol·un·tary
  de·hy·dra·tion
  hos·pi·tal
  mus·cle
  mut·ism
  nys·tag·mus
vo·lup·tu·ous
vo·lute
vol·u·tin
  gran·ules
Vol·vox
vol·vu·lo·sis
vol·vu·lus
  gas·tric v.
vo·mer
  v. car·ti·la·gi·ne·us
vo·mer·al
  groove
  sul·cus
vo·mer·ine
  ca·nal
  car·ti·lage
vo·me·ris
vom·er·o·bas·i·lar
  ca·nal
vom·er·o·na·sal
  car·ti·lage
  or·gan
vom·er·o·ros·tral
  ca·nal
vom·e·ro·vag·i·nal
  ca·nal
  groove
vom·i·ca
vom·i·cose
vom·i·cus
vom·it
  Bar·coo v.
  black v.
  cof·fee-ground v.

vom·it·ing
dry v.
ep·i·dem·ic v.
fe·cal v.
morn·ing v.
per·ni·cious v.
v. of preg·nan·cy
pro·jec·tile v.
psy·cho·gen·ic v.
re·ten·tion v.
ster·co·ra·ceous v.
vom·it·ing
gas
re·flex
vo·mi·tion
vom·i·tive
vom·i·to·ry
vom·i·tu·ri·tion
vom·i·tus
v. cru·en·tes
v. ma·ri·nus
v. ni·ger
von Economo's
dis·ease
von Gierke's
dis·ease
von Graefe's
sign
von Hippel-Lindau
dis·ease
syn·drome
von Kossa
stain
von Meyenburg's
dis·ease
von Recklinghausen's
dis·ease
von Spee's
curve
von Willebrand
fac·tor
von Willebrand's
dis·ease
syn·drome
Voorhoeve's
dis·ease
vor·tex
veins
vor·tex
v. coc·cyg·e·us
v. len·tis
Vor·ti·cel·la

vor·ti·ces
vor·ti·cose
veins
Vossius' len·tic·u·lar
ring
vous·sure
vox
v. cho·le·ra·i·ca
vox·el
voy·eur
voy·eur·ism
VS
vi·rus
vul·ga·ris
vul·ner·a·ble
pe·ri·od
pe·ri·od of heart
phase
vul·ner·a·ble child
syn·drome
Vul·pi·an's
at·ro·phy
ef·fect
vul·sel·la
for·ceps
vul·sel·lum
for·ceps
vul·va
vul·vae
vul·val
vul·var
slit
vul·vec·to·my
vul·vis·mus
vul·vi·tis
chron·ic atroph·ic v.
chron·ic hy·per·tro·phic v.
fol·lic·u·lar v.
leu·ko·plak·ic v.
vul·vo·cru·ral
vul·vo·u·ter·ine
vul·vo·vag·i·nal
anus
cys·tec·to·my
gland
vul·vo·vag·i·ni·tis
Vw
an·ti·gen
V-Y
pro·ce·dure
V-Y-plas·ty

W
chro·mo·some
fac·tor
pro·ce·dure
rays
W-
arch
"w"
her·nia
Waardenburg
syn·drome
Wachendorf's
mem·brane
Wachstein-Meissel
stain for cal·ci·um-mag·ne·
si·um-ATPase
Wada
test
wad·ding
wad·ding·to·ni·an
ho·me·o·sta·sis
wad·dle
wa·fer
Wagner's
dis·ease
syn·drome
Wagstaffe's
frac·ture
waist
w. of the heart
wait·er's
cramp
wak·ing
numb·ness
Walcher
po·si·tion
Waldenström's
mac·ro·glob·u·lin·e·mia
pur·pu·ra
syn·drome
test
Waldeyer's
fos·sae
glands
sheath
space
tract
Waldeyer's throat
ring

Waldeyer's zon·al
lay·er
walk
Walker
car·ci·no·ma
car·ci·no·sar·co·ma
trac·tot·o·my
Walker's
chart
walk·ing
ty·phoid
walk-through
an·gi·na
wall
an·te·ri·or w. of mid·dle
ear
an·te·ri·or w. of stom·ach
an·te·ri·or w. of va·gi·na
ax·i·al w.'s of the pulp
cham·bers
ca·rot·id w. of mid·dle ear
cav·i·ty w.
cell w.
chest w.
enam·el w.
ex·ter·nal w. of co·chle·ar
duct
in·fe·ri·or w. of or·bit
in·fe·ri·or w. of tym·pan·ic
cav·i·ty
jug·u·lar w. of mid·dle ear
lab·y·rin·thine w. of
mid·dle ear
lat·er·al w. of mid·dle ear
lat·er·al w. of or·bit
mas·toid w. of mid·dle ear
me·di·al w. of mid·dle ear
me·di·al w. of or·bit
mem·bra·nous w. of
mid·dle ear
mem·bra·nous w. of
tra·chea
w. of nail
pa·ri·e·tal w.
pos·te·ri·or w. of mid·dle
ear
pos·te·ri·or w. of stom·ach
pos·te·ri·or w. of va·gi·na
pul·pal w.

wall *(continued)*
splanch·nic w.
su·pe·ri·or w. of or·bit
teg·men·tal w. of mid·dle
ear
tho·rac·ic w.
tym·pan·ic w. of co·chle·ar
duct
ves·tib·u·lar w. of co·chle·
ar duct
Wallenberg's
syn·drome
wal·le·ri·an
de·gen·er·a·tion
law
wal·let
stom·ach
wall-eye
Walthard's cell
rest
Walther's
ca·nals
di·la·tor
ducts
gan·gli·on
plex·us
waltzed
flap
wan·der·ing
ab·scess
cell
er·y·sip·e·las
goi·ter
kid·ney
liv·er
or·gan
pace·mak·er
pneu·mo·nia
Wangensteen
drain·age
suc·tion
tube
Wang·i·el·la
Wang's
test
war
neu·ro·sis
war·ble
bot·fly
fly
Warburg-Lipmann-Dickens
shunt
Warburg's
ap·pa·ra·tus
the·o·ry
Warburg's old yel·low
en·zyme

Warburg's res·pi·ra·to·ry
en·zyme
ward
Wardrop's
dis·ease
meth·od
Ward's
tri·an·gle
ware·house·man's
itch
war·fa·rin so·di·um
warm
ag·glu·ti·nins
au·to·an·ti·body
warm-blood·ed
an·i·mal
warm-cold
he·mo·ly·sin
Warren
shunt
wart
an·a·tom·i·cal w.
as·bes·tos w.
cat·tle w.'s
com·mon w.
dig·i·tate w.
fig w.
fi·li·form w.
flat w.
fu·gi·tive w.
gen·i·tal w.
Henle's w.'s
in·fec·tious w.'s
moist w.
mo·sa·ic w.
nec·ro·gen·ic w.
Pe·ru·vi·an w.
pitch w.
plane w.
plan·tar w.
poin·ted w.
post·mor·tem w.
pro·sec·tor's w.
seb·or·rhe·ic w.
se·nile w.
soft w.
soot w.
tel·an·gi·ec·tat·ic w.
tu·ber·cu·lous w.
ve·ne·re·al w.
vi·ral w.
Wartenberg's
symp·tom
Warthin-Finkeldey
cells
Warthin's
tu·mor

Warthin-Starry sil·ver
stain
wart·pox
warty
dys·ker·a·to·ma
horn
ul·cer
wash
wash-bot·tle
washed
sul·fur
washed field
tech·nique
wash·er·man's
mark
wash·er·wom·an's
itch
wash·ing
so·da
wash·out
can·nu·la
test
Wasmann's
glands
Wassén
test
was·ser·hel·le
cell
Wassermann
an·ti·body
re·ac·tion
test
Wassermann-fast
wast·ed
ven·ti·la·tion
wast·ing
dis·ease
pal·sy
pa·ral·y·sis
wast·ing
salt w.
watch·mak·er's
cramp
wa·ter
as·pi·ra·tor
bath
bed
can·cer
can·ker
de·ple·tion
di·u·re·sis
dress·ing
gas
glass
im·mer·sion
in·tox·i·ca·tion
itch
sore

wa·ter
w. of ad·he·sion
al·ka·line w.
ar·o·mat·ic w.
ba·ry·ta w.
bit·ter w.
black w.
bound w.
bro·mine w.
cal·cic w.
car·bon·at·ed w.
car·bon di·ox·ide-free w.
car·bon·ic w.
cha·ly·be·ate w.
chlo·rine w.
w. of com·bus·tion
w. of con·sti·tu·tion
w. of crys·tal·li·za·tion
dis·tilled w.
earthy w.
free w.
gen·tian an·i·line w.
hard w.
heavy w.
in·dif·fer·ent w.
w. for in·jec·tion
w. of me·tab·o·lism
min·er·al w.
po·ta·ble w.
pu·ri·fied w.
sa·line w.
Selters w.
Selt·zer w.
soft w.
sul·fate w.
sul·fur w.
wa·ter-clear
cell of par·a·thy·roid
wa·ter·fall
wa·ter-ham·mer
pulse
Waterhouse-Friderichsen
syn·drome
wa·ter·ing-can
per·i·ne·um
scro·tum
wa·ter·pox
Waters'
op·er·a·tion
wa·ters
bag of w.
false w.
wa·ter·shed
in·farc·tion
wa·ter-sol·u·ble
chlo·ro·phyll de·riv·a·tives
Waterston
shunt

Waters' view
  roent·gen·o·gram
wa·ter-trap
  stom·ach
wa·ter wheel
  mur·mur
wa·ter-whis·tle
  sound
wa·tery
  eye
Watson-Crick
  he·lix
Watsonius wat·soni
Watson-Schwartz
  test
watt
wave
  A w.
  ac·id w.
  al·ka·line w.
  al·pha w.
  ar·te·ri·al w.
  B w.
  be·ta w.
  brain w.
  C w.
  can·non w.
  D w.
  del·ta w.
  di·crot·ic w.
  elec·tro·car·di·o·graph·ic w.
  ex·ci·ta·tion w.
  F w.
  f w.
  FF w.'s
  ff w.'s
  fi·bril·lary w.'s
  flat top w.'s
  flu·id w.
  flut·ter-fi·bril·la·tion w.'s
  mi·cro·e·lec·tric w.'s
  over·flow w.
  P w.
  per·cus·sion w.
  phren·ic w.
  post·ex·tra·sys·tol·ic T w.
  pulse w.
  Q w.
  R w.
  ran·dom w.'s
  re·coil w.
  ret·ro·grade P w.
  S w.
  son·ic w.'s
  su·per·son·ic w.'s
  T w.
  the·ta w.
  tid·al w.

Traube-Hering w.'s
U w.
ul·tra·son·ic w.'s
V w.
wave
  an·a·lyz·er
  form
  num·ber
wave·length
wave·num·ber
wave·shape
wax
  an·i·mal w.
  base·plate w.
  bleached w.
  bone w.
  box·ing w.
  Bra·zil w.
  car·nau·ba w.
  cast·ing w.
  Chi·nese w.
  ear w.
  earth w.
  emul·si·fy·ing w.
  grave w.
  Horsley's bone w.
  in·lay w.
  Ja·pan w.
  min·er·al w.
  palm w.
  par·af·fin w.
  veg·e·ta·ble w.
  white w.
  yel·low w.
wax
  ex·pan·sion
  form
  pat·tern
wax·ing
wax·ing-up
wax mod·el
  den·ture
wax-tipped
  bou·gie
waxy
  cast
  de·gen·er·a·tion
  fin·gers
  kid·ney
  liv·er
  spleen
WDHA
  syn·drome
wean
wean·ing
wean·ling
wear
  oc·clu·sal w.

wear-and-tear
pig·ment
weav·er's
cough
web
eye
web
esoph·a·ge·al w.
ter·mi·nal w.
Webb
an·ti·gen
webbed
fin·gers
neck
pe·nis
toes
web·bing
we·ber
Weber-Christian
dis·ease
Weber-Cockayne
syn·drome
Weber-Fechner
law
Weber's
ex·per·i·ment
glands
law
or·gan
par·a·dox
point
sign
syn·drome
test for hear·ing
tri·an·gle
Webster's
op·er·a·tion
test
Wechsler-Bellevue
scale
Wechsler in·tel·li·gence
scales
wed·del·lite
cal·cu·lus
Wedensky
ef·fect
fa·cil·i·ta·tion
in·hi·bi·tion
wedge
bi·op·sy
bone
pres·sure
re·sec·tion
spi·rom·e·ter
wedge
den·tal w.

wedge-and-groove
joint
su·ture
wedge-shaped
fas·cic·u·lus
tu·ber·cle
WEE
vi·rus
week·end
hos·pi·tal
Weeks'
ba·cil·lus
weep·ing
ec·ze·ma
Wegener's
gran·u·lo·ma·to·sis
Wegner's
dis·ease
line
Weibel-Palade
bod·ies
Weichselbaum's
coc·cus
Weidel's
re·ac·tion
Weigert-Gram
stain
Weigert's
law
stain for ac·ti·no·my·ces
stain for elas·tin
stain for fi·brin
stain for my·e·lin
stain for neu·rog·lia
Weigert's io·dine
so·lu·tion
Weigert's iron he·ma·tox·y·lin
stain
weight
atom·ic w.
birth w.
com·bin·ing w.
equiv·a·lent w.
gram-atom·ic w.
gram-mo·lec·u·lar w.
mo·lec·u·lar w.
weight·less·ness
Weil-Felix
re·ac·tion
test
Weill-Marchesani
syn·drome
Weil's
dis·ease
Weil's ba·sal
lay·er
zone

Weinberg's
  re·ac·tion
Weingrow's
  re·flex
Weir Mitchell
  treat·ment
Weir's
  op·er·a·tion
Weisbach's
  an·gle
weis·mann·ism
Weismann's
  the·o·ry
Weiss'
  sign
Weitbrecht's
  car·ti·lage
  cord
  fi·bers
  fo·ra·men
  lig·a·ment
Welch's
  ba·cil·lus
Welcker's
  an·gle
weld·er's
  con·junc·ti·vi·tis
  lung
well dif·fer·en·ti·at·ed lym·
  pho·cyt·ic
  lym·pho·ma
Wells'
  syn·drome
welt
Wenckebach
  pe·ri·od
  phe·nom·e·non
Wenzel's
  ven·tri·cle
Wepfer's
  glands
Werdnig-Hoffmann
  dis·ease
Werlhof's
  dis·ease
Wermer's
  syn·drome
Wernekinck's
  com·mis·sure
  de·cus·sa·tion
Werner's
  syn·drome
  test
Wernicke-Korsakoff
  en·ceph·a·lop·a·thy
  syn·drome
Wernicke's
  apha·sia

  ar·ea
  cen·ter
  dis·ease
  en·ceph·a·lop·a·thy
  field
  ra·di·a·tion
  re·ac·tion
  re·gion
  sign
  syn·drome
  zone
Wertheim's
  op·er·a·tion
Wer·ther's
  dis·ease
Wesselsbron
  dis·ease
  fe·ver
Wesselsbron dis·ease
  vi·rus
West Af·ri·can
  fe·ver
  try·pan·o·so·mi·a·sis
West Af·ri·can sleep·ing
  sick·ness
Westberg's
  space
Westergren
  meth·od
West·ern blot
  anal·y·sis
west·ern equine
  en·ceph·a·lo·my·e·li·tis
west·ern equine en·ceph·a·lo·
  my·e·li·tis
  vi·rus
West In·di·an
  small·pox
West Nile
  fe·ver
  vi·rus
Westphal-Erb
  sign
Westphal-Piltz
  phe·nom·e·non
Westphal's
  dis·ease
  phe·nom·e·non
  pseu·do·scle·ro·sis
  sign
Westphal's pu·pil·lary
  re·flex
Westphal-Strümpell
  pseu·do·scle·ro·sis
West's
  syn·drome
wet
  ber·i·beri

com·press
cup
dream
gan·grene
lung
nurse
pack
pleu·ri·sy
shock
tet·ter
wet cu·ta·ne·ous
leish·man·i·a·sis
wet and dry bulb
ther·mom·e·ter
wet·ta·ble
sul·fur
Wetzel
grid
Wever-Bray
phe·nom·e·non
Weyers-Thier
syn·drome
whar·ton·i·tis
Wharton's
duct
jel·ly
wheal
wheal-and-er·y·the·ma
re·ac·tion
wheal-and-flare
re·ac·tion
wheat
gum
wheat germ oil
wheat pas·ture
poi·son·ing
Wheatstone's
bridge
wheel
Burlew w.
Wheeler
meth·od
Wheeler-Johnson
test
Wheelhouse's
op·er·a·tion
wheeze
asth·ma·toid w.
whelp
whet·stone
crys·tals
whe·wel·lite
cal·cu·lus
whey
al·um
· pro·tein

whey
al·um
pro·tein
whip
bou·gie
whip·lash
in·ju·ry
Whipple's
dis·ease
op·er·a·tion
whip·worm
whis·key
whis·ky
whis·per
whis·pered
bron·choph·o·ny
pec·to·ril·o·quy
whis·per·ing
pec·to·ril·o·quy
whis·tle
Galton's w.
whis·tle-tip
cath·e·ter
whis·tling
de·for·mi·ty
rale
whis·tling face
syn·drome
white
ar·se·nic
bees·wax
bile
com·mis·sure
cor·pus·cle
di·ar·rhea
fat
fi·ber
fin·gers
gan·grene
graft
in·farct
lead
leg
line
line of anal ca·nal
lung
mat·ter
mus·cle
mus·tard
pe·tro·la·tum
pie·dra
pine
pitch
pulp
spot
sub·stance
throm·bus
tur·pen·tine

white *(continued)*
  wax
  yolk
white
  w. of eye
white blood
  cell
White·head
  de·for·mi·ty
white·head
Whitehead's
  op·er·a·tion
white mer·cu·ric
  pre·cip·i·tate
white mus·cle
  dis·ease
white-out
  syn·drome
white·pox
white pu·pil·lary
  re·flex
whites
white soft
  par·af·fin
white sponge
  ne·vus
white spot
  dis·ease
whit·ing
whit·low
  her·pet·ic w.
  mel·a·not·ic w.
  the·cal w.
Whitman's
  frame
Whitmore's
  ba·cil·lus
Whitnall's
  tu·ber·cle
whole
  blood
whole-body
  count·er
whole-body ti·tra·tion
  curve
whoop
  sys·tol·ic w.
whoop·ing
  cough
whoop·ing-cough
  vac·cine
whorl
  coc·cyg·eal w.
  dig·i·tal w.
  hair w.'s
whorled
  enam·el

Wickham's
  stri·ae
Widal's
  re·ac·tion
  syn·drome
wide
  plane
  spec·trum
wide field
  oc·u·lar
wide range
  au·di·om·e·ter
wid·ow's peak
width
  or·bi·tal w.
  win·dow w.
Wigand
  ma·neu·ver
wild
  gin·ger
  to·bac·co
  type
  yeast
Wildermuth's
  ear
Wilder's
  law of in·i·tial val·ue
  sign
  stain for re·tic·u·lum
Wildervanck
  syn·drome
Wilde's
  cords
  tri·an·gle
wild·fire
  rash
wild-type
  strain
Wilhelmy
  bal·ance
Wilkie's
  ar·tery
  dis·ease
Willett's
  clamp
  for·ceps
Williams
  syn·drome
Williams'
  stain
Willis'
  cen·trum ner·vo·sum
  cords
  pan·cre·as
  par·a·cu·sis
  pouch
Williston's
  law

wil·low
Wilms'
  tu·mor
Wilson
  block
Wilson-Mikity
  syn·drome
Wilson's
  dis·ease
  li·chen
  meth·od
  mus·cle
  syn·drome
wind
  con·tu·sion
wind·age
wind-broken
wind·burn
wind·gall
Win·di·go
  psy·cho·sis
win·dow
  lev·el
  width
win·dow
  aor·tic w.
  co·chle·ar w.
  oval w.
  round w.
  tach·y·car·dia w.
  ves·tib·u·lar w.
wind·pipe
wind·puffs
wine
  high w.
  low w.
  red w.
  sher·ry w.
wine
  spir·it
wing
  cell
  plate
wing
  an·gel's w.
  ash·en w.
  w. of cris·ta gal·li
  gray w.
  great·er w. of sphe·noid
    bone
  w. of il·i·um
  Ingrassia's w.
  less·er w. of sphe·noid bone
  w. of nose
  w. of sa·crum
  w. of vo·mer

winged
  cath·e·ter
  scap·u·la
Winiwarter-Buerger
  dis·ease
wink
  re·flex
Winkelman's
  dis·ease
wink·ing
  spasm
Winkler's
  dis·ease
Winslow's
  fo·ra·men
  lig·a·ment
  pan·cre·as
  stars
win·ter
  dys·en·tery of cat·tle
  ec·ze·ma
  itch
  sleep
Winterbottom's
  sign
win·ter·green oil
Winternitz'
  sound
Wintersteiner
  ro·settes
wire
  arch
  splint
wire
  Kirschner's w.
  lig·a·ture w.
  sep·a·rat·ing w.
  wrought w.
wire-loop
  le·sion
wir·ing
  cir·cum·fer·en·tial w.
  con·tin·u·ous loop w.
  cra·ni·o·fa·cial sus·pen·sion
    w.
  Gilmer w.
  Ivy loop w.
  per·i·al·ve·o·lar w.
  pyr·i·form ap·er·ture w.
  Stout's w.
Wirsung's
  ca·nal
  duct
wiry
  pulse
wis·dom
  tooth

Wiskott-Aldrich
  syn·drome
Wis·sler's
  syn·drome
Wistar
  rats
witch ha·zel
witch's
  milk
with·draw·al
  re·flex
  symp·toms
with·ers
  fis·tu·lous w.
wit·kop
Wit·ti·go
  psy·cho·sis
wit·zel·sucht
wob·ble
Wohl·fahr·tia
wohl·fahr·ti·o·sis
Wohlfart-Kugelberg-Welander
  dis·ease
wolf
  tooth
Wolfe
  graft
Wolfe-Krause
  graft
Wolfe's
  meth·od
Wolff-Chaikoff
  block
  ef·fect
wolff·i·an
  body
  cyst
  duct
  rest
  ridge
  tu·bules
wolff·i·an duct
  car·ci·no·ma
Wolff-Parkinson-White
  syn·drome
Wolff's
  law
Wölfler's
  gland
Wolf-Orton
  bod·ies
wolf·ram
wolf·ram·i·um
Wolfring's
  glands
wolfs·bane

Wollaston's
  dou·blet
  the·o·ry
Wolman's
  dis·ease
womb
  fall·ing of the w.
wood
  char·coal
  naph·tha
  spir·it
  sug·ar
  vin·e·gar
wood al·co·hol
wood·cut·ter's
  en·ceph·a·li·tis
wood·en
  res·o·nance
  tongue of cat·tle
wood·en-shoe
  heart
Wood's
  glass
  lamp
  light
wood wool
wool
  ball
  mag·got
wool al·co·hols
wool fat
  hy·drous w. f.
wool·ly
  hair
wool·ly-hair
  ne·vus
Woolner's
  tip
wool-sor·ters'
  dis·ease
  pneu·mo·nia
word
  blind·ness
  deaf·ness
word sal·ad
Woringer-Kolopp
  dis·ease
work·ing
  bite
  con·tacts
  oc·clu·sion
  side
work·ing oc·clu·sal
  sur·fac·es
work·ing out
work·ing side
  con·dyle
work·ing through

worm
  cad·dis w.
  fleece w.
  Manson's eye w.
  meal w.
worm
  ab·scess
  an·eu·rysm;
worm bark
wor·mi·an
  bones
Wormley's
  test
worm·seed
worm·wood
wort
Worth's
  am·bly·o·scope
Woulfe's
  bot·tle
wound
  clip
  de·his·cence
  fe·ver
  my·i·a·sis
wound
  abrad·ed w.
  avulsed w.
  blow·ing w.
  crease w.
  glanc·ing w.
  gun·shot w.
  gut·ter w.
  in·cised w.
  non·pen·e·trat·ing w.
  open w.
  pen·e·trat·ing w.
  per·fo·rat·ing w.
  punc·ture w.
  se·ton w.
  stab w.
  suck·ing w.
  tan·gen·tial w.
  trau·ma·top·ne·ic w.
wo·ven
  bone

W-plas·ty
Wr^a
  an·ti·gen
wreath
  cil·i·ary w.
Wright
  an·ti·gens
  res·pi·rom·e·ter
wright·ine
Wright's
  stain
  ver·sion
wrin·kle
wrin·kler
  mus·cle of eye·brow
Wrisberg's
  car·ti·lage
  gan·glia
  lig·a·ment
  nerve
  tu·ber·cle
wrist
  clo·nus
  joint
  sign
wrist clo·nus
  re·flex
wrist-drop
writ·er's
  cramp
writ·ing
  hand
wrought
  wire
wry
  neck
wry·neck
Wuch·er·e·ria
  W. ban·crofti
  W. ma·la·yi
wu·cher·e·ri·a·sis
Wurster's
  re·a·gent
  test
Wy·burn-Ma·son
  syn·drome

X
   body
   chro·mo·some
   dis·ease of cat·tle
   zone
X-
   stra·bis·mus
x-
   ray
xan·chro·mat·ic
xan·the·las·ma
   gen·er·al·ized x.
   x. pal·pe·bra·rum
xan·the·las·ma·to·sis
xan·the·las·moi·dea
xan·them·a·tin
xan·the·mia
xan·thene
   dyes
xan·thic
xan·thine
   x. de·hy·dro·gen·ase
   x. nu·cle·o·tide
   x. ox·i·dase
   x. ri·bo·nu·cle·o·side
xan·thi·nol ni·a·cin·ate
xan·thi·nol nic·o·tin·ate
xan·thi·nu·ria
xan·thism
xan·thi·u·ria
xan·tho·chroia
xan·tho·chro·mat·ic
xan·tho·chro·mia
xan·tho·chro·mic
xan·thoch·ro·ous
xan·tho·der·ma
xan·tho·dont
xan·tho·e·ryth·ro·der·mia per·
stans
xan·tho·gran·u·lo·ma
   ju·ve·nile x.
   nec·ro·bi·ot·ic x.
xan·tho·gran·u·lo·ma·tous
   cho·le·cys·ti·tis
   py·e·lo·ne·phri·tis
xan·tho·ma
   x. di·a·be·ti·co·rum
   x. dis·se·mi·na·tum
   erup·tive x.

   fi·brous x.
   x. mul·ti·plex
   nor·mo·li·pe·mic x. pla·
   num
   x. pal·pe·bra·rum
   x. pla·num
   x. tu·be·ro·sum
   x. tu·be·ro·sum sim·plex
   ver·ru·cous x.
xan·tho·ma·to·sis
   bil·i·ary x.
   x. bul·bi
   cer·e·bro·ten·di·nous x.
   fa·mil·i·al hy·per·cho·les·
   ter·e·mic x.
   nor·mal cho·les·ter·e·mic x.
xan·thom·a·tous
xan·thop·a·thy
xan·tho·phyll
xan·tho·pro·te·ic
xan·tho·pro·te·ic ac·id
xan·tho·pro·tein
xan·thop·sia
xan·thop·sin
xan·thop·sy·dra·cia
xan·tho·puc·cine
xan·tho·sine
   x. phos·phate
xan·tho·sis
xan·thous
xanth·u·ren·ic ac·id
xan·thu·ria
xan·thyl
xan·thyl·ic
xan·thyl·ic ac·id
xen·o·bi·ot·ic
xen·o·di·ag·no·sis
xen·o·gen·e·ic
   graft
xen·o·gen·ic
xe·nog·e·nous
xen·o·graft
xe·non
xe·non-arc
   pho·to·co·ag·u·la·tor
xen·o·par·a·site
xen·o·pho·bia
xen·o·pho·nia
xen·oph·thal·mia

Xen·o·psyl·la
xen·o·tro·pic
  vi·rus
xen·yl
xe·ran·sis
xe·ran·tic
xe·ra·sia
xer·o·chi·lia
xe·ro·der·ma
  x. pig·men·to·sum
xe·ro·gram
xe·rog·ra·phy
xe·ro·ma
xe·ro·mam·mog·ra·phy
xe·ro·me·nia
xe·ro·myc·te·ria
xe·ron·o·sus
xe·ro·pha·gia
xe·roph·a·gy
xe·roph·thal·mia
xe·roph·thal·mus
xe·ro·ra·di·o·graph
xe·ro·ra·di·og·ra·phy
xe·ro·sis
  x. pa·ren·chy·ma·to·sus
xe·ro·sto·mia
xe·ro·tes
xe·rot·ic
  de·gen·er·a·tion
  ker·a·ti·tis
xe·ro·to·cia
xe·ro·trip·sis
Xg
  an·ti·gen
Xg blood group
X-in·ac·ti·va·tion
xiph·i·ster·nal
  joint
xiph·i·ster·nal crunch·ing
  sound
xiph·i·ster·num
xiph·o·cos·tal
xiph·o·dyn·ia
xi·phoid
  car·ti·lage
  pro·cess
xi·phoi·dal·gia
xi·phoi·di·tis
xi·phop·a·gus
Xi·phoph·o·rus
  test
X-linked
  achro·ma·top·sia
  agam·ma·glob·u·lin·e·mia
  gene
  hy·po·gam·ma·glob·u·lin·e·
    mia

ich·thy·o·sis
in·her·i·tance
lo·cus
X-linked hy·po·phos·pha·tem·ic
  os·te·o·ma·la·cia
X-linked in·fan·tile
  hy·po·gam·ma·glob·u·lin·e·
    mia
XO
  fe·male
  syn·drome
XO go·nad·al
  dys·gen·e·sis
x-ra·di·a·tion
x-ray
  cap of Zinn
  do·sim·e·try
  mi·cro·scope
  ther·a·py
  tube
XX
  male
XX go·nad·al
  dys·gen·e·sis
XXX
  fe·male
XXY
  male
  syn·drome
XY go·nad·al
  dys·gen·e·sis
xy·lene
  x. cy·a·nol FF
xy·le·nol
xy·li·dine
xy·loi·din
xy·lo·ke·tose
xy·lol
xy·lo·met·az·o·line hy·dro·
  chlo·ride
xy·lo·py·ra·nose
xy·lose
  test
xy·lo·styp·tic
  ether
xy·lu·lose
ʟ-xy·lu·lo·su·ria
xy·lyl
  x. bro·mide
xy·lyl·ene
xy·ro·spasm
xys·ma
XYY
  male
  syn·drome

Y
body
car·ti·lage
chro·mo·some
fac·tor
Y-
ax·is
y-
an·gle
Ya·ba
tu·mor
Ya·ba mon·key
vi·rus
yang·go·na
Yang·tze
ede·ma
Yang·tze Val·ley
fe·ver
ya·qo·na
yaw
moth·er y.
yawn
yawn·ing
yaws
bosch y.
bush y.
crab y.
foot y.
for·est y.
guin·ea corn y.
ring·worm y.
year·ling
yeast
brew·ers' y.
com·pressed y.
cul·ti·vat·ed y.
dried y.
pri·mary dried y.
wild y.
yeast
fun·gus
RNase
yeast el·u·ate
fac·tor
yeast ex·tract
agar
yel·low
at·ro·phy of the liv·er
body

car·ti·lage
cor·al·lin
dis·ease
fe·ver
fi·bers
hep·a·ti·za·tion
lig·a·ment
mer·cu·ry io·dide
nail
pre·cip·i·tate
skin
spot
vi·sion
wax
yolk
yel·low
in·di·ca·tor y.
vi·su·al y.
yel·low bone
mar·row
yel·low fe·ver
vac·cine
vi·rus
yel·low root
yel·low soft
par·af·fin
yer·ba san·ta
Yer·sin·ia
Y. en·ter·o·co·li·ti·ca
Y. pes·tis
Y. pseu·do·tu·ber·cu·lo·sis
yer·sin·i·o·sis
pseu·do·tu·ber·cu·lar y.
yield
strength
stress
yin-yang
Y-linked
gene
in·her·i·tance
lo·cus
yo·ghurt
yo·gurt
yo·him·bine
yoke
al·ve·o·lar y.
yoke
bone

yolk
cells
cleav·age
mem·brane
sac
stalk
yolk
white y.
yel·low y.
yolk sac
tu·mor
Yorke's au·to·lyt·ic
re·ac·tion
Young-Helmholtz
the·o·ry of col·or vi·sion

Young pros·tat·ic
trac·tor
Young's
mo·du·lus
rule
yp·sil·i·form
Y-shaped
car·ti·lage
lig·a·ment
Yt^a
an·ti·gen
yt·ter·bi·um
yt·tri·um
Yvon's
test

Z
band
chro·mo·some
disk
fil·a·ment
line
pro·ce·dure
Zaglas'
lig·a·ment
Zahn's
in·farct
Zam·be·si
ul·cer
Zappert count·ing
cham·ber
Z-DNA
ze·a·tin
ze·bra
body
Zeeman
ef·fect
ze·in
Zeis'
glands
zeis·i·an
sty
Zeit·geist
Zellweger
syn·drome
ze·lo·pho·bia
ze·lo·typ·ia
Zenker's
de·gen·er·a·tion
di·ver·tic·u·lum
fix·a·tive
ne·cro·sis
pa·ral·y·sis
ze·o·lite
ze·o·scope
ze·ro
ab·so·lute z.
zero-
grav·i·ty
ze·ro de·gree
teeth
ze·ro end-ex·pi·ra·to·ry
pres·sure
ze·ro·grav·i·ty

ze·ro-or·der
re·ac·tion
ze·ta
po·ten·tial
ze·ta·crit
ze·ta sed·i·men·ta·tion
ra·ti·o
zeu·ma·tog·ra·phy
zi·do·vu·dine
Ziegler's
op·er·a·tion
Ziehen-Oppenheim
dis·ease
Ziehl-Neelsen
stain
Ziehl's
stain
Ziemann's
dots
stip·pling
Zieve's
syn·drome
Zi·ka
fe·ver
vi·rus
Zimmerlin's
at·ro·phy
Zimmermann
re·ac·tion
test
Zimmermann's
cor·pus·cle
gran·ule
Zimmermann's el·e·men·ta·ry
par·ti·cle
zinc
col·ic
gel·a·tin
zinc
z. ac·e·tate
z. cap·ry·late
z. chlo·ride
z. gel·a·tin
z. io·dide
me·dic·i·nal z. per·ox·ide
z. ox·ide
z. ox·ide and eu·ge·nol
z. per·man·ga·nate
z. per·ox·ide

zinc *(continued)*
z. phe·nol·sul·fo·nate
z. phos·phide
z. ste·a·rate
z. sul·fate
z. sul·fo·car·bo·late
z. su·per·ox·ide
z. un·dec·e·no·ate
z. un·dec·y·len·ate
z. white
zinc·if·er·ous
zinc·oid
zinc phos·phate
ce·ment
zinc sul·fate flo·ta·tion cen·trif·u·ga·tion
meth·od
zin·gi·ber
Zinn's
ar·tery
co·ro·na
lig·a·ment
mem·brane
ring
ten·don
zon·ule
Zinn's vas·cu·lar
cir·cle
zir·co·ni·um
gran·u·lo·ma
zo·ac·an·tho·sis
zo·am·y·lin
zo·an·throp·ic
zo·an·thro·py
zo·et·ic
zo·ic
zo·ite
Zollinger-Ellison
syn·drome
tu·mor
Zöllner's
lines
zo·me·pir·ac so·di·um
zo·na
z. ar·cu·a·ta
z. cil·i·ar·is
z. co·ro·na
z. der·ma·ti·ca
z. ep·i·the·li·o·se·ro·sa
z. fa·ci·a·lis
z. fas·ci·cu·la·ta
z. glo·mer·u·lo·sa
z. hem·or·rhoi·dal·is
z. ig·nea
z. me·dul·lo·vas·cu·lo·sa
z. oph·thal·mi·ca
z. pec·ti·na·ta
z. pel·lu·ci·da

z. per·fo·ra·ta
z. pu·pil·la·ris
z. ra·di·a·ta
z. re·tic·u·la·ris
z. ser·pi·gi·no·sa
z. stri·a·ta
z. tec·ta
z. vas·cu·lo·sa
zo·nae
zon·al
ne·cro·sis
zo·na·ry
pla·cen·ta
zon·ate
Zondek-Aschheim
test
zone
ab·dom·i·nal z.'s
an·dro·gen·ic z.
ar·cu·ate z.
Barnes' z.
cer·vi·cal z.
cer·vi·cal z. of tooth
cil·i·ary z.
com·fort z.
z.'s of dis·con·ti·nu·i·ty
do·lo·ro·gen·ic z.
en·try z.
ep·en·dy·mal z.
ep·i·lep·to·gen·ic z.
equiv·a·lence z.
erog·e·nous z.
ero·to·gen·ic z.
fe·tal z.
gin·gi·val z.
Golgi z.
grenz z.
Head's z.'s
in·ter·pal·pe·bral z.
in·ter·tu·bu·lar z.
iso·e·lec·tric z.
lan·guage z.
la·tent z.
Lissauer's mar·gi·nal z.
Looser's z.'s
man·tle z.
Marchant's z.
mar·gi·nal z.
mo·tor z.
neu·tral z.
nu·cle·o·lar z.
Obersteiner-Redlich z.
or·bic·u·lar z.
pec·ti·nate z.
pel·lu·cid z.
per·i·tu·bu·lar z.
po·lar z.
pro·tec·tive z.

pu·pil·lary z.
re·flex·o·gen·ic z.
sec·on·dary X z.
seg·men·tal z.
Spitzka's mar·gi·nal z.
sub·plas·ma·lem·mal dense z.
su·dan·o·pho·bic z.
ten·der z.'s
thy·mus-de·pen·dent z.
tra·bec·u·lar z.
tran·si·tion·al z.
trig·ger z.
troph·o·tro·pic z. of Hess
vas·cu·lar z.
ver·mil·ion z.
ver·mil·ion tran·si·tion·al z.
Weil's ba·sal z.
Wernicke's z.
X z.
zo·nes·the·sia
zo·nif·u·gal
zon·ing
zo·nip·e·tal
zo·no·skel·e·ton
zo·nu·la
z. ad·he·rens
z. oc·clu·dens
zo·nu·lae
zo·nu·lar
band
cat·a·ract
fi·bers
lay·er
sco·to·ma
spac·es
zon·ule
cil·i·ary z.
Zinn's z.
zo·nu·li·tis
zo·nu·lol·y·sis
zo·nu·ly·sis
zo·o·an·thro·po·no·sis
zo·o·blast
zo·o·der·mic
zo·o·e·ras·tia
zo·o·ful·vin
zo·o·gen·e·sis
zo·o·ge·og·ra·phy
zo·o·glea
zo·og·o·nous
zo·og·o·ny
zo·o·graft
zo·o·graft·ing
zo·oid
zo·o·lag·nia
zo·o·lite
zo·o·lith

zo·ol·o·gist
zo·ol·o·gy
zoom
zo·o·ma·nia
Zo·o·mas·tig·i·na
Zo·o·mas·ti·go·pho·ras·i·da
Zo·o·mas·ti·go·pho·rea
zo·om·y·lus
zo·o·no·sis
di·rect z.
zo·o·not·ic
in·fec·tion
po·ten·tial
zo·o·not·ic cu·ta·ne·ous
leish·man·i·a·sis
Zoon's
eryth·ro·pla·sia
zo·o·par·a·site
zo·o·pa·thol·o·gy
zo·oph·a·gous
zo·o·phile
zo·o·phil·ia
zo·o·phil·ic
zo·oph·i·lism
erot·ic z.
zo·o·pho·bia
zo·o·phyte
zo·o·plas·tic
graft
zo·o·plas·ty
zo·o·sa·dism
zo·os·mo·sis
zo·o·tech·nics
zo·ot·ic
zo·o·tox·in
zo·o·tro·phic
zos·ter
en·ceph·a·lo·my·e·li·tis
zos·ter·i·form
zos·ter im·mune
glob·u·lin
zos·ter·oid
zox·a·zo·la·mine
Z-plas·ty
Zsigmondy's
test
Z-tract
in·jec·tion
zuc·ker·guss·le·ber
Zuckerkandl's
bod·ies
con·vo·lu·tion
fas·cia
zwis·chen·fer·ment
zwit·ter
hy·poth·e·sis
zwit·ter·i·on·ic
zwit·ter·i·ons

zy·gal
  fis·sure
zyg·a·poph·y·se·al
zyg·a·poph·y·ses
zyg·a·poph·y·si·al
  joints
zyg·a·poph·y·sis
zyg·i·on
zy·go·dac·ty·ly
zy·go·ma
zy·go·mat·ic
  arch
  bone
  di·am·e·ter
  fos·sa
  mar·gin
  nerve
  pro·cess
  re·gion
zy·go·mat·i·co·au·ric·u·lar
  in·dex
zy·go·ma·ti·co·au·ri·cu·la·ris
zy·go·mat·i·co·fa·cial
  fo·ra·men
zy·go·mat·i·co·fron·tal
zy·go·mat·i·co·max·il·lary
  su·ture
zy·go·mat·i·co-or·bi·tal
  ar·tery
  fo·ra·men
zy·go·mat·i·co·sphe·noid
zy·go·mat·i·co·tem·po·ral
  fo·ra·men
zy·go·max·il·la·re
zy·go·max·il·lary
  point

Zy·go·my·ce·tes
zy·go·my·co·sis
zy·gon
zy·go·ne·ma
zy·go·po·di·um
zy·go·sis
zy·gos·i·ty
zy·go·sperm
zy·go·spore
zy·gote
zy·go·tene
zy·got·ic
zy·go·to·blast
zy·go·to·mere
zy·mase
zy·mo·deme
zy·mo·gen
zy·mo·gen·e·sis
zy·mo·gen·ic
  cell
zy·mog·e·nous
zy·mo·gram
zy·mo·hex·ase
zy·mol·o·gist
zy·mol·o·gy
Zy·mo·ne·ma
zy·mo·plas·tic
  sub·stance
zy·mo·san
zy·mo·scope
zy·mose
zy·mos·ter·ol
zy·mot·ic
  pap·il·lo·ma